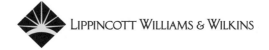

Introductory
Maternity
& Pediatric
Nursing

Introductory Maternity & Pediatric Nursing

N. Jayne Klossner, MSN, RNC
Director of Women's Services
North Central Baptist Hospital
Part of Baptist Health System
San Antonio, Texas

Nancy T. Hatfield, MAE, BSN, RN
Program Director, Chairperson
Albuquerque Public Schools
Practical Nursing Program
Albuquerque, New Mexico

LIPPINCOTT WILLIAMS & WILKINS
A **Wolters Kluwer** Company
Philadelphia • Baltimore • New York • London
Buenos Aires • Hong Kong • Sydney • Tokyo

Acquisitions Editor: Elizabeth Nieginski
Developmental Editor: Danielle DiPalma
Editorial Assistant: Josh Levandoski
Senior Production Editor: Sandra Cherrey Scheinin
Director of Nursing Production: Helen Ewan
Managing Editor/Production: Erika Kors
Art Director: Carolyn O'Brien
Senior Manufacturing Manager: William Alberti
Indexer: Coughlin Indexing Services, Inc.
Compositor: TechBooks
Printer: R.R. Donnelley-Willard

9 8 7 6 5 4 3 2

Library of Congress Cataloging-in-Publication Data

Klossner, N. Jayne.
  Introductory maternity and pediatric nursing / N. Jayne Klossner, Nancy
  T. Hatfield.
    p. ; cm.
  Includes bibliographical references and index.
  ISBN 10: 0-7817-3690-0
  ISBN 13: 978-0-7817-3690-9
    1. Maternity nursing.   2. Pediatric nursing.   I. Hatfield, Nancy T.   II. Title.
    [DNLM: 1. Maternal-Child Nursing—methods.   2. Nursing Process.
3. Pediatric Nursing—methods.   WY 157.3 K66i 2006]
  RG951.K565 2006
  618.92'00231—dc22   2004018127

Dedication

To Kevin

My husband, my partner, my friend—I love you with all my heart

To Katelyn

My "Baby Girl" for understanding all those nights I was at the computer during your

high school years. We made it!

To Joshua and Jonathan

My sons for the support and love you have given me from wherever you may be!

To John

My partner, my best friend; you are the light and love of my life

To Mikayla and Jeff

You taught me about children, caring, and happiness; my greatest joy in life is being your Mom

To Mom and Dad

Your unconditional love allowed me to be the child I was and the adult I am

Contributors

Martha Dianne DeBarros, BS. in Ed., LCCE, IBCLC
Coordinator
Family Education Services and Lactation Center
St. Luke's Baptist Women's Center
San Antonio, Texas

Karen Edmondson, RN
Instructor
University of South Carolina, Spartanburg
Mary Black School of Nursing
Spartanburg, South Carolina

Maryann Foley, RN, BSN
Independent Clinical Consultant
Flourtown, Pennsylvania

Margaret Dextraze Humm, RN, MSN, CNS
Clinical Nurse Specialist for Maternal-Child Health
St. Luke's Baptist Women's Center
San Antonio, Texas

Barbara Gonzalez Pino, PhD
Associate Professor
University of Texas at San Antonio
San Antonio, Texas

Cynthia Kincheloe RN, BSN, MSN
NICU Staff Nurse
Presbyterian Hospital
Albuquerque, New Mexico
Former Instructor
Albuquerque T-VI
Albuquerque, New Mexico

Frank Pino, PhD
Professor
University of Texas at San Antonio
San Antonio, Texas

Reviewers

Margaret D. Cole, RN, DSN
Associate Professor of Nursing
Spring Hill College
Mobile, Alabama

Karen R. Ferguson, RNC, BSN, MSN
Nursing Instructor
Calhoun Community College
Decatur, Alabama

Donna J. Gatlin, RN, BSN, MA
Nursing Instructor
Paris Junior College
Paris, Texas

Joy Green-Hadden, MSN, RN, FNP-C
Family Nurse Practitioner
Case Western University
Knoxville, Tennessee

Margaret J. Henry, RN, BSN
Assistant Professor of Nursing
Belmont Technical College
St. Clairsville, Ohio

Debra Lea Jenks, RN, MSN, PhD
Assistant Professor
Milwaukee School of Engineering
Milwaukee, Wisconsin

John A. McCarter, RN, BSN, MSN
Adjunct Pediatric Clinical Instructor
University of South Alabama College of Nursing
Mobile, Alabama

Audrey N. McLarty RN
Staff Nurse, Childbirth Educator
Huntsville Hospital for Women & Children
Huntsville, Alabama

Nancy Mizzoni, RN, MSN, CPNP
Associate Professor
Middlesex Community College
Lowell, Massachusetts

Vicki Nees, RNC, MSN, APRN-BC
Associate Professor
Ivy Tech State College
Lafayette, Indiana

Jan Peek, RN, MSN
Chairperson, Nursing Department
Calhoun Community College
Decatur, Alabama

Lisa Richwine, RN, BSN
LPN Instructor
Ivy Tech State College
Lafayette, Indiana

Gayle Sewell, RN, MN
Nursing Instructor
North Central Kansas Technical College
Beloit, Kansas

Russlyn A. St. John, RN, MSN
Associate Professor
St. Charles Community College
St. Peters, Missouri

Margaret C. Stone, RN (LPN), BSN, MSN
Associate Professor
North Shore Community College
Danvers, Massachusetts

Roselena Thorpe, RN, PhD
Professor and Department Chairperson Nursing
Community College of Allegheny County
Pittsburgh, Pennsylvania

Preface

This first edition of *Introductory Maternity and Pediatric Nursing* reflects the underlying philosophy of love, caring, and support for the childbearing woman, the child, and the families of these individuals. The content has been developed according to the most current information available. In this text we recognize that cultural sensitivity and awareness are important aspects of caring for the childbearing and child-rearing families. We also recognize that many children and pregnant women live in families other than traditional two-parent family homes and therefore refer to teaching and supporting the child bearing clients and family caregivers of children in all situations and family structures.

Maternal-child health care has seen a shift from the hospital setting into community and home settings. More responsibility has fallen on the family and family caregivers to care for the pregnant woman or ill child. We stress teaching the patient, the family, and the child, with an emphasis on prevention. The nursing process has been used as the foundation for presenting nursing care. Implementation information is presented in a narrative format to enable the discussion from which planning, goal setting, and evaluation can be put into action. The newest and most current NANDA terminology has been used for the possible nursing diagnoses for health care concerns.

Our goal in this text is to keep the readability of the text at a level with which the student can be comfortable. In recognition of the limited time that the student has and the frustrations that can result from having to turn to a dictionary or glossary for words that are unfamiliar, we have attempted to identify all possible unfamiliar terms and define them within the text. This increases the reading ease for the student, decreasing the time necessary to complete the assigned reading and enhancing the understanding of the information. A four-color format, current photos, drawings, tables, and diagrams will further aid the student in using this edition.

This text offers the instructor and student of maternity and pediatric nursing a user-friendly, comprehensive quick reference to features in the text, including the Family Teaching Tips, Nursing Care Plans, Nursing Procedures, and Personal Glimpses.

RECURRING FEATURES

In an effort to provide the instructor and student with a text that is informative, exciting, and easy to use, we have incorporated a number of special features throughout the text, many of which are included in each chapter.

Chapter Outlines

A basic outline of what will be covered in the chapter is presented at the beginning of each chapter. This roadmap helps students in recognizing the focus of the chapter.

Student Objectives

Measurable student-oriented objectives are included at the beginning of each chapter. These help to guide the student in recognizing what is important and why, and they provide the instructor with guidance for evaluating the student's understanding of the information presented in the chapter.

Key Terms

A list of terms that may be unfamiliar to students and that are considered essential to the chapter's understanding is at the beginning of each chapter. The first appearance in the chapter of each of these terms is in boldface type, with the definition included in the text. All key terms can be found in a glossary at the end of the text.

Nursing Process

The nursing process serves as an organizing structure for the discussion of nursing care covered in the text. This feature provides the student with a foundation from which individualized nursing care plans can be developed. Each Nursing Process section includes the nurse's role in caring for the patient and family and also includes nursing assessment, relevant nursing diagnoses, outcome identification and planning, implementation, and evaluation of the goals and expected outcomes. Emphasis is placed on the importance of involving the family and family caregivers in the assessment process. In the Nursing Process sections we have used current NANDA-approved nursing diagnoses. These are used to represent appropriate concerns for a particular condition, but we do not attempt to include all diagnoses that could be identified. The student will find the goals specific, measurable, and realistic and will be able to relate the goals to patient situations and care plan development. The expected outcomes and evaluation provide a goal for each nursing diagnosis and criteria to measure the successful accomplishment of that goal.

Nursing Care Plans

Throughout the text Nursing Care Plans are presented to provide the student with a model to follow in using the information from the nursing process to develop specific nursing care plans. To make the care plans more meaningful, a scenario has been constructed for each one.

Nursing Procedures

Needed equipment and step-by-step procedures are found to help the students understand the procedures. These can be easily used in a clinical setting to perform nursing procedures.

Family Teaching Tips

Information that the student can use in teaching the maternity patient, family caregivers, and children is presented in highlighted boxes ready for use.

Clinical Secrets

These present a recurring cartoon nurse who provides brief clinical pearls. The student will find these valuable in caring for patients in clinical settings. Safety concerns and important issues to consider are highlighted.

Personal Glimpse With Learning Opportunity

Personal Glimpses are presented in every chapter. These are actual first-person narratives, unedited, just as the individual wrote them. Personal Glimpses help the student have a view of an experience an individual has had in a given situation and of that person's feelings about or during the incident. These are presented to enhance the student's understanding and appreciation of the feelings of others. A Learning Opportunity at the end of each Personal Glimpse encourages students to think of how they might react or respond in the situation presented. These further enhance the student's critical thinking.

Cultural Snapshot

These boxes highlight issues and topics that may have cultural considerations. The student is encouraged to think about cultural differences and the importance of accepting the attitudes and beliefs of individuals from cultures other than his or her own.

Tables, Drawings, and Photographs

These important aspects of the text have been developed in an effort to help the student visualize the content covered. Many color photographs in a variety of settings are included.

Key Points

We have selected key points to help the student focus on the important aspects of the chapter. These provide a quick review of essential elements of the chapter. The Key Points are structured to recap each student objective stated at the beginning of the chapter.

References, Selected Readings and Websites

This section offers the student additional information on topics and conditions discussed in the chapter. The websites also provide resource information that the student can share with patients and families. Throughout the text, websites are included as resources for the student to access available sites discussing certain conditions, diseases and disorders, as well as offering support and information for families.

LEARNING OPPORTUNITIES

In order to offer students opportunities to check their understanding of material they have read and studied, many learning opportunities are provided throughout the text.

Test Yourself

These questions are found in each chapter and are designed to test understanding and recall of the material presented. The student will quickly determine if a review of what he or she just read is needed.

Workbook

At the end of each chapter the student will find a workbook section that includes

- **NCLEX–Style Review Questions** are written to test the student's ability to apply the material from the chapter. These questions use the client–nurse format to encourage the student to critically think about patient situations as well as the nurse's response or action. Innovative style questions have been included.
- **Study Activities** include interactive activities requiring the student to participate in the learning process. Important material from the chapter has been incorporated into this section to help the student review and synthesize the chapter content. The instructor will find many of the activities appropriate for individual or class assignments.
- **Internet Activities.** Many chapters include an Internet activity within the Study Activities that helps the student explore the Internet. Each activity takes the student step by step into a site where he or she can access new and updated information as well as resources to share with patients and families. Some include fun activities to use with pediatric patients. These activities may require the use of Acrobat Reader. This can be downloaded free of charge for the student to readily view the site.
- **Critical Thinking: What Would You Do?** Critical thinking real-life situations encourage the student to think about the chapter content in practical terms. These situations require the student to incorporate knowledge gained from the chapter and apply it to real-life problems. Questions provide the student with opportunities to problem solve, think critically, and discover his or her own ideas and feelings. The instructor also can use them as a tool to stimulate class discussion. Dosage Calculations are found in the Workbook section of each pediatric chapter where diseases and disorders are covered. This section offers the student practice in dosage calculations that can be directly applied in a clinical setting.

ORGANIZATION

The text is divided into nine units to provide an orderly approach to the content. The first unit helps build a foundation for the student beginning the study of maternity and pediatric nursing. This unit introduces the student to caring for the childbearing woman and for children in various settings.

The maternity section of the text begins with Unit 2. Foundational topics are presented in the first chapters of each unit followed by chapters that feature the application of knowledge within the nursing process. Maternity topics that address the low-risk woman are covered first in Units 2 to 5. Unit 6 addresses issues related to at-risk pregnancy, childbirth, and newborn care. The instructor may choose to teach the normal content of pregnancy followed by the at-risk pregnancy chapters, if desired. However, the author designed the content so that normal considerations would be covered first followed by discussion of the at-risk woman, fetus, and neonate. This grouping ensures that all normal content is covered before any at-risk topics are addressed, which cuts down on the need for parenthetical content in the at-risk chapters. It also encourages the student to review the normal chapters when studying the at-risk content. This repetition of content is designed to help cement the student's understanding of the material. In Unit 6 the at-risk disorders are organized so that an explanation of the disorder is covered first followed by a discussion of medical treatment and nursing care.

The basic approach to the study of caring for the child is organized within a unit discussing health promotion for normal growth and development. Principles of growth and development are discussed, and a chapter for each age group presents the developmental stages. Foundations of pediatric health care are included in a unit to include assessment and care of the child in various settings and situations. The specific health problems seen in children are covered using a body systems approach. This approach, which often is used in nursing education curriculums, provides a user-friendly approach to the study of nursing care of children.

Unit 1, Overview of Maternal and Pediatric Nursing Care

Unit 1 introduces the student in Chapter 1 to a brief history of maternity and pediatric nursing, and discusses current trends in maternal–child health care and maternal–child health status issues and concerns. A brief discussion of the nursing process is included. Chapter 2 follows with a discussion of the family, its structure, and family factors that influence childbearing and child rearing. The chapter introduces community-based health care and discusses the various settings in the community through which health care is provided for the maternity client and the child.

Unit 2, Foundations of Maternity Nursing

Unit 2 introduces the student in Chapter 3 to male and female reproductive anatomy, which is essential to the understanding of maternity nursing. The menstrual cycle and the sexual response cycle are also addressed. (Note: Pelvic anatomy is addressed in Chapter 8 and breast anatomy in Chapter 14.) Chapter 4 continues with a discussion of special reproductive issues to include family planning, elective termination of pregnancy, and issues of fertility.

Unit 3, Pregnancy

Unit 3 begins in Chapter 5 with a discussion of fetal development from fertilization through the fetal period. Chapter 6 introduces the student to diagnosis of pregnancy, physiologic and psychological adaptation of the woman during pregnancy. The chapter ends by outlining nutritional requirements of pregnancy. Chapter 7 covers the nurse's role in prenatal care and assessment of fetal well-being during pregnancy.

Unit 4, Labor and Birth

Unit 4 begins with a discussion of the labor process in Chapter 8. The four components of birth, the process of labor, and maternal and fetal adaptation to labor are covered. Female pelvic anatomy is discussed here. Chapter 9 introduces the student to concepts of pain management during labor and birth. The chapter begins with an overview of the characteristics and nature of labor pain as well as general principles of labor pain management. Nonpharmacologic and pharmacologic methods of pain management are reviewed. Chapter 10 covers the nurse's role during labor and birth to include assessment of the fetus through fetal monitoring and other methods. The nurse's role in each stage of labor is covered within the framework of the nursing process. The nurse-controlled delivery is also covered in this chapter. Chapter 11 discusses cesarean birth, version, cervical ripening procedures, induction and augmentation of labor, amnioinfusion, assisted delivery (including episiotomy, vacuum, and forceps delivery), and vaginal birth after cesarean.

Unit 5, Postpartum and Newborn

Unit 5 begins with a discussion of normal postpartum adaptation, nursing assessment, and nursing care in Chapter 12. Chapter 13 covers topics related to normal transition of the neonate to extrauterine life, general characteristics of the neonate, and the initial nursing assessment of the newborn. Chapter 14 delves into issues of infant nutrition. Breast-feeding and formula feeding are presented along with tips on choosing a feeding method, as well as advantages and disadvantages of each method. Physiology of breast-feeding, including breast anatomy, is covered here. The nurse's role in assisting the woman who is breast-feeding and the woman who is formula feeding is also discussed.

Chapter 15 presents the nurse's role in caring for the normal newborn and includes nursing care considerations in the stabilization and transition of the newborn, normal newborn care, assessment and facilitation of family interaction and adjustment, and discharge considerations. An emphasis is placed on teaching the new parents to care for their newborn.

Unit 6, Childbearing At Risk

Unit 6 begins with a focus on pregnancy at risk. Chapter 16 focuses on the pregnancy that is placed at risk by pre-existing and chronic medical conditions of the woman. This chapter covers the major medical conditions, such as diabetes and heart disease, as well as exposure to substances harmful to the fetus, threats from intimate partner violence, and age-related concerns on either end of the age spectrum. Chapter 17 introduces the student to the pregnancy that becomes at risk because of pregnancy-related complications and disorders. Threats from hyperemesis, bleeding disorders of pregnancy, hypertensive disorders, and blood incompatibilities are presented. Chapter 18 covers topics associated with the at-risk labor, such as dysfunctional labor, preterm labor, post-term labor, placental abnormalities, and emergencies associated with labor and birth. Chapter 19 looks at the postpartum woman at risk. Postpartum hemorrhage, subinvolution, infection, thrombophlebitis, malattachment, grief reaction, and postpartum depression and psychosis are addressed. In Chapter 20 gestational concerns and acquired disorders of the newborn are discussed. Chapter 21 addresses congenital disorders of the newborn, including congenital malformations, inborn errors of metabolism, and chromosomal abnormalities.

Unit 7, Health Promotion for Normal Growth and Development

Unit 7 includes Chapter 22, Principles of Growth and Development, which provides a foundation for discussion of growth and development in later chapters. The issues of children of divorce, latchkey children, runaway children, and homeless children and families are examined. Influences on and theories of growth and development are presented. The rest of this unit is organized by developmental stages, from infancy through adolescence. It includes aspects of normal growth and development.

Unit 8, Foundations of Pediatric Health Care

Unit 8 presents Chapter 28, Assessment of the Child (Data Collection), which covers collecting subjective and objective data from the child and the family. The chapter also includes interviewing and obtaining a history, general physical assessments and exams, and assisting with diagnostic tests. Care of the Hospitalized Child, Chapter 29, presents the pediatric unit, infection control in the pediatric setting, admission and discharge, the child undergoing surgery, pain management, the hospital play program, and safety in the hospital. Chapter 30, Procedures and Treatments, covers specific procedures for the pediatric patient as well as the role of the nurse in assisting with procedures and treatments. Chapter 31, Medication Administration and Intravenous Therapy, includes dosage calculation, administration of medications by various routes, and intravenous therapy. Chapter 32 discusses the concerns that face the family of a child with a chronic illness. The impact on the family of caring for a child with a chronic illness and the nurse's role in assisting and supporting these families is presented. Chapter 33 concludes this unit with the dying child. Included in this chapter is a teaching aid to help the nurse perform a self-examination of personal attitudes about death and dying, as well as concrete guidelines to use when interacting with a grieving child or adult.

Unit 9, The Child With a Major Illness

Unit 9 is structured according to a body systems approach as the basis for discussion of diseases and disorders seen in children. A brief review of basic anatomy and physiology of the body system discussed begins each chapter. Throughout the text, family-centered care is stressed. The nursing process and nursing care plans are integrated throughout this unit. Developmental enrichment and stimulation are stressed in the sections on nursing process. The basic premise of each child's self worth is fundamental in all of the nursing care presented.

Glossaries, Workbook Answers, and Appendices

The text concludes with a **Glossary** of key terms and an **English-Spanish Glossary** of maternity and pediatric phrases. Additionally, **Answers to Workbook Questions** are provided. Ten appendices are included at the back of the text and contain important information for the nursing student in maternity and pediatrics courses. Appendices include:

Appendix A: Standard and Transmission-Based Precautions
Appendix B: NANDA-Approved Nursing Diagnoses
Appendix C: JCAHO List of "Do Not Use" Abbreviations
Appendix D: Good Sources of Essential Nutrients
Appendix E: Breast-feeding and Medication Use
Appendix F: Cervical Dilation Chart
Appendix G: Growth Charts
Appendix H: Pulse, Respiration, and Blood Pressure Values in Children
Appendix I: Temperature and Weight Conversion Charts
Appendix J: Communicating With Children and Family Caregivers

TEACHING/LEARNING PACKAGE

Instructor's Resource CD-ROM

This essential resource for instructors offers a number of tools to assist you with teaching your course:

- The Instructor's Manual features Lecture Outlines, Teaching Strategies for both the classroom and clinical setting, and unique Critical Thinking Assignments with sample answers.
- PowerPoint presentations for every chapter provide an easy way for you to integrate the textbook with your students' classroom experience, either via slide shows or handouts.
- The Image Bank lets you use the photographs and illustrations from this textbook in your PowerPoint slides or as you see fit in your course.
- The Test Generator lets you put together exclusive new tests from a bank containing over 400 questions, spanning the book's topics in both maternity and pediatrics, to help you in assessing your students' understanding of the material.

Front-of-Book CD-ROM

This free Front-of-Book CD-ROM features video clips of labor and delivery and pediatric dosage calculation problems.

Contact your sales representative or visit LWW.com/Nursing for details and ordering information.

Acknowledgments

Many people were involved in the creation of this first edition of **Introductory Maternity and Pediatric Nursing.** We worked with some of these individuals on a frequent and ongoing basis, while others, we do not even know their names. With gratitude and appreciation we would like to thank every person on our team from Lippincott, Williams & Wilkins, whether they had a small or a large part in the process of publishing this textbook.

We especially want to express our appreciation to:

Danielle DiPalma, Developmental Editor, for being the solid foundation and support for this book. We thank her for her never-wavering belief that this text would be written and her dedication and commitment to ensure that would happen. Danielle, you are fantastic!

Sarah Kyle, Developmental Editor, for her attention to detail and excellent suggestions. We thank her for contributing material and for pitching in when the going got tough to help us meet our deadlines. Sarah, you are amazing!

Maryann Foley, Development Editor, for stepping in with her expertise and knowledge to help fine tune and complete the pediatric chapters.

Lisa Stead, Acquisitions Editor, for envisioning this project.

Elizabeth Nieginski, Senior Acquisitions Editor, for her support behind the scenes managing the business aspects of the project.

Katherine Rothwell and Josh Levandoski, Editorial Assistants, for their enthusiasm and help obtaining reviews and assisting with the many necessary administrative tasks.

Sandy Cherrey Scheinin, Senior Production Editor, for her help in the final editing process.

Michelle Clark, Ancillary Editor, for her work on the instructor's resource materials.

Cynthia Kincheloe for her excellent work writing two of the maternity chapters.

Doctors Frank and Barbara Pino for their wonderful work on the translation of the English-Spanish glossary, despite being asked at the last minute.

Heather Rojas for organizing, finding models, and working with us on the pediatric portion of the photo shoot.

Joe Mitchell for his patience and beautiful photography.

Peggy Humm for facilitating and organizing the photo shoot at St. Luke's Baptist Hospital.

Megan Klim, Development Editor, for her help with the photo shoot.

Doug Dobbs, if it weren't for him, I would never have known that Lippincott Williams & Wilkins wanted to do this project.

All of the women, children, families, and nurses who were models for the photos.

N. Jayne Klossner

Nancy J. Hatfield

Kevin, thank you from the bottom of the heart for all the support you have given me throughout this project. You have shown your love in so very many ways. Thank you for picking up the slack at home with the bills, chores, moving, and in the countless other ways that you have shown your support. Thank you for directly contributing to this project by taking photos and doing an initial edit of some chapters before I submitted them to Sarah. Thank you for making me laugh and helping me keep my sense of humor when it seemed the book would never be finished. Your encouragement and love have been my anchor. Thank you, Frannie Rettig, for your faith in me that I could do this project when I first took it on. And a special thanks to Donna Guenther for keeping everything together at work, and to Janeen Koti for taking the pager and other responsibilities, which enabled me to concentrate on the book when I needed to. Thanks to Kathy Eichner, Susan Monahan, Mark Clayton, and all my employees for your encouraging words and for understanding when I needed to rearrange my schedule to meet deadlines. I couldn't have done it without you!

I would like to thank my husband, John, for his never-ending confidence, patience and encouragement, and his sincere support of this project. His help with the everyday household responsibilities was invaluable in allowing me the time I needed to complete this text. I appreciate and thank my children, Mikayla and Jeff, and my parents, Edgar and Lucy Thomas, for their love, phone calls, and positive words of encouragement—always just when I needed them. My extended family and special friends offered support, listened to me, took pictures, and gave me insight and advice—always affirming this project could be accomplished. Thank you all.

Nancy

Contents

UNIT 7

Health Promotion for Normal Growth and Development   551

Quick Reference to Features

NURSING CARE PLANS

Overview of Maternal and Pediatric Nursing Care

The Nurse's Role in a Changing Maternal–Child Health Care Environment

1

STUDENT OBJECTIVES

On completion of this chapter, the student should be able to

1. Discuss factors influencing the development of maternity and pediatric care in the United States.
2. Describe how current trends in maternal–child care have affected the delivery of care to mothers, infants, and children in the United States.
3. Name three ways that nurses contribute to cost containment in the United States.
4. Examine the maternal–child health status in the United States.
5. Discuss the current health status of children and adolescents in the United States.
6. Discuss two possible reasons the United States ranks low compared with other developed countries in terms of infant mortality rate.
7. Discuss major objectives of Healthy People 2010 as they relate to maternal and pediatric nursing.
8. List new roles the nurse is expected to assume when providing maternal and pediatric nursing care.
9. Discuss how the nurse uses critical thinking skills in maternal and pediatric nursing.
10. List the five steps of the nursing process.
11. Explain the importance of complete and accurate documentation.

KEY TERMS

actual nursing diagnoses
capitation
case management
couplet care
critical pathways
dependent nursing actions
fetal mortality rate
independent nursing actions
infant mortality rate
interdependent nursing actions
maternal mortality rate
mortality rates
morbidity
neonatal
neonatal mortality rate
nursing process
objective data
outcomes
perinatal
perinatal mortality rate
prospective payment system
puerperal fever
risk nursing diagnoses
subjective data
utilization review
viable
wellness nursing diagnoses

The nurse preparing to care for today and tomorrow's childbearing and child-rearing families faces vastly different responsibilities and challenges than did the maternal and pediatric nurse of even a decade ago. Nurses and other health professionals are becoming increasingly concerned with much more than the care of at-risk pregnancies and sick children. Health teaching; preventing illness; and promoting optimal (most desirable or satisfactory) physical, developmental, and emotional health have become a significant part of contemporary nursing.

Scientific and technological advances have reduced the incidence of communicable disease and helped to control metabolic disorders such as diabetes. As a result, more health care is provided outside the hospital. Patients now receive health care in the home, at schools and clinics, and from their primary care provider. Prenatal diagnosis of birth defects, transfusions, other treatments for the unborn fetus, and improved life-support systems for premature infants are but a few examples of the rapid progress in child care.

Controversy continues to rage about choices in family planning. In January 1973, a Supreme Court decision declared abortion legal anywhere in the United States. In 1981, efforts were made to convince Congress that legislation should be passed to make all abortions illegal on the alleged grounds that the fetus is a person and, therefore, has the right to life. In the 1990s, bitter debate between "pro-life" and "pro-choice" groups raged and seems likely to continue for many years.

Tremendous sociologic changes have affected attitudes toward, and concepts in, maternal–child health. American society is largely suburban, with a population of highly mobile persons and families. The women's movement has focused new attention on the needs of families in which the mother works outside the home. Escalating divorce rates, changes in attitudes toward sexual roles, and general acceptance of unmarried mothers have increased the number of single-parent families. Many people have come to regard health care as a right, not a privilege, and expect to receive fair value for their investment. In addition, the demand for financial responsibility in health care has contributed to shortened hospital stays and alternative methods of health care delivery.

The reduction in the incidence of communicable and infectious diseases has made it possible to devote more attention to such critical problems as preterm birth, congenital anomalies, child abuse, learning and behavior disorders, developmental disabilities, and chronic illness. Research in these areas continues; as these findings become available, nurses will be among the practitioners who will help translate this research into improved health care for pregnant women, children, and families.

However, nurses' ability to translate the relevant medical research into practice is based on their understanding of the predictable but variable phases of pregnancy and of a child's growth and development, and on their understanding of and sensitivity to the importance of family interactions.

CHANGING CONCEPTS IN MATERNAL–CHILD HEALTH CARE

Maternity care has changed dramatically throughout the years as attitudes and opinions have altered. Historically, maternity care was a function of lay midwives, and most births occurred in the home setting. As knowledge increased about birth interventions and physicians developed methods of infection prevention, the family physician became the provider of choice for prenatal care, and hospitals, instead of homes, became the accepted place to give birth.

In today's society, as the health care consumer has become more knowledgeable, two different trends can be noted. On one hand, as lawsuits have become more common with large judgments being leveled against practitioners, maternity care has become increasingly specialized. Obstetricians often provide routine prenatal and delivery care. The at-risk client is frequently followed by a perinatologist, a physician who specializes in the care of women with high-risk pregnancies. Neonatologists provide expert specialized care to at-risk newborns. On the other hand, the consumer movement has pushed for birth to be viewed as a natural process in which little intervention is required. Therefore, the midwife has once again come to be accepted as a provider of maternity care, and some women elect to deliver at home or in birthing centers, which provide a home-like atmosphere.

Child health care has evolved from a sideline of internal medicine to a specialty that focuses on the child and the child's family in health and illness through all phases of development. Technologic advances account for many changes in the last 50 years, but sociologic changes, particularly society's view of the child and the child's needs, have been just as important. The development of, and current trends in, maternal and child health care are discussed briefly in the following sections.

Development of Maternity Care

In colonial times, most births occurred at home. The lay midwife, who had no formal education, attended the woman throughout labor and birth. Experience and knowledge about childbirth was shared among the women of the community. Childbirth was truly a woman's affair.

As physicians became educated in the practice of midwifery and began to use instruments such as forceps, to which the midwives had no access, physicians began to replace lay midwives as the attendant at deliveries. Few women became physicians because of the cultural pressures for a woman to fulfill the roles of housewife and mother.

Another change that occurred was that physicians began to increasingly rely on interventions to assist the natural process of labor and hasten delivery. Lay midwives mainly provided support and encouragement to a woman during her labor and relied on nature to take its course. Therefore, as more physicians began to attend deliveries, labor came to be viewed as an illness, or at the very least, a dangerous condition that required the skillful intervention of a physician. Two major developments greatly influenced the way maternity care was practiced in the United States—acceptance of the germ theory and development of anesthesia to decrease the pain of childbirth.

Acceptance of the Germ Theory

Before it was known how infection was transmitted, it was common for a woman to develop **puerperal fever**, an illness marked by high fever caused by infection of the reproductive tract after the birth of a child. Puerperal fever was often fatal. Although rates of infection and mortality were much higher in hospitals, women who delivered at home also were susceptible to puerperal fever.

In the late 1700s, Alexander Gordon, a Scottish physician, was the first to recognize that puerperal fever was an infection transmitted to patients by physicians and nurses as they moved between treating patients with puerperal fever and attending births or caring for women who had already delivered. The work of two other men, Oliver Wendell Holmes and Ignaz Philip Semmelweis, confirmed Gordon's infection theory and began the development of interventions to stop the transmission of puerperal fever.

In 1842, Oliver Wendell Holmes, the famous American poet, physician, and professor of anatomy and physiology at Harvard University, wrote an essay on puerperal fever based on conclusions he made after observing physicians in clinical practice. He strongly advocated that a physician who performed autopsies on individuals who died of infection[1] should not attend women during childbirth. Ignaz Philip Semmelweis (1818–1865), a German-Hungarian physician, made similar observations in his practice. He noticed a dramatic difference in rates of puerperal

fever between two maternity wards, one in which medical students practiced, the other run by midwives. The death rate in the ward attended by medical students was two to three times higher than that of the ward in which the midwives delivered. Semmelweis noticed that the only difference between the two wards was that the medical students would dissect cadavers, then go immediately to the maternity ward to examine patients. The midwives, of course, did not dissect cadavers. Then a physician friend of Semmelweis died from a cut he sustained while examining a woman who died of puerperal fever. These observations convinced Semmelweis that the infection was carried on the hands of the physicians. He began requiring medical students to wash their hands in a chlorinated lime solution between examinations. Immediately the mortality rate fell from approximately 18% to 1%, equivalent to the death rate in the midwives' ward.

The medical community largely ignored Holmes' advice and Semmelweis' work. Efforts to prevent the spread of infection did not begin in earnest until Louis Pasteur, a French chemist and microbiologist, proved that microorganisms cause infection. Joseph Lister, a British surgeon, embraced Pasteur's theory. Lister used carbolic acid as an antiseptic during surgery and greatly improved the survival rates of his surgical patients. His research and persistence led to general acceptance of the germ theory by physicians in Europe and the United States. As antiseptic techniques were applied to the childbirth process, maternal mortality rates fell.

Easing the Pain of Childbirth

The development and use of anesthesia during childbirth was the change that most influenced wealthy and middle-class women to begin delivering their children in hospitals, rather than at home. In the 1920s and 1930s, a method called "twilight sleep" greatly increased the number of women who chose to deliver in hospitals. Morphine and scopolamine were administered at the beginning of labor to induce twilight sleep. Morphine eased the pain of labor and scopolamine, an amnesiac, induced a hypnotic-like state and caused the woman to be unable to recall the pain of labor. This development allowed women to enjoy painless childbirth and gave the physician more control over the birth process. Therefore, the hospital came to be viewed as the safest and most humane place in which to deliver a baby.

Development of Pediatric Care

Pediatrics is a relatively new medical specialty, developing only in the mid-1800s. In colonial times, epidemics were common, and many children died in infancy or childhood. In some cases, disease wiped out entire families. Native American children, usually

---

[1] He specified puerperal fever, erysipelas, and peritonitis as types of infection that could be transmitted and cause puerperal fever in a woman who had just delivered.

cared for by medicine men, were exposed to new and fatal diseases. Children of slaves received only the care their slave owner cared to provide.

Families were large to compensate for the children who did not live to adulthood. Children were viewed as additional hands to help with the family farm chores. Sick children often were cared for by the adults in the family or by a neighbor with a reputation of being able to care for the sick.

The first children's hospital opened in Philadelphia in 1855. Until that point in Western civilization, children were not considered important, except as contributors to family income. Hospitalized children were cared for in hospitals as adults were, often in the same bed. Unfortunately, early institutions for children were notorious for their unsanitary conditions, neglect, and lack of proper infant nutrition. Well into the 19th century, mortality rates were commonly 50% to 100% among institutionalized children in asylums or hospitals.

Arthur Jacobi, a Prussian-born physician, has been recognized as the father of pediatrics. Under his direction, several New York hospitals opened pediatric units. He helped found the American Pediatric Society in 1888. During the early 1900s, intractable diarrhea was a primary cause of death in children's institutions. Initiation of the simple practices of boiling milk and isolating children with septic conditions lowered the incidence of diarrhea. This practice of pasteurizing milk was instrumental in decreasing the rate of death in children.

After World War I, a period of strict asepsis began. Babies were placed in individual cubicles, and nurses were strictly forbidden to pick up the children, except when necessary. Crib sides were draped with clean sheets, leaving infants with nothing to do but stare at the ceiling. The importance of toys in a child's environment appears not to have been recognized; besides, it was thought that such objects could transmit infection. Parents were allowed to visit for half an hour or perhaps 1 hour each week, and they were forbidden to pick up their children under penalty of having their visiting privileges revoked.

Despite these precautions, high infant mortality rates continued. One of the first people to suspect the cause was Joseph Brennaman, a physician at Children's Memorial Hospital in Chicago. In 1932, he suggested that the infants suffered from a lack of stimulation; other concerned child specialists became interested. In the 1940s, Ren Spitz published the results of studies that supported his contention that deprivation of maternal care caused a state of dazed stupor in an infant. He believed this condition could become irreversible if the child were not returned to the mother promptly. He termed this state "anaclitic depression." He also coined the term *hospitalism*, which he defined as "a vitiated condition of the body due to long confinement in the hospital" (*vitiated* means feeble or weak). Later the term came to be used almost entirely to denote the harmful effects of institutional care on infants. Another physician, Bakwin, found that infants hospitalized for a long time actually developed physical symptoms that he attributed to a lack of emotional stimulation and a lack of feeding satisfaction.

Working under the auspices of the World Health Organization, John Bowlby of London thoroughly explored the subject of maternal deprivation. His 1951 study, which received worldwide attention, revealed the negative results of the separation of child and mother due to hospitalization. Bowlby's work, together with that of associate John Robertson, led to a re-evaluation and liberalization of hospital visiting policies for children.

In the 1970s and 1980s, Marshall Klaus and John Kennell, physicians at Rainbow Babies and Children's Hospital in Cleveland, carried out important studies on the effect of the separation of newborns and parents. They established that this early separation may have long-term effects on family relationships and that offering the new family an opportunity to be together at birth and for a significant period after birth may provide benefits that last well into early childhood (Fig. 1-1). These findings also have helped to modify hospital policies. Hospital regulations changed slowly, but gradually they began to reflect the needs of children and their families. Isolation practices have been relaxed for children who do not have infectious diseases; children are encouraged to ambulate as early as possible and to visit the playroom, where they can be with other children. Nurses at all levels who work with children are prepared to understand, value, and use play as a therapeutic tool in the daily care of children.

● *Figure 1.1* The mother, father, and infant son soon after birth. Photo by Joe Mitchell.

CURRENT TRENDS IN MATERNAL–CHILD HEALTH CARE

Family-Centered Care

Childbirth came to be viewed as a safe and natural process as maternal and infant mortality rates began to fall. Women questioned the need for intense intervention in every birth. Also in question were the effects that medications and anesthesia had on the fetus. Many women began to insist on natural childbirth methods that allowed nature to take its course with minimal medical involvement. Some women voiced the desire for increased control over decisions about the timing and extent of interventions during labor and birth.

These efforts throughout the 1970s, 1980s, and 1990s led to family-centered maternity care, which eventually became the norm for American hospitals. Physicians and other health care providers began to respect the rights of women to participate in planning the type of care to be given during labor and birth. Husbands were at first allowed, and then encouraged, to participate in the birth process. Siblings were allowed greater access to their mother and the new baby. Birthing rooms and later labor, delivery, and recovery rooms (LDR) replaced the old assembly-line system of moving from a labor room, to a delivery room, to a recovery room. **Couplet care,** in which the mother and newborn remain together and receive care from one nurse, became the norm for postpartum care.

Family-centered pediatric nursing is a new and broadened concept in the health care system of the United States. No longer are children treated merely as clinical cases with attention given exclusively to their medical problems. Instead, health care providers recognize that children belong to a family, a community, and a particular way of life or culture and that their health is influenced by these and other factors (Fig. 1-2). Separating children from their backgrounds means that their needs are met only in a superficial manner, if at all. Even if nursing takes place entirely inside hospital walls, family-centered care pays attention to each child's unique emotional, developmental, social, and scholastic needs, as well as physical ones. Family-centered nursing care also strives to help family members alleviate their fears and anxieties and to cope, function normally, and understand the child's condition and their role in the healing process (see Chapter 2).

Regionalized Care

During the past several decades there has been a definite trend toward centralization and regionalization

External Factors
Physical Variables
Biologic Variables
Social Variables
Cultural Variables

Internal Factors
Personal Characteristics
Physiological Processes
Growth & Development
Behavior/Temperament

● *Figure 1.2* Internal and external factors that influence the health and illness patterns of the child.

of maternity and pediatric services. Providing high-quality medical care for the at-risk patient necessitated transporting the pregnant woman or the child to medical teaching centers with the best resources for diagnosis and treatment. To contribute to economic responsibility by avoiding duplication of services and equipment, the most intricate and expensive services and the most highly specialized personnel were made available in the centralized location: perinatologists, neonatologists, pediatric neurologists, adolescent allergy specialists, pediatric oncologists, nurse play therapists, child psychiatrists, neonatal and pediatric nurse practitioners, and clinical nurse specialists. In these large regional centers are found geneticists, at-risk antenatal units, neonatal intensive care units, computed tomography scanners, burn care units, and other highly specialized equipment and units.

Regionalized care often takes the maternity, neonatal, and pediatric patient far from home. Family caregivers must travel a longer distance to visit than if the patient were at a local suburban hospital. Family-centered care becomes even more important under these circumstances. Measures are taken to keep the hospitalization as brief as possible and the family close and directly involved in the patient's care. For the child in particular, separation from the family is traumatic and may actually retard recovery. Many of these regionalized centers (tertiary care hospitals) have accommodations where families may stay during the hospitalization of the pregnant woman, the neonate, or the child.

Advances in Research

Huge technological and scientific advances were made at the same time the movement for family-centered care was gaining momentum. It became possible to save premature and low–birth-weight infants who previously would not have survived. Diagnostic techniques were perfected. Surgical techniques to intervene on the fetus while in utero were developed. New research and techniques have made it possible to detect and treat children born with congenital problems and disorders almost immediately after birth. Pediatric specialists and specialty units add to the ability to treat childhood disorders sooner, thus decreasing the effect of the concern on the child and family. These are only a few examples of the research that has been done.

Questions that influence maternity care are guiding many biomedical research projects today. Two areas of intense scientific inquiry are the prediction and prevention of preterm labor and the causes, prevention, and treatment of pregnancy-induced hypertension, a condition exclusively found in pregnancy marked by high blood pressure, edema, and loss of protein in the urine. Progress in the prevention and/or treatment of these disorders would decrease maternal and infant mortality rates significantly.

Gene therapy is used to treat certain immune disorders. Scientists are studying ways to prevent and treat genetic disorders with gene therapy, which likely will be possible in the near future. Many animal, human, and stem cell studies are being done to better understand and treat a variety of obstetric disorders. Much progress has been made in understanding and treating infertility. Other examples of current studies include the identification of genes that are responsible for the unique characteristics of Down's syndrome and therapies to treat intrauterine growth retardation (IUGR), a condition in which the fetus fails to gain sufficient weight.

Bioethical Issues

An ethical issue is one in which there is no one "right" solution that applies to all instances of the issue. Ethical decision making is a complex process that should involve many groups of individuals with varying experiences and perspectives. Recent scientific and medical advances have raised bioethical issues that did not exist in times past. Examples of bioethical issues that are present in our world today include the Human Genome Project, prenatal genetic testing, surrogate motherhood, and rationing of health care.

The Human Genome Project (HGP) was started in 1990 with the purpose of studying all of the human genes and how they function. New concepts and ideas regarding many aspects of health and disease emerge as the project continues. Identification of gene mutations in people who may be carriers of genetic disorders or who may be at risk for developing inherited disorders later in life has been a big part of the research findings in the project. Genetic testing and counseling is one area that has been greatly affected by the HGP. A predisposition to certain diseases that become evident in adulthood is also being studied through the HGP. The ability to study the human gene and factors related to the inheritance of disease and disorders has an impact on the future health of all individuals.

Today it is possible to know many things about a child before the child is born. Ultrasound can reveal the gender of the fetus and certain abnormalities early in pregnancy. Amniocentesis and chorionic villus sampling show the entire genetic code of the fetus. In this way, many chromosomal abnormalities can be diagnosed during the first trimester. Decisions can be made about continuing with the pregnancy or preparing to cope with a child who has a genetic disorder. Some parents want to know everything possible before the child is born, whereas others do not wish to interfere with the natural order of things and decline any type of prenatal testing.

Many ethical questions can be raised regarding prenatal testing. Is it right to end a pregnancy because a child has a mild genetic abnormality? Will we become a society in which a child can be chosen or rejected for life based on his or her genetic code? Is it right to bring a child into the world with a severe defect, which may cause him and his caregivers untold pain and suffering? Is it OK to make life and death decisions based on quality of life? Or is any form of life sacred regardless of the quality? These and other questions have been raised in light of technology that makes prenatal diagnosis possible.

Surrogacy is an arrangement whereby a woman or a couple who is infertile contract with a fertile woman to carry a child. The fetus may result from in vitro fertilization techniques; embryos created from such techniques are subsequently implanted in the surrogate woman's womb to be carried to term. At other times the surrogate mother is impregnated by artificial insemination with the sperm of the man or with the sperm of an unknown donor.

Surrogate motherhood is a situation fraught with ethical dilemmas. Some of the questions that surround this issue include: Who has the right to make decisions about the pregnancy? Who is legally obligated for the unborn child? What if one or the other of the parties changes their minds before the end of the pregnancy? What if the infant is born with a genetic disorder that leaves him physically or mentally disabled?

Did you know? Many professional organizations have developed position statements that list guiding principles to be used when making certain ethical decisions. The American Academy of Pediatrics (AAP) has developed guidelines to be used when surrogacy options are being explored. For example, the AAP recommends that the rules surrounding adoption be used to guide decision making in surrogacy cases. This principle helps to safeguard the rights of the child in this unusual situation.

A phenomenon that some have referred to as "rationing of health care" is on the rise. On the one hand, there have been enormous advances in knowledge, technology, and the ability to intervene to change outcomes. Some conditions that were untreatable in the past can now be treated and even cured. On the other hand, individuals who live in poverty are less likely than persons of higher socioeconomic status to have access to these treatments and cures. Examples of ethical questions that arise in this situation include: To which services should all citizens have access regardless of ability to pay? What services are appropriate to exclude if the consumer cannot afford payment?

Demographic Trends

Several demographic trends are influencing the delivery of maternal–child health care in the United States. The aging of society and the tendency of American families to have fewer children have caused a shift in focus from the needs of women and children to those of the elderly. This trend has shifted fund allocation away from health care programs and research that enhance the health care of women and children.

The growing percentage of minority populations in relation to white, non-Hispanic populations in the United States will continue to affect health care. Nurses and other health care providers are expected to provide culturally appropriate care. The use of nontraditional methods of healing and over-the-counter herbal remedies must be assessed and integrated into the plan of care. More and more nurses are expected to accommodate the unique needs of these populations.

Poverty

One social issue that greatly influences maternity and pediatric care is the problem of poverty. A woman who lives in poverty is less likely to have access to adequate prenatal care. Poverty also has a negative impact on the ability of a woman and her children to be adequately nourished and sheltered. A woman who lives in poverty is at risk for substance abuse and exposure to diseases such as tuberculosis, human immunodeficiency virus /acquired immunodeficiency syndrome (HIV/AIDS), and other sexually transmitted infections. Each of these factors has been linked to adverse outcomes for childbearing women and their children.

Cost Containment

Cost containment refers to strategies developed to reduce inefficiencies in the health care system. Inefficiencies can occur in the way health care is used by consumers. For example, taking a child to the emergency department (ED) for treatment of a cold is inappropriate use. It would be more efficient for the child's cold to be treated at a clinic.

Inefficiencies also can relate to the setting in which health care is given. For example, in the past all surgical patients were admitted to the hospital the night, or sometimes even several days, before the scheduled procedure. This practice was found to be an inefficient use of the hospital setting. It was discovered that the patient could be prepared for surgery more efficiently on an outpatient basis without reducing quality.

Inefficiencies also can exist in the way health services are produced. For example, a neonatal intensive care unit (NICU) is a highly specialized, costly unit to operate. If every hospital in a large city were to operate a NICU, this would be an inefficient production of health services. It is more cost effective to have one large NICU for the entire region.

Cost Containment Strategies

There is no dispute that health care costs continue to increase at a rate out of proportion to the cost of living. This situation has challenged local, state, and federal governments; insurance payers; and providers and consumers of health care to cope with skyrocketing costs while maintaining quality of care. Some major strategies that have been implemented to help control costs include prospective payment systems, managed care, capitation, cost sharing, cost shifting, and alternative delivery systems.

Prospective Payment Systems. A **prospective payment system** predetermines rates to be paid to the health care provider to care for patients with certain classifications of diseases. These rates are paid regardless of the costs that the health care provider actually incurs. This system tends to encourage efficient production and use of resources. Prospective payment systems were developed by the government in an attempt to control Medicare costs. These systems include diagnosis-related groups (DRGs) for inpatient billing; ambulatory payment classifications (APCs); home health, inpatient rehabilitation facility, and skilled nursing facility prospective payment systems.

Managed Care. Managed care is a system that integrates management and coordination of care with financing in an attempt to improve cost effectiveness, use, quality, and outcomes. Managed care evolved from the old "fee-for-service" type of health insurance, in which providers of care were paid the amount they billed to provide a service. Under managed care plans, both the provider of service and the consumer have responsibilities to help control costs. The main types of managed care plans—health maintenance organizations (HMOs), preferred provider organizations (PPOs), and point-of-service (POS) plans—are discussed in the section "Payment for Health Services."

Capitation. **Capitation** is one method managed care plans have used to reduce costs. The health care plan pays a fixed amount per person to the health care provider to provide services for enrollees. This amount is negotiated up front, and the health care provider is obligated to provide care for the negotiated amount, regardless of the actual number or nature of the services provided.

Cost Sharing and Cost Shifting. Cost sharing refers to the costs that the patient incurs when using his health insurance plan. Examples of cost sharing are co-payments and deductibles. When costs go up, health insurance plans often increase the amount of deductibles and co-payments before they raise the price of the insurance premium. Cost shifting is a strategy in which the cost of providing uncompensated care for uninsured individuals is passed onto people who are insured. Often cost shifting results in higher premiums, co-pays, and deductibles.

Alternative Delivery Systems. Another way to control costs is to provide alternative delivery systems. In this situation, alternatives to expensive inpatient services are provided. Many hospitals found that it was more cost efficient to send a patient home earlier and provide follow-up care using a home health agency. Skilled and intermediate nursing and rehabilitation facilities and hospice programs are other examples of alternative delivery systems.

Nursing Contribution to Cost Containment

Specific cost containment strategies that nurses have been instrumental in implementing include health promotion, case management, and critical care paths.

Nurses are the primary providers of **utilization review**, which is a systematic evaluation of services delivered by a health care provider to determine appropriateness and quality of care, as well as medical necessity of the services provided.

Nurses have long advocated health promotion activities as a valuable way to maintain quality of life and control health care costs. Health promotion involves helping people to make lifestyle changes to move them to a higher level of wellness. Health promotion includes all aspects of health: physical, mental, emotional, social, and spiritual. Many nurses and nursing organizations lobby for increased spending on health promotion and illness prevention activities. For example, nurses may testify at a public hearing that it is more cost effective to provide comprehensive prenatal care for low income women than to pay high "back end" costs of highly specialized care in a NICU for a preterm baby. Nurses also may lobby for low-cost programs to provide periodic screening examinations in schools. The argument in this example is that it is cheaper to treat illness states when they are caught early in a screening program than to provide care when a disease is well advanced and harder to treat.

Although nurses are not the only licensed professionals qualified to provide case management, many case managers are nurses. **Case management** involves monitoring and coordinating care for individuals who need high-cost or extensive health care services. An at-risk pregnant woman with diabetes is a good candidate for case management because she requires frequent monitoring of blood sugars and coordination of several health care providers.

Concerns about cost containment, quality improvement, and managed care have led to the development of a system of standard guidelines, termed **critical pathways,** in many facilities. Critical pathways are standard plans of care used to organize and monitor the care provided. They include all aspects of care, such as diagnostic tests, consultations, treatments, activities, procedures, teaching, and discharge planning. Other names for clinical pathways are caremaps, collaborative care plans, case management plans, clinical paths, and multidisciplinary plans. To ensure success, the critical pathways must be a collaborative effort of all disciplines involved; all members of the health team must follow them.

The nursing process is part of the underlying framework of critical pathways. Nursing diagnoses and intermediate and discharge outcomes are necessary to avoid fragmenting care. Documentation of nursing interventions and outcomes is essential to the overall process. The nurse must thoroughly understand the nursing process to achieve accountability when providing care in a setting in which critical pathways are used (Table 1-1).

TABLE 1.1	Critical Path for School-ager With Long-Leg Cast After Fracture

A critical pathway is an abbreviated form of a care plan used by the entire multidisciplinary team. It provides outcome-based guidelines for goal achievement within a designated length of stay.

	Day One	Day Two
Diagnostic Tests	CBC X-ray left leg.	
Assessments	Establish baseline neurovascular status, then neurovascular checks every 2 hours. Inspect cast. Assess head, chest, and abdomen for other injuries. Assess skin integrity.	Perform neurovascular checks every 4 hours. Teach family to perform neurovascular checks. Inspect cast. Teach family cast inspection. Assess skin integrity. Teach family skin integrity assessment.
Diet	Diet as tolerated.	Diet as tolerated. Provide instruction on adding foods rich in protein.
Activity	Elevate leg when lying or sitting. Start nonweight-bearing crutch walking. Initiate safety precautions.	Elevate leg when lying or sitting. Assess ability to use nonweight-bearing crutch walking for discharge. Maintain safety precautions.
Medications	Tylenol with codeine for pain as ordered.	Tylenol with codeine for pain as ordered. Tylenol for pain as ordered.
Psychosocial	Assess developmental status. Promote self-care (bathing, dressing, grooming, etc.). Provide diversional activities. Assist in continuing school work. Teach safety.	Provide instruction on diversional activities for home. Instruct family on how to promote self-care. Reinforce safety teaching.
Discharge Planning	Teach cast care. Teach crutch walking. Arrange for home tutoring.	Provide written instructions and obtain feedback on cast care. Provide written instructions and obtain feedback on crutch walking. Provide written instructions for home tutoring. Include family and child in teaching. Arrange for follow-up appointment.

PAYMENT FOR HEALTH SERVICES

Access to and use of health care services often is facilitated by health care insurance. Typically, families with health care insurance are more likely to have a primary care provider and to participate in appropriate preventive care (Healthy People 2010, 2001). Statistics provided by Healthy People 2010 show that more than 44 million people in the United States do not have health insurance. Of this number, 11 million are children.

Most employment facilities provide some form of medical insurance for employees and their families; or families may elect to purchase their own insurance apart from an employer. This type of insurance is known as private insurance, whether it is provided by an employer or purchased directly by the health care consumer. For those who are uninsured, the federal and state governments have provided means to access health care services. In addition, specialized services are available, which may be funded by local, state, or federal governments or may be administered by private organizations.

Private Insurance

Private insurance can be acquired through work benefits or through individual means. The policyholder pays a monthly fee for the insurance coverage. The policyholder is responsible for paying the preset co-payment for any health services needed. Before the onset of managed care, medical services traditionally were paid for on a fee-for-service basis. Physicians billed for their services, and insurance providers paid whatever was charged. However, as technological advances were made and costs skyrocketed, managed care was created in an effort to contain costs and make

BOX 1.1	**Managed Care Plans**

Health Maintenance Organizations (HMOs)

With an HMO, contracts are made with selected health care providers and health care facilities to provide services to its policyholders for a fixed amount of money paid in advance for a specified set of time. The policyholder and insured family members choose health care providers and facilities from the list of those specifically associated with their HMO. The providers and facilities are closely evaluated for any unnecessary health care services.

Preferred Provider Organizations (PPOs)

PPOs consist of selected health care professionals and facilities who are under contract with insurance companies, employers, or third party payers to provide medical and surgical services to policyholders and insured family members. The policyholder has more choices for service providers when they choose a PPO versus a HMO. In addition, the services under a PPO are not fixed or prepaid. Should the policyholder choose to access services from a provider outside the PPO list of professionals and facilities, this may increase the policyholder's out-of-pocket expense for services rendered.

Some insurance companies provide physicians fixed amounts to provide health care to individuals, regardless of the actual costs involved. This system discourages physicians from ordering costly laboratory and diagnostic tests or from giving treatments of questionable therapeutic benefit. It has also encouraged physicians to see more patients, which decreases the amount of time available to individual patients.

Managed care has had multiple effects on individual consumers of health care. Consumers pay higher premiums with higher deductibles and co-payment amounts. At the same time, they have fewer choices. The consumer may choose from a limited number of providers that belong to a HMO or who are "in network" if the insurance plan is set up as a PPO. Review panels chosen by the HMO or PPO have the right to review and decline services deemed unnecessary. Usually the consumer cannot appeal these decisions. This situation has led to a consumer movement for the right to sue these companies when decisions negatively affect the individual's health.

This is not to say that all of the effects have been negative. Managed care has provoked the health care industry to be more cost conscious and fiscally temperate. Health care providers are less likely to order expensive tests and procedures unless there is an unmistakable benefit. However, health care costs, particularly pharmaceutical costs, have continued to increase out of proportion to other costs of living.

health care affordable. Managed care insurance plans include HMOs and PPOs (Box 1-1).

Federally Funded Sources

Medicaid

Medicaid was founded in 1965 under Title XIX of the Social Security Act. This federal program supplies block grants to states to provide health care for certain individuals who have low incomes. On average, the federal government contributes approximately 57% of the monies needed to finance the program. The states must fund the remaining 43% (National Association of State Budget Officers, undated). Under broad federal guidelines, each state develops and administers its own Medicaid program; therefore, eligibility requirements and application processes vary from state to state. Pregnant women and children who meet the income guidelines qualify for this program (Health Care Financing Administration, undated).

Although Medicaid has helped address the problem of access to health care for some childbearing women and some children, the process for applying is often complex and confusing. Many women and children who qualify do not benefit from the program. Concerned citizen groups in many states are working to modify the application process and find ways to assist eligible individuals to apply for and receive Medicaid.

State Child Health Insurance Program

Many families make too much money to qualify for Medicaid; however, health insurance is not available or affordable to them. Because of this problem, many pregnant women and children do not get adequate health care, particularly preventive care, such as prenatal care, well-child visits, and immunizations. In response to this need, the federal government instituted another block grant program to states under Title XXI of the Social Security Act. The State Child Health Insurance Program, also known by its acronym "SCHIP" or simply "CHIP," was enacted in 1997 as part of the Balanced Budget Act.

SCHIP provides health insurance to newborns and children in low-income families who do not otherwise qualify for Medicaid and are uninsured. Premiums and co-payment amounts are kept to a minimum and are based on a sliding scale according to total family income. Emphasis is placed on preventive care and health promotion in addition to treatment for illness and disease. One of the requirements for states to participate in SCHIP is that each state must develop an outreach program to inform and enroll eligible families and children.

Specialized Services

One federally funded program that continues to successfully meet its goal to enhance nutritional status for women and children is the Special Supplemental Nutrition Program for Women, Infants, and Children (WIC). WIC began serving low-income, nutritionally at-risk pregnant, breast-feeding, and postpartum women and their children (as old as 5 years) in 1974. The Food and Nutrition Service administers this grant program, which distributes monies to state agencies to provide benefits to eligible citizens.

WIC services are provided in local health departments, hospitals, and clinics in all 50 states. Women and their children must first meet income eligibility requirements, and then they are screened by a trained health professional (such as a nurse, social worker, or physician) for nutritional risk factors based on federal guidelines (Fig. 1-3). Nutritional risk factors are categorized as medically based risk and diet-based risk. Examples of medical risk factors include conditions such as young maternal age, anemia, poor pregnancy outcomes, and being underweight. Diet-based risk includes diets with deficiencies in any of the major food groups, vitamins, or minerals. Because there are not unlimited funds available, at-risk women are screened according to predetermined categories of priority.

The program is one of the federal government's success stories. It is currently estimated to be serving all eligible infants and 90% of all other eligible participants. Eligible women and their children receive food vouchers to redeem at participating grocery stores. The vouchers can be used to purchase foods that are high in at least one of the following nutrients: protein, iron, calcium, and vitamins A and C. Fortified cereals, milk, eggs, cheese, peanut butter, and legumes are examples of eligible foods. Although women are encouraged to breast-feed, if they choose to bottle-feed, their infants can receive formula assistance to 6 months of age.

Other institutions and organizations are available across the United States to provide health care services to children for special conditions regardless of the family's ability to pay. Two examples are the Shriners Hospital for Children and Easter Seals Early Childhood Intervention (ECI) program. The Shriners Hospital provides a wide variety of services to children with musculoskeletal disorders. Services provided to children include evaluation by specialists, diagnostic testing, surgical management, and provision of prostheses and other orthopedic devices for correction. The Shriners also have a "burn hospital" in Galveston, Texas. Children in serious need of complex treatment for burn injuries can come to this facility for complete service.

If a child is suspected of having a developmental delay that was identified during a routine clinic visit, Early Childhood Intervention (ECI), a program sponsored by Easter Seals, is available. This program can provide needed services for all children until the age of 3 years free of charge to any family in need of the service. The services provided include evaluation and weekly therapy for rehabilitation. A therapist also can go to the patient's home to provide needed therapy. A referral from the health care provider is all that is required to qualify for this type of assistance.

Here's how you can help!

Provide the patient and family with a list of available community health care resources before the patient leaves the hospital or the clinic. This information can be of great help, especially if the family needs financial assistance to afford adequate medical treatment.

Test Yourself

- Name two major developments that contributed to the modernization of maternity care in the United States.

- The work of which pediatric reformer led to the liberalization of hospital visiting policies for pediatric patients in the 1950s?

- Define "prospective payment system."

MATERNAL–CHILD HEALTH TODAY

One way to measure the health status of a nation is to determine **mortality rates** of childbearing women, infants, and children. Mortality rates are statistics recorded as the ratio of deaths in a given category to the number of individuals in that category of the population. The statistics that are of interest to the

● *Figure 1.3* A trained registered nurse screens a pregnant woman at a WIC clinic. If the woman meets income and nutritional eligibility requirements, she may receive vouchers to purchase nutritious foods.

maternity and pediatric nurse are maternal, fetal, neonatal, **perinatal** (the period surrounding birth, from conception throughout pregnancy and birth), infant, and child mortality rates. **Morbidity** refers to the number of person afflicted with the same disease condition per a certain number of population.

Maternal–Infant Health Status

Several definitions are required to better understand perinatal mortality rates. A **viable** fetus is one that is able to live outside of the uterus. In most states the law prescribes 20 weeks of gestation the arbitrary divider between viability and nonviability. The **fetal mortality rate** is calculated by dividing the number of deaths that occur in utero (during pregnancy) at 20 or more weeks of gestation (i.e., when the fetus is considered viable) by the number of live births plus fetal deaths.[2] **Neonatal** is the adjective used to describe the time period from birth through the first 28 days or 1 month of life. Therefore, the **neonatal mortality rate** is expressed as the number of infant deaths during the first 28 days of life for every 1,000 live births. **Perinatal mortality** encompasses the number of fetal/neonatal deaths that occur from 28 weeks of gestation through the first 7 days of life. The perinatal mortality rate is expressed as the number of deaths (as previously described) per 1,000 live births, plus fetal deaths that occur from 28 weeks of gestation and beyond. The **infant mortality rate** is the number of deaths during the first 12 months of life, which includes neonatal mortality. The **maternal mortality rate** refers to the number of maternal deaths per 100,000 live births caused by a pregnancy-related complication that occurs during pregnancy or during the 42 days after pregnancy. The leading causes of infant and maternal deaths are listed in Box 1-2. All death statistics relating to the fetus, neonate, and infant are reported as the number of deaths for every 1,000 live births. Maternal deaths are reported per 100,000 live births because they are uncommon.

Both infant and maternal mortality rates have fallen dramatically since the early 1900s (Figs. 1-4 and 1-5). At that time, for every 1,000 live births, approximately 100 infants died before they reached their first birthday. In 1999 that number had dropped to 7.1 deaths per 1,000 live births—a decline greater than 90%! Maternal mortality rates at the turn of the century were from 600 to 900 deaths per 100,000 live births and decreased to 7.7 deaths per 100,000 live births by 1997. This represents a greater than 99% decline in the maternal mortality rate (Centers for Disease Control, 1999).

Notwithstanding these remarkable advances, much work remains to be done. The United States lags behind 21 other industrialized nations in maternal

BOX 1.2	Leading Causes of Infant and Maternal Mortality in the United States

Infant Mortality

The three leading causes of infant death for the year 2000 (the latest year for which data are available) are listed in descending order.

1. Congenital malformations, deformations, and chromosomal abnormalities (21%)
2. Disorders related to short gestation and low birth weight (16%)
3. Sudden infant death syndrome (SIDS) (9%)*

Maternal Mortality

The three leading causes of pregnancy-related death for the years 1991 to 1999 (the latest year for which data are available) are listed in descending order.

1. Embolism (20%)
2. Hemorrhage (17%)
3. Pregnancy-related hypertension (16%)†

*Source: Centers for Disease Control. (2002). *National vital statistics report, 50*(12). Retrieved July 13, 2003, from http://www.cdc.gov/nchs/data/nvsr/nvsr50/nvsr50_12.pdf

†Source: Centers for Disease Control. (2003). *Fact sheet. Pregnancy-related mortality surveillance—United States, 1991–1999.* Retrieved July 13, 2003, from http://www.cdc.gov/od/oc/media/pressrel/fs030220.htm

mortality statistics. Since 1982, the maternal mortality rate has hovered between 7 and 8 deaths per 100,000 live births. The Healthy People 2000 goal[3] of 3.3 maternal deaths per 100,000 live births set in 1987 has not been reached (Centers for Disease Control, 1998).

● *Figure 1.4* United States infant mortality rate by year (1915–1997). Centres for Disease Control. (1999). Healthier mothers and babies. *MMWR: Morbidity and Mortality Weekly Report, 48*(38), 849–856. Retrieved March 3, 2002, from http://www.cdc.gov/mmwr/PDF/wk/mm4838.pdf

---

[2] Fetal deaths are often referred to as "stillbirths" in lay terminology.

[3] Healthy People 2000 were national health goals set in 1987. For further information on the Healthy People initiative see the website: http://www.health.gov/healthypeople/

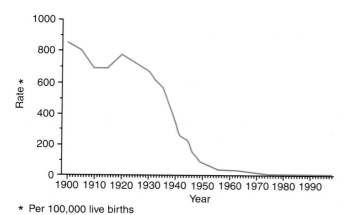

* Per 100,000 live births

● *Figure 1.5* United States maternal mortality rate by year (1900–1997).
Centres for Disease Control. (1999). Healthier mothers and babies. *MMWR: Morbidity and Mortality Weekly Report, 48*(38), 849–856. Retrieved March 3, 2002, from http://www.cdc.gov/mmwr/PDF/wk/mm4838.pdf

years of age. The lack of adequate financial resources, insurance, and education regarding birth control and health care in general contributes to this situation.

Child and Adolescent Health Status

In the first half of the 20th century, many children died during or after childbirth or in early childhood as a result of disease, infections, or injuries. Technological and socioeconomic changes have influenced the health care provided to children and also the health problems that confront today's children. Communicable diseases of childhood and their complications are no longer a serious threat to the health of children. As the 21st century begins, health problems for children focus much more on social concerns (Table 1-2). These issues are summarized below and discussed throughout the text.

Infectious diseases such as polio, diphtheria, scarlet fever, measles, and whooping cough once posed the greatest threat to children. However, today the largest risk to all children and adolescents is unintentional injury, frequently the result of motor vehicle accidents. Other unintentional injuries include drowning, falls, poisonings, and fires. Families, communities, and government agencies are minimizing the risks of injury-related death through protection and safety measures.

Morbidity rates among children often are associated with environmental and socioeconomic issues. According to the American Academy of Pediatrics (AAP), the increasing complexity in the environment seems to have created new morbidities that greatly affect the child's psychosocial development. These include:

In addition, there is a racial disparity in maternal mortality rates. The maternal mortality rate of black women for the years 1982 to 1996 hovers between 18 and 22 deaths per 100,000 live births, whereas white women have a mortality rate of 5 to 6 during the same period. A black woman is almost twice as likely as a white woman to experience a complication of pregnancy and is four times more likely to die of a complication of pregnancy. If the disparity were to be eliminated, the overall rate would fall from 7.5 to less than 6 per 100,000 live births (Centers for Disease Control, 1998).

The U.S. infant mortality rate lags behind that of many other industrialized nations. Preliminary statistics from 2002 indicate that the U.S. infant mortality rate is 6.69; nearly twice that of Iceland, the country with the lowest reported rate, which is 3.53 (*The World Factbook*, 2002). Many factors may be associated with high infant mortality rates and poor health. Low birth weight and late or nonexistent prenatal care are main factors in the poor rankings in infant mortality. Other major factors that compromise infants' health include congenital anomalies, sudden infant death syndrome, respiratory distress syndrome, and increasing rates of HIV. Low birth weight and other causes of infant death and chronic illness are often linked to maternal factors, such as lack of prenatal care, smoking, use of alcohol and illicit drugs, pregnancy before age 18 or after age 40, poor nutrition, lower socioeconomic status, lower educational levels, and environmental hazards.

Both infant and maternal mortality rates are much higher among nonwhite populations; studies repeatedly attribute high mortality rates to lack of adequate prenatal care and an increased birth rate among the high-risk group of adolescent girls and young women 15 to 19

- School problems, including learning disabilities and attention difficulties
- Child and adolescent mood and anxiety disorders
- Adolescent suicide and homicide, which is increasing alarmingly
- Firearms in home
- School violence
- Drug and alcohol abuse
- HIV and AIDS
- The effects of media on violence, obesity, and sexual activity.

Historically, disease conditions affecting children were very different from those affecting adults. Today, an increasing number of health conditions diagnosed in children used to be seen only among adults. For example, hyperlipidemia and hypercholesterolemia are becoming more frequently diagnosed in children. Statistics reveal an increase in the number of children older than 12 years of age identified with hypertension (elevated blood pressure). Obesity is another major health concern in children. According to the National Health

TABLE 1.2	Social and Health Concerns for Infants and Children

Every day in America the following occurrences take place:

	All US Children	Black Children	White Children	Latino Children	Asian American Children	Native American Children
Children and youths under 25 die from HIV infection	3	2	1	—	—	—
Children and youths under 20 commit suicide	6	1	5	—	—	—
Children and youths under 20 are homicide victims	13	6	5	—	—	—
Children and youths under 20 are killed by guns	15	5	7	—	—	—
Children and youths under 20 die from accidental injuries	34	6	28	—	—	—
Babies die before their first birthday	78	24	51	11	2	1
Babies are born at very low birth weight (<3 lb 4 oz)	156	49	92	21	5	1
Babies are born at low birth weight (<5.5 lb)	817	212	536	121	32	7
Babies are born to teenage mothers	1,354	372	959	334	24	22
Babies are born to mothers who had late or no prenatal care	410	114	275	124	18	9
Babies are born into poverty	1,951	723	13,231	679	—	—
Children and youths under 18 are arrested for drug offenses	351	143	270	—	4	3
Children and youths under 18 are arrested for violent crimes	186	105	126	—	4	2
Students drop out of high school each school day	2,911	500	2,144	672	—	—

Source: Children's Defense Fund, 2001.

Note: not all totals equal 100%.

and Nutrition Examination Survey (NHANES), from 1999 to 2000, 15% of children and adolescents between the ages of 6 and 19 years were found to be overweight or obese. In addition, children are now included in the statistics for patients experiencing depression. For example, major depressive disorder occurs in approximately 1% to 3% of children and dysthymic disorder (chronic depression with no clearly defined well periods) occurs in 1% of children and 8% of adolescents.

Developmental problems related to socioeconomic factors are on the rise, including mental retardation, learning disorders, emotional and behavioral problems, and speech and vision impairments. Lead poisoning appears to be a major threat to the child's developmental well-being. Although strict laws have minimized the amount of lead in gas, air, food, and industrial emissions, many children live and play in substandard housing areas, where they are exposed to chipped lead-based paint, dust, and soil.

Other prevalent factors that affect children's health include respiratory illness, violence toward children in the form of child abuse and neglect, homicide, suicide, cigarette smoking, alcohol and illicit drug use, risky sexual behavior, obesity, and lack of exercise.

Healthy living habits are established early in childhood. Many schools educate students about the hazards of tobacco, drugs, and the importance of exercise, nutrition, and safe sex. Many also provide immunization and screening programs. However, there is still a need for improvements and increases in the number of educational and support programs available to children, families, and communities. The program goals should be to alleviate many child health problems and provide children with adequate tools to make healthy living choices well into adulthood.

Addressing Maternal–Child Health Status

Box 1-3 shows the Centers for Disease Control (CDC) recommendations of ways to continue to decrease maternal and infant mortality. Other major steps toward addressing the issue of maternal–child health status are discussed in this chapter.

| BOX 1.3 | **Opportunities to Reduce Maternal and Infant Mortality** |

Prevention measures to reduce maternal and infant mortality and to promote the health of all childbearing-aged women and their newborns should start before conception and continue through the postpartum period. Some of these prevention measures include the following:

Before Conception
- Screen women for health risks and pre-existing chronic conditions, such as diabetes, hypertension, and sexually transmitted diseases.
- Counsel women about contraception and provide access to effective family planning services (to prevent unintended pregnancies and unnecessary abortions).
- Counsel women about the benefits of good nutrition; encourage women especially to consume adequate amounts of folic acid supplements (to prevent neural tube defects) and iron.
- Advise women to avoid alcohol, tobacco, and illicit drugs.
- Advise women about the value of regular physical exercise.

During Pregnancy
- Provide women with early access to high-quality care throughout pregnancy, labor, and delivery. Such care includes risk-appropriate care, treatment for complications, and the use of antenatal corticosteroids when appropriate.
- Monitor and, when appropriate, treat pre-existing chronic conditions.
- Screen for and, when appropriate, treat reproductive tract infections including bacterial vaginosis, group B streptococcus infections, and human immunodeficiency virus.
- Vaccinate women against influenza, if appropriate.
- Continue counseling against use of tobacco, alcohol, and illicit drugs.
- Continue counseling about nutrition and physical exercise.
- Educate women about the early signs of pregnancy-related problems.

During Postpartum Period
- Vaccinate newborns at age-appropriate times.
- Provide information about well-baby care and benefits of breast-feeding.
- Warn parents about exposing infants to secondhand smoke.
- Counsel parents about placing infants to sleep on their backs.
- Educate parents about how to protect their infants from exposure to infectious diseases and harmful substances.

From Centers for Disease Control. (1999). Healthier mothers and babies. *MMWR: Morbidity and Mortality Weekly Report, 48*(38), 849–856. Retrieved March 3, 2002, from http://www.cdc.gov/mmwr/PDF/wk/mm4838.pdf

National Commission to Prevent Infant Mortality

In 1986, Congress established the National Commission to Prevent Infant Mortality and charged it with the responsibility of creating a national strategic plan to reduce infant mortality and morbidity rates in the United States. In 1988, the Commission's first report, *Death Before Life: The Tragedy of Infant Mortality,* listed two primary objectives: to make the health of mothers and babies a national priority and to provide universal access to care for all pregnant women and children. The Commission concluded that educating the nation about the health needs of mothers and babies would cause a national response to the problem and that women would have to be given information and motivation to reduce infant mortality and morbidity rates. The Commission also stated that barriers of finances, geography, education, social position, behavior, and program administration problems must be eliminated to provide universal access to health care. In February 1990, the Commission published *Troubling Trends: The Health of the Next Generation,* which concluded that early prenatal care, along with smoking cessation, pregnancy planning, and nutrition counseling and food supplementation, would result in heavier and healthier infants. The Commission has been successful in its objective of decreasing infant mortality.

Healthy People 2010

In 1990, a national consortium of more than 300 organizations developed a set of objectives for the year 2000, *Healthy People 2000*. Prevention of illness, or health promotion, was the underlying goal of these objectives. States were encouraged to set their own objectives. Priority areas specifically affecting children were identified. These objectives were reviewed mid-decade; although there had been progress in some goals, much remained to be accomplished. The initiative has continued, and *Healthy People 2010* outlines two basic goals for health promotion and disease prevention. Goal one is to increase quality and years of healthy life; goal two is to eliminate health disparities (Healthy People 2010, 2001). These goals are divided further into focus areas and attainment objectives. Many of the focus areas and objectives directly relate to pregnant women and children and their health care (Box 1-4). Nurses caring for pregnant women and children use these objectives as underlying guidelines in planning care.

BOX 1.4	Healthy People 2010: Focus Areas Related to Childbearing Women and Children

Focus Area: Access to Quality Health Services
Goal: Improve access to comprehensive, high-quality health care services.
  Persons with health insurance
  Single toll-free number for poison control centers
  Special needs for children
  Early (starting in the first trimester) and consistent prenatal care
Focus Area: Educational and Community-Based Programs
Goal: Increase the quality, availability, and effectiveness of education and community-based programs designed to prevent disease and improve health and quality of life.
  School health education
  School nurse-to-student ratio
  Community health promotion programs
  Patient and family education
  Culturally appropriate and linguistically competent community health promotion programs
Focus Area: Environmental Health
Goal: Promote health for all through a healthy environment.
  Safe drinking water
  Elevated blood lead levels in children
  School policies to protect against environmental hazards
  Toxic pollutants
Focus Area: Family Planning
Goal: Improve pregnancy planning and spacing and prevent unintended pregnancy.
  Adolescent pregnancy
  Abstinence before age 15 and among adolescents age 15 to 17 years
  Birth spacing
  Contraceptive use
  Male involvement in pregnancy prevention
  Pregnancy prevention and sexually transmitted disease (STD) protection
  Insurance coverage for contraceptive supplies and services
  Problems in becoming pregnant and maintaining a pregnancy
Focus Area: HIV
Goal: Prevent HIV infection and its related illness and death.
  Condom use
  Screening for STDs and immunization for hepatitis B
  Perinatally acquired HIV infection
Focus Area: Immunization and Infectious Diseases
Goal: Prevent disease, disability, and death from infectious disease, including vaccine-preventable diseases.
  Hepatitis B and bacterial meningitis in infants and young children
  Antibiotics prescribed for ear infections
  Vaccination coverage and strategies
Focus Area: Injury and Violence Prevention
Goal: Reduce injuries, disabilities, and deaths due to unintentional injuries and violence.
  Child fatality review
  Deaths from firearms, poisoning, suffocation, motor vehicle crashes
  Child restraints
  Drownings
  Maltreatment and maltreatment fatalities of children
Focus Area: Maternal, Infant, and Child Health
Goal: Improve the health and well-being of women, infants, children, and families.
  Fetal, infant, child, adolescent deaths
  Maternal deaths and illnesses
  Prenatal and obstetric care
  Low birth-weight and very low–birth-weight, preterm births
  Developmental disabilities and neural tube defects
  Prenatal substance exposure
  Fetal alcohol syndrome
  Breast-feeding
  Newborn screening
Focus Area: Nutrition and Overweight
Goal: Promote health and reduce chronic disease associated with diet and weight.
  Overweight or obesity in children and adolescents
  Iron deficiency in young children and in females of childbearing age
  Anemia in low-income pregnant females
  Iron deficiency in pregnant females
Focus Area: Physical Fitness and Activity
Goal: Improve health, fitness, and quality of life through daily physical activity.
  Physical activity in children and adolescents
Focus Area: Sexually Transmitted Diseases
Goal: Promote responsible sexual behaviors, increase access to quality services to prevent STDs and their complications.
  Responsible adolescent sexual behavior
  STD complications affecting females
  STD complications affecting the fetus and newborn
  Screening of pregnant women
Focus Area: Substance Abuse
Goal: Reduce substance abuse to protect the health, safety, and quality of life for all, especially children.
  Adverse consequences of substance use and abuse
  Substance use and abuse
Focus Area: Tobacco Use
Goal: Reduce illness, disability, and death related to tobacco use and exposure to secondhand smoke.
  Adolescent tobacco use, age, and initiation of tobacco use
  Smoking cessation by adolescents
  Exposure to tobacco smoke at home among children
Focus Area: Vision and Hearing
Goal: Improve the visual and hearing health of the nation.
  Vision screening for children
  Impairment in children and adolescents
  Newborn hearing screening, evaluation, and intervention
  Otitis media
  Noise-induced hearing loss in children

Adapted from National Center for Health Statistics. (2001). *Healthy people 2010.* Hyattsville, MD, Author.

Test Yourself

- What deaths are covered under the term "perinatal mortality?"

- Name the number one cause of maternal mortality in the United States.

- Name the two basic goals for health promotion and disease prevention outlined by Healthy People 2010.

THE NURSE'S CHANGING ROLE IN MATERNAL–CHILD HEALTH CARE

The image of nursing has changed, and the horizons and responsibilities have broadened tremendously in recent years. The primary thrust of health care is toward prevention. In addition to the treatment of disease and physical problems, modern maternal–child care addresses prenatal care, growth and development, and anticipatory guidance on maturational and common health problems. Teaching also is an important aspect of caring for the childbearing and child-rearing family. Clients are educated on a variety of topics, from follow-up of immunizations to other, more traditional aspects of health.

Nurses at all levels are legally accountable for their actions and assume new responsibilities and accountability with every advance in education. Nurses practicing in maternity and pediatric settings at all levels must keep up to date with education and information on how to help their patients and where to direct families for help when other resources are needed. When the nurse functions as a teacher, adviser, and resource person, it is important that the information and advice provided be correct, pertinent, and useful to the person in need.

Advanced practice nurses, in particular the certified nurse midwife (CNM) and nurse practitioners—family, neonatal, and pediatric—have taken a significant place in caring for childbearing and child-rearing families. The family nurse practitioner (FNP) provides primary care for women and their families. When pregnancy occurs, the FNP usually refers the woman to a CNM or obstetrician for prenatal care. The neonatal nurse practitioner (NNP) specializes in the care of the neonate. NNPs are employed by hospital NICUs and by neonatologists to provide care for premature and other sick newborns. The pediatric nurse practitioner (PNP) specializes in primary care of the child. Some of these nurses specialize in school nursing or oncology, among other areas. In addition, clinical nurse specialists (CNS) are nurses with advanced education prepared to provide care at any stage of illness or wellness.

In many settings, nurses can provide health education to both children and their families. Such teaching may be concerned with safety, nutrition, health habits, immunizations, dental care, healthy development, and discipline. Some of these settings include schools, homes, and ambulatory settings. In schools, nurses have become much more than Band-Aid dispensers: they monitor well children, including their immunizations and their growth and development. School nurses often present or are consultants in classroom health education programs and often serve on committees that evaluate children with educational and social adjustment problems. For children with long-term or chronic illnesses, nurses can help provide care in the home. This home care often is part of a collaboration with other health care professionals. Ambulatory care settings help avoid separating the child from the family and provide a less costly means of administering health care to children. The pediatric nurse plays an important role in ambulatory settings. In addition, nurses are contributing to health care research that will help lead to more improvements in the care of children and their families.

Health teaching is one of the most important aspects of promoting wellness. Nurses are often in a position to do incidental teaching, as well as more organized formal teaching. Nurses also must be aware that they serve as role models to others in practicing good health habits. Some examples of possible teaching opportunities include those in a work environment, such as helping the child and family understand a diagnosis or proposed treatment, understanding medications, and providing teaching materials to children and families. In the community, the nurse can be an advocate for healthy living practices and policies or can serve as a volunteer in community organizations to promote healthy growth and development and anticipatory guidance. Nurses can become involved with their schools to offer knowledge and expertise in wellness practices. They should use every opportunity to contribute to and encourage healthy living practices.

Throughout this text, teaching opportunities are identified and teaching suggestions supplied. Nurses are encouraged to use these suggestions as a foundation for further teaching. However, during any teaching the nurse must be alert to the abilities of the child and the family to understand the material being presented. By using methods of feedback, questions and answers, and demonstrations when appropriate, the nurse can confirm that the information is understood. This also gives the nurse the opportunity to reinforce any areas of weak information. With experience, nurses can become very competent teachers.

A PERSONAL GLIMPSE

My Grandpa's eyes gave me my first vision of nursing. A licensed practical nurse, he filled my head with hospital stories and my belly with chocolate milk. He saw people hurt by pain and fear, and he made them feel better. I wasn't much bigger than the children I saw, but I knew I wanted to make them feel better too. So I went to nursing school in the same hospital where I shared chocolate milk with Grandpa.

My pediatric nursing career started at graduation 25 years ago. Back then, the community pediatric unit was always filled to capacity. Outpatient and critical care services for children were minimal, so disorders ranged from the mild to the severe. Newborns through teens were treated for everything from mild diarrhea to significant trauma. But two things remained constant regardless of age or diagnosis: the pain and the fear.

Soon, helping sick children feel better was no longer enough. I realized early in my career that the best way to help was to prevent children from getting sick in the first place. So I went back to school, through baccalaureate and masters' degrees, to become a pediatric nurse practitioner (PNP). Seventeen years later, I still practice as a PNP in a rural community.

Changes in health care have put more emphasis on the various nonhospital settings, where most children receive care. Healthy children are less likely to become ill and more likely to become healthy adults. Prevention and health promotion are essential. They should be part of the care of all children (and adults!), including those who are hospitalized. I always take the time to teach the importance of immunizations, proper nutrition, growth, and development. A little goes a long way, and there is tremendous satisfaction in knowing that I've helped to ease pain and fear before they have a chance to get started.

Mary

LEARNING OPPORTUNITY: What are the challenges for the nurse caring for the child in a community health setting? Describe the priorities of the pediatric nurse in health promotion and disease prevention.

CRITICAL THINKING

Along with teaching, it is important for the nurse to use clinical judgment and purposeful thought and reasoning to make decisions that lead to positive outcomes for the maternal and pediatric patient. This process is called critical thinking. The nurse takes data collected and uses skills and knowledge to make a conscious plan to care for the patient and family. As the plan is carried out, the nurse continues to evaluate and revise the care of the patient, keeping the desired outcomes always in mind. By using critical thinking, the nurse can be more proficient and effective at meeting the needs of the patient. Critical thinking is based on a systematic process and is used as the nurse follows and uses the nursing process.

THE NURSING PROCESS

The **nursing process** is a proven form of problem solving based on the scientific method. The nursing process consists of five components:

- Assessment
- Nursing diagnosis
- Outcome identification and planning
- Implementation
- Evaluation

Based on the data collected during the assessment, nursing diagnoses are determined, nursing care is planned and implemented, and the results are evaluated. The process does not end here but continues through reassessment, establishment of new diagnoses, additional plans, implementation, and evaluation until all the patient's nursing problems are identified and dealt with (Fig. 1-6).

Assessment

Nursing assessment is a skill that must be practiced and perfected through study and experience. The practical

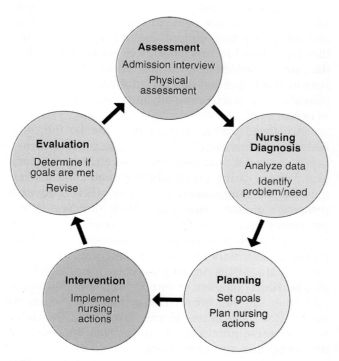

● *Figure 1.6* Diagram of the Nursing Process.

nurse collects data and contributes to the child's assessment. The nurse must be skilled in understanding the concepts of verbal and nonverbal communication; concepts of growth and development; anatomy, physiology, and pathophysiology; and the influence of cultural heritage and family social structure. Data collected during the assessment of the child and family form the basis of all the child's nursing care.

Assessment and data collection begin with the admission interview and physical examination. During this phase, a relationship of trust begins to build between the nurse, the child, and the family caregivers. This relationship forms more quickly when the nurse is sensitive to the family's cultural background. Careful listening and recording of **subjective data** (data spoken by the child or family) and careful observation and recording of **objective data** (observable by the nurse) are essential to obtaining a complete picture.

Nursing Diagnosis

The process of determining a nursing diagnosis begins with the analysis of information (data) gathered during the assessment. Along with the registered nurse or other health care professional, the practical nurse participates in the development of a nursing diagnosis based on actual or potential health problems that fall within the range of nursing practice. These diagnoses are not medical diagnoses but are based on the individual response to a disease process, condition, or situation. Nursing diagnoses change as the patient's responses change; therefore, diagnoses are in a continual state of re-evaluation and modification.

Nursing diagnoses are subdivided into three types: actual, risk, and wellness diagnoses. **Actual nursing diagnoses** identify existing health problems. For example, a child who has asthma may have an actual diagnosis stated as *Ineffective Airway Clearance related to increased mucous production as evidenced by dyspnea and wheezing.* This statement identifies a health problem the child actually has (ineffective airway clearance), the factor that contributes to its cause (increased mucous production), and the signs and symptoms. This is an actual nursing diagnosis because of the presence of signs and symptoms and the child's inability to clear the airway effectively.

Risk nursing diagnoses identify health problems to which the patient is especially vulnerable. These identify patients at high risk for a particular problem. An example of a risk nursing diagnosis is *Risk for Injury related to uncontrolled muscular activity secondary to seizure.*

Wellness nursing diagnoses identify the potential of a person, family, or community to move from one level of wellness to a higher level. For example, a wellness diagnosis for a family adapting well to the birth of a second child might be *Readiness for Enhanced Family Coping.*

The North American Nursing Diagnosis Association (NANDA) first published an approved list of nursing diagnoses in 1973; since then the list has been revised and expanded periodically. Nursing diagnoses continue to be developed and revised to keep them current and useful in describing what nurses contribute to health care.

Outcome Identification and Planning

To plan nursing care for the child, data must be collected (assessment) and analyzed (nursing diagnosis) and outcomes identified in cooperation with the child and family caregiver. These **outcomes** (goals) should be specific, stated in measurable terms, and include a time frame. For example, a short-term expected outcome for a child with asthma could be "The child will demonstrate use of metered-dose inhaler within 2 days." The goal must be realistic, child-focused, and attainable. After mutual goal setting has been accomplished, nursing actions are proposed. Although a number of possible diagnoses may be identified, the nurse must review them, rank them by urgency, and select those that require the most immediate attention.

After selecting the first goals to accomplish, the nurse must propose nursing interventions to achieve them. This is the planning aspect of the nursing process. These nursing interventions may be based on clinical experience, knowledge of the health problem, standards of care, standard care plans, or other resources. The interventions should be discussed with the child and family caregiver to determine if they are practical and workable. Proposed interventions are modified to fit the individual child. If standardized care plans are used, they must be individualized to reflect the child's age and developmental level, cognitive level, and family, economic, and cultural influences. Expected outcomes are set with specific measurable criteria and time lines.

Implementation

Implementation is the process of putting the nursing care plan into action. These actions may be independent, dependent, or interdependent. **Independent nursing actions** are actions that may be performed based on the nurse's own clinical judgment, for example, initiating protective skin care for an area that might break down. **Dependent nursing actions,** such as administering analgesics for pain, are actions that the nurse performs as a result of a physician's order. **Interdependent nursing actions** are actions that the nurse must accomplish in conjunction with other health team members, such as meal planning with the dietary therapist and teaching breathing exercises with the respiratory therapist.

Evaluation

Evaluation is a vital part of the nursing process. The practical nurse participates with other members of the health care team in the child's evaluation. Evaluation measures the success or failure of the nursing plan of care. Like assessment, evaluation is an ongoing process. Evaluation is achieved by determining if the identified outcomes have been met. The criteria of the nursing outcomes determine if the interventions were effective. If the goals have not been met in the specified time, or if implementation is unsuccessful, a particular intervention may need to be reassessed and revised. Possibly the outcome criterion is unrealistic and needs to be discarded or adjusted. The child and the family must be assessed to determine progress adequately. Both objective data (measurable) and subjective data (based on responses from the child and family) are used in the evaluation.

DOCUMENTATION

One of the most important parts of nursing care is recording information about the patient on the permanent record. This record, the patient's chart, is a legal document and must be accurate and complete. Nursing care provided and responses to care are included. In maternity and pediatric settings, documentation is extremely important because those records can be used in legal situations many years after they are written. These records include the nurse's observations and findings, and they help explain and justify the actions taken.

Documentation may be done in various forms, including admission assessments, nurse's or progress notes, graphic sheets, checklists, medication records, and discharge teaching or summaries. Many health care settings use computerized or bedside documentation records. Whatever the system or form used, concise, factual information is charted. Everything written must be legible and clear and include the date and time. Nursing actions such as medication administration must be documented as soon as possible after the intervention to ensure the action is communicated, especially in the care of childbearing women and children.

Test Yourself

- During the nursing process, analysis of information (data) gathered during the assessment is done in order to determine the _____ _____ (two words).

- In which part of the nursing process is it determined whether or not identified outcomes have been met?

- Name at least one important criterion that must be met when health information is documented.

KEY POINTS

- Two major developments that forever changed the way maternity care was given in the United States were acceptance of the germ theory that led to decreased deaths from infection and the development of obstetric anesthesia to ease the pain of childbirth.

- Many changes have taken place in the care of children in the past century. Until the early part of the 20th century, children were treated as miniature adults and were expected to behave that way.

- The concept of family-centered care developed in conjunction with the consumer movement that led childbirth to be viewed as a safe and natural process. Family-centered pediatric care recognizes that children should receive care within the context of their families and cultural norms.

- Regionalization of care contributes to economic responsibility by avoiding duplication of services and expensive equipment.

- Recent advances in research have led to new ethical dilemmas that must be addressed by health care providers. Examples include the Human Genome Project, prenatal genetic testing, surrogate motherhood, and rationing of health care.

- The increase in the number of older Americans, the tendency for American families to limit the number of children, and budget deficiencies have influenced a shift in focus away from programs for childbearing women and their infants.

- Poverty and the "rationing of health care" are social issues that have a negative impact on the health of childbearing women *and children* and increase the chance that complications will occur.

- Ethical dilemmas are by definition difficult to decide and involve complex choices and conflicts. Ethical decisions should always be made after careful consideration and with input from a variety of sources.

- Rising health care costs and shrinking budgets have led to attempts to reform health care. Managed care has become the norm of American health care. Attempts to contain health care costs have led to the development of prospective payment systems (such as HMOs and PPOs) and capitation. Nurses have been especially helpful with the cost-containment strategies of utilization review, critical pathways, and case management.

- Health care reform has led to changes in the Medicaid program and the development of SCHIP, low cost insurance for low-income children whose parents make too much money to qualify for Medicaid.

- One way in which the health status of a nation is measured is through morbidity (illness) and mortality (death) rates. Measures particularly useful to maternity and pediatric health include perinatal, maternal, and pediatric mortality rates.

- The three leading causes of infant mortality are congenital disorders, prematurity and low birth weight, and sudden infant death syndrome. The three leading causes of maternal mortality are embolism, hemorrhage, and pregnancy-induced hypertension.

- Although its infant mortality rate is improving, the United States still remains behind most other industrialized countries. Lack of or inadequate prenatal care is believed to be one major cause of this problem.

- Child health status has been influenced by technologic and socioeconomic changes. Many previous health concerns, such as communicable diseases of childhood, have been eliminated. Health problems for children today focus more on social concerns.

- *Healthy People 2010* sets goals for health care with a focus on health promotion and prevention of illness as the nation approaches the year 2010.

- The role of the nurse has changed to include the responsibilities of teacher, adviser, resource person, and researcher, as well as caregiver.

- The nurse uses critical thinking skills to take data collected and use it to develop a plan to meet the desired outcomes for the maternity and pediatric patient.

- The nursing process is essential in the problem-solving process necessary to plan nursing care. The five steps of the nursing process include assessment, nursing diagnosis, outcome identification and planning, implementation, and evaluation.

- Accurate and timely documentation is essential for providing a legal record of care given. This is particularly important to the maternity and pediatric nurse because legal action can occur many years after an event.

REFERENCES AND SELECTED READINGS

Books and Journals

Alden, E.R. (1999). The field of pediatrics. In C. DeAngelis, R. Feigin, & J. Warshaw (Eds.), *Oski's pediatrics: Principles and practice* (3rd ed.). Philadelphia: Lippincott Williams & Wilkins.

Butz, A. M., Pulsifer, M., Marano, N., Belcher H., Lears, M. K., & Royall, R. (2001). Effectiveness of a home intervention for perceived child behavioral problems and parenting stress in children with in utero drug exposure. *Archives of Pediatrics & Adolescent Medicine, 155*(9), 1029–1037.

Carr, I. (Undated). Dying to have a baby: The history of childbirth. Retrieved February 24, 2002, from http://www.umanitoba.ca/outreach/manitoba_womens_health/hist1.htm

Centers for Disease Control. (1999). Healthier mothers and babies. *MMWR: Morbidity and Mortality Weekly Report, 48*(38), 849-856. Retrieved March 3, 2002, from http://www.cdc.gov/mmwr/PDF/wk/mm4838.pdf

Cone, T. E. Jr. (1980). *History of American pediatrics.* Boston: Little Brown.

Centers for Disease Control. (1998). Maternal mortality—United States, 1982–1996. *MMWR: Morbidity and Mortality Weekly Report, 47*(34), 705–707. Retrieved March 3, 2002, from http://www.cdc.gov/mmwr/PDF/wk/mm4734.pdf

Corrarino, J. E., Williams, C., Campbell, W. S., Amrhein, E., LoPiano, L., & Kalachik, D. (2000). Linking substance-abusing pregnant women to drug treatment services: A pilot program. *Journal of Obstetric, Gynecologic, and Neonatal Nursing (JOGNN), 29*(4), 36976.

Eckenrode, J., Ganzel, B., Henderson, C. R., Smith, E., Olds, D. L., Powers, J., et al. (2000). Preventing child abuse and neglect with a program of nurse home visitation: The limiting effects of domestic violence [Abstract]. *The Journal of the American Medical Association (JAMA), 284*(11), 1385–1391.

Encyclopedia Britannica Article. (Undated). Pasteur, Louis. Retrieved February 24, 2002, from http://www.britannica.com/eb/article?idxref=55613

Encyclopedia Britannica Article. (Undated). Semmelweis, Ignaz Philipp. Retrieved February 24, 2002 from http://www.britannica.com/eb/article?eu=68445&tocid=0&query=%22puerperal%20fever%22

Health Care Financing Administration. (Undated). Overview of the Medicaid Program. Retrieved March 13, 2002, from http://www.hcfa.gov/medicaid/mover.htm

Healthy People 2010, A Systematic Approach to Health Improvement. (2001). Retrieved June 24, 2004 from www.health.gov/healthypeople.

Herrman, J. W. (2001). Updates & kidbits: Pediatric nursing and Healthy People 2010: A call to action. *Pediatric Nursing, 27*(1), 82–86.

Kleinpell, R. (2000). Healthy people 2010: The nation's new health agenda. *Nursing Spectrum.* Available at: http://-community.nursingspectrum.com/MagazineArticles.

NANDA Nursing Diagnoses: Definitions and Classification 2001–2002. (2001) Philadelphia: North American Nursing Diagnosis Association.

National Association of State Budget Officers. (Undated). *Medicaid.* Retrieved March 13, 2002, from http://www.nasbo.org/Policy_Resources/Medicaid/medicaid.htm

National Center for Health Statistics. Prevalence of overweight among children and adolescents: United States, 1999–2000. Retrieved May 25, 2004, from www.cdc.gov/nchs

University of Pennsylvania Health System. (Undated). *A century of obstetrics.* Retrieved January 20, 2002, from http://www.obgyn.upenn.edu/History/clinobhis.html

The World Factbook. (2002). Infant mortality rate. Retrieved July 13, 2003, from http://www.bartleby.com/151/a28.html

Wertz, R. W., & Wertz, D. C. (1989). *Lying-in: A history of childbirth in America, expanded edition.* Yale University Press: New Haven & London.

Websites
www.childstats.gov
www.health.gov/healthypeople
www.dhhs.gov
http://www.fns.usda.gov/wic/AboutWIC.htm

WORKBOOK

NCLEX-STYLE REVIEW QUESTIONS

1. Preventing and treating infections during childbirth have reduced maternal and perinatal mortality rates. Of the following, which scientific advancement has done the *most* to improve neonatal mortality statistics?

   a. Control of puerperal fever

   b. Use of anesthesia during labor

   c. Enforcement of strict rules in hospitals

   d. Treatment advances for preterm infants

2. The nursing process is a scientific method and proven form of which process?

   a. Cost containment

   b. Problem solving

   c. Oral communication

   d. Health teaching

3. The nurse collects data and begins to develop a trust relationship with the patient in which step of the nursing process?

   a. Assessment

   b. Planning

   c. Implementation

   d. Evaluation

4. The nurse carries out the nursing care for the patient in which step of the nursing process?

   a. Assessment

   b. Planning

   c. Implementation

   d. Evaluation

5. In caring for patients, a health care team often uses critical pathways. Which of the following are reasons critical pathways are used? (Select all that apply.) The critical pathway

   a. decreases cost for the patient and hospital.

   b. helps to establish a trusting relationship with patients.

   c. is followed by all members of the health team.

   d. provides organization for the care of the patient.

   e. includes all treatments and procedures.

STUDY ACTIVITIES

1. Choose the three social issues you think have the highest impact on health care concerns of children (use Table 1-1). Using these issues, complete the following table.

	How Does This Issue Affect Children's Health Care?	What Is the Nurse's Role in Dealing With This Issue?
Social issue Social issue Social issue		

2. Go to the following Internet site: http://web.health.gov/healthypeople/. At "Healthy People—Leading Health Indicators," click on "What are the Leading Health Indicators?"

   a. Make a list of the leading health indicators.

   b. Hit the back arrow and return to "Leading Health Indicators." Click on "Resources for Individual Action." What is a resource site you could share with a family caregiver regarding health care access?

   c. What is a resource site you could share with someone needing information on injury or violence?

CRITICAL THINKING: What Would You Do?

1. A new mother tells you that her husband makes a few dollars an hour over the minimum wage, so her new baby is not eligible for Medicaid. She sighs and wonders aloud how she is going to pay for the medical bills. What would you say to the new mother? Does she have any options? If so, what are they?

2. Describe sociologic changes that have affected child health concepts and attitudes.

3. Discuss how children were cared for in institutions in the 19th and early 20th centuries. Describe the hospital care of infants and children in the period immediately after World War I.

4. While working, you overhear an older nurse complaining about family caregivers "being underfoot so much and interfering with patient care." Describe how you would defend open visiting for family caregivers to this person.

Family-Centered and Community-Based Maternal and Pediatric Nursing

2

STUDENT OBJECTIVES

On completion of this chapter, the student should be able to

1. Identify the primary purpose of the family in society.
2. Discuss the functions of the family.
3. Discuss the types of family structure.
4. List four factors that have contributed to the growing number of single-parent families.
5. Describe how children are affected by family size and sibling order.
6. Explain the trend for families to spend less time together.
7. Identify the focus of community-based health care.
8. Describe advantages of community-based health care for the pregnant woman, child, and family.
9. Differentiate between primary, secondary, and tertiary prevention and give one example of each.
10. List the skills needed by a community health nurse.
11. Explain the information a nurse needs to successfully teach a group of individuals.
12. Describe how child advocacy helps children in community-based health care.

KEY TERMS

blended family
case management
client advocacy
cohabitation family
communal family
community-based nursing
cultural competency
extended family
nuclear family
primary prevention
secondary prevention
single-parent family
socialization
stepfamily
tertiary prevention

Each person is a member of a family and a member of many social groups, such as church, school, and work. Families and social groups together make up the fabric of the larger society. It is within the context of the family and the community that an individual presents herself to receive health care. It is critical for maternity and pediatric nurses to recognize the context of the patient's needs within the patient's family and community.

THE FAMILY AS A SOCIAL UNIT

The arrival of a baby alters forever the primary social unit—a family—in which all members influence and are influenced by each other. Each subsequent child joining that family continues the process of reshaping the individual members and the family unit. In addition, the community affects family members as individuals and as a family unit.

Nursing care of women and children demands a solid understanding of normal patterns of growth and development—physical, psychological, social, and intellectual (cognitive)—and an awareness of the many factors that influence those patterns. It also demands an appreciation for the uniqueness of each individual and each family. For nursing care to be complete and as effective as possible, the identified patient must be considered as a member of a family and a larger community.

Throughout history, family structure has evolved in response to ongoing social and economic changes. Today's families may only faintly resemble the nuclear families of 30 or 40 years ago, in which the father worked outside the home and the mother cared for the children. It is estimated that in 60% to 70% of today's families with school-age children, only one parent lives at home. More than 50% of American women with a child younger than age 1 year work outside the home. Changes such as these create bigger demands on parents and have contributed to the growing demands on public institutions to fill the gaps. "Blended" families or stepfamilies have created other major changes in family structure and interactions within the family. Divorce, abandonment, and delayed childbearing are all contributing factors.

Family Function

The family is civilization's oldest and most basic social unit. The family's primary purpose is to ensure survival of the unit and its individual members and to continue the society and its knowledge, customs, values, and beliefs. It establishes a primary connection with a group responsible for a person until that person becomes independent.

Although family structure varies among different cultures, its functions are similar. The family's func-

tions in relation to society are twofold: to reproduce and socialize offspring. For each family member the family functions to provide sustenance and support in the five areas of wholeness: physical, emotional, intellectual, social, and spiritual.

Physical Sustenance

The family is responsible for meeting each member's basic needs for food, clothing, shelter, and protection from harm, including illness. The family determines which needs have priority and what resources will be used to meet those needs. Sometimes families need help obtaining the proper resources. For instance, a pregnant woman's nutritional needs might be partially fulfilled through a community program. Some families need help learning to set priorities. For example, very young parents may benefit from parenting classes to help them set priorities for infant and child care.

The work necessary to meet the family's needs was once clearly divided between mother and father, with the mother providing total care for the children and the father providing the resources to make care possible. These attitudes have changed so that in a two-parent family, each parent has an opportunity to share in the joys and trials of child care and other aspects of family living. In the **single-parent family,** one person must assume all these responsibilities.

Don't be quick to judge! Sometimes it is difficult to remember how many responsibilities a single parent has. You may be able to help the parent find a Big Brother or Big Sister program in your community. In these programs an older teen or young adult "adopts" a child and provides special social opportunities for him. For instance, the Big Brother may take the child to a ball game.

Emotional Support

The process of parental attachment to a child begins before birth and continues throughout life. This process is enhanced when early interaction is encouraged between the new parents and the newborn.

Research studies continue to support the importance of early parent–child relationships to emotional adjustment in later life. As little as a few hours may constitute a critical period in the emotional bond between parent and child. Although specific results of these studies are controversial, it is generally agreed that young children are highly sensitive to psychological influences, and those influences may have long-range positive or negative effects.

Within the family, children learn who they are and how their behavior affects other family members.

Children observe and imitate the behavior of family members, learning quickly which behaviors are rewarded and which are punished. Participation in a family is a child's primary rehearsal for parenthood. How parents treat the child has a powerful influence on how the child will treat future children. Studies show that many abusive parents were abused by their parents as children.

Intellectual Stimulation

Many experts suggest that parents read to their unborn children and play music to provide early stimulation. It is unknown when the fetus can actually hear, but it is clear that the newborn recognizes and is comforted by his parents' voices.

The need for intellectual development continues throughout life. The small infant needs to have input through his five senses to develop optimally. Many parents buy brightly colored toys and play frequently with their infants to facilitate this stimulation. Talking and reading to the infant and small child is another way parents fulfill this function.

Socialization

Within the family, a child learns the rules of the society and the culture in which the family lives: its language, values, ethics, and acceptable behaviors. This process, called **socialization,** is accomplished by training, education, and role modeling. The family teaches children acceptable ways of meeting physical needs, such as eating and elimination, and certain skills, such as dressing oneself. The family educates children about relationships with other people inside and outside the family. Children learn what is permitted and approved within their society and what is forbidden.

Each family determines how goals are to be accomplished based on its principles and values. Family patterns of communication, methods of conflict resolution, coping strategies, and disciplinary methods develop over time and contribute to a family's sense of order.

Spirituality

Spirituality addresses meaning in life. The values and principles of each family are based in large part upon its spiritual foundation. Although spirituality may be expressed through religion, this is not the only way it is defined. Cultivating in children an appreciation for the arts (literature, music, theater, dance, and visual art) gives them the basis from which to begin their own spiritual journey.

Family Structure

Various traditional and nontraditional family structures exist. The traditional structures that occur in many cultures are the nuclear family and the extended family. Nontraditional variations include the single-

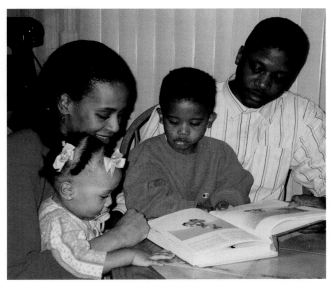

● *Figure 2.1* The nuclear family is an important and prominent type of family structure in American society. This nuclear family enjoys reading together.

parent family, the communal family, the stepfamily, and the gay or lesbian family. The adoptive family can be either a traditional or a nontraditional structure.

Nuclear Family

The **nuclear family** is composed of a man, a woman, and their children (either biological or adopted) who share a common household (Fig. 2-1). This was once the typical American family structure; now fewer than one-third of families in the United States fit this pattern. The nuclear family is a more mobile and independent unit than an extended family but is often part of a network of related nuclear families within close geographic proximity.

Extended Family

Typical of agricultural societies, the **extended family** consists of one or more nuclear families plus other relatives, often crossing generations to include grandparents, aunts, uncles, and cousins. The needs of indiviual members are subordinate to the needs of the group, and children are considered an economic asset. Grandparents aid in child rearing, and children learn respect for their elders by observing their parents' behavior toward the older generation.

Here's an important tip. In some cultures the extended family continues to play an important role in everyday life. It may be challenging, but when the extended family comes to visit the new mother and newborn, it is important to work with them to accommodate their needs.

A PERSONAL GLIMPSE

Living with both my mother and grandmother definitely has its advantages. Even though I had a male figure around me while I was growing up, it wasn't really the same as having a father who would always be there. I lived with my aunt and her family along with my mother and my grandmother. I had my uncle or cousin to turn to if I needed advice that my mother or my grandmother couldn't give me. However, my uncle wasn't always around, neither was my cousin, so a lot of my questions were left unanswered. Questions that I didn't think anybody else other than a man could answer. I learned a lot of things on my own, whether it was by experience or by asking somebody else.

Things are different now. It's only my mother, my grandmother, and myself. As I grow older, I'm finding that I can open up to the both of them a lot more. There is no reason to keep secrets. I can tell them anything and they understand. Actually they are a lot more understanding than I thought they would be about certain things. Every day I'm realizing that I can tell them anything.

People often ask me what it is like not knowing about my father. They ask me if I'm curious about my father. And I say, "Of course I'm curious. Who wouldn't be?" I also tell them that love is a lot stronger than curiosity. I love and care about my mother and grandmother more than anything in this world. No one father could ever give me as much love and devotion as the two of them give me. And I wouldn't give that up for anything.

Juan, age 15 years

LEARNING OPPORTUNITY: Where would you direct this mother in your community to go to find opportunities for her son to interact with male adults who could be positive role models for him? What are the reasons it would be important for this child to have appropriate adult male role models? If someone other than the biological parent has raised a child, What are some of the reasons these individuals seek their biological parents?

Single-Parent Family

Rising divorce rates, the women's movement, increasing acceptance of children born out of wedlock, and changes in adoption laws reflecting a more liberal attitude toward adoption have combined to produce a growing number of single-parent families. About 23% of households in the United States are included in this category, and most are headed by women (United States Bureau of Census, 2000). Although this family situation places a heavy burden on the parent, no conclusive evidence is available to show its effects on children. At some time in their lives, more than 50% of children in the United States may be part of a single-parent family.

Communal Family

During the early 1960s, increasing numbers of young adults began to challenge the values and traditions of the American social system. One result of that challenge was the establishing of communal groups and collectives, or **communal families.** This alternative structure occurs in many settings and may favor either a primitive or a modern lifestyle. Members of a communal family share responsibility for homemaking and child rearing; all children are the collective responsibility of adult members. Not actually a new family structure, the communal family is a variation of the extended family. The number of communal family units has decreased in recent years.

Gay or Lesbian Family

In the gay or lesbian family, two people of the same sex live together, bound by formal or informal commitment, with or without children. Children may be the result of a prior heterosexual mating or a product of the foster-child system, adoption, artifcial insemination, or surrogacy. Although these families often face complex issues, including discrimination, studies of children in such families show that they are not harmed by membership in this type of family (Gottman, 1990).

Did you know? The children of a gay or lesbian family are no more likely to become homosexual than are children of heterosexual families.

Stepfamily or Blended Family

The **stepfamily** is made up of the custodial parent and children and a new spouse. As the divorce rate has climbed, the number of stepfamilies has increased. If both partners in the marriage bring children from a previous marriage into the household, the family is usually termed a **blended family.** The stress that remarriage of the custodial parent places on a child seems to depend in part on the child's age. Initially there is an increase in the number of problems in children of all ages. However, younger children apparently can form an attachment to the new parent and accept that person in the parenting role better than can adolescents. Adolescents, already engaged in searching for identity and exploring their own sexuality, may view the presence of a nonbiological parent as an intrusion. When children from each partner's former marriage are brought into the family, the incidence of problems increases. Second marriages often produce children of that union, which contributes to the adjustment problems of the family members. However, remarriage may provide the stability of a two-parent family, which may offer additional resources for the child. Each family is unique and has its own set of challenges and advantages.

Cohabitation Family

In the nuclear family, the parents are married; in the **cohabitation family,** couples live together but are not married. The children in this family may be children of earlier unions, or they may be a result of this union. These families may be long lasting, and the cohabitating couple may eventually marry, but sometimes such families are less stable because the relationships may be temporary. In any family situation with frequent changes in the adult relationships, children may feel a sense of insecurity.

Adoptive Family

The adoptive family, whether a traditional or nontraditional family structure, falls into a category of its own. The parents, child, and siblings in the adoptive family all have challenges that differ from other family structures. A variety of methods of adoption are available, including the use of agencies, international sources, and private adoptions. Paperwork, interviews, home visits, long periods of waiting, and often large sums of money all contribute to the potential stress and anxiety a family who decides to adopt a child goes through. Sometimes adopted children have health, developmental, or emotional concerns. Many have been in a series of foster homes or have come from abusive situations. The family who adopts a child of another culture may have to deal with the prejudices of friends and family. These factors add to the challenges the adoptive family faces.

Some research shows that "open adoption," in which the identity of the birth and adoptive parents is not kept a secret, is less traumatic for the birth mother, child, and adoptive family. Legal issues must be worked out in advance to decrease the painful situations that can occur if a birth mother changes her mind about giving up her child for adoption.

The newly adopted child should be given a complete physical examination soon after the adoption. Basic information regarding the child's health, growth, and development is obtained so any problems or concerns can be discussed with the adoptive family. The feelings of the parents as well as the siblings need to be explored and support given. Throughout childhood and into adulthood adopted children often continue to have questions and need emotional support from health care personnel.

Test Yourself
- Name the two main purposes of the family in relation to society.
- What are the five areas of wholeness?
- What are the two traditional family structures?

Family Factors That Influence Childbearing and Child Rearing

Family Size

The number of children in the family has a significant impact on family interactions. The smaller the family, the more time there is for individual attention to each child. Children in small families, particularly only children, often spend more time with adults and, therefore, relate better with adults than with peers. Only children tend to be more advanced in language development and intellectual achievement.

Understandably a large family emphasizes the group more than the child. Less time is available for parental attention to each child. There is greater interdependence among these children and less dependence on the parents (Fig. 2-2).

Sibling Order and Gender

Whether a child is the firstborn, a middle child, or the youngest also makes a difference in the child's relationships and behavior. Firstborn children command a great deal of attention from parents and grandparents

● **Figure 2.2** Children from large families learn to care for one another. Many older children are expected to help with homework and prepare after-school snacks. Photo by Joe Mitchell.

and also are affected by their parents' inexperience, anxieties, and uncertainties. Often the parents' expectations for the oldest child are greater than for subsequent children. Generally firstborn children are greater achievers than their siblings.

With second and subsequent children, parents tend to be more relaxed and permissive. These children are likely to be more relaxed and are slower to develop language skills. They often identify more with peers than with parents.

Sexual identity in relation to siblings also affects a child's development. Girls raised with older brothers tend to have more male-associated interests than do girls raised with older sisters. Boys raised with older brothers tend to be more aggressive than are boys with older sisters (Craig, 1992).

Parental Behavior

Many factors have contributed to the change in the traditional mother-at-home, father-at-work image of the American family (Fig. 2-3). Sixty-five percent of American mothers of children younger than age 18 years work outside the home. Some mothers work because they are the family's only source of income, others because the family's economic status demands a second income, and still others because the woman's career is highly valued. More than half of all children between ages 3 and 5 years spend part of their day being cared for by someone other than their parents.

Many factors contribute to the trend for families to spend less time together. Both parents may work; the children participate in many school activities; family members watch television, rather than talking together at mealtime, or eat fast food or individual meals without sitting down together as a family; and there is an emphasis on the acquisition of material goods, rather than the development of relationships. All these factors contribute to a breakdown in family communication,

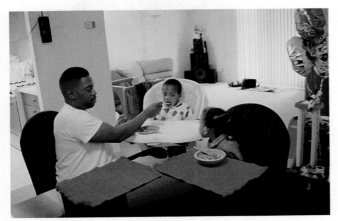

● **Figure 2.3** In some American families, traditional roles are being reversed. The father cares for the children while the mother is at work.

and they are typical of many families. Their impact on today's children, the parents of tomorrow, is unknown.

Divorce

From 1970 to 1990, the number of divorces increased every year. Although there has been a slight decrease in this number in recent years, more than 1 million children younger than age 18 years have been involved in a divorce each year. Although obviously these children are affected, it is difficult to determine the exact extent of the damage. Children whose lives were seriously disrupted before a divorce may feel relieved, at least initially, when the situation is resolved. Others who were unaware of parental conflict and felt that their lives were happy may feel frightened and abandoned. All these emotions depend on the children involved, their ages, and the kind of care and relationships they experience with their parents after the divorce.

Children may go through many emotions when a divorce occurs. Feelings of grief, anger, rejection, and self-worthlessness are common. These emotions may follow the children for years, even into adulthood, even though children may understand the reason for the divorce. In addition, the parents, either custodial or noncustodial, may try to influence the child's thinking about the other parent, placing the child in an emotional trap. If the noncustodial parent does not keep in regular contact with the child, feelings of rejection may be overwhelming. The child often desperately wants a sign of that parent's continuing love.

Culture

Each person is the product of a family, a culture, and a community. In some cultures, family life is gentle, permissive, and loving; in others, unquestioning obedience is demanded of children, and pain and hardship are to be endured stoically. The child may be from a cultural group that places a high value on children, giving them lots of attention from many relatives and friends, or the child may be from a group that has taught the child from early childhood to fend for oneself (Fig. 2-4).

The timing and number of children desired by the childbearing family are culturally influenced. Values and beliefs about birth control, abortion, and sexual practices influence the choices individuals and couples make about childbearing.

Culture also determines the family's health beliefs and practices. Respect for a person's cultural heritage and individuality is an essential part of nursing care. To plan culturally appropriate and acceptable care, nurses need to understand the health practices and lifestyle of families from various cultures. Rather than memorizing a list of generalized facts regarding different cultures, it is more useful for the nurse to develop **cultural competency,** the capacity to work effectively with people by integrating the elements of their culture into nursing

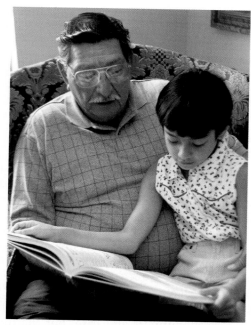

● **Figure 2.4** Many cultural preferences are seen in families. In some cultures, extended family members such as grandparents participate in raising children. Photo by Joe Mitchell.

care (Snow, 1996). To develop cultural competency, the nurse must first understand cultural influences on his or her life. The nurse must recognize surface cultural influences (e.g., language, food, clothing), as well as hidden cultural influences (e.g., communication styles, beliefs, attitudes, values, perceptions). Then the nurse may recognize and accept the different attitudes, behaviors, and values of another person's culture.

Integrating cultural attitudes toward food, cleanliness, respect, and freedom are of utmost importance. The nurse must be especially sensitive to the fears of the child who is separated from his or her own culture for the first time and finds the food, language, people, and surroundings of the health care facility totally alien. Cultural competency promotes cooperation from the child and family and minimizes frustration. These factors are essential in restoring health so that the child may once again be a functioning part of the family and the community, whatever the cultural background.

Test Yourself

- Name one way that family size affects a child's development.

- What are two factors that contribute to American families spending less time together?

- Define cultural competency.

HEALTH CARE SHIFT: FROM HOSPITAL TO COMMUNITY

In the last century, health care has gone through a number of changes. The sophisticated health care currently available is extremely expensive and has strained health care funding to a point where other health care approaches have become necessary. This need for change has led to the emergence of community-based health care and an emphasis on wellness and preventive health care.

The shift to community-based health care has impacted normal and at-risk maternity care. Many women with limited resources choose to obtain prenatal care from local health department clinics. A pregnant woman who develops complications can sometimes receive care at home with the assistance of a nurse case manager who helps to coordinate her care. This allows the woman to receive high quality care at a lower cost than if she were to require hospitalization. Community-based programs such as Women, Infants, and Children (WIC) provide nutritional screening and assistance for the low-income pregnant woman and her small children.

The shift to community-based health care also has been a positive factor in children's care. The child is no longer viewed simply as a person with an illness, but rather as a child who is a member of a family from a certain community with deep-seated cultural values, social customs, and preferences. Learning about the child's community and using that knowledge improves the level of care the child receives. In the community, the child can also receive preventive care and wellness teaching not usually available unless one is ill in the hospital setting.

Community-Based Nursing

Community-based nursing focuses on prevention and is directed toward persons and families within a community. The goals are to help persons meet their health care needs and to maintain continuity of care as they move through the various health care settings available to them.

The role of the nurse who works in the community is different from that of the hospital nurse. Generally the nurse in the community focuses on **primary prevention**, health promoting activities that help prevent the development of illness or injury. This level of prevention includes teaching regarding safety, diet, rest, exercise, and disease prevention through immunizations and emphasizes the nursing role of teacher and client advocate. Examples of primary prevention are a school nurse giving a drug education program to a fourth-grade class, and a nurse in a maternity clinic giving teaching tips on proper nutrition during pregnancy.

In some community settings, the nurse's role focuses on **secondary prevention**, health screening activities that aid in early diagnosis and encourage prompt treatment before long-term negative effects are realized. Such settings are clinics, home care nursing, and schools. The nurse participates in screening measures such as height, weight, hearing, and vision. During child assessments and follow-up, the nurse compiles a health history and collects data, including vital signs, blood work, and other diagnostic tests as ordered by the health care practitioner. One example of secondary prevention is when the school nurse identifies a child with pediculosis (head lice). The school nurse contacts the child's family caregivers and provides instructions on the care of the child and other family members to eliminate the infestation. Another example of secondary prevention is a community clinic nurse's identification of a pregnant adolescent who is gaining insufficient weight and is possibly anemic. The nurse works with the family caregiver to review the family's dietary habits and nutritional state. This would help determine if the problem is limited to the pregnant adolescent or if other family members are also malnourished and if there is lack of knowledge or inadequate means. After finding these answers, the nurse can help the family caregiver provide better nutrition for the family and focus on nutritional issues unique to the pregnant adolescent.

Tertiary prevention, health-promoting activities that focus on rehabilitation and teaching to prevent further injury or illness, occurs in special settings. For example, the at-risk infant or child might be helped through special intervention programs, group homes, or selected outpatient settings focusing on rehabilitation, such as an orthopedic clinic.

Another example of tertiary prevention is illustrated by a young rural family with a child who has spina bifida and who needs to be catheterized several times a day. The child is seen regularly at a specialized clinic at a major medical center. The family has no insurance, and the cost of catheters is such that the family caregivers feel they can no longer afford them. The nurse helps the family explore additional resources for financial help, such as an organization that will help fund their trips to the clinic for regular appointments. The nurse also finds a source to cover the costs of catheters and other incidental expenses.

Such a broad selection of settings and roles places the nurse in a remarkable situation. Pregnant women and children are seen in settings familiar to them—homes, schools, or community centers. In the community setting, the child's caregivers can more freely make choices; for instance, they may be more able to follow a child's medication regimen at home, rather than in the hospital, because the hospital may be perceived as a strange territory. Although involved in direct care, the nurse in the community spends a great part of his or her time as a communicator, teacher, administrator, and manager.

Community Care Settings for the Maternity Client

Prenatal and Postpartum Home Health Care

Nurses often made home visits in the early days of public health nursing. Through the years, it gradually became expected that patients would come to clinics and offices for care. Recently, in an effort to meet the challenges of cost-containment and poor access to care, some organizations and researchers have reinstituted home visits by nurses.

Current evidence shows that low-risk mothers and infants do not have better health outcomes when nurses or specially trained workers go to the home for follow-up social support and care, but the mothers report being happier with the care that they receive (Lieu et al., 2000; Morrell, Spiby, Stewart, Walters, & Morgan, 2000). The most positive results occur when nurses make in-home visits to at-risk populations, such as adolescent and poverty-stricken mothers.

When at-risk women are assessed and receive intervention from nurses in their homes during pregnancy and the postpartum period, some researchers have found both short- and long-term positive effects. In general these positive effects include a lower incidence of child abuse and neglect, longer periods of time between pregnancies, fewer overall pregnancies, less dependence on welfare, and fewer reports of criminal behavior and drug and alcohol abuse (Corrarino et al., 2000; Eckenrode et al., 2000; Kitzman et al., 2000; Olds et al., 1997). Some researchers have also found decreased incidence of preterm births and fewer infant hospitalization days when at-risk mothers receive planned nursing intervention, which includes home visits during pregnancy (Koniak-Griffin, Mathenge, Anderson, & Verzemnieks, 1999).

Settings for Birth

Choosing the setting in which to give birth has been guided by cultural beliefs, political beliefs, and personal preferences throughout the years. For example, on the United States western frontier during the mid- and late-1800s, women gave birth in their homes, attended by female family members or female neighbors. These women cared for the older children, helped with chores, and stayed with the new mother during the early postpartum period, when possible. Today, in most parts of the world, the choices of birth settings are primarily home, birthing centers, and hospitals (Fig. 2-5).

A

B

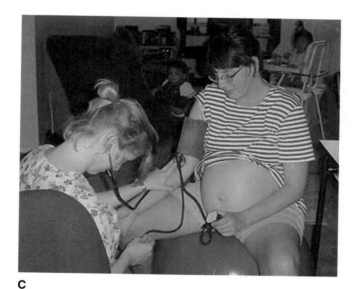

C

● *Figure 2.5* (Birth setting collage). There are many different settings in which a woman can choose to give birth. These decisions are influenced by preferences regarding methods of pain control and general beliefs about how a birth should be managed. (**A**) Hospital LDRP (**B**) Birthing center (**C**) Home setting. Photos by Joe Mitchell.

Home. In the early 20th century, home births were the norm before the availability of anesthesia and pain medication in the hospital setting. Today home births occur rarely. A woman may choose to deliver at home for a variety of reasons. She may desire a more comfortable setting, more control over birthing conditions and positions, or to prevent nonmedically indicated interventions. In addition, a woman may prefer to give birth at home so that she can take care of her healthy newborn, rather than experiencing periods of separation while her baby is cared for in a hospital nursery.

Midwives usually attend births at home; physicians rarely do. Some are lay midwives, often trained through apprenticeships with experienced lay midwives. Others are formally trained certified nurse midwives (CNMs) who practice independently in home settings and clinics with physician backup for consultation and referral. Laws in individual states regulate the practice of midwifery.

The safety of giving birth at home is debated. According to Ackerman-Liebrich, et al. (1996), "healthy low-risk women who wish to deliver at home have no increased risk either to themselves or to their babies." In a study of outcomes of 11,788 planned home births attended by CNMs (Anderson & Murphy, 1995), the researchers concluded that home birth can be an acceptable delivery option for low-risk women, if it is planned and attended by "qualified care providers." A newer study (Janssen et al., 2002) evaluating the safety of home births attended by trained midwives concludes that there are no increased risks with home births; however, the results of this study have been widely criticized for researcher bias. The American

College of Obstetricians and Gynecologists (2002) reports that newborns born at home tend to be at higher risk for very low Apgar scores; there is a strong association between newborn death and nulliparous women attempting to deliver at home; and that planned home births were associated with prolonged labor and postpartum hemorrhage. The latest Cochrane Review pertaining to home versus hospital birth (Olsen & Jewell, 2000) concluded that at present there is insufficient evidence indicating that one setting is superior to the other for low-risk women.

Birthing Centers. Since the early 1980s, birthing centers have increased in popularity and availability in some areas of the United States. The environment is usually comfortable with furnishings and lighting designed to make the laboring woman and her family feel welcome. There often are family areas (e.g., kitchens and sitting rooms) and bathrooms with showers and/or whirlpool tubs. A variety of health care professionals may be employed by a birthing center, including registered nurses (RNs), CNMs, licensed practical nurses (LPNs), and doulas (specialized birth attendants). Medical interventions are rarely done, so physicians are seldom present. However, birthing centers often are affiliated with a variety of obstetricians and pediatricians as consultants.

Only low-risk women are accepted as patients after being screened by the birthing center. Most birthing centers have medical equipment such as intravenous lines, fluids, oxygen, newborn resuscitation equipment, infant warmers, and local anesthesia for repair of tears or infrequently performed episiotomies. Mild narcotics are available, as is oxytocin for control of postpartum bleeding. If a laboring woman decides she wants an epidural anesthesia, or if she presents with complications determining her to be at risk, she is transported to a hospital.

Hospitals. Childbirth in a hospital setting began to be accepted as the norm by the 1920s. By 1950, the vast majority of births in the United States took place in hospitals. Today, 99% of births in the United States are in hospitals, with 92% attended by medical doctors (MDs). Doctors of osteopathic medicine (DOs) and midwives attend most of the other 8% of births in U.S. hospitals.

Until the 1970s giving birth in a hospital required enduring uncomfortable procedures (e.g., enemas, shaving); laboring, delivering, and recovering in separate rooms; and separation from the newborn until several hours after birth. Patients began to be more consumer oriented in the mid-1970s. They began to "shop around" for more family-centered maternity care, which included more time with their babies and less time moving from room to room. Hospital administrators and physicians began to listen to consumer needs, and hospital policies began to change. As a result, in many hospitals the trend is to promote family-centered maternity care in more home-like settings. Most hospitals today offer combination labor-delivery-recovery rooms (LDRs). The rooms are larger to accommodate family support and to allow health care professionals enough room to attend the birth. In addition, LDRs are aesthetically appealing, with home-like furnishings, wallpaper, softer lighting, and showers in the bathrooms.

Some hospitals have initiated combination labor-delivery-recovery-postpartum rooms (LDRPs), thus further reducing the number of locations to which a woman is moved during her hospital stay. Couplet care, another concept that some hospitals have embraced, places the healthy mother in the same room with her newborn as long as there is no medical indication for them to be separated. One nurse is responsible for the care of both. This practice encourages early bonding and provides time for new parents to learn to care for their newborns before discharge. Parents learn to recognize their newborns' cues and therefore are better prepared to care for their newborns at home.

Test Yourself

- Define primary prevention.
- Give one example of tertiary prevention.
- List three childbirth settings.

Community Care Settings for the Child

Care for a child is provided in a wide variety of community settings. Some settings provide primarily wellness care; others provide specialized care for children with a particular diagnosis or condition. These include outpatient settings, home care, schools, camps, community centers, parishes, intervention programs, and group homes.

Outpatient Settings

Outpatient settings for children are varied; as the health care delivery system continues to move into the community, more settings will be developed. Outpatient settings are organized according to who offers the services and who pays for them. Public (tax-supported) outpatient clinics may be an extension of a hospital's services or may be sponsored by a regional, county, or city health department. Private (based on fees charged) clinics are owned and operated by corporations or individuals and operate for a profit. A third system is the growing network of health maintenance organizations (HMOs). Some HMO plans

A PERSONAL GLIMPSE

The clinic is where you go when you're on the public access card and cannot afford real insurance. You hardly see the same doctor twice. A lot are interns working out their internship.

My baby was about 2 months old when he developed a bumpy rash on the crown of this head. I took him to the clinic because it was spreading and I didn't know what it could be. A doctor, who I could hardly understand, was on duty. This was the same doctor that told me I had chickenpox when I was pregnant (I didn't). He looked at the rash and looked at me very strange, then said, "This looks similar to a rash connected to HIV." He requested a test for AIDS! You cannot know the thoughts that go through your head. How? Where? Who? Why? Then I remembered that I had been tested when I first found out I was pregnant and it was negative. Since Jack, the baby's father, and I had not been with anyone else, I knew there must be another reason for this rash.

That doctor never took a sample to test or asked another doctor to come in and look at the rash. I took little Tommy home and started to use an ointment I'd heard about on his head every day for about a month. The rash went away and I've changed clinics since—like they're not all really the same. You get what you pay for.

Michelle

LEARNING OPPORTUNITY: What feelings do you think this mother might have been experiencing in this situation? What specific things could the nurse do to be of support and help to this mother?

charge a small co-payment for each visit. However, under the HMO system, the family is not free to choose the specialty care the child may receive. The child's primary care provider determines what, if any, specialized care is needed and who will administer that care (see Chapter 1).

Clinic services are based on community needs. Examples include a well-baby clinic offered by the county health department, an orthopedic clinic offered by a regional children's hospital, or a pediatric clinic of an HMO. Infants, children, and caregivers use the clinics for education, anticipatory guidance, immunizations, diagnosis, treatment, and rehabilitation.

A specialty clinic focuses on one aspect of an infant or child's well-being, for instance dentistry, oncology, sickle cell anemia, or human immunodeficiency virus/acquired immunodeficiency syndrome (HIV/AIDS). Some health department clinics specialize in at-risk infants born to drug-addicted mothers, children of

parents with a history of child abuse, or low birth-weight infants. Nurses in these clinics devote much of their efforts to parental education and guidance, as well as follow-up services for the child.

Home Health Care

Infants, children, and their families make up a significant proportion of the home health care population. Shortened acute care stays have contributed to the increasing number of children cared for by home nurses. Children are often more comfortable in familiar home surroundings (Fig. 2-6). Children and infants can be successfully treated for many conditions at home, where they and their caregivers are more comfortable and they can receive the love and attention of family members. The child's caregivers feel more confident about performing treatments and procedures when they have the guidance of the home nurse. Common conditions for which an infant or child may receive home care services include:

- Phototherapy for elevated bilirubin levels
- Intravenous antibiotic therapy for systemic infections
- Postoperative care
- Chronic conditions, such as asthma, sickle cell anemia, cystic fibrosis, HIV/AIDS, and leukemia and other cancers
- Respirator dependence
- Reconstructive or corrective surgery for congenital malformations
- Corrective orthopedic surgery

Other home health care team members may include a physical therapist, speech therapist, occupational therapist, home schooling teacher, home health aide, primary health care provider (physician or nurse practitioner), and social worker. Members of the team vary with the child's health needs.

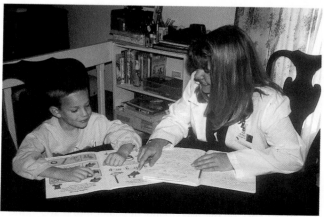

● **Figure 2.6** During a visit by the nurse, the child is comforted by the familiar surroundings of his home.

Schools and Camps

Health care has been practiced for many years in schools and camps, but the role of health care professionals in these settings has expanded (Fig. 2-7). The school nurse may be responsible for classroom teaching, health screenings, immunizations, first aid for injured children, care of ill children, administering medication, assisting with sports physicals, and identifying children with problems and recommending programs for them. Classroom teaching geared for each grade level can cover personal hygiene, sex education, substance abuse, safety, and emotional health.

Many mainstreamed children have chronic health problems that need daily supervision or care; for example, a child with spina bifida who needs to be catheterized several times during the day or a diabetic child who needs to perform glucose monitoring and administer insulin during school hours. Health records are maintained on each child. Some schools have clinics that provide routine dental care, physicals, screening for vision, hearing, scoliosis, tuberculosis, and follow-up on immunizations. Children learn to know the school nurse over a number of years and usually establish a comfortable, friendly relationship that often aids the nurse in helping the child solve his or her health problems.

The camp nurse knows the child for a much briefer time, but many camp nurses establish warm relationships with the children in their care. Camp nurses provide first aid for campers and staff, maintain health records, teach first aid and cardiopulmonary resuscitation (CPR), offer relevant health education, maintain an infirmary for ill campers, and dispense tender loving care to homesick children.

At camps for children with special needs, the campers' health care needs determine the type of nursing care required. For example, at a camp for diabetic children, the nurse may teach self-administration of insulin and the many aspects of diabetic care. Other camps may cater to children with developmental delays, physical challenges, or chronic illness such as asthma or cystic fibrosis. Others have specific purposes, such as weight control or behavior management. In each of these settings, the nurse provides basic health care with individualized health teaching based on the camp population. Each type of camp brings its own challenges and rewards; the benefits to the children and their families are often exceptional.

Community Centers, Parishes, and Intervention Programs

Community centers and parishes provide care relevant to a particular community. Parish centers may sponsor outreach programs in a church, synagogue, or other religious setting. The services offered by these centers are designed to meet community needs. For example, in areas with many homeless persons, centers may provide basic health care and nutrition. These centers may also provide food, clothing, money, or other resources. Other centers may provide childcare classes for new mothers or young families.

Some communities offer walk-in or residential clinics for special purposes such as teen pregnancy, alcohol and drug abuse, nutritional guidance, and family violence. Other specialized clinics offer programs on HIV/AIDS, cancer, and mental health; provide maternal and well-baby care; and offer day care services for children or the elderly.

Many communities also have services provided by volunteer service organizations such as the Lions, Rotary Club, Shriners, or Kiwanis. Some of these organizations have specific goals. For example, the Shriners sponsor clinics for children with orthopedic problems.

In any community center, there are people who can benefit from the services of health care professionals. Often the health services focus on education and other primary prevention practices. Nurses help design safety, exercise, and nutrition programs; provide basic immunization services; conduct parenting classes; organize crisis intervention programs for youth and teens; and help organize health fairs. The health care staff may be paid or may work on a volunteer basis, or there may be a combination of paid and volunteer staff.

Many services can be provided to smaller groups of infants and children with special needs. Such intervention programs may be supported by federal or state funds and offered through the school district or private associations for developmentally delayed, physically challenged, or emotionally disturbed children. The interventions are often multidisciplinary, consisting of a team of professionals who work together to meet the multiple needs of the child.

● **Figure 2.7** The school nurse cares for a young girl who injured her knee on the playground. In addition to first aid, the school nurse's duties include counseling, health education, and health promotion.

Professional teams may consist of a teacher, psychologist, neurologist, physical therapist, social worker, physician, and nurse. The most important team members are the family caregivers and the child, and it is essential to include them in planning meetings and program intervention development. The nurse's role as a team member involves interpreting diagnoses or medical orders to other team members and the family, teaching the family how to provide care for a medically fragile child, and effectively integrating the family into intervention programs.

Residential Programs

Residential programs, often called group homes, provide services for a number of health needs. Those geared primarily to children include chemical dependency treatment centers and homes for children with mental or emotional health needs, pregnant adolescents, and abused children. These homes vary in size and setup according to the children's needs.

Depending on the number of children a home serves, the nurse may be contracted to provide specific services. The nurse may work for the local health department or for a corporation that owns several group homes. For example, in a home with six children with minimal disabilities, the nurse may visit every 2 weeks to meet with and educate the staff, update health records, and provide immunizations. This may be all the health care service the home requires to maintain its group home license.

Homes that serve many children or that serve children with very complex needs may need to have nurses 24 hours a day. Often licensing standards require this complete coverage in addition to meeting the health care needs of the children. Some homes hire a multidisciplinary team of health care practitioners that may include nurses; medical social workers; psychologists; physical, speech, or occupational therapists; special education teachers; home health aides or attendants; and physicians. Not all the team members provide services to group homes on a full-time basis.

Skills of the Community-Based Nurse

The nursing process serves as the foundation of nursing care in the community, just as it does in a health care facility. Communication with the patient and family is essential. Teaching is a fundamental part of community-based care because of the emphasis on health promotion and preventive health care. Case management is necessary to coordinate care and monitor case progress through the health care system.

The Nursing Process

The focus of the community-based nurse is the patient within the context of the family. In the initial family assessment interview, the nurse determines how various family members affect the pregnant woman or the child and his condition. The nurse may obtain additional information by picking up on cues in the environment. Upon completion of data collection and assessment, the RN and health care team focus on identifying the nursing diagnoses based on the family's strengths, weaknesses, and needs. Family interaction and cooperation leads to collaborative goal setting and proposed interventions. The ongoing nursing process requires that these interventions be evaluated as the cycle continues.

Communication

Positive, effective communication is fundamental to the nursing process and the care of childbearing and child rearing families in the community. Establishing rapport with the child and the family, understanding and appropriately responding to cultural practices, and being sensitive to the needs of the child and family all require good communication skills.

Teaching

Teaching and health education are key components of community-based nursing care. Health care often involves teaching families, small groups of children, family caregivers, members of extended families, and large groups of children, on various topics that focus on primary prevention (Fig. 2-8).

Here's an idea. When teaching a group with which you are unfamiliar, ask the group leader for demographic information to help develop an appropriate teaching plan.

To teach a group successfully, the nurse must know the needs of the target population and have the

● **Figure 2.8** The nurse providing postpartum and newborn care in the home takes the opportunity to provide patient education.

appropriate teaching skills, strategies, and resources. When the nurse is familiar with the group, he already has important information, such as age, educational level, ethnic and gender mix, language barriers, and any previous teaching the group has had on the subject. The nurse should review growth and developmental principles to identify the appropriate level of information, learning activities, and average attention span. Additional information includes any available teaching resources, group size, seating arrangements, and other advantages or restrictions of the environment. For instance, the nurse may want to find out

- Are the chairs movable for small-group discussions?
- Is there a videocasette recorder to show a video?
- Can the children go outside?
- Will a lot of noise disturb others in the building?
- Will the classroom teacher or teacher's aide be in attendance?

A successful group teaching experience relies on a prepared nurse educator.

Case Management

Case management, a systematic process that ensures that a client's multiple health and service needs are met, may be a formal or an informal process. In formalized case management, the agency or insurer who pays for the health care services predetermines the contact with the client. In other settings, the nurse may determine the needed follow-up and either provide the services or assist with referrals to obtain services.

If case management is formalized, the insurer pays for nursing services. The case manager's role is clearly outlined with care plans, protocols, and limits to service determined by the insurer. In community agencies where nursing services are part of the overall service (for instance, schools or group homes), the intensity of follow-up is determined by the agency's philosophy, available resources, and the nurse's perception of the role and her individual skills.

Client Advocacy

Client advocacy is speaking or acting on behalf of others to help them gain greater independence and to make the health care delivery system more responsive and relevant to their needs. The nurse working in a community setting may often develop a long-standing relationship with childbearing and child rearing families because of the continuous nature of client contact in an outpatient, school, or other setting. This type of relationship may allow the nurse to discover broader health and welfare issues. Examples of interventions include

- Teaching a family about the services for which the pregnant woman or child is eligible.

● *Figure 2.9* A nurse advocate can help the child enter a school lunch program so that nutritional needs are met.

- Assisting the family to apply for Medicaid or other forms of health care reimbursement.
- Identifying inexpensive or free transportation services to medical appointments.
- Making telephone calls to establish eligibility for and to acquire special equipment needed by a physically challenged child.

Examples of client advocacy are limitless and include health and social welfare services that intertwine in ways that families cannot manage alone. One example is assistance with referrals and acquisition of needed resources. As a member of a team of health care professionals, the nurse assists with the referral process. This process focuses on the childbearing or child rearing family obtaining the appropriate services and resources. Actions taken are geared toward improving the childbearing or child rearing family's health or quality of life. The nurse must be knowledgeable about community resources, contact persons, details of appropriate applications, and other required documentation (Fig. 2-9).

The Challenge of Community-Based Nursing

There are differences between caring for childbearing and child rearing families in a hospital or clinic and caring for them in community settings. Community-based work requires a different set of skills.

The Unique Aspects of Community-Based Nursing

Community-based nursing practice is autonomous. The nurse must be self-reliant to be successful. There may not be many other health care practitioners with whom to consult; those available may be physically distant. To provide childbearing and child-rearing families with high-quality care, the nurse must have well-developed assessment and decision-making skills.

Community practice tends to be more holistic. The individual is viewed as an integrated whole mind, body, and spirit interacting with the environment. The community nurse must consider the effects of the mother's or child's health on family functioning, the child's educational progress, and the multiple services the family and child need to improve the quality of life.

A final difference is the focus on wellness. Some community settings have a population of at-risk pregnant women and children with an illness or diagnosis in common, such as diabetes or cerebral palsy. Working with these groups involves managing the disease or limitations with a wellness focus. For instance, the focus might be on teaching a group of pregnant women with diabetes about diabetic diets. Another example would be showing how the child with cerebral palsy can be included comfortably within the regular classroom.

In most areas where the community nurse works, the focus is on wellness. Women and children are basically well but may be going through a growth and developmental crises. The nurse intervenes to ease the transition from one developmental stage to another. The nurse provides anticipatory guidance to family caregivers and emphasizes preventive health practices. Teaching health-promotion practices to pregnant women and children is another activity of primary importance.

Issues Facing Pregnant Women, Children, and Families

Nurses who work in the community encounter the complex issues facing childbearing and child rearing families. Nursing care given to pregnant women, children, and families within their own environments allows the nurse to better understand their unique needs.

Poverty is a major issue that affects all aspects of recovery and responses to care. For many families, a lack of resources hinders compliance and takes its toll on the health of all family members. Services and resources may be inaccessible because of cost, location, or lack of transportation. Sometimes family caregivers see such services as unnecessary. Poverty, lack of information, questionable decisions about priorities, and ineffective coping skills affect the health of pregnant women, children, and families in significant ways. The results are often seen in emergency departments, neonatal intensive care units (NICUs), and in acute care beds of children's units.

The community nurse must explore these issues with the family caregivers. When a pregnant woman delays prenatal care, what issues surround this behavior? When a family does not follow up with an orthopedic appointment for a new cast application on the legs of a 6-month-old infant, what factors influenced their decision? When a family caregiver saves half of the antibiotic suspension for another child in the family with similar symptoms, what motivates this decision?

When a single parent keeps a physically disabled and developmentally delayed 9-year-old son at home in one room of the apartment, what types of care-giving services and information might be of benefit?

Test Yourself

- Name two conditions for which a child or infant could receive home health care.
- Define client advocacy.
- Name three unique aspects of community-based nursing.

Rewards of Community-Based Nursing

The nurse in community-based settings sees the client over a period of time. This allows the nurse to have a broader understanding of the context within which the individual and family lives. The clinic nurse may see the same family for different problems over a period of many years. The camp or school nurse watches children grow and gets to know siblings and families over time. A group-home nurse works intensely with a group of developmentally disabled children and learns to know each one and rejoice in their small triumphs. A nurse in a home for pregnant teens works with a young mother throughout her pregnancy and takes pleasure in the birth of a healthy baby.

For the community nurse, rewards come slowly and in different ways. For 4 months, a school nurse may diligently work with a child and family and a community service organization to obtain a pair of glasses for the child. This nurse may feel rewarded when the child no longer comes into the school nurse's office with headaches and is doing better in class work. The camp nurse may help a homesick new camper design a way to stay in touch with his or her parents and may encourage the camper to participate in camp activities. This nurse may also find reward when the camper returns each season. The nurse in a group home for teenage foster children with behavioral problems may help the teens develop a theater group that presents plays about safe sex and responsible teen dating to other group homes, high school classes, or community service organizations. This nurse may find reward after a year of work with the teens when they write the scripts, build the sets independently, and declare that they enjoy the theater group more than any other activity in the residence. This nurse may also find a deeper reward when he or she realizes that as a result of the theater group, there are fewer behavioral problems and the teens' self-esteem is high.

Community nurses work in many ways to prevent unnecessary hospitalization. Examples of health problems that the community nurse seeks to prevent include injuries to a child not appropriately secured in a car seat, severe burns to the face of a toddler from grabbing a tablecloth and spilling a cup of coffee, a near drowning in a backyard pool, an infant who fails to thrive because the parents do not know that infants need specific amounts of formula, or a pregnant teen who contracts HIV because she does not practice safe sex.

The community nurse helps families develop the skills and knowledge they need to make decisions that affect their lives and those of other family members. In this way, families can learn and practice preventive health care. With a focus on wellness, the community nurse provides a service that eventually improves the health of the entire community.

KEY POINTS

- The family is the basic social unit. It provides for survival and teaches the knowledge, customs, values, and beliefs of the family's culture.
- The basic functions of the family are to reproduce and socialize children to function within the larger society. To meet the needs of individual members, the family also functions to provide support in the five areas of wholeness: physical, emotional, intellectual, social, and spiritual.
- The nuclear family and the extended family are the two types of traditional family structures that exist in most cultures. The single-parent family, communal family, gay or lesbian family, and cohabitation family are four examples of nontraditional family structures.
- Mobility, changing attitudes about children born out of wedlock and divorce, women working outside the home, and changes in adoption laws all have contributed to an increase in single-parent families.
- Family size affects the child's development. Children from small families receive more individual attention and tend to relate better to adults. Children from large families develop interdependency skills.
- Birth order also influences development. First-born children tend to be high achievers. Subsequent children are often more relaxed and are slower to develop language skills.
- Families tend to spend less time together than in the past for many reasons—both parents may work, the children participate in many school activities, families often do not eat together, and there is an emphasis on acquisition of material goods, rather than the development of relationships.
- Community-based health care focuses on wellness and prevention and is directed toward helping persons and families meet their health care needs.

- Community-based health care is advantageous for the pregnant woman, child, and family because it allows the individual to receive care within the context of the community and culture. It also identifies and meets needs within the community, which may allow for less costly care than that provided in a hospital setting.
- Primary prevention focuses on preventing illness and injury. An example is a nurse in a maternity clinic giving teaching tips on proper nutrition during pregnancy.
- Secondary prevention involves health screening activities that aid in early diagnosis and encourage prompt treatment before long-term negative effects are realized. An example is a school nurse who identifies a child with head lice, then contacts the family caregivers with instructions on how to rid the child and family members of infestation.
- Tertiary prevention involves health-promoting activities that focus on rehabilitation and teaching to prevent additional injury or illness. An example is a child with spina bifida who requires frequent catheterizations and trips to a specialized clinic. The nurse assists the family to find resources so that proper care and medical monitoring can continue to prevent the development of additional problems.
- The community-based nurse needs to be able to use the nursing process to plan and provide care to families and groups, communicate effectively and teach individuals and groups, perform case management, and practice client advocacy.
- An effective community nurse educator must identify and assess the target population by determining the age, educational level, ethnic and gender mix, language barriers, and any previous teaching the group may have had. The nurse must assess each audience and gear the teaching appropriately. The teaching must be geared accordingly using appropriate materials.
- The community nurse functions as a child advocate by taking actions geared toward improving the child's health or quality of life. One example of child advocacy is when the nurse assists with the referral process to help the child and family obtain the services and resources needed to maintain health.

REFERENCES AND SELECTED READINGS

Books and Journals

Acherman-Liebrich, U., Voegli, T. Gunter-Witt, K., Kunz, I., Zullig, M., et al. (1996). Home versus hospital deliveries: Follow up study of matched pairs for procedures and outcome. Zurich study team. *BMJ: British Medical Journal,* 313(7068), 1313–1318.

Ahmann, E., & Johnson, B. H. (2001). Family matters: New guidance materials promote family-centered change in health care institutions. *Pediatric Nursing, 27*(2), 173–175.

Allender, J. A., & Spradley, B. W. (2000). *Community health nursing* (5th ed.). Philadelphia: Lippincott Williams & Wilkins.

American College of Obstetricians and Gynecologists. (2002, July 31). Home births double risk of newborn death. *ACOG News Release*. Retrieved June 7, 2003, from http://www.acog.org/from_home/publications/press_releases/nr07-31-02-3.cfm

Anderson, R. E., & Murphy, P. A. (1995). Outcomes of 11,788 planned home births attended by certified nurse-midwives: A retrospective descriptive study. *Journal of Nurse Midwifery, 40*(6), 468–473, 483–492.

Anonymous. (2001). Boost for children's healthcare. *Nursing Standard, 15*(24), 7.

Clayton, M. (2000). Health and social policy: Influences on family-centered care. *Pediatric Nursing, 12*(8), 31–33.

Corrarino, J. E., Williams, C., Campbell, W. S., Amrhein, E., LoPiano, L., Kalachick, D. (2000). Linking substance-abusing pregnant women to drug treatment services: A pilot program. *JOGNN: Journal of Obstetric, Gynecologic, and Neonatal Nursing, 29*(4), 369–376.

Craig, G. (1992). *Human development* (6th ed.). Englewood Cliffs, NJ: Prentice-Hall.

Eckenrode, J., Ganzel, B., Henderson, C. R., Smith, E., Olds, D. L., Powers, J., et al. (2000). Preventing child abuse and neglect with a program of nurse home visitation: The limiting effects of domestic violence. *The Journal of the American Medical Association (JAMA), 284*(11), 1385–1391.

Fuller, Q. (2000). Cultural competence in pediatric nursing. *Nursing Spectrum*. Available at: http://community.nursingspectrum.com/MagazineArticles.

Gottman, J. (1990). Children of gay and lesbian parents. In F. W. Bozett, M. Sussman (Eds.), *Homosexuality and family relations*. New York: Harrington Park.

Hunt, R. (2001). *Introduction to community-based nursing* (2nd ed.). Philadelphia: Lippincott Williams & Wilkins.

Janssen, P. A., Lee, S. K., Ryan, E. M., Etches, D. J., Farquharson, D. F., Peacock, D., Klein, M. C. (2002). *CMAJ: Canadian Medical Association Journal, 166*(3), 315.

Kitzman, H., Olds, D. L., Sidora, K., Henderson, C. R., Hanks, C., Cole, R., et al. (2000). Enduring effects of nurse home visitation on maternal life course: A 3-year follow-up of a randomized trial. *The Journal of the American Medical Association (JAMA), 283*(15), 1983–1989.

Koniak-Griffin, D., Mathenge, C., Anderson, N. L., & Verzemnieks, I. (1999). An early intervention program for adolescent mothers: A nursing demonstration project [Abstract]. *Journal of Obstetric, Gynecologic, and Neonatal Nursing (JOGNN), 28*(1), 51–59.

Lieu, T. A., Braveman, P. A., Escobar, G. J., Fischer, A. F., Jensvold, N. G., Capra, A. M. (2000). A randomized comparison of home and clinic follow-up visits after early postpartum hospital discharge. *Pediatrics, 105*(5), 1058.

Limerick, M., & Baldwin, L. (2000). Nursing in outpatient child and adolescent mental health. *Nursing Standard, 15*(24), 9.

McPherson, G., & Thorne, S. (2000). Children's voices, can we hear them? *Journal of Pediatric Nursing, 15*(1), 22–29.

Monsen, R. B. (2001). Raising kids, grandparents bear a burden. *Journal of Pediatric Nursing, 16*(2), 130–131.

Morrell, C. J., Spiby, H., Stewart, P., Walters, S., & Morgan, A. (2000). Costs and benefits of community postnatal support workers: Randomised controlled trial. *BMJ: British Medical Journal, 321*(7261), 593.

Newton, M. S. (2000). Family-centered care: Current realities in parent participation. *Pediatric Nursing, 26*(2), 164–168.

Olds, D. L., Eckenrode, J., Henderson, C. R., Kitzman, H., Powers, J., Cole, R., et al. (1997). Long-term effects of home visitation on maternal life course and child abuse and neglect: Fifteen-year follow-up of a randomized trial [Abstract]. *The Journal of the American Medical Association (JAMA), 278*(8): 637.

Olsen, O., & Jewell, M. D. (2000). Home versus hospital birth. *Cochrane Database of Systematic Reviews*. Retrieved June 1, 2003, from http://www.medscape.com/viewarticle/453976

Patterson, G. J. (1996). Lesbian and gay parenthood. *Handbook of parenting*. Hillsdale, NJ: Lawrence Erlbaum Associates.

Snow, C. (1996). Cultural sensitivity workshop. Philadelphia: Nationality Service Council, United Way.

Sperhac, A. M., & Strodtbeck, F. (2001). Advanced practice in pediatric nursing: Blending roles. *Journal of Pediatric Nursing, 16*(2), 120–126.

United States Bureau of Census. (2000). *Statistical abstract of the United States: 2000*. Washington DC: Superintendent of Documents.

Vessey, J. A. (2000). Primary care approaches: Coordinated school health. *Pediatric Nursing, 26*(3), 303–304, 307.

Woodring, B. C. (2000). Family matters: If you have taught, have the child and family learned? *Pediatric Nursing, 26*(5), 505–509.

Websites

Cultural Competence—available at www.air.org/cecp/cultural.

Minority Health—available at www.omhrc.gov/omh-home.htm.

Ethnic and Racial Health Disparities—available at http://raceandhealth.hhs.gov

www.health.discovery.com

www.kidshealth.org/kid

www.kinderstart.com

WORKBOOK

NCLEX-STYLE REVIEW QUESTIONS

1. In working with families, the nurse recognizes that different family structures exist. Which of the following examples best describes a blended family? A family in which

   a. the adult members share in homemaking as well as in child rearing.

   b. the partners in the marriage bring children from a previous marriage into the household.

   c. grandparents live in the same house with the grandchildren and their parents.

   d. partners of the same sex share a household and raise children together.

2. One role of the nurse in a community-based setting focuses on primary prevention. An example of primary prevention would be

   a. screening children for vision in a preschool.

   b. teaching bicycle safety in an after-school program.

   c. identifying head lice in a child in elementary school.

   d. exploring financial help for a client in a home setting.

3. One role of the nurse in a community-based setting focuses on secondary prevention. An example of secondary prevention would be

   a. screening children for vision in a preschool.

   b. teaching about nutrition in an after-school program.

   c. recommending a group home setting for an adolescent.

   d. administering immunizations to infants in a clinic.

4. One role of the nurse in a community-based setting focuses on tertiary prevention. An example of tertiary prevention would be

   a. testing children for hearing loss in a preschool.

   b. teaching bicycle safety in an after-school program.

   c. administering immunizations to infants in a clinic.

   d. exploring financial help for a client in a home setting.

5. A mother of a child being cared for in a home setting makes the following statements. Which statement *best* illustrates one of the positive aspects of home health care?

   a. "My family gets to visit once a week when my child is in the hospital."

   b. "I can do my child's care since you taught the procedure to me."

   c. "Our insurance pays for us to go to the well-child clinic."

   d. "The neighbor's child likes being in the group home."

6. When a nurse is doing teaching in a community-based setting, it is *most* important for the nurse to

   a. ask questions about the histories of those present.

   b. use posters that everyone in the group can read.

   c. tell the participants about the nurse's background.

   d. know the needs of the audience.

STUDY ACTIVITIES

1. Survey your community to discover the community-based health care providers available. Use the information you found to complete the following table.

Community-Based Health Care Providers	How Are They Funded?	What Types of Health Care for Children Do They Provide?

2. Using the information you obtained above, evaluate your community's health care services by answering the following:

   a. Does your community have adequate health care services for childbearing and child rearing families?

b. Are funding concerns an issue for your community? In what ways?

c. What other services do you think are needed to care for the childbearing and child rearing families in your community?

3. Select a community-based setting and outline the services that a nurse in that setting should ideally provide. Include the resources needed to provide the services.

4. Go to the following Internet site: http://www.culturediversity.org. At "Transcultural Nursing," click on "Cultural Competency."

a. What is the definition of cultural competence?

b. What are the five essential elements necessary for an organization to become culturally competent?

c. What are the four major challenges to attaining cultural competency?

5. Go to the following Internet site: http://www.faculty.fairfield.edu/fleitas/contents.html. At "Bandaides & Blackboards," click on "Kids." Go to "Lots of Stories" and click on the star.

a. In working with school-age children, what are some of the stories in this site you would encourage the children to read?

b. List the topics and diseases included in the stories that you could share with school-age children.

CRITICAL THINKING: What Would You Do?

Apply your knowledge of the family and the nurse's role in the community to the following situations.

1. Nine-year-old Shawn has become withdrawn, his school grades have fallen, and he complains of having headaches and stomachaches since his parents' divorce 3 months ago. He lives with his mother during the week and visits his father, who lives with a girlfriend, on weekends.

a. What concerns do you think Shawn's parents would have about his changes in behavior and his physical complaints?

b. What advice would you offer Shawn's parents regarding these concerns?

c. What could these parents do to help Shawn better adjust to the divorce?

2. You are making a home visit to the Andrews family because their newborn needs home phototherapy treatment for 3 to 5 days. You find 6-year-old Samantha ill with bronchitis. Both parents smoke. Outline a teaching plan for these caregivers regarding the health of their family.

3. Mrs. Perez, a second-grade teacher, asks you to teach a unit on personal hygiene to her class.

a. Identify the information you will need from Mrs. Perez.

b. Describe how you will present the lesson to these children.

Foundations of Maternity Nursing

Structure and Function of the Reproductive System

Male Reproductive System
    External Genitalia
    Internal Reproductive Organs
Female Reproductive System
    External Genitalia (Vulva)
    Internal Reproductive Organs
    Blood Supply for the Pelvic Organs

Reproductive Function
    Puberty
    Menstruation
    Menstrual Cycle
    Cervical Mucus Changes
    Menopause
Sexual Response Cycle

STUDENT OBJECTIVES

On completion of this chapter, the student should be able to

1. Explain two major functions of the reproductive system.
2. Label an anatomic drawing of the female and male reproductive systems, including external genitalia and internal anatomy.
3. Discuss major functions of each reproductive structure, gland, and organ.
4. Trace the path of sperm through the male reproductive system, from the site of formation to ejaculation from the body.
5. Describe the process of semen production.
6. Compare hormonal regulation of male reproductive function with that of the female.
7. Illustrate the inter-relationships of the ovarian and uterine cycles and the overall menstrual cycle.
8. Compare the sexual response cycle of the male to that of the female.

KEY TERMS

climacteric
corpus luteum
endometrium
epididymis
gametes
menarche
mons pubis
myometrium
ovulation
prepuce
seminiferous tubules
spermatogenesis
vas deferens
vestibule
vulva

The obstetric nurse is called upon to counsel prospective parents before and throughout pregnancy and childbirth. To accomplish this task, the nurse must have a working knowledge of reproductive anatomy and physiology and the menstrual cycle. This knowledge guides the nurse in choosing appropriate interventions for the childbearing woman and her family.

The main purpose of the male and female reproductive systems is to produce offspring. Male testes produce and female ovaries contain **gametes** or sex cells, spermatozoa (sperm) in the male and ova (eggs) in the female. Each gamete contains one half of the genetic material needed to produce a human baby. However, as you will see some of the structures in the reproductive tract serve dual purposes. Most often these alternate functions have to do with urinary elimination because the urinary system is connected closely with the reproductive system.

You will notice that most structures in the reproductive tract are paired (e.g., testes, ovaries, labia majora, labia minora) and that male and female reproductive systems are complementary; for example, male testes and female ovaries; male scrotum and female labia majora; and male glans penis and female clitoris. It is important to know that the pituitary gland governs reproductive hormone production and function (Fig. 3-1).

MALE REPRODUCTIVE SYSTEM

Sometimes the man's contribution to childbirth is not fully appreciated because of the focus on the pregnant woman and her growing fetus. However, the father's role is crucial to this process. His genetic material not only determines the sex of the unborn child, but also influences numerous other inherited traits. The male reproductive anatomy consists of external reproductive organs and internal reproductive organs. The purpose of the male reproductive tract is to allow for sexual intimacy and reproduction of offspring, and to provide a conduit for urinary elimination.

External Genitalia

The man's external reproductive organs, the external genitalia, consist of the penis and scrotum (Fig. 3-2).

Penis

The penis serves a dual role as the male organ of reproduction and as the external organ of urinary elimination. The penis is composed of a bulbous head, the glans penis or glans, and a shaft. The glans

Make a note of this. It is the prepuce that is removed in the surgical procedure called circumcision. Some parents choose to have this procedure done within the first few days of their son's life. Others choose to leave their male babies uncircumcised. Circumcision can be performed on adult males, usually for medical reasons; however, this procedure is not often done in adulthood.

is the most sensitive area on the penis because this is where the greatest concentration of nerve endings is found. This part of the penis is analogous to the clitoris in the female. At birth a layer of tissue, the **prepuce** or foreskin, covers the glans.

The shaft of the penis (Fig. 3-2) is made up of three columns of erectile tissue: the paired cavernous bodies (corpus cavernosa) and the spongy body (corpus spongiosum). The cavernous bodies are parallel, and the spongy body lies atop them in the midline. The spongy body is cradled in the channel created where the cavernous bodies meet. Each column is encased in a thick sheath called the tunica albuginea. Two layers of fascia encircle all three columns along the length of the shaft. The fascia gives the penis support, allowing it to become a firm structure during sexual stimulation.

The erectile tissue is well supplied with blood vessels and nerves. When the penis is stimulated sexually, parasympathetic nerves cause the veins in the shaft to dilate. The sinuses within the erectile tissue fill up with blood causing an erection. The erect penis is capable of penetrating the female vagina for the purposes of sexual fulfillment and intimacy. If the erect penis is stimulated to ejaculation within the vagina, the reproductive function of depositing sperm in the female reproductive tract occurs.

The urethra passes through the shaft of the penis within the spongy body. It functions to eliminate urine from the bladder and to transport semen to the woman's vagina during ejaculation.

Scrotum

The scrotum is an external sac that houses the testes in two internal compartments. The main functions of the scrotum are to protect the testes from trauma and to regulate the temperature within the testes, a process that is extremely important to the production of healthy male gametes. The ideal temperature within the scrotum is approximately 96°F, just slightly lower than normal body temperature. The skin of the scrotum is greatly pigmented and folded into furrows called rugae. When either the environmental or body temperature is hot, the cremaster muscle within the scrotal sac remains relaxed so that the testes dangle down, away

Female

Follicle-stimulating hormone

Anterior pituitary

Leutinizing hormone

Male

Follicle-stimulating hormone

Interstitial cell stimulating hormone

Stimulates the ovaries to produce estrogen

Causes ovulation and stimulates the ovaries to produce progesterone

Stimulates testes to secrete testosterone

Stimulates testes to produce sperm

Fallopian tube

Ovary

Endometrium

Urinary bladder

Ureter

Seminal vesicle

Vas deferens

Prostate gland

Bulbourethral (Cowper's) gland

Penile shaft

Urethra

Epididymis

Testis

● *Figure 3.1* Hormones of the anterior pituitary stimulate the reproductive system in the male and the female.

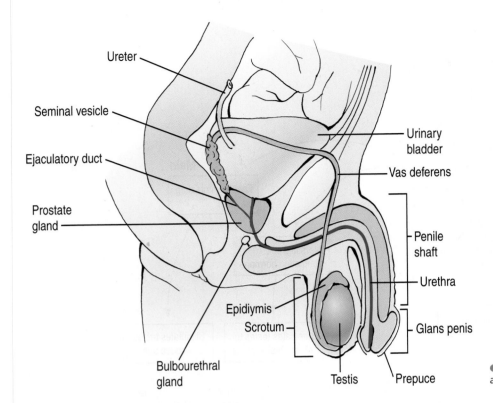

Ureter

Seminal vesicle

Ejaculatory duct

Prostate gland

Urinary bladder

Vas deferens

Penile shaft

Urethra

Glans penis

Epididymis

Scrotum

Bulbourethral gland

Testis

Prepuce

● *Figure 3.2* Male reproductive anatomy.

from the warmth of the body. If the temperature is cold, the cremaster muscle contracts, an action that pulls the scrotum in toward the man's body, thereby increasing the temperature in the testicles.

Internal Reproductive Organs

Male internal reproductive organs include the testes and a system of glands and ducts that are involved in the formation of nutrient plasma and the transport of semen out of the man's body (Fig. 3-3).

This is an important teaching tip. The temperature within the testes should be slightly lower than core body temperature. When the temperature is too hot, sperm are not produced efficiently. A simple act such as wearing constrictive clothing (e.g., tight jeans) for prolonged periods can lead to low sperm counts and male infertility because the scrotal contents are held too close to the body and the temperature within the testes becomes too hot for optimal sperm production.

Testes

The testes, two oval organs, one within each scrotal sac (Fig. 3-4), serve two important functions: production of male sex hormones, androgens, and formation and maturation of spermatozoa. Each testis is about 4 centimeters long by 2.5 centimeters wide and is di-

vided into lobes. The lobes contain **seminiferous tubules,** tiny coils of tissue in which **spermatogenesis,** production of sperm, occurs. Interstitial cells surround the seminiferous tubules and produce the androgen testosterone, which is necessary for the maturation of sperm. A system of tiny tubes called the rete testis lead from the seminiferous tubules to the **epididymis,** an intricate network of coiled ducts on the posterior portion of each testis that is approximately 6 meters (20 feet) in length. It is here that sperm mature. Refer to Table 3-1 for a summary of the hormones that influence male reproduction. Box 3-1 depicts how to perform testicular self-examination (TSE). This procedure is recommended monthly for all men age 15 years and older to detect early changes associated with testicular cancer.

Ductal System

The **vas deferens** is the muscular tube in which sperm begin their journey out of the man's body. It connects the epididymis with the ejaculatory duct. The vas deferens is sheathed in the spermatic cord, which also contains the blood vessels, nerves, and lymphatics that serve the testes. The left spermatic cord is usually longer than the right so that the left testis hangs lower than the right.

The spermatic cord (and vas deferens contained within it) leads into the abdominal cavity through the inguinal canal, arches over the urinary bladder, and then curves downward on the posterior side of the

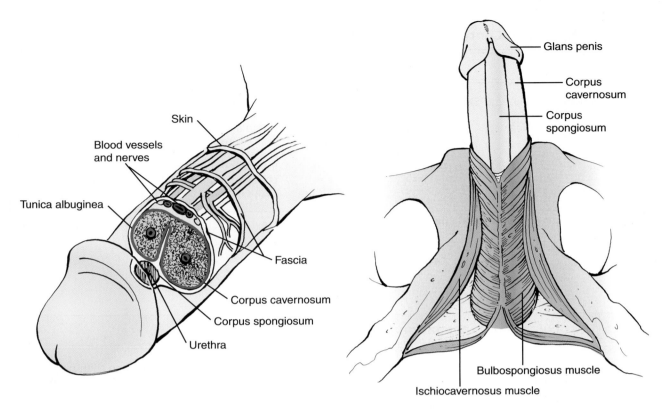

Notice the three columns of erectile tissue. These are well supplied with blood and nerve tissue. The cavernous bodies (corpus cavernosa) contain sinuses that fill with blood during an erection. The urethra traverses the shaft encased within the spongy body (corpus spongiosum).

● *Figure 3.3* Internal structure of the penis.

This view of the ventral aspect shows how the spongy body lies in relation to the cavernous bodies. Notice how the root of the penis is anchored to the pelvis by the tough connective tissue and muscle.

bladder. It is at this point that the vas deferens joins with the ejaculatory duct. The paired ejaculatory ducts then connect with the single urethra, which transports the sperm out of the man's penis during ejaculation.

Accessory Glands and Semen

The seminal vesicles are paired glands that empty an alkaline, fructose-rich fluid into the ejaculatory ducts during ejaculation. The prostate is a muscular gland that surrounds the first part of the urethra as it exits the urinary bladder. It is approximately the size of a chestnut. Prostatic fluid is alkaline and is secreted when the prostate contracts during ejaculation. The bulbourethral (Cowper's) glands secrete an alkaline fluid that coats the last part of the urethra during ejaculation.

The alkaline fluids secreted by these glands are nutrient plasmas with several key functions, including

- Enhancement of sperm motility (i.e., ability to move)
- Nourishment of sperm (i.e., provides a ready source of energy with the simple sugar fructose)

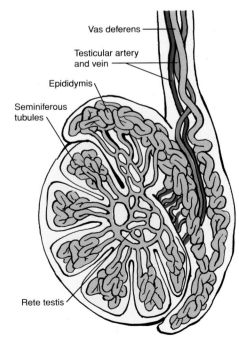

● *Figure 3.4* Internal structure of a testis.

TABLE 3.1	Hormonal Control of Male Reproductive Functions	
Hormone	Source	Reproductive Functions
Follicle-stimulating hormone (FSH)	Anterior pituitary	• Stimulates production of sperm in the seminiferous tubules
Interstitial cell-stimulating hormone (ICSH)[1]	Anterior pituitary	• Stimulates the interstitial cells to secrete testosterone
Testosterone	Interstitial cells	• Assists sperm to mature • Influences the development of secondary sex characteristics (facial and pubic hair growth, deepening of the voice, growth of the penis)

[1]Homologous to luteinizing hormone (LH) in the female.

BOX 3.1	Testicular Self-examination (TSE)

The National Institutes for Health recommend that men (starting at age 15) perform TSE once monthly for early detection of testicular tumors or abnormalities. The examination should be performed after a warm bath or shower. The warmth relaxes the scrotal skin, which makes it easier to detect abnormalities. There are four steps to a complete examination.

1. Inspection of scrotal sac. The man stands in front of a mirror and checks for swelling on the scrotal skin. It is normal for one testicle to hang lower than the other.
2. Palpation of testicles. The man examines each testicle with both hands. The index and middle finger are placed under the testicle, and the thumb is placed on top. The testicle is then rolled between the fingers and thumbs. The procedure is repeated on the other testicle. Pain should not be felt during the exam. Cancerous lumps are usually found on the sides of the testicle, but can also appear in the front.
3. Palpation of the epididymis. The man then palpates the epididymis, a cordlike structure found on the top and back of each testicle. Lumps on the epididymis are not cancerous.
4. Examination by a physician. If a suspicious lump or swelling is noted, the man is instructed to see a physician, preferably a urologist, as soon as possible. TSE should be done in association with annual health examinations.

Signs of testicular cancer include
• Small, painless lump in a testicle.
• Enlargement of a testicle. It is normal for one testicle to be slightly larger than the other.
• Significant loss in size of a testicle.
• A feeling of scrotal heaviness.
• A dull ache in the lower abdomen or groin.
• Testicular or scrotal pain or discomfort.
• Sudden accumulation of blood or fluid in the scrotum.
• Enlargement or tenderness of the breasts.

TABLE 3.2	A Sperm's Journey Through the Male Reproductive Tract
Event	**Site**
Formation of sperm	Seminiferous tubules (paired)
Maturation of sperm	Epididymis (paired)
Path into the abdominal cavity	Vas deferens (paired)
Connecting duct between vas deferens and urethra	Ejaculatory duct (paired)
Path out of the man's body	Urethra (single)

- Protection of sperm (i.e., sperm are maintained in an alkaline environment to protect them from the acidic environment of the vagina)

The alkaline fluids and sperm combination is a thick, whitish secretion termed semen or seminal fluid. An average human ejaculate has a volume of 1 to 5 mL and contains several hundred million sperm. Table 3-2 describes (in order) the journey of sperm from formation in the seminiferous tubules to the path out of the body via the urethra.

Test Yourself

- What is the general term that refers to male and female sex cells?

- Name two important functions of the testes.

- Trace a sperm through the male reproductive tract to outside of the body beginning at the seminiferous tubules. Name all the ducts and glands along the way.

FEMALE REPRODUCTIVE SYSTEM

The external genitalia, or **vulva,** and internal reproductive organs compose the female reproductive tract. The purpose of the female reproductive tract is to allow for sexual intimacy and fulfillment and to produce children through the processes of conception, pregnancy, and childbirth. Each part of the female reproductive tract contributes in some way to these purposes.

The mammary glands and bony pelvis are also part of female reproductive anatomy. Breast anatomy is discussed with infant nutrition and lactation in Chapter 14, and the bony pelvis is described in Chapter 8. Box 3-2

explains how to do a self-breast examination, an important procedure to detect breast cancer in the early stages.

External Genitalia (Vulva)

The external genitalia consist of the mons pubis, labia majora and minora, clitoris, vestibule, and perineum. Figure 3-5 illustrates these structures.

Mons Pubis

The **mons pubis,** or mons, is a rounded fatty pad located atop the symphysis pubis. Coarse pubic hair and skin cover the mons. The function of the mons is to protect the pelvic bones during sexual intercourse.

Labia Major and Minora

The labia majora (singular: labium major) are paired fatty tissue folds that extend anteriorly from the mons pubis and then join posteriorly to the true perineum. Labia majora are covered with pubic hair, are vascular, and contain oil and sweat glands. Inside the labia majora are the labia minora (singular: labium minor), paired erectile tissue folds that extend anteriorly from the clitoris and then join posteriorly to the fourchette, a tissue fold that is formed where the labia minora meet posteriorly. The labia minora are thinner than the labia majora, are hairless, contain oil glands, and are sensitive to stimulation.

Clitoris

At the apex of the labia minora is a hooded body composed of erectile tissue called the clitoris. The clitoris, similar to the glans penis, is highly sensitive and allows the woman to experience sexual pleasure and orgasm during sexual stimulation. The hooded structure over the clitoris is called the prepuce.

Vestibule

The area between the labia minora is called the **vestibule.** The urethral meatus (opening to the urethra),

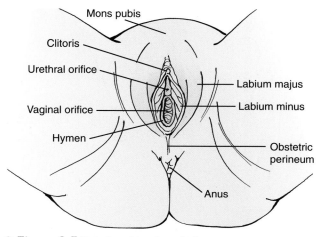

● **Figure 3.5** Female external genitalia.

BOX 3.2 | Breast Self-examination (BSE)

BSE is recommended once monthly for early detection of breast tumors or abnormalities. The examination should be performed approximately 1 week after the menstrual period ends, or if the woman is no longer having menstrual periods, then on a particular day each month that is easy for her to remember, such as the first day of the month. BSE is part of a comprehensive breast-screening program, which includes yearly clinical breast exams and mammography for women who are 40 years of age and older.

There are five steps to a complete examination.

1. Inspection of breast tissue with arms on hips. The woman stands in front of a mirror with the shoulders straight and the arms on her hips. She checks for any change in size, shape, or color, and for visible swelling or dimpling of breast tissue. It is normal for one breast to be slightly larger than the other.

2. Inspection of breast tissue with arms raised. The woman continues in front of the mirror and raises both arms. She looks for the same changes as described in Step 1.

3. Palpation of the nipple for discharge. The woman continues in front of the mirror, and then squeezes the nipple tissue, attempting to elicit a discharge. Any fluid (in a nonpregnant, nonlactating woman) is abnormal.

4. Palpation of breast tissue lying down. The woman lies down on a firm surface. She uses her right hand to exam her left breast and her left hand to examine her right breast. She should use a firm, smooth touch with the first few fingers of the hand. The fingers should be kept flat and held together.
   a. The entire breast should be covered, from the collarbone to the top of the abdomen, and from the armpit to the breast cleavage. (The armpit is an area that is frequently missed.)
   b. The woman should use a pattern to ensure that all breast tissue is covered. Some women use a circular pattern, beginning at the nipple and working outward in ever-larger circles until all breast tissue is palpated. Another method is to move the fingers up and down in vertical rows.
   c. The woman should use light palpation, then deep palpation in each area, so that superficial and deep abnormalities can be detected.

5. Palpation of breast tissue standing up. The entire process used in Step 4 is repeated in Step 5, only this time the woman is in the standing position. Many women find it helpful to perform this part of the exam in the shower.

Signs of breast cancer include
- Dimpling, puckering, or swelling of breast tissue.
- Breast pain.
- Nipple discharge.
- Change in position of a nipple.
- Breast lump or mass.

A PERSONAL GLIMPSE

For the first 12 years of my marriage I never experienced an orgasm. My husband and I married very young, just out of high school. In the early years of marriage sex was okay but never great for me. Then after three kids and no sleep, I really did not enjoy sex. I began to think there was something wrong with me. Why couldn't I enjoy sex when everyone else seemed to enjoy it? I began to speak confidentially with my nurse practitioner at my obstetrician's office. She had delivered two of my kids and I trusted her completely. I explained my concerns to her. She said that this is a very normal concern and that I was right to come see her. She said she would perform a physical examination to rule out any physical reasons for my lack of interest in, and enjoyment of, sex. A few days after the examination we sat in her office and talked. She told me that I was in great physical shape, my lab work looked fine, and my reproductive tract was healthy. She asked what kind of stimulation my husband provided before intercourse. I said none. She explained that this could be the reason I did not enjoy sex. She explained in detail how the female clitoris was designed and how it functions to bring sexual pleasure and orgasm during sexual stimulation. She showed me drawings of where it is located on my body and described how it changes during sexual stimulation. She encouraged me to locate it on my own body and ask my husband to stimulate that area during sexual intercourse. I took her advice and now I really enjoy sex with my husband. I wish someone had explained female reproductive anatomy to me earlier in my marriage.

Donna

LEARNING OPPORTUNITY: How does knowledge of the reproductive tract help nurses take care of women who desire greater sexual satisfaction?

physical exertion or with the use of tampons, so the appearance of this tissue is not a reliable method of ascertaining virginity.

Be careful! It is easy to confuse the clitoris with the urethral meatus. When you are preparing to catheterize a woman, use your finger and thumb to carefully part the labia minora, and then locate the urethral meatus below the clitoris and above the vaginal opening. If you touch the sensitive tissue of the clitoris with the catheter, you may cause the woman pain.

Perineum

The true perineum is a band of fibrous, muscular tissue that extends from the posterior portion of the labia majora to the anus. Several sets of superficial and deep muscle groups meet at the perineum to provide support for pelvic structures. The perineum and muscles of the pelvic floor are capable of great expansion during childbirth to allow for delivery of the fetus. These structures are also subject to the stresses and trauma of childbirth. The perineum is the site in which an episiotomy is sometimes done. Uncontrolled tearing and lacerations can also occur. If these are not properly repaired, or if they do not heal appropriately, the woman may experience stress incontinence or prolapse of pelvic organs later in life.

Internal Reproductive Organs

The internal reproductive organs include the vagina, uterus, fallopian tubes, and ovaries. Figure 3-6 illustrates the internal reproductive structures.

Vagina

The vagina, or birth canal, is a muscular tube that leads from the vulva to the uterus. The opening lies within the vestibule from which it slopes up and backward to the cervix. Because the walls of the vagina extend beyond the uterine cervix, the cervix dips into the

paraurethral (Skene's) glands, vaginal opening or introitus, and Bartholin glands are located within the vestibule. The paraurethral and Bartholin glands are each paired glands whose secretions moisten the delicate vaginal mucosa and raise the pH of vaginal fluid during sexual intercourse to enhance sperm motility.

The hymen is an avascular fold of tissue located around or partially around the introitus. It varies in shape from woman to woman and throughout an individual woman's reproductive life span. In times past an intact hymen was believed to be evidence of female virginity. However, the hymen can be torn in ways other than sexual intercourse, such as during heavy

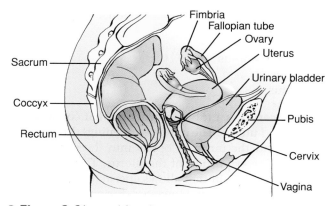

● *Figure 3.6* Internal female anatomy.

vagina and forms fornices, which are arch-like structures or pockets. The posterior fornix is largest because the posterior vaginal wall is longer than the anterior wall (approximately 9 and 7 centimeters long, respectively). Because of its location and size, the posterior fornix provides the physician ready access to the peritoneal cavity when invasive procedures are needed.

The vagina serves several important functions. The inner folds, or rugae, allow the vagina to stretch during birth to accommodate a full-term infant. In addition, normally, the vagina maintains an acidic pH of 4 to 5, which protects the vagina from infection. The vagina receives the penis during sexual intercourse and serves as the exit point for menstrual flow.

This is a good client teaching point. The acidic environment of the vagina is protective. Any change that alters the pH, particularly if the pH increases (becomes more alkaline), multiplies the risk for irritation and infection. Douching, tampons, or sanitary pads that contain deodorant, and antibiotic therapy (through the bloodstream) are examples of substances that can affect the pH of the vagina.

Uterus

The uterus, or womb, is a hollow, pear-shaped, muscular structure located within the pelvic cavity between the bladder and the rectum. The anterior surface is over the superior portion of the bladder, separated by the vesicouterine pouch, a fold of peritoneum. In the nonpregnant woman, the uterus is approximately 7.5 centimeters long by 5.0 centimeters wide (at the widest portion) and weighs approximately 40 grams. It is normally tipped forward and rests just above the urinary bladder (see Fig. 3-6). The main structures that provide support and hold the uterus in position are the broad ligaments laterally and the round ligament anteriorly. The functions of the uterus are to prepare for pregnancy each month, protect and nourish the growing child when pregnancy occurs, and to aid in childbirth. The uterus (Fig. 3-7) is divided into four sections:

- cervix
- uterine isthmus
- corpus
- fundus

The cervix is a tubular structure that connects the vagina and uterus. The outer os (opening) dips into the vagina, and the inner os opens into the uterine isthmus, the lower portion of the uterus. The cervix normally has a tiny slit that allows sperm to enter and the menstrual flow to exit. However, during childbirth the cervix must thin and open fully so that the baby can be born. The ciliated epithelium that lines the inner walls of the cervix produces mucus that lubricates the vaginal canal and serves to protect the uterus from ascending infectious agents.

The uterine isthmus is a narrow neck portion or corridor that connects the cervix to the main body of the uterus. During pregnancy and childbirth the uterine isthmus is referred to as the lower uterine segment. This is the thinnest portion of the uterus and does not participate in the muscular contractions of labor. Because it is the thinnest portion, this is the area of the uterus that is most likely to rupture during the stress of labor.

The corpus is the main body of the uterus, and the fundus is the topmost section. The walls of the corpus and fundus are made up of three layers. The perimetrium is the tough outer layer of connective tissue that supports the uterus. The middle layer is the **myometrium**, a muscular layer that is responsible for the contractions of labor. The muscle fibers of the myometrium wrap around the uterus in three directions: obliquely, laterally, and longitudinally. This muscle configuration allows for tremendous expulsive force during labor and birth. The vascular mucosal inner layer is called the **endometrium**. This is the tissue that changes under hormonal influence every month in preparation for possible conception and pregnancy.

The principal support for the uterus is provided by four paired ligaments (see Fig. 3-7), which anchor the uterus at the base (cervical region), leaving the upper portion (corpus) free in the pelvic cavity. The broad ligament is a sheet of peritoneum that attaches the lower sides of the uterus to the sidewalls of the pelvis. The right and left cardinal ligaments anchor the walls of the cervix and vagina to the lateral pelvic walls. The round ligaments are paired fibromuscular bands that tip the uterus forward and hold it in an anteflexed position. They extend from the anterior/lateral portions of the uterus to the labia majora. The round ligaments are homologous to the spermatic cord in the male. The uterosacral ligaments anchor the lower posterior portion of the uterus to the sacrum.

Fallopian Tubes

The paired fallopian tubes (also known as oviducts) are tiny, muscular corridors that arise from a lateral position on the superior surface of the uterus near the fundus and extend out on either side toward the ovaries. They are 8 to 14 centimeters in length. Each fallopian tube is divided into three sections. The isthmus, which means a neck or narrow section, is the medial one third of the tube that connects to the uterus. The ampulla, middle portion of the tube, connects the isthmus with the infundibulum, the outer portion that opens into the lower abdominal cavity. At the outer edges of the infundibulum are fimbriae,

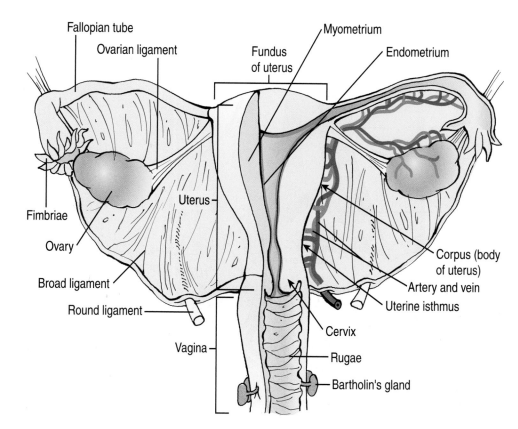

● *Figure 3.7* Anterior view of the female reproductive tract. The right fallopian tube and ovary, uterus, and vagina are shown in a cross-sectional view to demonstrate the internal structure of these organs.

fingerlike projections that undulate gently over the ovaries.

The tubes have a critical role in the process of conception. When an egg is released from the ovary, the undulating movements of the fimbriae attract the egg toward the fallopian tube. Once within the tube, muscular contractions and beating of tiny cilia propel the egg toward the uterus. If sperm are present, fertilization of the egg is possible. Fertilization most frequently occurs in the ampulla of the tube. The tubes secrete lipids and glycogen to provide nourishment to the fertilized egg as it makes its way to the uterus. The functions of the fallopian tubes are to provide a site for fertilization, a passageway, and a nourishing, warm environment for the fertilized egg to travel to the uterus.

You do the math. If one ovum matures every month during the childbearing years (from age 12 through 50), a woman would only use 456 ova. Even if that number were doubled to accommodate two eggs per cycle (a situation that sometimes results in twins), she would still use only 912 ova. Because on average a baby girl is born with 2 million immature ova, there are significantly more available than will ever be used.

Ovaries

The ovaries, two sex glands homologous to the male testes, are located on either side of the uterus. They are similar to almonds in size and shape. The ovaries are supported by the broad and ovarian ligaments. The female is born with all the ova (eggs) that she will ever have. Typically, females are born with approximately 2 million eggs, many of which will deteriorate during childhood. The remaining ova are usually released one per month during ovulation until the woman's reproductive years are over. The function of the ovaries is to produce the female hormones estrogen and progesterone, which are responsible for female secondary sex characteristics and for regulating the menstrual cycle in response to anterior pituitary hormones (see discussion in the Menstrual Cycle section).

Blood Supply for the Pelvic Organs

The pelvic organs have a rich blood supply (Fig. 3-8). The internal iliac artery arises from the common iliac artery and supplies the pelvic organs, gluteal region, hip, and medial thigh. The vagina and uterus are supplied by the vaginal and uterine arteries, respectively, both of which arise from the anterior division of the internal iliac artery. The ovarian artery, which supplies the ovaries and oviducts, branches directly from the abdominal aorta. The internal pudendal artery is the primary blood

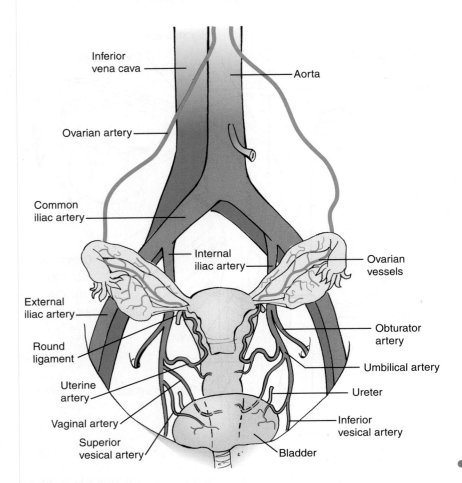

Inferior
vena cava

Aorta

Ovarian artery

Common
iliac artery

Internal
iliac artery

Ovarian
vessels

External
iliac artery

Round
ligament

Obturator
artery

Umbilical artery

Uterine
artery

Ureter

Vaginal artery

Inferior
vesical artery

Superior
vesical artery

Bladder

● *Figure 3.8* Pelvic blood supply.

supply to the perineum. This artery branches from the anterior division of the internal iliac artery and supplies the anus, superficial and deep perineal muscles, clitoris, and posterior aspect of the labia majora.

Several major veins drain the tissues of the pelvic organs. The ovarian vein, which drains the ovary, the distal part of the fallopian tube, and ureter, intersects directly with the inferior vena cava on the right and on the left connects with the left renal vein. The uterus, fallopian tubes, and vagina are drained by the uterine and vaginal venous plexus, respectively. A plexus is a network of veins that forms multiple tributaries. These plexuses connect with the uterine and vaginal veins to drain into the internal iliac vein. The external and internal pudendal veins allow deoxygenated blood from the perineal region to flow into the femoral, great saphenous, and internal iliac veins.

Test Yourself

- What structures are found in the vestibule?
- Name and describe the four divisions of the uterus.
- What important function do the ovaries fulfill?

REPRODUCTIVE FUNCTION

Puberty

Puberty is the time of life in which the individual becomes capable of sexual reproduction. Puberty occurs on average between the ages of 10 and 14 years. This phase is marked by maturation of the reproductive organs and development of secondary sex characteristics, external physical evidence of sexual maturity. Secondary sex characteristics include female breast development, growth of pubic and axillary hair, growth of external genitals (labia and penis), appearance of facial hair, and deepening of the voice in the male.

The changes associated with puberty happen in response to hypothalamic and pituitary hormones. Secondary sex characteristics develop in an orderly sequence, although the timing may be varied between individuals. Breast budding in the female is usually the first physical sign noted and occurs between the ages of 10 and 12 years on average. Appearance of pubic hair usually occurs just before **menarche**, the first menstrual period. Menarche is most frequently experienced between the ages of 12 and 14 years.

Menstruation

Menstruation, the casting away of blood, tissue, and debris from the uterus as the inner lining sheds, is variable in amount and duration. On average, flow lasts 4 to 6 days, with a total blood loss of 25 to 60 mL. Although this loss is seemingly negligible, with time it can contribute to low iron stores and anemia.

Menstrual Cycle

The menstrual cycle refers to the recurring changes that take place in a woman's reproductive tract associated with menstruation and intermenstruation. The menstrual cycle encompasses the events that transpire in the woman's reproductive organs between the beginnings of two menstrual periods. Hormones from the ovaries and the pituitary gland regulate these cyclical changes. The average cycle lasts 28 days, approximately one month; however, there are great variations between women, and an individual woman's cycle may vary in duration from cycle to cycle. For ease of understanding, the following discussion of the menstrual cycle is based on the average 28-day cycle.

Don't get lost in the details! The menstrual cycle is also referred to as the female reproductive cycle because the overarching goal is to produce human offspring. At any given time, a woman in her reproductive years is in some phase of the menstrual cycle unless pregnancy occurs, in which case the goal of the menstrual cycle has been met. When you understand the menstrual cycle, you will then be able to understand the process of conception, and you will be better prepared to counsel families on how to prevent pregnancy or how to increase the probability that pregnancy will occur.

There are two main components of the menstrual cycle, the changes that happen in the ovaries in response to pituitary hormones, the ovarian cycle, and the variations that take place in the uterus, the uterine cycle. We will discuss each cycle separately, but it is important to remember that both cycles work together simultaneously to produce the menstrual cycle (Fig. 3-9). Changes in cervical mucus also take place during the course of the menstrual cycle; these changes are discussed below.

Ovarian Cycle

Cyclical changes in the ovaries occur in response to two anterior pituitary hormones: follicle-stimulating hormone (FSH) and luteinizing hormone (LH). Each of the two phases of the ovarian cycle is named for the hormone that has the most control over that particular phase. The follicular phase, controlled by FSH, encompasses days 1 to 14 of a 28-day cycle. LH controls the luteal phase, which includes days 15 to 28.

Follicular Phase. At the beginning of each menstrual cycle, a follicle on one of the ovaries begins to develop in response to rising levels of FSH. The follicle produces estrogen, which causes the ovum contained within the follicle to mature. As the follicle grows, it fills with estrogen-rich fluid and begins to resemble a tiny blister on the surface of the ovary.

When the pituitary gland detects high levels of estrogen from the mature follicle, it releases a surge of LH. This sudden increase in LH causes the follicle to burst open, releasing the mature ovum into the abdominal cavity, a process called **ovulation**. Ovulation occurs on day 14 of a 28-day cycle. As the ovum floats along the surface of the ovary, the gentle beating of the fimbriae draws it toward the fallopian tube.

Remember, all of the ova already exist within the ovaries; however, they are in an immature state. In order to ripen, or mature, an ovum needs a stimulus. FSH is the messenger from the pituitary that provides the required stimulus.

Luteal Phase. After ovulation, LH levels remain elevated and cause the remnants of the follicle to develop into a yellow body called the **corpus luteum**. In addition to producing estrogen, the corpus luteum secretes a hormone called progesterone. If fertilization does not take place, the corpus luteum begins to degenerate, and estrogen and progesterone levels fall. This process leads back to day 1 of the cycle, and the follicular phase begins anew.

Test Yourself

- Which hormone is responsible for ovulation?
- What is the main purpose of FSH?
- What structure produces progesterone?

Uterine Cycle

The uterine cycle refers to the changes that are found in the uterine lining of the uterus. These changes come about in response to the ovarian hormones estrogen and progesterone. There are four phases to this cycle: menstrual, proliferative, secretory, and ischemic.

Menstrual Phase. Day 1 of the menstrual cycle is marked by the onset of menstruation. During the menstrual phase of the uterine cycle, the uterine lining is

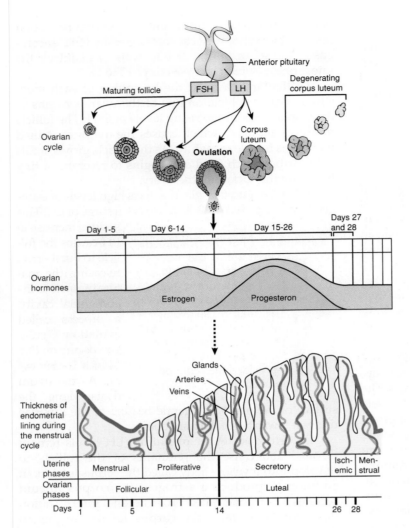

● *Figure 3.9* A 28-day (average) menstrual cycle. The anterior pituitary hormones control the ovarian cycle. The ovaries produce hormones that control the uterine cycle.

shed because of low levels of progesterone and estrogen. At the same time, a follicle is beginning to develop and starts producing estrogen. The menstrual phase ends when the menstrual period stops on approximately day 5.

Proliferative Phase. When estrogen levels are high enough, the endometrium begins to regenerate. Estrogen stimulates blood vessels to develop. The blood vessels in turn bring nutrients and oxygen to the uterine lining, and it begins to grow and become thicker. The proliferative phase ends with ovulation on day 14.

Secretory Phase. After ovulation, the corpus luteum begins to produce progesterone. This hormone causes the uterine lining to become rich in nutrients in preparation for pregnancy. Estrogen levels also remain high so that the lining is maintained. If pregnancy does not transpire, the corpus luteum gradually degenerates, and the woman enters the ischemic phase of the menstrual cycle.

Ischemic Phase. On days 27 and 28, estrogen and progesterone levels fall because the corpus luteum is no longer producing them. Without these hormones to maintain the blood vessel network, the uterine lining becomes ischemic. When the lining starts to slough, the woman has come full cycle and is once again at day 1 of the menstrual cycle.

Test Yourself

- What is the main function of estrogen during the menstrual cycle?

- Which hormone is active only during the secretory phase of the uterine cycle?

- What happens to the uterine lining during the ischemic phase?

- What causes the ischemic phase to occur?

Cervical Mucus Changes

Changes in cervical mucus take place over the course of the menstrual cycle. Some women use these characteristics to help determine when ovulation is likely to happen. During the menstrual phase the cervix does not produce mucus. Gradually, as hormonal changes transpire and the proliferative phase begins, the cervix begins to produce a tacky, crumbly type of mucus that is yellow or white. As the time of ovulation draws near, the mucus becomes progressively clear, thin, and lubricative, with the properties of raw egg white. At the peak of fertility (i.e., during ovulation), the mucus has a distensible, stretchable quality called spinnbarkheit (see Chapter 4 for further discussion of cervical mucus changes that indicate ovulation). After ovulation the mucus again becomes scanty, thick, and opaque.

Menopause

Menopause refers to the time in a woman's life when reproductive capability ends. Gradually the ovaries cease to function, and hormone levels fall. The woman begins to experience irregular menstrual cycles until finally they come to an end. The interlude surrounding menopause in which these changes take place is called the **climacteric**. The average age at which menopause occurs is between 47 and 55 years.

SEXUAL RESPONSE CYCLE

Sexuality is part of our human nature. We are sexual beings with sexual needs. Nature has provided us with the capacity to give and receive pleasure through the process of sexual stimulation. Therefore, a discussion of reproduction would be incomplete without mention of the physiology of sexual response.

There are two underlying physiologic responses to sexual stimulation in both men and women: vasocongestion and myotonia (muscular tension). These two processes are fundamental to almost all physiologic responses that take place during sexual arousal.

Vasocongestion occurs in the pelvic organs during sexual excitement because the arteries dilate, allowing inflow of blood that is greater than venous capacity to drain the area. The result is widespread congestion of the pelvic tissues. Vasocongestion leads to erection of the penis and clitoris, vaginal lubrication, and engorgement of the labia and testicles. Other tissue, such as the nipples and earlobes, may also be affected.

Myotonia is present throughout the body during sexual arousal and orgasm. It is evident in voluntary and involuntary contractions. Facial grimacing, spasmodic contractions of the hands and feet, and the involuntary muscular contractions during orgasm are the most notable examples of myotonia.

Four phases of the sexual response have been described: excitement, plateau, orgasm, and resolution. These phases occur in both sexes and follow the same general patterns regardless of the method of sexual stimulation.

During the excitement phase, the woman's clitoris becomes engorged and enlarged, the labia majora separate, and the labia minora increase in size. The uterus increases in size and begins to elevate. For the man, excitement leads to erection of the penis, thickening of the scrotal sac, and testicular elevation. In both sexes excitement is marked by an increase in heart rate, blood pressure, and respirations. Some individuals experience a "sex flush," reddening of the skin on the chest and neck. Duration of the excitement phase is from several minutes to several hours.

There is no set event that marks the beginning of the plateau phase. Vasocongestion and myotonia continue, and the heart rate and blood pressure remain elevated. For the female, the outer third of the vagina becomes engorged, the clitoris retracts behind its hood, and the labia minora deepen in color. The uterus is fully elevated in the pelvic cavity. The head of the penis in the male becomes further engorged, and the testes remain engorged and elevated. The plateau phase is typically a few seconds to several minutes in duration.

Orgasm, the climax of sexual response, is marked by a series of muscular contractions. The clitoris remains retracted behind the hood, and the outer third of the vagina, rectal sphincter, and uterus undergo rhythmic contractions. The male experiences contractions of the urethra, base of the penis, and rectal muscles, as well as emission and expulsion of semen.

During resolution, the muscles gradually relax and there is a reversal of vasocongestion. The heart rate, blood pressure, and breathing return to normal rates. The clitoris descends, and the labia and internal organs return to their prearoused positions and color. The male loses his erection, the testes descend, and the scrotum thins.

KEY POINTS

- Two major functions of the reproductive system are to produce offspring and to provide the experience of pleasure through physical intimacy.
- The testes and ovaries are responsible for the production of sex cells, or gametes.
- Male external genitalia include the penis and scrotum. The penis serves to eliminate urine from the bladder and functions to deposit sperm in the female reproductive tract for the purposes of reproduction. The scrotum regulates the temperature and protects the testes from trauma.

- The testes and ductal system compose the man's internal reproductive tract. Spermatogenesis occurs in the testes, and the ductal system serves as the exit route for sperm from the man's body.
- Sperm are formed in the seminiferous tubules and mature in the epididymis. During ejaculation, sperm travel from the epididymis through the paired vas deferens and ejaculatory ducts to the urethra and out of the body.
- Sperm need an alkaline environment and an energy source to be motile. The seminal vesicles (paired), prostate gland, and the bulbourethral glands (paired) contribute alkaline secretions to semen. The seminal vesicles also contribute fructose, an energy source for sperm.
- Testosterone, FSH, and interstitial cell-stimulating hormone (ICSH) are the male hormones responsible for production of sperm and the development of secondary sex characteristics.
- Female external genitalia, or vulva, includes the mons pubis, labia majora, labia minora, clitoris, urethral meatus, vaginal opening, and Bartholin glands. The vestibule is the area within the boundaries of the labia minora and includes the urethral meatus, vaginal opening, and Bartholin glands.
- The vagina is an internal reproductive organ that functions as the female organ for sexual intercourse, exit point for the menstrual flow, and as the birth canal. Rugae, or folds, allow for stretching during the birth process.
- The main divisions of the uterus are the cervix, isthmus, corpus, and fundus. The walls of the uterus have three layers: perimetrium (protective cover), myometrium (muscle), and endometrium (lining).
- The fallopian tubes lead from the uterus toward the ovaries. The isthmus is the narrow portion near the uterus. The ampulla is the middle portion, and the infundibulum is the outer portion close to the ovaries. Fimbriae on the infundibulum make wave-like motions over the ovary, a process that guides the ovum toward the fallopian tube.
- The ovaries are homologous to the male testes. The ovarian hormones, estrogen and progesterone, play a major role in the menstrual cycle and in the development of secondary sex characteristics in the female.
- The menstrual cycle begins with day 1, the start of menstrual flow. It encompasses the ovarian cycle and the uterine cycle. FSH and LH from the pituitary govern the ovarian cycle, and estrogen and progesterone from the ovaries guide the uterine cycle.
- The sexual response cycle is divided into four phases: excitement, plateau, orgasm, and resolution. Vasocongestion and myotonia are the primary physiologic processes that contribute to sexual response in both the male and female.

REFERENCES AND SELECTED READINGS

Books and Journals

Cunningham, F. G., Gant, N. F., Leveno, K. J., Gilstrap, L. C. III, Hauth, J. C., & Wenstrom, K. D. (2001). Anatomy of the reproductive tract. In *Williams obstetrics* (21st ed., pp. 31–61). New York: McGraw-Hill Medical Publishing Division.

Mattson, S., & Smith, J. E. (Eds.). (2000). *Core curriculum for maternal–newborn nursing*. AWHONN publication (2nd ed.). Philadelphia: WB Saunders.

Pillitteri, A. (1999). Reproductive and sexual health. In *Maternal & child health nursing: Care of the childbearing & childrearing family* (3rd ed., pp. 61–94). Philadelphia: Lippincott Williams & Wilkins.

Scanlon, V. C., & Sanders, T. (1999). *Essentials of anatomy and physiology* (3rd ed.). Philadelphia: F.A. Davis.

Websites
Male
http://www.healthac.org/male.html
http://www.nlm.nih.gov/medlineplus/ency/imagepages/1113.htm
Female
http://www.nlm.nih.gov/medlineplus/ency/imagepages/1112.htm
Menstrual Cycle
http://www.people.virginia.edu/~rjh9u/menscyc3.html
http://anatomy.med.unsw.edu.au/cbl/embryo/wwwhuman/MCycle/MCycle.htm
http://www.abington-repromed.com/cycle.html

WORKBOOK

NCLEX-STYLE REVIEW QUESTIONS

1. You are teaching a male client about the male reproductive system. You ask him which gland provides the sugar that gives the sperm energy to move. Which answer indicates that he correctly understands your teaching?

   a. Bartholin gland

   b. Bulbourethral gland

   c. Epididymis

   d Seminal vesicles

2. The vagina is a hostile environment for sperm. What characteristic of semen protects sperm from the vaginal environment?

   a. Acidic fluid

   b. Alkaline fluid

   c. Presence of testosterone

   d. Secretions from seminiferous tubules

3. You are preparing to perform a urinary catheterization on a female client. In which location will you expect to find the urinary meatus?

   a. Above the clitoris

   b. Below the vaginal opening

   c. On the true perineum

   d Within the vestibule

4. You are caring for a woman in labor. The doctor is concerned that the uterus might rupture. Which part of the uterus requires the closest assessment because it is the thinnest part of the uterus?

   a. Corpus

   b. Fundus

   c. Inner cervical os

   d. Lower uterine segment

5. Which ovarian hormone predominates during the proliferative phase of the uterine cycle?

   a. FSH

   b. LH

   c. Estrogen

   d. Progesterone

STUDY ACTIVITIES

1. In each row of the table you will find either a male or a female reproductive organ listed. In the column that is missing information, fill in the name of the homologous reproductive organ.

Male Reproductive Organ	Female Reproductive Organ
Glans penis	
	Round ligaments
	Ovaries
Foreskin or prepuce	

2. Go to the following Internet site: http://www-medlib.med.utah.edu/WebPath/webpath.html

   a. Click on "Systemic Pathology"

   b. Click on "Female Genital Tract Pathology"

   c. Look for pictures of a normal uterus, fallopian tubes, ovaries, and cervix.

3. Explain the step-by-step procedure for testicular self-examination. List important points to be covered when teaching TSE and why each step is important.

4. In your clinical group, have a discussion as to why it is important for a nurse to understand the menstrual cycle.

CRITICAL THINKING: What Would You Do?

Apply your knowledge of reproductive anatomy and physiology to the following situation.

1. Doug and Nancy, a young married couple, ages 26 and 22 years, respectively, have not been using any contraception for the past year, but Nancy has not become pregnant. Doug is a rancher and dresses in cowboy gear, including tight jeans. He works in a hot, humid environment for 10 to 12 hours almost every day.

   a. Using your knowledge about male reproductive anatomy, what is one possible reason pregnancy has not occurred?

   b. What advice might be helpful for Doug to increase the likelihood that pregnancy will occur?

2. Nancy complains of frequent vaginal infections. During an office interview, Nancy tells you that she douches at least once per week.

   a. What other questions should you ask regarding Nancy's hygiene habits?

   b. What advice might be helpful for Nancy to decrease her risk for vaginal infections?

Special Issues of Reproduction and Women's Health Care

WOMEN'S HEALTH ISSUES
Health Screening for Women
  Breast Cancer Screening
  Pelvic Examination and Pap Smear
  Vulvar Self-Examination
Common Disorders of the Female
  Reproductive Tract
  Menstrual Disturbances
  Infectious Disorders
  Disorders of the Uterus and Ovaries
  Pelvic Support Disorders
REPRODUCTIVE LIFE CYCLE ISSUES
Family Planning
  Planning Pregnancy
  Preventing Pregnancy
Nursing Process for Assisting the
  Couple to Choose a Contraceptive
  Method
  Assessment

Selected Nursing Diagnoses
Outcome Identification and
  Planning
Implementation
Evaluation: Goals and Expected
  Outcomes
Induced Abortion
Infertility
  Causes of Infertility
  Initial Evaluation of Infertility
  Comprehensive Evaluation and
    Diagnostic Testing
  Management of Infertility
  Psychological Aspects of Infertility
  Nursing Care
Menopause
  Clinical Manifestations
  Treatment
  Nursing Care

STUDENT OBJECTIVES

On completion of this chapter, the student should be able to

1. Describe recommendations for health screening for women.
2. Differentiate between dysmenorrhea and premenstrual syndrome (PMS).
3. Explain the clinical manifestations, treatment, and nursing care for endometriosis.
4. Discuss risk factors for pelvic inflammatory disease (PID).
5. Explain causes and risk factors for pelvic support disorders.
6. Discuss the significance of family planning.
7. Compare and contrast methods of contraception.
8. Explain advantages and disadvantages for each method of contraception.
9. List possible causes for fertility problems.
10. Identify diagnostic testing used related to fertility problems.
11. Discuss treatment options available for fertility problems.
12. Discuss the psychosocial sequelae related to fertility problems.
13. Identify major considerations for the perimenopausal and postmenopausal woman.

KEY TERMS

abstinence
amenorrhea
coitus interruptus
dysmenorrhea
dyspareunia
elective abortion
endometriosis
gestational surrogate
induced abortion
infertility
menorrhagia
metrorrhagia
perimenopause
postcoital test
spinnbarkeit
therapeutic abortion

The focus of this chapter is to examine issues related to women's health and reproduction. Women's health issues include preventive health care, menstrual disorders, pelvic infections, disorders of the uterus and ovaries, and pelvic support disorders. Issues related to the reproductive life cycle include family planning and contraception, elective termination of pregnancy, infertility, and menopause. Friends and family members often turn to the nurse as a resource for questions about women's health issues, becoming pregnant, contraception, or infertility. Therefore, the nurse's role in women's health and reproductive life cycle issues also is discussed.

Several Healthy People 2010 goals relate to the topics in this chapter. Selected goals include

- Reducing breast and cervical cancer deaths by increasing the number of females who comply with screening recommendations.
- Increasing the proportion of pregnancies that are intended from 51% to 70%.
- Promoting responsible sexual behaviors, strengthening community capacity, and increasing access to quality services to prevent sexually transmitted infections (STIs) and their complications. *Same as STD*
- Reducing the proportion of adults aged 50 years and older with osteoporosis from 10% to 8%.

WOMEN'S HEALTH ISSUES

Women's health issues encompass a broad variety of topics. Current research is highlighting the unique needs of women in relation to medical–surgical conditions, such as diabetes, heart disease, and stroke. Although these topics are critical to the overall health of women, this chapter focuses on conditions that occur universally, or near universally, in women.

HEALTH SCREENING FOR WOMEN

Health promotion is a broad concept that involves educating and assisting individuals to make behavior and lifestyle modifications for the prevention or early detection and treatment of disease. Because nurses are trusted health care professionals, individuals and families often turn to them for information and advice on health-related matters. As a result, health promotion for women is an area in which the nurse can have great influence.

Health screening is a component of a comprehensive health promotion plan. Screening tests do not diagnose disease. Instead, a positive result indicates the need for more thorough testing. The following discussion encompasses screening procedures that pro-

mote the early detection of disorders that are unique to, or occur commonly in, women.

Breast Cancer Screening

Breast cancer is the second most commonly diagnosed malignancy in women in the Western world.[1] Each year in the United States there are more than 200,000 new cases diagnosed and more than 40,000 deaths caused by breast cancer (American Cancer Society, 2004). A palpable mass is the most common "first" sign or symptom associated with breast disease. Recommended screening for early identification of breast cancer consists of a three-pronged approach: breast self-awareness, clinical breast examination, and mammography. Detection of breast cancer before axillary node involvement increases the chance for survival. It is the role of the nurse to educate women regarding the importance of each screening test and recommended techniques for breast self-examination.

The American Cancer Society (ACS) recommends that women get regular screening to detect signs of breast cancer in the very early stages, if possible. The recommendations vary according to age. The woman in her 20s and 30s should have a clinical breast examination at least every 3 years. When the woman reaches 40 years of age, she should schedule a yearly clinical breast examination, and she should have a yearly mammogram. Breast self-examination (BSE) is a self-scheduled, step-by-step approach the woman uses to check her breasts. In the past it was recommended that BSE be performed on a monthly basis. The ACS now presents BSE as optional because current research indicates that performing BSE does not decrease mortality associated with breast cancer. However, the ACS recommends that each woman know how her breasts normally look and feel, and if changes are found, to immediately report them to a physician. (Refer to Chapter 3, Box 3-2 for instructions on how BSE is done.)

Mammography is a screening tool that uses very–low-dose x-ray for examination of breast tissue. Mammography is useful in the early detection of cancer because it can detect a breast tumor 2 years before the woman or the primary care provider can palpate it. The ACS recommends yearly mammograms for women older than 40 years.

For this procedure the breast is placed on a platform and then compressed firmly between the platform and a plastic paddle (Fig. 4-1). Routine views include a top-to-bottom and a side view. The compression can be uncomfortable for some women. It is usually recommended to schedule the examination for the week after the menstrual period, when the breasts are less tender, to minimize discomfort.

---

[1] Nonmelanoma skin cancers are the most common type of cancer found in women.

● *Figure 4.1* Mammography. (**A**) Mammography equipment. (**B**) A top-to-bottom view of the breast. (**C**) A side view of the breast.

Pelvic Examination and Pap Smear

Every woman should have a yearly physical examination. A pelvic examination should be part of the total physical examination. A pelvic examination is done to detect changes associated with certain gynecologic conditions, such as infection, inflammation, pelvic pain, cancer, and other disorders. The Papanicolaou test (Pap smear) may be done in conjunction with the pelvic examination.

The pelvic examination begins with the woman in lithotomy position. The structures of the vulva are visualized and palpated. Then a speculum is inserted to visualize the walls of the vagina and the cervix. When the cervix is clearly visible, the primary care provider swabs the cervix. Secretions can be cultured to diagnose pelvic infection. Cell samples are obtained for the Pap smear. A bimanual examination follows the speculum examination. The practitioner inserts two lubricated fingers into the vagina with one hand and uses the other hand to palpate uterine and ovarian structures through the abdominal wall. A rectal examination to test for fecal occult blood and/or to palpate the rectovaginal wall is usually done at the end of the examination.

The Pap smear is an important screening tool for cervical cancer. In fact, the incidence of cervical cancer has decreased by 50% since practitioners began to routinely perform Pap smears in the 1970s (Katz, 2003) because precancerous changes are caught early and promptly treated. The American College of Obstetricians and Gynecologists' (ACOG's) newly revised guidelines recommend that the initial Pap smear be done approximately 3 years after the woman first has sexual intercourse or by 21 years of age, whichever comes first. Subsequent Pap smears should occur annually in women younger than 30 years of age. Healthy women age 30 and older may require a Pap smear only every 2 to 3 years. The woman who has the human immunodeficiency virus (HIV) or is otherwise immunocompromised, and the woman who was exposed to diethylstilbestrol (DES) in utero should continue to have annual Pap smears. ACOG continues to recommend annual pelvic examinations for all women, even when a Pap smear is not required.

Vulvar Self-Examination

Some primary care practitioners recommend that women older than 18 years (and those younger who are sexually active) should perform a monthly self-examination of the external genitalia. As with BSE, the major value of the monthly vulvar self-examination is that the woman will become familiar with her own normal anatomy. Using a hand mirror and an adequate light source, the woman should inspect her vulva for any lesions, growths, reddened areas, unusual discharge, or changes in skin color. Any changes in sensation, such as itching or pain, should also be noted. The woman should be cautioned that, although most changes are not cancerous, all changes should be reported to her primary care practitioner for evaluation.

COMMON DISORDERS OF THE FEMALE REPRODUCTIVE TRACT

There are several female reproductive tract disorders that occur commonly. Many involve disorders of menstruation. Others are related to or caused by infections or decreased support of the pelvic floor.

Menstrual Disturbances

Disturbances of the menstrual cycle may be related to increased or decreased frequency, and absent, excessive, or irregular bleeding. Pain may also be part of the symptomatology. Nursing intervention will depend on the cause and treatment of the disorder but may include providing information about recommended treatments or prescribed medications, caring for the woman before and after a procedure, and providing emotional support and reassurance.

Amenorrhea

Amenorrhea refers to the absence of menstruation. A 16-year-old girl, who is developing normally and yet does not experience menarche (the first menstrual period), is said to have *primary amenorrhea. Secondary amenorrhea* is defined as cessation of menstrual periods after they have occurred previously.

The presence of regular menstrual periods is a sign of health. Regular menses signal that the pituitary and ovarian connection are working together properly and that appropriate amounts of sex hormones are present.

Because pregnancy is the most common cause of amenorrhea in women of reproductive age, a pregnancy test is often the first test performed when a woman presents with this symptom. Once pregnancy is ruled out as a cause, a thorough review of systems is indicated.

Endocrine symptoms, such as hot flashes, night sweats, and vaginal dryness, associated with amenorrhea often indicate ovarian dysfunction. There are many factors that can cause the ovaries to stop working prematurely. These include history of radiation therapy or chemotherapy to treat cancer and unknown causes. Systemic symptoms may indicate disorders of the hypothalamus and pituitary. Factors that can interfere with normal hypothalamic function include excessive exercise; endocrine disorders, such as hyper- or hypothyroidism; human immunodeficiency virus/acquired immunodeficiency syndrome (HIV/AIDS); malnutrition; and major psychiatric disorders.

If there are no associated endocrine symptoms, the problem may be in the outflow tract. The ovaries may be functioning normally, but the endometrium may be scarred by adhesions (Asherman syndrome), so it does not respond to ovarian stimulation. Imperforate hymen or underdevelopment of the lower reproductive tract does not allow the menstrual flow to escape.

Medical intervention is based on a thorough assessment by physical examination, history taking, and laboratory testing to identify the underlying cause. Specific treatment is related to the underlying cause.

Atypical Uterine Bleeding

There are several types of atypical (abnormal) uterine bleeding. Heavy or prolonged bleeding, **menorrhagia**, is the most common menstrual complaint and can lead to anemia, if left untreated. **Metrorrhagia** refers to menstrual bleeding that is normal in amount but occurs at irregular intervals between menstrual periods. Metrorrhagia that occurs with hormonal contraceptives is called break-through bleeding. This type of bleeding frequently decreases over time.

Many of the factors that contribute to amenorrhea can also cause menorrhagia, including ovarian dysfunction. A thorough history and physical are indicated to rule out systemic causes. Other uterine conditions, such as polyps and fibroids, can cause menorrhagia. When causative factors cannot be found, a trial of oral progestin therapy may be initiated. If this therapy does not work, the primary care practitioner might insert an intrauterine device that releases progestin into the uterine cavity. The advantage of this therapy is that the hormones are released directly into the uterine cavity, so systemic levels remain low. Another therapy that may be used if traditional measures do not work is endometrial ablation, removal of the uterine lining. Hysterectomy, surgical removal of the uterus, remains a treatment option when other measures have failed.

This is worth noting. Pregnancy is the most common cause of abnormal bleeding during the reproductive years. Bear in mind that any woman of childbearing age who presents with atypical or irregular bleeding may be pregnant.

Dysmenorrhea

Dysmenorrhea is defined as painful or difficult menses. Primary dysmenorrhea refers to painful menstrual periods that cannot be attributed to a disease process. Secondary dysmenorrhea is painful menses secondary to pelvic pathology. This discussion focuses on primary dysmenorrhea, which is the more common of the two conditions. Secondary dysmenorrhea is discussed in conjunction with other disease states with which it occurs.

Don't get confused. Primary dysmenorrhea is not the same thing as premenstrual syndrome (PMS). A woman can have both conditions, but they are separate entities.

Primary dysmenorrhea is attributed to the action of prostaglandins on the uterus during ovulatory cycles. Prostaglandins contribute to dysmenorrhea in two ways. They cause the uterus to contract, which leads to painful cramping; and they decrease blood flow to the myometrium, which contributes to lactic acid buildup and additional pain.

Primary dysmenorrhea affects as many as 50% of women during their childbearing years (Alzubaidi, Calis, & Nelson, 2003). It occurs at a higher rate in younger women who have not borne children. As age and parity increase, the incidence of primary dysmenorrhea decreases. Risk factors that increase the severity of symptoms include earlier age at menarche, long and/or heavy menstrual flow, smoking, and a family history of the condition.

Clinical Manifestations

Primary dysmenorrhea typically begins within 6 months to 2 years after menarche. Severe intermittent cramping in association with constant pain in the lower abdomen, which may radiate to the lower back or upper thighs, is descriptive of the major symptoms. General malaise, fatigue, dizziness, nausea and vomiting, diarrhea, and headache frequently accompany the spasmodic cramping. Symptoms usually begin shortly before or with the onset of menstrual flow.

The primary care provider must rule out secondary dysmenorrhea before treatment can be initiated. A thorough history and physical and a pelvic examination are done, along with a variety of diagnostic procedures, to identify any underlying causes. If a causative factor is found, treatment is initiated to cure the underlying condition or control its symptoms. When no secondary cause is found, primary dysmenorrhea is diagnosed.

Treatment

The most effective treatments to date have been nonsteroidal anti-inflammatory drugs (NSAIDs) and oral contraceptives (birth control pills), given alone or in combination. NSAIDs, such as ibuprofen, naproxen, and meclofenamate, reduce symptoms by lowering prostaglandin levels and intrauterine pressure. NSAIDs are most effective when taken around the clock as soon as menstrual flow begins. They are less effective when taken on an as-needed basis. Gastrointestinal distress is the most common side effect.

Oral contraceptives relieve symptoms by inhibiting ovulation, which thins the endometrial lining and decreases prostaglandin production. Sometimes NSAIDs must be taken together with oral contraceptives to obtain adequate symptom control.

Alternative therapies that sometimes decrease dysmenorrhea include relaxation and massage, yoga, acupuncture, and herbal or homeopathic remedies.

Nursing Care

Nursing care of the woman with primary dysmenorrhea is directed toward education regarding the condition and its treatment and toward the effective relief of pain. Explain medication actions, common side effects, measures to reduce side effects, and timing of administration. Reassure the woman that sometimes medications have to be switched several times before the best therapy for her symptoms is determined. Reinforce that she should take her NSAIDs on a schedule, rather than waiting until the pain begins or becomes severe.

Several nonmedication interventions can help relieve the pain associated with dysmenorrhea. Heat can be soothing. Suggest the use of hot baths or heating pads. Sometimes changing positions can be helpful. Some women report relief when they assume a knee-chest position. Pain is usually less severe when the woman is in good general health. Encourage adequate exercise, diet, rest, and hygiene.

Test Yourself

- Define amenorrhea.
- What is the medical term for irregular menstrual flow?
- What is the difference between primary and secondary dysmenorrhea?

Premenstrual Syndrome

It is estimated that about 60% of all women experience premenstrual syndrome (PMS). PMS is characterized by physical and behavioral symptoms that occur cyclically during the last half of the menstrual cycle. Most likely to affect women in their 30s, it can occur as early as adolescence or as late as in the perimenopausal years.

Premenstrual dysphoric disorder (PMDD) is a more severe form of PMS. PMDD includes all of the physical symptoms of PMS with additional and more debilitating emotional symptoms. Approximately 5% of menstruating women are thought to experience PMDD.

Clinical Manifestations

PMS presents with a wide variety of symptoms, which may be physical, behavioral, or both (see Box 4-1). The symptoms can be highly distressing for the woman and her family. In making a diagnosis of PMS, the crucial component is the cyclical nature of the symptoms, as indicated in the following diagnostic criteria:

- Signs/symptoms must occur during the last half of the menstrual cycle.
- The woman should be asymptomatic before ovulation, and there must be at least 7 symptom-free days in each cycle.

BOX 4.1	Signs and Symptoms of Premenstrual Syndrome (PMS)

Physical Symptoms
- Edema
- Weight gain
- Abdominal bloating
- Abdominal cramping
- Constipation
- Hot flashes
- Breast swelling and pain
- Headache, migraine
- Acne
- Rhinitis
- Exacerbation of pre-existing conditions (e.g., arthritis, lupus, ulcers)
- Heart palpitations
- Hives
- Joint swelling and pain
- Sore throat
- Urinary difficulties
- Seizures
- Asthma
- Bruising
- Coordination difficulties
- Back pain
- Fainting
- Nausea
- Alcohol intolerance

Behavioral Symptoms
- Aggressive behavior
- Emotional lability
- Confusion
- Depression
- Increased appetite
- Food cravings (salt, sweet) and binges
- Fatigue, lethargy
- Poor concentration
- Sex drive changes
- Suicidal thoughts
- Withdrawal from others
- Anxiety
- Rage
- Sleeplessness

- Symptoms reported must be severe enough to affect relationships, work, and daily lifestyle.
- Diagnosis must be made based on symptoms charted as they occur, rather than depending on recall of past experiences. PMS diaries are used for this purpose.

Typically, the severity of symptoms progresses over time. In the early stages of PMS, women describe symptoms beginning a few days before their period that stop when bleeding begins. With time, symptoms begin to appear 1 to 2 weeks before the onset of menses. Some women describe a cluster of symptoms occurring at the time of ovulation, followed by a symptom-free week, then a recurrence of symptoms a week before menses. PMS should not be equated with dysmenorrhea. Many women with symptoms of PMS have pain-free periods.

Treatment

The cause of PMS remains unknown and is considered to be multifactorial, rather than arising from a single "cause." Pregnancy and menopause are the only true cures for PMS. Treatment is focused on alleviating the specific signs and symptoms. Vitamin B_6, calcium, and magnesium supplementation have been shown to be beneficial in some studies. Hormonal suppression of ovulation can be helpful, but side effects limit their long-term usefulness. Mild diuretics may reduce bloating. NSAIDs have been shown to relieve PMS symptoms. Naproxen sodium 500 mg/day is particularly beneficial. Antianxiety medications and stress-reduction techniques may also be prescribed.

PMDD responds to treatments similar to those used for PMS. In addition, low-dose antidepressant therapy during the last half of the cycle has been effective in treating the severe mood swings and other emotional problems that interfere with work productivity and social relationships.

Nursing Care

Assist the woman to find ways to decrease stress. Encourage regular exercise, even when she is experiencing symptoms. Exercise has been shown to decrease symptom severity. Encourage the reduction or elimination of caffeine and alcohol. Explain that limiting salt intake can decrease the symptoms of bloating. Family Teaching Tips: Relief Measures for PMS describes additional relief measures the nurse may recommend for the woman with PMS.

Endometriosis

Endometriosis is a painful reproductive and immunologic disorder in which tissue implants resembling endometrium grow outside of the uterus. The tissue implants respond to cyclic hormonal changes in a manner similar to that of endometrial tissue, causing menstrual-like internal bleeding that leads to inflammation,

FAMILY TEACHING TIPS

Relief Measures for PMS

DIET

- Reduce (or eliminate) caffeine intake (including coffee, tea, colas, and chocolate).
- Avoid simple sugars (as in candy, cakes, cookies).
- Reduce salt intake (pickles, fast foods, chips).
- Avoid alcohol.
- Drink 2 quarts of noncaffeinated fluid, preferably water, each day.
- Eat six small meals (to stabilize blood glucose levels).

EXERCISE

- Do aerobic exercise, such as walking or jogging, several times each week.

STRESS MANAGEMENT

- Note your pattern of PMS symptoms and alter your schedule to minimize stressors when symptoms are most severe.
- Utilize interventions such as relaxation techniques, massage, and warm baths.

SLEEP AND REST

- Maintain a regular sleep schedule.
- Drink a glass of milk before bedtime.
- Schedule exercise for early morning or early afternoon.
- Give yourself a quiet time to relax just before going to bed.

scarring, and adhesions in the pelvic and abdominal cavities. The condition occurs in 7% to 10% of women and is a leading cause of infertility and chronic pelvic pain. As many as 50% of the hysterectomies performed in the United States are done in an attempt to treat this debilitating disease.

Clinical Manifestations

Some women with advanced endometriosis are essentially asymptomatic and are unaware of the disease until the condition is observed during abdominal or pelvic surgery. Other women may experience debilitating, almost continuous pelvic pain, with only minimal abnormal tissue growth. Symptoms are typically most pronounced right before the onset of the period.

Cyclic pelvic pain that occurs in conjunction with menses is a classic symptom, as is menorrhagia. The pain and bleeding can involve the bladder, leading to hematuria, or can affect the bowel, leading to blood in the stools and painful defecation. Chronic pelvic pain, dysmenorrhea, and **dyspareunia**, painful intercourse, are

other common symptoms. Although endometriosis appears to play a role in infertility for some women, others experience no apparent difficulty with conception.

Physical examination reveals pelvic tenderness, particularly during menses. Laparoscopy is the primary diagnostic tool for endometriosis. Advantages are that the characteristic endometrial lesions can be directly visualized and biopsies taken. Disadvantages include that laparoscopy is an invasive surgical technique.

Treatment

Medical therapy is aimed at suppressing ovulation and inducing an artificial menopause, with resulting suppression of abnormal tissue and relief of pain and other associated symptoms. This objective can be accomplished through the use of oral contraceptives; gonadotropin-releasing hormone (GnRH) agonists, such as goserelin and leuprolide; or danazol, a synthetic steroid analog (androgen) that inhibits luteinizing hormone (LH) and follicle-stimulating hormone (FSH). Side effects include symptoms associated with menopause, such as labile emotions, hot flashes, and vaginal dryness.

Surgical intervention can be conservative (reproductive function is maintained), semiconservative (destroys reproductive function, but maintains ovarian function), or radical, which involves removal of the uterus and ovaries. The goal of conservative surgery is to destroy the abnormal tissue while preserving reproductive ability. Laser or electrodiathermy techniques are used to ablate (destroy) the lesions.

Nursing Care

Pain is a common nursing diagnosis for the woman with endometriosis. Evaluate the character and severity of pain. Assist the woman to find ways to cope with and decrease pain. Encourage the use of analgesics, as ordered.

Provide emotional support. Allow the woman to ventilate. She may particularly have this need if the endometriosis is causing infertility problems. Encourage the woman to ask questions. Assist the woman and her family to make treatment decisions by providing information regarding treatment options to include advantages, disadvantages, possible risks, and likely outcomes of each option.

Infectious Disorders

Infections of the reproductive tract can cause permanent damage, such as infertility and chronic pelvic pain. Organisms that are transmitted sexually cause many of these infections. Sexually transmitted infections (STIs) are discussed in the pediatric portion of the text and in Chapters 16 and 40. Toxic shock syndrome (TSS) and pelvic inflammatory disease (PID) are covered in this section.

Toxic Shock Syndrome

Toxic shock syndrome (TSS) is a rare illness caused by an exotoxin produced by the bacteria *Staphylococcus aureus*. TSS was first recognized in 1978; the majority of cases occurred in women who were using certain types of high-absorbency tampons. Shortly thereafter, changes were made to the composition and absorbency of tampons, and TSS cases declined dramatically. However, women who use tampons, diaphragms, or contraceptive sponges are still at risk for the illness.

TSS starts suddenly with a high fever (greater than 102°F), nausea, vomiting, abdominal pain, a rapid drop in blood pressure, watery diarrhea, headache, sore throat, and muscle aches. Within 24 hours, a sunburn-like rash develops. The mucous membranes may turn a deep red. Treatment requires hospitalization, often in an intensive care setting, intravenous (IV) fluids, and antibiotics.

Nurses can be helpful in the prevention of TSS. Teach the woman who uses tampons to wash her hands thoroughly before and after inserting or removing tampons. She should use the lowest absorbency that will handle her menstrual flow, change tampons frequently (at least every 2 to 3 hours), or alternate tampons with sanitary napkins. Between periods, tampons should be stored away from heat and moisture, to help prevent bacterial growth. Any vaginal device, such as a diaphragm or vaginal sponge, should be removed frequently and cleaned.

Pelvic Inflammatory Disease

Pelvic inflammatory disease (PID) is a broad term used to refer to inflammation of any portion of a woman's reproductive tract, such as uterus, fallopian tubes, or ovaries. PID occurs most commonly in association with untreated STIs, in particular gonorrhea and chlamydia. Untreated PID can lead to scarring, ectopic (tubal) pregnancy, and chronic pelvic pain. Peritonitis and sepsis are other life-threatening complications. Each year in the United States more than 1 million women will have an acute episode of PID. Rates are highest for adolescent girls who have multiple sexual partners and do not use condoms.

Clinical Manifestations

Major symptoms include lower abdominal pain and abnormal vaginal discharge. Other symptoms include chills, fever, vomiting, dyspareunia, menorrhagia, dysmenorrhea, fatigue, loss of appetite, backache, and painful or frequent urination. Some women are asymptomatic but can still experience permanent damage.

Diagnosis is made by history and physical to include a pelvic examination. Generally specimens are collected and cultured for STIs. Other tests that may be ordered include ultrasound, endometrial biopsy, or laparoscopy.

Treatment

Often the exact organism cannot be cultured, so primary care practitioners prescribe at least two wide-spectrum antibiotics. Sometimes two courses of antibiotics are necessary. Approximately 75% of cases of PID can be treated on an outpatient basis. Occasionally, the woman must be hospitalized for the administration of IV antibiotics. Sex partners of the woman with PID must also be treated with antibiotics, even if they have no symptoms.

Nursing Care

Patient teaching is an important nursing function for the woman with PID. Discuss the transmission, treatment, and prevention of infection. Encourage the woman to take all of her antibiotics, even after she starts to feel better. Explain the use of any pain medications that are prescribed. Explain how important it is for her partner to be treated, as well. Instruct the woman to avoid sexual intercourse until the full course of antibiotics has been taken and her partner has been treated.

Instruct her on ways to prevent STIs and PID in the future because the more frequently she experiences these infections, the more likely the infection will lead to scarring and infertility. The best way to prevent PID is to avoid sexual intercourse or to remain in a monogamous relationship—in which both partners are sexually faithful to the other. The next best way is for the woman's partner to use latex condoms for every act of sexual intercourse. Diaphragms and other barrier methods afford some protection but are not as reliable as condoms. Douching should be avoided because it can force bacteria into the reproductive tract.

Disorders of the Uterus and Ovaries

Cervical Polyps

Cervical polyps are benign tumors that hang on a stem-like pedicle and protrude through the cervical os. Cervical polyps are associated with infection and chronic inflammation. Postcoital (after intercourse) bleeding, metrorrhagia, menorrhagia, and leukorrhea (white or yellow vaginal discharge) are associated symptoms. Cervical polyps can be visualized during a speculum examination of the cervix and may be removed during the procedure. Tissue is sent to pathology for microscopic examination. Antibiotics are usually prescribed prophylactically after the polyps are removed.

Uterine Fibroids

Uterine leiomyomata, or fibroids, as they are commonly called, are benign estrogen-responsive tumors of the uterine wall that regress with menopause. Many are asymptomatic; however, the tumors can enlarge and cause pelvic pressure, pain, and menstrual irregularities. Diagnosis is made via transvaginal or abdominal ultrasound, hysterosalpingogram (injection of dye into the uterine cavity through a cannula in the cervix, followed by x-ray), or hysteroscopy (insertion of a scope through the cervical canal into the uterine cavity).

Therapy depends on the symptoms and whether or not the woman wishes to retain fertility. Because estrogen and progesterone stimulate fibroid growth, hormonal contraceptives are not recommended for treatment. The presence of uterine fibroids is the most common reason cited for hysterectomy and may be the treatment of choice if future pregnancy is not desired. A less radical procedure, myomectomy, can be done via a hysteroscopic procedure. Laparoscopy can also be used to remove multiple fibroids. Myomectomy and laparoscopy can preserve fertility in some patients. A newer procedure, uterine fibroid embolization, also known as uterine artery embolization, uses a technique similar to heart catheterization to introduce a catheter into the uterine artery and then inject a substance that flows to the arteries supplying the fibroids and blocks them. The fibroids shrink after the procedure because of decreased blood supply.

Ovarian Cysts

Two types of functional ovarian cysts can develop: follicular and luteal. The type is dependent upon when in the menstrual cycle the cyst develops. Most ovarian cysts develop during the childbearing years; however, cysts are possible at any time in the female life cycle.

Ovarian cysts are usually benign but can lead to complications, such as hemorrhage (which can be life threatening), ovarian torsion (twisting), inflammation, necrosis, and bacterial infection leading to septic shock. Pelvic adhesions, infertility, and chronic pelvic pain syndrome are chronic complications that can occur. Transvaginal and abdominal ultrasound done simultaneously is the most effective method for diagnosing an ovarian cyst. Laparoscopy allows for diagnosis and removal of cysts. Medical therapy is accomplished with oral contraceptives, which regulate the menstrual cycle and may cause regression of a cyst or prevention of additional cyst formation.

Pelvic Support Disorders

The pelvic organs are held in place by three types of support: endopelvic fascia, ligaments, and paired muscle groups of the pelvic floor. These support structures function like a hammock to support the urethra, bladder, small intestine, rectum, uterus, and vagina. Problems occur when these support structures relax or weaken, causing the organs to drop down or protrude through the vaginal wall.

Pelvic support disorders are named according to the affected organ:

- Cystocele occurs when the bladder bulges into the front wall of the vagina.
- Rectocele occurs when the rectum protrudes into the back wall of the vagina.
- Enterocele occurs when the small intestine and peritoneum jut downward between the uterus and rectum.
- Uterine prolapse occurs when the uterus drops down into the vagina.

Figure 4-2 illustrates pelvic support disorders.

The most common causes of pelvic support disorders are pregnancy, vaginal birth, and aging. Some medical experts think cesarean birth may be protective against pelvic support disorders, although this theory is controversial. Other causes include obesity, chronic coughing, frequent straining during bowel movements, heavy lifting, hysterectomy, nerve disorders, injuries, and tumors.

Clinical Manifestations

Pelvic support disorders are basically hernias in which organs prolapse (abnormally protrude) through the weakened tissues of the support structure. Common symptoms are a feeling of heaviness or pressure in the vaginal area, or a feeling that something is dropping out of the vagina. Symptoms tend to occur when the woman is upright and may be relieved when she is in the recumbent position. Dyspareunia is sometimes present. In mild cases, the woman may be asymptomatic. Some symptoms are specific to a certain type of prolapse. A cystocele may lead to urinary incontinence, whereas a rectocele may cause constipation.

Diagnosis of pelvic floor disorders is usually made during a pelvic examination. The primary care practitioner may ask the woman to cough or bear down during the examination. The woman may also be examined while standing. Other tests may be done to test bladder or bowel functioning.

Treatment

Treatment is based on the type of pelvic floor dysfunction, the severity of the dysfunction, and symptoms the woman is experiencing. For mild cases that are asymptomatic, no treatment may be necessary. Often, when treatment is recommended, it is helpful to start with less invasive techniques and then progress to more invasive techniques, as needed.

Kegel exercises can be done to strengthen pelvic floor muscles and improve tone. A pessary is a device that comes in various sizes and shapes that can be inserted into the vagina to hold pelvic organs in place. It must be fitted by the primary care practitioner and taken out periodically by the woman to be cleaned with soap and water and then reinserted.

Surgical techniques are often necessary to treat pelvic support disorders. Hysterectomy may be done

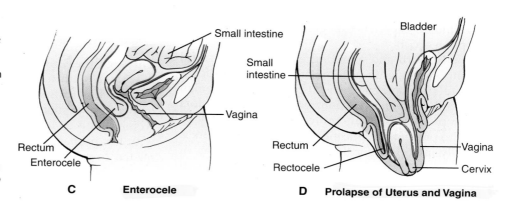

● **Figure 4.2** Pelvic support disorders. (**A**) Normal pelvic anatomy. (**B**) A cystocele occurs when the bladder bulges into the anterior vaginal wall. A rectocele develops when the muscles of the posterior vaginal wall weaken and the rectum and posterior vaginal wall protrude into the vagina. (**C**) An enterocele occurs when the small intestine and peritoneum protrude between the uterus and rectum into the posterior vaginal wall. (**D**) Prolapse of the uterus occurs when the uterus drops down into the vagina.

for uterine prolapse. During hysterectomy, other pelvic support disorders may also be repaired.

Nursing Care

Teach the woman to do Kegel exercises regularly. The muscles used to stop the stream of urine are tightly squeezed and held tightly while the woman counts to 10. The exercise is repeated 10 to 20 times in a row several times per day. A woman can perform Kegel exercises discreetly wherever she happens to be. They can be performed while sitting, standing, or lying down.

Teach the woman to recognize signs of urinary tract infection (UTI): pain or burning upon urination, urinary frequency and urgency, and cloudy urine. The woman with a cystocele is at higher risk for UTI. Other measures to prevent infection are to drink plenty of fluids, including fruit juices, to wipe from front to back after using the bathroom, and to get enough rest.

Test Yourself

- Name five symptoms of PMS.
- What is endometriosis?
- List three ways to prevent PID.

REPRODUCTIVE LIFE CYCLE ISSUES

Life cycle issues related to reproduction are present throughout the life span. Major milestones include prenatal differentiation of reproductive organs, growth and development of reproductive organs during childhood, maturation of the reproductive system in adolescence, reproductive capability during early and middle adulthood, declining reproductive capability during middle adulthood, and the end of reproductive capability in late middle to older adulthood. This section addresses issues directly related to reproductive functioning.

FAMILY PLANNING

Family planning consists of two complementary components: planning pregnancy and preventing pregnancy. Family planning gives the woman control over the number of children she wishes to have and allows her to determine when births will occur in relation to each other and in relation to her age and/or the age of the father. Women and couples can avoid unwanted pregnancies, bring about wanted births, and control the intervals between births. Family planning may be a component of the nurse's role for the nurse employed in a family planning clinic, physician or nurse—midwife practice, and in the acute care setting, such as in the postpartum or gynecology units.

Planning Pregnancy

For most women of childbearing age, planning a pregnancy can be accomplished simply by discontinuing the use of contraception. However, pregnancy planning should include "prepregnancy" planning. The condition of the woman before pregnancy affects pregnancy outcome. Therefore, a healthy pregnancy begins well in advance of conception. Pregnancy can be seen as a 12-month experience, beginning 3 months before conception occurs.

Good health and avoiding exposure to harmful substances are significant contributing factors for a successful pregnancy and a healthy baby. If the woman waits until pregnancy is confirmed to remedy factors that can put her or an unborn child at risk, it may be too late to prevent complications. Preconception care is especially important for the woman with a history of problems with a previous pregnancy, such as miscarriage or preterm labor or birth. In many cases causative factors can be identified and treated, reducing the risk for problems in subsequent pregnancies. Preconception care is equally important for the woman with a chronic medical condition, family history of genetic disorders, or any other factor that might increase the risk associated with pregnancy and childbirth.

Areas of Focus for Pregnancy Planning

Because a woman may not realize she is pregnant during the early and vulnerable weeks of fetal development, any woman of childbearing age should be aware of health problems or medication regimens that may adversely affect pregnancy and the birth of a healthy baby. There are several key areas upon which the woman and her partner should focus while planning for a pregnancy. These areas include nutrition and exercise, lifestyle changes, chronic illness and genetic disorders, and medications.

Nutrition and Exercise

It is recommended for women to optimize their intake of folic acid several months before becoming pregnant. Folate occurs naturally in foods such as dark green leafy vegetables and legumes. Ideally, daily dietary intake should supply a minimum of 400 micrograms. If needed, folic acid supplements can be taken to meet daily requirements.

Regular aerobic exercise conditions the heart, lungs, muscles, and other organs in preparation for the increased demands of pregnancy. Exercise can also be helpful in building up low-back and abdominal strength—two areas that can cause discomfort throughout pregnancy.

Lifestyle Changes

Smoking cessation is an important consideration when planning for pregnancy. Women who smoke are at higher risk for miscarriage, lower infant birth weight, sudden infant death syndrome, and infant respiratory illnesses.

Alcohol intake can affect the developing child, especially in the earliest weeks of pregnancy. Fetal alcohol syndrome is now recognized as a cause of serious and irreversible birth defects, particularly mental underdevelopment. The level of alcohol intake that causes birth defects to occur is unknown, so women of childbearing age are advised to abstain from alcohol before, as well as during, pregnancy.

Chronic Illness and Genetic Disorders

A woman with a chronic illness, such as diabetes, asthma, heart disease, or high blood pressure, is at higher risk for poor pregnancy outcome. Therefore, the woman with a chronic disorder will need to consult with her primary care physician about possible risks related to medications or therapies. Medication regimens often can be adjusted before pregnancy to decrease the risk to the woman and her fetus.

Referral for genetic counseling may be indicated for the following reasons: The woman or her partner has a genetic disorder. Either partner is known to be a carrier for a genetic condition. A previous child was born with a genetic syndrome or when there is a strong family history of a genetically transmitted disorder.

Medications

Be very careful! In no case should a woman discontinue or change her prescribed medication regimen without discussing it first with her primary care provider, even if she suspects she is pregnant. In some conditions, the risk to the baby or mother of an uncontrolled medical condition outweighs the possible risk of medication side effects.

Many medications cross the placenta easily and can cause birth defects. Prepregnancy planning includes assessment of medications the woman is taking. This assessment allows for timely adjustments in dosage or alterations in choice of medication.

Nursing Care

Nurses, especially those working in settings such as clinics or doctors' offices or in public health, play an important role in pregnancy planning and preconception care. A major nursing focus of preconception care is education and counseling, which may be offered

BOX 4.2	Nursing Assessment for Preconception Care

Nursing assessment for preconception care includes a complete health history for the woman and her partner, addressing specific concerns such as

- **Lifestyle:** tobacco, alcohol, caffeine, and drug use; prescription or over-the-counter medication use; exposure to toxins such as chemicals or radiation; exercise and rest patterns
- **Nutrition:** a 1- to 3-day meal diary; behaviors such as eating nonfood substances or binging or purging; special diets; dietary supplements; food intolerances; current weight and recent weight loss or gain
- **Medical history:** chronic diseases such as diabetes, hypertension, kidney disease, cardiac disease, asthma, and thyroid disease
- **Infectious disease history:** sexually transmitted infections (STIs); immune status related to rubella; risk for exposure to cytomegalovirus (CMV) or toxoplasmosis; risk for HIV/AIDS or hepatitis B
- **Reproductive history:** sexual history; menstrual, uterine, or cervical abnormalities; previous miscarriage or fetal deaths; previous preterm births; infants with birth weight less than 5½ pounds; infants requiring care in a neonatal intensive care unit (NICU); infants with birth defects or congenital anomalies
- **Family history:** genetic disease or birth defects such as cystic fibrosis, sickle-cell anemia, and phenylketonuria (PKU); consanguinity with partner; ethnic or racial background
- **Sociocultural history:** cultural/religious concerns; support systems; financial needs; the couples' relationship and readiness for parenting; availability of family or other support system; maternal age; socioeconomic status; readiness for pregnancy

FAMILY TEACHING TIPS

Pregnancy Planning

At least 3 months before attempting to conceive:
- Stop or considerably reduce smoking.
- Stop or considerably reduce alcohol consumption.
- Stop use of recreational drugs.
- Eat a healthy diet that is rich in protein, calcium, iron, and zinc.
- Avoid raw meats. Be sure to thoroughly wash your hands before and after handling raw meat.
- Take folic acid tablets (400 micrograms per day) to supplement the folate in a diet that includes leafy green vegetables, beans, and whole-wheat breads. Vitamin B complex is also beneficial.
- Begin a regular exercise program that includes aerobic conditioning.
- Share with your primary care provider any family history of genetic disorders or history of recurrent pregnancy loss.
- Know your rubella and varicella (chickenpox) immunity status and get vaccinated several months in advance of conception, if susceptible to either disease.
- Avoid exposure to X-rays.
- Consult your primary care provider about existing medical conditions or medications.

through individual counseling or in traditional classroom settings. The nurse also may be responsible for gathering the woman's and her partner's health histories, including current health status and lifestyle practices (Box 4-2).

Nursing interventions include anticipatory guidance or teaching, discussing issues such as risk behaviors or risk factors and corrective or preventative measures. Nutrition and exercise are important concerns for the woman planning to become pregnant. Advise the woman to consume a nutritious diet that provides all essential nutrients, with emphasis on calcium, iron, folic acid, protein, B-complex vitamins, vitamin C, and magnesium. Exercise that includes aerobic conditioning and muscle toning will improve circulation and general health. The woman should continue her current exercise plan or establish a routine beginning at least 3 months before she plans to become pregnant. Encourage the woman who is trying to become

pregnant to follow the recommendations in Family Teaching Tips: Pregnancy Planning.

Preventing Pregnancy

Planning pregnancy means that steps must be taken to prevent pregnancy when it is not desired. Serious negative health consequences may result from unplanned pregnancy. Also, it has been estimated that up to one-half of all unplanned pregnancies are terminated by induced abortion (Mishell, Burkman, Shulman, Westhoff, & Wysocki, 2002). Even so, approximately 50% of pregnancies in the United States are unplanned. Of those that are unplanned, more than half of the couples were using some form of contraception when conception occurred (Hutti, 2003).

When pregnancy happens despite contraceptive use, either the method is imperfect (method failure) or the individual does not use the method perfectly (user error). Contraceptive methods are graded based on their perfect use and typical use failure rates. Perfect use describes a contraceptive method that is used exactly as directed 100% of the time. Typical use accommodates humans' tendency to forget or make errors. Generally speaking, perfect use has a lower associated failure rate than does typical use. Table 4-1 compares the failure rates of major contraceptive methods.

TABLE 4.1 | **Comparison of Selected Contraceptive Methods: Failure Rates and STI Protection**

The failure rate is reported as a percentage. The number listed represents the number of women who become pregnant for every 100 women who use the method.

Contraceptive Method	Failure Rates With Typical Use*	Failure Rates With Perfect Use[†]	Protection From STIs When Used Correctly
Natural Methods			
Unprotected intercourse (leaving it to chance)	15%	15%	None
Abstinence	Unknown	0%	Completely protective
Coitus interruptus (withdrawal)	27%	4%	May offer some protection
Fertility awareness methods (FAM)	12%–22%	1%–5%	None
Barrier Methods			
Spermicides (nonoxynol-9)	2%–59%	6%	May actually increase risk by causing genital irritation
Male condom	15%	2%	Highly protective
Female condom	21%	5%	Offers fair protection
Diaphragm	16%	6%	Offers some protection
Cervical cap (nulliparous woman)	16%	9%	Offers some protection
Cervical cap (multiparous woman)	32%	26%	Offers some protection
Hormonal Methods			
Combination (estrogen/progestin) oral contraceptives (COCs)	5%	0.1%	None
Progestin-only pills (POPs or the "mini-pill")	5%	0.5%	None
Every-3-months hormonal injections (Depo-Provera)	3%	0.3%	None
Combined monthly hormonal injections (Lunelle)	3%	0.05%	None
Single rod hormonal implant (Implanon)	0%[‡]	0%	None
Hormonal implant (Norplant)	0.05%	0.05%	None
Transdermal patch (Ortho Evra)	0.8%	0.6%	None
Vaginal ring (NuvaRing)	0.65%	0.65%	
Intrauterine Devices			
IUD (copper)	0.8%	0.6%	None
IUD (levonorgestrel-releasing system)	0.1%	0.1%	None
Sterilization			
Female sterilization (tubal ligation)	0.5%	0.5%	None
Male sterilization (vasectomy)	0.15%	0.10%	None

* Typical use refers to percentage of women who have an accidental pregnancy during the first year of using the method in a typical manner.

[†] Perfect use refers to the percentage of women who experience an accidental pregnancy during the first year while using the method as directed 100% of the time.

[‡] No pregnancies have been reported to date with Implanon, although women are cautioned that no method of birth control is 100% effective (Hutti, 2003).

Table adapted from the following sources: Managing Contraception (produced by The Bridging the Gap Foundation) http://www.sexualetiquette101.com/[§]; Planned Parenthood website (www.plannedparenthood.org)[§]; Cwiak, C., & Zieman, M. (2003). New methods in contraception: A review of their advantages and disadvantages. *Women's Health in Primary Care, 6*(10), 473–478; Fehring, R. J. (2004). The future of professional education in natural family planning. *JOGNN, 33*(2), 34–43; Hutti, M. H. (2003). New and emerging contraceptive methods: Nurses can help women make wise choices. *AWHONN Lifelines, 7*(1), 32–39; Nissl, J. (2003). Healthwise knowledgebase topic: Hormone injections for birth control. Palo Alto Medical Foundation: A Sutter Health Affiliate. Melnikow, J., Hatcher, R.A., & Jones, K. (Medical reviewers). Retrieved April 10, 2004, from http://www.pamf.org/teen/healthinfo/index.cfm?section=healthinfo& page=article&sgml_id=hw239088.

[§]All website references were retrieved April 2004.

The woman who wishes to defer or avoid pregnancy has a wide variety of contraceptive methods from which to choose. An ideal method of contraception is one that is effective, easy to understand and use, and acceptable to both partners. There should be minimal side effects and low risk of sequelae. Ideally, the contraceptive should not be related directly with lovemaking and should not interfere with sexual pleasure. It should be inexpensive and easy to maintain. Protection from sexually transmitted infections (STIs) is an additional consideration. Reversible methods should allow the couple to conceive readily after discontinuing use of the method.

Natural Methods

A natural contraceptive method refers to any method that does not use hormones, pharmaceutical compounds, or physical barriers that block sperm from entering the uterus. Natural methods of birth control include abstinence, coitus interruptus, and natural family planning.

Abstinence

Abstinence, as related to birth control, means refraining from vaginal sexual intercourse. Abstinence can include other means of sexual stimulation, such as oral sex. Complete, or strict, abstinence refers to the avoidance of all sexual contact. Abstinence is a normal and acceptable alternative to sexual intercourse, especially for teens and singles in noncommittal relationships. The use of complete abstinence as a method of birth control has no cost, is readily available, and is the only 100% effective method for preventing pregnancy and STIs. A major drawback is that it can be difficult to maintain abstinence. A couple may make a rash decision during the heat of passion, which may leave the woman without a means of preventing pregnancy.

Coitus Interruptus

Coitus interruptus, also called withdrawal, requires the man to pull the penis out of the vagina before ejaculation to avoid depositing sperm in or near the vagina. However, the pre-ejaculate fluid may contain sperm, so pregnancy can occur. Effectiveness is dependent on the male partner's ability to withdraw his penis before ejaculation.

One advantage of coitus interruptus is that it provides some level of protection when no other method is available. However, the disadvantages are many. This is an unreliable method of birth control (see Table 4-1), and it offers no protection from STIs. This method requires a great deal of self-control on the part of the male partner and cannot be used if the man ejaculates prematurely. It is not recommended for sexually inexperienced men or adolescents (Planned Parenthood, Undated).

Fertility Awareness Methods

Fertility awareness methods (FAM) refer to all methods that use the identification of fertile and infertile phases of a woman's cycle to plan or prevent pregnancy. Such methods involve observing and charting the signs and symptoms of the menstrual cycle (e.g., menstrual bleeding, cervical mucus changes, and variations in basal body temperature) through the use of one or a combination of several methods to determine the woman's fertile period. Then abstinence or a barrier contraceptive method is used during days identified as fertile to reduce the risk of pregnancy. FAM is also used to plan pregnancy.

FAM is the only method of birth control that requires the cooperation of both partners. Many couples who prefer a natural, mutual method of preventing pregnancy find cooperation to be an empowering component of the method, giving them control of their fertility and encouraging shared responsibility. Advantages of these methods are that they are inexpensive, do not require the use of artificial devices or drugs, and have no harmful side effects. Disadvantages include that the method requires discipline to use and can seem cumbersome for a woman or couple with a busy lifestyle. It also has a high failure rate during the first year with typical use.

A foundational component for practicing FAM is knowledge about the menstrual cycle. Guidelines derive from the assumption that ovulation occurs exactly 14 days before the onset of the next menstrual cycle, and that the fertile window extends 3 to 4 days before and after ovulation, or in other words, between days 10 and 17 of the menstrual cycle. Four methods used to anticipate the fertile window are:

1. Calendar method
2. Basal body temperature method
3. Cervical mucus method
4. Symptothermal method

In addition to these four methods, some couples use an ovulation predictor test to determine ovulation and thus the fertile period.

Calendar Method. With the calendar method, fertile days are determined by an accurate charting of the length of the menstrual cycle over a period of 6 months. The number of days per cycle is counted, beginning on the first day of menses. The beginning of the fertile period is determined by subtracting 18 days from the length of the shortest cycle. The end of the fertile days is determined by subtracting 11 days from the length of the longest cycle. An example of how the fertile period is calculated using this method is found in Box 4-3. To avoid pregnancy, the couple abstains from sexual intercourse or uses a barrier method during the identified fertile period.

The major drawbacks of this method are that the couple is using data about past cycles to predict what

BOX 4.3	Calculation of Fertile Window Using the Calendar Method

A woman keeps track of the length of her menstrual cycles for at least 6 months. Then she calculates her fertile window by subtracting 18 days from her shortest cycle and 11 days from her longest cycle. For a woman whose shortest cycle is 24 days and longest cycle is 28 days, the calculation would be as follows:

Shortest cycle	Longest cycle
24	28
−18	−11
6	17

Therefore, the woman's fertile window would be days 6 to 17 of her menstrual cycle. She and her partner would then use abstinence or a barrier method to prevent pregnancy during the fertile window.

will happen in the future, and they are counting on the regularity of what can be an unpredictable event. In reality, the timing of the fertile period can be highly variable, even for women who consider their cycles to be regular. Wilcox, Dunson, and Baird (2000) found that more than 70% of women are in their fertile period before day 10 and/or after day 17 of their menstrual cycle. Thus, there are very few days during the menstrual cycle during which some women are not potentially fertile.

The method is contraindicated for women who do not have regular cycles, such as women who are anovulatory (absence of ovulation), adolescents, women approaching menopause, and women who have recently given birth.

Basal Body Temperature Method. The basal body temperature (BBT) is the lowest normal temperature of a healthy person, taken immediately after waking and before getting out of bed. The BBT method is based on the principle of identifying the shift in body temperature that occurs normally around the time of ovulation.

The BBT ranges from 36.2°C to 36.3°C during menses, and for about 5 to 7 days after. At about the time of ovulation, a slight drop in temperature may be observed, followed by a slight rise (approximately 0.2°C to 0.4°C) after ovulation in response to increasing progesterone levels. This temperature elevation persists until 2 to 4 days before menstruation. The BBT then drops to the lower levels recorded during the previous cycle, unless pregnancy occurs. The drop and subsequent rise in BBT is called the thermal shift.

To prevent conception, the couple avoids unprotected intercourse from the day the BBT drops through the fourth day of temperature elevation. The BBT must be charted daily on a graph for an entire month to

accurately perceive a pattern in BBT. Confounding factors such as fatigue, infection, anxiety, awakening late, getting fewer than 3 hours sleep, jet lag, alcohol consumption, and sleeping in a heated waterbed or using an electric heating blanket, may all cause temperature fluctuation, altering the expected pattern. Because so many factors can interfere, BBT alone is not a reliable method for predicting ovulation but should be used along with the calendar or cervical mucus methods.

Cervical Mucus Method. The cervical mucus method, also called the Billings method or the Creighton ovulation method, requires recognition and interpretation of characteristic changes in the amount and consistency of cervical mucus through the menstrual cycle. Accurate assessment of cervical mucus requires that the mucus be free of contraceptive gel or foam, semen, blood, or abnormal vaginal discharge for at least one full cycle.

Before ovulation cervical mucus is thick and does not stretch easily. This quality inhibits sperm from entering the cervix. Just before ovulation, changes occur that facilitate the viability and motility of sperm, allowing the sperm to survive in the female reproductive tract until ovulation. Cervical mucus becomes more abundant and thinner with an elastic quality. It feels somewhat slippery and can be stretched 5 centimeters or more between the thumb and forefinger, a quality referred to as **spinnbarkeit** (Fig. 4-3). These cervical mucus changes indicate the period of maximum fertility.

Observation begins on the last day of menses and is done several times a day for several cycles. Because

● **Figure 4.3** Spinnbarkeit refers to the stretchable, distensible quality of cervical mucus around the time of ovulation. Some fertility awareness methods (FAM) rely on this quality to help determine when ovulation has occurred.

mucus can be obtained at the vaginal introitus, there is no need to attempt to reach into the vagina to the cervix. Confounding factors include the presence of sperm, contraceptive gels or foam, vaginal discharge, use of douches or vaginal deodorants, sexual arousal, and medications such as antihistamines. Although self-evaluation of cervical mucus can help the woman to predict ovulation, the effectiveness of this method is enhanced when it is used in combination with the calendar and/or BBT methods. This method may be unacceptable for the woman who is uncomfortable touching her genitals.

Symptothermal Method. The symptothermal method is a combination of the calendar, BBT, and cervical mucus methods, along with an awareness of other signs of fertility. The woman acquires fertility awareness as she understands the secondary physiologic and psychological symptoms marking the phases of her cycle. These secondary symptoms include increased libido, midcycle spotting, mittelschmerz (unilateral lower abdominal pain in the ovary region associated with ovulation), pelvic fullness or tenderness, and vulvar fullness. The woman may palpate the cervix to assess for changes that normally occur with ovulation. The cervical os dilates slightly, the cervix softens and rises in the vagina, and cervical mucus becomes abundant with a slippery consistency. Calendar calculations and cervical mucus changes are used to approximate the beginning of the fertile period. Changes in cervical mucus and BBT are used to predict the end of the fertile period. Some studies have demonstrated a lower failure rate when multiple indicators are used to predict the fertile window (Fehring, 2004).

Ovulation Predictor Test. The Ovulation Predictor Test is a handheld device that detects metabolites of luteinizing hormone (LH) and estrogen in the urine. LH levels surge during the 12 to 24 hours before ovulation, and the test is designed to detect the increase. The home kit supplies testing materials for testing the urine over several days during a cycle. A positive reaction for LH is indicated by an easily read color change. Currently in the United States, the device is used to determine ovulation so that the woman can increase her changes of becoming pregnant. However, research is ongoing to determine the usefulness of the device as a contraceptive method.

Other Natural Methods

Other natural methods used to try to prevent pregnancy include douching after intercourse and breast-feeding. Douching is not reliable for preventing pregnancy; on the contrary, it may actually increase the chance of pregnancy by propelling sperm farther into the birth canal. Breast-feeding suppresses ovulation only if the woman is nursing at least 10 feedings per 24-hour period. Ovulation is suppressed by the release of prolactin, which stimulates milk production. Should the woman supplement with bottle feedings or solid foods, milk production and prolactin secretion will decrease, which may allow ovulation to occur.

Barrier Methods

Barrier methods of contraception provide a physical barrier, chemical barrier, or both to prevent sperm from entering the cervical os. Types of barrier methods of contraception include spermicidal gels or foams, condoms, diaphragms, and cervical caps. Spermicidal gels or foams are used frequently in conjunction with condoms, diaphragms, and cervical caps to increase effectiveness (see Table 4-1). Many barrier method contraceptives have the added benefit of providing at least some protection against STIs.

Spermicides

Spermicides provide a physical barrier that prevents sperm penetration and a chemical barrier that kills the sperm. The most commonly used chemical spermicide in the United States is nonoxynol-9 (N-9). Spermicides are available as aerosol foams, foaming tablets, suppositories, films, creams, and gels. Most of these products are designed to be inserted vaginally immediately before or within a few hours before engaging in vaginal sexual intercourse.

Although early research seemed to indicate that N-9 provided some protection against STIs, the World Health Organization (WHO) and Centers for Disease Control (CDC) recommend against relying on N-9 products for this protection. In fact, the WHO and CDC warn that spermicide use might actually increase the risk of STIs by creating irritation and breakdown of the protective vaginal or anal mucosa. N-9 is appropriate for contraceptive use in the woman who is at low risk for contracting HIV and who does not engage in multiple daily acts of vaginal or anal intercourse (Planned Parenthood, 2002). The effectiveness of spermicides can be greatly increased by combining them with other physical barrier methods, such as the condom, diaphragm, or cervical cap.

Advantages include that this method is readily available without a prescription. Spermicides can be inserted several hours before vaginal sexual intercourse and so can be used discreetly by the woman. Some disadvantages are that effectiveness rates are highly variable (see Table 4-1) and the method does not protect against (and may actually enhance) the transmission of STIs.

Male Condom

The male condom is a thin, stretchable sheath that covers the erect penis during sexual intercourse. A condom functions as a contraceptive by collecting semen before, during, and after ejaculation to prevent sperm from entering the vagina and causing pregnancy. The majority of condoms are made of latex rubber, although a small percentage is composed of other substances, such as natural membrane or polyurethane. Additional features in condoms manufactured in the United States include shape, and the addition of lubricants and spermicides. One feature related to shape is the presence or absence of a sperm reservoir tip. Some condoms are contoured, rippled, or have a roughened surface to enhance vaginal stimulation. A thinner sheath increases heat transmission and penile sensitivity. Some condoms are prelubricated with a wet jelly or a dry powder, and some have spermicide added to the interior or exterior surface. Effectiveness is dependent upon correct and consistent application and usage (see Table 4-1).

One significant advantage is the protection condoms afford against STIs. Condoms can be used as an additional protective measure against the transmission of HIV and other STIs, even when another method of contraception is used for birth control (such as oral contraceptives or barrier methods). Other advantages include low cost, easy availability, no prescription or physician visit needed, and condoms can be put on as part of sexual play. Some men find condom use helpful in preventing premature ejaculation or maintaining an erection for a longer period of time.

There are also disadvantages. The condom can break, which decreases its effectiveness. Some couples find that condoms decrease sexual sensation. Condom use can also be perceived as inhibiting spontaneity, or the man may feel self-conscious. Another potential disadvantage is latex allergy; however, polyurethane condoms can be used if this is an issue (see Family Teaching Tips: Safe Condom Use in Chapter 27).

Female Condom

The female condom, or vaginal sheath, is a thin tube made of polyurethane, with flexible rings at both ends. The closed end is inserted into the vagina and anchored around the cervix. The open end covers the labia. Like the male condom, the female condom collects sperm before, during, and after ejaculation to protect against pregnancy and STIs. The condom can be applied before intercourse, a feature that may increase spontaneity. Before intercourse, a spermicide can be added, if not already present. The female condom comes in one size and, like the male condom, is available without a prescription.

Advantages of the female condom are that it can be inserted before intercourse, an erection is not necessary to keep the condom in place, individuals who are allergic to latex can use it, and the external ring may supply clitoral stimulation. Reported disadvantages are that the condom may be difficult to apply, makes noise, causes vaginal or penile irritation, or it may slip into the vagina during vigorous intercourse, a condition that decreases its effectiveness.

Diaphragm and Cervical Cap

The diaphragm is a shallow dome-shaped latex rubber device with a flexible, circular wire rim that fits over the cervix. The wire rim may be flat, coiled, arcing, or wide seal. A diaphragm works by mechanically blocking sperm from entering the cervix. Spermicide, which must be used with the diaphragm to provide optimal protection, interferes with sperm motility.

Diaphragms are available by prescription in a wide range of diameters between 50 and 90 millimeters. They require special fitting by a trained practitioner. The woman must apply spermicidal jelly or cream to the rim and center of the diaphragm before inserting and positioning the diaphragm over the cervix (Fig. 4-4). A diaphragm may be inserted several hours before intercourse, and must be left in place over the cervix for at least 6 hours afterward to allow the spermicide time to destroy the sperm. If the device is inserted and more than 6 hours passes before sexual intercourse, or if intercourse is repeated, the woman should leave the diaphragm in place and insert another application of spermicidal cream, jelly, or foam into the vagina. A diaphragm should not be left in place for longer than 24 hours.

The cervical cap is much smaller than the diaphragm and is available in four sizes between 21 and 31 millimeters. Its rubber dome has a firm, pliable rim that fits snugly around the base of the cervix, close to the junction of the cervix and the vaginal fornices. The device should remain in place 6 to 8 hours after the last act of intercourse, but not longer than 48 hours. The seal of the cap provides a mechanical barrier. Spermicide applied in the center of the cap provides an additional chemical barrier.

The typical failure rates for both devices are similar for nulliparous women. However, the failure rate of the cervical cap in the multiparous woman is quite high (see Table 4-1). A primary health care provider must specifically fit the diaphragm or cervical cap to each woman. Both devices must be refitted after pregnancy (whether it ends in miscarriage, abortion, or delivery), abdominal or pelvic surgery, and weight gain or loss of 10 or more pounds. The woman must learn how to insert and remove the cap or diaphragm correctly and to verify proper placement. Before insertion, the woman should check either device for pinholes or weakened areas by holding it up to the light.

Here's a teaching tip for diaphragm use. Additional spermicidal jelly or cream must be inserted into the vagina if the woman has intercourse again within 6 hours. With the cervical cap, using additional spermicide for repeated episodes of intercourse is optional.

● **Figure 4.4** Application of a diaphragm. (**A**) To insert, fold the diaphragm in half, separate the labia with one hand, then insert upwards and back into the vagina. (**B**) To position, make certain the diaphragm securely covers the cervix. (**C**) To remove, hook a finger over the top of the rim and bring the diaphragm down and out.

Typical advantages for the use of diaphragms and cervical caps are that both devices offer some protection against STIs and pelvic inflammatory disease (PID). Both may be inserted ahead of time and are not easily felt by either partner, and therefore do not readily interfere with the spontaneity of love-making. Both methods can be used during breast-feeding and are immediately reversible.

Disadvantages unique to the diaphragm are that some sexual positions, penis sizes, and vigorous thrusting techniques can dislodge the device during intercourse, thus decreasing its effectiveness. Also, some women develop frequent bladder infections or cannot use the diaphragm because of poor vaginal tone. Disadvantages of both methods are that they can be difficult to insert and the woman must feel comfortable touching her genitals. Also, in rare instances women have developed toxic shock syndrome (TSS) with the use of these devices.

Hormonal Methods

Hormonal methods of contraception include oral contraceptives, implants, injections, vaginal ring, and transdermal patches. Depending on their hormonal composition, all hormonal methods prevent or suppress ovulation; thicken cervical mucus, making it resistant to sperm penetration; and create an inhospitable uterine environment, preventing implantation of any fertilized ovum, although this third mechanism of action is reported to occur rarely.

Advantages of hormonal contraceptives are that they are highly effective in preventing pregnancy (see Table 4-1) when used consistently and correctly. Several hormonal methods provide noncontraceptive health benefits, such as menstrual cycle improvements, management of perimenopause, and protection against certain cancers, ovarian cysts, ectopic pregnancy, pelvic inflammatory disease (PID), and acne (Davidson, 2003).

Although efficacious in preventing pregnancy, there are disadvantages to the use of hormonal methods of contraception. Sixty percent of new users discontinue hormonal methods during the first year of use because of experienced or perceived side effects (Hutti, 2003). In addition, hormonal contraceptives do not offer protection from STIs, including HIV, for either partner. Therefore, condoms should be used if STI protection is desired.

Combination Oral Contraceptives

Combination oral contraceptives (COCs), also known as "the pill," are the most commonly used reversible method of contraception (Mishell et al., 2002). COCs can be monophasic or phasic. Monophasic pills provide fixed doses of estrogen and progestin, whereas phasic pills (biphasic, triphasic, and multiphasic) are formulated to alter the amount of progestin, and in some cases, estrogen, within each cycle. Phasic preparations reduce the total dosage of hormones in a cycle, without sacrificing effectiveness. COCs are available in 21- or 28-day packs. If the woman uses a 21-day pack, she takes a pill each day for 21 days, then stops for 7 days. With the 28-day pack, a pill is taken daily throughout the cycle. The last 7 pills of the 28-pill pack are inert but help maintain the habit of taking the daily pill. Menstruation occurs during the time of pill withdrawal or when the inert pills are taken. Some practitioners are prescribing longer regimens of COCs to suppress menstruation while also providing birth control. COCs should be taken at the same time each day.

If taken daily as prescribed, COCs provide a high contraception effectiveness rate (see Table 4-1). In addition, COCs therapy offers many noncontraceptive benefits, in particular menstrual cycle improvements, including a decrease in menstrual blood loss, reduction in the occurrence of iron-deficiency anemia, regulation of irregular cycles, lessening of the symptoms of dysmenorrhea (painful menstrual periods), and lower incidence of premenstrual syndrome. COCs offer protection against endometrial adenocarcinoma and, perhaps, ovarian cancer. They are associated with a reduced incidence of benign breast disease, protection against the development of functional ovarian cysts and some types of pelvic inflammatory disease, and a decreased risk for ectopic pregnancy.

Disadvantages of COCs include no protection from HIV and other STIs. In addition, the woman must remember to take the pill every day. A large percentage of women stop using COCs because of side effects. Common side effects include nausea, headache, breast tenderness, weight gain, breakthrough spotting or bleeding, and amenorrhea. These side effects usually decrease over time and are less common with lower-dose preparations. COCs may promote growth of breast cancer, although they probably do not cause breast cancer. Another disadvantage is the expense. COCs require a visit to the primary care provider or clinic and are available by prescription only.

Some women should not use COCs, or use them only with great caution. Box 4-4 outlines contraindi-

---

This tip will be useful for the examination. The acronym "ACHES" can help you recall warning signs related to using oral contraception:

- **A**bdominal pain
- **C**hest pain, dyspnea, bloody sputum
- Severe **H**eadache, weakness or numbness in extremities
- **E**ye problems such as blurred vision, double vision, vision loss
- **S**peech disturbance, severe leg pain or edema

---

cations for their use. Instruct the woman to report any pre-existing health problems, any change in health that may affect her use of COCs, and the occurrence of any warning signs, including severe abdominal or chest pain, dyspnea, headache, weakness, numbness, blurred or double vision, speech disturbances, or severe leg pain and edema.

Progestin-Only Pills

Progestin-only pills (POPs), also referred to as the "mini-pill," contain only one hormone: progestin. Its major effect is to thicken the cervical mucus and make the endometrium inhospitable to implantation. POPs are slightly less effective than COCs in preventing ovulation.

Advantages include no estrogen side effects, so the woman is less likely to quit using the contraceptive. In addition, women for whom COCs are contraindicated (e.g., those older than 35 years who also smoke and those who have a history of thrombophlebitis) may take POPs. There are no "hormone-free" days or inert pills to take, so the woman can maintain a daily routine of taking the same pill every day. The woman who is lactating can take POPs after the newborn is 6 weeks old. POPs decrease dysmenorrhea and the pain sometimes associated with ovulation.

Menstrual irregularities are one disadvantage of POPs, although periods are usually very short and scanty, which some women find desirable. POPs must be taken every day at the same time of day without fail because their main action (thickening cervical mucus) lasts only 22 to 24 hours. As with COCs, POPs do not provide STI protection and require a primary care provider visit and a prescription.

Hormonal Injections

There are two types of hormonal injection therapies available: a progestin-only agent, depot medroxyprogesterone acetate (DMPA or Depo-Provera); and a combination estrogen/progestin product, medroxyprogesterone acetate with estradiol cypionate (MPA/E2C or Lunelle). Both products provide a level of contraceptive protection similar to that of COCs (see Table 4-1).

BOX 4.4	Contraindications for Using Combination Oral Contraceptives (COCs)

Women who should not use COCs include those who have any of the following conditions or lifestyle patterns:
- Thromboembolic disorders
- History of heart disease or cerebral vascular accident
- Estrogen-dependent cancer or breast cancer
- Impaired liver function
- Undiagnosed vaginal bleeding
- A confirmed pregnancy or a strong suspicion of pregnancy
- A smoking pattern of more than 15 cigarettes per day in women older than 35 years

As with other hormonal contraceptive methods, hormonal injections do not provide protection against STIs.

Depot Medroxyprogesterone Acetate: Depo-Provera. Depo-Provera consists of a slow-release form of progestin that prevents ovulation. Intramuscular injections are administered four times a year (i.e., each injection provides 3 months of protection). The first shot is given in the first 5 days of the menstrual period. After that the woman must schedule appointments every 11 to 13 weeks for an injection.

Advantages are that the woman does not have to remember to take a pill on a daily basis, and she does not have to use a product at the time of sexual intercourse. Depo-Provera provides the woman with a high level of privacy. No one has to know she is using this method of birth control, unless she chooses to share this information. Lactating mothers can use Depo-Provera. Other advantages include prevention of ectopic pregnancy, and improvement of premenstrual syndrome, depression, and the pain associated with endometriosis.

Take it easy! When administering an injection of Depo-Provera, do not massage the site. This could hasten absorption of the hormone and cause a shorter period of effective contraception.

Disadvantages include prolonged amenorrhea. Many women stop menstruating after the third Depo-Provera injection. This effect is not harmful, and some women may even consider it an advantage. In addition to menstrual irregularities, the most common side effects are weight gain, headache, and nervousness. Sometimes depression and premenstrual symptoms worsen. Another potential disadvantage is the length of time it takes (an average of 10 months) before fertility returns after discontinuing the method. Some women have allergic reactions, although this is rare. Depo-Provera may lower the woman's estrogen levels, leading to loss of bone mineral density and increased risk of fractures. Some research has shown an increase in LDL ("bad") cholesterol and a decrease in HDL ("good") cholesterol levels. Contraindications for using Depo-Provera include pregnancy, history of breast cancer, stroke, or liver disease.

Combined Monthly Injection (Lunelle). Lunelle is a combination progestin/estrogen product that is given via monthly intramuscular injection. Lunelle works by preventing ovulation and by causing cervical mucus to thicken and the endometrial lining to thin. Advantages to Lunelle as compared with Depo-Provera are that a regular menstrual pattern is maintained, estrogen levels remain within normal limits, and fertility returns within 2 to 3 months after stopping the method. As with Depo-Provera, Lunelle provides privacy for the woman's contraceptive choice.

Disadvantages include repeated injections and returning for an office visit every month. Lunelle may cause breast tenderness and is not recommended for breast-feeding women. Some menstrual irregularities are normal at first but usually resolve after the first month or two of use. Weight gain has been reported but less than with Depo-Provera.

Hormonal Implants

The hormonal implant currently available in the United States is Implanon, a single etonogestrel (progestin-only) rod implant. The implant is a small, flexible, plastic rod about the size of a matchstick. It is inserted under local anesthesia just under the skin on the inside of the upper arm. Insertion takes approximately 1 minute. Removal requires a small incision and takes about 3 minutes (Hutti, 2003). Contraceptive protection is provided for 3 years.

Implanon is an extremely effective method of birth control (see Table 4-1). Although no contraceptive method can claim to prevent pregnancy 100% of the time, in more than 70,000 cycles of use to date there have been no pregnancies reported with this method (Hutti, 2003). Other advantages include there are no daily pills to remember and no interference with sexual activity to use the method. Fertility returns quickly (within 3 months) after the implant is removed. Implanon frequently improves symptoms of dysmenorrhea and appears to be safe for lactating women.

Disadvantages include weight gain, which is the most common reason women stop using this method of birth control. Irregular bleeding patterns, acne, breast pain, vaginitis, pharyngitis, and headaches are other side effects sometimes experienced with Implanon. No protection from STIs is provided.

Norplant, a six-rod levonorgestrel implant system, was removed from the United States market in 2002. It was designed to last 5 years; therefore, some women continue to use this method of birth control until it must be removed after 5 years. Removal is a minor surgical procedure and may be difficult or painful. The rods have a tendency to break during removal. Common side effects include irregular menses, headaches, nervousness, mood changes, nausea, skin changes, and vertigo.

Transdermal Patch

The transdermal patch (Ortho Evra) supplies continuous levels of estrogen and progestin. It is available as a prescription and can be placed on the lower abdomen, upper outer arm, buttock, or upper torso, excluding the breasts. The patch is placed on the skin continuously for 3 weeks, and then removed for 1 week to allow menses to occur. Each new patch should be applied on the same day of the week. No more than one patch should be worn at a time.

Individuals who use the patch are more likely to be compliant with the method than with COCs or POPs because there is no daily requirement. It is a highly effective form of birth control (see Table 4-1). Disadvantages include decreased effectiveness in women who weigh more than 198 pounds. The most common side effects include breast symptoms, headache, application site reactions, nausea, upper respiratory tract infections, and dysmenorrhea (Hutti, 2003).

Vaginal Ring

The vaginal ring contraceptive (NuvaRing) is a soft, flexible ring, approximately 2 inches in diameter that contains estrogen and progestin. It is placed into the vagina once a month, during which time it releases low levels of hormones. Lower dosing is possible because it works in the vagina. The ring must be removed after 21 days to allow menstruation.

Advantages include low estrogen exposure with high effectiveness. There is a low incidence of hormone-related side effects, such as headaches, nausea, and breast tenderness. It is easy to insert and generally discreet to use. Disadvantages include that a woman must feel comfortable touching her genitals, some women or their partners may be able to sense the ring during intercourse, and the device may cause increased vaginal discharge.

Intrauterine Device

The intrauterine device (IUD) is a small T-shaped device that is inserted into the uterine cavity. Two types of IUDs are currently approved for use in the United States, each containing a chemically active substance (either copper or progestin). The copper-bearing device is effective for 4 to 10 years, and the progestin-releasing device for 5 to 7 years. As a safety measure, IUDs are also saturated with barium sulfate for radiopacity. Each month the woman must check for presence of the string in the vagina to confirm continued placement of the device.

The copper-bearing IUD acts by damaging sperm in transit through the uterus. Few viable sperm are able to reach the ovum, thus preventing fertilization. The progestin-bearing device affects the cervical mucus and endometrial development. The effect is local and causes no disruption of ovulation. The absence of estrogen makes the IUD a more appropriate contraceptive for women older than 35 years, heavy smokers, and for women with hypertension, vascular disease, or familial diabetes.

The IUD offers continuous protection from unwanted pregnancy without the need to remember a daily pill or engage in other manipulations between coital acts. The IUD can be placed at any time during the menstrual cycle after obtaining a negative pregnancy test. It can be placed immediately after childbirth or after an abortion. When pregnancy is desired, the care provider removes the device. The progestin-bearing device offers the added benefits of decreasing dysmenorrhea and is useful for decreasing bleeding in women with menorrhagia (abnormally long or heavy menstrual periods).

Side effects include cramping and bleeding upon insertion of the device. Common reasons for removal of the copper device include dysmenorrhea and increased menstrual flow. Headache, breast tenderness, and acne are common side effects of the progestin-releasing device. Risks include uterine perforation, pelvic inflammatory disease, bacterial vaginosis, and infection (the IUD offers no protection against STIs). Complications, which may transpire should pregnancy occur, include spontaneous abortion, ectopic pregnancy, or a preterm birth.

Here's another memory trick!

The acronym "PAINS" can help you remember the signs of potential complications related to IUDs.

- **P**eriod late, abnormal spotting or bleeding
- **A**bdominal pain, pain with intercourse
- **I**nfection exposure, abnormal vaginal discharge
- **N**ot feeling well, fever, chills
- **S**tring missing, shorter or longer

Sterilization

Sterilization is a permanent method of birth control obtained via a surgical procedure. Although in some instances reversal may be accomplished, the procedure to do so is expensive and often not successful. The incidence of successful pregnancy after reanastomosis of a tubal ligation is just 15%, and the fertility rate after vasectomy reversal is as low as 16%. Therefore, surgical sterilization procedures should be considered permanent.

Female Sterilization

Female sterilization, by tubal ligation or tubal occlusion, involves blocking or ligating (tying) the fallopian tubes. The procedure may be done immediately after giving birth (within 24 to 48 hours), at the time of an abortion, or during any phase of the menstrual cycle. It can be done using electrocautery or by application of bands or clips via a laparoscopic or minilaparotomy technique. In 2002, the Food and Drug Administration (FDA) approved injection of an occlusive material into the tubes using a transcervical approach (nonsurgical sterilization).

During a minilaparotomy, a small vertical incision is made in the abdominal wall near the umbilicus. The surgeon brings each tube through the incision and cauterizes the tube, which destroys the tissue. An alternative is to ligate and then cut each tube. The procedure may be done under regional anesthetic, or general anesthesia may be used. Oral analgesics are usually sufficient to relieve postoperative discomfort. Although female sterilization is considered a minor surgical procedure, the postoperative recovery period is about 1 to 2 days. The woman is instructed to report bleeding or signs of infection.

Nonsurgical sterilization (Essure Permanent Birth Control System) is accomplished by using hysteroscopy to guide a tiny metallic implant through the vagina, uterus, and into each fallopian tube. Flexible coils hold the implant in place, and mesh material embedded in the coils of the device causes irritation in the tubes, which respond by causing scar tissue to grow and eventually completely occlude the tubes. Alternative methods of birth control must be used for 3 months after the procedure to allow time for scar tissue to form and the method to be completely effective at preventing pregnancy.

Advantages of the Essure system include a less invasive procedure than a surgical approach and avoidance of general anesthesia. The procedure can be performed in a physician's office or clinic. The most common side effects are cramping and nausea and vomiting. Serious, but infrequently occurring, side effects include expulsion of the implant and uterine perforation.

Male Sterilization

Male sterilization, or vasectomy, can be done with a local anesthetic on an outpatient basis. The procedure takes about 20 minutes to perform. A small incision is made on each side of the scrotum over the spermatic cord. Each vas deferens is then ligated and cut. The surgeon may cauterize the cut ends of the vas deferens and then bury them in the scrotal fascia to reduce the chance of spontaneous reanastomosis. The skin incisions are closed, often with a single suture, and a dressing is applied.

Some pain, bruising, and swelling are to be expected after the surgery. Rest, the application of an ice pack, scrotal support, and a mild oral analgesic are effective comfort measures. Moderate inactivity may be recommended for 1 to 2 days because of scrotal tenderness. The skin sutures are removed about 4 to 7 days after surgery. The man should report any signs of bleeding or infection.

Sexual intercourse may be resumed as desired; however, with vasectomy, sterilization is not immediate because sperm remain in the system distal to the ligation. It takes approximately 1 month for the sperm to be purged from the man's system. Therefore, it is necessary for the couple to use another method of birth control until a negative sperm count verifies sterility. Vasectomy has no effect on the man's ability to achieve or maintain erection or on the volume of ejaculate. In addition, there is no interference with the production of testosterone, so secondary sexual characteristics are not affected.

Emergency Contraception

Emergency contraception refers to methods used to prevent pregnancy after unprotected intercourse. Emergency contraception was first used to protect rape victims from pregnancy. It can also be used if a condom breaks or unplanned unprotected sexual intercourse occurs. It is not recommended that emergency contraception be used as the only way of preventing pregnancy in sexually active individuals. It is much more effective to use a consistent form of birth control. It is also important to recognize that emergency contraception is not an "abortion pill." Emergency contraception works to prevent pregnancy from occurring.

Oral contraceptives or mifepristone (RU 486) may be prescribed as a "morning-after pill" to reduce the risk of pregnancy in the event of unprotected intercourse. A larger than usual dose is prescribed, with the exact dosage dependent upon the type of pill. The first dose is given within the first 72 hours after intercourse, followed by a second dose 12 hours after the first.

The copper IUD can be inserted as long as 5 days after unprotected intercourse. One advantage of this method is that it is very effective at preventing pregnancy. However, it should not be used in women who are at high risk for STIs because it can lead to infection, PID, and infertility in these women.

● Nursing Process for Assisting the Couple to Choose a Contraceptive Method

Providing care related to contraception is a collaborative process, involving a variety of health care personnel. The nurse often is working with a physician, certified nurse–midwife, nurse practitioner, family planning counselor, and social worker. Roles for each team member may vary across settings and may overlap within a specific setting. The nurse may be involved in history taking, teaching, and counseling, as well as assisting during physical assessment. Communication among team members and clear protocols for physical assessment, counseling, and teaching are essential to provide quality care. The quality of all family planning care is dependent on the ability of health care team members to work together as professional colleagues.

Steps toward developing excellence in practice include clarifying one's own feelings about family planning, maintaining a current knowledge base through independent study and continuing education activities, awareness of current standards of practice, evaluating current societal norms, and striving to avoid allowing personal prejudices to influence nursing care. Application of the nursing process provides a framework for the nurse working with women and their partners desiring a method of contraception.

ASSESSMENT

Assessment is an essential initial step for identifying the needs and desires of the woman and her partner regarding contraception. The assessment should be conducted in an unhurried and accepting atmosphere with adequate privacy to make the woman and her partner feel comfortable. It is important to treat the couple with respect, accepting their feelings and beliefs, even when these feelings and beliefs differ from the nurse's personal perspective. The assessment includes gathering physiologic, psychoemotional, sociocultural, and cognitive data related to the issue of preventing pregnancy.

The physician or nurse practitioner takes the patient's medical, reproductive, and contraceptive history. Examples of contraception-related questions include:
- What types of contraception were used in the past?
- What problems occurred?
- What did the couple like or dislike about the method?
- What were factors contributing to discontinuing use of the previous method?

The physician or nurse practitioner also performs a physical examination, which includes a general medical examination, a complete gynecologic examination, and routine diagnostic laboratory testing. This information assists in identifying any contraindications to a specific birth control method.

The nurse or family planning counselor often performs the psychoemotional, sociocultural, and cognitive assessments. Psychoemotional data should include information about the couple's feelings regarding their sexuality, family planning in general, and specific methods of contraception. To develop a long-range plan of care, it is important to discuss the couple's goals for their family, regarding the number of children they want and the preferred spacing of those children. Are both partners equally motivated? Studies have indicated that the woman's perception of her partner's support is a major predictor of her use or nonuse of any particular method.

Other important issues helpful in identifying the optimal contraceptive method include the woman's self-image, level of comfort with her body, and willingness to touch her genitals.

Sociocultural issues such as family background, religious beliefs, or cultural taboos may influence the couple's compliance with a particular method for contraception. It is important to identify myths or sexual practices related to culture. Social data that should be identified include information about the nature of the woman's sexual activity, such as the number of partners, and her desire for partner involvement in birth control. It is important to assess the relationship between the woman and her partner(s) and the level/quality of communication they share because this influences the choice and subsequent use of contraception. Financial issues may also have an influence on the choice of contraceptive method.

It is important to assess the couple's level of understanding about the reproductive cycle and their knowledge of varied types of birth control available. Many couples have a knowledge base regarding contraception gleaned from other sources, such as popular magazines, television, or the Internet. It is not unusual for new information to be disseminated by the lay media even before publication in professional journals. Identifying the couple's educational needs can be done as part of an interview or by using assessment questionnaires. Such assessment tools will help the nurse to quickly evaluate the couple's knowledge about birth control methods and identify educational needs, as well as personal preferences.

SELECTED NURSING DIAGNOSES

- Deficient Knowledge, lack of information related to reproductive cycle and birth control methods
- Decisional Conflict related to:
  - contraceptive alternatives
  - unwillingness of sexual partner to agree on birth control method
  - possibility of contraceptive method side effects
- Ineffective Sexuality Patterns related to interference with normal sexuality patterns or discomfort caused by the contraceptive method

OUTCOME IDENTIFICATION AND PLANNING

Appropriate goals may include that the woman and her partner will express adequate knowledge of the reproductive cycle and contraceptive methods; that a method of contraception suitable to their needs and lifestyle will be chosen; and that the woman and her partner will express satisfaction with their pattern of sexual expression. Other goals and interventions are planned according to the individual needs of the woman and her partner.

IMPLEMENTATION

Nursing interventions are chosen based on the assessment data, goals, and plan of care. The physician, or nurse practitioner will perform physical interventions, such as the fitting of diaphragms or cervical caps, or insertion of an IUD. Nursing interventions will be concerned primarily with psychoemotional, sociocultural, or cognitive needs of the woman and her partner.

Providing Teaching

Teaching must be presented in an unbiased manner, dispelling myths and misinformation, and providing needed information. Information may be presented through either group teaching sessions or individual discussion, depending on the needs and preferences of the couple. For example, if a couple has already decided on a specific method of contraception, a group session discussing all methods may not be appropriate. In any case, it is imperative to provide complete and accurate information, regardless of the teaching format. Any discussion of contraceptive methods should include the following information:

- A description of the method, including an example or illustration
- The mode of action, showing how the method acts to prevent pregnancy
- The effectiveness or failure rate of the method and causes for method failure
- Requirements for use, such as how to obtain the method, implementation, and necessary compliance
- How the method will affect love-making, such as when the method should be implemented in relation to coitus, and possible effects on coitus
- Medical and emotional advantages and disadvantages
- Risks, contraindications, side effects, drug interactions, warning signs, and any factors related to safe use
- Effectiveness of the method to protect against STIs and HIV
- Costs of the method, both initially and for the long term
- Reversibility or irreversibility of the method, including how to discontinue the method and the length of time until the return of fertility

Addressing Emotional or Sociocultural Needs

Discussion of emotional or sociocultural needs may be better addressed in private, individualized teaching sessions. This allows the couple to freely express feelings, opinions, and concerns, and ask questions about intimate, personal aspects of their lives. Religious, cultural, social, and financial concerns can be explored. In addition, the nurse will be better able to assess the couple's understanding and acceptance of the chosen method. The nurse should establish a trusting relationship with the couple, provide a warm and accepting atmosphere, and remain sensitive to their needs and concerns.

Assisting With Follow-up

After the woman and her partner have chosen a method, follow-up is important to determine satisfaction with the method and ability to use the method correctly. Often a follow-up telephone call is appropriate. Ask the woman how things are going using the chosen method. Inquire regarding adverse effects or any problems she is having that might cause her to quit using the method. Each office visit is another opportunity to explore with the woman regarding how she is doing and her satisfaction level. Periodically ask the woman to explain the steps of the chosen method and correct any misperceptions.

EVALUATION: GOALS AND EXPECTED OUTCOMES

- **Goal:** The woman and her partner will express adequate knowledge of the reproductive cycle and contraceptive methods.
  Expected Outcomes:
  - Describes the physical signs indicating fertile and infertile periods of the woman's menstrual cycle.
  - Verbalizes understanding about contraceptive methods.
- **Goal:** The woman and her partner will choose a method of contraception suitable to their needs and lifestyle.
  Expected Outcomes:
  - Discusses attitudes and feelings about contraception in general and about specific birth control methods.
  - Asks questions and expresses concerns related to using different birth control methods.
- **Goal:** The woman and her partner will express satisfaction with their pattern of sexual expression using the chosen birth control method.
  Expected Outcomes:
  - Voices satisfaction with the chosen method.

- Encounters no adverse reactions or complications related to the chosen birth control method.
- Demonstrates successful use of the selected birth control method through prevention of unplanned pregnancy.

INDUCED ABORTION

An **induced abortion** is the purposeful interruption of pregnancy before 20 weeks' gestation. A **therapeutic abortion** is a pregnancy termination performed for reasons related to maternal or fetal health or disease. The term **elective abortion** refers to an abortion performed at the woman's request that does not involve preservation of health. Most women who have abortions are Caucasian, younger than 24 years of age, and unmarried. Sixty percent of women who have abortions report using a contraceptive method that failed.

The type of abortion procedure used depends on the gestational age of the fetus. Table 4-2 briefly describes several of the more common abortion procedure techniques and special considerations associated with each procedure.

Nursing care roles and responsibilities vary, depending upon the setting, method of termination used, and the client's needs. In some settings, the nurse and physician may be the only health care providers involved. In others, care providers may include social workers or counselors. In either situation, the nurse's role is central to achieving optimal client care outcomes. It is important to examine personal beliefs and values related to abortion before assuming responsibility for the care of women choosing to have an abortion. The nurse must be able to provide compassionate and nonjudgmental care.

Document the amount and character of bleeding after the abortion procedure. Save anything that appears to be tissue or clots. A pad count with an estimation of pad saturation provides a more accurate record of blood loss. Assess the woman's vital signs frequently, as for other postoperative care, and observe for signs and symptoms of hypovolemic shock. Hematocrit testing is usually done before discharge. Rh immune globulin should be administered to the woman who is Rh negative.

Postabortion teaching should include information about signs and symptoms of possible complications, including elevated temperature, continued/excessive vaginal bleeding, malodorous vaginal discharge, and abdominal pain. Any adverse effects should be reported immediately. Advise the woman to delay sexual intercourse for 1 to 2 weeks. Contraception counseling and instructions about follow-up care and appointments are important.

Test Yourself

- Name the two complementary components to family planning.
- List one advantage and one disadvantage to the use of coitus interruptus as a birth control method.
- List one fertility awareness method and one barrier method of birth control.

INFERTILITY

Infertility is commonly defined as the inability to conceive after a year or more of regular and unprotected intercourse, or the inability to carry a pregnancy to term. Infertility affects approximately 10% to 15% of couples in the United States, a rate that has remained stable for the past 50 years (Garcia, Nelson, & Wallach, 2003). There are two main types of infertility: primary and secondary. A couple who has never been able to conceive is diagnosed with primary infertility; whereas, a couple who has been able to conceive in the past but is currently unable to do so is diagnosed with secondary infertility.

For the majority of couples who engage in frequent, unprotected intercourse, the chance for conception is about 60% at 6 months, 90% at 12 months, and 95% at 24 months. Because the chances of conception are affected by the frequency of intercourse, if a couple has intercourse only one time per week for 6 months, there is only a 15% chance of pregnancy. If the couple increases intercourse frequency to four times a week around the time of ovulation, the chance of conception increases to 83%. Research has shown that the optimal timing for sexual intercourse when conception is desired is every 48 hours at midcycle. Counseling about the timing and frequency of intercourse and the expected time of ovulation often can resolve problems of infertility.

Causes of Infertility

For conception to occur many factors have to work together perfectly. Viable sperm have to be deposited in the female reproductive tract. The passageway through the woman's cervix, uterus, and fallopian tubes has to be clear for sperm to negotiate the journey toward the egg. Ovulation has to occur. The egg must be swept into a fallopian tube. The egg must be fertilized within 12 to 24 hours after ovulation, before it begins to disintegrate. After fertilization, the egg must travel down the fallopian tube to the uterus and implant. Any factor that prevents the sperm and egg from meeting or interferes with the fertilized egg traveling to and implanting in the uterine lining can result in infertility.

TABLE 4.2	Selected Induced Abortion Techniques	
Method	Procedure	Special Considerations
Surgical techniques Menstrual aspiration	The endometrial cavity is aspirated with a flexible cannula and syringe within 1 to 3 weeks after a missed menstrual period.	• A positive pregnancy test must confirm pregnancy before the procedure is done. • Possible complications include implanted zygote missed during procedure, ectopic pregnancy not recognized, and uterine perforation (rare).
Dilatation and curettage (D&C)	1. Cervix is dilated with a blunt instrument or laminaria. 2. A sharp instrument, called a curette, is used to scrape the endometrium and remove uterine contents. 3. Suction may be used during the procedure to aspirate uterine contents.	• Primary procedure used in United States. • Used for 1st trimester terminations (up to 14 weeks). • Possible complications include uterine perforation, cervical laceration, hemorrhage, incomplete removal of products of conception, and infection.
Dilatation and evacuation (D&E)	Procedure is similar to D&C; however, wider dilation of the cervix is done to facilitate removal of the fetus and placenta.	• D&E is the surgical technique of choice for 2nd trimester abortions. • Complications are the same as for D&C.
Medical Techniques Mifepristone (RU 486)	One dose (600 mg) of this oral antiprogesterone is given alone or in conjunction with prostaglandins.	• Effective for 1st trimester (7 weeks and less) abortions. • Common side effects are nausea, vomiting, and gastrointestinal cramping. • Complications include hemorrhage secondary to incomplete expulsion of pregnancy or intra-abdominal hemorrhage secondary to rupture of an unrecognized tubal pregnancy.
Oxytocin	High-dose intravenous oxytocin is titrated until an effective uterine contraction pattern is established.	• Used for 2nd trimester abortions. • Oxytocin has an effectiveness rate similar to that of prostaglandins with fewer side effects. • The nurse must carefully monitor the uterine contraction pattern to avoid excessive stimulation.
Intra-amniotic hyperosmotic fluid infusion	Hyperosmotic saline or urea solutions are injected into the amniotic sac.	• Used infrequently to induce 2nd trimester abortions. • There is a high incidence of adverse side effects and complications associated with this procedure, including death.
Prostaglandins	Prostaglandins can be administered by • Vaginal suppository • Gel inserted by catheter into the cervical canal and lower uterus • Intramuscular injection • Injected into the amniotic sac • Oral route	• Frequently used to induce 2nd trimester abortions. • Side effects include fever, vomiting, diarrhea, and uterine hyperstimulation.

There are multiple factors that can contribute to the inability of a couple to conceive. Female factors alone account for approximately 48% of cases of infertility; whereas, male factors alone are causal in approximately 19% of cases. The interaction of both female and male factors is responsible for 17%, unknown factors for 10%, and other causes for 6% of the cases of infertility (Garcia et al., 2003).

If a couple is having trouble conceiving, it is helpful for them to review their health histories to identify risk factors for infertility (Box 4-5). Female-specific risk factors include any condition or situation that interferes

BOX 4.5	Risk Factors for Infertility

Risk Factors That Affect Both the Male and Female

Behavioral Factors
- Cigarette or marijuana smoking
- Alcohol use (even in moderation)
- Excessive exercise
- Being 10% to 15% over or under ideal body weight
- Multiple sexual partners (increases risk for STIs)

Occupational and Environmental Factors

Exposure to
- High environmental temperatures
- Certain chemicals
- Radiation
- Heavy electromagnetic or microwave emissions

Emotional Factors
- High stress levels
- Depression

Female-Specific Risk Factors

Factors That May Interfere With Ovulation
- Advancing age*
- Chronic medical conditions and/or associated treatments; examples include
  - Diabetes mellitus
  - Thyroid dysfunction
  - Systemic lupus erythematosus (SLE)
  - Rheumatoid arthritis
  - Hypertension
  - Asthma
- Hormonal imbalance, may be signaled by any of the following
  - Menstrual irregularities
  - Menorrhagia (prolonged or excessive bleeding)
  - Hirsutism
  - Acne
- Ovarian cysts

Factors That May Interfere With Travel of Sperm or Egg Through Female Genital Tract
- Surgical or invasive procedures involving the cervix or uterus, such as
  - Cone biopsy

- Cryosurgery
- Dilatation and curettage
- Myomectomy
- In utero diethylstilbestrol (DES) exposure
- Any surgical procedure directly involving the fallopian tubes (may cause scarring and narrowing of the lumen of the tube)
- Any pelvic surgery (could lead to adhesions and scarring)
- Endometriosis
- Ectopic pregnancy
- History of STIs or pelvic inflammatory disease (PID)

Factors That May Interfere With Implantation
- More than one induced abortion
- Using an IUD for contraception (can lead to scarring)
- Hormonal imbalance

Male-Specific Risk Factors

Factors That May Interfere With Sperm Viability
- Prescription medications for ulcers or psoriasis
- DES exposure in utero
- Exposure of the genitals to hot temperatures
  - Hot tubs
  - Steam rooms
  - Tight clothing
- Cryptorchidism
- Prostatitis
- Varicocele
- Genital tract infection
- Mumps after puberty

Factors That May Interfere With Sperm Deposit in Female Genital Tract
- Erectile dysfunction
- Retrograde ejaculation (semen is released into male bladder, rather than ejected from the penis during ejaculation)
- History of hernia repair
- Hypospadias
- Vasectomy

* Female fertility declines with advancing age. A woman in her 30s is 30% less fertile than one in her 20s.

with ovulation, patency of the cervix or fallopian tubes, or ability of the fertilized ovum to implant in the uterine lining. Male-specific risk factors include anything that can cause decreased or abnormal sperm production or any factor that prevents sperm from being deposited in the female reproductive tract.

Initial Evaluation of Infertility

Frequently the woman presents to her primary care provider with her concerns when she has been unable to conceive. The primary care provider or gynecologist performs the initial evaluation. If complex problems are found, or the problem is not readily identifiable, the woman and her partner are then referred to a

reproductive endocrinologist for additional evaluation and treatment.

Because of the high incidence of multiple contributing factors, evaluation of infertility should include both partners, even when the problem seems to be "obvious." Evaluation begins with a thorough history and physical examination for both partners to identify evidence of conditions that may be affecting fertility. Important health history information includes:

- The woman's menstrual pattern
- Number of pregnancies with the current partner or any other partner, and the pregnancy outcomes
- Identification of any sexual dysfunction for both partners

- History of STIs or genital tract surgery or trauma for both partners
- Lifestyle issues, such as alcohol consumption, tobacco use, recreational drug use, occupation, and patterns of physical activity for both partners
- Chronic medical conditions and treatment for both partners
- The couple's pattern of intercourse as related to the woman's ovulatory cycle
- Length of time the couple has had unprotected intercourse
- Natural techniques or home tests the couple has already used

In addition to the above-mentioned health history, the primary care practitioner will do a complete review of systems to help identify any endocrinologic or immunologic issues that might contribute to infertility. A thorough physical examination is done. A gynecologist may evaluate the female partner, whereas the male partner is frequently referred to an urologist for initial evaluation.

The woman's physical examination includes a pelvic examination, Pap smear, cultures for gonorrhea and chlamydia, and a bimanual examination (see Chapter 6). A pelvic ultrasound is part of the initial examination. The male examination includes determining if any genital tract abnormalities are present. Results of the initial evaluation are discussed with the couple. Plans for a more comprehensive evaluation, if needed, are explained.

Comprehensive Evaluation and Diagnostic Testing

Diagnostic testing for infertility usually begins with the simplest testing methods and moves toward the more complex and invasive methods. The couple should be told that diagnostic testing is done in relation to the woman's menstrual cycle. It may take up to two menstrual cycles to complete the testing (Garcia et al., 2003).

Frequently, male infertility factors are evaluated first because the testing is often simpler than that for female testing. The first diagnostic test is almost always a semen analysis. For this procedure, semen is collected via masturbation or in a special condom during intercourse if masturbation is unacceptable to the couple. Optimal results are obtained when the man has abstained from sexual release for 3 to 5 days before the test. The entire ejaculate is collected in a sterile container and must be delivered to the laboratory no later than 30 minutes after collection. The sample is examined for semen volume and quality, and for numbers, shape, motility, and viability of the sperm. Frequently two to three samples, collected at least 2 to 3 days apart, are analyzed. If the semen analysis results are normal, the diagnostic testing then focuses on the female partner.

A PERSONAL GLIMPSE

My husband and I had been married 5 years when we decided to start a family. I tried to get pregnant for 8 months without success. My aunt advised me to get a physical examination. Reluctantly I called to make an appointment. The physician couldn't see me for several months, so I booked the appointment with the Women's Health Nurse Practitioner. She performed a thorough physical exam. She told me that nothing appeared to be wrong with my reproductive tract. She said that many couples don't get pregnant right away. She instructed me that healthy living habits were good not only for a healthy heart, but also for a healthy reproductive tract. She advised me to start a regular program of exercise and to eat a well-balanced diet. She told me that stress can interfere with getting pregnant, and she referred me for yoga lessons after I indicated to her that I had always wanted to learn yoga. I followed her advice, and 6 months later I was pregnant.

Sylvia

LEARNING OPPORTUNITY: What advice can nurses give to couples who want to start a family? How does knowledge of the reproductive tract help nurses take care of women who want to get pregnant?

If the semen analysis results are abnormal, the analysis may be repeated 1 month later to rule out short-term causes or inadequate specimen collection. Additional tests of male fertility that may be performed include endocrine hormonal analysis. Serum levels of four hormones—follicle-stimulating hormone (FSH), luteinizing hormone (LH), testosterone, and prolactin—are evaluated. Transrectal (through the rectum) or scrotal ultrasonography may be done to identify structural abnormalities that could interfere with fertility. Sperm function tests are sometimes done to determine the ability of the sperm to penetrate and fertilize the egg. Testicular biopsy may be performed to obtain a sample of testicular tissue for analysis. The results of this analysis can often pinpoint the cause of male infertility.

Comprehensive fertility evaluation of the woman often begins with the least invasive techniques. The **postcoital test,** which evaluates the interaction of the man's sperm with the woman's cervical mucus, is frequently done. The timing of the test is critical for accurate results. The methods used to predict ovulation for FAM (i.e., BBT, cervical mucus changes, and/or a urinary LH kit) are used. When it has been determined that ovulation is about to occur, the couple is asked to have vaginal intercourse without lubricants. A sample of cervical mucus is collected 8 to 12 hours afterward and evaluated for mucus characteristics, a sperm count, and evaluation of sperm motility. Endocrine testing is useful. Serum hormone levels of estrogen, progesterone, thyroid-stimulating hormone, prolactin, and androgen are drawn to determine if endocrine abnormalities are present.

More invasive techniques include hysterosalpingogram, hysteroscopy, and laparoscopy. A hysterosalpingogram allows for identification of an obstruction anywhere along the tract. A hysteroscopy facilitates direct visualization of the endometrial cavity. This method can be used to diagnose and treat some endometrial conditions. Laparoscopy is usually the last test performed because it involves surgical and anesthetic risk and cost. This procedure provides for direct visualization of the pelvic cavity, which frequently allows for accurate diagnosis of the cause of infertility.

Management of Infertility

The appropriate therapy for infertility is chosen based on the underlying causes identified during diagnostic testing, duration of infertility, and the woman's age. As with testing, therapies begin with the simplest and least invasive and progress toward the more complex, as needed. Possible interventions include medication administration, surgical procedures, insemination techniques, advanced reproductive techniques, and other parenting/childbirth options.

Treatment of Cervical Factors

The easiest, most successful therapy for cervical abnormalities is intrauterine insemination. In this procedure, the physician inserts sperm directly into the uterus near the time of ovulation. More than one insemination may be performed to ensure that insemination coincides with ovulation. Sperm can be from the woman's partner, homologous insemination, or from a donor, heterologous insemination. The woman is placed in the dorsal lithotomy position and a speculum is inserted into the vagina. After the cervix is cleansed, the specimen is placed in a 1-mL syringe attached to a thin, flexible catheter, which is advanced through the cervix until it reaches the upper uterus. Care is taken not to injure the endometrium or induce bleeding. The semen specimen is injected slowly into the uterus, and the catheter is withdrawn. The woman is typically instructed to remain supine for at least 10 minutes after the insemination.

Treatment of Endometrial Factors

Most endometrial causes of infertility are treated by various surgical techniques. Hysteroscopy, laparoscopy, or laparotomy may be done, followed by a hysterosalpingogram to evaluate effectiveness of treatment. If the woman has endometriosis, it is treated as described previously in the chapter.

Treatment of Ovarian Factors

Medications to stimulate ovulation, also known as fertility drugs, are the treatment of choice when lack of ovulation is the cause of infertility. All have side effects and potential complications, which can be severe. Multifetal pregnancy is also common with these medications. Clomiphene citrate (Clomid, Serophene), human menopause gonadotropins (Pergonal, Humegon, Repronex), synthetic gonadotropin-releasing hormone (GnRH), and pure FSH are examples of fertility drugs used to treat ovarian dysfunction.

Treatment of Male Factors

If a varicocele is the cause of low sperm production, it is repaired surgically. If the cause of a low sperm count is unknown and FSH, LH, and testosterone levels are normal, then the man is treated with Clomid to increase sperm production. Alternatively, intrauterine insemination of the woman is done.

Assisted/Advanced Reproductive Therapies

The first advanced reproductive therapy (ART) to be successful in humans, in vitro fertilization, resulted in the 1978 delivery of Louise Brown. Since that time additional therapies have been developed, and indications for ARTs have been expanded to include conditions that heretofore would have been considered impossible to treat.

The four leading ARTs are in vitro fertilization (IVF), gamete intrafallopian transfer (GIFT), tubal embryo transfer (TET), and intracytoplasmic sperm injection (ICSI). The nurse's role in this area is to provide the couple with balanced and accurate information regarding the risks and benefits of the technologies available to facilitate their decision-making process (Box 4-6).

BOX 4.6   Ethical and Legal Issues Related to Advanced Reproductive Therapies (ARTs)

Research in the area of ARTs has resulted in additional technologies that, while giving new hope to couples who once considered their infertility irreversible, are also creating ethical and legal dilemmas for all concerned. Common ethical and legal questions include:

- Who should have the right to reproduce?
- Should ARTs be limited to married couples?
- Who owns the embryos produced?
- Should embryos be frozen for later use?
- Who are the parents?
- Do the biologic donors or surrogates have custodial rights?
- Should donors only be anonymous?
- Should fetal reduction techniques be done when ARTs results in multifetal gestation?

In Vitro Fertilization

IVF is a relatively common procedure that is used when the woman has absent or blocked fallopian tubes; when the man has a low sperm count; or when the etiology of infertility is unknown. IVF involves several steps. The procedure begins with administration of fertility drugs to the woman to stimulate ovulation. After one or more ova (eggs) are harvested from the ovary, the ova are fertilized by sperm in the laboratory and placed in a growth medium, where they develop for 48 to 72 hours. The embryos are then transferred to the uterus. In general, only three to four embryos are placed in the woman's uterus to reduce the risk of multifetal gestation.

Gamete Intrafallopian Transfer

In GIFT, the harvested ova are aspirated into a catheter containing prepared sperm. The ova are then transferred into the fallopian tube, where fertilization can take place. One prerequisite for the procedure is that the woman must have at least one patent fallopian tube. A success rate of 20% to 30% has been reported for this procedure.

Tubal Embryo Transfer

The TET procedure, also called zygote intrafallopian transfer (ZIFT), is a combination of IVF and GIFT. The ova are fertilized as in IVF; however, the embryos are returned to the fallopian tube versus the uterus. Success rates for TET are similar to the success rates for GIFT.

Intracytoplasmic Sperm Injection

ICSI is the latest development to give hope to the male with very low sperm counts. Fertilization is possible with only one sperm. The sperm is obtained by masturbation, testicular biopsy, or aspiration. Stroking the distal portion of the tail then paralyzes it. After the ovum is harvested, the sperm is placed into a microneedle (tail first), and then injected into the ovum. The fertilized ovum is placed into the woman's reproductive tract for implantation. Pregnancy rates are similar to those seen with IVF. An increased risk of congenital malformation and chromosomal abnormalities is associated with ICSI; however, some research studies do not demonstrate increased risk.

Surrogate Parenting

Surrogate parenting is a process by which a woman carries to term the infant of an infertile couple. A **gestational surrogate,** or surrogate mother, may donate only the use of her uterus, or she may also donate her ovum and agree to be inseminated with the male partner's sperm. Surrogate parenting has raised extensive legal and ethical issues that require counseling for both the infertile couple and the surrogate and possibly the surrogate mother's spouse and family.

Psychological Aspects of Infertility

Psychosocial sequelae related to infertility include shock, guilt, isolation, depression, and stress. The partner who has the identified problem is at most risk for feelings of guilt. It is important to avoid using words that imply blame when discussing the problem of infertility.

A couple who is having difficulty conceiving may feel isolated and "different" from others who are able to conceive. They may separate themselves from others in an attempt to avoid emotional pain. Infertility will challenge the couple's self-image, self-worth, and sense of command over events in their life. They may experience a "roller coaster" of emotions, ranging from hope to despair with each ovulatory cycle.

Infertility places stress on the couple's relationship. One or both may develop poor self-esteem and feel unworthy or unlovable. A man may find it difficult to perform sexually or provide semen specimens "on demand" at specific times. Intimacy, love, and support, essential components of a couple's sexual relationship, may be lost because intercourse takes on a "clinical" and mechanical tone.

Failure to achieve pregnancy may lead the couple to consider adoption. Adoption is a viable option for parenting, but the couple must consider some realities about pursuing this route. Many couples have preferences regarding the health status, race, and possibly other characteristics they desire in an infant. A couple may need to reflect on their willingness to adopt an older child, a child of another race, or a child with special needs. How will they feel about having minimal information about the child's background? How would they feel about knowing the child's birth mother or father? These and other questions must be asked and answered by the couple before deciding to adopt. The nurse should have information about adoption available and use positive language when discussing that option. Discussion should focus on sharing complete and balanced information and supporting the couples' feelings and decision.

Nursing Care

The major focus of nursing care related to infertility involves providing support for the couple as they undergo diagnosis and their chosen treatment option. Therapeutic communication skills are an essential component in nursing care. It is important to facilitate the couple's ability to communicate with each other and to encourage each partner to discuss his/her own feelings and be accepting of the other's. The nurse should reinforce the couple's coping strategies or assist them in exploring adaptive alternatives to poor coping, increasing their sense of control in this situation.

After the physician has told the couple about their diagnosis and potential treatment options, the nurse's major role is to provide additional information, helping them to make an informed decision. The nurse supports the couple through the decision-making process and helps them toward a resolution of infertility by either assisting with the grief process or through facilitating parenting. Providing emotional support is an essential component of care, especially when a treatment has been unsuccessful. The general goals for the couple with infertility will be aimed toward:

- Providing complete and accurate information about the diagnosis and treatment options available, including adoption, or child-free living.
- Education about human reproduction, including factors that interfere with normal conception.
- Providing support and counseling to the couple during the diagnostic and decision-making process.
- Assisting the couple during the process of treatment for infertility.
- Evaluating the need for referrals to other resources, such as psychological or pastoral counseling.

Test Yourself

- Define infertility.
- Which test of infertility is normally the first to be done?
- Describe two advanced reproductive technologies.

MENOPAUSE

Your perimenopausal patients will appreciate this tip! Encourage the woman in the perimenopausal period not to be lulled into a false sense of security. Although fertility declines, pregnancy can still occur. The woman in perimenopause should continue to use a reliable form of birth control.

Menopause, the cessation of menses, signals the end of the woman's reproductive capability. The climacteric, as defined in Chapter 3, refers to the gradual changes associated with declining ovarian function that are commonly called "the change of life."

Perimenopause refers to the time before menopause when vasomotor symptoms (hot flashes, night sweats) and irregular menses begin. Menopause is a normal part of the life cycle and is not a disease, although associated symptoms may be distressing and require treatment.

Menopause occurs when the ovaries no longer respond to stimulation from the pituitary. During the perimenopausal period, the woman begins to experience shorter menstrual cycles and irregular bleeding. Although these changes occur normally in response to hormonal changes, all irregular bleeding should be reported to the primary care practitioner for evaluation.

Clinical Manifestations

The perimenopausal woman typically experiences a set of symptoms that are together referred to as the "climacteric syndrome." These symptoms include hot flashes, insomnia, weight gain, bloating, emotional lability, irregular menses, and headache (Bachmann, 2002).

A hot flash is a sudden feeling of warmth or intense heat that may be accompanied by reddening of the skin on the upper body. The duration is anywhere from seconds to several minutes. The average length of symptoms in the perimenopausal woman is 2 years; however, some women experience hot flashes for 5 or more years. Although the physiology is not completely understood, a hot flash is linked to low estrogen levels and periodic surges of LH.

Physical changes associated with hormone depletion include changes to the reproductive organs. The vaginal mucosa thins and becomes pale and dry. Vaginal rugae disappear, and the vaginal walls become smooth. The uterus and ovaries decrease in size. Pelvic support muscles lose tone, and pelvic support disorders may become apparent. The skin loses its elasticity, and dense breast tissue is replaced with adipose tissue.

Decreased bone mineral density is one of the changes that can have life-threatening effects on the menopausal woman. The overall effect of decreased bone mineral density is loss of bone mass, with resulting reduction of bone strength and increased risk for fracture. This systemic condition is called osteoporosis. It is important to know the risk factors for osteoporosis (Box 4-7) because this disease often has no symptoms until a serious bone fracture occurs.

Treatment

The gold standard for prevention and treatment of perimenopausal symptoms as a whole has historically been hormone replacement therapy (HRT). However, recent research is showing the HRT may not be the best option for many women. The Women's Health Initiative (WHI) study was stopped early because of the adverse effects of HRT on women's health. An

BOX 4.7	Risk Factors for Osteoporosis

- Female gender
- Caucasian or Asian ethnicity
- Slender build
- Advanced age
- Estrogen deficiency because of menopause (especially if early or surgically induced)
- Low bone mass density
- Family history of osteoporosis
- Personal history of fracture as an adult
- Smoking
- Excessive alcohol intake
- Low dietary intake of calcium
- Vitamin D deficiency
- Inactive lifestyle
- Use of glucocorticoids
- Use of anticonvulsants

increased risk for coronary heart disease, stroke, venous thromboembolism, pulmonary embolism, and breast cancer was found with HRT therapy and no decrease in cardiovascular disease (one of the focuses of the study). Many health care professionals are advising that HRT be prescribed only for the control (not prevention) of perimenopausal symptoms, and that it be used at the lowest dose possible for the shortest time possible. Benefits of HRT shown by the WHI study are a decreased risk for colorectal cancer and osteoporotic fractures.

Treatment for Hot Flashes and Sweats

Hot flashes and sweats are the most common reasons that the perimenopausal woman seeks medical treatment. To date the most effective therapy for hot flashes continues to be HRT. Hormonal alternatives to HRT include progestins alone, which have been shown to be beneficial in treating hot flashes. Nonhormonal options that show promise include the antihypertensive agent lofexidine; the anticonvulsant gabapentin; and the antidepressants paroxetine and venlafaxine.

Treatment for Osteoporosis

Bone mineral density testing is recommended for postmenopausal women as follows: women at increased risk for osteoporosis should begin screening at age 60 years, and all other women should begin screening at age 65 years. Wallace, Rogers, Keenum, Shah, and Turner (2003) recommend that the primary care practitioner schedule bone mineral density testing with annual mammograms for postmenopausal women.

HRT continues to be beneficial for reducing the risk of osteoporosis and fractures in the peri- and postmenopausal woman. However, there are other treatment options that lower the risk for fractures. These options include raloxifene, calcitonin, and bisphospho-

nates. Calcium and vitamin D supplementation and regular weight-bearing exercise continue to be recommended as preventive measures.

Treatment for Vaginal Atrophy and Dryness

HRT continues to be an effective treatment, although the use of local applications of estrogen-containing vaginal creams, tablets, or suppositories brings relief of symptoms with minimal systemic absorption. The woman for whom estrogen use is contraindicated may benefit from nonestrogenic vaginal lubricants.

Nursing Care

Nurses have a large role to play in health promotion for the perimenopausal and postmenopausal woman. It is important to develop rapport with the woman and to let her know that you are available to talk about her concerns. Reassure the woman of the normality of menopause.

Give the woman factual information on HRT and other therapies. It may be helpful to give her a list of resources that she can read at home. It is important that the woman be informed of the risks and benefits of any therapy so that she can make an informed decision.

There are many nursing interventions that can help the perimenopausal woman. Suggest lifestyle modifications to decrease the discomfort of hot flashes. These include dressing in lightweight clothing and dressing in layers. Regular exercise and setting the thermostat to a lower temperature may also be helpful. Suggest that she avoid spicy foods, caffeine, and alcohol.

Some common sense guidelines to prevent osteoporosis can be helpful as well. Encourage regular weight-bearing activity, such as walking and stair climbing, at least three to four times per week. The postmenopausal woman should continue to take calcium and vitamin D supplements. She should take her calcium supplements with orange juice (or another vitamin C source) and avoid caffeine, which tends to interfere with the absorption of calcium.

Safety instructions can help prevent fractures from falls inside the house. Encourage the postmenopausal woman to have her bed lowered, if possible; to eliminate throw rugs and clutter from the floors; and to use night lights throughout the house. In the bathroom it is helpful to install safety tread and safety rails. Suggest that she keep a cordless or mobile telephone close by to eliminate the temptation to run to answer the phone. All of her slippers and shoes should have tread and should provide traction and stability.

Falls outside the home can be reduced if the woman will take extra precautions after dark. Advise her to use railings whenever possible. She should clear walkways of debris and avoid walking on ice.

FAMILY TEACHING TIPS

Reducing the Discomfort of Menopause

- Wear cotton clothes in layers.
- Avoid caffeine intake (e.g., colas, tea, coffee).
- Explore relaxation activities because stress exacerbates vasomotor symptoms.
- Discuss HRT with your caregiver.
- Consider nutritional supplements as recommended by your primary care practitioner to help reduce vasomotor symptoms.
- Use a water-soluble lubricant before intercourse.
- Nonprescription products, such as Replens and Lubrin, are effective for the relief of vaginal dryness.
- If using an estrogen vaginal cream, apply it at bedtime.
- Perform Kegel exercises to improve pelvic muscle tone.
- Drink at least 5 glasses of water per day. Do not count caffeine-containing drinks as part of this water intake.
- Urinate regularly; do not allow the bladder to become overdistended.
- Practice good hygiene, such as wiping from front to back, after toileting.

Review medications with the woman. She should understand how to take the medication and side effects that should be reported. She should also understand how often she should see the primary care practitioner and what routine screening examinations should be done, such as yearly mammograms and bone density measurements. Family Teaching Tips: Reducing the Discomfort of Menopause lists helpful tips to share with the woman and her family.

Test Yourself

- Define perimenopause.
- Name five symptoms that are part of the climacteric syndrome.
- Describe three things (nonpharmacologic) that the nurse can teach the older woman to do to treat or prevent hot flashes.

KEY POINTS

- Self-awareness of breast characteristics and yearly clinical breast examinations are recommended for women of all ages. Women older than 40 years should have yearly mammograms as well.
- Sexually active women younger than 30 years should have annual Pap smears. The healthy woman older than 30 years should have Pap smears every 2 to 3 years.
- Dysmenorrhea is defined as painful or difficult menses. Premenstrual syndrome (PMS) encompasses a constellation of symptoms that are cyclical in nature and progress with time.
- A classic symptom of endometriosis is cyclic pelvic pain that occurs in conjunction with menses. Therapy is aimed at suppressing ovulation and inducing an artificial menopause to suppress growth of abnormal tissue and relieve symptoms. The nurse's role is to help the woman find pain relief and provide support.
- The major risk factor for the development of pelvic inflammatory disease (PID) is untreated sexually transmitted infections (STIs). Treatment of the woman and her partner with antibiotics is recommended.
- Pelvic support disorders are caused by weakening of the structures that support the pelvic organs. Major risk factors include pregnancy, vaginal delivery, and aging.
- Family planning involves the two components of planning pregnancy and preventing pregnancy. Family planning should include prepregnancy planning, which involves focusing on nutrition and exercise, lifestyle changes, counseling and treatment for chronic illness and genetic disorders, and evaluation of medications.
- Natural methods of contraception do not use hormones or other physical barriers to prevent conception. These methods include abstinence, coitus interruptus, and fertility awareness methods (FAM). Natural methods do not require the use of artificial devices or hormones but require a great deal of education and discipline to be effective.
- Barrier methods provide a physical or chemical barrier or both to prevent pregnancy. These include spermicides, male and female condoms, the diaphragm, and cervical cap. Many barrier methods have the advantage of decreasing the risk for STIs.
- Hormonal methods of contraception include combination oral contraceptives (COCs), progestin-only pills (POPs), hormonal injections, hormonal implants, transdermal patch, and vaginal ring. Hormonal contraceptives are highly effective but do not provide reliable protection against STIs.
- Intrauterine devices (IUDs) are small objects that provide long-term pregnancy protection. They must be inserted by a primary care provider and require removal every few years. They do not provide protection against STIs.
- Female and male sterilization techniques are highly effective, permanent methods of contraception.

⬥ Emergency contraception refers to hormonal methods used to prevent pregnancy after unprotected intercourse.

⬥ Infertility is defined as the inability to conceive after a year of unprotected intercourse. Multiple factors contribute to infertility. Anything that interferes with the sperm and egg meeting or the fertilized egg from traveling to and implanting in the uterus can lead to infertility.

⬥ Evaluation of infertility begins with the least invasive and complex and progresses to the more invasive and complex techniques. All infertility evaluation begins with a thorough history and physical examination of both partners. Usually the first test is a sperm analysis, and the second test is a postcoital examination.

⬥ Treatment of infertility depends upon the identified cause. Therapeutic insemination techniques, surgical techniques to correct structural problems, medication to stimulate ovulation, and advanced reproductive therapies (ART) may all be used in the treatment of infertility.

⬥ If infertility treatment fails, surrogate parenthood, adoption, and childless living are options.

⬥ A couple undergoing evaluation and treatment for infertility may feel guilt, shock, isolation, depression, and stress. It is very stressful on a relationship to perform sexually "on demand," and intercourse often takes on a clinical and mechanical tone, rather than the desired traits of intimacy, love, and support.

⬥ Menopause is a natural part of the life cycle. It is not a disease; however, the associated symptoms may need medication or other interventions.

⬥ Hormone replacement therapy (HRT) used to be the gold standard of treatment for major menopausal-related symptoms; however, recent research has highlighted serious adverse effects that may be associated with HRT.

⬥ Hot flashes, osteoporosis, and vaginal atrophy and dryness are the major symptoms for which women need and desire treatment and nursing care during menopause.

REFERENCES AND SELECTED READINGS

Books and Journals

Alzubaidi, N., & Calis, K. A., & Nelson, L. M. (2003). Dysmenorrhea. In A. C. Sciscione, F. Talavera, A. D. Barnes, F. B. Gaupp, & L. P. Shulman (Eds.), *eMedicine*. Retrieved April 10, 2004, from http://www.emedicine.com/med/topic606.htm

American Cancer Society. (2004). *Detailed guide: Breast cancer*. Cancer Reference Information [online]. Retrieved April 15, 2004, from http://www.cancer.org/docroot/CRI/CRI_2_3x.asp?dt=5

Bachmann, G. (2002). Menopause. In R. K. Zurawin, F. Talavera, G. F. Whitman-Elia, F. B. Gaupp, & L. P. Shulman (Eds.), *eMedicine*. Retrieved April 10, 2004, from http://www.emedicine.com/med/topic3289.htm

Chandran, L. (2004). Menstruation disorders. In E. Alderman, R. Konop, W. Wolfram, P. D. Petry, & M. Strafford (Eds.), *eMedicine*. Retrieved April 15, 2004, from http://www.emedicine.com/ped/topic2781.htm

Cwiak, C., & Zieman, M. (2003). New methods in contraception: A review of their advantages and disadvantages. *Women's Health in Primary Care, 6*(10), 473–478.

Davidson, M. R. (2003). Contraception update: The latest hormonal options. *Clinician Reviews, 13*(6), 53–59.

Fehring, R. J. (2004). The future of professional education in natural family planning. *JOGNN, 33*(2), 34–43.

Garcia, J. E., Nelson, L. M., & Wallach, E. E. (2003). Infertility. In R. K. Zurawin, F. Talavera, A. D. Barnes, F. B. Gaupp, & L. P. Shulman (Eds.), *eMedicine*. Retrieved April 10, 2004, from http://www.emedicine.com/med/topic3535.htm

Hickey, M., & Farquhar, C. M. (2003). Update on treatment of menstrual disorders. *eMJA, 178*(12), 625–629. Retrieved April 15, 2004, from http://www.mja.com.au/public/issues/178_12_160603/hic10854.fm.html

Htay, T. T., Aung, K., Carrick, J., & Papica, R. (2004). Premenstrual dysphoric disorder. R. C. Albucher, F. Talavera, D. Chlmow, H. H. Harsch, & S. Soreff (Eds.), *eMedicine*. Retrieved April 9, 2004, from http://www.emedicine.com/med/topic3357.htm

Hutti, M. H. (2003). New and emerging contraceptive methods: Nurses can help women make wise choices. *AWHONN Lifelines, 7*(1), 32–39.

Katz, A. (Ed.). (2003). Conversations with colleagues: Cervical cancer screening. *AWHONN Lifelines, 7*(6), 512–514.

Kazzi, A. A., & Roberts, R. (2001). Ovarian cysts. In D. A. Stearns, F. Talavera, M. Zwanger, J. Halamka, & W. K. Mallon (Eds.), *eMedicine*. Retrieved April 10, 2004, from http://www.emedicine.com/EMERG/topic352.htm

McCrink, A. (2003). Evaluating the female pelvic floor. *AWHONN Lifelines, 7*(6), 516–522.

Mishell, D. R., Burkman, R. T., Shulman, L. P., Westhoff, C. L., & Wysocki, S. J. (2002). Understanding contraceptive effectiveness. *Dialogues in Contraception, 7*(2), special issue.

Nissl, J. (2003). Healthwise knowledgebase topic: Hormone injections for birth control. Palo Alto Medical Foundation: A Sutter Health Affiliate. J. Melnikow, R. A. Hatcher, & K. Jones (medical reviewers). Retrieved April 10, 2004, from http://www.pamf.org/teen/healthinfo/index.cfm?section=healthinfo&page=article&sgml_id=hw239088

Planned Parenthood Federation of America. (2002). *Fact sheet: Nonoxynol-9: Benefits and risks*. Katharine Dexter McCormick Library (publisher). Retrieved April 9, 2004, from http://www.plannedparenthood.org/library/birthcontrol/020926_non9.html

Planned Parenthood Federation of America. (Undated). *Birth control*. Retrieved April 9, 2004, from http://www.plannedparenthood.org/bc/index.html

Pradhan, A., & Bachmann, G. (2003). Today's therapeutic options for hot flashes: Treatment in the post-women's health initiative era. *Women's Health in Primary Care, 6*(11), 527–533.

Shaw, J. A., & Shaw, H. A. (2002). Menorrhagia. In T. M. Price, F. Talavera, A. D. Barnes, F. B. Gaupp, & L. P. Shulman (Eds.), *eMedicine*. Retrieved April 9, 2004, from http://www.emedicine.com/med/topic1449.htm

Shulman, L. P. (2003, September). Advances in contraception: Choices to improve quality of life [special edition]. *Patient Care for the Nurse Practitioner*, 3–12.

Taylor, D., & Hwang, A. C. (2003). Mifepristone for medical abortion: Exploring a new option for nurse practitioners. *AWHONN Lifelines*, 7(6), 524–529.

Wallace, L. S., Rogers, E. S., Keenum, A. J., Shah, A. R., & Turner, L. W. (2003). Promoting osteoporosis screening in postmenopausal women. *Women's Health in Primary Care*, 6(8), 380–391.

Wilcox, A. J., Dunson, D., & Baird, D. D. (2000). The timing of the "fertile window" in the menstrual cycle: Day specific estimates from a prospective study. *British Medical Journal*, 321(7271):1259–1262.

Websites

Endometriosis
http://www.endocenter.org/
http://www.endometriosis.org/

Ovarian Cysts (Laparoscopic Images)
http://www.pta.net.au/sgeg/ovcyst.htm

Family Planning
www.plannedparenthood.org/

Infertility
http://www.resolve.org/

Osteoporosis
http://www.nof.org/

WORKBOOK

NCLEX-STYLE REVIEW QUESTIONS

1. An adolescent girl asks the nurse when she should have her first "Pap test." How should the nurse reply?

   a. "I don't know. Ask the doctor."

   b. "When you first start having sex."

   c. "As soon as possible and every year thereafter."

   d. "Three years after you first have sex, or age 21, whichever comes first."

2. A 35-year-old female reports very heavy menstrual periods. How does the nurse chart this in the medical record?

   a. "Chief complaint: dysmenorrhea."

   b. "Complains of metrorrhagia."

   c. "Reports amenorrhea."

   d. "Reports menorrhagia."

3. A woman is having severe symptoms of PMS. She asks the nurse what she can do to obtain relief from symptoms. What reply by the nurse is most likely to be helpful?

   a. "Antibiotics are necessary to treat the underlying infection."

   b. "Diuretics tend to be the most helpful medications for PMS treatment."

   c. "Don't worry. The medication the doctor has prescribed will take care of your symptoms."

   d. "In addition to taking medications, stress reduction and regular exercise are beneficial."

4. A woman with a pelvic support disorder reports all of the following. Which statement by the woman should alert the nurse to instruct the woman to come in immediately for examination by a physician.

   a. "My urine is cloudy."

   b. "I forgot to do my Kegel exercises today."

   c. "Every time I cough a little bit of urine comes out."

   d. "I took my pessary out to wash it, and forgot to put it back in."

STUDY ACTIVITIES

1. Develop a 10-minute presentation on considerations a couple should make before deciding on a method of birth control.

2. Explain how natural family planning techniques can be used to enhance the chance that a couple will get pregnant. Why can these methods be used to both prevent and enhance pregnancy?

3. Using the table below, compare natural methods of contraception.

Method	How it Works to Prevent Pregnancy	Special Nursing Considerations

CRITICAL THINKING: What Would You Do?

Apply your knowledge of infertility and its treatments to the following situation.

1. Amanda Rodriguez is a 37-year-old woman who has never before been pregnant. She put off pregnancy to pursue her career as an attorney. Now she and her husband have been trying to conceive for 2 years without success. She has come to the clinic for initial evaluation.

   a. Explain to Amanda what she can expect from today's visit.

   b. If Amanda is experiencing infertility, what type is it?

   c. Amanda confides in you that she thinks God is punishing her for waiting to start a family. She says that she should have tried to have children several years ago when all her friends were having babies. How would you reply to Amanda?

2. The physician tells Amanda that her husband will need to have a semen analysis and then a postcoital test will be done.

   a. Explain both of these procedures to Amanda.

   b. The semen analysis reveals a low sperm count. The physician recommends ICSI. Amanda asks how that procedure is done. How will you answer Amanda?

3. Apply your knowledge of menopause to the following situation: Cindy McFarland, a 52-year-old woman, comes to the clinic because she has been experiencing hot flashes. She tells you that the hot flashes are very intense and seem to last "forever." She says that her sweat drenches her clothes and she is embarrassed to go out in public.

a. Explain the physiology of hot flashes to Cindy.

b. What treatments will the physician likely recommend for Cindy?

c. What other advice do you have for Cindy during this time of her life?

Pregnancy

Fetal Development

Every human being starts out as two separate germ cells, or gametes. The female gamete is the ovum, and the male gamete is the spermatozoon, or sperm for short. At conception the gametes unite to form the cell that eventually becomes the developing fetus. Human development is an ongoing process that begins at the moment of fertilization and continues even after birth. Many factors affect development. Some of these factors can cause abnormalities and birth defects. Others are part of the normal process of human development, such as gender determination. The major processes involved in human fertilization and development are discussed.

CELLULAR PROCESSES

It may seem contradictory to say that cellular division results in multiplication of cells, but that is exactly what happens in several stages of human conception and development. There are two major categories of cells and two major types of cellular division involved in the reproduction of human life.

Types of Cells

Cells are the building blocks of all organs. There are two major types of cells: soma cells, which make up the organs and tissues of the human body, and gametes, also known as germ cells or sex cells, which are found in the reproductive glands only.

The nucleus of each soma cell contains 46 chromosomes, arranged in 23 pairs. Each parent donates one chromosome of every pair. Each chromosome is composed of genes, which are defined as segments of DNA that control hereditary traits. Twenty-two of the 23 pairs of chromosomes are known as autosomes; the remaining pair determines an individual's gender.

The ovum and the sperm are, respectively, the female and male gametes. Each gamete has 23 chromosomes, exactly half of the 46 required chromosomes needed for human development.

Cellular Division

There are two types of cellular division involved in the creation of human life: mitosis and meiosis (Fig. 5-1).

● **Figure 5.1** **(A)** Mitosis of the soma cell. **(B)** Gametogenesis. The various stages of spermatogenesis are indicated on the left; one spermatogonium gives rise to four spermatozoa. On the right, oogenesis is indicated; from each oogonium, one mature ovum and three abortive cells are produced. The chromosomes are reduced to one-half the number characteristic for the general body cells of the species. In humans, the number in the body cells is 46, and that in the mature spermatozoon and secondary oocyte is 23.

Mitosis

Mitosis is the process by which somatic (body) cells give birth to daughter cells. Each daughter cell contains the same number of chromosomes as the parent cell. It is the process by which the body grows and somatic cells are replaced.

Meiosis

Meiosis is the process by which gametes undergo two sequential cellular divisions of the nucleus. It is in this way that the number of chromosomes of the gametes is halved. The formation and development of gametes or germ cells by the process of meiosis is known as **gametogenesis**. Remember, each gamete has only 23 chromosomes, which is half, also known as the haploid number, of the total number of chromosomes required for human cells.

The spermatozoon and the ovum are the male and female germ cells. The ovum undergoes meiosis just before ovulation, and the male germ cell divides in the seminiferous tubules of the testes. A **zygote**, or conceptus, results when an ovum and a spermatozoon unite. The zygote has the full complement of 46 chromosomes (also called the diploid number), arranged in 23 pairs. The process of meiosis occurs in either the testes or the ovaries.

Spermatogenesis. Spermatogenesis begins at puberty in the male. In the testes, primary spermatocytes, each containing 46 chromosomes, undergo the first meiotic division, which results in two secondary spermatocytes, each with 23 chromosomes. These spermatocytes then undergo a second meiotic division, resulting in a final number of four spermatids that contain the haploid number of chromosomes (23). The spermatids undergo a change in form to become mature spermatozoa but undergo no further meiotic divisions.

Oogenesis. In the ovaries, oogenesis begins before birth but is not fully complete until the childbearing years. At birth, the female ovaries contain primary oocytes, which have completed the prophase stage of the first meiotic division. The completion of the first meiotic division occurs before ovulation. The two cells that result from this division are not identical. They are called the secondary oocyte and the first polar body. The secondary oocyte contains the haploid number of chromosomes. The first polar body soon disintegrates because it contains almost no cytoplasm. The secondary oocyte begins its second meiotic division at ovulation but does not complete the process unless it is fertilized by a sperm.

Gender Determination

Gender determination occurs at the time of fertilization. Because the spermatozoon can have either an X or a Y chromosome, it is the male that is responsible for fetal gender determination. The Y chromosome is smaller

● **Figure 5.2** Inheritance of gender. Each ovum contains 22 autosomes and an X chromosome. Each spermatozoon (sperm) contains 22 autosomes and either an X chromosome or a Y chromosome. The gender of the zygote is determined at the time of fertilization by the combination of the sex chromosomes of the sperm (either X or Y) and the ovum (X).

and contains mainly genes for maleness. The female ovum always contains an X chromosome, which carries several genes for other traits besides femaleness.

This is worth noting! Many couples mistakenly believe that they can influence sex determination by using certain sexual positions, ingesting particular foods before intercourse, or timing sex to occur at specific times during the menstrual cycle. These beliefs are often rooted in folklore. Teach in a nonthreatening and respectful manner that cultural or family practices designed to control sex determination are not grounded in scientific principles.

A female fetus (XX) will develop when the ovum unites with a spermatozoon with an X chromosome. Conversely, fertilization with a spermatozoon that contains a Y chromosome will produce a male fetus (XY) (Fig. 5-2). Research states that there is an approximately 50-50 chance of either occurrence.

DEVELOPMENTAL STAGES OF PREGNANCY

The three different stages of human development during pregnancy are:

1. Pre-embryonic
2. Embryonic
3. Fetal

The pre-embryonic stage begins at fertilization and lasts through the end of the 2nd week after fertilization. The embryonic stage begins approximately 2 weeks after fertilization and ends at the conclusion of the 8th week after fertilization. By the end of the embryonic stage, all of the organ systems have begun development and the conceptus is distinctly human in form. The fetal stage begins at 9 weeks after fertilization and ends at birth. However, birth is not the end of human development. Human development is an ongoing process of transformation that begins with fertilization and continues through the teenage years and beyond. Figure 5-3 illustrates pre-embryonic, embryonic, and fetal development.

When discussing development during pregnancy in this chapter, time references are measured in the number of weeks after fertilization, not weeks of gestation. Table 5-1 shows the corresponding time frame for postfertilization and gestational dates.

Pre-embryonic Stage

The pre-embryonic stage begins with fertilization and encompasses the first 2 weeks thereafter. Cellular division and implantation occur during this stage of development.

TABLE 5.1	Comparison of Gestational Age to Fetal Developmental Age	
Stage of Development	Weeks After Fertilization	Gestational Age
Pre-embryonic	0–2 weeks	3–4 weeks' gestation
Embryonic	3–8 weeks	5–10 weeks' gestation
Fetal	9–38 weeks	11–40 weeks' gestation

Fertilization

Fertilization, also called conception, occurs when the sperm penetrates the ovum. The ovum is receptive to fertilization for approximately 24 to 48 hours after release from the ovary, and the sperm are viable for 24 to 72 hours after ejaculation into the female reproductive system. During the act of sexual intercourse, the man ejaculates approximately 300 to 600 million sperm. However, only one sperm will fertilize the mature ovum.

A   B   C

D   E

● *Figure 5.3* Pre-embryronic, embryronic, and fetal development. (**A**) Blastocyst 7 to 8 days after fertilization; (**B**) 4-week embryo; (**C**) 5-week embryo; (**D**) 6-week embryo; (**E**) 12- to 15-week fetus.

After the sperm are ejaculated into the vagina, they travel through the cervix, into the uterus, and then into the fallopian tube. Prostaglandins in the semen increase smooth muscle contractions of the uterus, thus facilitating the transport of sperm. Conception usually occurs when the ovum is in the ampulla (the outermost half) of the fallopian tube.

You do the math! If sperm are able to fertilize the ovum for as long as 72 hours after ejaculation, fertilization could potentially happen if coitus occurs 3 days before ovulation. Because the ovum can be fertilized only to a maximum of 48 hours after ovulation, fertilization can occur as long as 2 days after ovulation. Thus, the window of opportunity for conception to occur is between 3 days before until 2 days after ovulation.

Once a single sperm has penetrated the thick membrane that surrounds the ovum, called the zona pellucida, a chemical reaction occurs that causes the ovum to become impenetrable to other sperm. The chromosomes of the sperm merge with those of the ovum to complete the diploid number of 46.

Cellular Reproduction

The resulting single cell is now referred to as the zygote. The zygote begins the process of mitotic division known as **cleavage**. As the cells divide, the zygote transforms from one cell into two cells, and then each cell further divides to form a total of four cells. Each of these cells in turn divides to form a total of eight cells and so on. Each new cell contains the diploid number of chromosomes (46) beginning with the first mitotic division. All the while that cleavage is occurring, the zygote is traveling through the fallopian tube toward the uterus.

At about 3 days after fertilization, the total cell count has reached 32. The solid cell cluster is now referred to as a **morula**. The morula continues its journey toward the uterine cavity while cleavage and transformation of the cells continue. At about 5 days after fertilization, the dividing cell mass has developed a hollow, fluid-filled core and is now called a **blastocyst**. The blastocyst has an outer layer of cells, the trophoblast; a fluid-filled hollow core; and an inner cell mass. The trophoblast will go on to become the structures that nourish and protect the developing conceptus. By the end of the pre-embryonic period, the inner cell mass has become the embryonic disk, which will eventually become the fetus.

Implantation

On about the 6th day after fertilization, the trophoblast develops finger-like projections that help the blastocyst to burrow itself into the nutrient-rich endometrium. By the 10th day, the blastocyst is completely buried in the uterine lining. During the process of implantation, small cavities, called lacunae, develop around the blastocyst. Maternal blood pools in the lacunae, which allows nutrients from the woman to be exchanged for metabolic wastes from the blastocyst. The lacunae eventually become the intervillous spaces of the placenta. The tiny blastocyst begins to produce human chorionic gonadotropin (hCG), which signals the corpus luteum to continue producing progesterone to maintain the endometrial lining and the pregnancy.

Here is a teaching opportunity! Some women have a small amount of bleeding during the time of implantation, which is known as implantation bleeding. This bleeding can be mistaken for a scanty menstrual period and can lead to miscalculation of fetal age.

At this point in the woman's menstrual cycle, the endometrium is ready to support the pregnancy, and is now referred to as the **decidua**. The woman has not yet missed her menstrual period and is unaware of her pregnancy. Figure 5-4 illustrates the transport of the ovum from ovulation to fertilization and the transport of the zygote from fertilization to implantation.

Test Yourself

- Gametogenesis occurs by which type of cellular division: mitosis or meiosis?

- A male fetus carries which two sex chromosomes?

- What is the name of the single cell that results from fertilization?

Embryonic Stage

The embryonic stage lasts from the end of the 2nd week after fertilization until the end of the 8th week. This is also the time when the woman misses her first menstrual period. The developing conceptus is now called an **embryo**. By the end of the embryonic stage, all of the organ systems and major structures are present, and the embryo is fully recognizable as human in form.

During the embryonic period, the cells of the embryo multiply and tissues begin to assume specific functions, a process known as differentiation. It is

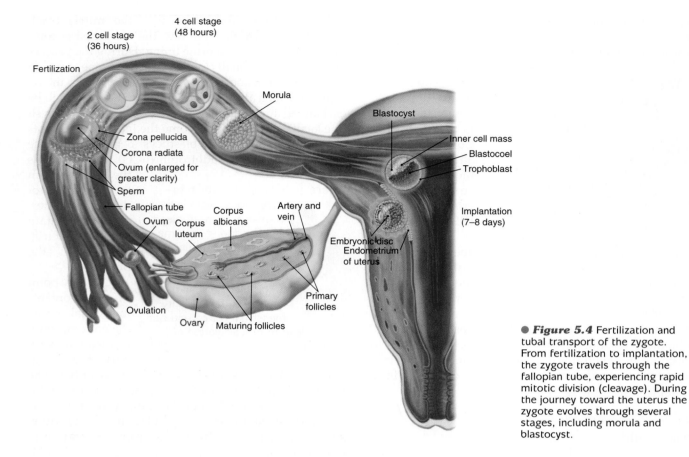

● **Figure 5.4** Fertilization and tubal transport of the zygote. From fertilization to implantation, the zygote travels through the fallopian tube, experiencing rapid mitotic division (cleavage). During the journey toward the uterus the zygote evolves through several stages, including morula and blastocyst.

through differentiation that tissues form rudimentary organs and organ systems.

In the 3rd week, three germ layers develop in the embryo. These layers are the ectoderm, mesoderm, and endoderm. The germ layers will become the different organs and tissues of the developing embryo. The ectoderm, which is the outer layer of cells, develops to form skin, hair, nails, and the nervous system. The mesoderm is the middle layer, which will form the skeletal, muscular, and circulatory systems. Lastly, the endoderm, which is the inner layer, will form the glands, lungs, and urinary and digestive tracts (Table 5-2).

Advise the woman who is trying to become pregnant to be very careful! Exposure to a **teratogen** (any substance or process that can interfere with normal development and lead to birth defects) during the embryonic stage produces the greatest damaging effects because it is during this time that cells are rapidly dividing and differentiating into specific body structures. (See "Teratogens and the Fetus.")

TABLE 5.2	**Body Structures Developing From the Primary Germ Cells**
Germ Layer	**Structure Formation**
Ectoderm	Skin
	Nervous system
	Nasal passages
	Crystalline lens of the eye
	Pharynx
	Mammary glands
	Salivary glands
Mesoderm	Muscles
	Circulatory system
	Bones
	Reproductive system
	Connective tissue
	Kidneys
	Ureters
Endoderm	Alimentary tract
	Respiratory tract
	Bladder
	Pancreas
	Liver

Fetal Stage

The fetal stage is from the beginning of the 9th week after fertilization and continues until birth. At this time, the developing human is referred to as the **fetus**. During the fetal stage, there is additional growth and maturation of the organs and body systems. At the beginning of this stage, the fetus is about 50 mm long and weighs about 8 grams. By the end of the fetal stage, the fetus will be about 36 cm long and weigh approximately 3,400 grams. Box 5-1 summarizes and illustrates the highlights of growth during the embryonic and fetal stages.

Test Yourself

- What is the name of the stage of development that occurs during weeks 3 to 8?
- List the three germ layers in the embryo.
- At the beginning of the fetal stage, how long is the fetus and how much does it weigh?

DEVELOPMENT OF SUPPORTIVE STRUCTURES

Fetal membranes surround the fetus in a protective sac filled with fluid that allows for protection and unrestricted growth. The fetus receives its nutrition from the woman's body, which also removes the metabolic wastes created by the fetus. This exchange is done at the placenta. The fetus and the placenta are connected by the umbilical cord. Table 5-3 summarizes characteristics of the supportive structures.

Fetal Membranes

A small space begins to form between the inner cell mass that will become the embryo and the tissue that has embedded into the endometrial lining. This space will become the amniotic cavity in which the fetus will grow. The amniotic cavity begins to develop around 9 days after conception. The amniotic cavity is surrounded by the **amnion**. The amnion is a thick fibrous lining, made up of several layers, that helps to protect the fetus and forms the inner part of the sac in which the fetus grows. This sac is filled with amniotic fluid. Lying against the amnion toward the exterior of the blastocyst is the **chorion**. The chorion is a second layer of thick fibrous tissue that surrounds the amnion. The amnion and chorion are not fused but lie in close contact with each other (Fig. 5-5). Together they make up the fetal membranes.

TABLE 5.3	Characteristics of Supportive Structures
Supportive Structure	**Characteristics**
Placenta	2–3 cm thick, thickness established by 20 weeks 15–20 cm in diameter 500–600 grams in weight Made up of 15–20 lobes called cotyledons
Amniotic fluid	About 1 liter at term Filtered and replaced every 3 hours Pale yellow to straw colored
Umbilical cord	50 cm long and 2 cm wide Blood flow through cord is about 400 mL/minute Two arteries, which carry deoxygenated blood to placenta from fetus One vein, which carries oxygen and nourishment from placenta to fetus Formed from the amnion

At the end of the 2nd week after fertilization, **chorionic villi** begin to appear on the chorion. These are finger-like projections that extend out from the chorion, giving it a rough appearance. Around 15 to 20 days after fertilization, cells in the chorionic villi form

● **Figure 5.5** The embryo is floating in amniotic fluid surrounded by the protective fetal membranes (amnion and chorion).

Labels: Uterine fundus, Amnion, Chorion, Umbilical cord, Placenta, Cervix

| BOX 5.1 | **Embryonic and Fetal Development** |

End of 4 Weeks

4 weeks

Chorionic villi form
The embryo is C-shaped
Length: 0.75 to 1 cm
Weight: 400 mg
Arms and legs are bud-like structures.
Rudimentary eyes, ears, and nose are discernible.
Foundations for nervous system, genitourinary
  system, skin, bones, and lungs are formed.

End of 8 Weeks

8 weeks

Length: 2.5 to 3 cm. (1 inch)
Weight: 8 grams
The head is disproportionately large as a result of
  brain development.
The heart, with a septum and valves, is beating
  rhythmically.
The fingers and toes are distinct and separated.
Sex differentiation begins.
Organogenesis is complete.

End of 12 Weeks

12 weeks

Length: 8 cm (3 inches)
Weight: 25 grams
Placenta is complete.
Divisions of the brain begin to develop.
The face is well formed.
The eyes are widely spaced and fused.
Heartbeat is audible by Doppler.
Kidney secretion has begun.
Spontaneous movements occur (may not yet be
  discernible by the woman).
Sex is discernible by outward appearance.

End of 16 Weeks

16 weeks

Length: 10 to 17 cm
Weight: 55 to 120 grams
Lungs are fully shaped.
Fetus swallows amniotic fluid.
Skeletal structure is identifiable.
Downy lanugo hair present on body.
Liver and pancreas are functioning.
Sex can be determined by ultrasound.

End of 20 Weeks

20 weeks

Length: 25 cm
Weight: 220 grams
Eyebrows and scalp hair are present.
Lanugo covers the entire body.
Vernix caseosa begins to form.
Heart sounds can be heard with a fetoscope.
Fetal movements are felt by the woman.

End of 24 Weeks

25 weeks

Length: 28 to 36 cm
Weight: 550 grams
Eyelids are now open.

BOX 5.1 (continued)	Embryonic and Fetal Development

Pupils are capable of reacting to light.
Active production of lung surfactant begins.
Exhibits a startle reflex.
Skin is red and wrinkled, with little subcutaneous fat.
Vernix caseosa covers the skin.
May survive if born in a facility with a fully equipped neonatal intensive care unit (NICU).

End of 28 Weeks

29 weeks

Length: 35 to 38 cm
Weight: 1,200 grams
Respiratory system is developed enough to provide gaseous exchange; however, the fetus needs care in a NICU in order to survive.
Adipose tissue begins to accumulate.
Male: The testes begin to descend into the scrotal sac.
Female: Clitoris is prominent and labia majora are small and do not cover the labia minora.

End of 32 Weeks

34 weeks

Length: 38 to 43 cm
Weight: 1,600 grams

The lungs are not yet fully developed, but the fetus usually does well, if born at this time.
Active Moro reflex is present.
Steady weight gain occurs.
Male: Testes descend into the scrotum. The scrotal sac has few rugae.

End of 36 Weeks

37 weeks

Length: 42 to 48 cm
Weight: 1,800 to 2,700 grams
Lanugo begins to thin.
Sole of the foot has few creases.
Birth position is usually assumed (vertex, head down).

End of 40 Weeks (Full Term)
Length: 48 to 52 cm
Weight: 3,000 grams
Vernix caseosa is evident in body folds.
Lanugo remains on the shoulders and upper back only.
Creases cover at least two thirds of the surface of the sole of the foot.
Female: The labia majora are well developed.

Adapted from: Pillitteri, A. (2003). *Maternal and child health nursing: Care of the childbearing and childrearing family* (4th ed.). Philadelphia: Lippincott Williams & Wilkins; Mattson, S., & Smith, J. E. (Eds.). (2000). *Core curriculum for maternal–newborn nursing.* AWHONN publication (2nd ed.). Philadelphia: WB Saunders; Reeder, S. J., Martin, L. L., & Koniak-Griffin, D. (1996). *Maternity nursing: Family, newborn, and women's health care* (18th ed.). Philadelphia: Lippincott-Raven; The Visible Embryo website, http://www.visembryo.com.

arterial-capillary-venous networks, which become fetal blood vessels. These capillaries pick up oxygen and nutrients from maternal blood that enters the intervillous spaces in exchange for waste products and carbon dioxide from the developing embryo.

Around the 8th week, some of the chorionic villi disintegrate, leaving a large area of the chorion that is smooth. The chorionic villi that remain increase in number and size and further branch out. The chorionic villi eventually become the fetal part of the placenta where the exchange of nutrients and wastes occurs.

Amniotic Fluid

The amniotic cavity is filled with a specialized fluid called **amniotic fluid**. Amniotic fluid serves four main functions for the fetus: physical protection, temperature regulation, provision of unrestricted movement, and symmetrical growth. Amniotic fluid is produced throughout the pregnancy by the fetal membranes. It also provides a medium that allows for fetal evaluation because it collects substances from the fetal alimentary, renal, and respiratory tracts. It is produced from maternal blood, fetal urine, and secretions from the fetal respiratory tract; 98% to 99% of amniotic fluid is water, whereas the remaining 1% to 2% is made up of electrolytes, creatinine, urea, glucose, hormones, fetal cells, lanugo (fine downy hair), and vernix caseosa (a cheesy substance that protects fetal skin).

The amniotic fluid acts as a cushion around the fetus. It protects the fetus from injury if the mother is bumped or falls. It helps to maintain a constant temperature around the fetus because the fetus is not mature enough to regulate its own temperature. Amniotic fluid allows for free movement of the fetus and aids in symmetrical growth. Lastly, it is a fluid source that the fetus drinks and then urinates. The swallowed amniotic fluid is absorbed by the fetal intestines and then urinated back into the amniotic sac.

The fetus also takes in and releases amniotic fluid when it practices fetal breathing movements. During the fetal exhalation, surfactant is released into the amniotic fluid. Surfactant is produced by the fetal lungs starting in the 28th week and helps to decrease the surface tension in the alveoli. Sampling of the amniotic fluid can help to determine if the fetal lungs are mature enough for birth.

The shed hair, epithelial cells, and sebaceous secretions from the fetus are swallowed by the fetus and help to make up the meconium that gathers in the fetal intestinal system. This is the first bowel movement the infant has after birth. If during pregnancy or labor the infant becomes stressed, the anal sphincter may relax and release meconium into the amniotic fluid. This action will cause the fluid to be stained a green color. Meconium staining of the amniotic fluid is said to have occurred if the amniotic fluid is green, instead of clear, at delivery. During the normal fetal process of swallowing and inhaling amniotic fluid in utero, the thick meconium particles can become trapped in the fetal lungs. The newborn is then at risk for meconium aspiration pneumonia.

Did you know? You can learn a lot from amniotic fluid! A procedure called amniocentesis can be performed to obtain a sample of amniotic fluid. The fluid can then be tested for surfactant, which reveals whether or not the lungs are mature enough to support respiration outside of the womb. The fluid can also be obtained for genetic testing because it contains fetal cells.

Placenta

The placenta is the organ that sustains and nourishes the growing pregnancy. The placenta has three main functions: to provide for the transfer and exchange of substances, to act as a barrier to certain substances, and to function as an endocrine gland by producing hormones. The placenta begins to develop during the 5th week after fertilization at the site of implantation. Most of the placenta is of embryonic origin, but about 20% is maternal in origin.

The placenta is made up of many lobes, or sections, called cotyledons. Each cotyledon consists of two or more main stem villi and their branches. A main stem villus consists of a branch of the umbilical vein and umbilical artery that branches out into the intervillous space. Maternal blood, from endometrial arteries, pools in the intervillous spaces.

The placenta is the exchange site for nutrients and wastes between the fetal and maternal circulatory systems. The maternal blood supply brings oxygen, water, electrolytes, vitamins, and glucose to the placenta. These nutrients are exchanged to the fetal circulation and taken to the fetus. The fetal circulation brings carbon dioxide, carbon monoxide, urea, and uric acid to be removed by the maternal circulatory system. These substances are carried across the placental membrane through simple or facilitated diffusion and active transport at the level of the chorionic villi.

The fetus receives passive immunity from the mother by transfer of maternal antibodies. Maternal antibodies to diphtheria, smallpox, and measles are transferred to the fetus. The fetus does not receive immunity to rubella, cytomegalovirus (CMV), varicella, or measles. If the woman is exposed to these infections during her pregnancy the fetus will be exposed and fetal infection may ensue. Some diseases are teratogenic (able to cause birth defects) to the fetus.

Don't pass up this teaching opportunity! Explain to the woman that she should consider that everything she takes in will pass to the fetus. Teach her to check with her primary care provider before taking any substance that is not specifically ordered for her. This warning extends to immunizations, as well.

The placenta acts as a barrier to some medications and hormones that are in the maternal blood supply. However, not all medications and substances are stopped by the placental barrier. Many of these substances cross over to the fetus.

The placenta also secretes hormones that help to sustain the pregnancy. These include progesterone, estrogen, human placental lactogen (hPL), and human chorionic gonadotropin (hCG). Progesterone is necessary to maintain the nutrient-rich endometrial lining (decidua). It also functions to keep the myometrium quiet, so that contractions do not occur prematurely, leading to loss of the pregnancy. Estrogen functions to provide a rich blood supply to the decidua and placenta. The main function of hCG is to sustain the corpus luteum at the beginning of the pregnancy. The main function of hPL is to regulate the glucose that is available for the fetus.

The well-being of the fetus is dependent upon free access of nutrients from the mother to the infant. Anomalies of the placenta or maternal–placental circulation impede fetal nourishment, which may lead to fetal growth restriction or death. Intrauterine growth restriction (IUGR) indicates fetal growth that has been slowed for some reason, resulting in a fetus that is smaller than expected for gestational age. IUGR can have many causes. Box 5-2 summarizes some of these common causes.

CULTURAL SNAPSHOT

Certain ethnic groups commonly produce offspring that are smaller than others. The fetuses of these ethnic groups are not referred to as IUGR. It is important to take into account the ethnicity and stature of both the mother and the father when evaluating an infant for IUGR.

Maternal hypertension, pregnancy-induced hypertension (PIH), or infectious agents can cause areas of infarction and subsequent calcification in the placenta. These areas lead to a decreased surface area, which decreases the amount of nutrients that can be delivered to the fetus at a given time. Vasoconstriction caused by hypertension, smoking, or illicit drug use also decreases the flow of blood to the fetus, which can lead to IUGR.

BOX 5.2	Common Causes of Intrauterine Growth Restriction (IUGR)

- Chromosomal abnormalities
- Fetal infection
- Placental infarcts
- Maternal nutritional deficiencies
- Maternal hypertension
- Pregnancy-induced hypertension (PIH)
- Maternal renal disease
- Maternal smoking
- Maternal illegal drug use
- Toxin/teratogen exposure
- Multifetal pregnancy

Umbilical Cord

The umbilical cord extends from the umbilicus of the fetus to the fetal surface of the placenta. In the cord are two arteries that bring deoxygenated blood from the fetus to the placenta and one vein that carries oxygenated and nourished blood from the placenta to the fetus. These three vessels are surrounded by a connective tissue called **Wharton's jelly,** which is a clear gelatinous substance that gives support to the cord and helps prevent compression of the cord, which could impair blood flow to the fetus.

Test Yourself

- The fetal membranes are composed of what two main structures?
- Name two functions of amniotic fluid.
- List three hormones produced by the placenta.

FETAL AND PLACENTAL CIRCULATION

Fetal Circulation

Fetal circulation differs from the pattern of human circulation that is present after birth. While in utero, the fetus is dependent upon the maternal circulation for its oxygenation, and the fetus does not use its lungs to oxygenate blood. Because the level of oxygen that is in the fetus' bloodstream is lower than maternal levels, fetal circulation aids in streaming oxygenated blood from the placenta to the major organs, especially the brain, liver, and kidneys. Fetal circulation is possible because of three major shunts that are present in the fetus but that close shortly after birth. These shunts are the ductus venosus, foramen ovale, and the ductus arteriosus.

Fetal blood flows to the placenta via the umbilical arteries. Each umbilical artery serves one half of the placenta. The arteries branch off into main stem chorionic villi that then branch down toward the decidua basalis in the intervillous spaces. The exchange of oxygen and nutrients from the woman's bloodstream for waste products from the fetus occurs at this level.

Fetal blood returns to the fetus from the placenta via the umbilical vein. In the umbilical vein, the saturation of fetal blood with oxygen is about 80%. The umbilical vein enters the fetus at the site that will be the umbilicus after birth. Approximately half of the oxygenated blood circulates from the umbilical vein to the liver, and the other half of oxygen-rich blood is shunted past the liver and flows directly into the inferior vena cava by way of the **ductus venosus**. The oxygenated blood in the inferior vena cava mixes with deoxygenated blood in the inferior vena cava that is returning to the heart from the lower limbs, abdomen, and pelvis, so that the oxygen saturation of the blood entering the right atrium is about 67%.

The majority of the blood in the right atrium is directed into the left atrium via the **foramen ovale**. The foramen ovale is a hole that connects the right and left atria so the majority of oxygenated blood can quickly pass into the left side of the fetal heart and be sent to the brain and the rest of the fetal body. Blood entering the right atrium from the superior vena cava is mostly deoxygenated. In the right atrium, this blood mixes with some of the well-oxygenated blood from the inferior vena cava, and this mixed blood enters the right ventricle, where it is then pumped to the fetal lungs via the pulmonary trunk.

In utero the fetus does not oxygenate its own blood in the lungs; therefore, blood supplied to the fetal lungs is for nourishment of the tissues only. The lungs are filled with fetal lung fluid and collapsed, which leads to high resistance. Because of this resistance, only 5% to 10% of the blood in the pulmonary artery enters the fetal lungs. The remainder of blood coming from the right ventricle enters the **ductus arteriosus**. The ductus arteriosus is a fetal shunt that links the pulmonary artery with the aorta.

In the left atrium the oxygenated blood is mixed with some deoxygenated blood that is returning to the heart from the lungs. The blood then travels to the left ventricle, where it is pumped to the aorta. The higher oxygenated blood from the ascending aorta is sent to the heart, head, and upper limbs by way of the aortic arch branch. The low oxygenated blood from the pulmonary artery enters the aorta via the ductus arteriosus below the aortic arch branch, which supplies the head and upper limbs with the highest oxygenated blood.

Blood in the abdominal aorta divides so that half of the blood supply returns to the placenta for reoxygenation while the other half goes to nourish the viscera and lower half of the body. The internal iliac arteries branch off to form the two umbilical arteries. The umbilical arteries then carry deoxygenated blood and waste products back to the placenta, which completes the fetal circulation circuit (Fig. 5-6).

At birth, when fetal blood stops being shunted to the placenta for oxygenation, rapid physiologic changes occur to allow the newborn to oxygenate his own blood by his lungs. After birth the ductus venosus, ductus arteriosus, and the umbilical vein and arteries constrict and eventually form ligaments, which remain present for the rest of the infant's life. It is possible for the ductus arteriosus to remain open, especially in premature infants or infants with hypoxia. When this shunt remains open, it is called a patent ductus arteriosus; medications or surgery may be required to close the duct. Refer to Chapter 13 for a detailed discussion of the circulatory changes that occur in the newborn.

Placental Circulation

The uterine arteries supply the uterus with maternal blood. The blood is then carried to the intervillous spaces by endometrial arteries, also known as spiral arteries. In the intervillous spaces, maternal blood flows around the chorionic villi, where nutrients and oxygen from the maternal circulation are transferred by diffusion and active transport across a thin membrane into the fetal circulation. Likewise, fetal wastes diffuse into the maternal bloodstream. Blood leaves the intervillous spaces by the endometrial veins and returns to the maternal circulatory system.

Test Yourself

- Name the three fetal shunts.
- Explain how the ductus arteriosus and foreman ovale aid the fetus in quickly getting oxygen-enriched blood to the tissues.
- By what processes do nutrients, oxygen, and wastes transfer between the pregnant woman's blood and fetal blood?

SPECIAL CONSIDERATIONS OF FETAL DEVELOPMENT

Teratogens and the Fetus

As described earlier in this chapter, teratogens are substances that cause birth defects. The severity of the defect depends upon when during development the conceptus is exposed to the teratogen (i.e., what body systems are developing at the time of exposure) and the particular teratogenic agent to which the fetus is exposed.

Effects of Teratogens on the Developing Fetus

During the pre-embryonic stage, exposure to a teratogen has an all-or-nothing effect. Either the exposure will cause death of the zygote, or there will be no effect because there is no connection between the maternal blood supply and the zygote.

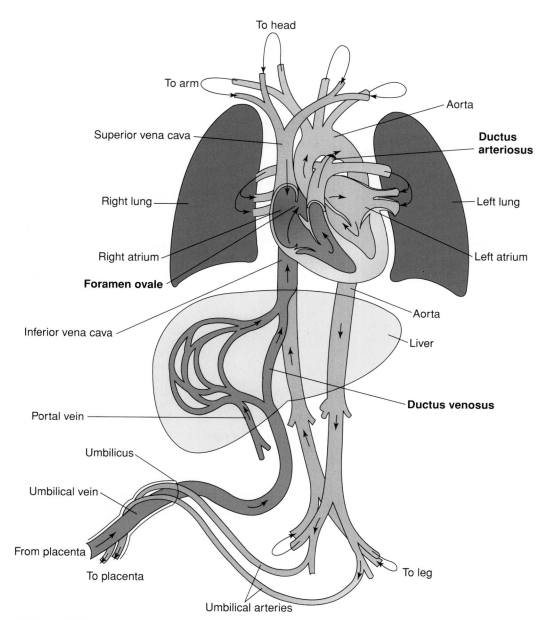

To head

To arm

Superior vena cava

Aorta

Ductus arteriosus

Right lung

Left lung

Right atrium

Left atrium

Foramen ovale

Inferior vena cava

Aorta

Liver

Ductus venosus

Portal vein

Umbilicus

Umbilical vein

From placenta

To placenta

To leg

Umbilical arteries

● **Figure 5.6** Fetal circulation. Arrows indicate the path of blood. The umbilical vein carries oxygen-rich blood from the placenta to the liver and through the ductus venosus. From there it is carried to the inferior vena cava to the right atrium of the heart. Some of the blood is shunted through the foramen ovale to the left side of the heart where it is routed to the brain and upper extremities. The rest of the blood travels down to the right ventricle and through the pulmonary artery. A small portion of the blood travels to the non-functioning lungs, while the remaining blood is shunted through the ductus arteriosus into the aorta to supply the rest of the body.

Exposure to a teratogen during the embryonic stage produces the greatest damaging effects. It is during this time that development of the primary structure and function of organs and tissues is initiated. Developing organs and body systems are highly susceptible to teratogens, and major abnormalities can result. Table 5-4 lists structures commonly affected by teratogen exposure during the embryonic period. Because the central nervous system (CNS) develops

continuously throughout pregnancy, these structures are always vulnerable to teratogens.

Exposure to a teratogen during the fetal stage will have less of an effect on the fetus than exposure during the embryonic period. The effect of a teratogen during this stage may cause physiologic defects and minor structural abnormalities. The CNS and brain continue to be susceptible to damage from teratogens during the fetal period.

TABLE 5.4	Structures Commonly Affected by Teratogens During the Embryonic Period

Week of Development (# of weeks after fertilization) in Which Exposure Occurs	Structures Commonly Affected
3	Heart and central nervous system (CNS)
4	Lip, heart, arm, leg, CNS
5	Heart, eye, arm, leg, CNS
6	CNS, heart, ear, teeth
7	CNS, ear, teeth, palate, heart
8	CNS, ear, palate, heart, external genitalia

TABLE 5.5	Common Teratogens and Associated Effects

Teratogen	Possible Effect
Medications	
Dilantin	Cleft palate
Chemotherapy agents	Major congenital malformations, especially of the CNS
Tetracycline	Damage to developing dental and osseous tissue
Alcohol	Fetal alcohol syndrome (FAS) with facial defects, low birth weight, affects brain
Infectious agents	
Varicella	Fetal varicella syndrome, which ranges in severity from generalized multiorgan damage to isolated defects, such as incomplete limb development or skin scarring
Rubella (German measles)	Cataracts, deafness, and cardiac malformations
CMV	Hearing loss, microcephaly
Environmental agents	
Mercury	Neurologic damage, blindness
Radiation	Congenital malformations, mental retardation (seen in large amounts of ionizing radiation)

Types of Teratogenic Agents

Teratogens usually fall into one of three categories: an ingested, infectious, or environmental substance. Table 5-5 summarizes some of the common teratogens and their effects.

Your sensitivity can make a big difference! Guilt is a common feeling in mothers whose infants are born with a birth defect. Many defects happen before the woman knows she is pregnant. Avoid statements that imply blame. For example don't say, "You shouldn't have been around x-rays while you were pregnant."

Ingested Teratogens. Most substances ingested by the pregnant woman pass to the fetus from the maternal bloodstream through the placenta and then into the fetal circulation. Commonly ingested teratogens include prescription medications, illicit drugs, and alcohol. Some medications may be therapeutic for the mother but also have teratogenic properties. For example, phenytoin (Dilantin) is therapeutic for preventing seizures in the mother but is also known to cause cleft palate and other abnormalities in the fetus. In such a circumstance, the risk to the mother must be weighed against the risk to the developing fetus. Not all medications are teratogenic. Acetaminophen (Tylenol) is an example of a medication that, when taken as directed, is nonteratogenic. Some medications, such as heparin, are known to be unable to cross the placental barrier and thus are safe to use during pregnancy.

In the 1950s many pregnant women were prescribed thalidomide to help control morning sickness. Thalidomide was discovered to cause limb deformities in the infants who were exposed to it in utero. Thalidomide use during pregnancy was discontinued when the teratogenic effects became known.

One of the fetus' main body systems affected throughout the embryonic and fetal period is the brain and CNS. Alcohol and illicit drugs such as marijuana, cocaine, and heroin are known to affect the CNS. Infants exposed to these substances during pregnancy may be born addicted to the substance to which they were exposed. Therefore, ingestion of these substances is strongly discouraged during pregnancy.

Infectious Teratogens. If the pregnant woman develops an infection during her pregnancy, the infection can pass to the fetus and affect fetal development. Some common infections that are known to have

A PERSONAL GLIMPSE

The worrying began when I found out I was pregnant with my oldest child. We hadn't been officially trying to get pregnant, and so right away I started thinking about all the things I had ingested while already pregnant. I was a 3-cup-a-day coffee drinker; I had taken several doses of Tylenol for headaches; and I remembered celebrating my birthday with a few glasses of wine. To top it all off, I hadn't been taking prenatal vitamins. I started panicking about the harm I had caused my developing baby. I immediately stopped drinking caffeine completely (which gave me very bad headaches); swore off wine for the duration; avoided taking any kind of medication for pain; never missed a day taking prenatal vitamins; and avoided eating fish, hot dogs, and lunch meat (I had heard that these foods were bad to eat during pregnancy). I was also concerned about microwave rays (and stopped using the microwave completely); cats and cat litter; gardening; being around my friends' children (they might have some lurking virus); and mold in the house. I was starting to drive my husband and myself crazy.

At my first prenatal appointment, I talked with the staff at my primary care provider's office. They gave me a brochure that listed things to avoid completely during pregnancy; things to limit during pregnancy; and things that were OK during pregnancy. It also contained practical advice for maintaining a healthy home environment during pregnancy and child rearing. I remained careful during my pregnancy, but I learned to relax a bit more and just use common sense.

Allison

LEARNING OPPORTUNITY: How can the nurse help the woman of childbearing age be aware of possible teratogens without unduly scaring her? How should the nurse advise the woman who is very worried that she may have done something to harm her unborn child before she was aware of the pregnancy?

teratogenic effects include varicella, cytomegalovirus (CMV), and rubella.

Environmental Teratogens. The pregnant woman may be exposed to substances in the environment that can have a teratogenic effect. Ionizing x-rays, radioactive substances, and certain chemicals can cause birth defects. The pregnant woman should take precautions to avoid these substances during her pregnancy. Avoiding unnecessary x-rays, or using a lead shield for unavoidable x-rays, and using gloves when handling chemicals are two ways the woman can help protect her developing fetus.

Ectopic Pregnancy

There are instances when the zygote implants in places other than the uterus. Of the implantations that occur outside of the uterine cavity, 95% occur in the fallopian tube. When the zygote implants outside the uterus, it is known as an **ectopic pregnancy**. An ectopic pregnancy that occurs in a fallopian tube is more specifically referred to as a tubal pregnancy. Usually tubal pregnancies are caused by blockage or scarring of the fallopian tubes, either from infection or trauma, such as a tubal ligation reversal. Ectopic pregnancy occurs in 19.7 of 1,000 pregnancies.

As the embryo grows in the confined space of the fallopian tube, it causes the tube to dilate. The tube will eventually rupture, unless the condition is caught in time. If the tube ruptures, it will result in maternal hemorrhage into the peritoneal cavity and can lead to maternal death. In the event of a tubal pregnancy, the affected tube and the products of conception are removed. Because there is no way to transplant the embryo into the uterine cavity and continue the pregnancy, tubal pregnancies always result in the death of the embryo. See Chapter 17 for a full discussion of ectopic pregnancy.

Multifetal Pregnancy

When a woman is carrying more than one fetus at the same time, the pregnancy is referred to as a multifetal pregnancy. Multifetal pregnancies can result in twins, triplets, or more. The rate of naturally occurring twin pregnancies is 1 in 50, and triplets naturally occur at a rate of 1 in 6,000 pregnancies. The overall rates of multifetal pregnancies have changed during the last few decades because of the increasing number of assisted reproductive procedures and the use of fertility medications.

Twins can be either identical or fraternal. Identical twins are derived from one zygote (one egg and one sperm divide into two zygotes shortly after fertilization), so identical twins are called **monozygotic** twins. They share the same genetic material and are always the same gender. Fraternal twins develop from separate egg and sperm fertilizations and are called **dizygotic** twins. Fraternal twins may or may not be the same gender, and their genetic material is not identical. In pregnancies that have more than two fetuses, they may have all developed from a single fertilized egg, also referred to as monozygotic, or they may have developed from separate eggs, or they may be a combination of both types (Fig. 5-7).

Twins can be classified one of three ways—diamniotic-dichorionic, diamniotic-monochorionic, and monoamniotic-monochorionic. Diamniotic-dichorionic twins each develop in their own amniotic sac. Their placentas do not share any vessels.

● *Figure 5.7* Twin pregnancy. (**A**) Fraternal (dizygotic) twins with two placentas, two amnions, and two chorions (diamniotic dichorionic). (**B**) Identical (monozygotic) twins with one placenta, two amnions, and one chorion (diamniotic monochorionic).

Diamniotic-monochorionic twins each have their own amniotic sac but share a common chorionic sac. They each have a separate placenta, but the placentas share some vessels. These types of twins are at risk for developing a condition referred to as twin-to-twin transfusion syndrome. In this syndrome, one fetus gives the other fetus part of its blood volume but does not receive any in return. Lastly, twins can be monoamniotic-monochorionic. These types of twins have one amniotic cavity that they both share. The greatest risk to these types of twins is cord entanglement. Conjoined twins occur in 1 in 50,000 to 80,000 deliveries.

Certain factors increase a woman's chance of becoming pregnant with dizygotic twins. She is more likely to have dizygotic twins if she is herself a twin or has twin siblings, if she recently stopped using oral contraceptives, if she is tall or has a large stature, or if she is of African-American heritage. The use of fertility medications, such as Clomid or Pergonal, increases a woman's chance of carrying a multifetal pregnancy. Multifetal pregnancies are at higher risk for certain conditions and need to be monitored closely (see Chapter 17).

Test Yourself

- Which organ system is susceptible throughout the pregnancy to teratogenic effects?
- Define ectopic pregnancy.
- Why are fraternal twins called dizygotic twins?

KEY POINTS

- Mitosis is the process of cell division by which two daughter cells are produced that have the diploid number of chromosomes (46). Meiosis is a special type of cell division in which cells with the haploid number of chromosomes (23) are formed.
- Spermatogenesis begins at puberty, whereas oogenesis starts during the fetal stage in the female infant and then stays in an arrested state until puberty. Spermatogenesis ends with four spermatids, each with 23 chromosomes. Oogenesis ends with one ova containing 23 chromosomes.
- Sex (or gender) determination occurs when the ovum and the sperm unite. The ovum always contributes an X chromosome, whereas the sperm contributes either an X or a Y chromosome. Two X chromosomes (XX) is female. An X and a Y chromosome (XY) is male.
- The pre-embryonic stage lasts from fertilization until the end of the 2nd week after conception. During this time the two sets of chromosomes combine, implantation occurs, and the beginning of maternal–fetal circulation occurs.
- The embryonic stage lasts from the end of the 2nd week until the end of the 8th week. During this time the organs and tissues begin to differentiate and assume specific functions. By the end of this stage all organs are developed and the embryo is distinctly human in appearance.
- The fetal stage lasts from the end of the 8th week until birth. During this time there is additional maturation and growth of already existing tissue.
- The fetal membranes are formed by the close union of the amnion and chorion. The amnion makes up the inner part of the membrane and is in contact with amniotic fluid and the fetus. The chorion is adjacent to (but not fused with) the amnion and has no contact with the fetus.
- Amniotic fluid serves as a cushion to protect the fetus from injury, a temperature control mechanism, and a medium that allows for free movement and unrestricted growth.

◆ The placenta transfers nutrients, such as oxygen and glucose, to the fetus while removing waste products, such as carbon dioxide and urea. The placenta acts as a barrier to some harmful substances but does not prevent most substances from passing to the fetus. The placenta has an endocrine function in that it secretes hormones that help to sustain the pregnancy. These hormones include hCG, hPL, estrogen, and progesterone.

◆ Maternal blood rich in oxygen and nutrients reaches the placenta at the level of the intervillous spaces that are surrounded by the chorionic villi. The chorionic villi contain the fetal blood vessels. Exchange of nutrients for wastes occurs by simple diffusion or active transport across a thin membrane that separates the fetal and maternal bloodstreams.

◆ Fetal blood that contains newly oxygenated blood and nutrients leaves the placenta via the umbilical vein and enters the fetal inferior vena cava via the ductus venosus. From there it travels to the right atrium, where most of the blood crosses the foramen ovale into the left atrium. The blood then travels to the aortic arch to the brain and the upper body. Some of the blood enters the right ventricle and goes to the lungs to nourish the tissues. Most of the blood that leaves the right ventricle is shunted to the aorta via the ductus arteriosus. Deoxygenated fetal blood returns to the placenta via the two umbilical arteries.

◆ Teratogens can be classified as ingested, infectious, or environmental. Ingested teratogens can be medications or illegal substances. Infectious teratogens include diseases such as cytomegalovirus (CMV) and rubella. Environmental teratogens include ionizing x-rays and chemicals.

◆ An ectopic pregnancy is one that develops outside of the uterus. Most ectopic pregnancies occur in a fallopian tube, which can rupture and lead to maternal hemorrhage and/or death. A tubal pregnancy always leads to death of the embryo, whether from tubal rupture or removal during surgery.

◆ Monozygotic twins are identical because they arise from one zygote and therefore share identical chromosomes. Dizygotic twins are fraternal because they arise from two separate zygotes and therefore do not share the same chromosomes.

REFERENCES AND SELECTED READINGS

Books and Journals

Blackburn, S. T., & Loper, D. L. (2002). *Maternal, fetal, and neonatal physiology: A clinical perspective* (2nd ed.). Philadelphia: WB Saunders.

Cunningham, F. G., Gant, N. F., Leveno, K. J., Gilstrap, L.C. III, Hauth, J. C., & Wenstrom, K. D. (2001). *Williams obstetrics* (21st ed.). New York: McGraw-Hill Medical Publishing Division.

Mattson, S., & Smith, J. E. (Eds.). (2000). *Core curriculum for maternal–newborn nursing*. AWHONN publication (2nd ed.). Philadelphia: WB Saunders.

Moore, K. L. (1998). *Before we are born: Essentials of embryology and birth defects*. Philadelphia: WB Saunders.

Pillitteri, A. (2003). *Maternal and child health nursing: Care of the childbearing and childrearing family* (4th ed.). Philadelphia: Lippincott Williams & Wilkins.

Potter, P. A., & Perry, A. G. (2000). *Fundamentals of nursing* (5th ed.). Oxford, UK: Elsevier Science.

Reeder, S. J., Martin, L. L., & Koniak-Griffin, D. (1996). *Maternity nursing: Family, newborn, and women's health care* (18th ed.). Philadelphia: Lippincott-Raven.

Robinson, J. N., & Abuhamad, A. Z. (2002). Determining chorionicity and amnionicity in multiple pregnancies. *Contemporary Ob/Gyn, 6,* 94–108. Retrieved November 28, 2003, from http://www.contemporaryobgyn.net

Yetter, J. F. (1998). Examination of the placenta. *American Family Physician, 57*(5), 1045. Retrieved November 28, 2003, from http://www.aafp.org/afp/980301ap/yetter.html

Websites
Visible Embryo
http://www.visembryo.com

IUGR
http://www.pediatrics.wisc.edu/childrenshosp/parents_of_preemies/IUGR.html

Teratogens
http://www.lpch.org/DiseaseHealthInfo/HealthLibrary/genetics/terathub.html
http://www.modimes.org/

Ectopic Pregnancy
http://www.aafp.org/afp/20000215/1080.html

WORKBOOK

NCLEX-STYLE REVIEW QUESTIONS

1. A mother ingests a teratogenic substance. At which stage of development will the most damage occur?

   a. Conception

   b. Pre-embryonic

   c. Embryonic

   d. Fetal

2. During which time frame does the embryonic stage last?

   a. Ovulation to conception

   b. 1 to 14 days after conception

   c. 3 through 8 weeks after conception

   d. 9 through 38 weeks after conception

3. What is the main purpose of the chorionic villi?

   a. To adhere the blastocyst to the endometrial lining

   b. To form the tissues that will become the placenta

   c. To produce amniotic fluid

   d. To provide an exchange site for the exchange of nutrients and wastes

4. Which one of the following is a fetal shunt that aids in fetal circulation?

   a. Foramen primum

   b. Foramen ovale

   c. Ductus deferens

   d. Septum secundum

5. Twins who share the same chromosomal material are classified as

   a. Monozygotic

   b. Dizygotic

   c. Fraternal

   d. Trizygotic

STUDY ACTIVITIES

1. Use the following table to compare major developmental milestones at each of the indicated gestational ages. Refer to this textbook and to the following website: http://www.visembryo.com

Gestational Age	Major Developmental Milestones
4 weeks	
8 weeks	
12 weeks	
16 weeks	
20 weeks	
28 weeks	
32 weeks	
36 weeks	

2. Talk to the following individuals in your community about teratogens. Have each person discuss several substances or processes that might be damaging to the fetus and how a pregnant woman can best protect her fetus from harm.

   a. Pharmacist

   b. Obstetrician

   c. Chemist

   d. Radiologist

3. Develop a teaching plan for an adolescent who is pregnant. Explain the processes of fertilization and development in language she will likely understand. Prepare the answers to three to four questions you anticipate she may ask you.

CRITICAL THINKING: What Would You Do?

Apply your knowledge of fetal development to the following situation.

1. Rebecca, a 25-year-old woman, has just discovered she is pregnant for the first time. She missed her first menstrual period 4 weeks ago and came to the office for a pregnancy test, which was positive.

   a. Rebecca asks you what her baby looks like right now. What will you tell her?

   b. Rebecca is worried because she has taken Tylenol several times during the past week for tension headaches. How will you advise her?

2. Rebecca comes in for her 12-week checkup. She measures larger than expected for dates, so the physician orders a sonogram.

a. Rebecca asks you to tell her what her baby looks like at this stage. How will you answer?

b. The sonogram shows that Rebecca is carrying twins. She wants to know whether they are identical or fraternal. How will you answer her?

Maternal Adaptation During Pregnancy

6

STUDENT OBJECTIVES

On completion of this chapter, the student should be able to

1. Differentiate between presumptive, probable, and positive signs of pregnancy.
2. Relate normal anatomy and physiology of the nonpregnant woman to that of the pregnant woman.
3. Explain expected changes in the major body systems during pregnancy.
4. Discuss maternal physiologic adaptation to pregnancy.
5. Discuss maternal psychological adaptation to pregnancy.
6. Outline components of a nutritious diet during pregnancy.

KEY TERMS

ballottement
Braxton Hicks contractions
Chadwick's sign
chloasma
colostrum
couvade syndrome
cretinism
diastasis recti abdominis
glycosuria
Goodell's sign
Hegar's sign
linea nigra
lordosis
Montgomery's tubercles
pica
pyrosis
scurvy
striae
supine hypotensive syndrome

Pregnancy is a time of adaptation and change, not only physically, but also psychologically as the woman and her partner prepare for parenthood. The body also must adapt and accommodate the needs of the growing fetus. This chapter explores the signs of pregnancy; the physiologic and psychological changes associated with pregnancy; and the changing nutritional requirements of pregnancy.

SIGNS OF PREGNANCY

The physician or certified nurse midwife (CNM) uses a combination of signs to diagnose pregnancy (Box 6-1). These signs can be categorized as presumptive, probable, and positive. The presumptive, or subjective, signs are the symptoms the woman experiences and

---

| BOX 6.1 | Signs of Pregnancy |

After each symptom, an alternative cause (if any) other than pregnancy is suggested. All symptoms and times can vary in occurrence between individuals.

Presumptive (Possible) Signs
- 3–4 weeks+: Early breast changes (e.g., prickling and tingling sensations). Could be caused by oral contraceptives.
- 4 weeks+: Amenorrhea (missed period). May be caused by hormonal imbalance, emotional stress, or illness.
- 4–14 weeks: Morning sickness. May be related to gastrointestinal disorders, pyrexial illness, and so on.
- 6–12 weeks: Bladder irritability. Can be associated with urinary tract infection or pelvic tumor.

Probable Signs
- 4–12 weeks: Presence of hCG in blood. May be caused by hydatidiform mole.
- 6–12 weeks: Presence of hCG in urine. Choriocarcinoma is a possible cause.
- 8 weeks+: Uterine growth. May be caused by tumors.
- 16 weeks: Braxton Hicks (painless contractions). May be caused by upset stomach.
- 16–28 weeks: Ballottement of fetus. May be elicited by a tumor.

Positive Signs
- 6 weeks+: Visualization of fetus by ultrasound.
- 20–24 weeks+: Fetal heart sounds by fetal stethoscope.
- 22 weeks+: Fetal movements palpable by a trained practitioner.
- Late pregnancy: Fetal movements visible.

Adapted from material by Ian Selth, BSc Midwife. Used with permission. Retrieved November 3, 2002, from http://www.midwifery.resources.btinternet.co.uk/midwifery.htm.

---

reports to the health care provider. Each of these signs, taken alone, can have causes other than pregnancy. The same is true for probable, or objective signs, the examiner finds and reports. The only signs that are 100% diagnostic of pregnancy are the positive signs, which also are objective data noted by the examiner.

Presumptive (Possible) Signs

Presumptive signs of pregnancy are subjective data that the woman reports. The most common presumptive sign of pregnancy is a missed menstrual period, or amenorrhea. There are many causes of amenorrhea. Some women have irregular periods. Emotional distress can cause a woman to skip a menstrual period. Some disorders, such as anorexia nervosa, can lead to amenorrhea. Women who perform intense exercise, such as marathon running, also can experience amenorrhea. Because so many factors, other than pregnancy, can cause a woman to miss a menstrual period, amenorrhea is classified as a presumptive or subjective sign of pregnancy.

Other presumptive signs include nausea, fatigue, swollen, tender breasts, and frequent urination. Nausea can be caused by emotional distress, a viral infection, gastritis, or a host of other problems. Anemia, lack of sleep, overexertion, or infection can lead to fatigue. Breast tissue can become swollen and tender just before a woman starts her menstrual period in response to hormonal changes. Frequent urination can result from a urinary tract infection, nervousness, or from taking in substances such as caffeine and alcohol that either act as urinary irritants or have diuretic properties.

Probable Signs

Probable signs of pregnancy are those detected by a trained examiner. These include objective data such as **Chadwick's sign**, the bluish-purplish color of the cervix, vagina, and perineum. The examiner also detects **Hegar's sign**, softening of the uterine isthmus, and **Goodell's sign**, softening of the cervix, during the speculum and digital pelvic examinations. Other objective signs include a change in the shape of the uterus, an enlarging uterus, and Braxton Hicks contractions. **Ballottement** occurs when the examiner pushes up on the uterine wall during a pelvic examination, then feels the fetus bounce back against the examiner's fingers. The reason these signs are considered probable, rather than positive, is that pelvic tumors and some types of cancers can cause similar signs.

Another probable sign is the pregnancy test. Although pregnancy tests performed in a laboratory are highly reliable (from 97% to 99%), there is still the small possibility for error. Pregnancy tests measure the

goes away after pregnancy

presence of human chorionic gonadotropin (hCG) in the urine or the blood. hCG levels can be elevated in conditions other than pregnancy, such as hydatidiform mole and choriocarcinoma.

A woman wants confirmation of pregnancy whether she is trying to get pregnant or thinks she might be pregnant when she was not planning a pregnancy. Many women use home pregnancy tests to determine if they are pregnant. These home pregnancy tests are approximately 95% reliable when they are performed correctly and done at least 10 days after the last menstrual period. It is important for the woman to know that the home pregnancy test is more likely to be correct when it reveals a positive result than when a negative result is obtained. In other words, if the home pregnancy test is negative, she should still monitor for signs of pregnancy and repeat the test or schedule an appointment with her physician.

Several types of pregnancy tests can be done in the practitioner's office. The enzyme immunoassays (EIA) utilizing monoclonal antibodies specific for hCG can be done in approximately 10 minutes and are reliable within 7 or 8 days after ovulation. EIA can be done on urine or the woman's serum. If urine is used, it is best to have the first voided specimen of the morning because this urine is highly concentrated, making detection of hCG easier. Serum radioimmunoassay beta subunit (RIA-hCG-b) testing measures only the beta subunit of hCG. RIA testing is highly sensitive and can help diagnose pregnancy even earlier than the EIA method.

Positive Signs

Positive signs are diagnostic of pregnancy because no other condition can cause the sign. The positive sign that can be elicited earliest in the pregnancy is visualization of the gestational sac or fetus. With transvaginal ultrasound the gestational sac can be seen as early as 10 days after implantation. The fetal outline and cardiac activity are visible by abdominal ultrasound at 7 to 8 weeks.

The fetal heart beat, heard at 9 to 10 weeks with Doppler technology and by 18 to 20 weeks with a fetoscope, is a positive sign of pregnancy. Palpation of fetal movements by a trained examiner is a positive sign of pregnancy after the 20th week.

PHYSIOLOGIC ADAPTATION TO PREGNANCY

The woman's body must make tremendous changes to accommodate a pregnancy (Table 6-1). While she is pregnant her body must maintain all her vital functions and those of the growing fetus. Some changes are structural and occur because of pressure exerted by the growing fetus and expanding uterus. Other changes are hormone related. The next section discusses the physiologic changes that occur during pregnancy by body system.

Reproductive Changes

Obviously, the reproductive system changes during pregnancy. Instead of shedding endometrial tissue every month, the decidua must be maintained. The myometrium (uterine muscle) must stay relatively relaxed. If it contracts too forcefully, the pregnancy will be lost. The uterus undergoes changes immediately after conception and continues to grow and change throughout the pregnancy. The cervix, vagina, perineum, and breasts also undergo changes.

Uterus

During the first weeks after conception, the uterine muscle cells begin to hypertrophy, causing the uterus to expand. It is thought that estrogen stimulates this muscle cell hypertrophy. At first the uterine walls become thicker, but as the pregnancy progresses, the growing fetus and accessory structures began to exert pressure so that the uterus enlarges and the uterine walls become thinner. By the end of the 12th week, the uterus expands upward into the abdominal cavity. At 16 weeks, the fundus can be palpated approximately halfway between the symphysis pubis and the umbilicus. At 20 weeks, the fundus reaches the level of the umbilicus. By the end of the pregnancy, the uterus occupies much of the abdominal cavity.

Beginning in the first trimester, the uterus begins to contract sporadically. These contractions are usually painless and do not cause cervical changes. By the second trimester these contractions can be palpated. **Braxton Hicks contractions**, the painless, intermittent, "practice" contractions of pregnancy, are named after the physician who first wrote about them, Braxton Hicks. During the third trimester as the pregnancy approaches term, Braxton Hicks contractions become more frequent and can sometimes cause discomfort. As the time for labor draws near, the contractions can become somewhat regular, causing the woman to think that she is in labor. This is the cause of so-called false labor.

Blood supply to the uterus increases dramatically throughout pregnancy. Under the influence of estrogen, new blood vessels grow in the placenta and uterine walls, and vasodilation occurs in maternal vessels to allow increased blood flow to the uterus and placenta. The diameter of the uterine artery increases during pregnancy. By 20 weeks, it doubles in diameter from the nonpregnant state.

TABLE 6.1	Anatomy and Physiology Comparison: Nonpregnant to Pregnant Woman	
System or Structure	Nonpregnant Characteristics	Pregnant Characteristics (At Term, Unless Otherwise Indicated)
Uterus	Weight: 70 grams Uterine cavity capacity: 10 mL Structure: Almost solid Shape: Pear shaped Location: Pelvis Percentage of cardiac output supplying all abdominal organs combined: 24%	Weight: 1,100 grams Uterine cavity capacity: 5 liters average, but may expand to as much as 20 liters Structure: Thin, muscular sac Shape: Globular Location: Fills the abdominal cavity Percentage of cardiac output supplying uterus/pelvic cavity alone: 20%
Breasts	Soft, nontender tissue Soft, nonprominent, relatively smooth areola	Tenderness in the first few weeks of pregnancy. Nodularity of breast tissue. Prominent areola with deepened pigmentation and prominent projections of Montgomery's tubercles.
Thyroid gland	Total gland volume: 12.1 mL	Total gland volume: 15.0 mL
Blood	Blood volume: 5 liters Red blood cell volume: 2 liters Plasma volume: 3 liters Hemoglobin: 12–16 g/100 mL Hematocrit: 36%–46% White blood cell count: 4,500–11,000/mm^3	Blood volume increases by 40%–50% (could be as high as 7.5 liters) Red blood cell volume increases by as much as 30% (2.6 liters) Plasma volume increases by 50% (4.5 liters) Hemoglobin: 11–12 g/100 mL Hematocrit: Decreases, particularly in the third trimester as plasma volume increases White blood cell (WBC) count: As great as 16,000 mm^3 (in labor the WBC count can reach as high as 25,000 mm^3)
Coagulation	Fibrinogen levels: 200–400 mg/dL Factors VII, VIII, and X: Normal	Fibrinogen levels: Values may be as high as 600 mg/dL Factors VII, VIII, and X: Increase by 20%–100% In general, pregnancy is considered to be a state of hypercoagulability.
Heart	Blood pressure in normal range: 90–140 mm Hg systolic and 60–90 mm Hg diastolic Heart rate 60–100 beats per minute Cardiac output: Approximately 5 liters per minute	Blood pressure decreases slightly, particularly in the second trimester Heart rate increases by 10–15 beats per minute Cardiac output increases (as much as 40%–50%) beginning by the fifth week gestation
Respiratory	Respiratory rate: 16–20 breaths per minute Nasal mucosa thin and moist Tidal volume (the volume of air moved during normal inspiration and expiration): 500 mL Oxygen consumption normal for adult female PaCO$_2$: 35–45 mm Hg	Respiratory rate: Unchanged or increased by 2–3 breaths per minute Nasal mucosa edematous due to vasocongestion. Tidal volume: 700 mL Oxygen consumption increases by 14% Average PaCO$_2$: 32 mm Hg

Cervix and Ovaries

The cervix undergoes characteristic changes under the influence of estrogen and progesterone. Vascularity is increased, and glandular tissue multiplies during pregnancy. The vascular congestion and increase in glandular tissue is responsible for Goodell's sign, Hegar's sign, and Chadwick's sign. Shortly after conception, a thick mucous plug develops in the opening of the cervix, which helps to protect the uterine cavity from infection. The mucous plug is expelled shortly before, or at the beginning of labor. Small capillaries break when the plug is expelled, causing a bloody show.

This will reassure your patient. Because the cervix increases in vascularity during pregnancy, a pelvic examination can rupture small capillaries and cause spotting afterward. After a pelvic examination, inform the woman that she can expect some spotting, particularly when she wipes after voiding. Reassure her that this spotting is normal unless the bleeding becomes heavy, like that of a menstrual period.

Follicles in the ovaries do not mature during pregnancy, and ovulation stops. The corpus luteum continues to function and produces progesterone for approximately 6 to 7 weeks. If the corpus luteum is removed or stops functioning before that time, a spontaneous abortion (miscarriage) will occur. After 7 weeks, the placenta produces enough progesterone to maintain the pregnancy.

Vagina and Perineum

The vagina and perineum are affected by hormonal changes and increased blood supply to the area. The vagina takes on a bluish-purplish hue, Chadwick's sign, because of vascular congestion. Copious secretions are produced in the vagina and cervix because of the increased blood flow to the area.

Breasts

In the first few weeks of pregnancy, the breasts become tender and the woman may feel tingling sensations. As pregnancy progresses, the breasts increase in size under the influence of estrogen. Prolactin, an anterior pituitary hormone, stimulates glandular production, causing the breast tissue to feel nodular. The areolas darken. **Montgomery's tubercles**, sebaceous glands on the areolas, produce secretions that lubricate the nipple. Montgomery's tubercles become more prominent during pregnancy. Tiny veins become visible on the surface of the breasts. **Striae**, stretch marks, sometimes appear. Striae appear reddish at first, then gradually fade to a light silvery color after childbirth.

As the mammary glands develop, the breasts begin to produce and secrete **colostrum**, a thick, yellow fluid that precedes milk production. Colostrum is sometimes referred to as the "foremilk." During the first 3 days of breast-feeding, colostrum is the nourishment the baby receives. It is rich in antibodies and protein.

Endocrine Changes

The hormonal changes that occur in pregnancy are tremendous. Rising levels of certain pregnancy hormones cause changes in almost every body system during pregnancy. The placental hormones are discussed in Chapter 5. Changes in the endocrine system itself occur during pregnancy. The pituitary gland enlarges by 135% compared with its nonpregnant size. In fact, pregnancy could not occur without the interaction of the pituitary hormones, follicle-stimulating hormone (FSH) and luteinizing hormone (LH).

Prolactin levels increase progressively during pregnancy. Although this hormone is not necessary for the successful completion of pregnancy, it is crucial for the initiation of lactation. Oxytocin, a posterior pituitary hormone, is responsible for the rhythmic uterine contractions of labor. Oxytocin stimulates the letdown reflex during breast-feeding and stimulates the uterus to continue contracting after delivery to control maternal bleeding.

Most endocrine glands are affected by the increased protein binding that occurs during pregnancy. Hyperplasia of glandular tissue and increased vascularity cause the thyroid gland to increase in size. The need for insulin is increased. Some women have borderline pancreatic activity when they are not pregnant. During pregnancy, these women develop gestational diabetes because the borderline pancreas cannot handle the increased demands placed upon it.

Test Yourself

- List three positive signs of pregnancy.
- Describe three changes that occur in breast tissue during pregnancy.
- What is the purpose of the hormone prolactin?

Hematologic Changes

Blood volume increases by approximately 40% to 45% above prepregnancy levels by the end of the third trimester. Blood plasma and red blood cells (RBCs) both increase in volume, although plasma volumes increase at a higher percentage (50%) than do RBCs (30%). This physiologic hemodilution causes a slight decrease in hemoglobin and hematocrit (H&H) levels.

The average hemoglobin level at term is 12.5 g/dL. Iron-deficiency anemia is not diagnosed until the hemoglobin levels fall below 11.0 g/dL. It is important to note that in the absence of sufficient iron, RBC volume increases by only 18%, rather than 30%.

Some blood clotting factors, such as fibrinogen and others, increase during pregnancy, making pregnancy a hypercoagulable state. However, clotting times and bleeding times remain within normal limits. As the uterus enlarges, blood return from the lower extremities is inhibited, a situation that can cause venous stasis. A combination of venous stasis and the state of hypercoagulability places the pregnant woman at risk for venous thrombosis (clot formation).

The increased blood volume and hypercoagulability of the blood serve protective functions during pregnancy. The expanded blood volume helps meet the needs of the enlarging uterus with its increased vascularity. It also helps protect the woman and the fetus from harmful effects of decreased venous return when the woman is standing or lying supine. The increased blood volume enhances the exchange of nutrients and respiratory gases between the pregnant woman and fetus. The increased blood volume and hypercoagulability serve to protect the woman from the blood loss that normally occurs during delivery.

Cardiovascular Changes

Tremendous demands are made upon the cardiovascular system during pregnancy. The heart has to handle the increased load of an expanded blood volume. It also must adjust to the demands of organ systems with increased workloads, such as the kidneys and uterus. In addition, the heart is physically pushed upward and to the left by the enlarging uterus, which may cause systolic murmurs.

Normally the blood pressure decreases slightly during pregnancy, particularly in the second trimester. The heart rate rises by 10 to 15 beats per minute on average. Cardiac output increases, beginning in the early weeks of pregnancy and continuing throughout pregnancy.

During late pregnancy the gravid uterus can compress the woman's vena cava and aorta causing the blood pressure to fall when the woman is in the supine position. This condition is called **supine hypotensive syndrome** (Fig. 6-1). The woman may feel light-headed and

An ounce of prevention. . .
Because of the danger of supine hypotensive syndrome in late pregnancy, advise the woman to avoid the supine position. If she wishes to lie on her back, instruct her to place a pillow under her right hip to keep the uterus away from the great vessels.

● **Figure 6.1** Supine hypotensive syndrome. When the woman lies flat on her back in the latter half of pregnancy, the uterus and its contents compress the aorta and vena cava against the spine. This compression decreases the amount of blood returned to the heart; therefore, the cardiac output and the blood pressure fall, leading to supine hypotensive syndrome. The cure (and prevention) is for the woman to rest on her side. As you can see in the illustration, when the pregnant woman is on her side, pressure is relieved from the great vessels and normal blood flow resumes.

dizzy; her skin may exhibit pallor and clamminess. The treatment for this condition is to reposition the woman to a lateral position. The traditional position is left side-lying.

Respiratory Changes

The respiratory system must accommodate to the changing needs and demands of pregnancy. Vasocongestion of the lining of the upper respiratory tract causes symptoms similar to that of the common cold. The nasal congestion and voice changes may persist throughout pregnancy. The nasal lining is more fragile, increasing the likelihood of nosebleeds. These characteristic changes to the respiratory tract lining are thought to occur under the influence of estrogen.

As the uterus enlarges, it pushes up on the diaphragm. The body compensates for this crowding by increasing the anteroposterior and transverse diameters of the chest so that total lung capacity stays approximately the same as it was before pregnancy. Ligaments that loosen under the influence of hormones (probably progesterone) allow for the increased thoracic diameters.

The woman becomes more aware of the need to breathe and may feel short of breath even when she is not. In the third trimester, pressure exerted on the diaphragm from the expanding uterus can also cause the woman to feel dyspneic.

Musculoskeletal Changes

Lordosis, an increased curvature of the spine, becomes more pronounced in the later weeks of pregnancy (Fig. 6-2) as the expanding uterus alters the center of gravity. The lordosis compensates by shifting the center of gravity back over the lower extremities.

12 weeks   20 weeks   28 weeks   36 weeks   40 weeks

● *Figure 6.2* Postural changes during pregnancy. Progressive lordosis, increased curvature of the spine, is characteristic during pregnancy. Notice how the lumbar and thoracic curves become more pronounced as pregnancy progresses. This occurs to counterbalance the effect of the protruding abdomen and to keep the center of balance over the lower extremities.

The increased curvature can result in low backache. Hormonal influences on pelvic joints cause them to increase in mobility, which contributes to lower back discomfort and causes the characteristic waddling gait of pregnancy.

As the uterus enlarges, increasing pressure is put on the broad and round ligaments that support the uterus. Prolonged pressure can lead to round ligament pain. A woman who has been pregnant several times or a woman who is carrying twins is more likely to experience **diastasis recti abdominis**, separation of the rectus abdominis muscle that supports the abdomen.

Test Yourself

- By what percentage does blood volume increase during pregnancy?
- By how much is cardiac output expected to increase?
- Define diastasis recti abdominis.

Gastrointestinal Changes

Nausea and vomiting are common in the first trimester under the influence of rising human chorionic gonadotropin (hCG) levels. Occasionally a large increase in saliva production (ptyalism) occurs. The gums may become tender and bleed easily. Current scientific evidence shows no increase in the rate of tooth decay during pregnancy.

As the uterus expands upward into the abdominal cavity, the intestines are displaced to the sides and upward. The stomach is pushed upward. The lower esophageal sphincter (LES) relaxes under the influence of hormones. Pressures in the esophagus are lower than in the nonpregnant state, while pressures within the stomach are increased. These changes lead to an increased incidence of **pyrosis**, heartburn caused by acid reflux through the relaxed LES.

Displacement of the intestines and possible slowed motility of the gastrointestinal tract under the influence of progesterone may lead to delayed gastric emptying and decreased peristalsis. As a result of these changes, the pregnant woman is predisposed to constipation. Constipation and elevated pressures in the veins below the uterus contribute to an increased incidence of hemorrhoid development during pregnancy.

Progesterone interferes with normal gallbladder contraction, leading to stasis of bile. Cholestasis and increased cholesterol levels increase the risk of gallstone formation during pregnancy. Cholestasis can occur within the liver and lead to pruritus (itching).

Urinary Changes

Renal and ureteral dilation occur as a result of hormonal changes and mechanical pressure of the growing uterus on the ureters. The dilation causes an increase in kidney size, particularly on the right side. Peristalsis decreases in the urinary tract, leading to urinary stasis and a resultant increase in the risk for pyelonephritis.

The glomerular filtration rate (GFR) rises by as much as 50% because of increased cardiac output and decreased renal vascular resistance. The rise in GFR occurs as early as the 10th week and is largely responsible for the increased urinary frequency noted in the first trimester. Urinary frequency is not a common complaint in the second trimester but occurs again in the third trimester because of the pressure of the expanding uterus on the bladder.

Glycosuria, glucose in the urine, may occur normally during pregnancy because the kidney tubules are not able to reabsorb as much glucose as they were before pregnancy. However, if the woman is spilling glucose in her urine, additional tests are warranted to rule out gestational diabetes. Protein is not normally found in the urine of a pregnant woman.

● *Figure 6.3* Linea nigra.

Integumentary Changes

Many skin changes in pregnancy result from hyperpigmentation. The so-called mask of pregnancy, known as **chloasma,** is evidenced by brown blotchy areas on the forehead, cheeks, and nose of the pregnant woman. This condition may be permanent, or it may regress between pregnancies. The condition can be stimulated with oral contraceptives. The skin in the middle of the abdomen may develop a darkened line called the **linea nigra** (Fig. 6-3). Striae (stretch marks) may develop on the abdomen in response to elevated glucocorticoid levels. As discussed in the section on breast tissue, the striae appear reddish and are more noticeable during pregnancy. After pregnancy they tend to fade and become silvery-white in color.

Test Yourself

- List two reasons the pregnant woman is predisposed to pyrosis.
- Name two urinary changes normally experienced during pregnancy.
- List two conditions that result from hyperpigmentation during pregnancy.

PSYCHOLOGICAL ADAPTATION TO PREGNANCY

While adapting to rapid changes in physiology, the pregnant woman also must come to grips with her new role as parent. No matter how many children the woman has, each new pregnancy brings with it a role change. Adjusting to the role of parenting is a process that occurs throughout the pregnancy and beyond.

How a woman adjusts to her role as parent is influenced by many factors. Societal expectations and cultural values may dictate the way a woman responds to pregnancy and the idea of parenthood. Family influences are usually very strong. The way the woman was raised and the values surrounding children and parenthood in her family of origin color the way a woman adapts to pregnancy. Her own personality and ability to adapt to change will influence her response. Even her past experiences with pregnancy have an effect on the way she deals with the current pregnancy. For example, if she has a history of a stillbirth, she may not fully accept the pregnancy or begin to bond with the baby until he is born.

Social support is critical during pregnancy. If the woman is in a long-term relationship and feels supported, she will be much better prepared to handle the demands of pregnancy than if she feels alone and isolated without support. If the woman does not have a supportive partner, it is important for her to identify someone with whom she can share the experience of pregnancy. Often this will be a female friend, or perhaps the woman's own mother.

First Trimester Task: Accept the Pregnancy

Pregnancy is a development stage, and as such, psychological tasks of pregnancy have been identified. The first task of pregnancy is to accept the pregnancy. This task is usually met during the first trimester, although some women have difficulty fully accepting the pregnancy until they can feel the baby move.

Initially the woman may be shocked that she is pregnant. Or she may be ecstatic or excited. There are a myriad of emotions that a woman may experience when she first hears the news that she is pregnant. Even if the pregnancy is desired intensely, a certain amount of ambivalence is a normal initial response to pregnancy. Ambivalence refers to the feelings of uncertainty most women must deal with in the early weeks of pregnancy. The woman may have tried to get pregnant for a while before conceiving, and now that the pregnancy has occurred she may have second thoughts or doubts about her ability to be a good parent. Or the pregnancy may have been unplanned, so she must sort through her feelings about this unexpected demand that has been placed upon her.

Acceptance can be healing.
Listen to your patient. Pregnancy and childbirth can stimulate many emotions. If the woman indicates that she wishes to talk, encourage her and use active listening skills. Let her know that it is normal to experience a wide array of feelings during pregnancy.

It may be helpful for her to hear that ambivalence is a healthy response because she may feel guilty about her uncertainty.

As the woman experiences the early physiologic changes of pregnancy, she gradually comes to accept that she is pregnant. She is usually introverted and focused on herself during the first trimester. The nausea associated with early pregnancy may leave her feeling sick and irritable. She may be fatigued. Often she is moody and sensitive.

It is important to be supportive of the woman's partner during this time. He (or she, if the woman is in a lesbian relationship) also must deal with feelings of ambivalence. In addition to accepting the pregnancy, the partner must learn to accept the pregnant woman as she changes with pregnancy. The mood swings, sensitivity, and irritability can make it difficult to cope. Jealousy of the unborn child can occur. It can be difficult to adjust to the introversion and self-focus of the woman. Often the partner is relieved to learn that the changes his partner is going through are normal responses to pregnancy.

A PERSONAL GLIMPSE

When I first found out that I was pregnant, I started shaking. I couldn't believe that I was pregnant. My husband and I didn't plan for this to happen so soon. We had wanted to wait about 8 more months before beginning our family. We weren't ready; we had only been married 5 months. We still had some financial debt to pay off and we had certain goals we wanted to meet.

We both wanted and loved children very much. In fact, we both wanted, and planned, to have three children. However, it was the timing that was wrong. I couldn't even tell my husband the news because he was away for several weeks. This added to my anxiety. Not only was I worried about my ability to be a mother, but I was worried that I may have eaten or been exposed to something harmful to my baby before knowing I was pregnant. I ended up confiding in my mother and best friends who truly helped me to calm down and get a grip.

I started to relax and accept the fact that, although my timing was off, this was pretty exciting. When I was finally able to tell my husband, he just beamed with joy. I knew in that moment that everything would be all right.

Sandra

LEARNING OPPORTUNITY: How would you advise this mother-to-be regarding her feelings when she found out that she was pregnant? How can the nurse help the woman and her family deal with the emotions that surround finding out about a pregnancy?

Second Trimester Task: Accept the Baby

Generally during the first trimester the woman is focused on the pregnancy and on accepting this new reality as being part of her identity. Gradually as the pregnancy progresses she comes to have a sense of the child as his own separate entity. This acceptance may be enhanced when she first hears the fetal heart beat, when she feels the baby move inside her, or when she sees the fetal image during a sonogram.

As she comes to accept the uniqueness of her baby, she may begin to shop for baby clothes or prepare the nursery. When ultrasound is done in the second trimester, it is generally possible to detect the sex of the child. The couple may name the baby once they know if it is a boy or a girl. But do not make the mistake of thinking that the woman has not yet accepted the baby if she does not name the baby during pregnancy. Some parents do not decide on a name until several days after the baby is born.

During the second trimester the woman may become more extroverted. She often feels much better since the nausea and fatigue of the first trimester have passed. She starts to show so that the pregnancy becomes apparent to those around her, and she may have the glow of pregnancy. Frequently the second trimester is a happy time. The woman may enjoy the extra attention and deference society gives to pregnant women.

It is important to remember that the partner is experiencing the pregnancy along with the woman. Some fathers actually experience some of the physical symptoms of pregnancy, such as nausea and vomiting, along with their partner. This phenomenon is called **couvade syndrome**. It may be easier for the man to accept his wife now that she is feeling better and is less introverted. In any event it is important to encourage the couple to communicate their needs effectively to each other. Each needs the support of the other.

Third Trimester Task: Prepare for Parenthood

Nesting instincts often begin in the third trimester. The couple may prepare the nursery and shop for baby furniture and clothes. A name may be chosen. It is during the third trimester that most childbirth classes are offered. The woman usually has a heightened interest in safe passage for herself and the baby during labor.

Toward the end of pregnancy most women begin to feel tired of being pregnant. Many discomforts of pregnancy show themselves during the third trimester. It may be difficult to get comfortable at night, and so it may be hard to get a good night's sleep. Backache and round ligament pain may be bothersome. Urinary frequency often returns as the gravid uterus presses down against the bladder. Braxton Hicks contractions may become uncomfortable and more frequent. It is important to be supportive of the woman and listen to her concerns.

It is helpful for the couple to attend childbirth preparation classes. Not only do they learn techniques to help them prepare for labor, but they are able to interact with other couples who are facing issues similar to their own. The social aspect of childbirth preparation can be a powerful source of support to the woman and her partner.

Test Yourself

- Describe two psychological characteristics normally associated with a woman in the first trimester of pregnancy.

- Which trimester of pregnancy is often the happiest for the woman?

- List two activities many women perform in the third trimester.

CHANGING NUTRITIONAL REQUIREMENTS OF PREGNANCY

Nutrition is an area that requires special attention during pregnancy, particularly during the second and third trimesters. The fetus needs nutrients and energy to build new tissue, and the woman needs nutrients to build her blood volume and maternal stores. There is an increased demand for energy and for almost every nutrient type. Most nutrient requirements can be met through careful attention to diet, although there are several nutrients that require supplementation during pregnancy.

Energy Requirements and Weight Gain

Energy requirements are increased during pregnancy because of fetal tissue development and increased maternal stores. During the first trimester, the recommended weight gain is 3 to 4 pounds total. Subsequently, for the remainder of pregnancy the recommendation is roughly 1 pound per week, for a total weight gain of 25 to 35 pounds for a woman who begins pregnancy with a normal body mass index (BMI).[1] Total weight gain recommendations vary depending upon the woman's prepregnancy BMI. A woman who is underweight when she enters pregnancy (low BMI) should gain 28 to 40 pounds, whereas a woman who has a high BMI (overweight) is recommended to gain 15 to 25 pounds during the pregnancy.

Failure to gain enough weight, and in particular gaining less than 16 pounds during pregnancy, has been associated with an increased risk of delivering a low birth-weight neonate (less than 2,500 grams or 5½ pounds). Low birth weight has consistently been associated with poor neonatal outcomes. Conversely, a woman who gains too much weight is at increased risk for delivering a macrosomic (greater than or equal to 4,000 grams or 8½ pounds) neonate. High birth-weight neonates experience complications and poor outcomes more frequently than do neonates with normal birth weights. A woman who gains too much weight also is at greater risk of requiring cesarean section.

Many women assume falsely that eating for two requires a significantly increased caloric intake. In fact, the required caloric increase during the first trimester is negligible. During the second and third trimesters, approximately 300 kilocalories per day are required above the woman's prepregnancy needs. It is important that the diet supply enough calories to meet energy needs; otherwise, protein will be broken down to supply energy, rather than to build fetal and maternal tissue.

Protein Requirements

Protein needs are increased during pregnancy because of growth and repair of fetal tissue, placenta, uterus, breasts, and maternal blood volume. It is recommended that the pregnant woman obtain adequate protein from animal sources, including milk and milk products. Milk is an excellent source of protein and calcium for the pregnant and breast-feeding woman. As stated previously, it is important for the woman to have adequate caloric intake to preserve protein stores for tissue building and repair. When protein is used to supply energy, there is less available for fetal, placental, and maternal tissue growth needs.

During the average pregnancy, approximately 1,000 grams of additional protein above the woman's basal needs are used. The fetus and placenta account for 500 grams of added protein. The other 500 grams is distributed among uterine muscle cells, mammary glandular tissue, and maternal blood in the form of hemoglobin and plasma proteins.

Mineral Requirements

Most minerals can be obtained from a varied diet without supplementation, even during pregnancy. However, it is important for a pregnant woman to get sufficient amounts of minerals to prevent deficiencies in the growing fetus and maternal stores. Table 6-2 compares the

---

[1] Body mass index (BMI) refers to body weight corrected for height of the person. The formula for determining BMI is: divide the person's weight (in kilograms or pounds) by her height squared (in meters or inches, respectively) then multiply by 100. Normal BMI is 19.8 to 26.

TABLE 6.2	Comparison of Recommended Daily Dietary Allowances (RDA) for Selected Vitamins and Minerals for Nonpregnant, Pregnant, and Lactating Women

Mineral/Vitamin	Function	RDA for Nonpregnant	RDA for Pregnant Women	RDA for Lactating Women	Selected Food Sources
Calcium (mg/day)	Essential role in blood clotting, muscle contraction, nerve transmission, and bone and tooth formation	1,000	1,000	1,000	Dairy products: milk, cheese, yogurt. Corn tortillas, calcium-set tofu, Chinese cabbage, kale, broccoli
Copper (µg/day)	Component of enzymes in iron metabolism	900	1,000	1,300	Organ meats, seafood, nuts, seeds, wheat bran cereals, whole grain products, cocoa products
Iodine (mg/day) Vitamin B_8	Component of thyroid hormones and prevents goiter and cretinism	150	220	290	Foods of marine origin, processed foods, iodized salt
Iron (mg/day)	Component of hemoglobin and numerous enzymes; prevents microcytic hypochromic anemia	18	27	9	Fruits, vegetables and fortified bread and grain products, such as cereal (nonheme iron sources), meat and poultry (heme iron sources)
Vitamin A (µg/day)	Required for normal vision, gene expression, reproduction, embryonic development and immune function	700	770	1,300	Liver, dairy products, fish (preformed Vitamin A sources); and carrots, sweet potatoes, mango, spinach, cantaloupe, kale, apricots (beta-carotene sources)
Vitamin B_1 (thiamin) (mg/day)	Coenzyme in the metabolism of carbohydrates and branched-chain amino acids	1.1	1.4	1.4	Enriched, fortified, or whole-brain products; bread and bread products, mixed foods whose main ingredient is grain, and ready-to-eat cereals
Vitamin B_2 (riboflavin) (mg/day)	Coenzyme in numerous redox reactions	1.1	1.4	1.6	Organ meats, milk, bread products, and fortified cereals
Vitamin B_3 (niacin) (mg/day)	Required for energy metabolism	14	18	17	Meat, fish, poultry, enriched and whole-grain breads and bread products, fortified ready-to-eat cereals

TABLE 6.2 (continued)	Comparison of Recommended Daily Dietary Allowances (RDA) for Selected Vitamins and Minerals for Nonpregnant, Pregnant, and Lactating Women				
Mineral/Vitamin	Function	RDA for Nonpregnant	RDA for Pregnant Women	RDA for Lactating Women	Selected Food Sources
Vitamin B$_6$ (pyroxidine) (mg/day)	Coenzyme in the metabolism of amino acids, glycogen, and sphingoid bases	1.3	1.9	2.0	Fortified cereals, organ meats, fortified soy-based meat substitutes
Vitamin B$_9$ (folacin, folate, folic acid) (μg/day)	Coenzyme in the metabolism of nucleic and amino acids; prevents megaloblastic anemia; in pregnancy folate deficiency is linked to an increased risk for neural tube defects	400	600	500	Enriched cereal grains, dark leafy vegetables, enriched and whole-grain breads and bread products, fortified ready-to-eat cereals
Vitamin B$_{12}$ (Cobalamine) (μg/day)	Coenzyme in nucleic acid metabolism; prevents megaloblastic anemia	2.4	2.6	2.8	Fortified cereals, meat, fish, poultry
Vitamin C (ascorbic acid) (mg/day)	Necessary for collagen synthesis and wound healing and as a protective antioxidant	75	85	120	Citrus fruits, tomatoes, tomato juice, potatoes, Brussels sprouts, cauliflower, broccoli, strawberries, cabbage, spinach
Vitamin D (calciferol) (μg/day)	Maintain serum calcium and phosphorus concentrations	5	5	5	Fish liver oils, flesh of fatty fish, liver and fat from seals and polar bears, eggs from hens fed vitamin D fortified milk products, fortified cereals
Zinc (mg/day)	Component of multiple enzymes and proteins; involved in the regulation of gene expression	8	11	12	Fortified cereals, red meats, certain seafood

Note: The RDA is that recommended for women of childbearing age (18–50 years). Requirements for teenagers and other special groups may differ. (Source: Food and Nutrition Board, 2002.)

Recommended Daily Dietary Allowances (RDA) of selected vitamins and minerals for nonpregnant, pregnant, and lactating women of childbearing age.

Iron

Iron is necessary for the formation of hemoglobin; therefore, it is essential to the oxygen-carrying capacity of the blood. If a woman's diet is iron deficient during pregnancy, her red blood cell volume will increase by only 18%; whereas, adequate supplementation of iron results in a 30% increase in red blood cell volume. This extra "cushion" of red blood cell volume increases the amount of oxygen available at the placenta for the fetus and helps protect the woman from the effects of blood loss after delivery.

Total iron requirements of pregnancy equal 1,000 milligrams. The fetus and placenta use 300 milligrams. Two hundred milligrams are lost through various routes of excretion, even when the woman is iron deficient. Five hundred milligrams are needed to supply the additional 450 milliliters of maternal red blood cells. Almost all of these additional iron requirements are needed during the second half of pregnancy, so the need for iron is increased dramatically after 20 weeks. If the woman is iron deficient, she will develop anemia. However, the fetus will get the iron needed to manufacture its red blood cells. This is one instance in which nature robs from the woman to adequately supply the fetus.

It is almost impossible for the woman to receive an adequate amount of iron from diet alone. Therefore, it is recommended that all pregnant women receive iron supplementation in the last half of pregnancy. Sometimes the physician will elect to omit the iron supplement during the first trimester because supplemental iron often intensifies the nausea and vomiting of early pregnancy. The dose will vary depending upon the individual needs of the woman. If she enters pregnancy with normal hemoglobin and hematocrit values, she will require lower doses of iron than if she is anemic when she becomes pregnant. A woman carrying twins or an obese woman will both require higher doses of supplemental iron.

Calcium

Calcium needs are not increased above prepregnancy levels (1,000 mg/day); however, it is important for the pregnant woman to obtain sufficient amounts of calcium. Calcium is needed for a variety of bodily processes, including nerve cell transmission, muscle contraction, bone building, and blood clotting. Although no direct link has been shown between low calcium levels and the development of gestational hypertension, some studies have demonstrated a reduction in risk of gestational hypertension when pregnant women take calcium supplements (Hofmeyr, Atallah, & Duley, 2002).

Calcium continuously moves between bone and blood because a precise amount is needed in the blood to maintain normal muscle contraction (including cardiac muscle contraction). Normally the movement of calcium in and out of bones is balanced, that is there is neither a net gain nor a net loss. However, if insufficient amounts are ingested, or if calcium is not absorbed from the gastrointestinal tract, the body will take calcium from the bones to maintain blood levels. This process will also occur to meet the calcium needs of the growing fetus.

Vitamin D is necessary for adequate absorption of calcium. The amount of vitamin D obtained from 10 to 20 minutes of exposure to sunlight per day is normally sufficient. If this source is not readily available, vitamin D is also present in fortified milk products.

Phosphorus

Phosphorus is readily available in a wide variety of foods. The pregnant woman normally has no trouble obtaining sufficient amounts of this nutrient. It is worth mentioning that intake of excessive amounts of phosphorus can inhibit calcium absorption. However, calcium metabolism requires a normal amount of phosphorus to build strong bones. The key to calcium and phosphorus consumption is to keep the two nutrients in balance.

Zinc

Zinc is needed during pregnancy to provide for fetal growth and during lactation for milk production. Milk production requires higher levels of zinc than the fetus demands during pregnancy. Absorption of this mineral increases during pregnancy and lactation. However, some studies show that zinc absorption does not increase in lactating women who are taking iron supplements. These findings suggest that taking iron supplements while breast-feeding may interfere with zinc levels. Foods that contain zinc include meat, seafood, and to a lesser extent, whole grains.

Iodine

Iodine is needed for normal thyroid activity. Women with severe iodine deficiencies deliver infants with **cretinism**, a congenital condition marked by stunted growth and mental retardation. Recent studies have linked subclinical hypothyroidism with increased rates of mental retardation.

Most women in the United States get sufficient amounts of iodine, but iodine intake has been declining in the past few years. Also, during pregnancy a woman loses larger amounts of iodine in the urine than when she is not pregnant. In light of these facts, the current recommendation is for all pregnant women to use iodized salt.

Vitamin Requirements

Vitamins are known to be catalysts for many chemical reactions in the body. A varied diet that includes adequate servings from each of the food groups on the Food Guide Pyramid should supply sufficient amounts of most vitamins during pregnancy. A brief description of the function and selected food sources for each vitamin are highlighted.

Folic Acid (Vitamin B$_9$)

The Centers for Disease Control report that more than 4,000 pregnancies per year are affected by neural tube defects, and that more than half of these defects could be prevented with adequate folic acid intake. Because formation of the nervous system occurs during the first few weeks of pregnancy, before a woman knows she is pregnant, all women of childbearing age are well advised to include at least 400 micrograms of folic acid per day in the diet.

There are several ways to meet the dietary requirement for folic acid. The Food and Drug Administration requires that enriched grain products, such as cereals, bread, rice, and pasta, be fortified with folic acid. Natural sources of dietary folic acid include dark green leafy vegetables, legumes, citrus fruits, and most berries. Of course, folic acid supplementation is also an option, either through folic acid tablets, or a multivitamin. Prenatal vitamins contain folic acid.

Vitamin A

Vitamin A is usually found in sufficient amounts in the diets of women who live in the United States. One concern is when a pregnant woman consumes too much vitamin A. In very large amounts (levels at or above 10,000 IU or 3,000 micrograms) preformed vitamin A, found in meats (primarily liver) and some fortified foods, can cause birth defects. For this reason pregnant women are encouraged to get the majority of their vitamin A intake from beta-carotene, a substance found in fruits and vegetables with yellow, orange, and red coloration, such as carrots and sweet potatoes. Beta-carotene is converted by the body to vitamin A and is much less toxic than preformed vitamin A. The key is balanced intake of this nutrient. Too much can be toxic to the fetus but too little can stunt fetal growth and cause impaired dark adaptation and night blindness.

Vitamin C

Vitamin C is essential in the formation of collagen, a necessary ingredient to wound healing. **Scurvy**, a disease characterized by spongy gums, loosened teeth, and bleeding into the skin and mucous membranes, results from severe vitamin C deficiency. Less severe deficiencies lead to easy bruising. Vitamin C is necessary for normal fetal growth and bone formation. This vitamin also helps the body to absorb iron. Recent research is highlighting a connection between mild vitamin C deficiency and the development of gestational hypertension (University of Pittsburgh Medical Center, 2002).

Fortunately most women in the United States get adequate amounts of vitamin C in their diets. Vitamin C is found in most fresh fruits and vegetables. The best sources include citrus fruits, papaya, and strawberries. Broccoli and tomatoes are good sources of vitamin C.

Vitamin B$_6$

Vitamin B$_6$, or pyridoxine, assists in the metabolism of the macronutrients (proteins, fats, and carbohydrates), helps convert amino acids, and forms new red blood cells. This vitamin is necessary for the healthy development of the fetus' nervous system. Although increased amounts of the vitamin are needed during pregnancy, a varied diet should supply all that is needed.

Vitamin B$_{12}$

Vitamin B$_{12}$, or cobalamine, is needed to maintain healthy nerve cells and red blood cells. It is also needed to form DNA. Vitamin B$_{12}$ occurs naturally only in animal sources, such as fish, milk, dairy products, eggs, meat, and poultry. This vitamin can also be found in fortified breakfast cereals. Most Americans get sufficient amounts of vitamin B$_{12}$ in the diet.

The two instances in which vitamin B$_{12}$ deficiency generally occurs are when a person lacks intrinsic factor or she is a vegan (see discussion of vegetarianism that follows). Persons who lack intrinsic factor cannot absorb vitamin B$_{12}$. Without intramuscular injections of the vitamin, these individuals experience pernicious anemia.

Dietary Supplementation During Pregnancy

Currently, routine multivitamin supplementation during pregnancy is not recommended by the American Academy of Pediatrics or the American College of Obstetricians and Gynecologists because it is thought that a diet that includes a variety of food types is sufficient to meet the needs of the pregnant woman. There are several exceptions. The woman who has nutritional risk factors requires a daily prenatal multivitamin supplement. Nutritional risk factors include multiple gestation, substance abuse, vegetarianism, and problems with hemoglobin formation. Some health care providers still recommend a daily vitamin supplement for all pregnant women.

Iron supplementation is recommended for all pregnant women after 28 weeks' gestation. If the woman has low hemoglobin, is obese, or is carrying twins, higher doses of iron are needed. Folic acid supplementation is also recommended during pregnancy to prevent neural tube defects. Recent studies support calcium supplementation for certain at-risk women. Women who are at risk for developing gestational hypertension and those who live in communities in which dietary calcium intake is low appear to benefit from calcium supplementation (Hofmeyr et al., 2002).

Special Nutritional Considerations

There are several situations that require unique nutritional considerations. These include vegetarianism, lactose intolerance, and pica.

Vegetarianism

There are several different categories of vegetarians. The lacto-ovo-vegetarian does not eat any flesh meats, but does include milk, eggs, and dairy products in the diet. The vegan is a strict vegetarian who does not eat milk, eggs, or any dairy product. A fruitarian only consumes fruits and nuts.

A lacto-ovo-vegetarian can easily get all of the required nutrients by careful attention to a few basic principles. Protein has always been a source of concern for vegetarian diets. Fortunately, a lacto-ovo-vegetarian can get sufficient protein by drinking milk, eating eggs, cheese, yogurt, and other dairy products, and by combining foods. Although vegetables and grains do not contain all of the essential amino acids, when they are skillfully combined, all of the essential amino acids can be obtained. The general rule is to combine a grain and a legume. For instance, a corn tortilla (grain) eaten with pinto beans (legume) provides all of the essential amino acids and qualifies as a complete protein. Other combinations include lentils and whole grain rice, peanut butter on whole wheat bread, and whole grain cereal with milk.

A vegan will need to take extra care to get enough protein because she does not use milk or dairy products. Food combining as discussed in the previous paragraph is an important nutritional strategy for the vegan. It can also help to suggest adding fortified soy milk and rice milk to the diet. Larger amounts of nuts and seeds can help offset the protein requirements. Vitamin B$_{12}$ must be supplemented for the pregnant vegan. A fruitarian

Don't get confused! A vegan can take oral forms of vitamin B$_{12}$. Only the woman who lacks intrinsic factor needs vitamin B$_{12}$ injections. Without intrinsic factor, the woman cannot absorb vitamin B$_{12}$ through the gastrointestinal system; therefore, she needs intramuscular injections.

will need intensive support from her health care provider and a dietitian to meet the nutritional requirements of a healthy pregnancy. Multivitamin supplementation is necessary in this situation.

Iron and zinc requirements are also of concern for the vegetarian. Nonmeat sources of iron are generally not absorbed as efficiently as meat sources. Therefore, the iron requirement for the vegetarian is higher. The same is true for zinc absorption and requirements.

Lactose Intolerance

Individuals of African, Hispanic, Native American, Ashkenazic Jewish, and Asian descent are more likely to have lactose intolerance than are those from a northern European heritage. Individuals with lactose intolerance lack the enzyme lactase that is necessary to break down and digest milk and milk products. Symptoms of lactase deficiency include abdominal distention, flatulence, nausea, vomiting, diarrhea, and cramps after consuming milk.

Some individuals who are lactose intolerant are able to tolerate cooked forms of milk, such as pudding or custard. Cultured or fermented dairy products, such as buttermilk, yogurt, and some cheeses may also be tolerated. Lactase may be taken with milk in the form of a chewable tablet and may allow the person to tolerate milk. Lactase-treated milk is available in most supermarkets and may be helpful.

Pica

Pica is the persistent ingestion of nonfood substances, such as clay, laundry starch, freezer frost, or dirt. It results from a craving for these substances that some women develop during pregnancy. These cravings disappear when the woman is no longer pregnant. Iron-deficiency anemia is associated with pica because many of these substances interfere with the absorption of iron. If you suspect or discover that a pregnant woman is practicing pica, tell the registered nurse (RN) or the health care provider immediately. Special counseling is indicated in this situation.

Test Yourself

- List the recommended weight gain (in pounds) for the woman with a normal body mass index.

- Describe two reasons it is important for the pregnant woman to get adequate amounts of protein.

- State the recommendations of the American Academy of Pediatrics regarding multivitamin supplementation during pregnancy.

KEY POINTS

- Presumptive signs of pregnancy, such as nausea and vomiting, can have many causes other than pregnancy. Probable signs of pregnancy are objective signs the examiner detects that point to pregnancy; however, they are not 100% indicative of pregnancy. Pregnancy tests and changes in the reproductive organs, such as Chadwick's and Hegar's signs, are probable signs of pregnancy.

- A positive sign of pregnancy is diagnostic because no other condition can cause the sign. Positive signs include visualization of the gestational sac or fetus with ultrasound, hearing the fetal heart beat with Doppler or fetoscope, and palpation of fetal movements by a trained examiner.

- Changes in anatomy and physiology that occur during pregnancy include the change of the uterus from a solid, pear-shaped, pelvic organ to a thin, globular shaped, muscular sac that fills the abdominal cavity. The thyroid gland increases in volume. Blood volume increases by 40% to 50%. Coagulation factors increase. Cardiac output increases by as much as 50%.

- The reproductive system undergoes significant changes during pregnancy. The uterus enlarges and the endometrial lining (decidua) is maintained. Blood supply to the uterus increases significantly. Increased vascularity to the reproductive tract is responsible for Goodell's, Hegar's, and Chadwick's signs.

- Endocrine system changes include enlargement of the pituitary gland, an increase in prolactin levels, and an increased need for insulin.

- Hematologic changes enhance the exchange of nutrients and gases between the woman and the fetus and protect the woman against blood loss during childbirth but predispose the woman to venous thrombosis.

- Cardiovascular changes predispose the woman to supine hypotensive syndrome if she lies on her back for prolonged periods late in pregnancy. The woman should lie on her side to prevent this syndrome.

- Respiratory system changes lead to nasal stuffiness and shortness of breath.

- Increasing lordosis, increased curvature of the spine, shifts the center of gravity and leads to a waddling gait in the last half of pregnancy.

- Gastrointestinal changes include nausea and vomiting in early pregnancy, pyrosis (heartburn) in mid and late pregnancy, constipation, and hemorrhoid formation.

- Changes in the urinary tract lead to an increased risk for pyelonephritis during pregnancy. Urinary frequency is common in the first trimester because of an increased glomerular filtration rate and again in the third trimester because of pressure of the gravid uterus on the bladder.

- Increased pigmentation, such as that seen in chloasma and the linea nigra, along with striae, are common integumentary changes.

- The psychological tasks of pregnancy include accepting the pregnancy during the first trimester, accepting the baby during the second trimester, and preparing for parenthood during the third trimester. Ambivalence is a normal feeling when pregnancy is first diagnosed. Couvade syndrome occurs when the father experiences some of the physical discomforts of pregnancy along with his partner.

- Nutritional requirements change during pregnancy. The woman needs nutrients to build extra blood volume and tissue, and the fetus needs nutrients to grow. Energy requirements are increased. A woman who enters pregnancy at normal weight should gain 25 to 35 pounds during pregnancy. A woman who is underweight should gain more, whereas a woman who is overweight should gain less. In no instance is it recommended for a woman to gain less than 15 pounds during pregnancy.

- Protein requirements increase during pregnancy. Most vitamins and minerals can be obtained without supplementation if the diet is adequate.

- After the first trimester, it is generally recommended for a woman to take an iron supplement because it is difficult to get adequate amounts of this mineral from diet alone. Although calcium needs do not increase, it is important for the pregnant woman to get sufficient amounts of this mineral.

- Folic acid supplementation is recommended to help prevent neural tube defects. Vitamin A can be toxic in large amounts. It is best to use beta-carotene (plant) sources to meet vitamin A needs during pregnancy.

- Vitamin C deficiency can lead to scurvy (severe), easy bruising, and possibly gestational hypertension.

- The woman who lacks intrinsic factor must take intramuscular injections of vitamin B_{12}, and the vegan must supplement this vitamin orally.

- Routine multivitamin supplementation is not currently recommended; however, the woman with nutritional risk factors should take prenatal vitamins. Iron and folic acid supplementation is generally recommended for all pregnant women.

- Vegetarians can receive an adequate diet with close attention to combining foods. The lacto-ovo-vegetarian can use milk and dairy products to obtain sufficient protein. The vegan can carefully combine foods (legumes and grains) to supply all of the essential amino acids and should take vitamin B_{12}

supplements. The fruitarian needs to be followed up closely by a dietitian and must take multivitamin supplements.

▶ When individuals lack the enzyme lactase, they are lactose intolerant. To get sufficient dairy products, these individuals can try taking lactase when they consume dairy products, or sometimes they can tolerate cooked forms of milk.

▶ Pica is ingestion of nonfood substances. This practice can lead to iron-deficiency anemia and other nutritional deficiencies and requires follow-up.

REFERENCES AND SELECTED READINGS

Books and Journals

Aguilera, P. A. (2001). Round ligament pain. *Emedicine*. Retrieved November 12, 2002, from http://www.emedicine.com/aaem/topic383.htm

Cunningham, F. G., Gant, N. F., Leveno, K. J., Gilstrap, L. C. III, Hauth, J. C., & Wenstrom, K. D. (2001). *Williams obstetrics* (21st ed., pp. 167—247). New York: McGraw-Hill Medical Publishing Division.

Food and Nutrition Board. (2002). *Dietary reference intakes tables*. The National Academies: Institute of Medicine. Retrieved November 11, 2002, from http://www4.nationalacademies.org/IOM/IOMHome.nsf/Pages/Food+and+Nutrition+Board

Hofmeyr, G. J., Atallah, A. N., & Duley, L. (2002). Calcium supplementation during pregnancy for preventing hypertensive disorders and related problems (Cochrane Review abstract). In The Cochrane Library, Issue 4, 2002. Oxford: Update Software. Retrieved November 11, 2002, from http://www.update-software.com/abstracts/ab001059.htm

Ladewig, P. W., London, M. L., Moberly, S., & Olds, S. B. (2002). *Contemporary maternal—newborn nursing care* (5th ed.). Upper Saddle River, NJ: Prentice Hall.

Le Hew, H. W., & Lemieux, J. (2000). Prenatal care. In A. T. Evans, & K. R. Niswander (Eds.), *Manual of obstetrics* (5th ed., pp. 19–39). Philadelphia: Lippincott Williams & Wilkins.

Mattson, S., & Smith, J. E. (Eds.). (2000). *Core curriculum for maternal—newborn nursing. AWHONN publication* (2nd ed.). Philadelphia: WB Saunders Company.

University of Pittsburgh Medical Center. (2002). Even mild vitamin C deficiency may have negative effect on vascular function. *Science Daily*. Retrieved November 11, 2002, from http://www.sciencedaily.com/releases/2002/06/020605073010.htm

Websites

Pregnancy
http://www.cfsan.fda.gov/~dms/wh-preg2.html

Pregnancy signs
http://www.thebabycorner.com/pregnancy/signs.html
http://www.fda.gov/cdrh/oivd/homeuse-pregnancy.html

Nutrition during pregnancy
http://www.4woman.gov/faq/preg-nutr.htm
http://www.vrg.org/nutrition/pregnancy.htm

WORKBOOK

NCLEX-STYLE REVIEW QUESTIONS

1. Amanda is 2 weeks late for her menstrual period. She has been feeling tired and has had bouts of nausea in the evenings. What is the classification of the pregnancy symptoms Amanda is experiencing?

   a. Positive

   b. Presumptive

   c. Probable

   d. No classification

2. Amanda makes an appointment with an obstetrician. During the exam, the obstetrician notes that the uterine isthmus is soft. What is the name of this sign, and how is it classified?

   a. Chadwick's sign; presumptive

   b. Goodell's sign; presumptive

   c. Goodell's sign; probable

   d. Hegar's sign; probable

3. Amanda is now 16 weeks pregnant. If the pregnancy is progressing as expected, where would the practitioner find the uterine fundus?

   a. Just above the pubic bone.

   b. Halfway between the pubic bone and the umbilicus.

   c. At the umbilicus.

   d. The uterine fundus would not be palpable at 16 weeks.

4. You are teaching Amanda about a proper diet during pregnancy. If Amanda understands your instructions, how will she reply when you ask her approximately how many calories per day does she need over her normal prepregnant needs?

   a. "About 300."

   b. "Approximately 500."

   c. "I need to double my calories because I'm eating for two."

   d. "I should not increase my calories while I'm pregnant."

STUDY ACTIVITIES

1. Devise a 3-day meal plan for a vegan who is pregnant. How will you meet her needs for protein, iron, calcium, and vitamin B_{12}?

2. Perform an Internet search using the key terms "pica" and "pregnancy." Share your findings with your clinical group.

3. Develop a teaching plan on the importance of folic acid for a group of women who wish to become pregnant. Be sure to address why women of childbearing age should get enough of this nutrient, how much is required, and examples of food sources.

CRITICAL THINKING: What Would You Do?

Apply your knowledge of maternal physiologic and psychological adaptation to pregnancy to the following situation.

1. Carla is 20 weeks pregnant. You are assisting the midwife during this prenatal visit.

   a. Where do you expect to find Carla's uterine fundus?

   b. You attempt to listen to the fetal heart beat with a Doppler. Do you expect to be able to hear the heart beat?

   c. Carla reports that she is excited about the pregnancy and that she and her husband have been shopping for the nursery. What do you chart regarding Carla's psychological adaptation? Is she showing evidence that she is completing the appropriate task for the trimester?

2. Carla is in the office for her 32-week checkup. She has gained a total of 20 pounds so far during her pregnancy. When you enter the room to check her vital signs you notice that she is lying on her back and she looks pale. Her blood pressure is 70/40 mm Hg.

   a. What is the likely cause of Carla's symptoms?

   b. What action do you take first, and why?

   c. How should you advise Carla regarding her weight gain?

3. Monica has just found out that she is pregnant. She is a vegan.

   a. How would you advise Monica to get enough protein in her diet?

   b. Monica complains that the iron pills her doctor prescribed are causing constipation. She asks you why she needs to take iron. How do you reply?

   c. Monica loves carrot juice, but she has heard that too much vitamin A could be unhealthy for the baby. How would you advise her?

Prenatal Care

STUDENT OBJECTIVES

On completion of this chapter, the student should be able to

1. Explain the goals of early prenatal care.
2. Explain to a pregnant woman what to expect during the first prenatal visit.
3. Examine components of the obstetric history.
4. Assist the practitioner with a pelvic examination and a Papanicolaou (Pap) smear.
5. Delineate the laboratory tests that will be done during the first prenatal visit.
6. Use Nagele's rule to calculate the due date.
7. Recognize factors that put the pregnancy at risk.
8. Describe components of subsequent prenatal visits.
9. For each fetal assessment test, outline the nursing care and implications.
10. Identify common nursing diagnoses for a pregnant woman.
11. Choose appropriate nursing interventions for the pregnant woman.
12. Teach the woman how to deal with the common discomforts of pregnancy.
13. Explain to the woman normal self-care during pregnancy.
14. Assist the woman and her partner to prepare for labor, birth, and parenthood.
15. Evaluate the effectiveness of care given during pregnancy.

KEY TERMS

amniocentesis
biophysical profile
chorionic villus sampling
cordocentesis
doula
estimated date of confinement
estimated date of delivery
gravida
microcephaly
multigravida
Nagele's rule
nulligravida
parity
percutaneous umbilical blood
  sampling
teratogens

Early prenatal care is crucial to the health of the woman and her unborn baby. In fact, the best strategy is for the woman to seek care before she conceives, as was discussed in Chapter 4. In the year 2000, according to the March of Dimes Perinatal Data Center (2002), approximately 83% of pregnant women began prenatal care in the first trimester, 13% in the second trimester, whereas approximately 4% received late or no prenatal care. Although this statistic falls short of the Healthy People 2000 goal that 90% of pregnant women would begin care in the first trimester, it does show a significant increase compared with 1990 statistics, which indicated 75% of women received early prenatal care.

The goal of early prenatal care is to optimize the health of the woman and the fetus and to increase the odds that the fetus will be born healthy to a healthy mother. Early prenatal care allows for the initiation of strategies to promote good health and for early intervention in the event a complication develops. As a trusted health care provider, the nurse has a large role to play in teaching women about the importance of early and continued prenatal care.

Assessment of maternal and fetal well-being during pregnancy is the focus of prenatal care. The nurse has a large role to play with a heavy emphasis on the teaching role throughout the pregnancy. At each prenatal visit the nurse screens the woman, monitors vital signs, performs other assessments as delegated by the primary care provider, answers questions, and provides appropriate teaching.

ASSESSMENT OF MATERNAL WELL-BEING DURING PREGNANCY

First Prenatal Visit

Ideally the first prenatal visit occurs as soon as the woman thinks she might be pregnant. Often the event that signals the woman to seek care is a missed or late menstrual period. She also may be experiencing some of the signs associated with pregnancy, such as nausea, fatigue, frequent urination, or tingling and fullness of the breasts. The utmost question on the woman's mind, regardless of whether the pregnancy was planned or not, is "Am I pregnant?" If the woman obtained a positive pregnancy test at home, she will want to confirm the results. If she did not, then she may feel anxious, nervous, excited, or any number of emotions until the primary care provider confirms the diagnosis of pregnancy.

The first prenatal visit is usually the longest because the baseline data to which all subsequent

assessments are compared are obtained at this visit. The woman may not be mentally prepared for all the questions and tests that must be done, particularly because her main goal at the first visit is to determine whether or not she is, in fact, pregnant. The major objectives of this visit are to confirm or rule out a diagnosis of pregnancy, ascertain risk factors, determine the due date, and provide education on maintaining a healthy pregnancy. These objectives are met through history taking, a physical examination, laboratory work, and teaching. Refer to The Nursing Process for Prenatal Care at the end of the chapter for discussion of teaching topics.

History

The history is one of the most important elements of the first prenatal visit. The woman may be asked to fill out a written questionnaire; the nurse or physician will then confirm the answers. Some health care providers may prefer to obtain the history exclusively by face-to-face interview. Whatever method is chosen, review the history thoroughly and call the primary care provider's attention to any abnormal or unusual details. There are several parts to the history, including chief complaint, reproductive history, medical-surgical history, family history, and social history.

Chief Complaint. The chief complaint will be elicited, which is usually a missed menstrual period. Ask the woman about presumptive and probable signs of pregnancy.

Reproductive History. Note the time of menarche, as well as a summary of the characteristics of the woman's normal menstrual cycles. Common questions include, "Are your periods regular?" "How frequently do your periods occur?" The first day of the last menstrual period (LMP) is noted, if the woman knows this information. Details of each pregnancy are reviewed, including history of miscarriages or abortions and the outcome of each pregnancy (i.e., how many weeks the pregnancy lasted and whether or not the pregnancy ended with a living child).

Here's a tip that should increase the accuracy of the history. If a partner or other family members accompany the woman, find a tactful way to separate them for at least part of the history collection. A woman may have a history of a previous pregnancy, an abortion that she may not wish to reveal to her family members, or she may be the victim of domestic violence. In any of these instances, it is necessary to interview the woman alone if truthful answers are to be expected. Assure her that all information is held in strict confidence and shared only with other members of the health care team on a need-to-know basis.

A problem the woman had in a previous pregnancy may manifest itself again in the current pregnancy or increase the chance that she will develop another type of complication.

The obstetric history is a part of the reproductive history and is recorded in a specific format that is a type of medical shorthand. The word "gravid" means pregnant. The number of pregnancies the woman has had (regardless of the outcome) is recorded as the **gravida**. For example, a woman who has had one pregnancy is a gravida 1, whereas a woman who has had five pregnancies is a gravida 5. A woman who has never been pregnant is a **nulligravida**, whereas a woman who has had more than one pregnancy is a **multigravida**.

Once the total number of pregnancies has been determined and recorded, the next part of the obstetric history is parity. **Parity**, or para, communicates the outcome of previous pregnancies. If a gravida 1 delivers a live-born infant, or an infant who is past the age of viability (greater than 20 weeks), she is then referred to as a gravida 1, para 1. Nonviable fetuses that are delivered before the end of 20 weeks' gestation are considered abortions (either spontaneous or induced) and are not counted in the parity. For example, if a woman had a pregnancy that ended at 17 weeks, another at 26 weeks, and another at 40 weeks, and she is currently pregnant, she is a gravida 4 para 2 abortus 1. The parity refers to the outcome of the pregnancy and is counted as 1, even if the woman delivers twins or triplets.

One of the most common methods of recording the obstetric history is to use the acronym GTPAL. "G" stands for gravida, the total number of pregnancies. "T" stands for term, the number of pregnancies that ended at term (at or beyond 38 weeks' gestation); "P" is for preterm, the number of pregnancies that ended after 20 weeks and before the end of 37 weeks' gestation. "A" represents abortions, the number of pregnancies that ended before 20 weeks' gestation. "L" is for living; the number of children delivered who are alive as of the time the history is taken. Some primary care providers further divide abortions into induced and spontaneous and note multiple births and ectopic pregnancies. Box 7-1 defines terms associated with the obstetric history.

It also is important to obtain information regarding complications that may have occurred with other pregnancies. If a woman hemorrhaged after a previous delivery, she has a higher risk of hemorrhaging after subsequent deliveries. If she develops gestational diabetes with a pregnancy, she will likely develop the condition again with subsequent pregnancies. If she has a history of preterm delivery, her risk is increased that she will deliver another baby prematurely. Any abnormality that presented itself in a previous pregnancy must be noted.

BOX 7.1 | Obstetric History Terms

- *Gravida*: Total number of pregnancies a woman has had, including the present pregnancy.
- *Para*: The number of fetuses delivered after the point of viability (20 weeks' gestation), whether or not they are born alive.
- *Nulli* (null or none), *primi* (first or one), and *multi* (many): Prefixes used in front of the terms "gravida" and "para" to indicate whether or not the woman has had previous pregnancies and deliveries.
- GTPAL: Acronym that represents the obstetric history.
    Gravida
    Term deliveries
    Preterm deliveries
    Abortions
    Living children

Medical–Surgical History. After a thorough reproductive history is elicited, the primary care provider must obtain a detailed medical–surgical history of the woman. If she has any major medical problems, such as heart disease or diabetes, she will require closer surveillance throughout the pregnancy. All medications the woman is taking, including over-the-counter medications and herbal remedies, should be noted in the prenatal record.

The medical history also involves determining if there are risk factors for infectious diseases. Exposure to anyone with tuberculosis indicates the need for further screening to rule out the disease. The immunization status should be assessed. Although most immunizations are contraindicated during pregnancy, the woman who is at risk for an infectious disease can take precautions to decrease the chance she will contract infection during pregnancy. Risk factors for human immunodeficiency virus/acquired immunodeficiency syndrome (HIV/AIDS) and other sexually transmitted infections (STIs) must be determined (Box 7-2).

Family History. A family history also is important because it may highlight the need for genetic testing or

---

BOX 7.2 | Risk Factors for Sexually Transmitted Infections (STIs)

- Sex with multiple partners
- Sex with a partner who has risk factors
- Intravenous drug use (needle sharing)
- Anal intercourse
- Vaginal intercourse with a partner who also engages in anal intercourse
- Unprotected (no condom) intercourse

TABLE 7.1	Genetic Disorder Screening Criteria by Ethnicity
Ethnicity	Genetic Disorders for Which Screening May Be Recommended
African-American, Indian, Middle Eastern	Sickle cell anemia; thalassemia
European Jewish, French Canadian	Tay-Sachs disease
Mediterranean, Southeast Asian	Thalassemia
Caucasian	Cystic fibrosis

counseling. Inquiry will be made regarding the health status of the father of the baby and any close relatives of the woman and her partner. If there is a family history for cystic fibrosis or hearing loss, genetic screening may be indicated. The ethnic background of the woman and relatives of the unborn child are important factors to note. For instance, many people of African-American descent are carriers for sickle cell anemia; people of Mediterranean descent are at increased risk for thalassemia. See Table 7-1 for examples of ethnic-related genetic diseases.

Social History. The social history focuses on environmental factors that may influence the pregnancy. A woman who has strong social support, adequate housing and nutrition, and greater than a high school education is less likely to develop complications of pregnancy than is a woman who lives with inadequate resources. The type of employment may also have a bearing on the health of the pregnancy. A job that requires exposure to harmful chemicals is less safe for the woman and fetus than is a job that does not involve this type of exposure.

Smoking, alcohol, and illicit and over-the-counter drug use can all potentially harm a growing fetus, so it is important to determine the woman's consumption patterns, particularly since conception. If the woman owns a cat or likes to garden, she is at increased risk for contracting toxoplasmosis, an infection that can cause the woman to lose the pregnancy or can result in severe abnormalities in the fetus.

Physical Examination

The physical examination covers all body systems and is completed by the primary care provider. The nurse provides assistance, as needed. The head-to-toe physical is done first. The examiner is looking for signs of disease that may need treatment and for any evidence of previously undetected maternal disease or other signs of ill health. A breast examination is part of the

physical. Although it is rare, breast cancer in a young pregnant woman is a possibility.

The head-to-toe physical is followed by a vaginal speculum examination and a bimanual examination of the uterus. During the speculum examination, a Papanicolaou test or Pap smear is done, and some signs of pregnancy, such as Chadwick's sign, can be noted (see Nursing Procedure 7-1). The bimanual examination (Fig. 7-1) allows the practitioner to feel the size of the uterus and to elicit Hegar's sign.

Laboratory Assessment

There are many laboratory tests that will be done during the course of the pregnancy. A complete blood count (CBC) gives the health care provider an indication of the overall health status of the woman. Anemia will be manifested as a low blood count and low hemoglobin and hematocrit. Anemia is one indication of suboptimal nutritional status and is associated with poor pregnancy outcomes, unless it is caught and treated early. A woman who is at risk for sickle cell anemia or thalassemia is given a hemoglobin electrophoresis test.

Other laboratory tests routinely ordered include a blood type and antibody screen. This test helps identify women who are at risk of developing antigen incompatibility with fetal blood cells. A, B, and O incompatibilities can develop, as well as $Rh_o(D)$ incompatibilities. If an

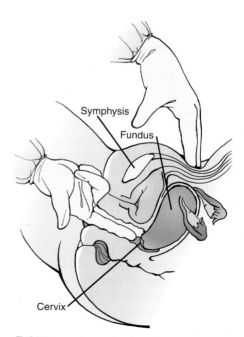

● *Figure 7.1* Bimanual examination. The fundus (top portion) of the uterus is palpated through the abdominal wall while the hand in the vagina holds the cervix in place. In this way the examiner can determine the size of the uterus, which helps date the pregnancy.

Nursing Procedure 7.1
Assisting the Practitioner With a Pelvic Examination and Collection of the Pap Smear

EQUIPMENT

Examination table with stirrups or foot pedals
Drapes
Sterile gloves for the examiner
Speculum
Swab for the Pap test
Glass slide
Fixative
Sterile lubricant (water-soluble)

PROCEDURE

1. Explain procedure to the patient.
2. Instruct the patient to empty her bladder before the procedure.
3. Wash hands thoroughly.
4. Assemble equipment, maintaining the sterility of the equipment.
5. Position patient on stirrups or foot pedals so that her knees fall outward.
6. Drape the patient with a sheet or other draping for privacy, covering the abdomen and legs, leaving the perineal area exposed.
7. Open packages as needed throughout the procedure.
8. After the practitioner obtains the specimen and swipes the slide, spray the fixative on the slide.
9. Place the sterile lubricant on the practitioner's fingertips, when indicated for the bimanual examination.
10. Wash hands thoroughly.
11. Label specimen according to facility policy.
12. Send sample to laboratory with appropriate request form.
13. Rinse reusable instruments and dispose of waste appropriately.
14. Wash hands thoroughly.

Note: A full bladder interferes with the pelvic examination and causes discomfort for the woman.

---

antigen incompatibility develops, the fetus may suffer from hemolytic anemia as the mother's antibodies cross the placenta and attack his red blood cells (refer to Chapter 20 for further discussion of antigen incompatibilities).

Other tests screen for the presence of infection. The woman will be tested for hepatitis B, HIV, syphilis, gonorrhea, and Chlamydia. Each of these infections can cause serious fetal problems unless they are treated. A rubella titer will be drawn to determine if the woman is immune. If she is not, this fact will be noted in her chart, and she will need a rubella immunization immediately after delivery because the rubella vaccine cannot be given safely during pregnancy. A urine culture will screen for bacteria in the urine, a situation that can lead to urinary tract infection and premature labor if it is not treated. The Pap smear is evaluated to screen for cervical cancer.

Determining the Due Date

One important aspect of the first visit is to calculate the due date, or the **estimated date of delivery** (EDD). An older term that is sometimes still used is **estimated date of confinement** (EDC). Both terms refer to the estimated date that the baby will be born. This is critical information for the primary care provider to know because she will manage problems that may arise during the pregnancy differently, depending on the gestational age of the fetus. Therefore, it is essential to have an accurate due date.

There are several means by which to date a pregnancy. The most common way to calculate the EDD is to use **Nagele's rule**. To determine the due date using Nagele's rule, add 7 days to the date of the first day of the LMP, then subtract 3 months. This is a fairly simple way to estimate the due date, but it is dependent upon knowing when the first day of the LMP was. Sometimes this date is impossible to determine, particularly if the woman experiences irregular menstrual cycles, or if she just cannot remember the date.

During the pelvic examination, the practitioner can feel the size of the uterus to get an idea of how far along the pregnancy is. For instance, a uterus that is the size of a hen's egg is approximately 7 weeks. If the uterus feels to be the size of an orange, the pregnancy is approximately 10 weeks along, and at 12 weeks the uterus is the size of a grapefruit. Other ways to validate the gestational age are to note landmarks in the pregnancy. The fetal heart beat can first be detected by Doppler ultrasound between 10 and 12 weeks. Quickening typically occurs around 16 weeks for multigravidas and 20 weeks for primigravidas.

One of the most common and reliable ways to date the pregnancy is for the practitioner to order an obstetric sonogram. During this procedure, high frequency sound waves reflect off fetal and maternal pelvic structures and allow them to be visualized in real time. Fetal structures, such as the femur and the head, are measured. The measurements allow the practitioner to estimate the gestational age of the fetus, and thereby determine a due date. The earlier in the pregnancy the sonogram is done, the more accurate the due date. If there is a discrepancy between the EDD calculated using Nagele's rule and the EDD determined by sonogram, the results of the sonogram (if it is done early in the pregnancy) will be used to base treatment decisions.

Risk Assessment

The risk assessment is done by taking into account all of the information gathered from the history, physical examination, and laboratory tests. There are many factors that put a pregnancy at risk. These factors include a negative attitude of the woman toward the pregnancy (e.g., an unwanted pregnancy), seeking prenatal care late in the pregnancy, and maternal substance abuse (alcohol, tobacco, or illicit drugs). A history of complications with previous pregnancies or poor outcomes, and the presence of maternal disease also put the current pregnancy at risk. Social factors that increase the risk of poor outcomes include inadequate living conditions and domestic violence or physical abuse. If the woman is unaware of the adverse effects of tobacco and alcohol, the benefits of folic acid, or the risk of HIV, the pregnancy is at increased risk for complications and poor outcomes. Age also plays a factor. Young teens and women older than 35 years of age are at higher risk for a complicated pregnancy. An unplanned pregnancy or a pregnancy when the woman is unsure of her LMP date may also be at risk.

Test Yourself

- What is the obstetric term used to indicate the number of pregnancies a woman has had?

- List four laboratory tests that are routinely ordered during the first prenatal visit.

- State how to calculate the due date using Nagele's rule.

Subsequent Prenatal Visits

Traditionally women are seen once monthly from weeks 1 through 32. Between weeks 32 and 36, prenatal visits are biweekly. From week 36 until delivery the woman is seen weekly in the primary care provider's office. Current research shows that fewer visits for low-risk pregnancies and more visits for at-risk pregnancies may be more beneficial overall than a rigid adherence to the traditional schedule of visits. In any event, the woman needs encouragement to keep her appointments and maintain regular prenatal care throughout the pregnancy.

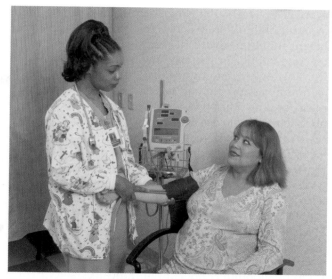

● *Figure 7.2* The Practical Nurse measures the blood pressure at a prenatal visit.

Most subsequent visits include specific assessments. Weight, blood pressure (Fig. 7-2), urine protein and glucose, and fetal heart rate are all data that may be collected by the practical nurse. At every visit, inquiry should be made regarding the danger signals of pregnancy (discussed in the The Nursing Process for Prenatal Care). The woman should be asked about fetal movement, contractions, bleeding, and membrane rupture. Normally the pelvic examination is not repeated until late in the pregnancy, close to the expected time of delivery.

At each office visit the practitioner will measure the fundal height in centimeters (Fig. 7-3). This measure provides a confirmation of gestational age between weeks 18 and 32. In other words, between weeks 18 and 32, the fundal height in centimeters should match the

● *Figure 7.3* The Certified Nurse Midwife (CNM) measures the fundal height. Between 18 and 32 weeks' gestation there is a good correlation between the gestation in weeks and the fundal height in centimeters.

number of weeks the pregnancy has progressed. For example, if the woman is 18 weeks pregnant, the fundal height should measure 18 centimeters. If there is a discrepancy between the size and dates, a sonogram is usually done to determine the cause of the discrepancy. A fundal height that is larger than expected could mean, among other things, that the original dates were miscalculated, that the woman is carrying twins, or that there is a molar pregnancy (Chapter 17).

The woman undergoes screening at particular times during the pregnancy. Sometime between 15 and 20 weeks' gestation, a maternal serum alpha-fetoprotein (MSAFP) should be drawn (see the discussion in the section on fetal assessment). Between 24 and 28 weeks, all women should be screened for gestational diabetes. At 28 weeks, a woman who is $Rh_o(D)$-negative should be screened for antibodies and given anti-D immune globulin (RhoGam), if indicated (see Chapter 23 for further discussion of hemolytic disease of the newborn). The woman should be screened for Group B streptococcus (GBS) after 35 weeks and before the end of 37 weeks. Positive cultures indicate the need for antibiotics for the woman during labor and close observation of the newborn for 48 hours after birth.

Test Yourself

- How often is a woman with an uncomplicated pregnancy seen in the office from weeks 1 through 32?

- What purpose does measuring the fundal height serve during prenatal visits?

- List the time during pregnancy when a woman is normally screened for gestational diabetes.

ASSESSMENT OF FETAL WELL-BEING DURING PREGNANCY

Throughout the pregnancy the primary care provider may order tests to assess the well-being of the fetus. Some of the most common tests and procedures are described in the discussion that follows. Not every woman will receive every test, although some screening tests are recommended for all pregnant women at certain points during the pregnancy.

Fetal Kick Counts

A healthy fetus moves and kicks regularly, although the pregnant woman usually cannot perceive the movements until approximately gestational week 16 to 20. The primary care provider or the nurse instructs the

Don't forget. "Routine" for the nurse is not at all routine for the woman. She will need careful explanation of all testing that is planned, whether or not it is a normal part of prenatal care or performed for some other reason. If a screening test result is "suspicious," or further testing is indicated, remember that the woman will need emotional support. It is scary not knowing what to expect while waiting for test results. Accept and let her talk through her feelings.

woman to monitor her baby's movements on a daily basis. Instruct the woman to choose a time each day in which she can relax and count the baby's movements. Each kick or position change counts as one movement. Using a special form, or a blank sheet of paper, instruct the woman to note the time she starts counting fetal kicks, then she is to keep counting until she counts 10 movements. A healthy fetus will move at least 10 times in 2 hours. If it takes longer than 2 hours for the fetus to move 10 times, or if the woman cannot get her baby to move at all, she should immediately call her health care provider. The primary care provider will want to do additional tests to determine the well-being of the fetus.

Ultrasonography

Ultrasound has been used for many years in the United States to determine gestational age, observe the fetus, and diagnose complications of pregnancy. Because it appears to be a safe and effective way to monitor fetal well-being, the procedure is performed frequently (Fig. 7-4). One result of monitoring virtually every pregnancy with ultrasound is that most parents know the gender of their child before she is born. Many sonographers take a still picture of the fetus and provide this to the parents, if desired.

● *Figure 7.4* Ultrasound is used to identify fetal and placental structures during pregnancy.

● **Figure 7.5** Fetus viewed via ultrasound. The outline of the fetal head and trunk can be clearly seen in the transverse position.

As stated earlier in the chapter, ultrasound uses high frequency sound waves to visualize fetal and maternal structures (Fig. 7-5). The developing embryo can first be visualized at about 6 weeks' gestation. An ultrasound performed at this stage is usually done to diagnose the pregnancy. The fetus is visualized in real time, so that his cardiac activity and body movements can be monitored. Box 7-3 lists ways ultrasound technology is used to monitor the pregnancy and fetal well-being.

BOX 7.3	Uses for Ultrasound Technology During Pregnancy

- Diagnose pregnancy: intrauterine and ectopic (outside the uterine cavity).
- Diagnose multifetal pregnancies (twins, triplets).
- Monitor fetal heart beat and breathing movements. The fetus makes "practice" breathing movements in utero as early as 11 weeks gestation.
- Take measurements of the fetal head, femur, and other structures to determine gestational age or diagnose fetal growth restriction.
- Detect fetal anomalies.
- Estimate the amount of amniotic fluid that is present. Either too much (hydramnios) or too little (oligohydramnios) can indicate problems with the pregnancy.
- Identify fetal and placental structures during amniocentesis or umbilical cord sampling.
- Detect placental problems, such as abnormal placement of the placenta in placenta previa or grade the placenta (determine the age and functioning).
- Diagnose fetal demise (death). Absence of cardiac activity is used to diagnose fetal death.
- Verify fetal presentation and position.
- Estimate the birth weight, particularly if the fetus is thought to be abnormally large (macrosomic).

Most abnormalities of the fetus, placenta, and surrounding structures are best detected between 16 and 20 weeks' gestation. Detailed sonograms can diagnose severe congenital heart, spine, brain, and kidney defects. However, ultrasound cannot pick up all abnormalities. Some anomalies, such as Down syndrome, have subtle characteristics that often cannot be picked up until late in the pregnancy. However, a skilled practitioner can detect 70% to 80% of Down syndrome cases when observing for nuchal translucency (fetal neck thickness) on ultrasound between weeks 11 and 14. There are two main ways an ultrasound can be done–the transabdominal approach, in which the transducer is placed on the abdomen to visualize the pregnancy, and the endovaginal approach, in which a specialized probe is inserted into the vagina to visualize the cervix and fetal structures.

Transabdominal Ultrasound

It is important for the woman to have a full bladder for the procedure, particularly during the first trimester. A full bladder pushes the uterus up so that the contents can more easily be seen. Instruct the woman to drink several large glasses of water 2 hours before the procedure and not to empty her bladder.

If you are assisting during the procedure, make certain that a small wedge or sandbag is placed under one hip to prevent vena-caval hypotension. Explain to the woman that a special gel will be used on her abdomen and that it probably will be cold. She should not feel any discomfort during the procedure, other than the discomfort of a full bladder. The procedure is performed in a darkened room. Although the technician performing the sonogram can see fetal structures and obvious defects during the sonogram, it will take several hours to get the official results because the radiologist must review the films and dictate the diagnosis. After the procedure, clean the excess gel off of the woman's abdomen and assist her to the bathroom.

Endovaginal Ultrasound

The endovaginal approach allows for clearer image because the probe is very close to fetal and uterine structures. The pregnancy can usually be visualized sooner than with the transabdominal method. The endovaginal method has been used to predict or diagnose preterm labor because the cervix can be measured and analyzed for changes.

The woman's bladder can be empty for the endovaginal examination. Assist the woman into lithotomy position (as for a pelvic examination) and drape her for privacy. A female attendant must be present in the room at all times during the procedure. The examiner covers the probe (which is smaller than a speculum) with a specialized sheath, a condom, or the finger of a glove; applies ultrasonic transducer gel to the covered probe; and inserts the probe into the vagina. The woman will feel the probe being moved about in different directions during the test. The probe may cause mild discomfort but generally is not painful.

Doppler Flow Studies

Another test that uses ultrasound technology is a Doppler flow study, or Doppler velocimetry. A specialized ultrasound machine is used to measure the flow of blood through fetal vessels. The ultrasound transducer is placed on the woman's abdomen, and blood flow can be assessed in the umbilical vessels, fetal brain, and fetal heart. If the test shows that blood flow through fetal vessels is less than normal, the fetus may not be receiving enough oxygen and nutrients from the placenta, and additional studies will most likely be ordered. Preparation and nursing care for a Doppler flow study are the same as for ultrasonography.

Maternal Serum Alpha-fetoprotein Screening

Alpha-fetoprotein is a protein that is manufactured by the fetus. The protein is found in small amounts in the pregnant woman's bloodstream. Many physicians recommend measuring MSAFP between 16 and 18 weeks' gestation because abnormal levels may indicate a problem and the need for additional testing.

MSAFP levels are elevated in several conditions. Higher-than-expected levels of MSAFP may indicate that the pregnancy is farther along than was predicted initially. When the woman is carrying multiple fetuses, such as twins or triplets, or when the fetus has died, MSAFP levels will be elevated. The main reason physicians screen MSAFP is to check for neural tube defects, such as anencephaly (failure of the brain to develop normally) or spina bifida (failure of the spine to close completely during development). MSAFP levels are usually elevated if the fetus has either of these anomalies or omphalocele or gastroschisis (failure of the abdominal wall to close). Low MSAFP levels may also indicate a problem, in particular Down's syndrome.

It is important for the parents-to-be to understand the reasons for and implications of MSAFP testing. Even when the levels are abnormal, approximately 90% of the time the woman will be delivered of a healthy baby. However, abnormal results increase the likelihood that the fetus has an abnormality, and additional testing with ultrasound and/or amniocentesis is usually indicated. Even when the follow-up ultrasound is normal, there is no guarantee that the fetus will be healthy. An elevated MSAFP in the presence of a normal ultrasound increases the risk that the woman will develop a complication of pregnancy such as preeclampsia or intrauterine growth restriction.

Some women want to have the test done so that they can decide whether or not to end the pregnancy before the age of viability. Other women feel strongly that abortion is not an option, but they may want to know if an anomaly is present so that they can deliver in a hospital with high-level care and have specialists immediately available to resuscitate and care for the baby. Other women may decide against testing because a false-positive test might be needlessly worrisome and lead to more invasive, riskier tests, such as amniocentesis, even though the baby might be healthy. These are issues each woman must consider in consult with her partner and physician. No matter what decision the woman makes regarding testing, it is critical that she be supported in her decision.

Triple-Marker (or Multiple-Marker) Screening

The sensitivity of MSAFP testing is increased when the levels of two other hormones are measured in conjunction with MSAFP. When MSAFP, human chorionic gonadotropin (hCG), and unconjugated estriol (uE3) levels are measured from the same maternal blood sample, the test is called a triple-marker screen. A low MSAFP, low estriol, and elevated hCG suggests that the baby has Down syndrome; whereas low levels of all three hormones increases the risk the fetus has trisomy 18, a more severe and less common chromosomal defect. A fourth biochemical marker in maternal serum, inhibin A, has been found to increase the ability of blood tests to predict chromosomal abnormalities of the fetus, so some practitioners add this fourth screen. The test is then known as a multiple-marker screen.

Sometimes the physician will order serial estriol levels in the third trimester to monitor the well-being of the fetus. Falling estriol levels in the third trimester may indicate that the fetus is in jeopardy, in which case an emergency cesarean delivery may be done to save the fetus' life. Nursing care for MSAFP or triple marker screening is the same as that for any venous blood sampling of the woman.

Amniocentesis

An **amniocentesis** is a diagnostic procedure whereby a needle is inserted into the amniotic sac and a small amount of fluid is withdrawn. A variety of biochemical, chromosomal, and genetic studies can be done using the amniotic fluid sample.

The procedure is usually performed between 15 and 20 weeks' gestation, and genetic studies are done to identify fetal abnormalities. Because early amniocentesis (<14 weeks) is associated with a higher rate of pregnancy loss (abortion) and fetal foot deformities, most practitioners will not perform amniocentesis

> **BOX 7.4** **Selected Indications for Chromosomal Studies by Amniocentesis or Chorionic Villus Sampling**
>
> - Advanced maternal age (generally accepted as older than 35)
> - Previous offspring with chromosomal anomalies
> - History of recurrent pregnancy loss
> - Ultrasound diagnosis of fetal anomalies
> - Abnormal MSAFP, triple marker screen, or multiple marker screen
> - Previous offspring with a neural tube defect
> - Both parents known carriers of a recessive genetic trait (such as cystic fibrosis, sickle cell anemia, or Tay-Sachs disease)

before 14 weeks. Early and second trimester cases are done to determine the genetic makeup of the fetus. This can be done because fetal cells are found within the amniotic fluid. Box 7-4 lists indications for first and second trimester amniocentesis. Third trimester amniocentesis is usually done to determine fetal lung maturity to allow for the earliest possible delivery in certain at-risk pregnancies.

Because amniocentesis is an invasive procedure that carries a small risk of spontaneous abortion, injury to the fetus, and chorioamnionitis (infection of the fetal membranes), informed consent is required. The physician explains the procedure and risks to the woman and answers her questions. If you are asked to witness the consent, be certain that the woman has had all her questions answered before she signs. Explain the procedure to her so that she knows what to expect. Many women are worried that the procedure will be painful. Although pain is a subjective feeling that is experienced differently for each person, most women find that the procedure is much less painful than they anticipated. Usually women report feeling a slight pinching sensation or vague cramping.

Ultrasonography is done before amniocentesis to locate a pocket of amniotic fluid. Without ultrasound to guide the needle, there is a high risk that the needle could puncture the placenta or the fetus. After the pocket of fluid is located (usually on the upper portion of the uterus), the site is prepared with Betadine or alcohol, and sterile drapes are placed on the abdomen around the site. The ultrasound transducer is also covered with sterile drapes. Next the practitioner inserts a 20- to 22-gauge spinal needle into the chosen site. The practitioner watches the ultrasound picture and guides the needle along the chosen path into the pocket of fluid. The first 0.5 cc of fluid is discarded to avoid contamination of the specimen with maternal

cells. Then 20 mL of fluid is withdrawn, and the needle is removed. At this point the practitioner monitors the fetal heart rate by ultrasound to ensure fetal well-being. Then the fluid, which is normally straw colored, is placed into sterile tubes, labeled, and sent to the laboratory for analysis. Results are usually available within 2 to 3 weeks and are highly accurate (approximately 99%).

The woman should remain on bed rest the day of the procedure. Attach continuous electronic fetal monitoring to observe the fetal heart rate and contractions, if they should occur. Women who are $Rh_0(D)$-negative should receive anti-D immunoglobulin (RhoGam) after the procedure. The site should be monitored for leakage of amniotic fluid (a rare complication), and the woman's temperature should be monitored. Any temperature elevation, leaking of fluid from the site or from the vagina, vaginal bleeding, cramps, or contractions should be immediately reported to the RN or the attending practitioner. After several hours of monitoring, the woman may be sent home. Instruct her to remain on bed rest for the rest of the day. The following day she may do light housework chores, and the third day she may resume regular activities. Warning signs that should be reported to the attending practitioner immediately include fever, amniotic fluid leakage, vaginal bleeding, and/or cramping.

As with any medical procedure that carries risk, amniocentesis has advantages and disadvantages that each woman and her partner must consider carefully before submitting to the procedure. The most common reason for undergoing amniocentesis is to determine if there is a fetal abnormality so that the pregnancy might be ended (elective abortion) before the age of viability. Many women will not consider an abortion under any circumstances. In these cases, there are still benefits to amniocentesis. If the fetus does have a chromosomal abnormality, knowing in advance allows for the medical team and the parents to prepare for the birth. It also allows the physician to make better decisions about managing the pregnancy. Every woman who is contemplating amniocentesis should have genetic counseling. Then, no matter what decision the woman makes, it is critical that the health care team be supportive of her decision.

Chorionic Villus Sampling

Chorionic villus sampling (CVS) is a newer procedure that can provide chromosomal studies of fetal cells similar to amniocentesis. Indications for CVS are the same as for amniocentesis (see Box 7-4). One advantage of CVS testing is that it is done earlier in the pregnancy than is amniocentesis, which allows for a decision about elective abortion to be made sooner in the pregnancy. Elective abortions are safer for the woman the earlier they are performed. CVS is typically performed at 10 to 12 weeks' gestation. Because CVS is an invasive procedure, informed consent is required.

Just before the procedure, ultrasonography is performed to confirm fetal well-being, the location of the placenta, and gestational age. For the transcervical approach, the woman is placed in lithotomy position in stirrups, and her vagina and cervix are cleaned with Betadine or other antiseptic fluid. Using ultrasound guidance, a small catheter is inserted into the woman's vagina and through the cervix. Placental tissue is then extracted into a syringe to obtain fetal cells for chromosomal analysis. The procedure can also be done transabdominally with a needle, similar to the procedure for amniocentesis. The woman usually experiences minimal discomfort and may resume normal activities after the test. Anti-D immunoglobulin (RhoGam) should be administered after the procedure to $Rh_o(D)$-negative women.

One advantage of CVS testing is that the results are available in 7 to 10 days, much faster than with amniocentesis. However, there are disadvantages to this technique. First, some authorities report a higher rate of pregnancy loss[1] with transcervical CVS versus transabdominal CVS and second trimester amniocentesis. Other authorities indicate that the risk for pregnancy loss with CVS is comparable with that of amniocentesis. The risk is lowered for both procedures as the skill level of the practitioner increases. A second potential disadvantage is that because no amniotic fluid is withdrawn in CVS, the amniotic alpha-fetoprotein cannot be evaluated, as it can with amniocentesis. This would mean the woman would need to have MSAFP levels drawn at 16 to 18 weeks' gestation to test for neural tube defects. A woman who has amniocentesis performed does not need the MSAFP test because the fetal alpha-fetoprotein level, which is a more accurate predictor of spinal defects than maternal serum levels, is already known. The third disadvantage of CVS is that there is a small risk that the cells taken from the placenta will be different than fetal cells. If this happens, a situation called "placental mosaicism," the test results would be abnormal, even if the fetus were normal. Some authorities suggest if CVS is performed before 9 weeks' gestation, it can cause fetal limb and digit deformations.

Percutaneous Umbilical Blood Sampling

Percutaneous umbilical blood sampling (PUBS), also known as **cordocentesis**, is a procedure similar to amniocentesis, except that fetal blood is withdrawn, rather than amniotic fluid. The woman is prepared in the same manner as for amniocentesis, informed consent is obtained, and ultrasound is performed to locate the placenta and fetal structures and to confirm gestational age and viability. A thin needle is inserted transabdominally under ultrasound guidance, and blood is withdrawn from the umbilical cord close to its insertion with the placenta. Alternatively blood can be withdrawn from the fetal heart or from the umbilical vein within the liver, although these sites are not commonly chosen. The blood is then sent for testing.

Sometimes PUBS is done specifically to diagnose and treat certain diseases of the blood, such as von Willebrand's disease, alloimmune thrombocytopenia, and hemolytic disease. It is also used to diagnose and treat cases of fetal infection, such as toxoplasmosis, rubella, cytomegalovirus, varicella zoster, human parvovirus, and HIV. Through the technology of cordocentesis, the fetus with thrombocytopenia can receive weekly infusions of platelets until delivery. The fetus with hemolytic disease can receive exchange transfusions (part of the fetus' blood is withdrawn and the same amount replaced with healthy blood). The fetus found to be have an infection can be treated with antibiotics or receive other therapies, depending upon the type of infection. The blood obtained from cordocentesis can also be sent for rapid chromosomal studies. Results are back within 48 to 72 hours. The risks associated with PUBS are approximately the same as those of amniocentesis.

Nonstress Test

The nonstress test (NST) is a noninvasive way to monitor fetal well-being. Usually around 28 weeks and onward, the fetal nervous system is developed enough so that the autonomic nervous system works to periodically accelerate the heart rate. Therefore, the woman can be attached to an electronic fetal monitor (EFM), and the fetal heart can be observed for accelerations.

The woman requires no special preparation other than placement of EFM (refer to Chapter 10 for in-depth discussion of fetal monitoring). She may or may not be given an event marker to hold.[2] If she is given

---

[1] The latest report available from the Centers for Disease Control (CDC) is 1995. In that report, a pregnancy loss of 0.5% to 1.0% (1/200 to 1/100) was found with transcervical CVS, as compared with a 0.25% to 0.50% (1/400 to 1/200) risk with amniocentesis. These data are probably no longer valid because the technique has been perfected over time.

[2] In the past it was very important to monitor the fetal heart rate in conjunction with fetal movement. Now it is generally felt that spontaneous accelerations with or without fetal movement are indicative of fetal well-being, so it is not necessary to have the woman track fetal movements, although some practitioners may prefer this.

one, she is instructed to push the button every time she feels the fetus move. The fetal monitor strip is evaluated after 20 minutes. If there are at least two accelerations of the fetal heart in a 15×15 window, that is the fetal heart accelerates at least 15 beats above the baseline for at least 15 seconds, the NST is said to be "reactive" provided that the baseline and variability are normal and that there are no decelerations of the fetal heart rate. In the presence of a reactive NST,[3] fetal well-being is assumed for at least the next week.

If, however, there are no accelerations or less than 2 occur within 20 minutes, the strip is said to be "nonreactive." In this case the monitoring would continue for another 20 minutes in the hopes of obtaining a reactive NST. This decision is made based on knowledge of fetal sleep cycles, which last for approximately 20 minutes. During fetal sleep, it is expected that there will be no accelerations, so waiting an additional 20 minutes is indicated. Sometimes the nurse will attempt to stimulate the fetus. She may clap loudly close to the woman's abdomen or may manipulate the fetus through the abdomen with her hands, or she may give the woman something cold to drink. Any of these activities might stimulate a sleeping fetus to wake up, and a reactive tracing may be obtained. If the tracing remains nonreactive or equivocal (results cannot be positively interpreted), additional testing is warranted. In these instances the practitioner will frequently recommend vibroacoustic stimulation or a contraction stress test.

Vibroacoustic Stimulation

Vibroacoustic stimulation of the fetus is obtained with an artificial larynx placed a centimeter from or directly on the maternal abdomen. The sound stimulates the fetus to wake up, and in healthy fetuses a reactive NST will be obtained. Some practitioners use vibroacoustic stimulation for all NSTs because it decreases the length of time needed to obtain a reactive tracing and decreases the number of false-nonreactive tracings. Other practitioners use vibroacoustic stimulation as the second step after obtaining a nonreactive NST.

Contraction Stress Test

Uterine contractions cause a momentary reduction of uteroplacental blood flow. This situation stresses the fetus. A contraction stress test (CST) monitors the fetus' response to contractions to determine his well-being. The woman is placed on EFM as for the NST. There are three ways to obtain uterine contractions for a CST. If the woman is having spontaneous Braxton Hicks contractions, the fetal response to these contractions can be assessed. Another way is to induce uterine contractions through nipple stimulation. Nipple stimulation is thought to cause a release of oxytocin from the posterior pituitary gland. The oxytocin then stimulates the uterus to contract. The third way is to start an intravenous drip of Pitocin (synthetic oxytocin) to induce contractions.

No matter what way is used, the goal is to have three contractions of at least 40 seconds' duration within a 10-minute period of time. Then the fetal monitor strip is reviewed to determine the reaction of the fetus to the stress of the contractions. If there are no late decelerations (decelerations that occur after the contractions—refer to chapter 10 for detailed information on decelerations) after any of the contractions, the CST is said to be negative, which is a reassuring sign. A negative CST indicates that the fetus is not suffering from hypoxia and does not need immediate delivery. An equivocal CST occurs when there are late decelerations after some, but not all, of the uterine contractions. This result is suspicious of fetal hypoxia and may cause the physician to decide to perform a cesarean delivery of the fetus. A positive CST, late decelerations after every contraction, is indicative of fetal hypoxia and requires delivery of the fetus. An unsatisfactory CST occurs when there are insufficient contractions. The test must then be repeated within 24 hours, or a biophysical profile might be ordered.

Biophysical Profile

Biophysical profile (BPP) uses a combination of factors to determine fetal well-being. Five fetal biophysical variables are measured. Fetal heart rate acceleration is measured by performing the NST. Then breathing, body movements, tone, and amniotic fluid volume are measured using ultrasound. Each variable is given a score of 0 or 2 for a maximum score of 10. A score of 8 to 10 indicates fetal well-being. A score of 6 means possible fetal asphyxia, whereas a score of 4 indicates probable fetal asphyxia. Scores of 0 to 2 are ominous and require immediate delivery of the fetus.

Test Yourself

- How many times should the fetus move in a 2-hour period of time?

- What three tests are included in the triple-marker screening test?

- What tissue is extracted for study when chorionic villus sampling is used?

---

[3] Some authorities define a reactive NST based on the gestational age of the fetus. In these cases, a reactive test is defined as gestational age >34 weeks: ≥15 bpm for ≥15 secs, and gestational age <34 weeks: ≥10 bpm for ≥15 secs.

● The Nursing Process for Prenatal Care

The nurse is in a unique position to positively influence behaviors of the pregnant woman and to increase the chance she and her baby will stay healthy. Through consistent use of the nursing process, the nurse can detect problems early in order to intervene, or assist the primary care provider to intervene, and support the woman through her pregnancy. Of course teaching remains the primary nursing intervention throughout pregnancy.

ASSESSMENT

Ongoing assessment and data collection are essential components of prenatal visits. During the first prenatal visit, pay close attention to cues the woman may give regarding her feelings toward the pregnancy. Ambivalence is normal. The woman may express feelings of doubt about the pregnancy or her ability to be a good parent. These are normal reactions when a woman first finds out she is pregnant, and she needs reassurance that her responses are normal. Withdrawal or consistently negative remarks are warning signs that should be brought to the attention of the registered nurse (RN) or primary care provider.

If you are asked to administer the initial questionnaire, show the woman all the pages and assist her to complete it, if necessary. Review the document carefully when she is done to ensure completeness. Look for answers that indicate the need for further assessment. Alert the RN or the primary care provider when possible risk factors are identified in the history.

Assess for signs of nervousness and anxiety. She may express her nervousness by being restless or tense or by being quiet and withdrawn. Be attuned to signals she is giving regarding her comfort level. Inquire carefully regarding current medications, food supplements, and over-the-counter remedies she is using. This assessment should be done at every visit.

Note if the woman has been experiencing nausea and vomiting. Pay close attention to signs that might indicate poor nutritional status. Weight is an obvious clue. If the woman is overweight or underweight, she will need special assistance with nutritional concerns throughout the pregnancy. Other warning signs of poor nutritional status include dull, brittle hair; poor skin turgor; poor condition of skin and nails; obesity; emaciation; or a low hemoglobin level. Ask the woman

Don't make unfounded assumptions. Teaching is important no matter how many babies the woman has delivered. Don't make the mistake of assuming that just because this is not the woman's first baby, or because she is educated, or even that she is a nurse, that she has the information she needs to maintain a healthy pregnancy. Assess her knowledge level by asking her questions and entertaining her questions.

to write down a typical day's food consumption pattern, and then compare her normal intake to the food guide pyramid to determine if her diet is adequate for her nutritional needs.

Determine her education level and knowledge of pregnancy and prenatal care. If she is highly knowledgeable, she may ask high-level questions that indicate an understanding of basic issues. Conversely, she may ask basic questions, or no questions at all, which could indicate a knowledge deficit.

During subsequent visits, you may be asked to assess for signs of fetal well-being. These include obtaining fetal heart tones (FHTs) with an ultrasonic Doppler device (Fig. 7-6) beginning in week 10, and soliciting reports of active fetal movements after quickening. Pay close attention to vital signs, particularly the blood pressure. Monitor for danger signs of pregnancy (Box 7-5).

SELECTED NURSING DIAGNOSES

- Anxiety related to uncertainty regarding pregnancy diagnosis and not knowing what to expect during the office visit

● **Figure 7.6** The nurse listens to fetal heart tones with a Doppler device.

BOX 7.5	Danger Signs of Pregnancy

Inquire regarding these warning signals at every visit. Instruct the woman to report any of these signs, if she should experience them, to her health care provider right away.
- Fever or severe vomiting
- Headache, unrelieved by Tylenol or other relief measures
- Blurred vision or spots before the eyes
- Pain in the epigastric region
- Sudden weight gain or sudden onset of edema in the hands and face
- Vaginal bleeding
- Painful urination
- Sudden gush or constant, uncontrollable leaking of fluid from the vagina
- Decreased fetal movement
- Signs of preterm labor
  - Uterine contractions (four or more per hour)
  - Lower, dull backache
  - Pelvic pressure
  - Menstrual-like cramps
  - Increase in vaginal discharge
  - A feeling that something is not right

- Health-seeking behaviors related to maintaining a healthy pregnancy and concerns regarding the common discomforts of pregnancy
- Deficient Knowledge of self-care during pregnancy
- Risk for Injury related to complications of pregnancy
- Fear related to the unknown of childbirth, concerns regarding safe passage of self and infant through the delivery experience, and concerns related to assuming the parenting role

OUTCOME IDENTIFICATION AND PLANNING

Maintaining the health of mother and fetus is the primary goal of nursing care during the prenatal period. Specific goals are that the woman's anxiety will be reduced, she will manage the symptoms and discomforts associated with pregnancy; that she will feel confident in her ability to care for herself throughout the pregnancy; that she nor the fetus will experience injury from complications of pregnancy; that she will have sufficient knowledge to adequately meet her needs and those of the growing fetus throughout the pregnancy; and that she will express confidence in her ability to go through the labor and birth experience and assume the parenting role.

IMPLEMENTATION

Relieving Anxiety

Escort the woman to the examination room and explain the normal procedure and what she can expect during the visit. Much anxiety can be alleviated when the woman knows what to expect. Maintain a calm, confident demeanor while giving care. Protect the woman's privacy during invasive examinations.

Try to understand the woman's perspective. Note if her anxiety level increases. Anticipate concern when fetal testing is planned. Solicit questions and correct misconceptions the woman may have. Provide factual information concerning the treatment plan. Use active listening. Encourage positive coping behaviors.

Relieving the Common Discomforts of Pregnancy

Pregnant women tend to experience similar discomforts because of the significant bodily changes they undergo. Some discomforts tend to occur in early pregnancy, some toward the end, and others continue throughout. Selected discomforts are listed in Table 7-2 along with hints for helping the woman cope with these discomforts.

Nasal Stuffiness and Epistaxis

A pregnant woman is prone to nasal stuffiness and epistaxis (nosebleeds). Estrogen is the hormone most likely culpable for this discomfort because it contributes to vasocongestion and increases the fragility of the nasal mucosa. Sometimes the woman may have symptoms of the common cold that persist throughout pregnancy. Nasal decongestants, other than normal saline nasal sprays, are generally not recommended. In any event, the woman should consult with her primary care provider before taking any medications, including over-the-counter remedies. Menthol applied just below the nostrils before bedtime might help relieve some discomfort from congestion.

Avoiding vigorous nose blowing may prevent nosebleeds. It is also helpful to keep the nasal passages moist. Using a humidifier in the house and staying well hydrated can accomplish this. If a nosebleed occurs despite precautions, instruct the woman to pinch the nostrils and hold pressure for at least 4 minutes until the bleeding stops. Ice may help stop the bleeding. If the bleeding is heavy or does not stop with pressure, instruct the woman to consult with her primary care provider.

Nausea

Morning sickness, or nausea, is a common complaint of early pregnancy. Rising levels of human chorionic gonadotropin (hCG) are thought to be a

TABLE 7.2	Common Discomforts of Pregnancy	
Discomfort	**Contributing Factor or Cause**	**Hints for Relieving the Discomfort**
Bleeding gums	Stimulating effects of estrogen on the gums	• Visit the dentist • Use rinses and gargles to freshen the oral cavity • Use a soft-bristled toothbrush
Nasal stuffiness	Effects of estrogen on the nasal mucosa cause vasocongestion and stuffiness.	• Use a cool-air vaporizer • Try normal saline nasal sprays • Try to avoid commercial medicated nasal sprays because initial relief may be followed by rebound stuffiness
Nosebleeds	The tiny veins of the nasal lining are prone to breaking and causing nosebleeds. Dry nasal passages increase the risk.	• Avoid vigorous nose blowing • Use a humidifier • Drink plenty of fluids
Breast tenderness	Progesterone and estrogen are thought to contribute to the tingling or heavy sensations in the breasts that come and go throughout pregnancy.	• Wear a well-fitted support bra • Wearing a bra at night might be helpful if breast discomfort is interfering with restful sleep.
Nausea	Rising levels of hCG are thought to contribute to nausea.	• Begin the day with a high-carbohydrate food, such as melba toast, saltines, or other crackers. • Eat small high-carbohydrate meals frequently throughout the day. • Avoid noxious odors. • Take a walk outside in the fresh air. • Delay iron or vitamin supplementation until the second trimester.
Feeling faint	Postural hypotension can easily develop with the hemodynamic changes that occur in a normal pregnancy as the blood vessels in the periphery relax and dilate.	• Change positions slowly. • Avoid abrupt position changes. • Eat small, frequent, high-carbohydrate meals.
Fatigue	Cause is unknown. Progesterone may contribute.	• Plan for daily naps. • Take frequent rest breaks throughout the day. • Go to bed early.
Shortness of breath	In early pregnancy the effects of progesterone can create a sense of shortness of breath. In later pregnancy the uterus pushes on the diaphragm.	• Sit up straight to increase diameter of the chest. • If shortness of breath is interfering with sleep, prop up with pillows.
Heartburn	Relaxation of the LES under the influence of progesterone and increased intra-abdominal pressure due to the growing uterus cause acid reflux into the lower esophagus.	• Eat small, frequent meals • Avoid substances that increase acid production, in particular cigarette smoking. • Avoid substances that cause relaxation of the LES, such as coffee, chocolate, alcohol, and heavy spices. • Avoid lying down after a meal. • Avoid lying flat.
Stretch marks (striae gravidarum)	Stretch marks can occur on the breasts and abdomen. They are thought to be caused by increased levels of glucocorticoids. Stretch marks appear red during pregnancy, then gradually fade to a silvery white color.	• It may help to gain weight gradually over time, sudden bursts of weight may contribute to formation of stretch marks. • Regular exercise may also be helpful in preventing stretch marks.

TABLE 7.2 (continued)	Common Discomforts of Pregnancy	
Discomfort	Contributing Factor or Cause	Hints for Relieving the Discomfort
Low back pain	Changes in the center of gravity and loosened ligaments	• Avoid gaining too much weight. • Avoid high-heeled shoes. • Always bend at the knees, not the waist. • Avoid standing for too long at one time. • Keep one foot on a stool when standing. Frequently change the foot that is resting on the stool.
Round ligament pain	Sharp, severe pain, usually on the right side brought on by stretching of the round ligaments that support the uterus.	• Avoid sudden changes in positions or sudden movements. • Apply heat. • Lie on the side opposite the pain.
Leg cramps	Imbalanced calcium/phosphorus ratio; pressure of the uterus on the nerves; and circulatory changes in the lower extremities	• Avoid plantar flexion. • Eat foods high in calcium. • Try taking Tums (high in calcium). • Rest frequently with the feet elevated. • When cramps occur, extend the affected leg and dorsiflex the foot.
Varicose veins	Increased pelvic pressure, vasodilation in the lower extremities and vagina, along with pooling of blood in the lower extremities can contribute to varicosities of the legs and vagina.	• Exercise daily. • Rest with the legs elevated several times daily. • Wear compression stockings. Put them on before getting out of bed in the morning. • Avoid prolonged periods of standing or sitting. Move around frequently. Stretch and take small walks. • When you must stand for a time, frequently exercise the leg muscles and change positions frequently. • Keep within the recommended weight range during pregnancy.
Ankle edema	Progesterone effects, increased pressure in the lower extremities, increased capillary permeability	• Avoid prolonged periods of standing. • Rest frequently with the feet elevated. • Soak in a warm pool or bath. • Avoid constrictive garments on the lower extremities.
Flatulence	Relaxation of the gastrointestinal tract under the influence of progesterone, pressure of the uterus on the intestines, air swallowing	• Avoid gas-producing foods. • Chew foods thoroughly. • Get plenty of exercise. • Maintain regular bowel habits.
Constipation and hemorrhoids	Slowing of the gastrointestinal tract under the influence of progesterone and increased blood flow and pressure in the pelvic area	• Drink at least 8 glasses of non-caffeinated beverages per day. • Eat plenty of fiber. • Get adequate exercise. • Use a stool softener, if prescribed by the health care provider. • Use topical anesthetic agents to treat the pain of hemorrhoids.
Trouble sleeping	Many discomforts of pregnancy, as well as the increase in size of the abdomen, can all contribute to sleepless nights in the third trimester.	• Get adequate exercise. • Try different positions and use pillows to support and wedge. • Try sleeping in a sitting position. • Drink a glass of warm milk before retiring. • Have a late-night, high-carbohydrate snack • Try progressive muscle relaxation or guided imagery.

cause. Although "morning sickness" is the lay term for the nausea of pregnancy, many women experience nausea at other times during the day, or even throughout the day.

Fortunately, caloric intake during the first trimester is not as crucial as it is in the second and third trimesters, so the nausea is usually not harmful to the pregnancy. Some helpful suggestions include advising the woman to place a high-carbohydrate snack, such as melba toast or saltine crackers, at the bedside before retiring. In the morning before getting out of bed, she should eat the snack. This can help prevent early morning nausea. Other helpful hints are to encourage the woman to eat small amounts frequently throughout the day, instead of consuming three, heavy meals hours apart, and to never let the stomach become completely empty. It also helps for her to avoid strong odors. Sometimes it is easier for the woman to eat when someone else prepares the meal. Persistent vomiting may be a sign of hyperemesis gravidarum, a complication of pregnancy that can lead to dehydration and electrolyte imbalances. If the vomiting is severe or prolonged, the primary care provider should be consulted. Fortunately, nausea generally subsides by the end of the first trimester.

Feeling Faint

Sometimes women feel faint during the first few weeks of pregnancy. This could be caused by postural hypotension and is aggravated by low blood sugar levels. Advise the woman to change positions slowly and to avoid abrupt position changes. Eating frequent high-carbohydrate meals helps to keep blood sugar levels up. If she feels faint, a walk outside might help. Or she might need to lie down with her feet elevated or sit with her head lower than her knees until the feeling passes.

Frequent Urination

Frequent urination can be bothersome and interfere with sleep. It is thought that frequent urination in the first trimester is caused by the increasing blood volume and increased glomerular filtration rate. Frequency usually diminishes during the second trimester, only to reappear in the third trimester because of pressure of the enlarging uterus on the bladder.

Increased Vaginal Discharge

Leukorrhea, or increased vaginal discharge, is common during pregnancy. Increased production of cervical glands and vasocongestion of the pelvic area contribute to the discharge. If the discharge causes itching or irritation, or if there is a foul smell noted, the health care provider should be contacted because these are signs of infection.

Douching should be avoided. Sanitary pads can be worn to absorb the discharge.

Shortness of Breath

Shortness of breath may occur during the first trimester because of the effects of progesterone. The woman may feel an increased sense of the need to breath. This sensation can be uncomfortable and is often perceived as shortness of breath. During the latter half of pregnancy as the uterus pushes upward on the diaphragm, shortness of breath can occur.

Advise the woman to take her time and rest frequently. If shortness of breath occurs during exercise, she may need to decrease the level of intensity. During late pregnancy, shortness of breath may interfere with sleep. Propping up with pillows can help expand the chest and decrease the sensation of being unable to catch her breath. Shortness of breath accompanied by chest pain or coughing up blood or a smothering sensation with fever are danger signs that indicate the need for medical intervention. The former is a sign of pulmonary embolism; the latter is a sign of severe respiratory infection, such as pneumonia.

Heartburn

Heartburn, or pyrosis, is a common complaint during pregnancy. Several factors contribute to this discomfort. Progesterone causes a generalized slowing of the gastrointestinal tract and can cause relaxation of the lower esophageal sphincter (LES). When the LES is relaxed, acid content from the stomach can back up into the lower part of the esophagus and cause a burning sensation, known as heartburn. The increased pressure in the abdomen from the enlarging uterus contributes to the problem.

Prevention is generally the best way to treat heartburn. Several factors aggravate the condition. Smoking increases the acid content of the stomach and should be avoided. Certain foods and beverages, such as coffee, chocolate, peppermint, fatty or fried foods, alcohol, and heavy spices, can contribute to LES relaxation and exacerbate heartburn.

The woman should be advised to eat smaller meals more frequently and to avoid drinking fluids with meals. Filling the stomach with a heavy meal or with food and fluid increases the pressure and contributes to gastric reflux. It is best if the woman avoids lying down after meals. If she must lie down, suggest that she lie on her left side with her head higher than her abdomen. Placing 6-inch blocks under the head of the bed, or propping pillows at night to keep the chest higher than the abdomen can also help prevent heartburn. The physician may prescribe an antacid. If so, vitamins should not be taken within 1 hour of taking antacids. Sodium bicarbonate should not be used as an antacid during pregnancy.

Backaches
About one half of all pregnant women experience low back pain at some point during pregnancy. Obesity and previous history of back pain are risk factors. Softening and loosening of the ligaments supporting the joints of the spine and pelvis can contribute to low back pain, as can the increasing lordosis of pregnancy and the changing center of gravity.

Low back pain is best prevented by advising the woman to use good body mechanics, such as bending the knees to reach something on the floor, rather than stooping over from the waist. She should also avoid high-heeled shoes. Good pelvic support with a girdle might be helpful for some women. Severe back pain is usually associated with some type of pathology and should be investigated.

Round Ligament Pain
The round ligaments support the uterus in the abdomen. As the uterus expands during pregnancy, pressure is applied to the round ligaments and they stretch and thin. Some women experience round ligament pain as a result of this stretching. The pain most frequently occurs on the right side and can be severe. The pain can occur at night and awaken the woman from sleep, or exercise can bring it on.

Helpful hints to treat round ligament pain include the application of heat. A heating pad or warm bath might be soothing. Sometimes lying on the opposite side can relieve some of the pressure on the ligament and reduce the pain. Avoiding sudden movements may help prevent round ligament pain. If fever, chills, painful urination, or vaginal bleeding accompanies the pain, the woman should seek emergency care because the pain is likely caused by a medical condition.

Leg Cramps
Leg cramps are a common occurrence during pregnancy. An imbalanced calcium/phosphorous ratio, pressure of the uterus on nerves, and circulatory changes in the lower extremities can all contribute to leg cramps. Preventive measures include getting enough rest, resting several times per day with the feet elevated, walking, wearing low-heeled shoes, and avoiding constrictive clothing. Another preventive measure is for the woman to avoid plantar flexion (pointing the toes forward). Making certain that the diet includes enough calcium is also important to prevent leg cramps. When cramps occur, the woman's partner can help by assisting her to extend her leg, then dorsiflex the foot so that the toes point toward the woman's head. If she is alone, she can extend her leg and dorsiflex the foot until the cramp resolves.

Constipation and Hemorrhoids
The natural slowing of the gastrointestinal tract under the influence of hormones can lead to constipation during pregnancy, and constipation can lead to hemorrhoids. The best way to treat constipation is to prevent it. The same common sense approaches to preventing constipation that are advisable under normal situations are also helpful during pregnancy. These include drinking at least 8 glasses of noncaffeinated beverages each day. Advise the woman to get adequate exercise. Adding fiber to the diet or a bulk-forming supplement such as Metamucil to the daily routine are also helpful hints.

Hemorrhoids can become a problem during pregnancy because of the increased blood flow in the rectal veins and pressure of the uterus that prevents good venous return. Elevating the legs and hips intermittently throughout the day can help counteract this problem. Constipation aggravates the condition. Pain and swelling can be relieved by applying topical anesthetics, such as Preparation H or Anusol cream, and compresses such as witch hazel pads.

Trouble Sleeping
Many of the discomforts discussed previously, such as heartburn and shortness of breath, can contribute to restlessness at night and trouble sleeping. As the pregnancy progresses, it becomes increasingly difficult to find a position of comfort in bed. Suggest that the woman try lying on her side with plenty of pillows to support her back and legs. If that position doesn't help, she may find it easier to sleep in an armchair. Sleep may be easier in the sitting position. Urinary frequency returns during the third trimester and can contribute to sleeplessness because of frequent trips to the restroom. Drinking the majority of fluids early in the day and limiting fluids in the evening hours can reduce this problem. Heartburn can contribute to reduction in sleep, as can the movements of an active fetus. Some degree of sleeplessness and restlessness at night is to be expected in the third trimester.

Teaching Self-Care During Pregnancy
The woman is usually too distracted during the first visit to absorb and retain much information that is given to her. Keep teaching sessions brief and give her printed materials to read at home. The primary care provider should have a list of

resources, such as books and websites, that could be put in a handout format to give to the woman. Teaching topics should be tailored to the individual needs of the woman during subsequent visits. Important self-care topics are discussed below. Family Teaching Tips: Major Topics to Cover During Prenatal Care highlights key topics that should be covered with the pregnant woman during the course of prenatal care.

Maintaining a Balanced Nutritional Intake

During the first trimester the fetus' demands on maternal stores are less than at other times during the pregnancy. This is helpful because sometimes it is difficult for the woman to eat a well-balanced diet when she is coping with nausea. Focus on assessing the adequacy of her diet and answering her questions during the first visit. Emphasize the importance of taking the prenatal

FAMILY TEACHING TIPS

Major Topics to Cover During Prenatal Care

The pregnant woman should be taught to:
- Avoid alcohol. Alcohol harms the fetus; no amount of alcohol is safe during pregnancy.
- Avoid smoking. Smoking harms the fetus. It can lead to lower birth weight and increase the incidence of preterm labor.
- Eat a healthy, well-balanced diet. If you consume a variety of nutritious foods daily, you will likely get the nutrients you need.
- Consume approximately 300 calories more per day than before pregnancy.
- Take an extra 400 micrograms of folic acid per day. If the doctor ordered prenatal vitamins, the recommended dose will be met.
- Avoid dieting during pregnancy. Every pregnant woman with a normal body mass index should gain 25 to 30 pounds during the pregnancy.
- Continue to exercise during pregnancy. However, do not exercise to the point of exhaustion or start a grueling new workout that you were not doing before pregnancy.
- Avoid handling raw meat and cat litter. Wear gloves when gardening to prevent contracting toxoplasmosis from animal droppings, an infection that is very harmful to the baby.
- Handle cold cuts carefully. Heat thin slices of meat in the microwave until steaming hot. Wash hands with hot soapy water after handling deli meats to avoid listeriosis, a bacterial infection that is harmful to the baby.
- Avoid douching. Douching during pregnancy can cause a fatal air embolism.
- Avoid taking any medication (other than Tylenol) or over-the-counter herbal remedy unless your primary care provider has approved it.

vitamins the primary care provider ordered for her. On subsequent visits, assist the woman to assess her own diet for adequacy by using the food guide pyramid (Fig. 7-7). Teach principles of adequate nutritional intake during pregnancy.

The key to healthy nutrition during pregnancy is quality and variety. Some pregnant women may be overwhelmed by detailed nutritional guidelines. In general it is safe to counsel the pregnant woman about the following general strategies. Make certain there is enough food to eat and then advise the woman to eat the amount and type of food that she wants, salting it to taste. The Food Guide Pyramid can assist the pregnant woman achieve a balanced diet. Monitor weight gain throughout pregnancy. There should be a steady increase in weight throughout pregnancy, for a total increase of 25 to 35 pounds. Sudden weight gain often is associated with fluid retention and may be a sign of developing preeclampsia. Periodically assess the diet by asking the woman to do a 1- to 3-day food recall. Encourage the woman to take her iron and folic acid supplement. Monitor the hemoglobin and hematocrit at the 28-week checkup for any decreases.

Dental Hygiene

A pregnant woman needs to continue regular dental checkups and practice excellent dental hygiene. This includes at least twice daily brushing, once daily flossing, and a nutritious diet. If pregnancy gingivitis is a problem, then regular dental checkups are a must. Untreated gingivitis can damage the gums and result in bone and tooth loss.

Vomiting in association with morning sickness can be hard on teeth. Stomach acids in the vomitus can make the teeth more susceptible to injury from the toothbrush. To reduce the impact of this problem, instruct the woman to rinse with water after vomiting, followed by a fluoride rinse or sugarless chewing gum to help neutralize the stomach acid. She should avoid brushing her teeth for at least 1 hour after vomiting to decrease the risk of enamel loss.

Exercise

Exercise is healthy during pregnancy. A woman may generally maintain her normal exercise routine during pregnancy, as long as she does not become overheated or excessively fatigued. Conditioned women have safely run marathons during pregnancy. In fact, women who exercise during pregnancy experience shorter labors, have fewer cesarean deliveries, and have fetuses that experience fewer episodes of fetal distress.

The American College of Obstetricians and Gynecologists recommends that a well-conditioned

FOOD GUIDE PYRAMID
A guide to daily food choices

● Fat (naturally occurring and added
○ Sugars (added)

These symbols show fat and added sugar in foods.

Fats, oils, and sweets
USE SPARINGLY

Milk, yogurt, and cheese group
2-3 SERVINGS

Meat, poultry, fish, dry beans, eggs, and nuts group
2-3 SERVINGS

Vegetable group
3-5 SERVINGS

Fruit group
2-4 SERVINGS

Bread, cereal, rice, and pasta group
6-11 SERVINGS

● *Figure 7.7* The food guide pyramid.

Source: U.S. Department of Agriculture/U.S. Department of Health and Human Services

woman continue her pattern of aerobic exercise during pregnancy. If the woman is sedentary before pregnancy, she should not start a vigorous aerobic routine. In this situation, walking is the preferred exercise. There are some high-risk conditions, such as premature rupture of membranes, pregnancy-induced hypertension, vaginal bleeding, or incompetent cervix, in which exercise is contraindicated.

General common sense guidelines include advising the woman to listen to her body. If she is feeling fatigued, she should slow down or stop. She should not allow her heart rate to exceed 140 beats per minute. In the last trimester as the center of gravity changes, extra care should be taken to avoid injury during exercise.

Hygiene

Perspiration and vaginal discharge increase during pregnancy, making personal hygiene a concern for some pregnant women. In general, tub baths or showers can continue throughout pregnancy with an eye toward safety. The following general considerations should be given to hygiene during pregnancy.

• Bathe in warm, not hot, water. Extreme temperature elevations associated with hot show-

ers, baths, saunas, hot tubs, and fever are dangerous to the developing fetus and should be avoided.

• Take care, particularly in the third trimester, when getting in and out of the tub or shower. Fainting can occur. This situation is enhanced if the water is too hot. Because the center of gravity changes, balancing can become problematic. Handrails in the shower or tub are ideal. Rubber bath mats are also helpful.

• Avoid douching during pregnancy. This practice is dangerous and can result in an air embolism due to the increased vascularity of the genital area. Gentle cleansing of the genital area with warm water and soap are sufficient to control discomfort from increased vaginal secretions.

Breast Care

A pregnant woman is well advised to wear a bra that fits well and supports the breasts. She should be taught to use only clean water to wash the nipples. Soap dries the nipples and can lead to cracking.

Some women wish to condition their nipples for breast-feeding. Exposing the nipples to air and sunlight for a portion of each day is helpful.

Manually stimulating the nipples by rolling them between the fingers or oral stimulation of the nipple by the partner as a part of sexual expression are additional ways to toughen the nipples. These practices are acceptable as long as there is no history of preterm labor because nipple stimulation can stimulate labor.

Clothing

Clothing should be loose and comfortable. Constricting garments around the waist or on the legs should not be worn. If finances are tight, the woman might try borrowing clothes from a friend or relative, rather than investing in expensive maternity clothes. She might also buy used maternity clothes. High heels exacerbate backache and can be a safety hazard for the pregnant woman who has problems with balance. Shoes should fit comfortably.

Sexual Activity

Many couples are fearful that sexual activity during pregnancy might hurt the fetus. Unless there is a history of preterm labor, vaginal bleeding, ruptured membranes, or other medical contraindication, intercourse and other sexual activities can be safely continued throughout pregnancy. Many factors influence the woman's desire for sexual activity. During the first trimester she may feel nauseous and tired, so her interest in sex might be low. During the second trimester, she often feels better and may have a heightened interest in sex. The increased blood flow to the pelvic area can intensify the sexual experience for the pregnant woman. Some women experience orgasm for the first time during pregnancy. During the third trimester, fatigue may reduce her desire. Or she might fear hurting the fetus.

A word of caution: If the couple practices anal intercourse, it is important to warn them not to proceed to vaginal intercourse after engaging in anal intercourse. The danger is that the bacteria *Escherichia coli* will be introduced into the vagina and cause an ascending infection.

The partner's sexual desire is also dependent on several interrelated factors. Some men find the pregnant body sexually appealing and desirable. Others may have trouble adjusting to their partner's changing body shape. Some men are afraid of hurting their partner or the unborn child during intercourse. It may be helpful to have a tactful discussion regarding sexual concerns with the woman and the partner. During the third trimester the male superior position may become difficult to accomplish. A side-lying or woman superior position might be easier.

Sometimes the woman might be content with kissing, cuddling, and caressing as forms of sexual expression. If her partner needs more release, the woman might stimulate him to ejaculation, or he may prefer to masturbate. The essential ingredient is ongoing respectful communication between the partners regarding their sexual needs and desires.

Employment

How long a woman can remain safely employed during pregnancy is dependent on several factors. In general, a woman with a low-risk pregnancy can continue working until she goes into labor, unless there are specific hazards associated with her job. Research demonstrates that women in physically demanding jobs, such as working in the fields (day laborers), experience a higher incidence of low birth-weight infants, preterm delivery, and hypertension during pregnancy. A woman who is required to stand for long periods as part of her job also is at increased risk for preterm delivery.

When a woman chooses to work during pregnancy, it is most helpful if she can take frequent rest periods. If she must stand for prolonged periods, suggest that she shift her weight back and forth, and that she take frequent breaks to walk around and to sit with her feet elevated. Of course she should avoid excessive fatigue.

Exposure to **teratogens**, substances capable of causing birth defects, is always a concern when a woman works during pregnancy. The woman should investigate the type of chemicals or other substances she is exposed to during the course of her work and then work with her employer to limit exposure to harmful substances.

Travel

Travel is generally not limited during the first trimester and can be carried out safely in the second and third trimesters with careful planning. One concern when traveling long distances is the chance that labor will occur while the woman is away from her health care provider. It is advisable for the woman to carry copies of her prenatal records with her when she travels. In this way, appropriate care can be rendered if she must seek health care away from home.

When travel by car is permitted, the woman should be encouraged to make frequent stops (at least every 2 hours) so that she can empty her bladder and walk about. Sitting for prolonged periods in one position can predispose the woman to clot formation. Decreasing fluid intake to avoid having to stop to void is not recommended. Insufficient fluids can lead to dehydration and increase the risk for clot formation, constipation, and hemorrhoids. There is no increased risk with air travel, other than the risk of developing complications in an area remote from the help needed.

The greatest risk to the fetus during an automobile crash is death of the mother. Therefore, it is recommended that all pregnant women use three-point seat belt restraints when traveling in the car. The lap belt should be under her abdomen and over her thighs. The shoulder harness should fit between her breasts. Safety belts should be snugly and comfortably applied. The use of airbags is controversial. Some authorities suggest that airbags are safe to use during pregnancy. Others have encountered stillbirths after airbag deployment in a car crash (Cunningham et al., 2001).

Test Yourself

- List three suggestions for reducing nausea in early pregnancy.

- Name three actions the pregnant woman can take to reduce heartburn.

- Why should the pregnant woman avoid hot showers or baths?

Medication Use

The general principle regarding medication use during pregnancy is that almost all medications cross the placenta and can potentially affect the fetus. No medication, including over-the-counter medications and herbal remedies, should be used during pregnancy without the express approval of the primary care provider. Before any medication is taken, a careful appraisal of risk versus benefit should be made. There are some diseases and conditions for which the pregnant woman must continue to receive treatment, such as epilepsy, asthma, diabetes, and depression.

The problem with most medications is that they are known to cross the placenta, but it is not always known what affect the medication has on the fetus or pregnancy. Because of ethical concerns, controlled trials of medication use during human pregnancy are usually not possible. The little that is known about medication effects during pregnancy comes from animal trials and from experience over the years in treating chronic maternal conditions. The problem with animal studies is that there is no guarantee that human pregnancies or fetuses will respond in the same way as the animal that is being studied responds. Box 7-6 describes the Food and Drug Administration's five pregnancy categories for medications.

Substance Use and Abuse

Substance use is a term that simply refers to use of a substance, whereas the term *substance abuse* specifically identifies that a problem is identified with the use of the substance. Although many substances have the potential for abuse, this

---

| **BOX 7.6** | **FDA Pregnancy Categories of Medications** |

The Food and Drug Administration (FDA) has delineated five categories for medication use during pregnancy. Each category details the overall threat, if any, the drug in that category might pose to the fetus or pregnancy. The categories are differentiated according to the type and reliability of documentation available and the risk-versus-benefit ratio. The categories are as follows:

Category A: Adequate studies in pregnant women have not demonstrated a risk to the fetus in the first trimester of pregnancy, and there is no evidence of risk in later trimesters.

Category B: Animal studies have not demonstrated a risk to the fetus, but there are no adequate studies in pregnant women. Or animal studies have shown an adverse effect, but adequate studies in pregnant women have not demonstrated a risk to the fetus during the first trimester of pregnancy, and there is no evidence of risk in later trimesters.

Category C: Animal studies have shown an adverse effect on the fetus, but there are no adequate studies in humans; the benefits from the use of the drug in pregnant women may be acceptable despite its potential risks. Or there are no animal reproduction studies and no adequate studies in humans.

Category D: There is evidence of human fetal risk, but the potential benefits from the use of the drug in pregnant women may be acceptable despite its potential risk.

Category X: Studies in animals or humans demonstrate fetal abnormalities or adverse reaction; reports indicate evidence of fetal risk. The risk of use in a pregnant woman clearly outweighs any possible benefit.

In any case, no drug should be given during pregnancy unless there is a clear benefit for its use.

section covers caffeine, tobacco, alcohol, and recreational drug use. More extensive coverage regarding potential fetal effects is given to this topic in Chapter 20.

Caffeine. There is controversy and uncertainty regarding the role of caffeine use during pregnancy. Current recommendations are that coffee and caffeine in moderation may be safely used during pregnancy without risk of adverse effects. Caffeine in large doses, such as that found in 5 cups of coffee or more per day, increases the risk of spontaneous abortion.

Tobacco. Smoking is contraindicated during pregnancy. Smoking increases the risk for low birth weight, preterm delivery, abortions, stillbirths, sudden infant death syndrome (SIDS), birth defects, and neonatal respiratory disorders, including asthma. Smoking poisons the fetus with carbon monoxide and nicotine, leading to fetal hypoxia. It also affects the placenta, causing it to age sooner than normal, a condition that reduces blood flow to the fetus, contributing to hypoxia and stunted growth.

In 1998, 12% of American women smoked during pregnancy. These 12% delivered 20% of the low birth-weight neonates born that year (Cunningham et al., 2001). It is clear that reducing the number of women who smoke during pregnancy will decrease the number of low birth-weight infants. As mentioned, low birth-weight infants are at much higher risk for neonatal morbidity and mortality. Although nicotine gum is classified as a pregnancy Category C (see Box 7-6) drug and the transdermal patch is in pregnancy Category D, the risk of harm caused by smoking may outweigh the risk of harm from these aids to stop smoking.

Alcohol. There is no safe amount of alcohol consumption during pregnancy. A pregnant woman is strongly advised not to drink any alcoholic beverages during pregnancy or when she thinks she might be pregnant because alcohol is a known teratogen. For years, the risk of fetal alcohol syndrome (FAS) has been linked to the use of large amounts of alcohol during pregnancy. This syndrome is characterized by **microcephaly**, a very small cranium, facial deformities, growth restriction, and mental retardation. Although smaller amounts of alcohol may not lead to a full-blown case of FAS, subtle features of the syndrome might present to include milder forms of mental retardation.

Marijuana. There is conflicting data about the effects of marijuana on pregnancy. However, infants born to women who smoke marijuana during pregnancy show evidence of stressed nervous systems. These infants tend to have high-pitched cries, tremulousness, and reduced response to visual stimuli. As they grow, these children tend to have lower IQs, impaired cognitive function, and deficits in language, behavior, and performance of visual-perceptual tasks. One study shows an increased risk of SIDS when the father uses marijuana during and after the pregnancy.

Cocaine. Cocaine has many negative effects on pregnancy. Cocaine use is associated with a higher rate of spontaneous abortion and premature labor. Infants born to women who use cocaine during pregnancy tend to be small and have a higher incidence of low birth weight. Cocaine use during pregnancy can cause the placenta to pull away from the uterine wall prematurely (placental abruption), leading to fetal and maternal hemorrhage. These infants exhibit withdrawal behaviors after birth and must receive special treatment for the withdrawal (refer to Chapter 20).

Maintaining Safety of the Woman and Fetus

Monitor the woman at every visit for warning signs of pregnancy (see Box 7-5). If she reports experiencing any of the warning signs, notify the RN or primary care provider immediately. If at any time during the pregnancy an elevated blood pressure is noted, report this finding immediately to the RN or primary care provider, particularly if it is accompanied by a headache, epigastric pain, or blurred vision.

Preparing the Woman for Labor, Birth, and Parenthood

The woman who is well prepared for labor, birth, and parenting is likely to feel confident and use positive coping measures. There are many ways to prepare for the birth and parenting experience. Many women search the Internet for information and to find resources. There are many books available that address these issues. The primary care provider should provide lists of resources available in the local community.

Packing for the Hospital or Birthing Center

As the woman prepares for the birth of her baby, she will begin to gather items she will need at the hospital or birthing center. She should pack one bag of items she will need for labor and another bag of things for her postpartum stay and the trip home from the hospital (Box 7-7).

Communicating Expectations About Labor and Birth

It is important for the woman to feel comfortable communicating her desires regarding labor and birth. Some women feel very strongly about

BOX 7.7 | What to Pack for the Hospital or Birthing Center

Labor Items
- Lotion for massage or effleurage
- Sour lollipops (counteracts nausea, moistens mouth, gives energy)
- Mouth spray or toothbrush and toothpaste
- Chapstick or lip balm
- Socks
- Tennis ball, ice pack, back massager (for pressure for back labor)
- Picture or object for focal point
- Camera with good batteries and plenty of film (check with hospital regarding policies on cameras during delivery)
- CD player and CDs for relaxation music
- Contact lens case and solutions
- Hair brush and hair ribbon or band to get hair off neck
- Hand fan
- Favorite pillows

Postpartum Items
- Nursing gowns
- Robe and slippers
- Nursing bras
- Toilet articles (toothpaste and toothbrush, deodorant, tissues)
- Cosmetics
- Pen and paper
- Baby book
- Personal address book with telephone numbers
- Loose fitting clothes for the trip home
- Socks for baby
- Clothes for baby to wear home
- Baby blankets appropriate for weather

Be careful. It isn't helpful to make promises that you can't keep. If a woman or her partner is communicating unrealistic expectations about the birth process, be honest and tell her that it is unlikely her expectation will be met. The woman will appreciate if you are up-front with her. This will give her the opportunity to decide if her expectation is negotiable or if she needs to go elsewhere to get her needs met.

having natural childbirth or breast-feeding. Others want an epidural as soon as possible after they go into labor. These are only three examples of expectations a woman may have. Encourage the woman to write down her questions and expectations and to communicate these to her primary care provider. Some women develop written birth plans (Box 7-8) to communicate their desires. These can be helpful to the woman and the primary care provider. If the expectations are communicated early, there is time for the woman to find another provider if her current provider cannot or will not meet her expectations.

Choosing the Support Person

The expectant mother may have choices involving her labor support team if she delivers in the hospital or birthing center. Some hospitals limit her to one or two persons for labor support. Other women may have the option of having more support persons for labor. The woman may have the father of the baby as her main support person. In other situations, the primary support person might be her mother, sister, other family member, or friend.

The mother also may choose to have a **doula** with her as a support person. The word "doula" is Greek for servant. DONA, an acronym for Doulas of North America (founded in 1992), is an international association of doulas who are trained "to provide the highest quality emotional, physical and educational support to women and their families during childbirth and postpartum." A doula may be contracted to provide support for labor and birth and help with establishing breast-feeding. Other doulas are contracted to provide support for the postpartum period. Many doulas provide both prenatal and postnatal support. The doula's role may include assisting the woman and her partner in preparing for and carrying out their plans for the birth, providing emotional support, physical comfort measures, and an objective viewpoint, as well as helping the woman get the information she needs to make good decisions. A woman may choose to hire a doula because she wants to decrease the likelihood of needing pharmacologic pain management, Pitocin, forceps, vacuum extraction, or cesarean birth and because she wants an advocate at a time when she feels unable to vocalize her needs adequately.

Childbirth Education Classes

Since the 1970s, many parents have begun to prepare for labor and childbirth by attending classes (Fig. 7-8). Today, classes are offered by childbirth educators in private practice, not-for-profit organizations, and hospitals. Some classes adhere to the philosophy of one method of unmedicated childbirth (Box 7-9). Others combine philosophies of two or more methods of childbirth. Still others tend to teach the woman little about birthing a baby without medical pain management and focus on what medical procedures and routines she can expect

● **Figure 7.8** The nurse is teaching couples in a childbirth class.

when she is admitted to the hospital. Some programs combine information about birth, baby care, and breast-feeding in one series of classes. Others offer separate classes for which the woman and her partner can register. Box 7-10 lists common topics included in childbirth education classes.

Other Birth and Parenthood Preparation Classes

In addition to labor and birth preparation, other educational offerings include pregnancy and postpartum exercise classes, baby care classes, breast-feeding classes, and sibling preparation classes. In some communities, childbirth educators in private practice or not-for-profit childbirth education organizations provide classes to clients who seek and pay for these classes. In other communities, hospital-based family education programs dominate the parenting education arena.

Pregnancy and Postpartum Exercise Classes. The purpose of these classes is to enhance endurance, as well as strengthen arms, legs, pelvic floor, back, and abdomen. A certified childbirth educator or a nurse usually offers these classes. Some fitness centers also offer pre- and postnatal exercise classes. Basic pregnancy exercises, such as the pelvic tilt, Kegel, tailor sit and tailor stretch, and stretches as comfort measures for the discomforts of pregnancy, should be included, as well as exercises that allow the woman to be able to utilize beneficial labor positions comfortably. Postnatal exercise classes strengthen muscles affected by the pregnancy. Sometimes, they incorporate the baby as part of the exercise.

Baby Care Classes. These classes are usually offered to the pregnant woman and her partner. Basics such as infant bathing, diapering, and feed-

ing are featured. Parents-to-be are also presented with information on newborn sleeping and waking patterns and infant comforting and rousing techniques. Safety information including proper handling of the baby, car seat safety, and safety proofing the home is included. Signs of illness and guidelines for when to call the pediatrician are an important part of this class. Items needed for the layette are usually discussed or a list of the items needed is provided in handouts (Box 7-11).

Breast-feeding Classes. This class is usually taught by an International Board Certified lactation consultant but also may be conducted by certified breast-feeding educators or specially trained nurses. Usually offered in the last trimester of pregnancy, this class is designed to educate the woman and her partner on the benefits of breast-feeding, signs of good latch and position, and establishing a good milk supply. Selection of and using a breast pump and milk storage are topics of interest in this class as many women plan to return to work and continue to nurse their infants. Attendance of this class by the woman's partner increases his support and ability to provide assistance, thus contributing to the success of breast-feeding. Usually, telephone numbers for community resources for lactation support are offered.

Siblings Classes. Many hospitals provide sibling classes for children who are soon to be big brothers and big sisters. Siblings' class goals include preparing children for the time of separation from mother while she is in the hospital and helping the children accept the changes resulting from the arrival of the new baby in the family. Basic infant care is demonstrated, with emphasis on how the child can be included or help with the tasks related to baby care. Tours of the maternal–child areas of the hospital are usually included. Suggestions are shared with parents on ways to help the older siblings accept changes in the household after the baby arrives.

In hospitals where siblings are allowed to attend births, siblings classes may include information on how to help prepare the older child for being present at delivery. Most hospitals require an adult to be responsible for children at birth, in addition to the partner who is caring for the laboring woman.

EVALUATION: GOALS AND EXPECTED OUTCOMES

- **Goal:** The woman's anxiety is reduced.
  Expected Outcomes: The woman will verbalize a reduction in anxiety and will name at least two outlets for dealing with her anxiety.

(text continues on page 167)

BOX 7.8 | Sample Birth Plan

Birth plan for Rachel Thompson
Due date: March 23, 2005
Patient of Dr. Maria Martinez
Scheduled to deliver at Metropolitan Medical Center

January 10, 2005

Dear Dr. Martinez and Staff at Metropolitan Medical Center,

I have chosen you because of your reputations for working with parents who feel strongly about wanting as natural a birth as possible. I understand that sometimes birth becomes a medical situation. The following is what I would prefer as long as medical interventions are not indicated. I would appreciate you working with me to have our baby in the way described in our birth plan, if possible.

Sincerely,

Rachel Thompson

Laboring
I would prefer to avoid an enema and/or shaving of pubic hair.
I would like to be free to walk around during labor.
I prefer to be able to move around and change position at will throughout labor.
I would like to be able to have fluids by mouth throughout the first stage of labor.
I will be bringing my own music to play during labor.
I do not want an IV unless I become dehydrated.
I need to wear contact lenses or glasses at all times when conscious.

Fetal Monitors
I do not want to have continuous fetal monitoring unless it is required by the condition of my baby.

Stimulation of Labor
If labor is not progressing, I would like to have the bag of water ruptured before other methods are used to augment labor.
I would prefer to be allowed to try changing position and other natural methods before oxytocin is administered.

Medication/Anesthesia
I do not want to use drugs if possible. Please do not offer them. I will ask if I want some.

C-section
If a cesarean delivery is indicated, I would like to be fully informed and to participate in the decision-making process.
I would like my husband present at all times if my baby requires a cesarean delivery.
I wish to have regional anesthesia unless the baby must be delivered immediately.

Episiotomy
I am hoping to protect my perineum. I am practicing ahead of time by squatting, doing Kegel exercises, and perineal massage.
If possible, I would like to use perineal massage to help avoid the need for an episiotomy.

Pushing
I would like to be allowed to choose the position in which I give birth, including squatting.
Even if I am fully dilated, and assuming my baby is not in distress, I would like to try to wait until I feel the urge to push before beginning the pushing phase.

Immediately After Delivery
I would like to have my baby placed on my chest.
I would like to have my husband cut the cord.
I would like to hold my baby while I deliver the placenta and any tissue repairs are made.
I plan to keep my baby with me following birth and would appreciate if the evaluation of my baby can be done with my baby on my abdomen unless there is an unusual situation.
I would prefer to hold my baby skin to skin to keep her warm.
I want to delay the eye medication for my baby until a couple hours after birth.
I have made arrangements to donate the umbilical cord blood if possible.

Postpartum
I would like a private room so my husband can stay with me.
Unless required for health reasons, I do not wish to be separated from my baby.

Nursing My Baby
I plan to nurse my baby very shortly after birth if baby and I are OK.
Unless medically necessary, I do not wish to have any formula given to my baby (including glucose water or plain water). If my baby needs to be supplemented, I prefer an alternative method to using a bottle.
I do not want my baby to be given a pacifier.
I would like to meet with a lactation consultant.

Photo/Video
I would like to make a video recording of labor and/or the birth and want pictures of the doctor and the baby.

Labor Support
My support people are my husband, Owen, and friends Judy and Margaret and I would like them to be present during labor and/or delivery.
I would like my other children (ages 4 years and 6 years) to be present at the birth. My physician has approved this. Judy and Margaret will take care of the other children during the birth.

BOX 7.9	Methods of Prepared Childbirth

Dick-Read Method

The work of Dr. Grantly Dick-Read has been recognized as fundamental to most methods of prepared childbirth. Dr. Dick-Read was a British obstetrician who practiced from 1919 to 1940. Dr. Dick-Read regarded fear as the basis of pain in childbirth and believed that civilization had culturally conditioned women to expect childbirth to be painful. He described a fear–tension–pain cycle and was convinced that women expected birth to be painful. Therefore, when labor began, the laboring woman tensed in fear at the beginning of each contraction. This tension resulted in the increase of pain; the pain reinforced the belief that labor was painful; and thus the cycle continued. He believed that pregnant women could interrupt this fear–tension–pain cycle with prenatal education and knowledge to reduce fear of the birth process and conscious relaxation during labor.

Lamaze Method

This method is based on Dick-Read's ideas and Pavlov's experiments with conditioned response. It is named after the French obstetrician Dr. Fernand Lamaze, who studied the Pavlov method in Russia and brought back his newfound knowledge to his patients in Paris. The Lamaze instructor teaches the pregnant woman to rehearse conditioned positive responses (i.e., relaxation, breathing, and attention focusing) to a stimulus (i.e., beginning of a contraction). Then, when she is in labor, the goal is for her to respond with the helpful conditioned responses, instead of natural responses (e.g., panic, breath holding, and increased tension) that can slow the progress of labor and increase the level of pain perceived by the woman. Her partner is trained to respond by supporting the laboring woman with encouragement and praise; providing focus and offering physical comfort measures, such as position changes, controlling the environment, massage, talking her through the contractions, enhancing her relaxation, and instilling confidence (Bing, 1994).

Bradley Method

Dr. Robert Bradley also based his obstetric practice on the work of Dick-Read. Dr. Bradley became convinced that the way to make childbirth an enjoyable experience was to copy what animals do naturally. The Bradley method of childbirth is explained in Dr. Bradley's book *Husband Coached Childbirth*. The principles of the Bradley method include:

- The need for darkness and solitude. Animals usually choose to birth babies in dark secluded places, therefore the room should be darkened.
- The need for quiet. Loud or unexpected noises are disturbing.
- The need for physical comfort. Comfort measures, such as controlling the room temperature, pillows for support, positioning, nonconstricting clothing, and familiar objects, contribute to the laboring woman's needs.
- The need for physical relaxation. Conscious relaxation on the part of the laboring woman increases her comfort and allows her uterus to work more effectively and quickly. Tensing up during contractions produces increased pain.
- The need for controlled breathing. Slow, deep, sleep-like breathing by mouth is encouraged throughout labor.
- The need for closed eyes and the appearance of sleep. Shutting the eyes enhances concentration on deep breathing by shutting out visual stimuli.

Underwater Birth Method

During the 1980s, the concept of giving birth in water began to gain popularity. In written accounts of these births, often published in lay magazines, women read of laboring and delivering in tubs of warm water at home or in birthing centers and also in shallow natural bodies of water, such as seas or bays near a beach. Those who encourage water births cite that humans begin life surrounded by liquid in the womb. Moreover, soaking in a warm bath enhances relaxation. Free from gravity's pull on the body, and with reduced sensory stimulation, the laboring woman's body is less likely to secrete stress-related hormones, thus allowing production of endorphins. As a result, there is believed to be an analgesic effect on the laboring woman. In Belgium, Dr. Serge Weisel studied the effects of laboring in water on hypertension and states that women experience a drop in blood pressure within 10 to 15 minutes after entering the water. An apparent benefit of birthing in water is the increased elasticity of the perineum, reducing the frequency of and severity in tearing of the perineum.

In 1989, Barbara Harper, RN, founded Waterbirth International/GMCHA (Global Maternal Child Health Association). This organization provides information and facilitates networking among those who are interested in learning more about birthing in water.

Hypnotherapy for Birth

Some women use traditional hypnosis with posthypnotic suggestions during labor and delivery. Others use forms of self-hypnosis, incorporating the basics of Drs. Dick-Read and Lamaze, such as deep relaxation and breathing for each phase of labor. A recent article in the *Journal of Family Practice* (Martin, Schauble, Surekha, & Curry, 2001) concludes that using hypnosis to prepare for labor can have positive clinical outcomes by reducing the number of complications, surgical interventions, and length of postpartum stay.

BOX 7.10	Common Topics Included in Childbirth Education Classes

- Psychological and emotional aspects of pregnancy
- Fetal development
- Anatomic and physiologic changes involved in pregnancy and childbirth
- Induction of labor: indications for induction and what to expect
- Stages/phases of labor: physical and emotional changes of each
- Partner's role in providing support for each stage/phase of labor
- Comfort measures for labor: relaxation, movement, breathing, focus, massage, pressure, encouragement, and support
- Medication and anesthesia options for labor and birth
- Back labor: causes, physical signs, and comfort measures
- Communication with obstetrician/pediatrician: verbal and written birth plans
- What to pack for the hospital
- Hospital admission routine
- Medical procedures and interventions, such as vaginal examinations, routine laboratory work, fetal monitoring, artificial rupture of membranes (AROM), IVs, vacuum extraction, and forceps
- Cesarean birth
- Choosing a pediatrician
- Physical and emotional aspects of the postpartum period

BOX 7.11	Suggested Items for the Layette

Clothes
- 4 to 6 "onesies"
- Gowns
- Sleepers
- 2 to 3 Blanket Sleepers
- 4 to 6 Undershirts
- 4 to 6 Pairs of socks
- 4 to 6 Receiving blankets
- 3 to 4 Hooded towels
- 4 to 6 Washcloths
- 4 to 6 Bibs
- 4 to 6 Burp cloths
- Several packages of newborn size diapers and wipes or washcloths

Baby Supplies
- Baby lotion
- Baby shampoo
- Zinc oxide ointment
- Cotton swabs
- Rubbing alcohol
- Cradle or bassinet
- Crib
- Changing pad or table
- Sling
- Swing
- Stroller
- Baby bathtub

Expected Outcomes: Expresses realistic expectations regarding plans for labor and birth; schedules and attends childbirth education and/or parenting classes; prepares the home for arrival of the baby.

- **Goal:** The woman's symptoms and discomforts of pregnancy are manageable.
  Expected Outcomes: Voices feeling relaxed and confident in her ability to deal with the common discomforts of pregnancy, and demonstrates the use of effective strategies for coping with the discomforts of pregnancy.
- **Goal:** The woman will feel confident in her ability to care for herself throughout pregnancy.
  Expected Outcomes: Verbalizes understanding of how to modify lifestyle to accommodate the changing needs of pregnancy; answers questions regarding self-care appropriately; asks informed questions.
- **Goal:** The woman and fetus remain free from preventable injury throughout the pregnancy.
  Expected Outcomes: Schedules and attends prenatal visits; describes warning signs to report; calls with questions and concerns; calls if warning signs are experienced.
- **Goal:** The woman will express confidence in her ability to go through the labor and birth experience and assume the parenting role.

Test Yourself

- Identify at least five ways smoking increases pregnancy risk.

- How much alcohol is it OK for a pregnant woman to drink?

- What is a doula?

KEY POINTS

- The goal of early prenatal care is to increase the chances that the fetus and the mother will remain healthy throughout pregnancy and delivery.

- The first prenatal visit is the longest one. The main goals are to confirm a diagnosis of pregnancy, identify risk factors, determine the due date, and provide education regarding self-care and danger signs of pregnancy.

- The obstetric history looks at previous pregnancies and their outcomes. Determining the gravida and parity of the woman is an important part of the obstetric history. The parity is usually further subdivided into the number of term deliveries, preterm deliveries, abortions (spontaneous or induced), and living children.

- A complete physical examination will be done during the first visit to include a breast exam, a speculum examination with a Pap test, and a bimanual examination of the uterus.

- The most common laboratory assessments (in addition to the Pap test) done on the first visit include a CBC, blood type and screen, hepatitis B, HIV, syphilis, gonorrhea, Chlamydia, rubella titer, and a urine culture.

- Nagele's rule is used to determine the due date. Add 7 days from the first day of the last menstrual period, then subtract 3 months to obtain the due date.

- Any abnormal part of the history, physical examination, or lab work can put the pregnancy at risk. A history of difficult pregnancy or pregnancy complications puts subsequent pregnancies at risk.

- Subsequent prenatal visits are shorter and focus on the weight, blood pressure, urine protein and glucose measurements, fetal heart rate, and fundal height. Inquiry is made regarding the danger signals of pregnancy at each prenatal visit.

- Ultrasonography uses high frequency sound waves to visualize fetal and maternal structures. Ultrasound is done to determine or confirm gestational age, observe the fetus, and diagnose fetal and placental abnormalities.

- Maternal serum alpha-fetoprotein testing is recommended for every pregnant woman between 16 and 18 weeks. Elevated levels are associated with various defects, in particular fetal spinal defects.

- Amniocentesis involves aspiration of amniotic fluid through the abdominal wall to obtain fetal cells for chromosomal analysis. Amniocentesis is usually done between 15 and 20 weeks' gestation.

- Chorionic villus sampling is similar to amniocentesis, but it can be performed earlier, usually at 10 to 12 weeks. Placental tissue is aspirated through a catheter that is introduced into the cervix.

- The nonstress test measures fetal heart rate acceleration patterns. A reactive NST is reassuring. The contraction stress test exposes the fetus to the stress of uterine contractions. A negative CST is reassuring. A positive CST indicates probable hypoxia or fetal asphyxia.

- The biophysical profile combines the NST and several ultrasound measures, breathing, movements, tone, and amniotic fluid volume to predict fetal well-being.

- Common nursing diagnoses during the pregnancy are anxiety, health-seeking behaviors, risk for injury, and deficient knowledge.

- Nursing interventions are tailored to the needs of the individual woman. Nursing care is focused on relieving anxiety and the common discomforts of pregnancy, such as nausea and heartburn. Assisting the woman to maintain a balanced nutritional intake occurs throughout the pregnancy. Maintaining safety is done by monitoring the blood pressure and weight and inquiring regarding the danger signals at each visit. Teaching is ongoing throughout the pregnancy.

- Helping the woman prepare for labor, birth, and parenting is an important nursing task. The nurse can refer the woman to community resources, such as childbirth education or sibling classes.

- Nursing care has been successful if the woman is less anxious, reports that pregnancy discomforts are tolerable, consumes a balanced diet, and verbalizes an understanding of self-care.

REFERENCES AND SELECTED READINGS

Books and Journals

Bing, E. (1994). *Six practical lessons for an easier childbirth* (3rd rev. ed.). New York: Bantam Books.

Brundage, S. C. (2002). Preconception care. *American Family Physician, 65*(12), 2507–2514. Retrieved October 12, 2002, from http://www.aafp.org/afp/20020615/2507.pdf

Cunningham, F. G., Gant, N. F., Leveno, K. J., Gilstrap, L. C. III, Hauth, J. C., & Wenstrom, K. D. (2001). *Williams obstetrics* (21st ed.). New York: McGraw-Hill Medical Publishing Division.

Drugan, A., Feldman, B., Johnson, M. P., & Evans, M. I. (1999). Prenatal diagnosis: Procedures and trends. In Avery, G. B., Fletcher, M. A., & MacDonald, M. G. (Eds.), *Neonatology: Pathophysiology & management of the newborn* (5th ed., pp. 161–171). Philadelphia: Lippincott Williams & Wilkins.

Ferber, A., & Sicherman, N. (2001). The amniocentesis report: A decision guide for expectant parents and health care professionals. Retrieved October 27, 2002, from http://www.amniocentesis.org/1233asdflkjabasopir-woier55876985/thankyoudownload.html

Martin, A. A., Schauble, P. G., Surekha, H. R., & Curry, R. W. (2001). The effects of hypnosis on the labor processes and birth outcomes of pregnant adolescents. *The Journal of Family Practice, 50*(5), 441–443.

North American Nursing Diagnosis Association (NANDA). (2001). *NANDA nursing diagnoses: Definitions & classification 2001–2002.* Philadelphia: Author.

Olney, R. S., Moore, C. A., Khoury, M. J., Erickson, J. D., Edmonds, L. D., & Atash, H. K. (1995). Chorionic villus sampling and amniocentesis: Recommendations for prenatal counseling. *MMWR, 44*(RR-9), 1–12. Retrieved October 27, 2002, from http://aepo-xdv-www.epo.cdc.gov/wonder/prevguid/m0038393/m0038393.asp

Wilkinson, L. D. (2000). Prenatal care for the family physician, Part 1: Preconception and early pregnancy care. *Family Practice Recertification, 22*(10), 37–58.

Websites
Prenatal care

http://www.nlm.nih.gov/medlineplus/prenatalcare.html

Prenatal teaching

http://www.midwife.org/focus/sharewithwomen.cfm
http://www.2bparent.com/pregnancy.htm

Nutrition

http://www.pueblo.gsa.gov/cic_text/food/food-pyramid/main.htm

Doulas

http://dona.org/
http://www.doula.com/

WORKBOOK

NCLEX-STYLE REVIEW QUESTIONS

1. A woman reports that her LMP occurred on January 10, 2005. Using Nagele's rule, what is her due date?

   a. October 17, 2005

   b. October 17, 2006

   c. September 7, 2005

   d. September 7, 2006

   [handwritten: add 7 days to 1st day of LMP + subt 3 mos ÷10 +7 17th Oct]

2. A woman presents to the clinic in the first trimester of pregnancy. She has three children living at home. One of them was born prematurely at 34 weeks. The other two were full term at birth. She has a history of one miscarriage. How do you record her obstetric history on the chart using GTPAL format?

   a. G3 T2 P1 A1 L3

   b. G4 T3 P0 A1 L3

   c. G4 T2 P1 A1 L3

   d. G5 T2 P1 A1 L3

3. A woman who is 28 weeks' pregnant presents to the clinic for her scheduled prenatal visit. The nurse midwife measures her fundal height at 32 centimeters. What action do you expect the midwife to take regarding this finding? The midwife will

   a. order a multiple marker screening test.

   b. order a sonogram to confirm dates.

   c. schedule more frequent prenatal visits to monitor the pregnancy closely.

   d. take no action. This is a normal finding for a pregnancy at 28 weeks' gestation.

4. A G1 at 20 weeks' gestation is at the clinic for a prenatal visit. She tells the nurse that she has been reading about "group B strep disease" on the Internet. She asks when she can expect to be checked for the bacteria. How does the nurse best reply?

   a. "I'm glad that you asked. You will be getting the culture done today."

   b. "The obstetrician normally cultures for group B strep after 35 weeks and before delivery."

   c. "You are only checked for group B strep if you have risk factors for the infection."

   d. "You were checked during your first prenatal visit. Let me get those results for you."

5. Results of an early CVS test show that a woman's baby has severe chromosomal abnormalities. When the obstetrician explains the findings to her, she becomes tearful. She shares with you that it is against her religious beliefs to have an abortion. How would you best respond to her?

   a. "Abortion is really the best thing for the baby. He has no chance of a normal life."

   b. "I agree with you. It is against my religious beliefs, too."

   c. "It is dangerous to carry a fetus with chromosomal abnormalities to term. You really should consider an abortion to protect your health."

   d. "You don't have to decide what to do today. Take some time to talk this over with your family. I will support you whatever decision you make."

STUDY ACTIVITIES

1. Do an Internet search on "genetic counseling." Make a list of at least three genetic counselors in your area to which a pregnant woman could be referred.

2. Using the following table, fill in key points for each topic regarding self-care during pregnancy. Note any special precautions for that topic that would be important to emphasize to the pregnant woman.

Topic	Key Points	Special Precautions
Nutrition		
Dental hygiene		
Exercise		
Hygiene		
Breast care		
Clothing		
Sexual activity		
Employment		
Travel		
Medication use		

3. Develop a teaching plan for pregnant women who are 20 weeks and greater. Address common discomforts of pregnancy that the women are likely to encounter during the last half of pregnancy.

CRITICAL THINKING: What Would You Do?

Apply your knowledge of the nurse's role during pregnancy to the following situations.

1. Theresa Martinez presents to the clinic because she thinks she might be pregnant.

   a. What nursing assessments should be completed?

   b. During the history, Theresa reports that there is a history of type II diabetes in her family, and that her mother delivered large babies (10 and 11 pounds). What should you do with this information?

   c. The obstetrician asks you to assist her during the physical examination. What equipment and supplies will you gather?

2. Amanda Jones calls the clinic. She is a G2 P1 at 28 weeks' gestation. She is worried because she thinks the baby is moving less than usual.

   a. What should you tell Amanda to do first?

   b. Amanda comes to the office to be checked because she is still worried about the baby. What is the priority nursing assessment that should be completed at this time? Why?

   c. Because Amanda has decreased fetal movement, the physician orders a biophysical profile (BPP). How would you explain this test to Amanda? Which part of this test would you normally expect to be a nursing function?

3. Rebecca Richards is pregnant for the first time. She is 40 years of age. The obstetrician has suggested chromosomal studies.

   a. Explain the advantages and disadvantages of chorionic villus sampling (CVS) versus amniocentesis.

   b. Rebecca tells you that she is opposed to abortion for any reason. She asks why she should go through CVS because she will not accept an abortion. How would you respond to Rebecca?

   c. Halfway through the pregnancy, Rebecca's fetus is diagnosed with thrombocytopenia. What therapy will likely be ordered for the fetus? Explain this therapy to Rebecca.

Labor and Birth

The Labor Process

8

STUDENT OBJECTIVES

On completion of this chapter, the student should be able to

1. Explain the four essential components of the labor process.
2. Illustrate how the four components of labor work together to accomplish birth.
3. Identify three current theories regarding causes of labor onset.
4. Differentiate between Braxton Hicks contractions and true labor contractions.
5. Outline the seven mechanisms of a spontaneous vaginal delivery.
6. Classify the stages and phases of labor.
7. Discuss ways the woman physiologically and psychologically adapts to labor.
8. Describe fetal physiologic responses to labor.

KEY TERMS

android pelvis
anthropoid pelvis
caput succedaneum
cardinal movements
diagonal conjugate
effacement
engagement
false pelvis
fetal attitude
fetal lie
fetal presentation
gynecoid pelvis
molding
obstetric conjugate
platypelloid pelvis
station
true pelvis

t is essential for the nurse to understand the components of labor, how these components work together in the process of labor, and how the woman and fetus adapt to labor (in normal situations). This knowledge allows the nurse to support the laboring woman appropriately and assist her through a safe labor and delivery. In this chapter, each component of labor and birth is explored separately, followed by a discussion of the combined components during the process of labor. Normal maternal and fetal adaptation to labor also are explored.

THE FOUR ESSENTIAL COMPONENTS OF LABOR

Four essential components of labor have been identified. These factors are sometimes referred to as the "four Ps" of labor: passageway, passenger, powers, and psyche. A problem in any of these four areas will negatively influence the labor process.

Passageway

The bony pelvis forms the rigid passageway through which the fetus must navigate to be delivered vaginally. The basic shape and dimensions of the pelvis may favor a vaginal birth or may interfere with the ability of the fetus to descend and be delivered vaginally. The soft tissue of the cervix and vagina form the birth canal and also are part of the passageway.

The flared upper portion of the bony pelvis is referred to as the **false pelvis**. The false pelvis is not considered part of the bony passageway. The portion of the pelvis below the linea terminalis is called the **true pelvis**. The true pelvis is the bony passageway through which the fetus must pass during delivery. Important landmarks of the true pelvis include the inlet (entrance

to the true pelvis), midpelvis, and outlet (exit point). Figure 8-1 illustrates important parts of the pelvis.

Pelvic Shape

It is the shape of the inlet that determines the pelvic type. There are four basic pelvic shapes: gynecoid, anthropoid, android, and platypelloid (Fig. 8-2). The **gynecoid pelvis** is most favorable for a vaginal birth. This pelvic type is categorized as a typical female pelvis, although only about half of all women have a gynecoid pelvis. The rounded shape of the gynecoid inlet allows the fetus room to negotiate the dimensions of the bony passageway.

The **anthropoid pelvis** is elongated in its dimensions and is sometimes referred to as apelike. The anterior-posterior diameter is roomy, but the transverse diameter is narrow compared with that of the gynecoid pelvis. However, a vaginal birth often can be accomplished in the approximately 25% of women who have an anthropoid pelvis (Mattson & Smith, 2000).

Take note of this detail. The shape and dimensions of the inlet cannot be determined by the size of the woman. A woman might be small in stature but have a roomy gynecoid pelvis. A larger woman may have a small, contracted platypelloid or android pelvis.

The **android pelvis** is the typical male pelvis. The heart shape of the android pelvis is not favorable to a vaginal delivery. The fetus often gets stuck in this type of pelvis and must be delivered by cesarean section. Approximately 20% of women have an android pelvis.

The least common type is the **platypelloid pelvis**. This pelvis is flat in its dimensions with a very narrow anterior-posterior diameter and a wide transverse diameter. This shape makes it extremely difficult for the fetus to pass through the bony pelvis. Therefore,

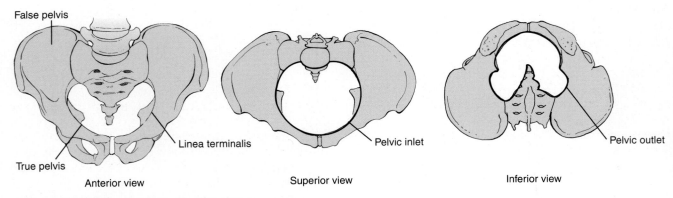

● **Figure 8.1** Important landmarks of the pelvis.

most favorable

need to be 9 cm to get head thru

A Gynecoid

B Anthropoid

C Android

D Platypelloid

● *Figure 8.2* Pelvic shapes. (**A**) Gynecoid, (**B**) anthropoid, (**C**) android, and (**D**) platypelloid.

women with a platypelloid pelvis (about 5% of women) usually must deliver the fetus by cesarean section.

Pelvic Dimensions

Early in the pregnancy, particularly if a woman has never delivered a baby vaginally, the health care provider may take pelvic measurements to estimate the size of the true pelvis. These measurements can help predict if the pelvis is adequate for a vaginal delivery.

The most important measurement of the inlet is the **obstetric conjugate** because this is the smallest diameter of the inlet through which the fetus must pass. However, the obstetric conjugate cannot be measured directly; therefore, the health care provider must estimate the size. The estimate is obtained by measuring the **diagonal conjugate**, which extends from the symphysis pubis to the sacral promontory. Then, 1.5 to 2.0 centimeters are subtracted from the measurement of the diagonal conjugate to approximate the dimensions of the obstetric conjugate. An obstetric conjugate measurement of 11 centimeters is considered to be adequate to accommodate a vaginal delivery.

Measurements of the midpelvis are taken at the level of the ischial spines. If the ischial spines are prominent and extend into the midpelvis, they can

Here's an interesting fact. A woman's pelvis might be roomy enough for a vaginal delivery in one portion, but too small in another portion. That is to say that just because the inlet and the outlet are adequate for delivery does not mean that the midpelvis is adequate. The midpelvis might be contracted and too small to allow the fetus to pass through that section of the bony passageway.

reduce the diameter of the midpelvis and might interfere with the journey of the fetus through the passageway during labor. One important measurement of the outlet is the angle of the pubic arch. This angle should be at least 90 degrees.

Soft Tissues

The cervix and vagina are soft tissues that form the part of the passageway known as the birth canal. In early pregnancy, the cervix is firm, long, and closed. As the time for delivery approaches, the cervix usually begins to soften. Then, when labor begins, uterine contractions affect the cervix in two ways. First, the cervix begins to get shorter, a process called

effacement. Cervical effacement is recorded as a percentage. The cervical canal measures approximately 2 centimeters when it is uneffaced. At a length of 1 centimeter, the cervix is 50% effaced. When the cervix is paper thin, the effacement is recorded as 100%.

The second cervical change that occurs during normal labor is dilation. The cervix must open to allow the fetus to be born. Dilation is measured in centimeters. When the cervix is dilated completely, it measures 10 centimeters. Normally, a primiparous woman will experience effacement before dilation. For a multiparous woman, both processes usually occur at the same time. Often, the multipara will be dilated 1 to 2 centimeters for several weeks before labor begins. Figure 8-3 illustrates the processes of cervical dilation and effacement as they normally occur for the primipara.

The vaginal canal participates in childbirth via passive distention. The rugae of the vaginal walls are obliterated during birth, which allows for considerable expansion. The muscles and soft tissues of the primipara provide greater resistance to stretching and distending than do those of the multipara. This is one reason the first baby often takes longer to be born than do subsequent babies.

● *Figure 8.3* Cervical dilation and effacement.

Before labor

Early effacement

Complete effacement

Complete dilation

Passenger

The "passenger" refers to the fetus. Although the fetus basically has a passive role to play, the size of the fetal skull and fetal accommodation to the passageway (i.e., fetal lie, presentation, attitude, position, and station) can significantly affect labor progress. Each concept is defined and discussed in relation to its influence on the progression of labor.

Did you know? One very important consideration of the passenger is the relationship between the size of the fetal head and pelvic dimensions. The diameters of the fetal skull, as well as the way the fetus positions himself in relation to the pelvis, have a major impact on the process of labor and the type of delivery that results.

Fetal Skull

The skull is the most important fetal structure in relation to labor and birth because it is the largest and least compressible structure (Fig. 8-4). The diameters of the fetal skull must be small enough to allow the head to travel through the bony pelvis. Fortunately, the fetal skull is not entirely rigid. The cartilage between the bones allows for the bones to overlap during labor, a process that reduces the diameter of the head. **Molding**, or elongation of the fetal skull, is another way that the head accommodates to the birth canal. Molding may be particularly pronounced for the newborn of a primipara.

Fetal Accommodation to the Passageway

Fetal Lie. Fetal lie describes the long axis of the fetus in relation to the long axis of the pregnant woman. Basically, there are three ways that the fetus can situate itself in the uterus: in a longitudinal, transverse, or oblique position (Fig. 8-5). A longitudinal lie, in which the long axis of the fetus is parallel to the long axis of the mother, is the most common. When the fetus is in a transverse lie, the long axis of the fetus is perpendicular to the long axis of the woman. An oblique lie is in between the two.

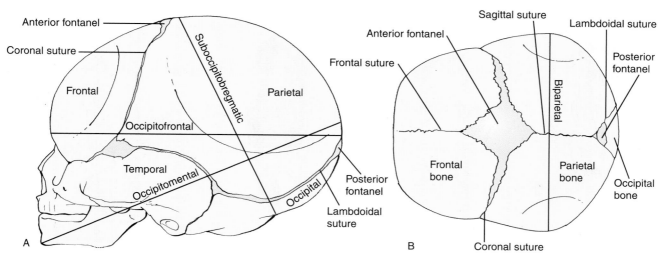

● **Figure 8.4** Clinically important landmarks of the fetal skull. **(A)** Side view showing important diameters in a cephalic presentation. **(B)** Top view showing sutures and fontanels.

Fetal Presentation. Fetal presentation refers to the foremost part of the fetus that enters the pelvic inlet. There are three main ways that the fetus can present to the pelvis: head (cephalic presentation), feet or buttocks (breech presentation), or shoulder (shoulder presentation). Approximately 96% of fetuses are in a cephalic presentation at the end of pregnancy (Cunningham et al., 2001).

Breech presentations occur in approximately 3.5% of term pregnancies (Cunningham et al., 2001).

Figure 8-6 illustrates different types of breech presentations. Shoulder presentations are the least common, occurring in less than 0.5 % of all term pregnancies (Cunningham et al., 2001). This presentation is associated with a transverse lie.

Fetal Attitude. Fetal attitude refers to the relationship of the fetal parts to one another. In a cephalic presentation, there are several different ways the head can present to the maternal pelvis, depending on fetal attitude. The most common attitude, and the one that is

● **Figure 8.5** Longitudinal versus transverse lie. The drawing on the left illustrates a breech presentation in a left sacrum posterior (LSP) position. The lie is longitudinal (the fetus lies parallel to the maternal spine). The drawing on the right is a transverse lie (the fetus lies crosswise to the maternal spine).

Frank breech presentation. Right sacrum posterior (RSP) position. Well-flexed attitude.

Complete breech presentation. Left sacrum posterior (LSP) position. Well-flexed attitude.

Single footling (incomplete) breech presentation. Presenting part: one foot. Right sacrum anterior (RSA) position. Partially extended attitude.

Double footling (incomplete) breech presentation. Presenting part: both feet. Sacrum posterior (SP) position. Attitude of extension.

● *Figure 8.6* Types of breech presentations. Each fetus is in a longitudinal lie.

most favorable for a vaginal birth, is an attitude of flexion, also called a vertex presentation. When the fetus curls up into an ovoid shape, she presents the smallest diameters of her skull to the bony pelvis. When the fetus is neither flexed nor extended, she is in a military presentation and a larger head diameter presents. If the fetus demonstrates an attitude of partial extension, the brow (or frontum) becomes the presenting part. In an attitude of full extension the face presents. Figure 8-7 shows variations of cephalic presentation in association with fetal attitude.

Position. The fetal position is determined by comparing the relationship of an arbitrarily determined reference point on the presenting part to the quadrants of the maternal pelvis (Table 8-1). To determine position, the nurse must first establish the presenting part and locate the appropriate reference point. Then a determination is made as to which pelvic quadrant the reference point is facing.

When position is being documented, the side of the maternal pelvis the presenting part is facing is named first, followed by the reference point. The last

Well-flexed attitude: Vertex presentation Smallest diameter presents—9.5 cm

No flexion or extension: Military presentation Occipitofrontal diameter presents—11 cm

Partial extension: Brow presentation Largest diameter (occipitomental) presents—13.5 cm

Full extension: Face presentation Submentobregmatic diameter presents—9.5 cm

● *Figure 8.7* Relationship of fetal attitude and the diameter of the fetal skull that presents to the maternal pelvis. All of the fetuses are in a cephalic presentation and are exhibiting a longitudinal lie. The presentations can be further differentiated as vertex, military, brow, and face presentations, respectively. Notice the varying degrees of fetal flexion.

TABLE 8.1	Reference Points for Determining Position
Presenting Part	Reference Point
Vertex	Occiput
Brow	Frontum (brow)
Face	Mentum (chin)
Breech	Sacrum
Shoulder	Scapula (acromial process)

part of the designation is used to specify whether the presenting part is facing the anterior or the posterior portion of the pelvis or whether it is in a transverse position. For instance, the occipital bone, or occiput, is the reference point in a vertex presentation. If the occiput is facing the right anterior quadrant of the pelvis, the position is recorded as right occiput anterior (ROA). Box 8-1 describes how to determine the abbreviation used to document fetal position in the clinical record. Figure 8-8 illustrates different positions in a vertex presentation. (See Figure 8-6 for examples of different positions in a breech presentation.)

BOX 8.1	Recording Fetal Position

For each presentation there are eight possible positions. Record the notation as an abbreviation using the following criteria:

First Designation
Refers to the side of the maternal pelvis in which the presenting part is found*
  Right (R)
  Left (L)

Second (Middle) Designation
Reference point on the presenting part
• Occiput (O)—vertex and military presentations
• Frontum or brow (Fr)—brow presentation
• Mentum or chin (M)—face presentation
• Sacrum (S)—breech presentation
• Scapula (Sc)—shoulder presentation

Third (Last) Designation
Refers to the front, back, or side of the maternal pelvis in which the reference point is found
• Anterior (A)—front of the pelvis
• Posterior (P)—back of the pelvis
• Transverse (T)—side of the pelvis

* This designation is not included in the notation if the reference point is exactly in the middle and is turned neither to the left nor to the right.

Be careful! A transverse position is not the same as a transverse lie. The lie refers to the general way the fetus is positioned (lying) in the uterus; whereas, position refers to the way the landmark on the presenting part is facing a specific quadrant of the pelvis. Therefore, in a transverse lie, the shoulder presents to the pelvis; however, a fetus could be in a breech or a cephalic presentation, with the presenting part in a transverse position in reference to the pelvis.

Think about this. When the fetus is floating, he is said to be high in the pelvis. A high station is recorded as a negative (minus) number. On the other hand, if the fetus has moved deep into the pelvis, his station is low and is recorded as a positive (plus) number. As the fetus is being born, his station is a plus four (+4).

Station. Station refers to the relationship of the presenting part to the ischial spines (Fig. 8-9). When the widest diameter of the presenting part is at the level of the ischial spines, the station is recorded as zero (0). If the presenting part is above the level of the ischial spines, the station is recorded as a negative number and is read "minus." If the presenting part is below the level of the ischial spines, the station is recorded as a positive number and is read "plus." For example, in a cephalic presentation, if the vertex is 1 centimeter above the level of the ischial spines, the station is reported as a minus one and recorded as −1. If, on the other hand, the presenting part is 1 centimeter below the level of the ischial spines, the station is reported as a plus one and recorded as +1.

When the station is a minus four (−4) or higher, the fetus is said to be floating and unengaged. When the fetus is floating, the presenting part has not yet entered the true pelvis. When the presenting part has settled into the true pelvis at the level of the ischial spines, the fetus is at a station of zero (0) and engaged.

Test Yourself

• What term is used to describe the fetal part that enters the birth canal first?

• When the nurse describes the relationship of fetal parts to one another, what term does she use?

• How is fetal lie described if the fetus is lying perpendicular to the maternal spine?

Left occiput posterior
(LOP)

Left occiput transverse
(LOT)

Left occiput anterior
(LOA)

Right occiput posterior
(ROP)

Right occiput transverse
(ROT)

Right occiput anterior
(ROA)

● *Figure 8.8* Examples of fetal position in a vertex presentation. The lie is longitudinal for each illustration. The attitude is one of flexion. Notice that the view of the top illustration is seen when facing the pregnant woman. The bottom view is that seen with the woman in a dorsal recumbent position.

● *Figure 8.9* Fetal station.

Powers

The primary force of labor comes from involuntary muscular contractions of the uterus. These labor contractions cause dilation and effacement of the cervix during the first stage of labor. Secondary powers are voluntary muscle contractions of the maternal abdomen during the second stage of labor that help expel the fetus.

Each involuntary uterine contraction is composed of three phases—increment, acme, and decrement—followed by a relaxation period (Fig. 8-10). The increment, or building up of the contraction, is the longest phase. During the increment, the contraction gains strength until the acme, or peak, of the contraction is reached. The decrement is the letting-up phase, as the contraction relaxes gradually to baseline.

The rhythmic, intermittent nature of contractions is documented using three descriptors: frequency, duration, and intensity (see Fig. 8-10). Frequency refers to how often the contractions are occurring and is measured by counting the time interval from the beginning of one contraction to the beginning of the

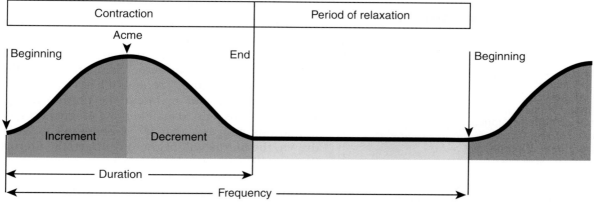

● *Figure 8.10* Anatomy of a uterine contraction. The three phases of a contraction are the increment (building up in intensity), acme (peak intensity), and decrement (decreasing intensity). The contraction is normally followed by a period of relaxation. The nurse assesses the contraction pattern by measuring duration (length of time from the beginning to the end of one contraction), intensity (strength of the contraction, measured at the acme, or peak), and frequency (length of time from the beginning of one contraction to the start of the next contraction).

following contraction. Duration is the interval from the beginning of a contraction to its end. Intensity refers to the strength of the contraction. This characteristic is most often estimated by palpating the fundus at the peak of the contraction and is documented as mild, moderate, or strong. Intensity can also be measured directly with an intrauterine pressure transducer, although this technique is not used routinely.

It is extremely important to the well-being of the mother and the fetus that there is a period of relaxation between contractions (see Fig. 8-10). The blood vessels that supply the placenta are compressed with each contraction, thereby decreasing the amount of oxygen that flows to the fetus. The relaxation period allows for the vessels to fill with oxygen-rich blood to supply the uterus and placenta. Relaxation also is necessary so that maternal muscles do not become overly fatigued and to allow the laboring woman momentary relief from the pain of labor.

This is an important point. Because blood flow to the placenta is interrupted temporarily with each contraction, oxygen to the fetus is decreased. It is as if the fetus must hold his breath during each contraction. Obviously, the fetus cannot tolerate contractions that last too long, are too strong, or that have no rest period between them for any prolonged period of time.

Psyche

Many factors affect the psychological state or psyche of the laboring woman (Box 8-2). When the woman feels confident in her ability to cope and finds ways to work with the contractions, the labor process is enhanced. However, if the laboring woman becomes fearful or has intense pain, she may become tense and fight the contractions. This situation often becomes a cycle of fear, tension, and pain that interferes with the progress of labor.

Test Yourself

- From where does the primary force of labor come?

- How is the frequency of uterine contractions measured?

- What is the purpose of the relaxation period between uterine contractions?

THE PROCESS OF LABOR

The discussion thus far has centered on the individual components of the labor process. However, it is the interplay between the components that allows for labor to progress so that the fetus can be born. The following section illustrates how the labor process works to accomplish birth.

The Onset of Labor

Scientists often search for reasons why things work as they do. One question that intrigues scientists is, "What is the trigger that causes labor to begin?" As

BOX 8.2	Factors That May Affect the Maternal Psyche

Factors that may affect the woman's psyche during labor include the woman's:
- Current pregnancy experience
  - Unplanned versus planned pregnancy
  - Amount of difficulty conceiving
  - Presence of risk factors
  - Complications of pregnancy
- Previous birth experiences
  - Complications of delivery
  - Mode of delivery (cesarean versus vaginal)
  - Birth outcomes (e.g., fetal demise, birth defects)
- Expectations for current birth experience
  - View of labor as a meaningful or a stressful event
  - Realistic and attainable goals versus idealistic views that conflict with reality (a situation that can lead to disappointment)
- Preparation for birth
  - Type of childbirth preparation
  - Familiarity with institution and its policies and procedures
  - Type of relaxation techniques learned and practiced
- Support system
  - Presence and support of a birth companion
    - Husband
    - Mother
    - Lesbian partner
    - Friend
    - Doula
- Culture
  - A woman's culture influences and defines
    - The childbirth experience
      Shameful versus joyful
      Superstitions and beliefs about pregnancy and birth
      Prescribed behaviors and taboos during the intrapartum period
    - Relationships
      Interpersonal interactions
      Parent–infant interactions
      Role expectations of family members
      Support person involvement
    - Pain
      Meaning and context of pain
      Acceptable responses to pain
    - The significance of touch
      Soothing versus intruding
      May be a symbol of intimacy

Adapted from Mattson, S., & Smith, J. E. (Eds.). (2000). *Core curriculum for maternal–newborn nursing* (2nd ed., pp. 227–229). AWHONN publication. Philadelphia: WB Saunders.

pregnancy nears term, the pregnant woman is more concerned with when labor will begin than with what causes labor to begin. She often asks the physician, "When will I go into labor?" This section explores both sets of questions.

Theories of Labor Onset

There are several hypotheses regarding what causes labor to begin. One theory of labor initiation is called the progesterone-withdrawal theory. As stated in previous chapters, progesterone is referred to as the "hormone of pregnancy" because it has a tendency to relax the uterus and maintain the uterine lining. These functions help to maintain the pregnancy. This hypothesis suggests that if progesterone is withdrawn, the uterus will begin to contract, the uterine lining will begin to slough, and labor will result. However, research to date seems to indicate that blocking progesterone does not by itself induce labor.

Oxytocin theory is another hypothesis regarding the cause of labor. Because the hormone oxytocin causes the uterus to contract, some scientists have proposed that a rise in oxytocin levels may be responsible for initiating labor. However, blood levels of oxytocin do not measurably increase before labor begins; therefore, some researchers have concluded that oxytocin is probably not the main factor that stimulates labor to begin. Finally, much research has been done regarding the prostaglandin theory of labor. It has been determined that prostaglandins influence labor in several ways, which include softening the cervix and stimulating the uterus to contract. However, evidence supporting the theory that prostaglandins are the agents that trigger labor to begin is inconclusive.

Because a single causative factor of labor initiation has not yet been determined, the most likely answer seems to be that labor results from a combination of factors working together that stimulates the onset of labor (Ruiz, 1998).

Anticipatory Signs of Labor

Although it cannot be said with certainty what factors actually initiate labor, nature usually provides clues as to the nearness of labor. Approximately 2 weeks before labor the presenting part may settle into the pelvic cavity, causing the pregnant woman to sense that the baby has "dropped." This subjective feeling is called "lightening." The woman will be able to breathe more easily, and she may need to urinate more frequently because of the pressure of the fetus on the urinary bladder. Not all women experience lightening before the onset of labor. Multiparous women often do not experience lightening until labor begins.

Braxton Hicks contractions occur more frequently and are more noticeable as pregnancy approaches term. These irregular, false labor pains usually decrease in intensity with walking and position changes. The woman may experience gastrointestinal disturbances, such as diarrhea, heartburn, or nausea and vomiting as labor approaches. Sometimes the mucous plug will be expelled a week or two before labor ensues.

Frequently the woman will experience a burst of energy 24 to 48 hours before the onset of labor. She may have the energy and desire to do spring cleaning or some other big project in anticipation of the baby's arrival, a phenomenon known as the nesting urge. The nurse should caution the woman regarding the nesting urge and advise her to conserve her energy for the work of labor.

Clinical signs that labor is approaching include ripening or softening and effacement (thinning) of the cervix. Dilation of the cervix may accompany softening and effacement, particularly in multiparous women. The practitioner will inform the woman of these changes when a pelvic examination is done during a scheduled office visit.

Differences Between False and True Labor

Here's a helpful hint. The definition of true labor contains the core information needed to tell the difference between true and false labor. By definition, true labor results in progressive dilation and effacement of the cervix to bring about the birth of the fetus. If contractions are occurring but the cervix is not getting thinner (effacing) or opening (dilating), the woman is not in true labor.

At the end of pregnancy, Braxton Hicks contractions increase in frequency and become more noticeable. These practice contractions can be quite uncomfortable, making it difficult to distinguish true labor from false labor (Table 8-2). Sometimes a woman presents to the labor suite because she thinks she is in labor. After the initial assessment, the woman may be asked to walk for an hour or two. Then a vaginal examination is performed to determine any cervical changes. If there are changes, true labor is diagnosed and the woman is admitted to the hospital. If there are no changes, she may be sent home with instructions to return if the contractions become stronger, more regular, or if other signs of true labor occur, such as increased bloody show or rupture of the membranes.

Mechanisms of a Spontaneous Vaginal Delivery

For a vaginal birth to occur, the passenger must pass through the passageway. The turns and movements made during the journey are referred to as the mechanisms of delivery or the **cardinal movements**, and include engagement, descent, flexion, internal rotation, extension, external rotation, and finally, expulsion (Fig. 8-11). Although the movements will be discussed separately, it is important to understand that these mechanisms may overlap or occur simultaneously.

Initial descent of the fetal head may result in **engagement** (presenting part descends to the level of the ischial spines). Engagement may occur as much as

You may want to make a note of this! Traditionally it has been said that if the primigravida begins labor before engagement has occurred, she has a higher likelihood of having a cesarean birth. However, a study published in the *Journal of Nurse Midwifery* reports that an unengaged vertex in the nullipara in early labor does not by itself predict whether or not a vaginal birth can be accomplished (Diegmann, Chez, & Danclair, 1995).

TABLE 8.2	Characteristics of False Versus True Labor	
	True Labor	**False Labor**
Cervical changes	Progressive dilation and effacement	No change
Membranes	May bulge or rupture spontaneously	Remain intact
Bloody show	Present	Absent; may have pinkish mucous or may expel mucus plug
Contraction pattern	Regular (may be irregular at first) pattern develops in which contractions become increasingly intense and more frequent	Pattern tends to be irregular, although the contractions may seem to have a regular pattern for a time
Pain characteristics	Often starts in the small of the back and radiates to the lower abdomen; may begin with a cramping sensation	May be described as a tightening sensation; usually the discomfort is confined to the abdomen
Effects of walking	Contractions continue and become stronger	May decrease the frequency or eliminate the contractions altogether

1. Head floating, before engagement

2. Engagement; descent, flexion

3. Further descent, internal rotation

4. Complete rotation, beginning extension

5. Complete extension

6. Restitution (external rotation)

7. Delivery of anterior shoulder

8. Delivery of posterior shoulder

● **Figure 8.11** The cardinal movements (or mechanisms) of delivery.

2 weeks before labor or not until after the onset of labor. Engagement is more likely to occur earlier in the primigravida and later in the multigravida.

Flexion is the attitude that presents the smallest diameters of the fetal head to the dimensions of the pelvis. As the head descends during labor, the fetus often is coaxed into and assumes an attitude of flexion as the head encounters resistance from the muscles of the pelvic floor.

Frequently in early labor the fetal head presents to the pelvis in a transverse position because the pelvis is widest from side to side. During active labor, the fetal head typically rotates from a transverse position to an anterior position that is most favorable for a vaginal delivery. This movement is called internal rotation. Labor can be prolonged if the fetus does not rotate because the widest diameters of the fetal head present to the pelvis, resulting in a less than optimal fit

Think this through. If the fetal head enters the pelvis in a transverse position, the fetus has to rotate only 45 degrees to the anterior position. However, if the fetal head enters the pelvis in an occiput posterior position, the fetus must rotate 90 degrees to the preferable anterior position. Several things may happen in this scenario. The labor may be unusually prolonged and painful while the baby rotates, and/or the birth may be painful and traumatic if the fetus delivers face up, a condition referred to as a persistent posterior position. It is typical for a woman to complain of back labor when the fetus is in the posterior position. Sometimes a cesarean delivery is needed if the fetus does not rotate to the anterior position.

between the head and the bony passageway.

Extension must occur for the fetal head to pass under the pubic arch. The head is usually well flexed on the chest as the fetus travels through the birth canal, but when the fetus reaches the pubic arch, it must extend under the symphysis pubis. As the newborn's head is born, external rotation (restitution) lines the head up with the shoulders. Expulsion (birth) occurs after delivery of the anterior and posterior shoulders.

Test Yourself

- List three anticipatory signs of labor.
- What is the main difference between true and false labor?
- List the cardinal movements of labor.

Stages and Duration of Labor

Labor is categorized into four stages, and the first stage is divided further into three phases. Each stage and phase of labor has unique characteristics that help the nurse and physician or midwife determine if labor is progressing as expected. It is important to note that individual labors vary greatly with regard to length. Many factors affect the progress of labor, such as use of agents to soften the cervix, labor induction techniques, and type of anesthesia (if any) used. These factors are discussed in other chapters.

Pay attention! This can be confusing. Although technically a woman who has never delivered a viable child is considered a nullipara, when she goes into labor, she is usually referred to as a primipara.

The following discussion focuses on the physical characteristics of each stage of labor and approximate time periods of each stage. Because parity influences labor progress, typical differences between the primiparous woman and the multiparous woman are noted.

First Stage: Dilation

The first stage of labor begins with the onset of true labor and ends with full dilation of the cervix at 10 centimeters. This stage is subdivided into three phases: latent, active, and transition.

Early Labor (Latent Phase). Early labor begins when the contractions of true labor start and ends when the cervix is dilated 4 centimeters. Contractions during this phase are of mild intensity and may occur as infrequently as every 30 minutes, although the frequency typically ranges between 5 and 10 minutes with a duration of 30 to 45 seconds. In a normal labor, the pattern of contractions during the latent phase becomes increasingly regular with shorter intervals between contractions.

This advice may be helpful on a test! It is easy to confuse phases of the first stage of labor with stages of labor. Be sure you are able to clearly define each stage and phase so that you do not confuse the phases with the stages during an examination.

This phase lasts on average approximately 8 to 9 hours for a primiparous woman but generally does not exceed 20 hours in length. Multiparous women usually experience shorter labors. The average length of the latent phase for a multipara is approximately 5 hours, with an upper limit of 14 hours.

Here's a tip for encouraging the woman. Sometimes nulliparous women become discouraged during the early phase of labor, particularly if the length approaches the 20-hour mark and the cervix is still dilated less than 3 cm. The woman should be told that the cervix of a woman who has never delivered a child effaces before it dilates. The contractions during early labor thin the cervix, whereas the contractions of active labor tend to cause more rapid dilation.

Active Labor (Active Phase). The active phase begins at 4 centimeters cervical dilation and ends when the cervix is dilated 8 centimeters. Contractions typically occur every 2 to 5 minutes, last 45 to 60 seconds, and are of moderate to strong intensity. This stage is characterized normally by progressive cervical dilation and fetal descent.

For primiparas, dilation should occur at approximately 1.2 centimeters/hour. Multiparas progress at a slightly faster pace of 1.5 centimeters/hour. These designations are only approximations and may vary a great deal if the woman receives medication, anesthesia, or other medical intervention during labor. Fetal descent is often slow in the first stage of labor regardless of parity. Occasionally the fetus does not descend during active labor.

Transition (Transition Phase). Transition is considered to be the most difficult part of labor. This phase of the first stage of labor starts when the cervix is dilated 8 centimeters and ends with full cervical dilation. The contractions are of strong intensity, occur every 2 to 3 minutes, and are of 60 to 90 seconds in duration.

Frequently the woman will experience a strong urge to push as the fetus descends. It is important for the woman to resist the urge to push until the cervix is dilated completely. Pushing against a partially dilated cervix can cause swelling, which slows labor, or the cervix can develop lacerations, leading to hemorrhage.

Second Stage: Birth

The second stage begins when the cervix is dilated fully and ends with the birth of the infant. The contractions usually continue at a frequency of every 2 to 3 minutes, last 60 to 90 seconds, and are of strong intensity. The average length of the second stage is 1 hour for primiparas and 20 minutes for multiparas, although it is considered normal for a primipara to be in this stage for 2 hours or longer.

During the second stage, the woman is encouraged to use her abdominal muscles to bear down during contractions while the fetus continues to descend and rotate to the anterior position. Fetal descent is usually slow but steady for the primipara. Frequently the fetus of a multipara, after not making significant downward progress for several hours during active labor, will suddenly descend and be born with one push. When the fetus is at a station of +4, he proceeds to move through the cardinal movements of extension and external rotation, followed by delivery of the shoulders and expulsion of the rest of the body.

Third Stage: Delivery of Placenta

Stage three begins with the birth of the baby and ends with delivery of the placenta. A time frame of 5 to 20 minutes is considered normal for both primiparas and multiparas. Signs that indicate the placenta is separating from the uterine wall consist of a gush of blood, lengthening of the umbilical cord, and a globular shape to the fundus.

The placenta usually delivers spontaneously by one of two mechanisms. Expulsion by Schultze's mechanism indicates that the fetal or shiny side of the placenta delivers first. Delivery by Duncan's mechanism specifies that the maternal or rough side of the placenta presents first.

Fourth Stage: Recovery

Because of the tremendous changes that the new mother's body goes through during the process of labor and delivery, the period of recovery after delivery of the placenta is considered to be a fourth stage of labor. This recovery stage may last from 1 to 4 hours. The woman is observed frequently for signs of hemorrhage or other complications.

MATERNAL AND FETAL ADAPTATION TO LABOR

Maternal Physiologic Adaptation

Labor has an effect on the woman as if she were engaged in moderate to vigorous aerobic exercise. There is an increased demand for oxygen during the first stage of labor, attributable in part to the energy used for uterine contractions. To meet the demand, there is a moderate increase in cardiac output throughout the first stage of labor. During pushing (second stage), cardiac output may be increased as much as 40% to 50% above the prelabor level. Immediately after birth, it may peak at 80% above the prelabor level.

The pulse is often at the high end of normal during active labor. These normal increases in the heart rate are accentuated if the woman becomes dehydrated or exhausted with the work of labor. Blood pressure, however, does not change appreciably during normal labor, although the stress of contractions may cause a 15-mm Hg increase in the systolic pressure. The increased demand for oxygen and the pain of uterine contractions cause the respiratory rate to increase, which puts the laboring woman at risk for hyperventilation. Mouth breathing and dehydration contribute to dry lips and mouth.

Labor prolongs the normal gastric-emptying time. This change often leads to nausea and vomiting during active labor and increases the woman's risk for aspiration, particularly if general anesthesia is required. Traditionally, the laboring woman has been given intravenous (IV) fluids while solid food and fluids are withheld. However, research shows that the risk for aspiration remains high, even if the woman is maintained on a nothing by mouth (NPO) status because gastric secretions become more acidic during periods of fasting. The newer recommendations are to allow the laboring woman to have clear liquids, unless there is a high likelihood that she will deliver by cesarean.

Pressure on the urethra from the presenting part may cause overfilling of the bladder, a decreased sensation to void, and edema. A full bladder is uncomfortable and slows the progress of labor. As the bladder fills, it rises upward in the pelvic cavity, which puts pressure on the lower uterine segment and prevents the head from descending. Sometimes the use of an in-and-out (straight) urinary catheter becomes necessary to empty the bladder.

Some laboratory values are affected by labor. The stress of vigorous labor may cause an increase in the white blood cell (WBC) count to as high as 30,000/mm³. This increase is the body's normal response to inflammation, pain, and stress. Frequently the urine specific gravity is high, indicating concentrated urine, and there may be a trace amount of urinary protein because of increased metabolic activity. Gross proteinuria is never considered normal during labor and is a sign of a developing complication.

Maternal Psychological Adaptation

Labor is hard work that puts a demand on the woman's coping resources. The woman's response changes as labor progresses. During early labor the woman is often excited and talkative, although anxiety and apprehension are common responses. As labor becomes active, the woman becomes more introverted and focuses her energies on coping with the stress of contractions. Women who are unprepared psychologically for labor lose control easily during the active phase and may resort to crying, screaming, or thrashing about during contractions. This response may impede the labor process by causing muscular tension. Tense muscles work against cervical dilation and fetal descent.

Transition is the most intense phase of the first stage of labor, and many women, even ones who have had natural childbirth classes, have a difficult time maintaining positive coping strategies during this phase of labor. Many women describe feeling out of control during this phase of labor. A woman in transition needs support, encouragement, and positive reinforcement. Once pushing efforts begin, the woman usually feels more in control and is better able to cope.

CULTURAL SNAPSHOT

The laboring woman's culture influences her response to pain. In some cultures the woman is expected to accept pain stoically. In other cultures loud expressions of pain are accepted. It is important to perform a careful assessment of a woman's discomfort and to determine measures the laboring woman thinks would be helpful to relieve the pain. Just because the woman is quiet during labor does not mean that she is not experiencing pain. (Refer to Chapter 9 for an in-depth discussion of pain management during labor.)

BOX 8.3	Evaluating Fetal Scalp pH

Fetal pH
- Greater than 7.25
  - Reassuring
  - Associated with normal acid-base balance
- Between 7.20 and 7.25
  - Worrisome
  - May be associated with metabolic acidosis
- Less than 7.20
  - Critical
  - Represents metabolic acidosis
- Less than 7.0
  - Damaging
  - Frequently associated with fetal neurologic damage

Maternal responses to the actual birth vary widely. Many mothers are excited and eager to see and hold the baby. Others are exhausted and may doze intermittently. Most new mothers are anxious about the baby's health. When the woman holds the baby for the first time, it is normal for her to use fingertip touching and for her to explore the infant and count his fingers and toes.

Fetal Adaptation to Labor

Normal labor stresses the fetus in several ways. Intracranial pressure is increased as the fetal head meets resistance from the birth canal. Sometimes this increased pressure results in a slowing of the fetal heart rate at the peak of a contraction—a normal phenomenon described in Chapter 10. Placental blood flow, the source of oxygen for the fetus, is temporarily interrupted at the peak of each contraction. Placental blood flow is interrupted for longer periods during pushing efforts. Because of these changes, even the healthy fetus experiences a slowly decreasing pH throughout labor. Box 8-3 describes normal and abnormal changes in fetal pH. Although the fetal cardiovascular system is stressed, a healthy fetus is able to compensate and maintain the heart rate within normal limits.[1] This ability to compensate demonstrates the presence of a healthy neurologic system.

The act of passing through the birth canal is beneficial to the fetus in two ways. The process of labor stimulates surfactant production to promote respiratory adaptation at birth, and as the fetus descends, maternal tissues compress the body, a process that helps clear the respiratory passageways of mucus.

---

[1] An in-depth discussion of fetal heart rate changes is presented in Chapter 10.

Infants who are born by cesarean section usually require more frequent suctioning because they have not had the benefit of this "vaginal squeeze."

Pressure on the fetus caused by progress through the birth canal may result in areas of ecchymosis or edema, particularly on the presenting part. Pressure on the vertex may cause formation of a **caput succedaneum**, swelling of the soft tissue of the head, or development of a cephalohematoma, collection of blood under the scalp.

Test Yourself

- How many centimeters must the cervix dilate before a woman is considered to be in active labor?
- Which stage requires the woman to help by pushing?
- In which stage of labor does birth occur?

KEY POINTS

- Four essential components of the labor process are the passageway (maternal pelvis and soft tissues), passenger (fetus), powers (involuntary and voluntary muscle contractions), and psyche (psychological state of the woman).
- The bony pelvis is the rigid passageway through which the fetus must pass. There are four basic pelvic shapes: gynecoid, anthropoid, android, and platypelloid. The gynecoid type is the most favorable for vaginal birth. The diameters of the inlet, midpelvis, and outlet are important in determining the adequacy of the pelvis for vaginal delivery.
- The cervix, part of the soft tissue of the passageway, must completely efface (thin) and dilate (open) for the fetus to be born. Full dilation is equal to 10 centimeters.
- The fetal skull is the most important fetal structure because it is the largest and least compressible. A comparison of the diameters of the true pelvis to the diameters of the fetal skull is important when the physician is attempting to determine if a vaginal delivery is possible.
- Fetal lie refers to the relationship of the long axis of the fetus to the long axis of the mother. A longitudinal lie is the most favorable to a vaginal birth.
- The large majority of fetuses enter the pelvis head first, a condition referred to as a cephalic presentation. When the feet or buttocks present first, it is called a breech presentation. A shoulder presentation is uncommon.

- A flexed fetal attitude presents the smallest diameters of the fetal head to the pelvis.
- The part of the fetus that is closest to the cervix is the presenting part. Presentation and attitude together determine the presenting part.
- To determine fetal position, the nurse must first verify the presenting part and locate the reference point: occiput, frontum, mentum, sacrum, etc. Then the relationship of the reference point to maternal pelvic quadrants is determined to confirm fetal position.
- Station is a determination of the relationship of the presenting part to the ischial spines. Zero station occurs when the presenting part is at the level of the ischial spines. When the fetus is high in the pelvis (above the ischial spines), the station is recorded as a negative number. A low station (below the ischial spines) is recorded as a positive number.
- The primary power of labor comes from involuntary uterine contractions, which serve to efface and dilate the cervix. Secondary powers are supplied by maternal pushing efforts during the second stage of labor.
- The contraction pattern (frequency, duration, and intensity) and the resting interval are important to assess because the fetus can become hypoxic if contractions are too close together, too strong, or do not have a rest period.
- Maternal psyche is an important influence on the labor process. Nursing interventions can help break the cycle of fear, tension, and pain that can interfere with labor.
- Theories of what causes labor to begin include progesterone withdrawal theory and the oxytocin and prostaglandin theories. It is most likely that all three of these influences, along with other factors, work together to initiate labor.
- Anticipatory signs of labor include lightening, Braxton Hicks contractions, a burst of energy, and cervical ripening and dilation.
- True labor results in progressive effacement and dilation. It is characterized by contractions that become progressively stronger and occur more frequently. Walking does not cause true labor contractions to stop.
- Engagement, descent, flexion, internal rotation, extension, and external rotation are the mechanisms of delivery or cardinal movements by which the fetus is born.
- Labor is categorized in four stages: first stage, dilation; second stage, birth; third stage, expulsion of placenta; and fourth stage, recovery. The first stage is composed of three phases: latent, active, and transition. Each phase and stage has unique characteristics that differentiate it from other phases and stages.

- Labor affects the mother in much the same way as vigorous exercise does. The heart rate, cardiac output, and respiratory rate increase to meet the body's increased oxygen need. Other systems, notably the gastrointestinal and urinary, are also affected.
- The healthy fetus is able to withstand the stress that labor makes on the cardiovascular system. A vaginal birth helps mature the respiratory system and clears mucus from the respiratory tract

REFERENCES AND SELECTED READINGS

Books and Journals

Cunningham, F. G., Gant, N. F., Leveno, K. J., Gilstrap, L. C. III, Hauth, J. C., & Wenstrom, K. D. (2001). Section IV: Normal labor and delivery. In *Williams obstetrics* (21st ed., pp. 249–330). New York: McGraw-Hill Medical Publishing Division.

Diegmann, E. K., Chez, R. A., & Danclair, W. G. (1995). Station in early labor in nulliparous women at term. *Journal of Nurse-Midwifery, 40*(4), 382–385.

Mattson, S., & Smith, J. E. (Eds.). (2000). *Core curriculum for maternal–newborn nursing* (2nd ed.). AWHONN publication. Philadelphia: WB Saunders.

Ruiz, R. J. (1998). Mechanisms of full-term and preterm labor: Factors influencing uterine activity. *JOGNN: Journal of Obstetric, Gynecologic, & Neonatal Nursing, 27,* 652–660.

Simpson, K. R., & Creehan, P. A. (2001). *AWHONN Association of Women's Health, Obstetric and Neonatal Nurses: Perinatal nursing.* Philadelphia: Lippincott Williams & Wilkins.

Wolcott, H. D., & Conry, J. A. (2000). Normal labor. In A. T. Evans & K. R. Niswander (Eds.), *Manual of obstetrics* (6th ed., pp. 392–424). Philadelphia: Lippincott Williams & Wilkins.

Websites

http://www.emedicine.com/aaem/topic284.htm

http://www.ecc.cc.mo.us/ecc/library/web/reserves/normallabor.htm

http://www.ecc.cc.mo.us/ecc/library/web/reserves/normal_labor2.htm

http://www.methodisthealth.com/pregnancy/labor.htm

http://www.pelvicfloor.com/library/library.html?show=yes&subcategoryid=18

http://www.avc.edu/alliedhealth/documents/LaborandDeliveryII.ppt

WORKBOOK

NCLEX-STYLE REVIEW QUESTIONS

1. A 32-year-old woman is dilated 4 centimeters. The physician states that she has a roomy pelvis and the baby is in a right occiput anterior (ROA) position at a +1 station. Her contractions are occurring every 10 minutes, lasting 30 to 40 seconds, and palpate mild in intensity. She is calm and relaxed. Given these data, which essential component of labor is unexpected and likely to slow the progress of labor at this time?

   a. Passageway

   b. Passenger

   c. Powers

   d. Psyche

2. A woman near the end of pregnancy comments to the nurse, "I'm curious. What causes labor to begin?" Which reply by the nurse is best?

   a. "It is a mystery. No one knows."

   b. "It is believed that several factors work together to stimulate labor to begin."

   c. "The pituitary gland in the brain releases a special hormone that signals labor to begin."

   d. "You don't need to worry about that. The baby will come when he is ready."

3. The fetus is in a cephalic presentation. His occiput is facing toward the front and slightly to the right of the mother's pelvis and he is exhibiting a flexed attitude. How does the nurse document the position of the fetus?

   a. LOA

   b. LOP

   c. ROA

   d. ROP

4. A woman has just delivered a healthy baby girl, but the placenta has not yet been delivered. What stage of labor does this scenario represent?

   a. First

   b. Second

   c. Third

   d. Fourth

STUDY ACTIVITIES

1. Using the table below, write a brief definition or explanation of each of the "four Ps" of labor. List critical nursing observations/assessments that should be made for each area and briefly describe what should be documented.

Four Ps of Labor	Definition or Explanation	Observations (What to Look for)	Documentation
Passageway			
Passenger			
Powers			
Psyche			

2. Develop a teaching aid or poster explaining the stages of labor to a first-time pregnant woman.
3. Have a discussion with your clinical group about the way culture affects behaviors and choices regarding labor and birth. Compare different rituals and taboos of which your classmates are aware that relate to labor and birth.

CRITICAL THINKING: What Would You Do?

Apply your knowledge of the components of labor to the following situation.

1. Anna, a 25-year-old gravida 2, has been in labor for several hours, but her cervix is not dilating. The physician says that Anna's pelvis is roomy and adequate for a vaginal delivery.

   a. In what way do you anticipate the journey of the fetus through the passageway will be affected because Anna's cervix is not dilating?

   b. Discuss two possible causes of the failure of Anna's cervix to dilate.

2. Anna's midwife performs a vaginal examination and states the fetus is "occiput posterior."

   a. Anna asks you, "What does it mean that the baby is occiput posterior?" How would you explain this situation to Anna?

   b. What will you tell Anna's partner regarding the probable progress of labor because the fetus is in a posterior position?

3. Anna has been in active labor for 7 hours. She has been quietly coping with contractions with the help of her partner. Now she begins to cry, "I can't stand it anymore!" She screams at her partner, "This is all your fault. You're not helping me at all!"

 a. The nurse performs a pelvic examination. How far do you expect Anna to be dilated? What stage and phase of labor is most likely represented in this scenario?

 b. How will you advise Anna's partner? How can he continue to be helpful and understanding during this difficult part of labor?

4. Anna progresses to the second stage of labor, but the fetus has not rotated to an anterior position, so the baby is delivered face up.

 a. What does the physician document in the delivery note regarding the position of the baby at birth?

 b. How would you expect the baby's head to look after his long journey through the birth canal?

 c. How do you expect Anna will react to the birth of her baby?

Pain Management During Labor and Birth

9

The Pain of Labor and Childbirth
  Uniqueness of Labor and Birth Pain
  *Physiology and Characteristics of Labor
  Pain*
  Factors Influencing Labor Pain

*Principles of Pain Relief During
  Labor*
Pain Management Techniques
  Nonpharmacologic Interventions
  Pharmacologic Interventions

STUDENT OBJECTIVES

On completion of this chapter, the student should be able to

1. Describe sources of labor pain.
2. Discuss principles of labor pain management.
3. Explain various relaxation techniques that help a woman cope with labor.
4. Compare nonpharmacologic interventions to manage labor pain.
5. Differentiate analgesia from anesthesia.
6. Describe advantages and disadvantages of opioid administration.
7. Compare methods of regional anesthesia.
8. Explain major complications associated with epidural and spinal anesthesia.
9. Discuss reasons general anesthesia is risky for a pregnant woman and her fetus.
10. List life-threatening complications associated with general anesthesia.

KEY TERMS

analgesia
anesthesia
effleurage
intrathecal
opioids

Pain is an individual, subjective, sensory experience. However, a complex interplay of physiologic, psychological, emotional, environmental, and sociocultural factors influences the way a person perceives and responds to pain. A woman's response to labor pain is influenced by all of the aforementioned factors to include her expectations about labor and her confidence in her ability to cope with labor. The licensed practical nurse (LPN) assists the registered nurse (RN) to manage the pain associated with labor and birth.

THE PAIN OF LABOR AND CHILDBIRTH

Uniqueness of Labor and Birth Pain

The pain of labor and birth is different from other types of pain in several ways. In most instances, pain is a warning sign of injury, but labor pain is associated with a normal physiologic process. In other types of pain, greater intensity is often associated with greater injury. During labor, intensity increases as the woman approaches birth, which is the desirable and positive outcome. Although the pain of labor begins without warning, once it is established it occurs in a predictable pattern with respite from pain between contractions. This characteristic is different than most other types of pain. Because it is predictable, the woman can prepare for and better cope with the pain.

Physiology and Characteristics of Labor Pain

There are two general concepts related to pain that are helpful to understand: threshold and tolerance. The pain threshold is the level of pain necessary for an individual to perceive pain. Pain tolerance refers to the ability of an individual to withstand pain once it is recognized. Each woman has her own pain threshold and tolerance of pain. Each woman responds to labor in a unique way, and the experience of labor is reported differently among women. In addition, each labor is experienced uniquely in a woman who bears more than one child.

Pain sensations associated with labor originate from different places, depending on the stage of labor. During the first stage of labor, stimulation of pain receptors in the cervix and lower uterine segment predominates in response to the stretching required to thin and open the cervix. Some researchers hypothesize that labor pain is associated with ischemia to the uterus, in much the same way that ischemia causes angina. However, this theory is debated because blood flow to the uterine muscle is actually increased during a contraction, whereas blood flow to the placenta is decreased. During the second stage of labor the main source of pain is from pressure on the perineum and birth canal as the fetus descends.

Caution! Don't assume that the woman who reports severe pain has low pain tolerance. Always do a thorough assessment because pain that is not manageable with normal interventions may be a signal that something else, other than labor, is occurring. For instance, severe unrelenting abdominal pain in conjunction with a uterus that does not relax may indicate placental abruption. Severe pain may occur with uterine rupture. Epigastric pain is often present in severe preeclampsia just before a seizure. And don't forget that the pregnant woman may also have an undetected medical condition, such as perforated bowel or appendicitis.

Labor pain in the first stage of labor has characteristics similar to other types of abdominal pain. It is often diffuse in nature, occurs in the lower abdomen, and may be referred to the lower back, buttocks, and thighs. It is often described as occurring in waves, with some "waves" more powerful than others. The contraction begins as a sensation of cramping in the lower abdomen or lower back and gradually increases in strength to the peak of the contraction, and then it slowly abates until pain is no longer perceived.

The pain of birth is sometimes described as the most intense sensation of pain. It is generally experienced as an intense sensation of burning in the perineum as the tissues stretch in response to the fetus pressing against them during descent. Often the sensation is so intense that an episiotomy can be done without anesthesia, and the woman does not perceive it.

Factors Influencing Labor Pain

Many factors influence the pain of labor and birth, making it a multidimensional experience. Examples of psychosocial influences include the level of the woman's fear and anxiety, her culture, and the circumstances surrounding the birth experience, such as whether or not the pregnancy is planned or unplanned, the child is wanted or unwanted, the birth is preterm or term, and the fetus is living or dead.

The perceived intensity of labor pain is affected by many variables. The younger the woman, the more likely she is to report severe pain. Women bearing children for the first time also report more intense levels of pain. High levels of anxiety and fear correlate with high levels of perceived pain. A woman who has experienced significant nonobstetric forms of pain usually reports lower levels of pain during labor than does a woman who does not have prior experience with severe pain.

There also are physiologic variables that affect the experience of labor pain. A woman who is physically conditioned usually reports lower levels of pain during labor and birth. The stress of labor causes the body to release endorphins, natural pain-killing substances similar to morphine. Interestingly, levels of endorphins rise as labor progresses and peak immediately after birth. When pharmacologic methods are used to treat the pain of labor, the levels of endorphins circulating in the woman's bloodstream are decreased.

Physiologic factors directly related to the birthing process also affect the perception of pain. In general, the longer the labor the more likely the woman is to report extreme pain. Obstructed labor is usually perceived as being more painful. Obstructed labor can result from fetopelvic disproportion and abnormal fetal positions. Labor that is induced with oxytocin often is reported to be extremely strong. The contractions may be described as intense and lacking the gradual ebb and flow of naturally occurring contractions. Back labor usually is perceived as being intensely painful, even excruciating. Some women report that back labor feels as if the back is literally breaking in two. In addition, when a woman experiences back labor, her pain may not completely resolve between contractions.

Principles of Pain Relief During Labor

There is no one "perfect way" to control labor pain. Each woman responds to the experience uniquely. Research has shown that women report higher levels of satisfaction with their labor experience when they feel a high degree of control over the experience of pain (McCrea & Wright, 1999). The nurse owes it to the woman to inform her of pain management options and to be supportive of the choices that she makes. It is also important to remember that the woman has the right to change her mind about the acceptability of any particular pain management technique at any time before or during labor.

Rarely is there a completely pain-free labor. Even

Sensitivity and understanding go a long way! It is important for the nurse to be nonjudgmental when assisting a woman to cope with pain. Too often, nurses project their own values regarding labor pain onto the woman. Some nurses feel very strongly that a woman should have a "natural" childbirth without pharmacologic intervention. Other nurses don't understand why any woman would want to "suffer" through labor without an epidural. In both situations, the nurse is in danger of not providing the support that the laboring woman needs and deserves.

when a woman receives an epidural, she frequently reports severe pain before the epidural is administered. Caregivers commonly underrate the severity of pain when compared with the woman's ratings (Leeman et al., 2003a). It is important to accept the woman's description of the severity of the pain, even when she may not appear to be in pain.

CULTURAL SNAPSHOT

A woman's cultural values influence the way that she responds to pain. Some women are very vocal. They may cry or moan with pain. Some women display a stoic response to pain. They may be very quiet or appear to be resting. Caregivers frequently underestimate the pain of both types of women. The woman who is vocal may be labeled a "difficult" patient who does not handle pain well. The stoic woman may be labeled a "good" patient. However, neither of them is likely to get the pain control that they need, unless the nurse does a careful pain assessment.

Ideally the woman will discuss labor pain management with her primary care provider during the pregnancy and will attend prenatal classes. The woman who enters labor knowing what to realistically expect usually copes better and reports a more satisfying labor experience than does one who is not as well prepared. However, if the woman is not prepared, the nurse can teach the woman what to expect and assist her to cope when she presents in labor.

PAIN MANAGEMENT TECHNIQUES

Labor pain management techniques can be divided into two major categories: nonpharmacologic interventions and pharmacologic interventions. Safety considerations for the woman and her fetus are an important part of the nursing care plan for both categories.

Nonpharmacologic Interventions

Almost every woman uses some type of nonpharmacologic pain intervention during labor, even when pharmacologic methods are used. Most commonly, a woman uses a combination of techniques to cope with labor. She may need assistance coping before medication is used or in conjunction with medication.

There are numerous methods of nonpharmacologic pain relief. Some interventions have been researched and are known to be effective. Some have not been well

TABLE 9.1	Comparison of Selected Nonpharmacologic Interventions for Relief of Labor Pain		
Intervention	**Effectiveness to Relieve Labor Pain**	**Advantages**	**Disadvantages**
Continuous labor support	Highly effective throughout labor. May increase the woman's perception of personal control, a factor that correlates with higher satisfaction with the labor experience.	• Low technological/high-touch intervention • Addresses the emotional and spiritual aspects of labor and birth.	Most busy labor and delivery hospital settings cannot provide this level of support for the laboring woman, so the woman and her husband must usually hire a doula if they desire this level of support.
Patterned breathing	Can be very effective when the woman has practiced before labor and has an attentive labor coach.	• Does not require any special tools. • Promotes relaxation. • Basic patterns can be taught by the nurse when the couple presents in labor.	Requires training and practice before labor to be most effective.
Effleurage	Can be helpful during early labor to decrease the sensation of pain.	• Is easy to learn and simple to perform. • Does not require any special tools.	Is less effective during active labor as the contractions become more intense.
Water therapy	Highly effective to promote relaxation and decrease the sensation of pain, especially during the 1st hour or two of use.	• Many women find water very comforting during labor. • Promotes relaxation.	• Requires availability of a tub—equipment that is not always available in the hospital setting. • May slow labor if used too early. • The woman may notice decreased effectiveness over time.
Imagery	Can be very effective for some women.	• Is noninvasive. • Requires no special tools. • Incorporates spirituality with the birthing process.	• Requires discipline and practice to achieve maximum benefit. • May not be appropriate for individuals with mental illness or history of emotional trauma.
Hypnosis	Carefully selected women can benefit from hypnosis during labor.	• Requires no special tools. • Promotes the woman's sense of control over her pain. • Involves a holistic approach to labor.	• Special training by a therapist is required. • Can be expensive and may not be covered by insurance. • Does not work for all women. • Severe anxiety and psychosis is a possible side effect.
Intradermal water injections	Very effective to relieve back pain during labor.	• Can be administered by the nurse.	• Invasive (requires an injection). • Not effective for abdominal discomfort associated with contractions.
Acupressure and acupuncture	Anecdotal reports suggest that these therapies may be helpful to reduce the pain of labor.	• Addresses the holistic nature of labor and incorporates spiritual and emotional aspects. • Acupressure is noninvasive.	• Requires a trained practitioner to perform. • Acupuncture is invasive and requires special needles.

researched. However, the intervention that works for the woman is frequently the best one to use. Typically a woman will need a variety of interventions throughout labor. As labor becomes more intense, she frequently needs to try different methods. For example, effleurage and distraction are often helpful in early labor, but not as effective in active labor and transition. Table 9-1 compares selected nonpharmacologic interventions.

Continuous Labor Support

Continuous labor support with a trained nurse or doula (trained lay person who supports and coaches a woman during labor) has been shown to be effective to increase the coping ability of the laboring woman. Additional benefits include a decrease in requests for pain medication, fewer obstetric interventions, and a lower cesarean delivery rate. The same benefit is not afforded when nurses provide intermittent labor support, as is typical for busy labor and delivery settings. The nurse can encourage the woman to hire a doula, particularly if childbirth is desired with minimal medical intervention.

Comfort Measures

Don't underestimate the need for comfort measures during labor. Encourage the use of lip balm to keep the lips hydrated during labor. Ice chips, lollipops, and clear liquids (if allowed) can be helpful to moisten the mouth. Mouth breathing during labor can lead to dry mouth.

Change the linens when they become soiled with perspiration or body fluids. Most facilities have pads that are placed under the buttocks to catch bloody show and amniotic fluid during labor. Explain to the woman that it will be impossible to keep her completely dry, but reassure her that you will change the pads frequently. Give perineal care with warm water after she uses the restroom and before changing the linens.

Relaxation Techniques

Relaxation is the objective of almost every nonpharmacologic intervention. When the woman becomes anxious or apprehensive, she tenses her muscles. This action can slow the labor process and decrease the amount of oxygen reaching the uterus and the fetus. When the woman maintains a state of relaxation during and between contractions, she is actually working with her body to facilitate the labor process. The following discussion highlights several techniques that may help the woman to relax during labor. Some of these methods should be learned from a trainer and practiced before labor to be most effective, although the nurse can teach the woman and her partner some of the basic techniques when she presents to the delivery suite.

Patterned Breathing. In times past, very structured breathing techniques were taught during childbirth classes. Now the trend is to teach basic principles of patterned breathing without emphasizing strict patterns. In general the woman begins with a slow-paced breathing pattern. She maintains the slow-paced pattern until it is no longer working to enhance relaxation, and then she switches to a higher level. Table 9-2 describes the basic breathing patterns that are often taught in childbirth preparation classes.

All breathing patterns should begin and end with the woman taking a cleansing breath. A cleansing

TABLE 9.2	Patterned Breathing Techniques for Labor*
Breathing Pattern	**Description**
Slow-paced breathing	The woman takes slow, deliberate breaths while she focuses on maintaining a relaxed stance. She may use effleurage, music, or any technique that encourages relaxation while using slow-paced breathing. The rate is approximately 6 to 10 breaths per minute.
Modified-paced breathing	The woman begins taking slow, deep breaths at the beginning of the contraction. She then increases the rate while decreasing the depth of respirations as she reaches the contraction peak, after which she slows the rate and increases the depth.
Patterned-paced breathing or the "pant-blow" technique	This technique is similar to modified-paced breathing with the addition of a rhythmic pattern. There are several rhythms that can be taught; however, the 4-to-1 rhythm is a popular one. The woman takes 4 light breaths and then blows out through her lips, as if she is blowing out a candle. Different rhythms can be used, such as 4-to-1, followed by 6-to-1 and repeating through the peak of the contraction.

* Note that each pattern begins and ends with a cleansing breath.

breath is a deep, relaxed breath that signals the woman to relax and provides deep ventilation. Breathing may be done through the nose or through the mouth, whichever is most comfortable and natural for the woman. If she breathes through her mouth, pay particular attention to measures to keep the mouth moist.

Breathing should be comfortable to the woman and should not cause her to hyperventilate. If she feels short of breath, she may need to take deeper breaths. If she begins to tingle in her hands and around her mouth, she is probably hyperventilating. She should slow her breathing and breathe into her cupped hands or a paper bag until the tingling stops.

Attention Focusing. Many childbirth classes teach methods of attention focusing, or concentration. Women attending Lamaze-oriented classes are encouraged to focus internally or externally, whichever is more effective. Bradley classes advocate an internal focus because Dr. Bradley, the method's founder, believed that external focus distracts the woman from the job of "listening to her body" while laboring. Attention focusing, or concentration, helps the woman to work with her body, instead of panicking.

Another name for internal focus is imagery. Imagery is a technique used to help the woman associate positive thoughts with the birth process. The method engages the senses and promotes relaxation. The woman is encouraged to visualize a positive, healing situation during contractions. For example, some childbirth educators encourage the woman to visualize each contraction as a wave. As the contraction strengthens, the tide rises. As the contraction fades away, the tide ebbs. Or the woman may visualize her body opening and allowing the fetus to pass through. Sometimes the woman visualizes herself at a favorite relaxing place, such as the beach or in a comfortable chair at a vacation cabin. Music is sometimes used in association with imagery to help the woman focus and relax.

The woman who focuses externally opens her eyes and focuses on a picture, person, or object that is helpful to her. For example, one woman used a picture of her grandmother as her focus. As she looked into her grandmother's face during her contractions, she drew strength remembering that her grandmother had birthed 11 babies, all at home without drugs. Another used as her focus a picture of a mountain she and her husband had climbed. As she labored, she remembered her feelings as she overcame the challenges of the ascent of the mountain and likened it to the challenge of her labor. Knowing the feeling of accomplishment she felt as she reached the peak of the mountain, she felt strengthened knowing she would have a strong sense of achievement when she felt her baby slide from her body and held him in her arms. Focusing on sounds, music, voices, relaxation, and breathing may also benefit the laboring woman.

● **Figure 9.1** A woman uses a birthing ball to position herself during labor.

Movement and Positioning. Changing positions frequently can be helpful during labor. Any position of comfort is acceptable, as long as the fetal heart rate stays within the normal range. If the woman wants to be on her back, be certain to place a pillow or a wedge under one hip to prevent supine hypotension. The woman may find a birthing ball to be helpful (Fig. 9-1). The ball allows her to rock and move to a position of comfort. Women who are encouraged to ambulate and reposition themselves, as needed, during labor report higher satisfaction levels with the birthing process.

Touch and Massage. Effleurage, a form of touch that involves light circular fingertip movements on the abdomen, is a technique the woman can use in early labor (Fig. 9-2). The theory is that light touch stimulates the nerve pathways to the brain and keeps them busy, thereby blocking the pain sensation. As contractions become stronger during active labor, effleurage becomes less effective. At that point, deeper pressure can be used. Direct pressure may be applied with the hands over the area of greatest pain intensity, often above the pubic bone or on the upper thighs. Abdominal pressure may be applied by the woman or by her partner/coach.

If the woman is experiencing intense back labor, it is often helpful for the nurse or partner to give the woman a massage over the lower back or to use the fists or palms of the hands to apply counter-pressure (Fig. 9-3). Alternately, a tennis ball can be used to massage the lower back.

Water Therapy. Exposure to warm water either by showering or bathing in a tub or whirlpool can signifi-

● *Figure 9.2* Effleurage. The woman uses her fingertips to lightly touch her abdomen using circular strokes. This form of light touch often decreases the sensation of pain in early labor.

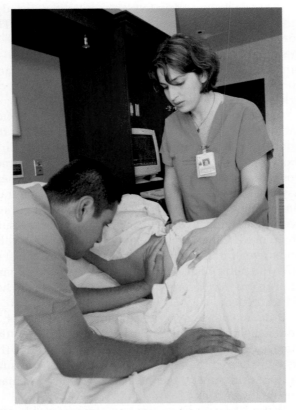

● *Figure 9.3* The woman's partner uses the palm of his hand to apply counter-pressure to the woman's lower back.

cantly increase the ability of the laboring woman to cope with uterine contractions. In fact, some women use water not only to provide labor pain relief, but they also deliver in water. Figure 9-4 shows a woman using water to help her relax during labor.

Suggestions for using water safely during labor differ slightly between authors. Leeman et al. (2003a) recommend that the water temperature be maintained at or lower than body temperature, that the woman be in active labor (at 5 centimeters) before using water, and that the bath be limited to 1 to 2 hours in length. Waterbirth International (undated) recommends using a water temperature of 95°F to 100°F (not to exceed 101°F). This organization also suggests that the woman get in the water whenever she chooses to do so, with the caveat that entering water before 5 centimeters of cervical dilation may cause labor to progress more slowly. There is no time limit given for bathing, although the organization does suggest that the 1st hour in the water is usually the most relaxing and helpful for the laboring woman.

There are differing opinions in the medical establishment regarding the safety and advisability of using water during labor and birth. Current research confirms the safety and efficacy of this intervention. However, more research is needed to establish guidelines for practice and to encourage more hospital settings to provide water therapy during labor.

Hypnosis. Hypnosis has been successfully used to help a woman relax and decrease the pain of labor. The woman attends several sessions with a trained therapist during pregnancy. At each session she learns how to induce a trance-like state that she can use during labor. Hypnosis can induce intense states of anxiety or psychosis in certain individuals.

● *Figure 9.4* A woman at full dilation waits for the urge to push while relaxing in water at home. The woman reports that although this was her largest child, this labor and birth was the easiest for her. She attributes this to the water therapy. Photo by Kaye Bullock, CPM.

● **Figure 9.5** Location of intradermal water injections. The nurse administers four sterile water injections to relieve the pain of back labor.

Intradermal Water Injections

Intradermal injections of sterile water have been found to be effective in relieving the pain of back labor (Leeman et al., 2003a). The technique is most effective when two caregivers administer the injections simultaneously. Four injections of 0.1 mL sterile water are given into the intradermal space in the lower back (Fig. 9-5). The injections significantly reduce back pain for 45 to 90 minutes after they are given.

Acupressure and Acupuncture

Acupressure and acupuncture are two similar techniques used in traditional Chinese medicine. The goal is to restore balance by promoting the flow of energy, which decreases muscle tension, promotes relaxation, and decreases the sensation of pain. Acupuncture involves the use of needles, whereas acupressure is a noninvasive form of massage. Both methods involve stimulating energy points. Research has demonstrated that both forms of treatment can be helpful in the treatment of pain; however, research is limited regarding the usefulness of these methods for treating labor pain (Koehn, 2000).

Test Yourself

- Name two general principles of pain relief during labor.
- List three nonpharmacologic methods of labor pain management.
- Describe three relaxation techniques that help increase the woman's ability to cope with labor pain.

Pharmacologic Interventions

One reason women began to choose the hospital as a place to deliver babies was for the pharmacologic pain relief methods that were available. The pendulum has swung back and forth regarding the favor in which pharmacologic methods are viewed. In the 1950s women were given strong medications that caused them to forget the pain of labor. Beginning in the 1960s and 1970s, women demanded to have more control and more say over the birth process, and natural childbirth came into favor as the "best" way to experience labor and birth. Currently, many women choose to deliver in hospitals so that they can get pain relief from epidural analgesia.

It is important to understand the difference between analgesia and anesthesia, although the terms are sometimes used interchangeably. **Analgesia** is the use of medication to reduce the sensation of pain. **Anesthesia** is the use of medication to partially or totally block all sensation to an area of the body. Anesthesia may or may not involve loss of consciousness. Table 9-3 compares pharmacologic medications used to relieve labor pain.

Analgesia and Sedation

Sedatives are given to promote sedation and relaxation; however, they do not provide direct pain relief (analgesia). Barbiturates, such as secobarbital (Seconal) and pentobarbital (Nembutal), may be given in early labor to promote sleep. These medications can cause respiratory and central nervous system depression in the newborn if given within 12 to 24 hours of birth (Poole, 2003).

Opioids, medications with opium-like properties (also known as narcotic analgesics), are the most frequently administered medications to provide analgesia during labor. Opioids, such as meperidine (Demerol) and fentanyl (Sublimaze), blunt the pain sensation but do not completely relieve the pain. These medications frequently assist the woman to better tolerate labor

Be very careful! Always warn the woman and her support person to call the nurse before she tries to get up after IV sedation has been administered. Women have experienced falls when attempting to ambulate after IV sedation. Women have delivered their babies unattended in the bathroom after being sedated because they mistake the urge to push for the need to have a bowel movement. Physical injury can occur to the newborn when the delivery is unattended. For example, the cord can break, leading to hemorrhage. Or the newborn can be physically injured from falling and hitting the floor.

TABLE 9.3	Comparison of Selected Pharmacologic Interventions for Relief of Labor Pain

Medication Class	Associated Side Effects	Advantages	Disadvantages
Sedatives	• Excessive sedation and/or central nervous system depression • Decreased FHR variability	• Promote sleep in the early stage of labor. • Decrease anxiety. • Promethazine (Phenergan) and hydroxyzine (Vistaril) may be administered with an opioid to decrease nausea and vomiting. • May increase effectiveness of uterine contractions.	• Do not provide pain relief. • Can produce neonatal respiratory depression if given within 12–24 hours of birth.
Opioids (narcotic analgesics)	• Nausea and vomiting • Pruritus • Delayed gastric emptying • Dysphoria • Drowsiness • Hypoventilation • Decreased FHR variability • Neonatal depression (Poole, 2003)	• Increases the woman's ability to cope with uterine contractions. • May be nurse administered.	• Reduces but does not eliminate pain sensations. • Associated with neonatal central nervous system and respiratory depression. • Inhibits neonatal sucking and delays effective feeding. • May decrease neonatal alertness (Leeman et al., 2003b).
Paracervical block	• Fetal bradycardia • Maternal complications are uncommon but include fainting, laceration of the vaginal mucosa, local anesthetic toxicity, hematomas, postpartum neuropathy, paracervical or subgluteal abscesses (Poole, 2003)	• Provides excellent pain relief for the first stage of labor. • Does not interfere with maternal mobility.	• Requires multiple injections because the duration of pain relief is short. • Cannot be used for pain relief in the second stage of labor. • Rapidly crosses the placenta, which can lead to fetal central nervous system depression. • Can cause constriction of the uterine artery, with resultant decrease in blood flow to the placenta. • Is not used frequently because of the association with fetal bradycardia.
Epidural analgesia/ anesthesia	• Hypotension, which often requires administration of medication to raise the blood pressure • Maternal fever • Shivering • Itching (if opioids are used) • Inadvertent injection of anesthetic into the bloodstream • Accidental intrathecal block with possible spinal headache • Inadequate pain relief or failed block • Fetal distress	• Relieves pain better than do opioids. • Often completely eliminates pain sensation. • Anesthesia can be continued indefinitely • If the woman needs a cesarean section, the epidural can be used to provide anesthesia, which saves time in an emergency situation. • Serious side effects are rare.	• Often impairs motor function, which decreases the ability to walk during labor. • Women frequently require urinary catheterization. • Increases the need for labor augmentation with oxytocin, particularly when administered before 5 cm of dilation. • Increases the duration of the second stage of labor. • Vacuum assistance and forceps are more frequently required.

TABLE 9.3 (continued)	Comparison of Selected Pharmacologic Interventions for Relief of Labor Pain		
Medication Class	**Associated Side Effects**	**Advantages**	**Disadvantages**
			• Increases the likelihood of maternal fever, which increases neonatal sepsis evaluation and antibiotic treatment (Leeman et al., 2003b). • Must be administered by an anesthetist or anesthesiologist. • Requires complex nursing care.
Intrathecal anesthesia (spinal block)	• Hypotension • Shivering • Spinal headache	• Rapid onset of analgesia. • Provides excellent pain relief. • It's the anesthetic method of choice for planned cesarean birth.	• A complete block results in the woman's lower extremities being temporarily paralyzed. • Used alone for labor, the dose might wear off before labor is completed. • Must be administered by an anesthetist or anesthesiologist. • Requires complex nursing care.
General anesthesia	• Hypertension during intubation • Hypotension during maintenance • Difficult or failed intubation • Aspiration of stomach acid/contents • Malignant ~~hypothermia~~ *Malig hyperthermia* • Uterine atony	• Especially useful in emergency situations because total anesthesia can be accomplished rapidly. • Provides total pain relief.	• Requires intubation, which is more challenging during pregnancy. • All agents used to induce and maintain general anesthesia cross the placenta and can cause severe neonatal depression.

contractions and may induce relaxation and sleep between contractions. Opioids are most frequently given by the intravenous (IV) route because this route provides fast onset and more consistent drug levels than do the subcutaneous or intramuscular routes.

Timing of analgesia administration is important to the safety of the woman and her fetus. If analgesia is given too early in the labor process, the contractions may decrease in frequency and intensity, which can actually prolong labor. If opioids are given too close to delivery, the fetus may be born with respiratory depression, which can interfere with the vital first breaths. Given at the appropriate time, opioids can promote relaxation and cause labor to progress more quickly.

Test Yourself

- What is the difference between analgesia and anesthesia?

- What is another name for opioids?

- What side effect is likely to occur when opioids are given too close to delivery?

Anesthesia

There are three basic types of anesthesia: local, regional, and general. Local anesthesia is used to numb the perineum just before birth to allow for episiotomy and repair.

Keep this tidbit in mind. In general, neonatal respiratory depression is more likely to occur if opioids are administered between 1 and 3 hours before birth occurs. Respiratory depression occurs infrequently when analgesia is timed within 1 hour of birth or at least 4 hours before delivery (Poole, 2003). However, it is not always possible to time medications this precisely. Therefore, be prepared to administer naloxone (Narcan) to the newborn whenever maternal analgesia has been given during labor.

induce regional anesthesia/analgesia. The types of regional anesthetics that may be used during labor are pudendal block, paracervical block, epidural anesthesia, combined epidural/spinal anesthesia, and spinal block.

Anytime an anesthetic is administered using any of the techniques described, there is a chance that the local anesthetic agent will inadvertently enter the bloodstream and cause a toxic reaction in the woman. Fortunately, this situation rarely occurs; however, the nurse must be prepared to assist with a full resuscitation, if one is needed. Every facility in which regional anesthetics are administered must have emergency equipment available, including oxygen, oral airway, equipment for emergency intubation and cardiac monitoring, and emergency medications.

It is the nurse's role to assist the anesthesia provider and to closely monitor the woman and her fetus during and after administration of anesthesia. Most of these techniques require IV access. Vital signs must be closely monitored during the procedure and afterward until the vital signs are stable and the effects of the anesthetic have abated.

Pudendal Block. A pudendal block is given just before the baby is born to provide pain relief for the birth. Two injections are given bilaterally into the vaginal wall to block pain sensations to the pudendal nerve. A pudendal block can be helpful when vacuum extraction or forceps are needed to assist the delivery. This method is most effective when administered by an experienced practitioner. If an incomplete block occurs, the practitioner may have to inject additional local anesthesia for episiotomy repair.

Paracervical Block. A paracervical block involves the injection of a local anesthetic in the area close to the cervix. This method provides significant pain relief during the first stage of labor. It cannot be used once

Several types of regional anesthesia are discussed here. In general, regional anesthesia, rather than general anesthesia, is preferred for cesarean births.

Regional Anesthesia. Regional anesthesia involves blocking a group of sensory nerves that supply a particular organ or area of the body. Local anesthetics and opioids are given to

complete dilation is attained. The procedure must be repeated frequently because the duration of action is short. One advantage of the technique is that it does not block sensation and movement in the lower extremities, as does epidural anesthesia. Many practitioners do not perform paracervical blocks because of the risk of fetal bradycardia.

Test Yourself

- List three types of regional anesthesia.
- Why is it critical for all facilities in which regional anesthesia is provided to have emergency equipment available?
- Describe a pudendal block.

Epidural Anesthesia. Epidural anesthesia for the management of labor pain has become increasingly popular in the United States. This method usually provides excellent pain relief, often completely blocking pain sensation. The anesthesiologist or nurse anesthetist places a small catheter into the epidural space and then injects the catheter with local anesthetics or opioids to provide pain relief. Sometimes a one-time dose of medication is placed into the spinal fluid (in the subarachnoid space), which is called an **intrathecal** injection, in conjunction with epidural anesthesia. The advantage of the combined epidural/intrathecal technique is that the intrathecal dose is effective almost immediately. It provides pain relief until the epidural begins to work.

Although its use is popular, epidural anesthesia is not without risk. There is significant risk of maternal hypotension that often must be treated with vasopressors (medication to raise the blood pressure). Before a woman receives epidural anesthesia, an IV line must be in place. She must receive 500 to 2,000 mL of IV fluid bolus before medications are administered to reduce the risk of hypotension. Because it is an invasive procedure, informed consent is required.

The anesthetist must evaluate the woman before placing an epidural. The anesthetist reviews the medical history and laboratory results and interviews the woman. The procedure is explained, questions answered, and informed consent obtained. The nurse gives the IV fluid bolus and positions the woman for epidural placement. The woman can be sitting up on the edge of the bed with her feet dangling, or she may be side lying. In either case, it is important for her spine to be arched because this position opens up the spaces between the vertebrae and allows for easier insertion of the catheter. The nurse holds the woman in position or assists the support person to do so (Fig. 9-6). The pulse and oxygen saturation are monitored continuously during the procedure using pulse oximetry. The blood pressure is monitored frequently (sometimes every 3 to 5 minutes) during the procedure.

When the woman is positioned properly, the anesthetist prepares a sterile field with the supplies and medications that will be needed. The woman's back is prepared with alcohol and Betadine. A local anesthetic is used to numb the planned insertion area. A needle is used to enter the epidural space (just outside the dura mater) and a test dose is administered (see Figure 9-6). The anesthetist questions the woman regarding how she feels and what she is experiencing to detect any adverse reaction. If there is none, the anesthetist proceeds to place the epidural catheter, remove the needle, and tape the catheter securely to the woman's back. At this point the nurse assists the woman to a position of comfort. The supine position is avoided, or a wedge is placed under the right hip.

Once the epidural catheter is in place, the anesthetist may intermittently bolus the catheter when the woman begins to feel pain, or a continuous infusion can be set up and connected to the catheter. In either case, it is critical that the epidural catheter be clearly marked so that medications are given by the right route. Management of the epidural is the role of the anesthetist. The nurse monitors for, reports, and treats any untoward effects.

After delivery, the RN stops the continuous infusion and removes the epidural catheter. A sterile pressure dressing is applied to the site. Nursing care during recovery from epidural anesthesia includes assessment of return of sensory and motor function to the lower extremities, and monitoring for urinary retention. The nurse should instruct the woman not to ambulate without assistance. It is a good idea to allow the woman to dangle her legs for a while before she attempts to ambulate. The nurse should be available to provide immediate assistance, if needed, during initial ambulation attempts.

Intrathecal Anesthesia. Intrathecal anesthesia, also known as a spinal block, is similar to epidural anesthesia. The main difference is the location of the anesthetic. Instead of injecting local anesthesia and/or opioids into the epidural space, these medications are placed in the subarachnoid space into the spinal fluid (see Figure 9-6). This type of anesthesia is most frequently used for planned cesarean deliveries. The disadvantage to using

A

● *Figure 9.6* Epidural or intrathecal anesthesia. **(A)** The woman is correctly positioned for epidural anesthesia. **(B)** Location of epidural catheter. Note that the epidural space is located just outside the dura mater. No spinal fluid is present in the epidural space. The epidural catheter is left in place to allow for intermittent or continuous infusion of medications to relieve the pain of labor and birth. **(C)** Location of intrathecal injection. Notice that the needle has a drop of spinal fluid at the hub to indicate the subarachnoid space has been entered. The local anesthetic or narcotic is then injected into this space.

A PERSONAL GLIMPSE

I was 37 weeks' pregnant with my first baby. I started to have some contractions while I was at work. Nothing big; I wasn't even sure they were contractions because they didn't hurt, but I was able to time them at 10 to 15 minutes apart. I went home at lunchtime and called my husband to tell him that I thought I was in labor. He hurried home to be with me. I stayed home the rest of the day and did some light housework. Around 6 p.m. the contractions started to get more intense. I ran some warm water and soaked in the tub. It made me feel better for a while. My husband kept timing the contractions until they were 5 minutes apart. Then I called the hospital, and the nurse told me to come on in. We arrived at the hospital at about 8 p.m. The nurse checked me and said I was at 4 cm and 95% effaced. The nurse suggested that we walk the hallways to speed things along. Sure enough, 45 minutes later, I was a good 5 cm. She asked me if I wanted anything for the pain, and I said no. I was hanging in there just fine. The pain wasn't as bad as I thought it would be. After approximately 45 minutes, the contractions became more intense, and I begged my husband to call the nurse. The nurse checked me and I was 7 cm. By now I was begging for an epidural. The anesthesiologist came in and asked me some questions and told me about some risks. I didn't care. I just wanted the epidural. I had to sit very still through several contractions while the doctor put in the epidural, but it was worth it because the pain went away right away. An hour after the epidural was inserted I was dilated to 8 cm. I was very excited, but then I got stuck at 8 cm for several hours. The doctor thought that the epidural must have slowed down my labor. They were having a hard time monitoring my baby with the external device so they had to insert an internal monitor. Then the nurse started me on Pitocin to help me progress. Sure enough, after an hour of Pitocin I was completely dilated and ready to push. For me, pushing was the hardest part. I still felt no pain because of my epidural, so the nurse had to tell me when I was having a contraction so that I could start pushing. I threw up several times from pushing so hard. However, the baby just didn't come down. After 2 hours, I was totally exhausted. The nurse asked if I wanted her to call the doctor and have her come and use the vacuum to help get the baby out. I was just so tired that I said yes. Elizabeth Michelle was born after just two pushes with the vacuum. She didn't cry at first, so the nurse rushed her to the warming table and gave her some oxygen. Then I heard the most beautiful sound in the world, a cry. My husband and I were thrilled. After the nurse dried the baby, I got to hold her for a while before they took her to the nursery. The baby weighed 7 pounds even, and was 19 1/2 inches long. She was worth everything I went through to have her.

Laura

LEARNING OPPORTUNITY: What questions should the nurse ask the woman about pain relief during labor? What should the nurse tell the woman about pain management options when she presents to the birthing facility in labor?

---

a spinal block during labor is that the anesthetic might wear off while the woman is still in labor. Nursing care is similar to that provided for epidural anesthesia.

Complications Associated With Epidural and Intrathecal Anesthesia. Hypotension is the most frequent side effect seen with epidurals or intrathecal anesthesia. Low blood pressure occurs in approximately one-third of women who receive epidural or spinal anesthesia. As noted, prehydration with IV fluids helps to prevent or decrease the severity of this side effect. If the blood pressure falls dramatically, ephedrine may be given intravenously to raise the blood pressure.

Spinal headaches occur rarely because of advanced techniques and smaller needle sizes than those used in the past. A spinal headache is suspected when the woman has an intense headache in the upright position that is relieved when she lies still. Treatment involves hydration and having the woman lie flat. Sometimes caffeine is prescribed. Usually the headache will resolve spontaneously in several days. If it does not resolve, an epidural blood patch may be done. In a procedure similar to that used to provide epidural anesthesia, the anesthesia provider injects 20 mL of the woman's blood into the epidural space. The headache is relieved in 95% of women who have the patch.

When narcotics are used in addition to anesthetics, pruritus is a common side effect. Most women tolerate the itching, particularly because the pain relief is generally excellent for the first 24 hours after surgery. Nalbuphine (Nubain), a narcotic agonist-antagonist, and diphenhydramine (Benadryl), an antihistamine, are two medications that may be ordered to treat severe pruritus.

Respiratory depression is another possible side effect when narcotics are used for spinal and/or epidural anesthesia. For this reason, it is recommended that naloxone (Narcan) be readily available to be given intravenously if respiratory depression occurs. Sometimes the anesthesiologist may order continuous pulse oximetry for the first 24 hours. In all cases it is prudent to take vital signs at least every 2 hours and to check on the woman frequently during the first 24 hours after spinal or epidural narcotics have been administered. Nursing Care Plan 9-1: The Woman With Labor Pain describes pain management for a woman in labor.

General Anesthesia. General anesthesia is not used frequently in obstetrics because of the risks involved. The pregnant woman is at higher risk for aspiration. It requires more skill to intubate a pregnant woman because of physiologic changes in the trachea and thorax. In fact, failed intubation is the leading cause of anesthesia-related maternal mortality (Poole, 2003). In addition, general anesthetic agents cross the placenta and can result in the birth of a severely depressed neonate who requires full resuscitation.

When general anesthesia is to be used, the anesthetist usually orders preoperative medications to reduce the risk of aspiration. Bicitra 30 mL may be given orally. Antacids often are ordered to be given intravenously before surgery.

The anesthetist may use an inhalation agent, an IV agent, or more commonly both to induce anesthesia. The woman is preoxygenated with 100% oxygen and then rapidly put to sleep. The RN gives cricoid pressure (pressure with the thumb and forefinger over the cricoid cartilage in the trachea), which closes off the esophagus and decreases the risk of aspiration. Cricoid pressure is maintained until the woman is intubated and the cuff inflated. The anesthetist then manages the airway and continues to administer anesthetic agents and muscle relaxants as needed throughout surgery. Every attempt is made to deliver the baby as quickly as possible after the woman is anesthetized to avoid neonatal depression. The nurse is prepared to resuscitate the newborn, if necessary.

When the surgery is completed, the anesthetist removes the endotracheal tube when the woman is awake and has regained her protective reflexes (swallowing and gagging). The woman is then taken to the postanesthesia care unit (PACU). The RN completes a full assessment; administers oxygen; and monitors oxygen saturation, vital signs, and the continuous electrocardiogram. The RN must be especially vigilant to monitor for hypoventilation after general anesthesia.

Life-threatening complications can occur with general anesthesia. These include failed intubation, aspiration, and malignant hyperthermia. The nurse must be prepared to act quickly in any of these situations.

Because failed intubation is the leading cause of anesthesia-related maternal deaths, the anesthetist must have a variety of tools readily available to use in the event that the woman cannot be intubated quickly. The woman is preoxygenated before every intubation attempt to give the anesthetist time to perform the procedure. If attempts to intubate are unsuccessful, the anesthetist may try to ventilate without intubating the woman. Other options include reversing the anesthesia (i.e., waking the woman) and performing an emergency tracheostomy.

Aspiration is a real threat for the pregnant woman undergoing general anesthesia. Upward pressure of the pregnant uterus on the stomach increases the risk for reflux of stomach contents with subsequent aspiration. Often preoperative medications are ordered to reduce the risk of aspiration. In addition, cricoid pressure by the trained RN during intubation attempts can help prevent this life-threatening complication.

Malignant hyperthermia is a rare, but potentially life-threatening, complication of general anesthesia. It is an inherited condition in which sustained muscle contractions occur when specific anesthetic agents are administered. For this reason, a thorough history is important before general anesthesia is given. Ideally, a pregnant woman with a family history of malignant hyperthermia will be identified in the prenatal period so the health care team can be prepared to care for the woman if general anesthesia becomes necessary. In these cases, it is best for the woman to receive epidural anesthesia during labor. This practice allows for safe anesthesia if a cesarean delivery is performed. If cesarean delivery is planned, the woman usually receives spinal anesthesia.

The nurse must be alert to the development of signs and symptoms of the disorder. Early signs include severe muscle rigidity, tachycardia, irregular heart rhythm, decreased oxygen saturation, and cyanosis. Body temperature can rapidly increase to lethal levels; however, this may be a late sign. Dantrolene sodium is given intravenously to treat malignant hyperthermia. This medication must be readily available in any area in which general anesthesia is administered.

Postoperative nursing care of the woman who receives general anesthesia is similar to that of the woman who receives regional anesthesia. However, careful assessment for hypoventilation and uterine atony are indicated.

Test Yourself

- Describe the procedure for epidural placement.

- List four complications associated with epidural or spinal anesthesia.

- Name two ways to reduce the threat of maternal aspiration when general anesthesia is used.

NURSING CARE PLAN 9.1

The Woman With Labor Pain

CASE SCENARIO:
Patricia (Pattie) Smith is a 29-year-old gravida 1, para 0 at term. She attended childbirth preparation classes with her husband, Ed. Pattie says that she wants to try natural childbirth, but that she might change her mind and request an epidural if the pain becomes unbearable. She is admitted to the hospital in active labor at 4 centimeters dilation. Admitting vital signs are BP 120/76 mm Hg, T 98.7°F, P 70 bpm, R 20 per minute. She describes her pain as starting in the small of her back and then radiating to her lower abdomen with each contraction. She says that the intensity is strong, particularly at the peak of the contraction. Her contractions are occurring every 5 minutes, last 50 to 60 seconds, and palpate moderate intensity. The fetal heart rate is in the 140s to 150s and is reactive.

NURSING DIAGNOSIS
Acute Pain related to uterine contractions.

GOAL: Reports ability to tolerate the pain of labor.

EXPECTED OUTCOMES:
• Uses nonpharmacologic interventions.
• Uses pharmacologic interventions, if desired.
• Expresses satisfaction with pain control.

NURSING INTERVENTIONS	*RATIONALE*
Perform a pain assessment at least every hour during labor to include pain description, location, duration, and intensity (measured by a pain scale).	A thorough pain assessment will reveal the need for more intensive interventions to control the pain of labor.
Note reports of continuous, severe pain. If this occurs, report it to the RN in charge immediately.	Severe, unrelenting pain may be associated with a complication of labor.
Assess general comfort at least every hour. Note the condition of the lips and offer lip balm PRN. Offer ice chips and lollipops to relieve complaints of dry mouth. Give perineal care as indicated, and change the under-buttock pad frequently. Change the linen when it becomes moist with perspiration or other body fluids.	Comfort measures increase the ability of the woman to cope with labor. It is more difficult to cope if the woman has dry, cracked lips, a dry mouth, moist linens, and is in need of perineal care.
Encourage the use of relaxation techniques that are helpful for Pattie.	The more relaxed the woman can remain during labor, the better she will be able to cope with the pain of labor.
Reinforce the use of patterned breathing. Encourage her to switch to a more complex pattern of breathing when simpler patterns are no longer helpful.	Patterned breathing techniques are learned during childbirth classes. Use of these techniques can facilitate relaxation and increase the woman's ability to cope.
Assist Pattie to change positions frequently.	Position changes can help the woman to better cope. If she remains "frozen" in one position, she is more likely to become tense, which increases the perception of pain.
Encourage the use of effleurage, for as long as it is helpful. Encourage the use of pressure when effleurage is no longer helpful.	The use of touch, such as effleurage and pressure, can interrupt the sensation of pain.

Pattie progresses to 8 centimeters dilation. At this point she is having difficulty maintaining control. She thrashes about at the peak of contractions and says that nothing is helping the pain. She begs for an epidural. The obstetrician agrees, and the anesthesiologist is called.

NURSING DIAGNOSIS
Acute Pain related to advanced progress of labor.

GOAL: Ability to cope with labor.

NURSING CARE PLAN 9.1 continued

The Woman With Labor Pain

EXPECTED OUTCOMES:
- Uses nonpharmacologic and pharmacologic interventions.
- Expresses satisfaction with pain control.

NURSING INTERVENTIONS	RATIONALE
Remain supportive of Pattie's decision to use an epidural for pain relief.	The woman has the right to change her mind about pain relief interventions and to choose interventions that will best help her to cope.
Reassure Ed that this is a normal response to this phase of the labor process, and that Pattie's request does not represent a failure on his part as her coach.	There is a danger that the coach may feel that he has somehow "failed" when pharmacologic interventions are requested.
Continue to perform a pain assessment every 30 minutes after the epidural is placed.	Frequent assessment of pain will allow for rapid detection of the onset of pain.
Report new complaints of pain to the anesthesiologist.	New reports of pain may signal the need for a bolus of medication through the epidural catheter.

NURSING DIAGNOSIS
Risk for Injury related to possibility of hypotension associated with epidural anesthesia.

GOAL: Maintenance of adequate blood pressure to support perfusion to vital organs, including the placenta.

EXPECTED OUTCOMES:
- Blood pressure will not drop below 90/60 mm Hg.
- Oxygen saturation will remain above 96%.
- Fetal monitor strip baseline will remain above 120 with reactive patterns noted.

NURSING INTERVENTIONS	RATIONALE
Prehydrate Pattie with 1,000 cc of lactated Ringer's solution, as ordered.	Prehydration with IV fluid will decrease the risk of hypotension.
Monitor oxygen saturation with pulse oximetry.	A decrease in oxygen saturation can be quickly detected and treated, which will help prevent adverse fetal affects.
Monitor fetal heart tones and reactivity.	Monitoring is done to detect decreases in the fetal heart rate, which may indicate inadequate placental perfusion.
Assist Pattie to a sitting position with her feet dangling over the side of the bed. Demonstrate to Ed how to hold Pattie in the proper position for catheter insertion.	When the woman is in the proper position, the epidural is placed more easily.
Monitor the blood pressure, pulse, and oxygen saturation every 3 to 5 minutes during the procedure.	Frequent monitoring allows for early detection of changes that may indicate the development of a complication.
Once the epidural catheter is taped in place, assist Pattie to a side-lying position.	The side-lying position enhances blood pressure and placental perfusion.
Monitor for signs of urinary retention and insert a Foley catheter, as ordered, if needed.	Epidural anesthesia frequently causes urinary retention, which may interfere with the progress of labor.
Check for progress of labor shortly after the epidural takes effect.	Rapid progress of labor sometimes occurs because the woman relaxes after the pain is relieved.
Monitor for ability to push effectively in the second stage of labor. Report this finding to the anesthesiologist.	Sometimes, epidural anesthesia can interfere with the ability to push effectively. The anesthesiologist may decrease the amount of medication given to allow for partial return of sensation with an increased ability to push.

EVALUATION:
Pattie pushes well and delivers a healthy baby boy 3 hours after she receives her epidural. Her blood pressure remains above 90/60 mm Hg. She reports that she is very satisfied with her labor experience and does not regret getting the epidural.

KEY POINTS

- Sources of pain during the first stage of labor are the thinning and stretching of the cervix in response to uterine contractions. Sources of pain during the second stage of labor are the stretching of tissues in the perineum as the fetus descends.

- Major principles of labor pain management include that women are more satisfied when they have control over the pain experience; caregivers commonly underrate the severity of pain; and women who are prepared for labor usually report a more satisfying experience than do women who are not prepared.

- Nonpharmacologic interventions to relieve labor pain include continuous labor support, comfort measures, various relaxation techniques, intradermal water injections, and acupressure and acupuncture.

- Relaxation techniques that help a woman cope with labor include patterned breathing, attention focusing, movement and positioning, touch and massage, water therapy, and hypnosis.

- Most nonpharmacologic interventions are noninvasive, address emotional and spiritual aspects of birth, and promote the woman's sense of control over her pain. Disadvantages include that many of the interventions require special training and/or practice before birth, and these methods are not effective for every woman.

- Analgesia reduces the sensation of pain. Anesthesia partially or totally blocks all sensation to an area of the body.

- Advantages of opioid administration during labor include an increased ability for the woman to cope with labor, and the medications may be nurse administered. Disadvantages include frequent occurrence of uncomfortable side effects, such as nausea and vomiting, pruritus, drowsiness, and neonatal depression; and pain is not eliminated completely.

- Types of regional anesthesia include pudendal block, paracervical block, epidural anesthesia, combined epidural/spinal anesthesia, and spinal block. A pudendal block provides pain relief for the birth. Paracervical blocks and epidurals provide pain relief during labor.

- Complications associated with epidural and spinal anesthesia include hypotension, maternal fever, shivering, pruritus, inadvertent injection into the bloodstream, spinal headache, and fetal distress.

- General anesthesia is risky for the pregnant woman because of the increased risk for aspiration. It is risky for the fetus because the medications cross the placenta and may result in severe neonatal depression that requires intensive resuscitation.

- Life-threatening complications associated with general anesthesia include failed intubation, aspiration, and malignant hyperthermia. Preoperative antacids and cricoid pressure reduce the incidence of aspiration. Dantrolene sodium is used to treat malignant hyperthermia.

REFERENCES AND SELECTED READINGS

Books and Journals

Cunningham, F. G., Gant, N. F., Leveno, K. J., Gilstrap, L. C. III, Hauth, J. C., & Wenstrom, K. D. (2001). *Williams obstetrics* (21st ed.). New York: McGraw-Hill Medical Publishing Division.

Hawkins, R. M. F. (2001). A systematic meta-review of hypnosis as an empirically supported treatment for pain. *Pain Reviews, 8*, 47–73.

Koehn, M. L. (2000). Alternative and complementary therapies for labor and birth: An application of Kolcaba's theory of holistic comfort. *Holistic Nursing Practice, 15*(1), 66–77.

Leeman, L., Fontaine, P., King, V., Klein, M. C., & Ratcliffe, S. (2003a). The nature and management of labor pain: Part I. Nonpharmacologic pain relief. *American Family Physician, 68*(6), 1109–1112.

Leeman, L., Fontaine, P., King, V., Klein, M. C., & Ratcliffe, S. (2003b). The nature and management of labor pain: Part II. Pharmacologic pain relief. *American Family Physician, 68*(6), 1115–1120.

Mattson, S., & Smith, J. E. (Eds.). (2000). *Core curriculum for maternal–newborn nursing.* AWHONN publication (2nd ed.). Philadelphia: WB Saunders.

McCrea, B. H., & Wright, M. E. (1999). Satisfaction in childbirth and perceptions of personal control in pain relief during labour. *Journal of Advanced Nursing, 29*(4), 877–884.

Poole, J. (2003). Analgesia and anesthesia during labor and birth: Implications for mother and fetus. *JOGNN, 32*(6), 780–793.

Vincent, R. D., & Chestnut, D. H. (1998). Epidural analgesia during labor. *American Family Physician, 58*(8), 1785–1792.

Waterbirth International. (Undated). FAQs: All about Waterbirth. Retrieved March 6, 2004, from http://www.waterbirth.org/spa/content/category/5/65/40/

Websites
http://www.childbirth.org/articles/labor/painrelief.html
http://www.reddinganesthesia.com/labor.htm
http://www.painfreebirthing.com/anatomy.htm

WORKBOOK

NCLEX-STYLE REVIEW QUESTIONS

1. A 22-year-old gravida 2 para 0 is in the doctor's office for a checkup at 36 weeks' gestation. Which comment by the woman indicates that she needs additional information about pain relief during labor?

   a. "I have discussed pain relief options with the doctor and my childbirth educator."

   b. "I'm so glad that I won't have any pain because I'm going to have an epidural."

   c. "I've been practicing the relaxation exercises I learned in my childbirth class."

   d. "I want to have medications through the IV if the pain gets so bad that I can't handle it."

2. The labor nurse reports to the nurse on the on-coming shift, "The woman in labor room 2 is handling her pain very well. She smiles whenever I go in to talk to her, and she doesn't complain at all!" What assessments by the on-coming labor nurse would best reveal if the off-going labor nurse's observations were correct?

   a. Asking the woman to describe her pain and rate it on a scale of 0 to 10.

   b. Observing for grimacing, moaning, and other nonverbal indicators of pain.

   c. Taking the woman's vital signs and observing her interactions with visitors.

   d. No additional assessments are indicated until the woman begins to report pain.

3. A woman asks the nurse during a doctor's visit, "What pain relief method is best?" What answer by the nurse best answers the question?

   a. "Epidurals are best because they provide complete pain relief."

   b. "Most women need IV pain medications at some point during labor."

   c. "It is best to learn and use several methods of pain relief to find the one that works best for you."

   d. "There is no one best way. However, natural childbirth is best for the baby."

4. A 34-year-old gravida 3 para 2 is experiencing severe back pain with each contraction. She is extremely uncomfortable and upset because she never had this type of pain with her other labors. What interventions are most likely to help in this situation?

   a. Comfort measures, intermittent labor support by the nurse, and reassurance that the pain is temporary

   b. Counter-pressure with a fist or tennis ball to the lower back and intradermal water injections

   c. Effleurage, ambulation, and frequent position changes

   d. Hypnosis, imagery, and slow chest breathing

5. The nurse is preparing a woman for epidural anesthesia. The woman asks, "Why is my IV running so fast? It feels cold!" What reply by the nurse is best?

   a. "Don't worry. This is a routine procedure in preparation for an epidural."

   b. "I'll slow the IV down so you won't feel so cold."

   c. "IV fluids help prevent spinal headaches."

   d. "IV hydration helps prevent the blood pressure from dropping too low."

STUDY ACTIVITIES

1. Use the following table to compare advantages and disadvantages of pain relief methods for labor.

Method	Advantages	Disadvantages
Natural childbirth		
IV analgesia		
Epidural anesthesia		
General anesthesia		

2. Develop a teaching plan on the advantages and disadvantages of epidural anesthesia to present to a childbirth education class.

3. Interview the following caregivers in the community regarding their recommendations for pain relief during labor: a doula, a nurse-midwife, a family practice physician, and an

obstetrician. What similarities did you find in their answers? In what ways did they disagree? Which argument did you find most convincing? Share your findings with your clinical group.

CRITICAL THINKING: What Would You Do?

Apply your knowledge of pain management during labor to the following situation.

1. Betty, a 30-year-old gravida 1, reports that she wants to try natural childbirth.

   a. What recommendations will you make to increase the chances that she will be able to experience natural childbirth?

   b. About what will you caution her to decrease the likelihood that she will have unrealistic expectations about pain relief during labor?

2. Betty presents to the labor suite in labor. She is 3 cm dilated, 90% effaced, and at a -1 station. Her contractions are every 3 to 5 minutes apart and of moderate intensity.

   a. What nonpharmacologic pain interventions are most helpful at this point in Betty's labor?

   b. Several hours later, Betty is 5 cm dilated, 100% effaced, at a 0 station. She is requesting IV analgesia. How will you reply?

   c. When Betty reaches 8 cm, she is screaming at the peak of contractions. She says, "I can't stand the pain anymore. I want an epidural." How will you reply?

Nursing Care During Labor and Birth

STUDENT OBJECTIVES

On completion of this chapter, the student should be able to

1. Discuss the assessments and procedures the nurse performs during the woman's admission to the hospital.
2. Illustrate how to apply the external fetal monitor.
3. Compare and contrast advantages and disadvantages of external fetal monitoring with that of internal fetal monitoring.
4. Identify the role of the practical (vocational) nurse in the interpretation of fetal heart rate patterns.
5. Define three major deviations from the normal fetal heart rate baseline.
6. Differentiate between early, variable, and late decelerations with regard to appearance, occurrence in relation to uterine

KEY TERMS

acceleration
amnioinfusion
early deceleration
late deceleration
lochia
long-term variability
nadir
open-glottis pushing

contractions, causes, and whether or not the pattern is reassuring or nonreassuring.
7. Outline appropriate nursing interventions for each major periodic change: early, variable, and late deceleration patterns.
8. Discuss advantages and disadvantages of intermittent auscultation, fetal stimulation, fetal scalp sampling, fetal pulse oximetry, and continuous electronic fetal monitoring for monitoring fetal status.
9. Assess a laboring woman for progress of labor and birth throughout each stage and phase of labor.
10. Identify common nursing diagnoses associated with each stage of labor and birth.
11. Choose appropriate nursing interventions for each stage of labor and birth to facilitate safe passage of the mother and fetus.
12. Evaluate the effectiveness of care given during labor and birth.

periodic changes
ritual
short-term variability
urge-to-push method
uteroplacental insufficiency
variability
variable deceleration
vigorous pushing

The onset of labor heralds the transition from pregnancy to motherhood, and the transformation of the fetus to a newborn. The process is experienced on many dimensions, including physiologic, psychological, social, and spiritual. When the powers, passageway, passenger, and psyche work together harmoniously, the miracle of birth progresses in an orderly and predictable sequence.

The practical nurse's role in labor and delivery is to provide care to the laboring woman under the supervision of a registered nurse (RN). The licensed practical nurse (LPN) must have a basic understanding of the processes of labor and birth to provide care to the woman and her family. It is important for the LPN to be able to recognize deviations from the "normal" or expected sequence of labor and birth and to report deviations immediately. The LPN is expected to answer the woman's and her support person's questions regarding labor and birth. Although the LPN does not independently perform many of the procedures and assessments described in this chapter, a basic understanding of these procedures and assessments is necessary for the LPN to effectively assist the RN or physician.

The role of the obstetric nurse is central to the care of the laboring woman and her family. The nurse facilitates the labor process and ensures safe passage of the laboring woman and fetus through this critical life event. The effective obstetric nurse has an attitude of acceptance of the mother's preferences during labor and birth, utilizes supportive actions, and develops keen assessment skills to detect subtle changes in maternal or fetal status.

Although labor and birth are normal physiologic events, the nurse must be prepared to recognize and manage complications that may arise during the process. It also is critical that the nurse be prepared to give intensive support to the laboring woman and her partner or coach. Assisting the family during the miracle of labor and birth is a challenging but ultimately satisfying and rewarding experience.

Every woman's labor is unique, and if a woman bears more than one child, each birth is experienced differently. This chapter focuses on the nursing care of a first-time mother undergoing normal progression of labor and birth who does not experience complications. Common deviations associated with the nursing care of the multiparous woman are noted. For purposes of this chapter, it is assumed that the delivery environment is a labor, delivery, and recovery room (LDR) in a hospital setting. Similar nursing interventions apply to other settings, and the labor process is the same regardless of the environment in which birth occurs.

THE NURSE'S ROLE DURING ADMISSION

The woman may present to the birthing suite at any phase of the first stage of labor. Therefore, it is important for the nurse to immediately assess birth imminence, fetal status, risk factors, and maternal status. If birth is not imminent and the fetal and maternal conditions are stable, the nurse performs additional admission assessments, including the status of labor, the full admission health history, and a complete maternal physical assessment.

IMMEDIATE ASSESSMENTS

Birth Imminence

Nursing assessment for signs that birth is imminent begins from the moment the woman arrives in the labor and delivery unit. If the woman is introverted and stops to breathe or pant with each contraction, the nurse infers that she is in an advanced stage of labor. In addition, if the woman makes statements such as, "I feel a lot of pressure," or "The baby is coming," or "I want to have a bowel movement," it is likely the woman is in the second stage of labor, and the baby will be born directly. Other signs that birth is imminent include sitting on one buttock (if the woman is brought to the unit in a wheelchair) and bearing down or grunting with contractions. When any of these signs is present, it is prudent to quickly move the woman to a labor bed, perform a vaginal examination if the presenting part is not yet visible, and be prepared to assist with the birth.

Nursing judgment is in order. If the woman presents to the hospital in an advanced stage of labor, and it appears that delivery is imminent, the admission history and physical is abbreviated to focus on current status. The history can be completed later, even after delivery, if necessary.

Occasionally the nurse is the only person available to deliver the baby. Figure 10-1 illustrates the steps to follow for an emergency birth. You may not have time to perform all the steps listed. Do the best you can with the time and equipment there is available to you. It is helpful to instruct the woman to remain calm and reassure her that you know what to do to assist with the delivery. Instruct her to blow out through her lips in little puffs (as if she were blowing out candles) so that she won't forcefully expel the baby in an uncontrolled manner. Then follow the steps in Figure 10-1 to assist with the birth.

Once the baby is delivered it is not necessary to cut the cord immediately. However, in most facilities the protocol is to double clamp the cord and cut between the clamps. Dry the infant thoroughly to prevent heat loss and place him under a radiant warmer for resuscitation, or place the newborn in skin-to-skin contact with his mother and cover them both with a blanket.

The birth attendant usually arrives before delivery of the placenta. However, if signs of placental separation occur (a gush of blood, lengthening of the cord at the introitus), allow the placenta to deliver, and then massage the uterus to help it contract. Another way to prevent excessive blood loss immediately after delivery of the placenta is to place the infant to the woman's breast. The suckling action of the newborn will stimulate the woman's body to release oxytocin, which helps her uterus to contract and control bleeding.

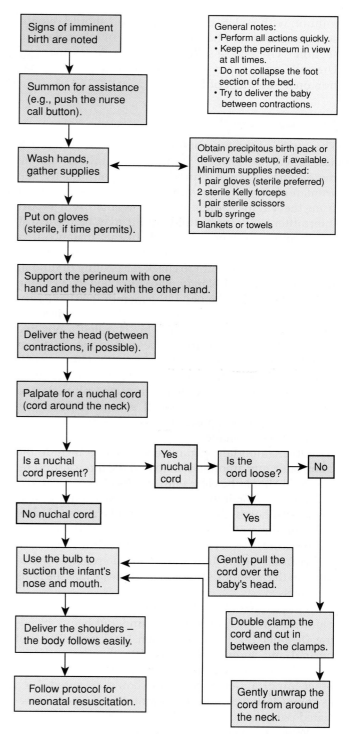

● **Figure 10.1** Emergency delivery by the nurse.

Fetal Status

When the woman arrives at the hospital, perform an immediate assessment of fetal status. In most delivery suites the woman is placed on the fetal monitor for continuous monitoring, but it is within accepted standards of care to check the fetal heart rate (FHR) by fetoscope or by Doppler ultrasonography for the low-risk woman. The FHR should be strong and regular, with a baseline between 110 and 160 beats per minute[1] with no late decelerations and should remain so throughout all phases and stages of labor. See the section "The Nurse's Role: Ongoing Assessment of Uterine Contractions and FHR" for in-depth information on assessment of FHR.

Risk Assessment

The status of the membranes is one of the initial risk assessments performed. Symptoms indicating that the membranes have ruptured include reports by the woman of a gush or continual leaking of warm fluid from the vagina. Sometimes the woman will report intermittent leaking of fluid, and it may be unclear if the membranes have ruptured. In this instance it is important to look for objective signs of rupture. The RN may use a speculum to check for pooling of fluid in the vagina. Or the RN may place nitrazine paper in the fluid to determine the pH. If the membranes have ruptured, the nitrazine paper will turn dark blue, indicating that the fluid is alkaline. This is called a positive nitrazine test. If the status of the membranes is still in doubt, a fern test may be done. The RN will collect a fluid sample and smear it on a slide. The slide is then taken to the laboratory or given to the physician to observe under a microscope. If a ferning pattern is seen, the fern test is positive, and a diagnosis of membrane rupture is made.

Other important parameters to assess include the color, odor, and amount of fluid and the time of rupture. The fluid should be clear with specks of vernix caseosa and no foul odor. If the membranes have been ruptured for several hours, the woman should be assessed carefully for signs of infection, such as elevated maternal temperature, cloudy or foul-smelling fluid, and fetal tachycardia. Green fluid signals the presence of meconium in the amniotic sac and may indicate that the fetus is distressed.

Assess for vaginal bleeding. The presence of bloody show is an expected finding, but heavy bleeding (heavier than a normal menstrual period) is not normal and should be reported to the charge nurse immediately. In addition to the amount of bleeding, other important characteristics should be noted, such as color (dark or bright red), amount and type of associated pain, and time that the bleeding began.

When delivery is imminent, it is important to ask the woman if she experienced any problems with this pregnancy, such as bleeding, high blood pressure, or diabetes. Determine if any prenatal fetal assessment tests were done and if any complications were diagnosed.

Some nurses find this approach helpful. If the woman presents to the labor unit complaining of "bleeding," ask her how many times she has changed sanitary napkins. Her answer will guide your determination of the approximate amount of bleeding and allow you to teach the woman about expected versus abnormal amounts of bleeding during labor.

Verify the expected due date. Ask if any complications were experienced with previous pregnancies. Establish the approximate number of times the woman saw the health care provider for prenatal care and during what month of pregnancy prenatal care began. Each of these assessments is important to determine if risk factors are present that might require a specialist to be present at the delivery.

Maternal Status

A quick physical assessment of the woman's status upon admission to the hospital is crucial. Assess the woman's vital signs, including temperature, pulse, respiration, and blood pressure, for signs of infection, hypertension, or shock. If there is not enough time before delivery to do a full assessment of vital signs, the blood pressure is the most critical immediate measurement.

ADDITIONAL ASSESSMENTS

Maternal Health History and Physical Assessment

The admission health history is taken as part of the initial assessment and includes an obstetric history, determination of current status, a medical–surgical history, social history, desired plans for labor and birth, and desires/plans for the newborn. Box 10-1 lists examples of data that are obtained routinely for each category in the admission health history. Review the prenatal record to obtain baseline vital signs

This is critical to remember. Monitoring for the development of pregnancy-induced hypertension (PIH) is an important nursing function throughout pregnancy and childbirth. Signs of PIH that should be reported immediately include elevated blood pressure (greater than 140/90 mm Hg), brisk DTRs or presence of clonus, protein in the urine, edema of the hands or face, sudden weight gain, and reports of headache or blurred vision.

---

[1]In the past the baseline FHR was expected to be between 120 and 160 beats per minute. Newer standards list 110 as the lower acceptable limit of normal.

BOX 10.1	Components of the Admission Health History

- Obstetric history
  - Number and outcomes of previous pregnancies in GTPAL (gravida, term, preterm, abortions, living) format (refer to Chapter 9 for a detailed explanation of using these terms to describe an obstetric history)
  - Estimated delivery date (EDD)
  - History of prenatal care for current pregnancy
  - Complications during pregnancy
  - Dates and results of fetal surveillance studies, such as ultrasound or nonstress test (NST)
  - Childbirth preparation classes
  - Previous labor and birth experiences
- Current status
  - Time of contraction onset
  - Contraction pattern
  - Status of membranes
  - Description of bloody show or bleeding
  - Current fetal movements
- Medical–surgical history
  - Chronic illnesses
  - Current medications
    - Prescribed
    - Over-the-counter
    - Herbal remedies
- Social history
  - Drug and alcohol use during pregnancy
  - Amount of smoking during pregnancy
  - Marital status
  - Support system
  - Domestic violence screen
  - Cultural/religious considerations that affect care
- Desires/plans for labor and birth
  - Presence of a partner, coach, and/or doula (refer to Chapter 8 for discussion of doulas)
  - Pain management preferences
  - Other personal preferences affecting intrapartum nursing care
- Desires/plans for newborn
  - Plans for feeding—breast or formula
  - Choice of pediatrician
  - Circumcision preference, if the infant is male
  - Rooming-in preference

● *Figure 10.2* The nurse measures the woman's weight during the admission process to labor and delivery. Photo by Joe Mitchell.

Assist the RN to perform a head-to-toe physical assessment. Critical measurements include lung sounds, the presence or absence of right upper quadrant (RUQ) pain or tenderness, deep tendon reflexes (DTRs), clonus, and amount and location of any edema.

Labor Status

Assess the woman's contraction pattern to include frequency, duration, and intensity (see the section "The Nurse's Role: Ongoing Assessment of Uterine Contractions and FHR" for in-depth information on monitoring uterine activity).

It also is important to determine fetal lie, presentation, attitude, position, and station when the laboring woman first presents to a birthing facility. This process begins through the use of Leopold's maneuvers. Fetal presentation, position, and attitude often can be determined using this technique. The four steps are outlined and illustrated in Nursing Procedure 10-1.

The initial vaginal examination is done to assess dilation and effacement of the cervix and allows for specific information to be gathered regarding the

and weight and to identify other pertinent information.

Obtain the woman's current weight and compare it with her weight at her most recent prenatal visit (Fig. 10-2). Sudden weight gain indicates fluid retention and may signal the onset of pregnancy-induced hypertension (PIH). Measure vital signs, which should be similar to the woman's baseline. It is normal for the pulse to increase slightly during labor, but the blood pressure, measured during the relaxation phase of a contraction, should not be elevated. Collect a urine specimen to screen for the presence of protein, ketones, glucose, blood cells, or bacteria.

Nursing Procedure 10.1
Leopold's Maneuvers

Leopold's maneuvers are a noninvasive method of assessing fetal presentation, position, and attitude. This technique can also be used to locate the fetal back before applying the fetal monitor.

EQUIPMENT

Warm, clean hands

PROCEDURE

1. Determine presentation.
   Stand beside the woman, facing her. Place both hands on the uterine fundus and palpate the contents of the fundus. If the buttocks are in the fundus indicating a vertex presentation (which is true 96% of the time), you will feel a soft, irregular object that does not move easily. However, if the head is in the fundus indicating a breech presentation, you will palpate a smooth, hard, round, mobile object.

2. Determine position.
   Place both hands on the maternal abdomen, one on each side. Use one hand to support the abdomen while you palpate the opposite side with the other hand. Repeat the procedure so that both sides of the

abdomen are palpated. Try to determine the location of the fetal back and extremities in relationship to the maternal pelvis. The back will feel hard and smooth and the extremities will be irregular and knobby.

3. Confirm presentation.
   Place one hand over the symphysis pubis and attempt to grasp the part that is presenting to the pelvis between your thumb and fingers of one hand. In the vast majority of cases you will feel a hard, round fetal head. If the part moves easily, it is unengaged. If the part is not movable, engagement probably has occurred. If the breech is presenting, you will feel a soft, irregular object.

4. Determine attitude.
   Begin the last step by turning to face the woman's feet. Using the finger pads of the first three fingers of each hand, palpate in a downward motion in the direction of the symphysis pubis. If a hard bony prominence is felt on the side opposite the fetal back, you have located the fetal brow, and the fetus is in an attitude of flexion. If the bony prominence is found on the same side as the fetal back, you are palpating the occiput, and the fetus is in an attitude of extension.

passenger's progress through the birth canal. In addition to confirming presentation, position, and attitude, fetal station can be established. In the full-term primigravida, the fetus is usually engaged, although it is not uncommon for the fetus to be unengaged and ballottable for the multipara during early labor.

As the LPN, it is your role to assist with vaginal examinations. There is no firm rule that establishes how frequently vaginal examinations should be performed during labor. The RN observes for cues that labor is advancing, so that vaginal examinations will only be done as frequently as is necessary to evaluate labor progress. Because vaginal examinations are invasive, performing them too frequently increases the risk for infection. Vaginal examinations are done when other labor assessments indicate labor is advancing, before administering pain medications, when the water bag breaks, or for the sudden onset of deep variable decelerations. Vaginal examinations should never be done if the woman presents with bright red painless bleeding until placenta previa is ruled out (see Chapter 17 for a description of placenta previa).

Record the results of the initial vaginal examination in the woman's clinical record. These results can then be compared with the results of subsequent examinations to demonstrate progress of labor or to diagnose arrest of dilation or descent. One example of a form used to graph results of cervical examinations is the partograph (Fig. 10-3). This graph gives a visual representation of the progress of labor and allows for documentation of parameters indicating maternal and fetal status. Each time a vaginal examination is done, the cervical dilatation and location of the fetal head is plotted on the graph. The "alert" line on the graph allows for the nurse or physician to quickly determine if labor is not progressing as expected. No cervical change in 2 hours when the woman is in active labor is called "arrest of dilatation." Failure of the fetus to descend (the station does not change) in a primigravida is a sign that labor is not progressing as expected, even if cervical dilation is occurring. The fetus of a multigravida may not descend until full dilation has occurred and then may move down the birth canal rapidly. The physician or nurse midwife should be notified when labor does not progress as expected.

Balance is the order of the day. Vaginal examinations should be done frequently enough to adequately assess labor progress but not frequently enough as to cause infection. Usually the practitioner or RN does not perform a vaginal examination unless there are indications that labor progress has been made (e.g., increased bloody show, increased restlessness and introversion of the laboring woman, or a desire to push) or there are signs of umbilical cord compression. In this instance a vaginal examination is done to check for a prolapsed cord.

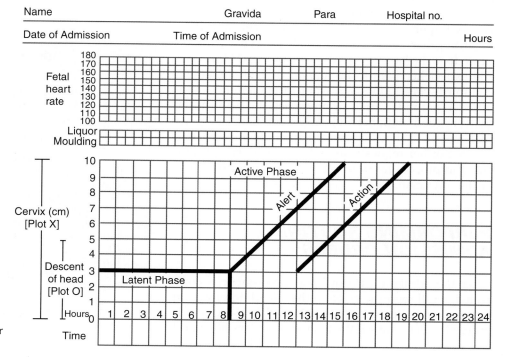

● *Figure 10.3* Partograph for recording labor progress.

CULTURAL SNAPSHOT

A woman's culture has a tremendous impact on the type and quantity of support she needs and on her methods of coping with the stress of labor. Some cultures frown on the presence of men during the labor and birth process. In these cases, it would be counterproductive for the nurse to pressure the man to be the support person.

Ask the woman to identify who should provide support. Inquire regarding the relationship of the support person to the woman. Ask the woman to identify any special methods that might help her cope with labor. This information will help you to individualize care while taking into account the woman's culture.

Labor and Birth Preferences

One very important part of the assessment is to determine if the woman and her partner have special requests for labor and birth. Some women go to great lengths to plan the birth. Ask if the woman has a written birth plan. It is hoped she has reviewed the plan with her physician well ahead of time and the physician has approved the document. Read through the plan and notify the RN of the contents. Birth plans often contain preferences regarding such things as mobility during labor, intravenous (IV) fluids during labor, episiotomy, presence of friends and family at the birth, fetal monitoring, pain management, and food and fluids during labor.

Many women do not have birth plans. However, it is very important to ask the woman specific questions regarding her preferences and needs. What expectations does she have about the labor process? How does she expect her pain to be managed? Did she attend childbirth class? Does she want to try natural childbirth? What individuals, if any, does she want in the delivery room with her? It is important to reassure her that she can change her mind at any time during labor. If some of her requests are outside the normal protocols and procedures used at the facility, inform the RN or the physician.

PERFORMING ROUTINE ADMISSION ORDERS

After the admission history and assessment is completed, a full report is given to the attending physician or nurse midwife. Sometimes additional observation is ordered to determine if the woman is in true labor, or if she should be sent home to wait until active labor

ensues. If the woman is to be admitted, the nurse carries out routine admission orders, which may include a perineal shave preparation or clip or Fleet enema if the membranes are intact. However, these procedures are no longer considered to be a routine part of labor care. In most facilities, some type of IV access is started. Usually a liter of the ordered IV solution is hung and titrated to the specified rate. Alternatively, a saline lock may be inserted to allow for IV access if needed for medication administration or fluid bolus. Some practitioners and facilities do not routinely insert an IV as part of the admission procedure.

Laboratory studies are part of the routine admission orders. The results are compared with the prenatal record to determine if changes have occurred during pregnancy. For example, a VDRL or RPR serology test is drawn to determine if the woman has developed a syphilis infection during pregnancy so that mother and baby can be treated, if necessary. Box 10-2 lists laboratory work that is ordered routinely when a woman is admitted to the delivery suite.

A little sensitivity is in order. If the woman is not in true labor and is to be discharged, she may feel embarrassed. Reassurance and acceptance can help relieve her anxiety. Instruct the woman regarding when to return to the hospital. It is a good idea to provide the telephone number to the delivery suite. This may be comforting for the woman, particularly if she is encouraged to call with concerns or questions.

BOX 10.2	Admission Laboratory Studies

- Complete blood count (CBC)
  - Monitor hemoglobin and hematocrit for signs of iron-deficiency anemia (hemoglobin levels below 11 g/dL).
  - White blood cell count (WBC) may increase to 20,000/mm^3 with the stress of labor. Levels above 20,000/mm^3 may indicate infection.
- Blood type and Rh factor
- Serologic studies, such as VDRL or RPR, to test for syphilis
- Rubella titer (not done if prenatal record indicates the woman is immune)
- ELISA to detect HIV antibodies (requires informed consent)
- Vaginal or cervical cultures
  - Gonorrhea
  - Chlamydia
  - Group B streptococcus
- Urinalysis (clean-catch specimen)

THE NURSE'S ROLE: ONGOING ASSESSMENT OF UTERINE CONTRACTIONS AND FHR

The nurse makes frequent assessments of uterine activity and FHR during labor. These assessments are necessary to determine adequacy of the labor pattern and to detect signs of fetal well-being or distress. Table 10-1 compares the advantages and disadvantages of each of the methods discussed in the text for monitoring uterine and fetal status during labor.

MONITORING UTERINE CONTRACTIONS

The uterine contraction pattern should be evaluated every time the FHR is assessed (see Box 10-5 for frequency of assessment). The contraction pattern can be evaluated using external or internal methods.

External Methods

If intermittent assessment techniques are used, the pattern is evaluated by palpation. If electronic fetal monitoring (EFM) is used, a tocodynamometer (toco) is used to measure contraction frequency and duration. The toco is a transducer with a sensor that works like a moveable button. It is placed on the fundus with the sensor facing down and then strapped securely to the abdomen with a belt (see Nursing Procedure 10-3). As the uterus contracts, the sensor is displaced; an action that sends a signal to the microprocessor. The signal is converted by the microprocessor into a graphic representation of the uterine contraction on the video display and printout along with the FHR pattern tracing. In this way the health care provider can monitor the FHR pattern in conjunction with the uterine contraction pattern.

Here's a helpful hint. It is difficult for inexperienced nurses to determine the intensity of uterine contractions by palpation. One suggestion is to touch the tip of your nose, if the fundus can be indented as far as the tip of your nose at the peak of a contraction, the contraction can be recorded as mild. If the fundus feels firmer, as when you touch your chin, the contraction is of moderate intensity. A fundus that cannot be indented, one that feels like you are pushing on your forehead, is indicative of a strong contraction.

Contraction frequency and duration are determined by evaluating the EFM tracing. However, unless the woman has an internal uterine pressure catheter, the contractions must be palpated manually to evaluate intensity. As you will recall from Chapter 8, the height of the contraction is an estimate of its intensity. However, many factors affect the height of the contraction on an external tracing. For example, a small woman with minimal adipose tissue may be having mild contractions, but on the monitor strip the contractions appear tall and pronounced. On the other hand, an obese woman may be having strong contractions that barely register on the tracing. For these reasons, palpation is the most accurate way to estimate intensity when using external monitoring. Nursing Procedure 10-2 describes how to palpate uterine contractions.

Internal Method

Infrequently, an intrauterine pressure catheter is used. The physician places the catheter tip above the presenting part in a pocket of amniotic fluid, and then the catheter is connected to the fetal monitor. In addition to recording the frequency and duration of contractions, the internal catheter accurately measures the intensity of uterine activity. This information is particularly useful when the woman is undergoing labor after a previous cesarean delivery or when she is receiving oxytocics to induce labor.

Test Yourself

- Name three signs that indicate that birth is imminent.
- List the four parameters that must be charted regarding ruptured membranes.
- How do you evaluate the uterine contraction pattern when external EFM is used?

MONITORING FHR

Labor is not only stressful for the woman, but it stresses the fetus as well. If there is decreased blood flow to the placenta, or the fetus is subjected to chronic hypoxia, the fetus may not be able to withstand the stress of labor. General characteristics of the FHR and any changes that occur with uterine contractions give clues as to fetal status. For these reasons the fetal heart rate is monitored in relation to the contraction pattern.

TABLE 10.1	Comparison of Monitoring Techniques During Labor		
Technique	**Description**	**Advantages**	**Disadvantages**
Intermittent FHR auscultation	Fetoscope, Doppler, or EFM used to periodically check FHR	• Noninvasive • Increases maternal comfort and mobility • Focus of health care provider is the laboring woman, rather than technology	• Requires one-to-one nurse-to-patient staffing ratios • Subtle signs of distress may be overlooked
Continuous external EFM	External transducer placed on maternal abdomen with straps to detect the FHR via ultrasound technology	• Noninvasive • Provides a continuous tracing of FHR • Allows for detection of signs of fetal compromise	• Cannot accurately detect short-term variability • An active fetus or maternal movement can interfere with the continuity of the tracing • Generally confines the laboring woman to bed, unless telemetry unit is used
Continuous external monitoring of uterine contractions	External toco placed on maternal abdomen with straps to detect uterine contraction	• Noninvasive • Shows the frequency and duration of uterine contractions • Allows for comparison of FHR pattern with uterine contraction pattern	• Does not accurately depict the intensity of uterine contractions • Tends to be confining and limits maternal movement
Continuous internal EFM	Electrode is placed on the fetal scalp and connected to a reference electrode on the maternal thigh to record electrical activity of the fetal heart	• Yields accurate information regarding variability • Allows for continuous monitoring of active fetus • Allows for continuous monitoring even if laboring woman is restless and changes positions frequently	• Invasive; requires that the membranes be ruptured and the cervix be at least partially dilated • Requires a specially trained practitioner for insertion • Increased risk for complications, such as chorioamnionitis, fetal scalp cellulites, or osteomyelitis (rare)
Continuous internal monitoring of uterine contractions	Intrauterine pressure catheter inserted into a pocket of amniotic fluid to detect pressure changes within the uterus and record the contraction pattern	• Allows for more accurate determination of contraction intensity than external techniques • Useful for labors in which there is a risk for uterine rupture (e.g., previous uterine incision or induction with oxytocics)	• Invasive; requires that the membranes be ruptured and the cervix be at least partially dilated • Requires a specially trained practitioner for insertion • Increased risk for complications, such as chorioamnionitis
Fetal scalp sampling	Small sample of fetal scalp blood is taken during a special vaginal examination and tested for pH level	• Gives direct evidence of fetal status • Allows for better practitioner decisions regarding continuation of labor	• Invasive; requires that the membranes be ruptured and the cervix be at least partially dilated • Requires a specially trained examiner to collect the specimen • Increased risk for infection, blood incompatibilities, and fetal anemia
Fetal scalp pulse oximetry	Sensor placed on the fetus' cheek or brow to detect oxygen saturation	• Does not require a blood sample to be taken • Allows for continuous reading of fetal oxygenation status • Gives direct evidence of fetal status	• Invasive; requires that the membranes be ruptured and the cervix be at least partially dilated • Requires a specially trained practitioner for insertion • Fetal oximetry is fairly new technology; equipment expense may prohibit its use.

Nursing Procedure 10.2
Palpation of Uterine Contractions

EQUIPMENT

Warm, clean hands

PROCEDURE

1. Explain procedure to the woman and her partner.
2. Wash hands thoroughly.
3. Locate and place one hand on the uterine fundus.
4. Use the tips of your fingers to feel changes in the uterus as it contracts.
5. At the beginning of the contraction you will feel the muscle begin to tighten.
6. Note the time the contraction begins.
7. Use your fingertips to evaluate how strong the contraction gets before the muscle begins to relax. Intensity is measured at the strongest point (the acme) of the contraction.
8. Note the time the contraction ends to determine duration.
9. Continue with your hand on the fundus through the next three contractions. Note if the uterus completely relaxes by becoming soft between contractions.

10. Note the time from the beginning of one contraction to the beginning of the following contraction to determine frequency. Frequency is documented as a range when appropriate (e.g., every 3–5 minutes, or every 2–3 minutes), unless they are occurring regularly (e.g., every 2 minutes, every 5 minutes).
11. Wash hands.
12. Chart the contraction pattern (frequency, duration, and intensity) in the labor record. Document whether or not the uterus is fully relaxing between contractions.

Note: It is best to time several contractions consecutively before charting frequency because it is rare for contractions to be exactly "x" minutes apart. It is more common that the contraction pattern occurs every "x" to "y" minutes apart (e.g., every 3 to 5 minutes). Palpation is a method that takes practice. It is best to learn to palpate contractions in conjunction with the use of EFM. In this way, you can see the contraction begin and concentrate on perceiving the tightening of the uterus with your fingertips. You can also see the acme, which lets you know when to evaluate intensity.

Intermittent Auscultation of FHR

An acceptable method for monitoring FHR in a low-risk pregnancy is to use intermittent auscultation. Usually the woman is placed on external EFM for 20 minutes to get a baseline evaluation of the FHR. If the pattern is reassuring, then a fetoscope, hand-held Doppler device, or the external EFM is used to monitor the FHR at intermittent intervals. The FHR is auscultated with the same frequency as is recommended for continuous monitoring methods (see Box 10-5). The FHR is monitored for at least 1 full minute and is auscultated throughout at least one uterine contraction. If any abnormalities are noted, or if there is slowing of the FHR with or after contractions, the woman is placed on a fetal monitor for continuous monitoring.

There are several advantages to the use of intermittent auscultation. The woman has more freedom to move about than when she is strapped continuously to a fetal monitoring device, and nurses are encouraged to focus on the laboring woman and her support person, rather than on the technology.

There are also disadvantages to the use of intermittent auscultation. This approach takes more of the nurse's time than does continuous EFM, a situation that requires higher staffing levels. Therefore, intermittent auscultation may not be practical in a busy labor and delivery unit. Another drawback is the potential that an ominous FHR pattern might be missed. Although intermittent auscultation is recommended only for low-risk

pregnancies, it is possible for a complication to develop during labor in a heretofore low-risk pregnancy. A non-reassuring FHR pattern might be the only indication that a complication has developed. If this pattern is not recognized quickly, the fetus could become severely compromised before interventions are initiated.

Continuous EFM

As with monitoring uterine contractions, there are two ways the FHR can be monitored using a continuous fetal monitoring device. Continuous EFM can be accomplished using external (indirect) methods or through the use of internal (direct) monitoring techniques.

External EFM

The most common way to assess fetal status during labor is with the use of an external EFM. Although fetal monitors are manufactured by several companies and vary in shape and size, the basic components are the same and include a microprocessor, transducer, tocodynamometer (toco), audio capability, and graphic printout. The external monitor works on the principle of ultrasound. The transducer releases ultrasonic waves that are intercepted by the movement of fetal heart valves as the heart beats. The signal is then interpreted by the microprocessor, with results sent to the recording units. Characteristics of the fetal heart rate pattern can then be monitored continuously via a video display

Nursing Procedure 10.3
Application of External Fetal Monitors

EQUIPMENT

Electronic fetal monitor
Tocodynamometer (toco)
Transducer
Two belts
Ultrasonic gel
Monitor paper

PROCEDURE

1. Thoroughly wash your hands.
2. Locate the fetal back through the use of Leopold's maneuvers (see Nursing Procedure 10-1).
3. Assist the woman to a position of comfort. If she wishes to be on her back, a wedge should be placed under one hip to tilt the uterus off of the great vessels.
4. Place ultrasonic gel on the transducer and turn on the power to the fetal monitor.
5. Place the transducer on the woman's abdomen over the fetal back.
6. Turn up the volume and move the transducer over the abdominal wall until the heartbeat is clearly heard.
7. When the monitor is consistently recording the FHR, secure the transducer in place with a belt.

8. Next locate the hardest part of the uterine fundus.
9. Place the toco over the fundus and secure it to the maternal abdomen with a belt (see figure).
10. Check to make sure the paper is recording the FHR and uterine contraction pattern.

11. Label the EFM strip with the laboring woman's identification data, the date and time the EFM was applied, and maternal vital signs and position.
12. Be sure the call light is within reach before you leave the room.
13. Thoroughly wash your hands.

Note: It is important to position the woman comfortably before attempting to locate the fetal heart. If you wait until after you locate the FHR to reposition, you may lose the FHR and need to relocate the transducer.

and/or a continuous printout. As stated, the toco is used to monitor the contraction pattern, which allows for monitoring of the FHR pattern in conjunction with the uterine contraction pattern. See Nursing Procedure 10-3: Application of External Fetal Monitors.

External EFM is used to screen for signs of fetal compromise. It is noninvasive and used widely. However, the information gleaned from external monitoring is less precise than that of internal monitoring. Sometimes it is difficult to get a consistent tracing if the fetus is small or extremely active or if the woman is obese. Maternal positioning can adversely affect the quality of the tracing, and many women find external monitoring uncomfortable and confining.

Some EFM manufacturers have developed telemetry units, which provide wireless transmission of FHR patterns and uterine activity to the monitoring device so that the woman is not attached by cables to the EFM. These units allow for continuous EFM while the woman ambulates, alternates her position, or uses a birthing ball. Telemetry units have even been developed that allow for the woman to submerse her body in water to soothe the discomfort of labor.

Internal EFM

Internal EFM is an invasive procedure in which a spiral electrode is attached to the presenting part just under the skin (Fig. 10-4). A wire that extends from the

● *Figure 10.4* Internal fetal scalp electrode in place on the fetal scalp, connected to the reference electrode on the maternal thigh and to the EFM. Internal monitoring techniques allow for more precise measurement of the electrical activity of the fetal heart.

spiral electrode is connected to a reference electrode that is placed on the laboring woman's inner thigh. The signal is interpreted by the microprocessor, and a graphic representation of the electrical activity of the fetal heart is recorded. This method gives more precise results than does external monitoring and is more reliable for detecting signs of fetal compromise. It is easier to obtain a consistent tracing regardless of fetal activity and is not usually affected by maternal position changes. When internal techniques are used, the most frequent combination is that of internal fetal scalp electrode with an external toco to record the contraction pattern. Infrequently, an intrauterine pressure catheter is used (refer to the previous discussion). Because internal techniques are invasive, the fetal membranes must be ruptured and the cervix must be adequately dilated to use them. Accordingly, these procedures increase the risk of maternal and fetal infection and injury.

This is important! All invasive procedures carry risks, particularly increased risk for infection. In this instance, both the woman and the fetus can become ill with infection because of the use of the internal monitor. Chorioamnionitis is a serious uterine infection that requires intravenous antibiotics and a lengthened hospital stay. Newborns have experienced cellulitis of the scalp and even the dangerous bone infection osteomyelitis after internal scalp monitoring was used during labor. Fortunately this situation rarely occurs (Wolcott & Conry, 2000).

Evaluating FHR Patterns

Baseline FHR

The obstetric nurse is responsible for monitoring FHR patterns. Not only must the pattern be assessed and interpreted accurately, but the nurse also must know how to intervene and when to notify the physician or certified nurse midwife (CNM). The LPN is not expected to make a final decision about an FHR pattern; that is the responsibility of the trained RN. However, the LPN must be able to differentiate reassuring and nonreassuring signs in order to get help when it is indicated.

When you are asked to interpret a fetal monitor tracing, the first element that must be evaluated is the baseline FHR. The baseline rate is measured between uterine contractions during a 10-minute period. The normally accepted baseline rate is between 120 beats per minute (bpm) and 160 bpm, although the lower limit is considered to be 110 bpm by some researchers. Rates between 110 and 120 bpm are usually acceptable if all other signs are reassuring.

The baseline **variability**, fluctuations in FHR, also is evaluated. There are two types of variability: **short-term variability** (STV) and **long-term variability** (LTV). STV (sometimes called "beat-to-beat" variability) refers to the moment-to-moment changes in FHR that result in roughness of the EFM tracing. LTV refers to the wider fluctuations that make the EFM tracing look wavy over time. LTV is considered to be normal if the fluctuations are greater than 6 bpm and less than 25 bpm (Fig. 10-5). Box 10-3 gives definitions of LTV.

A word of caution is in order. Make certain that a nonreassuring pattern is not attributable to medical intervention. For example, fetal bradycardia may result from maternal hypotension that arises when the woman receives epidural anesthesia. Or a narcotic analgesic administered to the woman may cause decreased variability. In these examples, correcting the maternal condition may be all that is needed to correct the nonreassuring pattern.

BOX 10.3	Fetal Heart Rate (FHR) Long-Term Variability (LTV) Definitions

- Absent: No fluctuations of FHR
- Minimal: Less than or equal to 5 bpm
- Moderate: 6 to 25 bpm (normal)
- Marked: Greater than 25 bpm

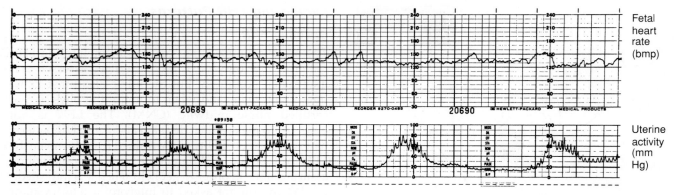

● **Figure 10.5** The EFM tracing shows moderate (normal) LTV.

FHR variability results from the interplay between the sympathetic and parasympathetic branches of the autonomic nervous system. The sympathetic division nudges the FHR higher, whereas the parasympathetic division tugs the FHR downward. Therefore, variability in the tracing is a reassuring sign that the fetal nervous system is intact.

There are three major deviations from a normal FHR baseline: tachycardia, bradycardia, and absent or minimal variability. Fetal tachycardia is defined as a baseline rate of greater than 160 bpm. When the baseline FHR falls below 110 bpm, the condition is identified as fetal bradycardia. Tachycardias and bradycardias are diagnosed if the abnormal rate continues for at least 3 minutes. The absence of variability also is a non-reassuring sign. Examples of conditions that can cause fetal tachycardia, bradycardia, and absent variability are listed in Table 10-2.

Periodic Changes

The next step after evaluating the baseline is to check for **periodic changes**, variations in the FHR pattern that occur in conjunction with uterine contractions. Periodic changes are designated as reassuring, benign, or nonreassuring. Figure 10-6 illustrates the appearance and causes of certain periodic changes.

TABLE 10.2	Conditions That Can Influence the FHR Baseline
Baseline FHR Deviation	**Possible Causes**

Tachycardia (>160 bpm)
  Mild 161–180 bpm
  Severe >180 bpm
	• Maternal or fetal infection
	• Dehydration
	• Fever
	• Hyperthyroidism
	• Fetal hypoxemia (acute or chronic) or anemia
	• Premature fetus
	• Fetus with congenital anomalies
	• Certain medications given to the woman in labor, particularly tocolytics (medications used to stop preterm labor), and any drug that causes maternal tachycardia (e.g., caffeine, epinephrine, or theophylline)
	• Street drugs

Bradycardia (<110 bpm)
  Moderate 80–100 bpm
  Severe < 80 bpm
	• Maternal hypotension
	• Supine hypotensive syndrome
	• Vagal stimulation
	• Fetal decompensation

Decreased or absent variability	• Medications
	  • Narcotics
	  • Magnesium sulfate (to treat preterm labor or PIH)
	  • Tocolytics (medications to stop labor)
	• Fetal sleep (normal fetal sleep cycle is 20 minutes)
	• Prematurity
	• Fetal hypoxemia

● **Figure 10.6** Appearance and causes of periodic changes: early, variable, and late decelerations.

Reassuring Periodic Changes. Spontaneous elevations of the FHR, **accelerations**, above the baseline by at least 15 bpm for at least 15 seconds (15 × 15 window) are considered to be reassuring. In fact, as stated in Chapter 7, accelerations are the basis for the nonstress test (NST).

Benign Periodic Changes. Sometimes instead of accelerations, you will notice slowing of the FHR. If the dip in the FHR tracing occurs in conjunction with and mirrors a uterine contraction, it is called an **early deceleration.** This type of deceleration is shaped like a U on the EFM tracing, like that of a contraction. Three criteria must be met for the deceleration to be classified as early. The FHR begins to slow as the contraction starts. The lowest point of the deceleration, the **nadir**, coincides with the acme (highest point) of the contraction. The deceleration ends by the end of the contraction.

Current scientific evidence indicates that early decelerations are caused by pressure on the fetal head as it meets resistance from the structures of the birth canal. The contraction pushes the fetal head downward,

causing pressure, which in turn leads to a slowing of the FHR. As long as the baseline remains within normal limits and the variability is good, early decelerations are considered benign. Therefore, no specific nursing intervention is indicated other than to continue to monitor the tracing and observe closely for the development of nonreassuring patterns.

Nonreassuring Periodic Changes. A **variable deceleration** is so named because it may occur at any point during a contraction, and it has a jagged, erratic shape on the EFM tracing. The FHR suddenly drops from the baseline and then recovers. A variable deceleration may be shaped like a U, V, or W.

The presence of variable decelerations, or *variables*, as labor and delivery personnel commonly call them, indicates some type of acute umbilical cord compression. Often it will be found at delivery that the umbilical cord is wrapped around a body part, such as the neck (nuchal cord) or foot. At other times the cause of compression is oligohydramnios (decreased amount of amniotic fluid), or it occurs as the result of an occult (hidden) cord prolapse.[2] It is important to note that the cord compression is not continuous. The compression occurs when the uterus is contracting and squeezing the cord against the fetus. It is relieved when the uterus relaxes between contractions.

Variable decelerations require careful observation. If the baseline is within normal limits, variability is present, and the variables recover quickly (within the space of a normal contraction), there is no immediate cause for alarm. However, you should be aware that the fetus is being stressed whenever the cord is compressed because the umbilical cord is his lifeline to oxygen. It is as if he must hold his breath while the cord is being compressed during the contraction. Therefore, nursing interventions are aimed at relieving the compression.

Pay attention to the details! Here's how to tell if variable decelerations indicate distress. A healthy fetus that is coping well with the stress of cord compression will show small "shoulders" (accelerations) on either side of the deceleration. As hypoxia develops, the shoulder on the recovery side will get larger (this is called "overshoot"), followed by loss of shoulders altogether and loss of variability. Finally, the variable deceleration will develop a late component, seen as a slow recovery to baseline. Any variable deceleration that lasts longer than 1 minute or dips deeper than 60 bpm below the baseline is worrisome.

First assist the woman to change positions. Try to find a position that is comfortable for the woman that relieves the compression. If the variables stop after the position change, you will know that the compression has been relieved. However, if the variables continue, try a variety of position changes, including the knee-chest position.

Other interventions for persistent or prolonged variables include stopping any oxytocic infusion, increasing the rate of IV fluids (if they are infusing), starting oxygen via face mask at 10 to 12 liters per minute, and notifying the charge nurse and physician. The charge nurse may perform a vaginal examination to rule out a prolapsed cord. Sometimes the physician will order an **amnioinfusion**, infusion of normal saline into the uterus, to cushion the umbilical cord and relieve compression.

The most ominous type of periodic change is a pattern of **late decelerations**. Like early decelerations, these decelerations appear smooth and U shaped on the EFM tracing, but unlike early decelerations, they are offset from the contraction. Late decelerations begin late

Don't forget the importance of your observation skills. It is easy to be so concerned about the fetal monitor tracing that the skills of inspection and palpation are overlooked or downplayed. Always begin your assessment by looking at the laboring woman and performing a quick visual inspection of the environment. If there are no immediate problems, then you may turn your focus to reading the EFM strip. Technology does not replace the need for your assessment skills.

in the contraction and recover after the contraction has ended. The slope and size of the deceleration mirrors the intensity of the contraction. Figure 10-7 compares early and late decelerations on a fetal monitor tracing.

Late decelerations are associated with **uteroplacental insufficiency**, diminished or deficient blood flow to the uterus and placenta. This pattern occurs when the blood supply is interrupted chronically, rather than acutely, as is the case with variable decelerations. This is a grave situation because the placenta is the fetus' sole source of oxygen. Interventions are aimed at improving blood flow to the placenta.

When late decelerations are detected on the monitor, the following interventions are indicated. Position the woman on her right or left side[3] to relieve compression on the maternal great vessels. Discontinue the infusion of oxytocics (if present). Apply oxygen via a face mask at 10 to 12 liters per minute. Immediately notify the charge nurse and physician. Sometimes the physician will order tocolytics (medications to relax the uterus) in an attempt to improve blood flow to the placenta. Box 10-4 lists signs of an increasingly distressed fetus.

Test Yourself

- What are the components of the electronic fetal monitor?
- What is the baseline fetal heart rate?
- How does a late deceleration appear on the fetal monitor tracing?
- What interventions should be taken when a pattern of late decelerations is detected?

---

[2]A cord prolapse is an obstetric emergency that is discussed in Chapter 18.

[3] Research shows that positioning the woman on either side relieves pressure on the abdominal aorta and inferior vena cava and improves blood flow to the placenta. Previously it was thought that positioning on the left side afforded the best blood flow. Some health care providers may still prefer to use the left side when late decelerations are detected.

● **Figure 10.7** An early deceleration mirrors the contraction, is caused by head compression, and is benign, requiring no intervention. A late deceleration mirrors the contraction but is offset because a late deceleration begins after the contraction has started and ends after the contraction has ended. The cause is uteroplacental insufficiency, and interventions are aimed at improving blood flow to the placenta.

Measures Used to Clarify Nonreassuring FHR Patterns

When a nonreassuring FHR pattern is detected with EFM, more accurate methods for determining fetal hypoxia and acidosis are sometimes necessary. Some techniques currently in use include fetal stimulation, fetal scalp sampling, and fetal scalp pulse oximetry.

Fetal Stimulation

Because the presence of a nonreassuring pattern does not always correlate with fetal compromise, the physician or CNM may elect to try fetal stimulation. For this procedure the fetus is stimulated indirectly with an acoustic vibrator through the abdominal wall or is stimulated directly on the scalp by the gloved fingers of the examiner's hand during a vaginal examination. If the fetus responds by accelerating the heart rate, fetal acidosis is not present. If FHR accelerations do not occur after stimulation, fetal acidosis is a strong possibility.

BOX 10.4	Signs of an Increasingly Distressed Fetus

As the fetus becomes hypoxic, certain physiologic signs can be noted. These signs are listed in order of least distress to most distress. As you move down the list, the signs are indicative of ever-worsening hypoxia.
1. Absent accelerations
2. Gradual increase in FHR baseline
3. Loss of baseline variability
4. Late deceleration pattern develops
5. Decelerations gradually increase in length and take longer to recover to baseline
6. Persistent bradycardia
7. Death

Fetal Scalp Sampling

Fetal scalp sampling, a technique for checking fetal status, was developed in the late 1960s to verify fetal distress. Many physicians continue to use fetal scalp sampling to determine fetal pH when nonreassuring FHR patterns are detected with EFM.

For this procedure the physician places a cone-like device into the vagina through the dilated cervix and holds it on the fetal scalp. The scalp is cleaned; a tiny cut is made (like a finger stick to check for blood sugar); a small amount of blood is collected in a tube; and pressure is placed on the fetal head wound until the bleeding stops. The blood sample is tested immediately to determine the pH. A fetal pH within the normal range (between 7.20 and 7.25) is reassuring. If, however, the pH is abnormally low (less than 7.20), the fetus is acidotic. Fetal acidosis indicates that the fetus is truly in distress and needs to be delivered quickly so that the newborn can be resuscitated outside of the womb.

Although the risk is low, complications can result from fetal scalp sampling. The fetus can get an infection from the cut on the scalp; fetal and maternal blood may intermingle, potentially leading to blood incompatibilities; and the fetus can experience anemia from blood loss.

Fetal Scalp Pulse Oximetry

Because of the possibility of complications associated with fetal scalp sampling, a newer technique is sometimes used to monitor fetal oxygenation: fetal scalp pulse oximetry. This technology uses the same principles of pulse oximetry as those used to measure oxygen saturation in adult patients. In this instance, the sensor must be inserted into the uterus and placed next to the fetal cheek or temple. The sensor detects fetal oxygen saturation levels. The signal is then interpreted by a microprocessor, which sends the information to a monitor that gives a continuous readout. In this way, the physician or nurse midwife can make a better decision about fetal status than with EFM alone. Research is being done to determine if fetal pulse oximetry reduces the number of cesarean deliveries for fetal distress.

Test Yourself

- What evidence does fetal scalp sampling reveal regarding fetal status?
- What is fetal scalp pulse oximetry?

THE NURSE'S ROLE DURING EACH STAGE OF LABOR

● The Nursing Process During the First Stage of Labor (Dilation)

The first stage of labor is traditionally divided into three phases: latent, active, and transition. The first stage begins with the onset of labor and ends when the cervix is 10 cm dilated and 100% effaced. The nurse's role during this stage of labor focuses on assessment, providing physical care to the mother and fetus, providing psychological care to the mother, and keeping the physician informed about labor progress (Box 10-5).

Latent Phase (Early Labor)

ASSESSMENT

During the latent phase of labor, assess fetal status at least once every hour. Evaluate labor status every 60 minutes. Contractions during early labor are typically 5 to 10 minutes apart, last 30 to 45 seconds, and are of mild intensity. The cervix is dilated from 1 to 3 cm, and effacement has begun. Additional assessment parameters include maternal status and the status of the membranes.

It is also important to assess the woman's psychosocial state during the latent phase of labor. She may be talkative and express feelings of confidence and excitement. Conversely, she may be fearful, particularly if she is not prepared for the event; or she may experience anticipatory anxiety.

SELECTED NURSING DIAGNOSES

- Risk for Injury (fetal and maternal) related to possible complications of labor

- Anxiety related to uncertainty of labor onset and insecurity regarding ability to cope
- Acute Pain related to contractions
- Deficient Knowledge of labor process related to inadequate preparation for delivery or unexpected circumstances of labor

OUTCOME IDENTIFICATION AND PLANNING

Maintaining the safety of the laboring woman and her fetus throughout the latent phase of the first stage of labor are primary goals when planning care. Other goals and interventions are planned according to the individual needs of the laboring woman and her partner. Appropriate goals may include that fetal and maternal injury will be avoided; that the laboring woman's anxiety will be reduced and her pain will be manageable; and that the woman and her partner will have adequate knowledge of the labor process.

IMPLEMENTATION

Preventing Fetal and Maternal Injury
Monitor the woman's vital signs every hour. The temperature may be taken every 4 hours unless the water bag is not intact, which requires hourly monitoring. Mild tachycardia may be associated with anxiety or the stress of labor contractions. Immediately report elevations in the blood pressure or temperature.

Check the fetal monitor tracing frequently. Record FHR and uterine contraction pattern at least hourly during the latent stage of labor. Report extended periods of reduced variability, FHR decelerations, or other signs of fetal distress.

Relieving Anxiety
Encourage the woman to verbalize her fears and uncertainties. It may be helpful to ask what most concerns her about labor. Often anxiety is measurably decreased once fears are verbalized. When the source of anxiety is determined, specific measures can be implemented to decrease the anxiety. For example, if the woman is unsure she will be able to withstand the pain of labor, a discussion of pain relief options may be helpful. If she does not know what to expect, she may benefit from a brief explanation of the normal process of labor.

The woman also may fear losing control. In this instance, it may be appropriate to involve the partner in developing a plan to assist her if she starts to lose control. Verbal cues and position changes can be suggested as part of the plan. It is always advisable to inquire regarding coping behaviors that have been helpful to her

BOX 10.5	Nursing Care for the First Stage of Labor

Caring for the Woman

Assess the woman's vital signs.
- Temperature
  - If membranes are intact, monitor and record every 4 hours.
  - If membranes are ruptured, measure every 2 hours.
  - An elevated temperature may be associated with dehydration or infection.
- Blood pressure, pulse, and respirations
  - Measure every 60 minutes during the latent phase of labor.
  - Measure every 30 minutes during active labor and transition.
  - Measure every 15 minutes during the second stage of labor.
  - When certain procedures are done, such as induction of labor or placement of epidural anesthesia, the vital signs will be taken more frequently.

Monitor hydration status.
- Maintain strict intake and output.
- Maintain and monitor IV fluids, if present.
- Offer ointment for dry lips.
- Provide frequent mouth care.
- Offer fluids and ice chips if allowed/desired.
- Encourage voiding every 2 hours.
- Check for the presence of glucose or protein in the urine.

Remain attuned to the maternal psyche.
- Provide ongoing assessment of maternal coping status.
- Assess effectiveness of partner coach, or doula in supporting and comforting the woman.
- Promote positive coping.
  - Teach/reinforce patterned breathing techniques (Chapter 9).
  - Encourage frequent position changes.
  - Encourage rituals and creative approaches to dealing with contractions.
  - Administer analgesia appropriately, if desired by the woman.
  - Assist with the administration of anesthesia as ordered, if desired by the woman.
- Provide supportive care.
  - Provide privacy.
  - Provide a relaxing environment.
    - A fan may helpful if the woman is hot.
    - Soft lighting or darkening the room promotes relaxation.
    - Keep noise to a minimum.
      - Some women need absolute quiet during a contraction.
      - Some women find music to be soothing.
  - Provide for personal hygiene needs.
    - Absorbent pads are placed under the hips and buttocks to catch the continual drainage associated with labor.
    - Frequent perineal care and pad changes promote comfort.

- Some women find a shower comforting.
- Keep the woman and her partner or coach informed of labor progress and purpose of procedures.
- Be a role model for the support person.
  - Actively involve the partner or coach, if so desired by the laboring woman. Remember some cultures discourage participation by the father in the birthing process.
  - Encourage the support person to take breaks as needed.

Caring for the Fetus

Assess FHR* (*Note:* The recommendations apply to both intermittent and continuous monitoring techniques):
FHR of the low-risk laboring woman should be evaluated every
- 1 hour during latent phase of the first stage of labor
- 30 minutes during active phase of the first stage of labor
- 15 minutes during the second stage of labor
FHR of the at-risk laboring woman should be evaluated every
- 30 minutes during latent phase of the first stage of labor
- 15 minutes during the active phase of the first stage of labor
- 5 minutes during the second stage of labor
Additional times for monitoring and documenting the FHR pattern
- Immediately after artificial or spontaneous rupture of the membranes
- Before and after medication administration during labor and at time of peak medication action
- Before and after any invasive procedure (e.g., vaginal exam, enema expulsion, urinary catheterization, amnioinfusion)
- Before and after ambulation
- After any increase in frequency, duration, or intensity of uterine contractions

Management of the Labor Process

Observe for spontaneous rupture of the membranes, or assist when the birth attendant performs an artificial rupture of the membranes.
- Observe the color of the fluid (should be clear); green or cloudy fluid should be reported.
- Record the time of rupture, the characteristics and amount of fluid, and an assessment of the FHR.
Monitor for signs of umbilical cord prolapse (this labor complication is discussed in Chapter 18).
- Immediately after the membranes rupture, when the risk for prolapse is greatest, assess the FHR for 1 full minute.
- If fetal bradycardia is present, perform a vaginal examination to check for a prolapsed cord.
- Continue ongoing fetal assessments because prolapse can occur anytime after the membranes rupture.

(box continues on page 232)

BOX 10.5 (continued)	**Nursing Care for the First Stage of Labor**

Assess uterine contraction pattern each time the FHR is assessed.
- Pattern should generally correlate with the phase of labor.
- Uterus should relax completely between contractions.
- Tetanic contractions (lasting longer than 90 seconds and of strong intensity) or failure of the uterus to relax should be reported.

Assess bloody show.
- An increase may be a sign of advancing labor.

- Heavy bleeding is a sign that a complication of labor is developing.

Assist the RN or childbirth attendant with vaginal examinations to determine progress of dilatation, effacement, and descent. To decrease the risk of infection:
- Sterile technique should be used.
- The number of examinations should be kept to a minimum.

Note maternal and fetal response to interventions.
Document all assessments and procedures.

* Recommendations of the American College of Obstetrics and Gynecology (ACOG) and Association of Women's Health, Obstetric, and Neonatal Nurses (AWHONN).

during other stressful situations. In this way, the couple can be assisted to adapt successful coping strategies to assist coping efforts during labor.

Promoting Comfort

It is important to support the woman and her partner in their attempts to cope with the discomfort and stress of labor. If the membranes are intact, encourage the woman to ambulate. Even if the membranes are ruptured, she may ambulate with a support person or nurse, if the fetus is engaged and well applied to the cervix. If the membranes are ruptured she should not ambulate alone or leave the nursing unit. Ambulation and upright positions are frequently helpful throughout the labor process. If the woman chooses not to ambulate, assist with comfort measures and position changes. However, at no time should the woman be allowed to remain flat on her back.

If the woman and her coach are well prepared for labor, they may decide to stay at home during the latent phase. This practice is permissible as long as the membranes are intact, and some nurses encourage it to allow the woman more control over the early labor process. Encourage distraction techniques. Engaging in conversation, watching television, and shopping are examples of diversionary activities that may be helpful during the latent phase of labor. Food and beverage intake during labor is a subject of debate (Box 10-6).

Providing Patient Teaching

The latent phase of labor is an excellent time to teach the woman and her partner or coach about the process of labor. Important teaching points include what the woman and her coach can expect to experience during each phase and stage of labor. Pain relief options and appropriate timing of analgesia and anesthesia should be explained and discussed. Briefly describe the frequency and purpose of nursing assessments and interventions common to each stage of labor.

It is important that the woman and her partner understand how to work with the labor

BOX 10.6	**Food and Fluid Intake During Labor**

For the past 50 decades in the United States the normal practice has been to withhold food and fluids from the laboring woman. This practice was recommended to prevent the woman from aspirating in the event that anesthesia would be needed for a cesarean delivery. Now there are a wide range of practices and opinions on the issue.

Nurse midwives who deliver patients at home or in birthing centers often allow food and fluid intake during the latent phase of labor and then restrict the woman to clear fluids during active labor. Fluids are needed during labor to prevent dehydration. Because the woman who delivers at home rarely has an IV, she is usually encouraged to take fluids by mouth. Many midwives who deliver in birthing centers give IV fluids to the woman in active labor. In this instance the woman is usually allowed clear liquids as a comfort measure.

Practices regarding food and drink during labor vary widely at hospitals across the country. Many physicians prefer to give IV fluids to every woman in active labor and allow only ice chips, while others allow clear liquids. Currently, more research is needed before updated recommendations can be made. The nurse is well advised to follow the practitioner's recommendations regarding food and fluid intake during labor.

process and how to avoid fighting against it. If the woman has not attended childbirth preparation classes, use this time to quickly teach basic relaxation techniques. Otherwise, review and reinforce breathing and relaxation techniques that the couple learned in class (refer to Chapter 9 for discussion of breathing and relaxation techniques).

The partner or coach needs encouragement regarding the importance of his or her role during labor. Give information regarding measures the woman may find comforting during each stage of labor, and encourage the partner to take breaks periodically to conserve energy for the duration of labor. Explain the importance of using the nurse as a resource and source of support for the partner and the woman throughout labor. Anxiety and fear are reduced and the labor process is enhanced if the woman knows what to expect and is supported during labor.

Evaluation: Goals and Expected Outcomes
- **Goal:** Fetal and maternal injury is avoided.
  Expected Outcomes: Maternal vital signs are stable.
  - Blood pressure is not elevated above baseline levels.
  - The woman is afebrile.
  - Fetal heart tones are within the expected range without decelerations or other signs of distress.
- **Goal:** The woman's anxiety is reduced.
  Expected Outcomes: She verbalizes confidence in her ability to cope with labor.
- **Goal:** The woman's pain is manageable.
  Expected Outcomes: She is relaxed and coping with contractions.
  - Demonstrates the use of effective strategies for coping with labor.
  - Expresses the ability to cope with her pain.
- **Goal:** The woman and her partner have adequate knowledge of the labor process.
  Expected Outcomes: The woman and her partner express realistic expectations regarding the duration, intensity, and process of labor.

Test Yourself

- What assessment findings would lead the nurse to keep the low-risk laboring woman on bed rest?
- Describe four important nursing interventions during the latent phase of labor.

Active Phase (Active Labor)

ASSESSMENT

Assess the woman's psychosocial state. Note if the woman is becoming more introverted, restless, or anxious; if she is feeling helpless or fears losing control; or if distraction techniques are failing to promote coping. These behaviors signal that the woman is moving into the active phase of labor.

Assessment of Labor Progress
During the active phase, evaluate the contraction pattern every 30 minutes. Typically, contractions occur every 2 to 5 minutes, last 45 to 60 seconds, and are of moderate to strong intensity. The cervix should dilate progressively from 4 to 8 cm. The fetus should descend steadily, although descent does not typically progress as rapidly as does cervical dilation. As the fetus descends below the level of the ischial spines, station is described in positive numbers. Plot cervical changes and fetal descent on a labor graph to evaluate labor progress. It is also critical to assess whether the uterus is relaxing completely between contractions. An adequate relaxation period allows for sufficient blood flow to the placenta and promotes oxygenation of the fetus.

Assessment of Fetal Status
Fetal status must be assessed and documented at least every 30 minutes. Record the baseline FHR every 30 minutes, and evaluate the strip for signs of distress. Variability should be present, except for brief periods of fetal sleep or when narcotics or other medications are administered, and no late decelerations should be present. Accelerations of the FHR are reassuring.

Assessment of Maternal Status
Maternal status should be assessed with the same frequency as fetal status. The woman becomes more introverted during active labor because the contractions are closer together, of a stronger intensity, and last longer than during early labor. Blood pressure may rise slightly but should be lower than 140/90 mm Hg. It is important to take the blood pressure between contractions because the stress of a uterine contraction can cause the blood pressure to rise briefly, resulting in an inaccurate measurement.

Pulse and respirations may also increase with the work of labor. Monitor for signs of tachycardia and hyperventilation. A falling blood pressure and a rising pulse could indicate the onset of shock and must be reported immediately. There are several labor complications that can cause shock, including hemorrhage or uterine rupture.

Assess the presence and character of pain at least hourly during active labor. Ask the woman to rate her pain on a standardized pain scale to make pain assessments measurable. Anxiety and tension often decrease the woman's ability to cope with contractions; therefore, it is important to document how the woman and her partner are coping and to determine if the coping strategies are helpful. For example, if the woman is using patterned breathing techniques to manage contractions, she may hyperventilate and need assistance to regain control of her breathing technique.

Evaluate breathing patterns frequently. Assess for signs of hyperventilation, which include tachypnea, feelings of light-headedness or dizziness, complaints of tingling around the mouth or in the fingers, and carpopedal spasms (Fig. 10-8).

Exercise caution! When the membranes rupture, whether it be spontaneously or artificially, check the FHR for 1 full minute immediately afterward. If fetal bradycardia occurs, or deep variable decelerations are noted on the EFM tracing, assist the woman to the knee-chest position and call the RN immediately to perform a vaginal examination to check for a prolapsed cord.

Check for dry cracked lips, thick saliva, and a coating on the tongue that may be caused by mouth breathing and lack of oral intake (if restricted). Measure the temperature every 4 hours if the water bag is intact and hourly after the membranes have ruptured. Mon-

● *Figure 10.8* Carpopedal spasms.

BOX 10.7 Danger Signs During Labor

If any of the following signs occur during labor, immediately notify the RN, physician, or nurse midwife.
- Elevated maternal blood pressure (BP) (≥140/90 mm Hg)
- Low or suddenly decreased maternal BP (≤90/50 mm Hg)
- Elevated maternal temperature (>100.4°F)
- Amniotic fluid that is green, cloudy, or foul smelling
- Nonreassuring FHR patterns
- Prolonged uterine contractions (>90 seconds duration)
- Failure of the uterus to relax between contractions
- Heavy or bright red bleeding
- Maternal reports of unrelenting pain, right upper quadrant pain, or visual changes

itor for signs of infection, such as elevated temperature, fetal and maternal tachycardia, and cloudy, foul-smelling amniotic fluid. Box 10-7 lists danger signs to watch for during labor.

SELECTED NURSING DIAGNOSES

- Risk for Trauma to the woman or fetus related to intrapartum complications or an undetected full bladder
- Acute Pain related to the process of labor
- Anxiety related to fear of losing control
- Ineffective Coping related to situational crisis of labor
- Ineffective Breathing Pattern: hyperventilation related to anxiety and/or inappropriate application of breathing techniques
- Impaired Oral Mucous Membrane related to dehydration and/or mouth breathing
- Risk for Infection related to invasive procedures (e.g., vaginal examinations) and/or rupture of amniotic membranes

OUTCOME IDENTIFICATION AND PLANNING

In addition to maintaining maternal and fetal safety during the active phase of the first stage of labor, appropriate goals may include that the laboring woman will verbalize her ability to cope with pain; exhibit lessened anxiety; demonstrate effective strategies for coping with labor; display effective breathing patterns; maintain an intact oral mucosa; and remain free of signs of infection.

IMPLEMENTATION

Preventing Trauma During Labor

It is important to continue to closely monitor the fetus during active labor. Any signs of fetal distress that do not respond to position changes should be reported immediately. Abnormal vital signs should also be reported. Immediately report heavy bleeding or failure of the uterus to relax well between contractions.

Another source of trauma that can interfere with the progress of labor is a full bladder. Every 2 hours palpate the area just above the symphysis pubis feeling for a rounded area of distention, which indicates the bladder is full. Failure of the fetus to descend is another sign that the bladder might be full. Offer the bedpan every 2 hours or assist the woman to the restroom, if allowed. If the woman is unable to void, perform a sterile in-and-out catheterization procedure.

Providing Pain Management

The active phase of labor is the time when pain relief measures are most often implemented. Epidural anesthesia may be initiated, or narcotic analgesia may be administered (pain relief options are discussed in greater detail in Chapter 9); however, it is critical to respect the woman's preferences for pain control. If the woman desires a natural childbirth, you will be challenged to provide intensive support throughout the active phase of labor.

Implementing general comfort measures can help to manage the pain and discomfort of labor. Work closely with the coach to demonstrate distraction and relaxation techniques, such as effleurage, back rubs, or application of pressure to the lower back during contractions, as discussed in Chapter 9. A cool, damp washcloth to the forehead is often comforting.

Linens and gowns are soiled frequently during active labor with perspiration, amniotic fluid, and bloody show. Linen savers, such as chucks or other under-buttocks pads, should be placed under the hips and replaced as needed. Provide frequent perineal care. At a minimum, perineal care should be done after any invasive procedure involving the vagina and after elimination.

Reducing Anxiety

During active labor, assist the woman and her partner to implement the anxiety reduction plan that was agreed upon during early labor. Continue to encourage the woman to verbalize her concerns. If her chosen method of pain relief is not working, remind her that she can change her mind about pain relief options. You may need to repeat earlier instruction and reassure the couple that it does not represent a failure on the woman's part if she chooses an alternate method of pain management. If she starts to lose control, assist the labor coach to use verbal cues and position changes to help the laboring woman regain control.

Promoting Effective Coping Strategies

It is important to support the woman and her partner in their attempts to cope. Some women do not benefit from the use of patterned breathing techniques. Frequently these women will develop personalized "rituals" to help them cope with contractions.

A **ritual** is a routine; a repeated series of actions that the woman uses as an individualized way of dealing with the discomfort of labor. For example, one woman might find it helpful to close her eyes and attempt to visualize a peaceful scene during contractions. Another woman might involve her partner by squeezing his hands throughout each contraction. Still another woman might assume a particular position during contractions. As long as these creative approaches to coping are helpful, encourage and support their use. When the ritual is not working to promote adaptation, assist the woman in trying other approaches.

Here's a helpful hint. Vigorous application of breathing techniques can lead to hyperventilation. Hyperventilation can cause respiratory alkalosis. Breathing into a paper bag retains CO_2, reverses alkalosis, and relieves associated symptoms.

Promoting Effective Breathing Patterns

Frequently reinforce breathing techniques appropriate to the active phase of labor (see Chapter 9). Often it helps to make eye contact and perform the breathing patterns with the woman during her contraction to help keep her focused (Fig. 10-9). If hyperventilation occurs, breathing into cupped hands or a paper bag usually relieves the problem.

Maintaining Integrity of the Oral Mucosa

Frequent mouth care stimulates saliva production, which helps to keep the oral mucosa moist. Suggest that the woman brush her teeth or gargle with normal saline when her mouth feels dry. Chewing gum also stimulates saliva production and leaves a pleasant taste in the mouth. Providing ice chips, sips of clear liquids, flavored ice, or hard candy (if allowed) can be soothing. Lip balm is comforting if the lips are dry or chapped. If the

● **Figure 10.9** The nurse instructs the labor coach to maintain eye contact and breathe with his partner during contractions to help keep her focused. Photo by Joe Mitchell.

woman does not have lip balm, the water-soluble lubricant available in most labor rooms can be used to moisten the lips.

Preventing Infection

Handwashing remains the number one way to prevent the spread of infection. Wash your hands thoroughly be- fore and after providing care. Encourage the woman and her partner to wash their hands before and after any contact with the perineum and after using the restroom.

Frequent vaginal examinations are discouraged, particularly if the membranes are ruptured. Nursing judgment is indicated to determine frequency. Usually it is best not to examine the cervix unless there is a clear indication that labor is progressing. Assist the examiner to maintain sterile technique when it becomes necessary to perform a vaginal examination.

Invasive procedures, such as the application of an internal fetal monitor or insertion of a urinary catheter, should be kept to a minimum and done only if there are clear indications for their use. Strict adherence to sterile technique when performing an invasive procedure is critical.

Check out this tip. A full bladder may interfere with fetal descent. Encourage the woman to void at least every 2 hours during labor.

EVALUATION: GOALS AND EXPECTED OUTCOMES

- **Goal:** Fetal and maternal trauma is avoided.
  Expected Outcomes: Maternal vital signs are stable.
  - Blood pressure is not elevated above baseline levels.

- The woman is afebrile.
- Bladder distention does not occur.
- The uterus is relaxing well between contractions.
- Fetal heart tones are within the expected range without decelerations or other signs of distress.
- **Goal:** Pain is manageable.
  Expected Outcomes: The woman is relaxed and coping with contractions.
  - States that the pain of labor is tolerable.
  - States pain relief techniques are effective.
- **Goal:** Anxiety is reduced.
  Expected Outcomes: The woman reports decreased anxiety.
- **Goal:** Coping is effective.
  Expected Outcomes: The woman demonstrates individualized rituals to cope with labor.
  - Uses social supports (partner, coach, relative, or doula) to help cope with labor.
- **Goal:** Breathing techniques are effective.
  Expected Outcomes: The woman uses slow and accelerated breathing techniques during contractions.
  - Does not hyperventilate.
- **Goal:** Oral mucosa remains intact.
  Expected Outcomes: Lips and mucous membranes remain moist and intact.
- **Goal:** Exhibits no signs of infection.
  Expected Outcomes: The woman remains afebrile.
  - White blood cell count remains within expected limits.
  - Amniotic fluid remains clear and odorless.
  - No foul-smelling drainage.
  - No fetal tachycardia.

Test Yourself

- Why is it important for the laboring woman to void frequently?
- What assessment findings are associated with the nursing diagnosis Ineffective Breathing Pattern: hyperventilation?
- List five nursing interventions appropriate for the active phase of labor.

Transition Phase

ASSESSMENT

Assess for signs that the woman has reached the transition phase of the first stage of labor. Look for an increase in the amount of bloody show and a strong urge to push if fetal station is low. It is important to assess the woman's ability to cope. She will often express irritability, restlessness, and will feel out of control. She may tremble, vomit, or cry. It is important to assess for hyperventilation during this phase.

Do you know the why of it?

Nausea and vomiting are common occurrences during labor because of decreased gut peristalsis and delayed gastric emptying time. If vomiting occurs, assist the woman to turn to her side to help prevent aspiration.

Check the contraction pattern at least once every 30 minutes; contractions should occur every 2 to 3 minutes, last 60 to 90 seconds, and be of strong intensity. The uterus should relax completely between uterine contractions. Cervical examination during transition re-veals dilation between 8 and 10 cm.

It is important to continue to evaluate fetal status at least every 30 minutes. The FHR baseline should remain between 110 and 160 bpm and should not significantly increase or decrease. It may be normal to see variable decelerations as the fetal head descends. Variability should be present. There should be no late decelerations or other signs of fetal distress.

SELECTED NURSING DIAGNOSES

- Acute Pain related to intense uterine contractions and pressure of the descending fetal head
- Ineffective Breathing Pattern: hyperventilation related to intense uterine contractions and loss of control of breathing techniques
- Powerlessness related to intensity of the labor process
- Fatigue related to energy expended coping with the intensity of labor

OUTCOME IDENTIFICATION AND PLANNING

Major goals for the transition phase of the first stage of labor include that the woman's pain will be manageable; she will exhibit effective breathing patterns; she will maintain a sense of control; and she will rest between uterine contractions.

IMPLEMENTATION

Managing Pain

The woman should be assured that although this period of labor is the most intense, it is usually short in duration. Narcotics are not given at this advanced stage of labor to prevent delivery of a neonate who is too sleepy to take his first breath. Continue to assist the coach to provide comfort and support during uterine contractions. Frequent position changes, breathing with the woman during contractions, and providing other comfort measures may help decrease the intensity of the pain stimulus.

Promoting Effective Breathing Patterns

If the woman has been trained in patterned breathing techniques, encourage her to switch to a more advanced technique when the pattern she is using is no longer working. Assist the coach to breathe with her and to assess for signs of hyperventilation. She may feel the urge to push. Explain the importance of resisting the urge to push until the cervix is fully dilated.

This advice could save the day. If the woman is feeling a strong urge to push, assist her to blow at the peak of the contraction when the urge is most intense. Pushing efforts before the cervix is fully dilated can result in cervical lacerations or can cause edema of the cervix and slow dilatation.

Promoting a Sense of Control

Accepting behavioral changes of the laboring woman is an important nursing intervention during this forceful period of labor. You will need to provide intensive psychological support. If the woman falls asleep between contractions, awaken her at the beginning of a contraction so that she can begin her coping strategy before the contraction reaches full intensity.

Supporting the Woman Through Fatigue

Relaxing with contractions may be almost impossible; assist the woman to achieve relaxation or even sleep between contractions. Help her to find a position that is comfortable. Support her position with pillows. Placing a cool cloth to her forehead or giving her a back rub may help her relax between contractions (Fig. 10-10). Some women find music to be soothing. When she is able to relax between contractions she conserves energy that she will need during the next stage in order to push effectively. The partner/coach is often fatigued as well; encourage him or her to take breaks as necessary.

Preparing the Room for Delivery

Often the nurse prepares the room for delivery during the transition phase (Fig. 10-11). Many delivery units have physician preference cards so that the nurse can prepare the equipment and

● *Figure 10.10* The labor coach provides comfort measures, such as a cool washcloth to the face and forehead, to help the woman relax as much as possible during the transition phase of labor. © B. Proud.

supplies most often needed by the attending physician. Prepare the table maintaining surgical asepsis so that a sterile field is available during delivery. It is important to ensure that supplies and medications needed for the birth are readily available. Check the infant resuscitation area and replace any missing supplies or malfunctioning equipment.

EVALUATION: GOALS AND EXPECTED OUTCOMES

- **Goal:** The woman's pain is manageable.
  Expected Outcomes: She tolerates the pain of contractions and pressure from the fetal head without pushing.
- **Goal:** The woman's breathing pattern is effective.

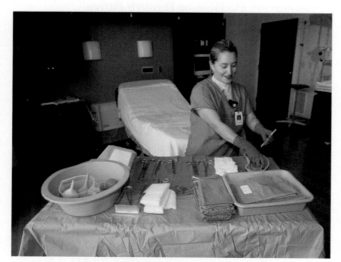

● *Figure 10.11* The nurse prepares the labor room for delivery. Photo by Joe Mitchell.

Expected Outcomes: She uses accelerated breathing techniques during contractions.
- Does not hyperventilate.
- **Goal:** The woman maintains a sense of control.
  Expected Outcomes: She expresses ability to deal with contractions.
- **Goal:** The woman rests between uterine contractions.
  Expected Outcomes: She sleeps or rests with eyes closed between uterine contractions.
  - Remains quiet and calm between uterine contractions.

Test Yourself

- Discuss the five signs associated with the transition phase of labor.

- What responsibilities does the nurse have for supporting the partner or coach?

- Why is it important that the woman refrain from pushing until the cervix is completely dilated?

● The Nursing Process During the Second Stage of Labor: Expulsion of the Fetus

The second stage of labor begins when the cervix is 10 cm dilated and 100% effaced and ends with the birth of the newborn. Nursing care during this stage of labor focuses on providing physical and psychological support to the woman while she pushes the fetus through the birth canal. Assessment of maternal and fetal well-being during this stage is crucial.

ASSESSMENT

During the second stage of labor, close observation of the laboring woman and her fetus is indicated. Monitor the blood pressure, pulse, and respirations every 15 to 30 minutes. Cervical examination reveals that the cervix is fully dilated (10 cm) and completely effaced. The fetal station is usually 0 to + 2.

Assess the contraction pattern every 15 minutes. The pattern will be similar to that found in the transition phase (i.e., contractions occur every 2 to 3 minutes, last 60 to 90 seconds, and are of strong intensity). Assess for the woman's report of an uncontrollable urge to push, which is caused by pressure from the descending fetal head.

Assessment of the fetus during the second stage is essential. As the fetus descends into the pelvis, the pressure on his head is very intense. There may also be pressure on the cord during contractions. It is not uncommon for the fetal monitor strip to reveal early or variable decelerations. Variables are usually not ominous at this stage as long as the FHR returns quickly to baseline as the contraction relaxes, the baseline remains between 110 and 160 bpm, and variability is present. Check the FHR every 15 minutes for low-risk women and every 5 minutes for women determined to be at risk for labor complications.

Evaluate the woman's psychosocial status; the laboring woman may find it less difficult to cope with the contractions now that she can push. Often she is less irritable and more cooperative. Assess the woman's level of fatigue. If the second stage is prolonged, she may become extremely fatigued and experience difficulty finding the energy to push.

SELECTED NURSING DIAGNOSES

- Fatigue related to pushing efforts
- Risk for Trauma related to pushing techniques and positioning for delivery.

OUTCOME IDENTIFICATION AND PLANNING

Appropriate goals for the second stage of labor include that the woman will push effectively despite fatigue and that she will give birth with minimal or no trauma to the fetus and herself.

IMPLEMENTATION

Promoting Effective Pushing Despite Fatigue
All of the comfort measures appropriate to active labor continue to apply during the second stage, particularly while the woman is pushing. Using comfort measures such as applying a cool cloth to the forehead and offering ice chips and mouth care can promote relaxation between contractions, which helps to conserve energy and prevent exhaustion.

Assist the woman to the chosen position for pushing and provide support throughout each pushing effort. For instance, if the woman is using the sitting position to push, the nurse and coach can assist her to the sitting position when the contraction starts and support her back while she pushes.

If the woman has experienced a prolonged labor and is having a difficult time pushing effectively, it may be appropriate to position her on her side for comfort and allow her to rest for 30 minutes to an hour in order to regain her strength. As long as there is no evidence of fetal distress on the monitor tracing, allowing for a break from pushing is acceptable. In fact, if the woman is able to push more effectively after the break, often the fetus will descend and birth will occur soon afterward.

Reducing the Risk for Trauma: Using Effective Pushing Techniques and Positions
The LPN assists the RN to ensure the safety of mother and baby during the second stage by promoting effective pushing techniques and positions for pushing.

Effective Pushing Techniques. Once the cervix is fully dilated, the woman can begin pushing

A PERSONAL GLIMPSE

After 2 days of doctors trying to induce labor, I was about ready to request a cesarean section. Although I truly desired a vaginal birth, my husband and I were at our wits' end after having tried every measure available to start labor. During those frustrating days, the nurses I had were so supportive. They encouraged me to think positively and hold onto hope that I would eventually have a vaginal birth. When I was finally able to push, my labor and delivery nurse, Mary Ellen, was so supportive. Somehow, she convinced me that every push was the first one. With her gentle guidance, I believed I could get my baby out, even when it seemed it would never happen. I will never forget how helpful and tender she was. She told me time and again that I was "almost there" while my doctor shook his head in disagreement. Having spent more time with Mary Ellen than with the doctor who would eventually deliver my child, I believed her assessment far more than his! I don't think I even remember his name, but I will always remember Mary Ellen for her reassurance and gentle care.

Sara

LEARNING OPPORTUNITY: Describe three supportive nursing behaviors that can encourage a woman to not give up when labor seems overwhelming.

Why do you think the nurse's support is beneficial to prevent unnecessary cesarean deliveries?

efforts. Traditionally, obstetric nurses have taught women to use vigorous pushing techniques. When **vigorous pushing** is used, the woman is told to take a deep breath, hold the breath and push while counting to 10. She is encouraged to complete three "good" pushes in this manner with each contraction. However, recent research has revealed that vigorous pushing techniques that employ the Valsalva maneuver are associated with changes in the mother's heart rate and blood pressure, and the FHR may be adversely affected.

Based on research, two natural forms of pushing are advocated: open-glottis pushing and the urge-to-push method. Encourage the woman to use **open-glottis pushing,** which is characterized by pushing with contractions using an open glottis so that air is released during the pushing effort.

Watch out! When the mother is pushing effectively, delivery can occur rapidly. Monitor for signs of imminent delivery, which include grunting, bulging of the perineum, crowning of the fetal head, and exclamation that "the baby is coming!"

The nurse also may encourage the woman to use the **urge-to-push method,** in which the woman bears down only when she feels the urge to do so using any technique that feels right for her. No matter what pushing technique is used, never leave the woman alone during pushing efforts.

Positions for Pushing. There are many different positions that are acceptable for pushing and for delivering the baby. However, in this country most deliveries are accomplished in a modified dorsal recumbent position in which the woman's legs are on foot pedals and the head of the bed is elevated approximately 45 degrees. Occasionally the practitioner will ask for the legs to be positioned in stirrups (lithotomy position). The nurse removes the bottom part of the bed to allow easy access to the perineum. Dorsal recumbent and lithotomy positions allow for greater control by the attendant but are not necessarily the most comfortable or effective positions for enhancing delivery.

Don't forget! Prevention of supine hypotension remains a priority during delivery. If a lithotomy position is used, place a wedge under the woman's hip to tilt the uterus away from the major vessels.

One major disadvantage of the lithotomy position is that gravity is not used to assist the birth.

● *Figure 10.12* Bulging of the perineum is an indicator of imminent delivery. © B. Proud.

Other positions use gravity to aid in the pushing process, which conserves energy during the second stage of labor. Some positions, such as hands and knees, encourage rotation of the fetus, which shortens the second stage of labor. The hands and knees position enhances blood flow to the placenta, resulting in less fetal distress. Table 10-3 illustrates and compares positions used for pushing and delivery of the baby.

Preparing for Delivery of the Newborn
Nursing judgment is necessary to decide when to prepare the woman for delivery. The nurse may observe bulging of the perineum or crowning of the fetal head, which indicate imminent delivery (Fig. 10-12). Preparation of the primipara is typically done when the fetus is crowning, whereas preparation of the multipara may be done when the fetus reaches a +2 or +3 station. However, preparation may be done sooner in both cases if the fetus is descending rapidly.

If the woman has been laboring in a birthing bed and the semisitting or lithotomy position is to be used for delivery, the bed is "broken"—the lower part of the bed is removed to allow room for the birth attendant to control the delivery. Often the woman's feet are placed on foot pedals. If stirrups are used, take care to position the stirrups properly, then lift both legs together and place them in the stirrups. Clean the woman's perineum with an antiseptic solution (Fig. 10-13, p. 243); often a Betadine scrub is used. Position the instrument table close to the birthing bed and uncover it. If necessary, an in-and-out catheterization of the urinary bladder is done.

Prepare the equipment necessary to receive the baby in anticipation of the birth. This preparation involves turning on the radiant warmer and placing a warm blanket under the warmer. Be sure that the forms to begin the baby's chart

TABLE 10.3	Comparison of Positions for Pushing and Delivery

Position	Advantages	Disadvantages
Lithotomy: This was the position used by the majority of physicians in the 1960s to 1980s. It is still used occasionally. The woman is positioned on a flat delivery bed with her legs in stirrups.	Easy access to the perineum and greater control of delivery by birth attendant	Greater risk of supine hypotensive syndrome and positioning injuries (e.g., clot formation from compression or muscle strain from improper placement in stirrups)
Modified dorsal recumbent or semi-sitting: This is a common pushing position. When it is time for delivery, the woman's feet are placed on foot pedals and the birthing bed is "broken" in preparation for delivery.	Easy access to the perineum and good control of delivery by birth attendant	May be uncomfortable for the woman. May not be the best position to facilitate expulsion of the baby.
Side-lying	May increase comfort of the woman.	Decreases access to the perineum by the birth attendant. Requires high degree of cooperation from the woman and possible assistance of the nurse or support person to hold the upper leg during delivery.

(table continues on page 242)

TABLE 10.3 (continued)	Comparison of Positions for Pushing and Delivery	
Position	Advantages	Disadvantages

Squatting

Highly likely to increase the comfort of the woman. Uses gravity to facilitate expulsion of the baby.

Difficult access to the perineum. Requires a birth attendant who is flexible and willing to use this approach. The woman may lose her balance in this position. A pushing bar can help maintain balance, or a birthing stool may be used.

Hands and knees: The woman is assisted to her hands and knees on the birthing bed to push and deliver the baby.

Encourages rotation of the fetal head, which hastens delivery. Enhances placental blood flow, which decreases fetal stress. Allows for the perineum to stretch better than other positions so that an episiotomy is less often required. Allows for greater access to the perineum by the birth attendant than some of the other alternative positions.

May be more tiring for the woman. Does not allow for the use of instruments to assist delivery.

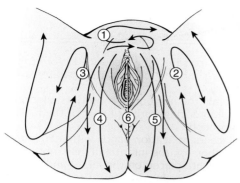

● **Figure 10.13** Perineal scrub in preparation for delivery. An antiseptic solution is used to clean the perineum just before delivery. The numbers represent the order in which each stroke is completed. The arrows represent the direction of the scrub. A new sponge is used for each stroke.

are in the room, and check the resuscitation equipment once more before delivery.

The RN is responsible for overseeing events in the delivery room. Surgical terms are used to describe the role of the RN; therefore, she is referred to as the circulator. The RN should remain in the delivery room until after the infant is born, the placenta is delivered, and mother and baby are stable. Box 10-8 lists the major responsibilities of the nurse in the delivery room, including immediate care of the newborn (see Chapters 13 and 15 for comprehensive coverage of newborn care). Figure 10-14 (pp. 246–247) shows a delivery sequence from crowning through birth of the newborn.

This advice could be a life-saver! The risk of splashing of bodily fluids is high during a delivery. Strictly follow universal precautions. Eye shields, gowns, and gloves may be necessary for protection from contact with bodily fluids.

EVALUATION: GOALS AND EXPECTED OUTCOMES

- **Goal:** The woman will push effectively despite fatigue.
  Expected Outcomes: She maintains the energy to push effectively with contractions.
  - The partner or coach retains a supportive, active participant role.
- **Goal:** Trauma to the woman and her fetus are avoided.
  Expected Outcomes: Maternal vital signs remain stable.
  - Fetal heart rate remains within acceptable limits.

● The Nursing Process During the Third Stage of Labor: Delivery of Placenta

The third stage of labor begins with the birth of the newborn and ends with delivery of the placenta. Nursing care during this stage of labor focuses on monitoring for placental separation and providing physical and psychological care to the woman.

ASSESSMENT

Assess the woman's psychosocial state after she gives birth. Immediately after birth the new mother often experiences a sense of relief that the birth has been accomplished and contractions have ceased. Monitor for signs of placental separation, which generally occur within 5 to 20 minutes of delivery. These signs begin with a uterine contraction, then the fundus rises in the abdomen, the uterus takes on a globular shape, blood begins to steadily trickle from the vagina, and the umbilical cord lengthens as the placenta separates from the uterine wall.

The placenta may deliver in one of two ways (Fig. 10-15, p. 246). The most common way is for the smooth, shiny fetal side to deliver first (Schultze's mechanism). Sometimes the edge of the placenta appears at the introitus, revealing the rough maternal surface (Duncan's mechanism). The latter mechanism of delivery is more frequently associated with retained placental fragments. After the placenta is delivered, the birth attendant inspects it for completeness. Palpate the fundus to make certain the uterus is well contracted, and monitor the perineum for excess bleeding.

SELECTED NURSING DIAGNOSES

- Risk for Deficient Fluid Volume related to blood loss in the intrapartum period
- Risk for Trauma: Hemorrhage, amniotic fluid embolism, or uterine inversion related to separation of the placenta during the third stage of labor

BOX 10.8	Responsibilities of the Nurse in the Delivery Room

Closely monitor the laboring woman.
- Record vital signs and status assessments per facility protocol.
- Assess for maternal response to anesthesia.

Closely monitor the fetus. Assess FHR
- Every 15 minutes for low-risk labors.
- Every 5 minutes for at-risk labors.

Maintain accurate delivery room records.
- Note and record the time of delivery.
- Record all nursing procedures performed and maternal/newborn response.

Provide immediate newborn care (refer to Chapters 13 and 15 for in-depth discussion of newborn adaptation and care).
- Maintain warmth.
  - Immediately dry the newborn on the woman's abdomen or under the radiant warmer.
  - Wrap the newborn snugly and place a cap on the head when not in skin-to-skin contact with the woman or when not under a warmer.
- Assess adaptation to extrauterine life.
  - Assess and record Apgar scores (see Chapter 15 for a discussion of Apgar scoring).
- Maintain a patent airway.
  - Position the newborn to facilitate drainage.
  - Suction secretions with a bulb suction device or with wall suction.

- Provide for safety and security. Before the newborn and the mother are separated after delivery
  - Obtain the newborn's footprints and mother's thumb or fingerprint (if part of the facility protocol).
  - Place identification bands with matching numbers on the infant and new mother. Two bands are placed on the infant and one on the new mother. In some facilities a band is also placed on the new father or support person.

Promote parental-newborn bonding.
- Allow/encourage the woman and her partner to hold the newborn.
- Allow/encourage breast-feeding immediately after delivery.
- Encourage skin-to-skin contact with the newborn.
- Point out positive characteristics of the newborn.

Assist the birth attendant.
- Perform sponge and instrument counts.
- Ensure that supplies are available for episiotomy and repair, if needed.
- Obtain additional supplies as needed, such as forceps or vacuum extractor for difficult deliveries, or extra suturing material.

OUTCOME IDENTIFICATION AND PLANNING

The major goals during the third stage of labor are that the new mother will maintain adequate fluid volume and that she will remain free of trauma.

IMPLEMENTATION

Preventing Fluid Loss

Monitor the woman's vital signs at least every 15 minutes during the third stage of labor to detect signs of dehydration. Tachycardia and a falling blood pressure are signs of impending shock and should be reported immediately. Note how much time has passed since the birth of the newborn. The placenta normally separates within 20 minutes of delivery. If a longer period of time has passed, the woman may be experiencing retained placenta, which can lead to acute fluid loss from hemorrhage. Monitor intravenous fluids to ensure patency and prevent the development of dehydration.

Maintaining Safety and Preventing Trauma

Monitor the woman for any sudden change in status. Complaints of shortness of breath, chest pain, or tachypnea may indicate the development of an amniotic fluid embolism (a discussion of this complication is found in Chapter 18).

Administer oxytocin as soon as the placenta is delivered. Oxytocin causes the uterus to contract, which puts pressure on the open blood vessels at the former placenta site. When the placenta separates from the uterine wall, it leaves an open wound that is subject to hemorrhage if the uterus does not contract effectively. Oxytocin is most frequently added to the IV fluids, but some physicians and midwives prefer that it be given using the intramuscular method. It is important not to give an oxytocic medication before the placenta is delivered because the drug given at this time will increase the risk of a retained placenta.

EVALUATION: GOALS AND EXPECTED OUTCOMES

- **Goal:** The woman will maintain an adequate fluid volume.
  Expected Outcomes: Blood pressure does not fall and the pulse does not rise.
- **Goal:** The woman remains free of trauma.
  Expected Outcomes: The placenta is delivered intact with less than 500 milliliters of blood loss.
  - Respirations remain unlabored.
  - Lung sounds are clear.
  - Fundus remains firm.

A

B

C

D

E

F

● **Figure 10.14** Delivery sequence from crowning through birth of the newborn. (**A**) Early crowning of the fetal head. Notice the bulging of the perineum. (**B**) Late crowning. Notice that the fetal head is appearing face down. This is the normal OA position. (**C**) As the head extends, you can see that the occiput is to the mother's right side—ROA position. (**D**) The cardinal movement of extension. (**E**) The shoulders are born. Notice how the head has turned to line up with the shoulders—the cardinal movement of external rotation. (**F**) The body easily follows the shoulders.

(figure continues on page 246)

G

● ***Figure 10.14*** (continued) (**G**) The newborn is held for the first time! © B. Proud.

A

B

● ***Figure 10.15*** A healthy placenta after delivery. (**A**). Notice the shiny surface of the fetal side. The umbilical cord is inserted in the center of the fetal surface. (**B**). The maternal side is rough and divided into segments (cotyledons). Photos by Joe Mitchell.

● The Nursing Process During the Fourth Stage of Labor

The fourth stage of labor begins with delivery of the placenta and ends when the woman's physical condition has stabilized (usually within 2 hours). Nursing care during this stage focuses on continued assessment and care of the woman and promoting parental–newborn bonding.

ASSESSMENT

Continue to assess the woman for hemorrhage during the fourth stage of labor. The new mother is at highest risk for hemorrhage during the first 2 to 4 hours of the postpartum period. Monitor the woman's vital signs, and palpate the fundus for position and firmness. The fundus should be well contracted, at the midline, and approximately one fingerbreadth below the umbilicus immediately after delivery. Assess the **lochia** (vaginal discharge after birth) for color and quantity. The lochia should be dark red and of a small to moderate amount.

Monitor for signs of infection. The temperature may be elevated slightly, as great as 100.4°F, because of mild dehydration and the stress of delivery. Any elevation above that level may indicate infection and should be reported. The lochia should have a fleshy odor but should not be foul smelling.

The woman should void within 6 hours after delivery. Trauma from the birth may have caused edema in the perineal area or anesthesia may persist, leading to an inability to sense a full bladder. Both conditions can lead to urinary retention. Monitor for suprapubic distention and a high fundus that is displaced to the right. These signs indicate that the urinary bladder is full.

Assess the woman's comfort level. There are many sources of pain during the immediate postpartum period. Cramping from uterine contractions and perineal pain from edema or episiotomy repair are common sources of pain for the new mother. Ask the woman to describe the location of the pain and to rate it on a standardized pain scale.

Assess the mother's psychosocial state during the fourth stage. Typically, the mother is fatigued and ravenously hungry. It is normal for her to be self-absorbed and demonstrate dependent behaviors. She also has an intense need to talk about the labor and delivery experience.

Assess initial bonding behaviors of the new family. It is normal for parents to want to hold and touch the newborn as soon as it is born. You may notice that the parent begins initial inspection of the newborn with the fingertips; this is normal behavior and indicates positive beginning attachment.

Be careful not to be too hasty to diagnose inadequate bonding. Some mothers are so fatigued that they may not desire prolonged interaction with the newborn beyond the initial inspection. Behaviors that indicate a risk for inadequate attachment include turning away from the newborn or making disparaging comments about the newborn.

Perhaps this advice will be useful. Many nurses use a numbered scale from 0 to 10 to assess their patients for pain. Explain that "0" indicates no pain, whereas "10" indicates the worst pain imaginable, and then ask the woman to choose a number that most closely matches her pain level. In this way you can easily evaluate the effectiveness of your interventions by asking her to rate her pain again on the same scale after intervening.

SELECTED NURSING DIAGNOSES

- Risk for Impaired Parent–Infant Attachment related to disappointment regarding the gender of the newborn or an unwanted pregnancy
- Risk for Deficient Fluid Volume related to possibility of hemorrhage from the former site of placenta attachment
- Risk for Infection related to invasive procedures and vaginal examinations during labor
- Impaired Urinary Elimination related to perineal trauma during delivery
- Acute Pain related to episiotomy, birth trauma, and/or afterpains
- Fatigue related to energy expended during labor

OUTCOME IDENTIFICATION AND PLANNING

Appropriate goals for the new mother during the fourth stage of labor (recovery) are that the parents will begin a positive bonding process with their newborn, and that the woman will maintain adequate fluid volume, remain without signs of infection, fully empty the bladder at the first voiding, report a tolerable pain level, and report the ability to rest and sleep during the immediate postpartum period.

IMPLEMENTATION

Providing Care Immediately After Delivery

After the birth attendant has completed his or her duties, inspect and cleanse the perineum. Remove the soiled drapes and linen and place an absorbent pad under the buttocks with two sterile perineal pads against the perineum. Place a warm blanket over the new mother. Reassemble the birthing bed. If stirrups were used, remove both legs from the stirrups at the same time.

Promoting Parent–Newborn Attachment

While the birth attendant is suturing any lacerations or episiotomy and making a final inspection of maternal tissues, it is important to promote parental bonding with the newborn. Hand the newborn to the woman as soon as it is determined that he does not need extraordinary resuscitation. If the father is present at the delivery, encourage him to hold and interact with the newborn (Fig. 10-16). This is a good time for the new mother to attempt breast-feeding for the first time. If the woman permits it, place the newborn skin-to-skin against her body and place several blankets over them. This technique (called kangaroo care) keeps the infant warm and promotes bonding.

Maintaining Adequate Fluid Volume

Continue to monitor the woman for signs of fluid volume deficit or hemorrhage. Take vital signs every 15 minutes during the fourth stage of labor. Falling blood pressure and tachycardia may indicate fluid volume deficit or hemorrhage and should be reported. Massage the fundus

● **Figure 10.16** The father and mother bond with their newborn son soon after birth.

every 15 minutes and inspect the lochia for amount and color. The fundus should be firm or should quickly become firm when gently massaged. Continue to monitor IV fluids and offer food and fluids to the new mother.

Preventing Infection

Continue to use excellent handwashing technique. Hands should be washed before and after care, between patients, and any time bodily fluids are contacted. Of course, it is critical to use standard precautions. Wear gloves at all times when you perform procedures anywhere near the perineum or dirty linens. Anything that comes in direct contact with the perineum should be sterile. The perineal pads should be handled from the ends and not touched in the middle area.

Promoting Urinary Elimination

If the woman has the urge to void, assist her to the bathroom unless she is still under the effects of anesthesia and does not have complete control of her legs. It is much easier for her to void sitting on a toilet than it is on a bedpan. Have her dangle her feet at the bedside for several minutes before assisting her to a standing position. Once she is safely in the bathroom, run water or let her soak her hands in warm water if she is having difficulty getting the stream of urine started. An in-and-out catheterization is usually not done unless there is significant suprapubic distention or discomfort from the full bladder or until 6 hours have passed without voiding.

Minimizing Pain

Nonsteroidal anti-inflammatory drugs (NSAIDs) and oral narcotic analgesics, such as codeine, often are prescribed for pain after delivery. The NSAIDs are quite effective at reducing painful uterine cramping. Many providers order large doses (600 to 800 mg) of ibuprofen to be given every 6 to 8 hours around the clock. This type of dosing is often more effective at keeping pain under control than is an "as needed" schedule, in which the woman must ask for the medication before it is given.

Combination medications consisting of a mild analgesic, such as acetaminophen, with a narcotic such as codeine, may be ordered on an as-needed basis for breakthrough pain. Sometimes codeine is ordered for perineal pain, and the NSAIDs are given to control cramping. Assess the woman's pain frequently and administer medications before the pain becomes intolerable.

Warmth to the abdomen may be helpful in reducing the discomfort of uterine cramping. Position changes may also be helpful. If the pain is

Watch out! Extreme perineal pain may indicate the development of a perineal hematoma. Inspect the perineum with each vital sign check. Inquire further regarding perineal pain if the new mother becomes restless, is unable to find a comfortable position, tilts to one side when sitting, or reports unbearable pain in the perineum. The RN in charge should be notified immediately if any of these signs is present.

from an episiotomy or edema of the perineum, it is helpful to apply ice packs. Most labor units have combination perineal pads/ice packs. These are convenient for the nurse, but a clean glove filled with ice also works as an ice pack. If used, it should be applied between the two perineal pads so that a nonsterile object does not come in direct contact with the perineum.

Reducing Fatigue

After the initial bonding period, it may be helpful to discourage visitors and promote rest for the new mother. Her partner can stay with her to care for the newborn if the newborn is rooming-in or if the hospital provides couplet care. If the newborn is to be stabilized in a newborn nursery, this is a good time for both the new mother and her partner to get some much-needed rest and sleep, if possible.

EVALUATION: GOALS AND EXPECTED OUTCOMES

- **Goal:** The parents begin a positive bonding process.
  Expected Outcomes: They inspect the newborn immediately after birth.
  - They make positive comments about the newborn.
- **Goal:** The woman maintains an adequate fluid volume.
  Expected Outcomes: Blood pressure and pulse remain within expected limits.
  - Fundus remains firm.
  - Vaginal bleeding remains small.
- **Goal:** The woman remains free of signs of infection.
  Expected Outcomes: She remains afebrile.
  - Lochia has a normal fleshy odor and is not malodorous.
- **Goal:** The woman empties her bladder effectively.
  Expected Outcomes: She expresses the ability to void without difficulty.
  - No suprapubic distention.

- **Goal:** The woman expresses a tolerable pain level.
  Expected Outcomes: She reports that interventions are effective at relieving pain.
- **Goal:** The woman avoids extreme fatigue.
  Expected Outcomes: She reports the ability to rest and sleep in the immediate postpartum period.

Test Yourself

- Identify four signs of placental separation.

- How often are vital signs checked during the fourth stage of labor?

- Name three parameters that should be assessed with each vital sign check during the fourth stage of labor.

KEY POINTS

- Continuous support of a skilled obstetric nurse facilitates the labor process and the woman's satisfaction with the birth experience.

- Throughout the labor process, the nurse is responsible for monitoring maternal and fetal status and labor progress. Frequent assessment of vital signs and FHR are critical nursing functions.

- When a woman arrives at the labor unit, immediate assessment involves observing for signs that birth is imminent, in which case admission procedures are abbreviated until after delivery.

- If the birth is not imminent, admission assessment includes a thorough obstetric, medical–surgical, and social history and a complete physical assessment. Fetal, maternal, and labor statuses are determined, and a report is made to the birth attendant.

- Intermittent auscultation of FHR allows for freedom of maternal movement and focuses the nurse's attention on the woman, rather than the technology. Disadvantages are that subtle signs of fetal distress may be missed.

- External fetal monitoring is noninvasive and allows for evaluation of baseline FHR and long-term variability. However, it is less precise than internal monitoring, which can detect short-term variability and provides a more consistent tracing. Internal monitoring requires that the membranes be ruptured and the cervix be at least partially dilated.

- To apply the fetal monitor, first locate the fetal back, and then apply the transducer using ultrasonic jelly. Next locate the fundus and place the

toco on the firmest part of the fundus. Both the toco and transducer are secured to the abdomen with straps.

- The LPN must be able to detect nonreassuring FHR patterns so that he can notify the charge nurse and/or the primary health care provider, who then makes a final decision regarding care of the patient.

- No intervention is required for early decelerations, other than continued monitoring. Nursing interventions for variable decelerations are aimed at relieving cord compression and include maternal position change or amnioinfusion. Late decelerations require aggressive management. The woman is positioned on either side, oxygen is started via face mask, and any oxytocin infusion is discontinued. Sometimes tocolytics are prescribed to decrease the frequency and duration of uterine contractions, which improves blood flow to the placenta.

- Fetal stimulation is another way to measure how well the fetus is tolerating the stress of labor. It can be done noninvasively with an acoustic vibrator or invasively during a vaginal examination. An increase in the FHR with stimulation is reassuring.

- Fetal scalp sampling is an invasive procedure that provides direct evidence of fetal status via the pH. Disadvantages include that it requires that the membranes be ruptured and there is a small chance that fetal and maternal blood will intermingle and lead to incompatibilities. Fetal pulse oximetry gives direct evidence of fetal oxygenation without being directly invasive to the fetus. It does, however, require that the membranes be ruptured.

- The latent phase of the first stage of labor is marked by feelings of excitement and also by anticipatory anxiety and fear. Teaching about the labor process can help reduce anxiety. Distraction techniques are helpful in facilitating coping.

- Contractions become more frequent and stronger during the active phase of labor. Distraction techniques typically do not help during active labor. Support of the woman and her partner include encouragement to continue behaviors that promote coping and assistance in finding alternative approaches when coping is ineffective. Reinforcing breathing techniques and rituals can be helpful.

- The transition phase is the most intense phase of labor. The woman becomes irritable and less cooperative. The challenge for the nurse is to assist the woman to rest between contractions and to avoid pushing efforts until the cervix is fully dilated.

- Full dilation of the cervix marks the beginning of the second stage of labor. Because the woman can now participate actively by pushing, she often feels re-energized to deal effectively with the labor. The open-glottis method of pushing is recommended. Encouragement and reinforcement of pushing techniques are helpful nursing interventions.

♦ The placenta is delivered in the third stage of labor. The nurse monitors for signs of placental separation and ensures that the fundus remains contracted after the placenta delivers. Risk for trauma from birth-related complications is an appropriate nursing diagnosis.

♦ During the fourth stage of labor, or the recovery period, the risk for hemorrhage is high. Close monitoring of the fundus, lochia, and vital signs is warranted. Risk for deficient fluid volume and risk for birth-related trauma are priority nursing diagnoses.

REFERENCES AND SELECTED READINGS

Books and Journals

Association of Women's Health, Obstetric and Neonatal Nurses (AWHONN). (2000). *Fetal assessment. AWHONN Position Statement*. Retrieved September 14, 2001, from http://www.awhonn.org/resour/POSITION/psresp.html

Association of Women's Health, Obstetric and Neonatal Nurses (AWHONN), Mattson, S., & Smith, J. E. (Eds.). (2000). *Core curriculum for maternal–newborn nursing* (2nd ed.). Philadelphia: W. B. Saunders Company.

Berkowitz, K., & Nageotte, M. P. (2000). Intrapartum fetal monitoring. In A. T. Evans & K. R. Niswander (Eds.), *Manual of obstetrics* (6th ed., pp. 313–329). Philadelphia: Lippincott Williams & Wilkins.

California College of Midwives. (1999). *Intermittent auscultation augmented with episodic electronic fetal monitoring (EEFM) for community-based midwives. Technical Bulletin No. 2*. Retrieved January 20, 2002, from http://www.goodnewsnet.org/college99/efm99bb.htm

Cuervo, L. G., Rodriguez, M. N., & Delgado, M. B. (1998). Enemas during labor. *Cochrane Review Abstract*. Retrieved September 14, 2001 from http://www.medscape.com/cochrane/abstracts/ab000330.html

Cunningham, F. G., Gant, N. F., Leveno, K. J., Gilstrap, L.C. III, Hauth, J. C. & Wenstrom, K. D. (2001). *Williams obstetrics* (21st ed.). New York: McGraw Hill Medical Publishing Division.

Hodnett, E. (1996). Nursing support of the laboring woman. *Journal of Obstetric, Gynecologic, and Neonatal Nursing (JOGNN), 25*(3), 257–264.

Mozurkewich, E., & Wolf, F. M. (2000). Near-infrared spectroscopy for fetal assessment during labour. From *Cochrane Abstracts*. Retrieved January 20, 2002, from http://search.medscape.com/Cochrane/abstracts/ab002254.html

Nettina, S. M. (2001). Nursing management during labor and delivery. In *The Lippincott Manual of Nursing Practice* (7th ed., pp. 1124–1151). Philadelphia: Lippincott Williams & Wilkins.

University of Pennsylvania Health System. (Undated). A century of obstetrics. Retrieved January 20, 2002, from http://www.obgyn.upenn.edu/History/clinobhis.html

Wolcott, H. D., & Conry, J. A. (2000). Normal labor. In A. T. Evans & K. R. Niswander (Eds.), *Manual of obstetrics* (6th ed., pp. 392–424). Philadelphia: Lippincott Williams & Wilkins.

Websites
http://www.childbirth.org/
http://www.childbirth.org/articles/labor.html
http://www.thebabycorner.com/pregnancy/labor.html

Doulas
http://doulanetwork.com/

WORKBOOK

NCLEX-STYLE REVIEW QUESTIONS

1. A woman presents to the labor suite and states, "I have water leaking down my legs." What assessment is most appropriate in this situation?

   a. DTRs

   b. Fern test

   c. Blood pressure check

   d. Urine test for protein

2. A primipara is dilated 8 cm and is completely effaced at a +1 station. She tells the nurse, "I can't keep myself from pushing when I have a contraction." What intervention is most appropriate in this situation?

   a. Offer comfort measures.

   b. Reapply the fetal monitor.

   c. Assist the woman to blow at the peak of contractions.

   d. Tell the coach that it is not good for the baby if she pushes right now.

3. A G1 P0 is in the active phase of labor. She is a low-risk patient. You evaluate the fetal monitor strip at 10:00 a.m. Moderate variability is present. The FHR is in the 130s with occasional accelerations, no decelerations. At what time do you need to re-evaluate the FHR?

   a. 10:05 a.m.

   b. 10:15 a.m.

   c. 10:30 a.m.

   d. 11:00 a.m.

4. A G3 P2 with no apparent risk factors presents to the labor and delivery suite in early labor. She refuses the fetal monitor. She says that she delivered her second baby at home without a monitor and everything went well. How do you plan to handle this situation?

   a. Explain that she will need to be on the monitor for a few minutes to be certain this baby is doing well. After this initial assessment the baby can then be monitored intermittently.

   b. Insist that the fetal monitor be used because there are not enough staff members to adequately monitor her using any other method.

   c. Request that the charge nurse reassign you to another patient because you do not want to be responsible if anything were to happen to her baby during labor.

   d. Tell her that it is her decision, but continuous EFM is the only recommended way to monitor how well her baby is doing during labor.

5. In which situation is it most likely that the physician would consider performing an amnioinfusion? The EFM tracing shows

   a. consistent early decelerations, variability present, and occasional accelerations.

   b. flat line without variability and no decelerations.

   c. occasional mild variable decelerations and moderate variability present.

   d. deep variable decelerations with every contraction.

STUDY ACTIVITIES

1. Choose what you think are the three most important nursing assessments and interventions during labor. Using the table below, compare your top three picks for the laboring woman during the active phase, transition phase, and the second stage of labor. Include the frequency of the interventions. What similarities do you see? What differences are apparent?

	Active Phase	Transition	Second Stage
Major nursing assessments			
Major nursing interventions			

2. Run a search on the Internet using the key words "birth plans." How many sites returned? After exploring some of the sites, what are the main issues covered in a birth plan? Does a birth plan seem realistic to use if the woman intends to deliver in the hospital? Why or why not?

3. Interview a labor and delivery nurse. Ask her how her facility handles birth plans. Does she recall a time when parts of the birth plan could

not be honored? How was the situation handled? What was the outcome?

CRITICAL THINKING: What Would You Do?

Apply your knowledge of the labor process and the nurse's role during labor and birth to the following situation.

1. Priscilla, a 26-year-old G1 P0, presents to the birthing center because her "labor pains" have begun. She talks excitedly with her husband, who is to be her coach. She says that she is pleased that the happy day is finally here, but she is afraid that she will "lose it" when the contractions get stronger. She and her husband have attended childbirth preparation classes.

   a. What nursing assessments should be completed?

   b. What phase/stage of labor do you suspect Priscilla is in?

   c. What do you expect the vaginal examination will reveal?

   d. What nursing interventions will you implement for Priscilla and her husband?

   e. How would your care be different if the couple had not attended childbirth classes?

2. Several hours after admission to the birthing center, Priscilla is dilated 5 cm and the cervix is completely effaced. When a contraction begins, Priscilla kneels on the bed, rests her upper body against her husband, closes her eyes and sways slowly while humming softly. At the end of the contraction her husband gently places her on her side and she rests with her eyes closed until the next contraction begins.

   a. What phase/stage of labor is Priscilla in?

   b. What nursing assessments need to be completed at this time?

   c. What is your assessment of Priscilla's coping technique?

   d. What nursing actions are appropriate for Priscilla and her partner at this point in her labor?

3. Three hours later, Priscilla becomes agitated and snaps at her husband and the nurse. She exclaims, "I can't stand this anymore! I want to go *home*!"

   a. What nursing assessments should be completed at this time? Why?

   b. What nursing interventions are appropriate for Priscilla and her husband now?

   c. How would you decide whether or not your interventions had been effective?

4. It is the beginning of your shift. The charge nurse gives you report on Martha Brown, a 29-year-old G2 P1. The fetus is in a vertex presentation and the water bag is intact. A vaginal examination was done 1 hour previously. At that time her cervix was 4 cm dilated and 80% effaced. The station was +1 and the position was LOT. Continuous EFM is ordered, and IV fluids are infusing into her left arm.

   a. What assessments do you make, in what order, when you enter Martha's room?

   b. How do you evaluate the contraction pattern?

5. A few hours later, you go to check on Martha. You notice that she is much more restless than she has been. The fetal monitor tracing shows the FHR baseline in the 140s. Moderate variability is present. During each contraction the FHR dips into the 120s. The dip is smooth with a gentle slope on both sides, like a contraction, only upside down. The FHR is back to 140 by the end of the contraction. You do perineal care because Martha has a lot of bloody show.

   a. How do you interpret the FHR pattern? Is the pattern reassuring or nonreassuring? Defend your answer.

   b. What should your next action be? Why?

Assisted Delivery and Cesarean Birth

11

STUDENT OBJECTIVES

On completion of this chapter, the student will be able to

1. Describe external version to a patient who is scheduled for the procedure.
2. Identify at least four medical indications for induction of labor.
3. Explain the Bishop score and its usefulness in predicting the likelihood of induction success.
4. Contrast mechanical methods for hastening cervical readiness with pharmacologic methods.
5. Outline essential steps and possible complications associated with oxytocin induction.
6. Describe the procedure of amnioinfusion.
7. Compare mediolateral and midline episiotomies.
8. Differentiate between vacuum extraction and forceps-assisted delivery.
9. Explain maternal and fetal complications of cesarean delivery.
10. Name two of the most common and three less common indications for cesarean birth.
11. Differentiate between vertical and transverse skin and uterine incisions.
12. Compare nursing interventions needed to prepare a family for a planned cesarean birth with those for a family who is to undergo emergency cesarean delivery.
13. Explain important aspects involved with attempted VBAC.

KEY TERMS

amnioinfusion ✓
amniotomy ✓ AROM
Bishop score ✓
cesarean birth ✓
chorioamnionitis ✓ infect am fluid
elective induction ✓
episiotomy ✓
fetal fibronectin ✓
forceps ✓
laminaria ✓
version ✓

There are many tools and techniques available to the birth attendant to decrease the risk of labor and/or birth to the woman and her fetus.[1] Some procedures, such as repositioning the fetus, are done before labor. Induction techniques are used to initiate labor, if delivery is indicated. Some tools allow the primary care provider to intervene during labor when conditions arise that threaten the safety of the woman or her fetus. The birth attendant also has tools that are used to assist the delivery. Many of these options help avoid cesarean delivery, which subjects the woman and her fetus to all the hazards of major surgery.

Before the advent of surgical asepsis and antibiotics, if a laboring woman could not deliver a child vaginally, there were few options available to the physician or midwife. Sometimes the woman died. Other times extreme measures were taken and the unborn child's life was sacrificed to save the life of the mother (*Encyclopaedia Britannica*, 2002). Today, cesarean birth is frequently done if other options do not work or the risk of vaginal delivery outweighs the risk of surgical intervention.

● *Figure 11.1* External version. One or two physicians manipulate the fetus through the abdominal wall to coax the fetus to turn to a vertex presentation.

VERSION

Version is a process of manipulating the position of the fetus while in utero. There are two types of version: external and internal.

External Version

External version is a procedure that is most frequently done to reposition a fetus that is breech or shoulder presentation near term (37 weeks and beyond). It must be done in a facility that has full capacity to perform an emergency cesarean delivery, if one should become necessary. The procedure is uncomfortable and occasionally has to be stopped because of discomfort of the woman.

The fetal monitor is connected, and a nonstress test (NST) performed by the registered nurse (RN). If the NST is reactive, the process can begin. An intravenous (IV) line is started, and laboratory work drawn in the event an emergency cesarean delivery becomes necessary. An ultrasound examination is performed to confirm the presentation and lie of the fetus, note placental location, determine if enough amniotic fluid is present, and rule out congenital anomalies and nuchal

cord (umbilical cord around the fetus' neck). Some physicians have better success when a tocolytic, such as SQ terbutaline, is given to relax the uterus. The physician's hands are then placed on the abdomen in an attempt to manipulate the fetus to turn to a vertex presentation (Fig. 11-1). Often (approximately 65% of the time) the maneuvers are effective, and the fetus turns. Occasionally, the fetus will turn around again (revert) to a breech position, although this is more likely to occur if the fetus is premature. The ultrasound examination is repeated afterward to determine if the maneuvers were successful.

Nursing care includes assisting the woman to empty her bladder just before the procedure. Position the woman supine with a pillow or wedge under the right hip. If ordered, the RN administers tocolytics. Take and record vital signs before and after the procedure. Afterward the RN monitors the fetus for 30 minutes to an hour. You may be instructed to administer Rho (D) immune globulin (RhoGAM) to the Rh-negative woman.

Internal Version

Internal version is done infrequently and is usually reserved to turn a second twin when she is breech. The physician inserts his fingers through the cervix (which must be sufficiently dilated to allow the procedure) and manipulates the fetus to turn. Alternatively, the

---

[1] The student should be aware that all of the procedures discussed in this chapter carry risk. Many of these procedures are done to correct problems discussed in Chapter 18. Although many of these techniques are frequently used, they should not be considered routine.

physician may do an internal podalic version by bringing down the fetal legs into the maternal pelvis.

INDUCTION OF LABOR

When a condition exists that could endanger the life of the woman or the fetus, the physician may elect to induce labor, rather than wait for nature to take its course. The rate of induced labors has risen dramatically over the past few years (Martin et al., 2003). There are many reasons for this rise, although one contributing factor seems to be an increase in the number of elective inductions. An **elective induction** is one in which the physician and woman decide to end the pregnancy in the absence of a medical reason to do so. Simpson and Atterbury (2003) caution against elective induction unless the woman understands that elective inductions often result in more interventions, longer labors, higher costs, and possible cesarean birth.

There are several ways to induce labor. Stripping the membranes and cervical ripening procedures may be used to encourage the onset of labor or to prepare the cervix for oxytocin-induced labor. Artificial rupture of membranes is a common practice used to induce labor or to augment a naturally occurring labor. Pitocin, a synthetic form of oxytocin, given intravenously is another common method used to induce or augment labor.

Indications

Any condition that endangers the life of the woman or the fetus if the pregnancy were to continue is considered a medical indication for induction of labor. There are many such conditions. Postdate pregnancy, a pregnancy that persists beyond the expected due date, is probably the most common reason that labor is induced. Premature rupture of membranes (PROM);

spontaneous rupture of membranes (SROM) without the onset of spontaneous labor; **chorioamnionitis**, infection of the fetal membranes; pregnancy-induced hypertension; and preeclampsia are obstetric complications that often require labor induction. Other examples include severe intrauterine fetal growth restriction or maternal medical conditions such as diabetes mellitus or gestational diabetes. Sometimes labor is induced in an attempt to avoid an unattended delivery. For example, a woman who has a history of rapid labors and who lives far away from the hospital or birthing center may have labor induced at or near term. In any case, the risks of allowing the pregnancy to continue are weighed against the risks of labor induction before a decision is made to induce labor.

Contraindications

Conditions in which spontaneous labor is contraindicated are also contraindications for the induction of labor. For example, complete placenta previa, history of a classical uterine incision, or more than two previous low transverse uterine incisions are contraindications for both spontaneous and induced labor. Fetal contraindications include certain anomalies, such as hydrocephalus, fetal malpresentations, and fetal compromise. Structural abnormalities of the pelvis and invasive cervical cancer are maternal contraindications. Certain medical conditions that necessitate a cesarean delivery, such as active genital herpes, preclude labor induction.

Labor Readiness

Cervical readiness is generally a prerequisite for successful labor induction. A cervix that is favorable for induction is called a "ripe" cervix. One commonly used scoring method to determine cervical readiness is the **Bishop score** (Table 11-1). Five factors are evaluated: cervical consistency, position, dilation, effacement, and

TABLE 11.1	Bishop Scoring System				
	Factor				
Score	Dilatation (cm)	Effacement (%)	Station*	Cervical Consistency	Cervical Position
0	Closed	0–30	−3	Firm	Posterior
1	1–2	40–50	−2	Medium	Midposition
2	3–4	60–70	−1.0	Soft	Anterior
3	≥5	≥80	+1, +2		

*Station reflects a −3 to +3 scale.

Adapted with permission from Bishop, E. H. (1964). Pelvic scoring for elective induction. *Obstet Gynecol, (24)*, 266–268.

fetal station. Each factor is given a score of 0 to 3: the higher the score, the greater the chance that induction will be successful. In general, a score of 9 or greater is associated with a favorable response to oxytocin-induced labor; that is the cervix is soft, in an anterior position, partially dilated and effaced, with an engaged fetus. A Bishop score of 5 or less indicates an unripe or unfavorable cervix, and labor induction is less likely to be successful.

One relatively new method for predicting labor readiness is determination of cervical length by endovaginal ultrasound. A cervix that measures 28 millimeters in length (or less) is associated with a favorable induction rate, even in the presence of a low Bishop score. Refer to Chapter 7 for a description of this diagnostic procedure.

Another newer method for determining labor readiness is measurement of fetal fibronectin levels. **Fetal fibronectin** is a protein found in fetal membranes and amniotic fluid. Its presence in cervical secretions is associated with labor readiness. The test consists of swabbing the cervical area during a speculum examination to obtain a secretion sample. The sample is then sent to a laboratory to test for fetal fibronectin levels. However, this test is not done widely to determine labor readiness at term; it is more often used as a predictor of preterm labor risk.

In addition to cervical readiness, the fetus should be mature before labor is induced, unless a condition exists in which the risks of prematurity are outweighed by the risks of continued pregnancy. Maturity can be assessed in several ways. If the pregnancy has completed at least 38 weeks' gestation (as determined by reliable dating methods), the fetus is considered to be mature. Fetal lung maturity is the most important factor to be considered. Measuring the lecithin/sphingomyelin (L/S) ratio via amniocentesis assesses lung maturity. An L/S ratio greater than 2.0 or a positive phosphatidyl glycerol test indicates fetal lung maturity.

Cervical Ripening

Frequently labor induction is indicated, but the cervix is not ready. In this situation a procedure to ripen the cervix may be used before induction with oxytocin is started. The following discussion explores mechanical and pharmacologic methods used to ripen a cervix in preparation for labor induction.

Mechanical Methods

One of the most common mechanical methods used to hasten cervical readiness is a procedure called "membrane stripping." The primary care provider inserts a gloved finger through the internal cervical os and sweeps the finger 360 degrees to separate the membranes from the lower uterine segment. Plasma levels of prostaglandins (one substance associated with the onset of labor) are measurably higher after membrane stripping. Several research studies support the efficacy of membrane stripping to initiate spontaneous labor and decrease the use of oxytocin without increasing the risk of maternal infection or likelihood of cesarean birth (Cunningham et al., 2001, p. 474).

Mechanical dilation of the cervix is sometimes attempted by inserting a catheter into the cervix and inflating the balloon. Mechanical dilation can be accomplished with or without infusion of normal saline, a procedure known as extra-amnionic saline infusion, although the addition of saline does not increase the likelihood of success. The risk of uterine hyperstimulation and the risk for cesarean birth are both reduced with the use of mechanical dilation as compared with the use of pharmacologic methods to induce labor (Boulvain, Kelly, Lohse, Stan, & Irion, 2003).

Laminaria, or cervical dilators, are sometimes used to soften and dilate the cervix. Laminaria are made from the root of seaweed. The cylindrical material is placed in the cervix and works by absorbing moisture, which causes it to expand slowly. As the material expands, it dilates the cervix gradually. Laminaria are most frequently used to induce abortion for therapeutic and elective reasons, or to induce labor when the fetus has died in utero. Few scientific studies have been done to evaluate their use for induction of labor at term, although some practitioners use them for this purpose.

Pharmacologic Methods

Locally applied prostaglandins have been found to be effective in preparing an unripe cervix for labor. There are two main preparations, although the only substance approved by the United States Food and Drug Administration (FDA) for this purpose is prostaglandin E_2 gel or vaginal inserts (dinoprostone). Prostaglandin E_1 (misoprostol) is used frequently for cervical ripening, although it is not approved for this use.

Prostaglandin E_2 (Dinoprostone)

There are two preparations of prostaglandin E_2 available for use: prostaglandin E_2 gel (Prepidil) and prostaglandin E_2 vaginal inserts (Cervidil). Prepidil comes in a 2.5-mL syringe that dispenses 0.5 mg of dinoprostone. The practitioner injects this preparation into the cervix. Cervidil is available as a 10-mg vaginal insert that is placed into the posterior fornix during a vaginal examination. If uterine hyperstimulation occurs, Cervidil can be removed by pulling on the string that is left in the vagina.

The woman receiving dinoprostone should be in a facility that has continuous fetal monitoring capabilities. Assist the RN to place the fetal monitor and run a tracing for at least 20 minutes to obtain a reactive NST.

When the practitioner is ready, bring the medication to the bedside and assist with a vaginal examination. Instruct the woman about the importance of lying in a recumbent position (do not forget to put a wedge under one hip) for at least 30 minutes. Continue the fetal monitor tracing, as ordered (usually for 30 minutes to 2 hours), and monitor for signs of uterine hyperstimulation or fetal distress.

Prostaglandin E_2 is usually administered in the evening. Sometimes the woman is allowed to go home and return when labor ensues. However, some physicians prefer to keep the woman in the delivery suite overnight and begin oxytocin induction of labor in the morning (6 to 12 hours after dinoprostone is applied).

Prostaglandin E_1 (Misoprostol)

The synthetic prostaglandin E_1 analog misoprostol (Cytotec) is an antiulcer agent whose properties promote cervical ripening. It is available in a 100-microgram tablet that is usually divided. The practitioner or a specially trained nurse places one quarter of the tablet (25 micrograms) in the posterior vaginal fornix. The dose can be repeated every 4 to 6 hours (Goldberg & Wing, 2003). Sometimes a higher dosing protocol (1/2 tablet or 50 micrograms) is used. However, the higher dose is associated with more cases of uterine hyperstimulation and fetal distress and is not recommended. Misoprostol (Cytotec) can be given orally. Results similar to the 25-microgram vaginal dose are obtained when one tablet (100 micrograms) is given by mouth. Nursing care for the woman receiving misoprostol is similar to that described for dinoprostone.

Artificial Rupture of Membranes

Artificial rupture of membranes (AROM), also known as an **amniotomy**, can be done to induce labor or to augment labor that has already begun. A hard plastic instrument with a hook on the end, an Amnihook, is introduced into the vagina during a digital examination. The practitioner then guides the instrument through the cervix with two fingers and uses the hook to snag a hole in the membranes. At this point amniotic fluid is usually expelled. This process causes the body to release prostaglandins, which enhances labor.

Oxytocin Induction

Labor is often induced through the use of intravenous oxytocin (Pitocin), a synthetic form of the posterior pituitary hormone that causes the uterus to contract. The woman is admitted to a labor and delivery suite and the external fetal monitor is attached. After at least 20 minutes of fetal monitoring to obtain a baseline fetal heart assessment, a mainline IV is started. Then a secondary IV line that contains oxytocin is started via an infusion pump so that the dose of the medication can be controlled carefully. One common protocol is to place 10 units of oxytocin in 1,000 mL of IV fluid. Using this protocol, 6 mL/hour is equal to a dose of 1 milliunit/minute. The dose is usually titrated up by 1 to 2 milliunits every 15 to 20 minutes until an adequate contraction pattern is obtained.

Several potential complications are associated with the use of oxytocin for inducing labor. There is a higher risk that a cesarean birth will become necessary whenever labor is induced. This is particularly true for primigravidas (Simpson & Atterbury, 2003). There is also a risk that the uterus will be hyperstimulated. Hyperstimulation leads to contractions that occur one after the other without a sufficient rest period in between. This can lead to fetal distress and even uterine rupture. Another potential complication is water intoxication. Because oxytocin is a posterior pituitary hormone, it is chemically related to antidiuretic hormone. Therefore, oxytocin can have an antidiuretic effect, causing the kidneys to retain water. Symptoms of water intoxication include hyponatremia, confusion, convulsions, or coma. Congestive heart failure and death also can occur.

Nursing Care

The licensed practical nurse's (LPN's) role during induction depends upon the procedure. The RN maintains responsibility for monitoring the woman and her fetus during pharmacologic cervical ripening procedures and oxytocin induction and augmentation. However, the LPN may be asked to assist the birth attendant during a pelvic examination in which mechanical methods of cervical ripening are used (i.e., membrane stripping and laminaria insertion) or during amniotomy. When amniotomy is done, document the fetal heart rate before and after the procedure. Notify the RN or birth attendant if the rate drops precipitously. Sometimes the birth attendant will ask for suprapubic or fundal pressure during the procedure. It is permissible to give this assistance, if you have been properly trained to do so.

Test Yourself

- True or false: External version always requires the use of a tocolytic to relax the uterus.

- Name two medical indications for the induction of labor.

- Which locally applied prostaglandin is approved by the FDA to be used for cervical ripening?

AMNIOINFUSION

Amnioinfusion is infusion of sterile fluid into the uterine cavity during labor. This procedure is done to relieve persistent deep variable decelerations associated with cord compression. It is also done to dilute thick meconium-stained amniotic fluid in an effort to decrease morbidity and mortality from meconium aspiration syndrome. Prerequisites for this procedure include ruptured membranes and adequate cervical dilation to allow introduction of the intrauterine pressure catheter (IUPC) into the uterus. Only physiologically compatible fluid is to be used. Lactated Ringer's and 0.9% normal saline are suitable. Never use a dextrose solution. It is recommended that the fluid be warmed using a blood warmer when the fetus is preterm. Term fetuses can tolerate room temperature fluids.

Exercise caution! Fluids should never be placed in a baby blanket warmer or in the microwave. Doing so is against manufacturer's recommendations and could result in serious burns.

Contraindications and Possible Complications

Contraindications include any situation in which placement of the IUPC is inadvisable, such as placenta previa, abruptio placenta, and so on. Other contraindications include multiple gestation, malpresentation of the fetus, absent/diminished fetal heart rate variability or other signs of fetal distress, fetal anomalies incompatible with life, uterine anomalies, and chorioamnionitis.

Possible complications of this procedure include polyhydramnios from trapped amniotic fluid, high intrauterine pressure readings, placental abruption, chorioamnionitis, and problems caused by solution temperature issues, e.g., maternal chilling from fluid that is too cold or fetal tachycardia from fluid that is too warm.

Nursing Care

The RN is responsible for monitoring the woman who receives an amnioinfusion. The solution is connected to IV tubing and primed. The RN will assist the physician or nurse midwife to insert the IUPC according to manufacturer's guidelines. After the IUPC is in place, the IV tubing is attached to the infusion port. A fluid bolus of 250 mL (or the amount ordered) is given. Then the tubing is connected to an IV pump and the rate decreased to approximately 150 mL/hour or as ordered.

The RN will monitor the resting tone of the uterus at least every 30 minutes. The resting tone should not exceed 25 mm Hg. You may be asked to assist the woman with perineal care. Assess and record the amount, color, and odor of the fluid that is being expelled onto the under-buttocks pad. If no fluid is returning at all, notify the RN immediately.

ASSISTED DELIVERY

Sometimes a problem develops in one of the essential components toward the end of labor. The fetus may descend to the pelvic floor without rotating to the anterior position. Or the mother may become tired and stop pushing effectively. In cases such as these, the birth attendant may elect to use an operative technique or device to hasten the delivery. Types of assisted delivery include episiotomy, vacuum-assisted delivery, and forceps delivery.

Episiotomy

An **episiotomy** is a surgical incision made into the perineum to enlarge the vaginal opening just before the baby is born. In the recent past, physicians performed episiotomies on virtually all primigravidas delivered in the United States. This procedure is no longer considered to be routine, although episiotomies are still performed in approximately 40% of all deliveries (Simpson & Creehan, 2001, p. 326).

It was commonly believed that an episiotomy was less painful and healed faster than a jagged tear that might result if an episiotomy were not performed. However, research has not validated these assumptions. In fact, research studies demonstrate that an episiotomy increases the risk that the perineum will tear into the anal sphincter (Carroli & Belizan, 2004), a condition that increases maternal discomfort as well as the risk of infection and long-term consequences, such as anal incontinence. In addition, women on whom an episiotomy is performed may lose more blood than women who are delivered over an intact perineum (Simpson & Creehan, 2001, p. 326). Box 11-1 lists several measures that can reduce the need for episiotomy.

There are, however, situations in which an episiotomy may be indicated. These include:

- The baby's shoulders are stuck in the birth canal after the head is born (shoulder dystocia).
- The head will not rotate from an occiput-posterior position (persistent occiput-posterior).
- The fetus is in a breech presentation.
- Forceps or vacuum-assisted delivery is used to shorten the second stage of labor.

BOX 11.1	Methods to Minimize the Need for Episiotomy

- Kegel exercises during pregnancy to strengthen perineal muscles
- Using natural pushing techniques, particularly in the side-lying position
- Patience with the delivery process
- Protection of the perineum immediately before birth (by the birth attendant) to avoid uncontrolled delivery of the fetal head

There are two basic types of episiotomies (Fig. 11-2). A median or midline episiotomy extends from the fourchette straight down into the true perineum. This type of episiotomy increases the risk for extension into the anal sphincter but is easier for the physician to repair and causes less discomfort for the woman than a mediolateral episiotomy, which is angled to the right or left of the perineum.

Repair of the perineum is needed if an episiotomy is performed. If the woman had epidural anesthesia, she may not need additional anesthesia for repair. Often, local anesthesia is used to numb the perineum for repair. Have suture readily available according to the physician or nurse midwife preference. Reassure the woman that the sutures are absorbable and do not need to be removed.

Vacuum-Assisted Delivery

A device sometimes used to hasten delivery is the vacuum extractor. In this procedure the birth attendant places a suction cup (some are soft silicone cups and others are hard metal cups) on the fetal head; then suction is applied, and the device is used to gently guide the delivery of the infant (Fig. 11-3). The nurse provides

A PERSONAL GLIMPSE

When I was pregnant with my second child, I re-read everything about the experience: the pregnancy, the delivery, the recovery, and nursing. Having had one healthy baby before this one, I felt like I was prepared for what was going to happen in the whole process of delivering a baby.

When my water broke at 4 a.m. on a Saturday, my husband and I rushed to the hospital. The vaginal delivery went well and quickly. However, after our little girl was born, I was told that I had been given an "episiotomy." Of course during the delivery, I was numb from the epidural, and I really had no idea what had gone on other than being told to push numerous times. The nurse left me some cotton pads, and told me to keep myself clean until the stitches "melted."

The area of the episiotomy caused me a lot of pain. Every time I sat on the toilet to urinate, my vaginal area would hurt. I would avoid having bowel movements, as those were very painful as well. When I told the nurses about how much it hurt, they would tell me to clean myself better after urinating, and got a doctor to prescribe me a stool softener to take home.

It wasn't until I was discharged and my mother was staying at home with me to help out, that we figured out what the problem was. I asked my mother to look at my vaginal area, and she saw that one of the stitches had a knot that had irritated the skin around it and caused a sore.

It would have been better if one of the nurses had looked for me (with my giant belly after the delivery, I couldn't see a thing) and figured out what the problem was before I had left the hospital.

Shelly

LEARNING OPPORTUNITY: Discuss two actions the nurse could take to better prepare this new mother to understand how to take care of her episiotomy. What assessments do you think the nurse should make for a patient with an episiotomy?

A

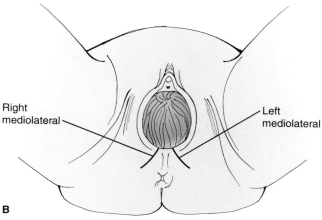

Right mediolateral

Left mediolateral

B

● **Figure 11.2** Two basic types of episiotomy. **(A)** Midline episiotomy extends straight down into the true perineum. **(B)** Mediolateral episiotomy angles to the right or the left of the perineum.

A

B

● **Figure 11.3** Delivery assisted by vacuum extraction. (**A**) The birth attendant has just placed the suction cup on the fetal head and is using the hand pump to increase the pressure. (**B**) Gentle traction is placed on the fetal head to assist it through the last maneuvers of delivery.

the necessary equipment, connects and regulates the suction as instructed by the birth attendant, monitors fetal status, and supports the laboring woman during the procedure by keeping her informed of the procedure and progress.

Forceps-Assisted Delivery

Forceps are metal instruments with curved, blunted blades (somewhat like large hollowed-out spoons) that are placed around the head of the fetus by the birth attendant to facilitate delivery (Fig. 11-4). Low and outlet forceps are used more frequently than are midforceps. Outlet forceps are applied when the fetal head can be seen at the introitus; low forceps are used when the station is equal to or greater than + 2, but the head is not yet showing on the perineum; whereas, midforceps are used when the fetal head is well engaged but still relatively high in the pelvis (higher than +2).

Midforceps are most often used to assist the fetus to rotate to an anterior position.

Indications and prerequisites for use of forceps and the vacuum extractor are similar. Any problem that causes the second stage of delivery to be prolonged or any situation of concern that is likely to be relieved by delivery of the infant may be an indication for assisted delivery. Maternal indications include fatigue (the woman may become exhausted while pushing), certain chronic conditions such as heart or lung disease, and prolonged second stage of labor. If fetal distress is evident and the criteria for forceps delivery are met, then forceps may be used to rapidly deliver the infant and relieve the cause of distress.

Nursing Care

During an assisted delivery the nurse obtains needed equipment and supplies; monitors maternal and fetal

● **Figure 11.4** Forceps-assisted delivery.

status before, during, and after the procedure; assists the birth attendant; provides support for the woman; and documents the type of procedure, as well as maternal and fetal response. The nurse is aware that use of a technique to assist vaginal delivery may not work and anticipates the possibility of cesarean delivery. Episiotomy care after delivery is discussed in Chapter 12.

For both vacuum-assisted and forceps-assisted deliveries (operative vaginal deliveries), inspect the infant carefully for signs of trauma. This could include cephalhematoma, retinal hemorrhage, bruising, edema, exaggerated caput (chignon), forceps mark, and transient facial paralysis. Reassure the parents that forceps marks and exaggerated caput from vacuum-assisted deliveries will subside in a few days.

Maternal soft tissue trauma may also result from an operative vaginal delivery. Inspect the perineum for bruising and edema. Monitor closely for excessive bleeding or development of a hematoma. (Refer to Chapter 19 for nursing care of the woman with postpartum hemorrhage.)

Test Yourself

- Name two indications for amnioinfusion.
- Name two situations in which an episiotomy is helpful.
- List at least two fetal complications and one maternal complication of forceps or vacuum-assisted delivery.

CESAREAN BIRTH

A **cesarean birth** is the delivery of a fetus through abdominal and uterine incisions: laparotomy and hysterotomy, respectively. Cesarean comes from the Latin word "caedere," meaning, "to cut." Sometimes the term "cesarean section" is used. This discussion uses the terms "cesarean birth" and "cesarean delivery" because the focus for the nurse and the woman is the birth experience.

Indications

There are many indications for cesarean birth. The majority (more than 85%) are done for the following four reasons:

1. History of previous cesarean
2. Labor dystocia (difficult labor)
3. Fetal distress
4. Breech (buttocks or feet first) presentation (Cunningham et al., 2001)

Other less common obstetric indications include placenta previa (placenta covers the cervix), abruptio placentae (placenta separates from the uterus before birth), cephalopelvic disproportion (fetal head cannot fit through the pelvis), active vaginal herpes lesions, prolapse of the umbilical cord, and ruptured uterus. Sometimes medical and obstetric conditions necessitate early delivery of the fetus and require cesarean delivery. Examples include maternal diabetes mellitus, pregnancy-induced hypertension, and erythroblastosis fetalis.

Incidence

Cesarean birth was rarely done before the development of antibiotics and antiseptic surgical techniques because of high maternal mortality rates from infection. This method of delivery has become increasingly accepted in modern times. The rate of cesarean deliveries quadrupled (from 4.5% to 22.8%) between 1965 and 1988 (Cunningham et al., 2001). There are multiple contributing factors to this dramatic increase, which include an increase in the percentage of pregnant women who are carrying their first child,[2] a rise in the number of older pregnant women, almost universal use of continuous electronic fetal monitoring, a trend toward delivering breech presentation through the abdomen, and an increasing concern regarding malpractice litigation. From 1988 to 1996 the rate fell, attributable in large part to a decrease in the rate of primary cesarean births and an increase in the number of vaginal births after cesarean (VBAC). From 1996 through the year 2000, overall cesarean rates steadily rose from 14.6% to 16.1% (Joseph et al., 2003). In 2002, the rate rose to 26.1%, the highest cesarean delivery rate ever reported in the United States. Much of this overall increase is probably related to a dramatic decrease in the rate of VBACs, from 23% in 2001 to 12.6% in 2002 (Martin et al., 2003).

Risks

Cesarean birth is a major surgery and carries with it all the risks associated with surgery combined with the risks of birth itself. A woman who is delivered by cesarean is up to four times more likely to die than is a woman who delivers vaginally (*ACOG News Release*, 2003), although death is a rare occurrence in obstetrics. Some surgical risk factors are increased because of the normal physiologic changes of pregnancy. For example, thrombophlebitis is a complication of both surgery and pregnancy, so the risk is compounded during cesarean delivery. There are risks to the fetus, as well. A fetus delivered by cesarean may inadvertently be delivered

---

[2] A primigravida is more likely to experience cesarean delivery than a multigravida.

prematurely, and he is more likely to have respiratory distress. For these reasons the American College of Obstetricians and Gynecologists (ACOG) recommends that cesarean delivery be performed only when the risks of vaginal delivery clearly outweigh the risks of surgery.

Because of the higher morbidity and mortality rates associated with cesarean delivery versus vaginal delivery, attempts have been made to decrease the cesarean delivery rate. Much research has focused on determining ways to safely deliver a woman vaginally after a previous cesarean birth and on methods to treat labor dystocia. These treatment modalities are discussed elsewhere in this chapter.

Maternal Complications

Maternal complications that can occur during the operation include laceration of the uterine artery, bladder, ureter, or bowel; hemorrhage requiring blood transfusion; and hysterectomy. The most common postoperative complication associated with cesarean birth is infection. Two common infection sites are the uterus and the surgical wound, although sepsis, urinary tract infection, and other infections also can occur. Pneumonia, postpartum hemorrhage, thrombophlebitis, and other surgical-related complications may be experienced during the postoperative period.

Fetal Complications

The most common fetal complications are unintended delivery of an immature fetus because of miscalculation of dates and respiratory distress because of retained lung fluid. Because a fetus delivered by scheduled cesarean birth does not go through labor, he does not have the chance to get most of the amniotic fluid squeezed out of his lungs, as does a baby born vaginally. Therefore, respiratory distress is seen more frequently in these newborns. In addition, the fetus' respiratory drive can be depressed if the mother is given general anesthesia, making it difficult for the newborn to take her first breath. Less commonly, the fetus can be injured, that is, the scalpel cutting through the uterine wall can nick the baby. Usually these wounds are superficial and require minimal intervention.

Incision Types

There are two major incisions made during cesarean birth: one through the abdominal wall and the other into the uterus.

Abdominal Incisions

Abdominal incisions can be done using a vertical approach. These are done in the midline of the lower abdomen. A low transverse incision also can be performed. This type is called *Pfannenstiel's* incision, commonly known as a "bikini cut." Although a low transverse incision slightly increases the risk for bleeding, this is usually the preferred method for cosmetic reasons.

Uterine Incisions

Uterine incisions can be vertical or low transverse (Fig. 11-5). There are two types of vertical uterine incisions: classical and low cervical. The classical incision extends through the body of the uterus to the fundus. This incision is used only in severe emergencies, when it is critical to deliver the fetus immediately or when the fetus is unusually large. Bleeding during surgery is more likely with a classical uterine incision. It carries a higher risk for abdominal infection and the highest risk for uterine rupture in subsequent pregnancies. The low

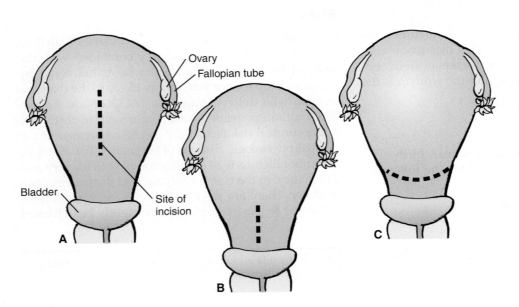

● **Figure 11.5** Types of uterine incisions used for cesarean delivery. (**A**) Classical approach. This incision is only used in extreme emergencies when it is critical to deliver the fetus, or when the fetus is too large to use a smaller incision. (**B**) Low (cervical) vertical approach. This incision is used infrequently. It has the advantage of allowing for extension of the incision into the body of the uterus, if the surgeon has difficulty extracting the fetus. (**C**) Low (cervical) transverse approach. This incision is used most frequently. The scar has a lower risk of rupturing during subsequent pregnancies and is associated with fewer complications.

Ovary
Fallopian tube
Bladder
Site of incision

cervical vertical incision is smaller and carries a lower risk for uterine rupture than does the classical approach, but it is infrequently used because it is more complicated to perform, carries higher risk of maternal injury, and is associated with a higher risk of uterine rupture than is the low cervical transverse incision. The low cervical transverse incision is the preferred method. This incision is associated with the least risk of uterine rupture, is easier to repair, and is least likely to cause adhesions.

Don't get confused. The type of skin incision does not indicate the type of incision used on the uterus. If the woman is not known by the surgeon, he will ask for the previous surgical record, if it is available, to determine the type of uterine incision.

● *Figure 11.6* The scrub nurse sets up the back table in preparation for cesarean delivery.

Test Yourself

- Cesarean delivery involves incisions into what two structures?

- Name three possible complications of cesarean birth.

- What is Pfannenstiel's incision?

Steps of a Cesarean Delivery

Because cesarean delivery involves major surgery, the time period encompassing the procedure is referred to as the perioperative period, which is divided into three phases: preoperative, intraoperative, and postoperative. Care of the woman during the preoperative and intraoperative phases is completed using a team approach, sometimes referred to as collaborative management. The LPN is frequently involved in some of the preoperative care to prepare the woman for surgery. The LPN may also be a part of the intraoperative care by functioning in the scrub nurse role. The immediate postoperative care in the postanesthesia care unit (PACU) is usually carried out by the RN. The LPN may assume care of the woman during the postoperative phase, after she has sufficiently recovered from anesthesia. The major steps of a cesarean delivery are delineated in the following sections and Figures 11-6, 11-7, and 11-8.

Preoperative Phase

Preparing the woman for the cesarean birth is the focus of preoperative care. Nursing duties during the preoperative phase are discussed in the Nursing Care section. The anesthesiologist interviews the woman; explains the planned anesthesia to include risks; obtains verbal consent; reviews laboratory results; and orders preoperative medications, such as antacids and, less frequently, a sedative.

The scrub technician or nurse opens the sterile cesarean delivery pack and instruments, puts on a sterile gown and gloves, and proceeds to prepare the back table and mayo instrument stand (Fig. 11-6). The circulating RN fastens the back of the scrub nurse's gown, and together the circulating RN and scrub nurse perform an initial instrument, sponge, and sharp count.

The support person changes into attire (usually disposable scrub suit or a disposable gown that covers the clothes) appropriate for the operating room (OR). A surgical cap and mask are also provided. The preoperative checklist and chart are reviewed for completeness. A surgical cap is placed on the woman's head to cover her hair, and she is transported to the OR suite by wheelchair or stretcher, or she may ambulate to the OR.

Intraoperative Phase

The intraoperative phase begins once the woman enters the OR. The woman is positioned on the operating table for regional anesthesia.[3] She may be placed in the sitting position with her legs dangling to one side, or she may be placed in the side-lying position. The nurse supports the woman so that her back remains in a C-shaped curve during placement of regional anesthesia by the anesthesiologist (Fig. 11-7A).

The nurse and anesthesiologist assist the woman to the supine position on the OR table. At this point, the Foley catheter is inserted, if not already placed in the preoperative area. The nurse places a wedge under one hip, and then places a warm blanket and a safety strap on the woman's legs. The fetal heart rate is checked for at least 1 minute. A grounding pad is placed

---

[3] It is uncommon for general anesthesia to be performed. Nursing care variations for this type of anesthesia are addressed in Chapter 9.

A

B

C

D

E

● *Figure 11.7* Cesarean birth–intraoperative phase.

on the woman's thigh. The anesthesiologist places electrocardiogram leads, a blood pressure cuff, and pulse oximeter device and connects them to the monitoring equipment. The woman's arms are positioned on arm boards and gently restrained with soft restraints.

Meanwhile, the surgeon and the assistant perform a surgical scrub. The circulating RN performs a sterile abdominal preparation with alcohol, or Betadine, as per facility policy (Fig. 11-7B). Then, the surgeon and assistant place sterile drapes on the woman. During the draping procedure, the RN calls for the individuals who will be attending the newborn. The RN also calls for the support person, who is seated at the woman's head behind the surgical drapes.

The surgeon uses small pickup forceps to test the level of anesthesia before proceeding (Fig. 11-7C). Once the surgeon is satisfied that the anesthesia level is sufficient, the surgeon makes the initial cut and proceeds to cut through the layers of skin, fascia, and muscle until the lower segment of the uterus is exposed (Fig. 11-7D).

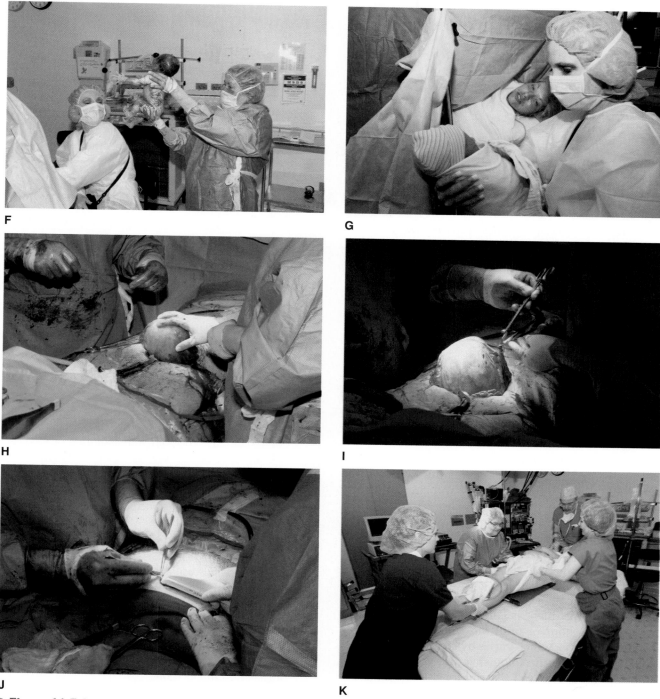

● *Figure 11.7* Continued

Then the surgeon makes the incision into the uterus. The newborn's head is delivered (Fig. 11-7E), followed by the body. The umbilical cord is double clamped and cut, and the newborn is briefly shown to the mother and support person (Fig. 11-7F) before being taken to the warmer for assessment and resuscitation, as needed. The placenta is delivered manually shortly after the baby is born.

When the newborn is breathing well and the skin color is pink, he is double-wrapped in prewarmed blankets, a cap is placed on his head, and he is taken to the woman and support person for initial bonding (Fig. 11-7G).

The fundus and body of the uterus are brought through the incision (Fig. 11-7H), and the inside is cleaned thoroughly by the surgeon; then the uterine incision is sutured close. The circulating RN and scrub technician perform the second OR count. If the woman desires a tubal ligation, it is performed at this time. The tubes are tied and ligated (Fig. 11-7I), and the specimens handed to the circulating RN, who labels them to

● *Figure 11.8* Cesarean birth—postoperative phase.

be sent to the laboratory. The uterus is then placed back in the pelvic cavity.

Repair of muscle and fascia layers is done with absorbable suture while the third OR count is done. The skin is closed with staples (Fig. 11-7*J*) or suture. A sterile dressing is placed, the drapes are removed, the uterine fundus is massaged, and a sterile perineal pad is placed. The woman is then moved from the OR table to a stretcher (Fig. 11-7*K*), and she is transported to the PACU for initial recovery from anesthesia.

Postoperative Phase

The woman is placed in the PACU, where the PACU RN receives report from the circulating RN (in labor and delivery units, the PACU RN and circulating RN may be the same individual). The RN places the woman on a cardiac monitor, an automatic blood pressure device, and a pulse oximeter (Fig. 11-8). A thorough assessment is done to include level of consciousness, cardiac and respiratory status, condition of the dressing, fundal and lochia status, urinary output, condition and patency of IV site, and a full set of vital signs. This assessment is completed at least every 15 minutes for 1 hour or until the woman meets PACU discharge criteria, which varies by facility and anesthesiologist. The anesthesiologist writes orders for pain control in the PACU and usually for the first 24 hours after surgery.

Nursing Care

Providing Family Teaching for a Planned Cesarean Birth

The focus of nursing intervention for a planned cesarean is family education (see Family Teaching Tips: Preparing for a Planned Cesarean Birth). Each time you encounter the woman before surgery is an opportunity to explore with the woman and her partner what they know about cesarean delivery. Do they

FAMILY TEACHING TIPS

Preparing for a Planned Cesarean Birth

Explain or demonstrate to the pregnant woman and partner
- How and where to preregister and have blood work drawn.*
- Where and when to meet the anesthesiologist for preoperative evaluation.
- Date, time, and location to which to present before the surgery.
- The amount of time she is to remain NPO before surgery.
- Procedures for partner participation in the birth process.
- That an IV will be placed in the preoperative holding area and will remain in place for approximately 24 hours after the procedure, when she is tolerating liquids by mouth.
- That regional anesthesia (epidural or spinal) is usually performed to decrease the risk to mother and baby associated with general anesthesia.
- That a Foley catheter will be inserted into her urinary bladder and will remain in place for approximately 24 hours after surgery.
- How long after the surgery until she will likely be transferred to her postpartum room.
- How to turn, cough, and deep breathe every 1 to 2 hours after surgery.
- The importance of early and frequent ambulation to decrease the pain and distention of gas and to decrease risks associated with major surgery, such as respiratory complications, infection, thrombophlebitis, and so on.
- Methods of pain control most frequently ordered and the importance of requesting pain medications before pain becomes severe.
- Likely sources of pain and the appropriate type of pain control for each (e.g., gas build-up responds best to ambulation and simethicone; incisional pain is usually best treated with narcotics; and uterine cramping often responds well to nonsteroidal anti-inflammatory drugs).
- Nursery procedures, including when she and her partner may reasonably expect to interact with their newborn.
- Ways to cope with breast-feeding after cesarean, such as use of the football hold to decrease pressure on the incision.

* Some of these procedures will be done the morning of surgery, depending upon the protocols of the facility at which the woman has chosen to deliver.

know the procedural steps to take, such as where to preregister, when and where to have laboratory work drawn, and when and where to present for surgery? Do they know what to expect during the surgical experience? Does the woman know how to help avoid complications in the postoperative period, such as the how and why of taking deep breaths and turning frequently while in bed, and why it is important to ambulate as soon as possible after surgery? Does she know the principles of postoperative pain control and what options are available to her for pain relief? Teaching is more effective when it occurs over time, is repeated, and focuses on topics in which the family is interested.

Providing Preoperative Care

Nursing interventions to help the woman and her partner prepare for cesarean birth depend on many factors, including whether or not the procedure was planned and whether or not the woman has experienced cesarean delivery in the past. Ideally, the woman and her partner will have attended childbirth classes. Part of class discussion centers on the possibility of cesarean birth. When a woman is prepared psychologically for the experience, coping is enhanced.

Whether the cesarean is planned or emergent, several preparations are critical. Always check to see if informed consent has been given and that a signed consent form documents it (Fig. 11-9). Ask the woman when she last had anything to eat or drink. She should have nothing by mouth (NPO) for at least 8 hours before surgery. Frequently an antacid, such as Bicitra 30 mL, is given before surgery to reduce the risk of aspiration while the woman is under the effects of anesthesia. An IV must be in place with a large-bore (generally 18-gauge or lower) catheter. Lactated Ringer's is a commonly

Remember: A patient can always change her mind. If she signed an informed consent but then states she has changed her mind, she's not sure, or she needs more information, alert the charge nurse or physician immediately so that her concerns can be addressed.

● *Figure 11.9* The nurse witnesses signing of the informed consent form.

ordered IV fluid. Sometimes an abdominal shave preparation is done immediately before surgery, although it is becoming more common to use clippers to remove hair from the abdomen and perineal area. Clippers do not cause skin nicks like razors can, so clippers are the preferred tool to use. A Foley catheter must be in place before the surgery begins to decrease the risk that the surgeon might inadvertently cut or puncture a full bladder during surgery. Sometimes the catheter is placed in the preoperative area. Alternately, the circulating nurse may place it after anesthesia has been administered, which is more comfortable for the woman.

Certain laboratory studies must be done. The routine complete blood count is important, as is the blood type and screen. When a type and screen is done, the laboratory holds at least 2 units of blood that matches the woman's blood type. In the event of an emergency, the final steps of cross matching are done, so that the appropriate blood can be transfused. Most physicians also order other laboratory studies, such as electrolytes. When the woman is ready for surgery, assist the RN to transfer her to the operating suite and then to the operating table.

Providing Support During an Unplanned or Emergency Cesarean Birth

When a cesarean birth becomes necessary because of an unplanned or emergency situation, the nurse must move quickly to prepare the patient for surgery. The woman and her family are often anxious and worried about the baby. She may be fearful of the surgery or anesthesia, particularly if she has never had surgery before. There is usually not much time for education; therefore, support of the woman and her family becomes paramount (Nursing Care Plan 11-1).

Support is shown in many ways. Explain procedures as you are doing them. If the RN or physician says the fetal monitor tracing is reassuring, reinforce this important fact to the woman and her partner. Explain what sensations she can expect to experience and what to expect next. Be empathic. Acknowledge her feelings and let her know that these feelings are normal considering the situation with which she must cope.

Providing Care in the Immediate Recovery Phase

Nursing care in the postoperative period is influenced by many factors. Some of these are the type of anesthesia that was given, complications that occurred during surgery, the outcome and condition of the neonate, and stability of maternal condition.

Assist the RN to transfer the woman from the operative suite to the PACU. The RN will connect her

NURSING CARE PLAN 11.1

The Woman Undergoing an Unplanned (Emergency) Cesarean Delivery*

CASE SCENARIO

Rene Truitt is a 28-year-old primigravida who went into spontaneous labor at 40 weeks' gestation. She received an epidural when her cervix progressed to 4 centimeters dilation and reported adequate pain relief. She progressed to full dilation and pushed for 2 hours, but the fetal head did not descend below 0 station. The fetal monitor tracing is now showing occasional late decelerations. The physician has ordered a primary cesarean delivery. Rene is voicing concern over the welfare of her baby and is crying softly. Her husband is attempting to comfort her.

NURSING DIAGNOSIS

Anxiety related to fetal status and unexpected surgical procedure.

GOAL: Rene will demonstrate positive coping behaviors to deal with her anxiety.

EXPECTED OUTCOMES:
- Seeks information to reduce anxiety.
- Accepts her husband's offered support.
- Voices acceptance of the situation.

NURSING INTERVENTIONS	*RATIONALE*
Remain with Rene while preparing her for surgery.	Presence of the nurse can be reassuring in a stressful situation.
Display a calm and confident manner.	Promotes trust.
Explain procedures as you perform them.	Understanding what is happening helps decrease anxiety.
Emphasize the qualifications of the surgical team (i.e., surgeon, circulating nurse, anesthesiologist).	Promotes trust and confidence.
Briefly describe what Rene and her husband will experience throughout the procedure.	Understanding what to expect helps decrease anxiety.
Encourage Rene's husband to participate throughout (e.g., holding her hand, remaining with her whenever possible).	The presence of a support person can be comforting.

NURSING DIAGNOSIS

Risk for injury related to major surgical procedure.

GOAL: Rene will not experience preventable injury throughout the perioperative period.

EXPECTED OUTCOMES:
- Gives informed consent for cesarean delivery.
- Urinary output remains at least 30 cc/hour.
- Urine color remains clear yellow.
- Maintains adequate fluid volume.

NURSING INTERVENTIONS	*RATIONALE*
Check the chart for signed informed consent for cesarean delivery. Obtain signed consent, if not already completed.	Although it is primarily the physician's responsibility to obtain informed consent, the signed form is evidence that Rene has consented.
Make certain that Rene and her husband have had any questions or concerns they have about the procedure addressed. If there are additional questions, notify the RN or physician immediately.	It is imperative that Rene understand the risks involved for cesarean delivery, as well as the risks involved for continuing to attempt vaginal birth.
Check the chart for laboratory results. If they are not on the chart, place them in the chart before surgery.	The surgical team will refer to lab results to help determine if extra safety precautions are needed.
Make certain that at least 2 units of packed red blood cells are on hold in the lab, as ordered. Alternatively, the blood should at least be typed and screened.	Rene is at increased risk for bleeding because she will be experiencing major surgery. It is imperative that blood be immediately available, in the event hemorrhage should occur.

NURSING CARE PLAN 11.1 continued

The Woman Undergoing an Unplanned (Emergency) Cesarean Delivery*

NURSING INTERVENTIONS	RATIONALE
Check the IV line for patency before surgery. Inform the RN immediately if the IV needs to be restarted.	A patent IV line with a large-bore needle must be in place before Rene can go to surgery.
Check to see if a Foley catheter is in place. If not, insert the catheter before transporting Rene to the OR suite.	A urinary catheter is necessary to keep the bladder drained. This will decrease the chance of bladder injury during surgery.

NURSING DIAGNOSIS
Risk for aspiration (maternal) related to gravid uterus pressing upward on the stomach and anesthesia for cesarean delivery.

GOAL: Rene will not experience respiratory compromise.

EXPECTED OUTCOMES:
- Maintains a respiratory rate between 16 and 22 breaths/minute
- Maintains a regular respiratory rhythm
- Remains free from adventitious breath sounds

NURSING INTERVENTIONS	RATIONALE
Report to anesthesiologist the date and time of last oral intake (solid and liquid).	This information allows the anesthesiologist to plan how to best protect the airway during surgery.
Administer IV or PO antacids, as ordered before surgery.	Antacids decrease the acidity of stomach contents, which reduces the potential for injury from aspiration.
Assess respiratory status before and after surgery.	Preoperative assessment will determine baseline respiratory status. Postoperative assessment is done to detect changes that might be associated with aspiration.

* *Note:* This care plan addresses preoperative care of a woman who experiences an unplanned cesarean delivery. Postoperative nursing care is addressed in Chapter 12.

---

to monitoring devices that will record the electrocardiogram, blood pressure, pulse, and oxygen saturation of the blood. The RN will also take vital sign and pulse oximetry readings every 5 minutes until the readings are stable, and then every 15 to 30 minutes until the patient has met predetermined criteria. The RN will monitor the patient's urinary output to make certain it is at least 30 cc/hour.

In addition to normal PACU activities, postpartum assessments must be done. The condition of the fundus must be evaluated and recorded along with vital signs. The nurse's hand or a pillow can support the incision while the fundus is gently massaged to determine if it is firm. A firmly contracted uterus will minimize bleeding. In conjunction with the fundal check, an assessment of the amount and type of lochia flow is made. These assessments are performed and recorded

A word of caution is in order. During cesarean birth the surgeon is able to thoroughly clean the inside of the uterus. Therefore, there should be less lochia flow than is present after a vaginal delivery. Moderate amounts of lochia after a cesarean delivery should alert the nurse to the possibility of postpartum hemorrhage.

at the same time interval as the vital signs. (Refer to Chapter 12 for a full discussion of postpartum assessment and nursing care.)

The timing and process of recovery is influenced in large part by the type of anesthesia given. Chapter 9 discusses the different types of anesthesia, including recovery considerations.

VAGINAL BIRTH AFTER CESAREAN

In times past the adage "once a cesarean, always a cesarean" guided the practice of obstetricians, and most women who had experienced a primary cesarean birth were scheduled for repeat cesareans. During the 1980s, a push was made to decrease the number of cesarean births in the United States by reducing the number of repeat cesarean births. Many obstetricians encouraged their patients to attempt a vaginal birth after one or more cesarean births (VBAC). However, recent studies and experience have shown that the risk for uterine rupture during VBAC often outweighs the benefits of a vaginal birth, and many obstetricians no longer offer this procedure for their patients. However, there are women who may be potential candidates for VBAC. These women are counseled by their physician regarding the benefits and risks.

Prerequisites

ACOG recommendations regarding trial of labor for a woman who has previously delivered by cesarean include an adequate pelvis, no previous uterine ruptures, personnel and facilities available to perform an immediate cesarean delivery, and no more than two previous low transverse uterine scars (Cunningham et al., 2001, p. 542). In 2002, ACOG added stipulations to include signed informed consent that lists benefits and risks; surgeon, anesthesia provider, and operating room personnel in the hospital; ability to perform a cesarean delivery in less than 18 minutes after the order is given; sufficient blood in the hospital; and a practitioner (this is often the RN) at the bedside who can read and interpret EFM tracings and who can recognize the signs and symptoms of uterine rupture (Dauphinee, 2004).

Contraindications

The risk for uterine rupture during VBAC is much higher when a classical incision was previously done on the uterus; therefore, VBAC is contraindicated when this type of scar is present. It is also contraindicated if the woman has a history of previous uterine rupture.

Procedure

If VBAC is determined to be a valid option, the woman is given what is called a "trial of labor." Generally she is allowed to go into labor on her own. Then her progress is monitored carefully. The

BOX 11.2	Signs of Uterine Rupture

- Dramatic onset of fetal bradycardia or deep variable decelerations
- Reports by the woman of a "popping" sensation in her abdomen
- Excessive maternal pain (can be referred pain, such as to the chest)
- Unrelenting uterine contraction followed by a disorganized uterine pattern
- Increased fetal station felt upon vaginal examination (e.g., station is now −3 when it has been −1)
- Easily palpable fetal parts through the abdominal wall
- Signs of maternal shock

woman is attached to continuous EFM throughout labor, and the nurse must be vigilant to monitor for signs of uterine rupture (Box 11-2). The use of oxytocin during labor is not contraindicated absolutely, but its use requires monitoring that is even closer than usual.

Nursing Care

It is outside the scope of the LPN to care for a laboring woman who has a history of a previous cesarean delivery. An experienced RN will manage the labor. Special written informed consent that outlines the risks and benefits of VBAC is required. The woman may verbally withdraw her consent at any time during the course of labor. At the time she withdraws her consent, the trial of labor is discontinued, and the woman is prepared for a cesarean delivery (Dauphinee, 2004).

During the labor the RN continuously monitors the EFM tracing. Any nonreassuring patterns are immediately reported because a nonreassuring pattern is the most significant sign of a ruptured uterus. The specially trained LPN may function as the scrub nurse if a cesarean is indicated during trial of labor.

Test Yourself

- What is the primary focus of nursing intervention when a cesarean delivery is planned?
- What is the primary focus of nursing intervention when a cesarean birth is emergent?
- What is one contraindication for a trial of labor after previous cesarean delivery?

KEY POINTS

◗ External version is done in an attempt to reposition a fetus in a breech or shoulder presentation to a more favorable vertex presentation.

◗ Medical indications for the induction of labor include postdate pregnancy, PROM, chorioamnionitis, pregnancy-induced hypertension, intrauterine fetal growth restriction, or certain medical conditions such as maternal diabetes.

◗ The Bishop score is used to help determine cervical readiness for labor. Five factors are evaluated: cervical consistency, position, dilatation, effacement, and fetal station.

◗ Mechanical methods to enhance ripening of the cervix include membrane stripping and mechanical dilation of the cervix with either a catheter or laminaria.

◗ Pharmacologic methods to ripen the cervix require closer monitoring of the woman and include local application of prostaglandin gel or vaginal inserts, or insertion of a prostaglandin tablet.

◗ Oxytocin induction requires continuous fetal monitoring, a mainline IV, and a secondary IV line that contains the oxytocin, which is connected to an IV pump. Oxytocin is titrated up until an adequate contraction pattern is obtained.

◗ Complications associated with the use of oxytocin include higher risk for cesarean delivery, hyperstimulation of the uterus with possible fetal distress, and uterine rupture. Water intoxication is another potential complication.

◗ Amnioinfusion involves infusing fluid via an IUPC into the uterine cavity after the membranes have ruptured and the cervix is at least partially dilated. This procedure is done to relieve signs of cord compression and to dilute thick meconium-stained fluid.

◗ An episiotomy is a surgical incision made in the perineum to enlarge the vaginal opening just before delivery. A midline episiotomy extends straight downward into the true perineum. A mediolateral episiotomy is angled to the right or the left of the perineum.

◗ Vacuum extraction uses a suction cup that is attached to the fetal head, which allows the physician to provide gentle downward traction to assist delivery.

◗ In a forceps-assisted delivery, hard metal tools shaped something like large hollowed-out spoons are applied to the fetal head. Midforceps are used to rotate the fetus to an anterior position. Low and outlet forceps are more frequently used to shorten the second stage of labor.

◗ Cesarean delivery is a major surgical procedure. It carries with it all the risks and complications associated with abdominal surgery in addition to those associated with normal birth.

◗ The four most common indications for cesarean delivery are history of previous cesarean, labor dystocia, fetal distress, and breech presentation. Other less common indications include placenta previa, abruptio placentae, cephalopelvic disproportion, active vaginal herpes lesions, prolapse of the umbilical cord, ruptured uterus, and certain medical and obstetric conditions.

◗ Both skin and uterine incisions can be vertical or transverse. The uterine incision is the most important of the two. The classical uterine incision is associated with the highest risk for rupture in subsequent pregnancies. The low cervical transverse uterine incision is the preferred method.

◗ Nursing interventions for a planned cesarean birth are focused on education to prepare the family for the birth. Interventions for an emergency cesarean include mostly supportive behaviors, such as explaining procedures as they are done and providing appropriate reassurance.

◗ A woman who wishes to experience VBAC must be given a trial of labor. Because of the risk for uterine rupture, the woman is carefully screened for this procedure. History of a classical uterine incision or a previous uterine rupture is a contraindication for VBAC.

REFERENCES AND SELECTED READINGS

Books and Journals

ACOG News Release. (2003). Weighing the pros and cons of cesarean delivery. The American College of Obstetricians and Gynecologists (ACOG). Retrieved March 20, 2004, from http://www.acog.org/from_home/newsrel.cfm (Scroll down and click on the article).

Boulvain, M., Kelly, A., Lohse, C., Stan, C., & Irion, O. (2003). Mechanical methods for induction of labour (Cochrane Review). *The Cochran Library, Issue 1*(2003). [Abstract]. Retrieved April 6, 2003, from http://www.cochrane.org/cochrane/revabstr/ab001233.htm

Carroli, G., & Belizan, J. (2004). Episiotomy for vaginal birth (Cochrane Review). *The Cochrane Library, Issue 1*(2004). [Abstract]. Retrieved March 7, 2004, from http://212.49.218.202/abstracts/ab000081.htm

Caughey, A. B., & Mann, S. (2002). Vaginal birth after cesarean delivery. In: S. D. Spandorfer, F. Talavera, C. V. Smith, F. B. Gaupp, & L. P. Shulman (Eds.). *eMedicine*. Retrieved April 24, 2003, from http://www.emedicine.com/med/topic3434.htm

Coco, A. S., & Silverman, S. D. (1998). External cephalic version. *American Family Physician*. Retrieved April 24, 2003, from http://www.aafp.org/afp/980901ap/coco.html

Cunningham, F. G., Gant, N. F., Leveno, K. J., Gilstrap L. C. III, Hauth, J. C., & Wenstrom, K. D. (2001). *Williams obstet-*

rics (21st ed.). New York: McGraw Hill Medical Publishing Division.

Dauphinee, J. D. (2004). VBAC: Safety for the patient and the nurse. *Journal of Obstetric, Gynecologic, and Neonatal Nursing (JOGNN), 33*(1), 105–115.

Encyclopaedia Britannica (Eds.). (2002). Cesarean section. Retrieved January 28, 2002, from http://www. britannica. com/eb/article?eu=22509

Goldberg, A. B., & Wing, D. A. (2003). Induction of labor: The misoprostol controversy [Abstract]. *Journal of Midwifery & Women's Health, 48*(4), 244–248.

Harman, J. H., & Kim, A. (1999). Current trends in cervical ripening and labor induction. *American Family Physician, 61*(August), 477–488. Retrieved April 5, 2003, from http://www.aafp.org/afp/990800ap/477.html

Joseph, K. S., Young, D. C., Dodds, L., O'Connell, C. M., Allen, V. M., Chandra, S., & Allen, A. C. (2003). Changes in maternal characteristics and obstetric practice and recent increases in primary cesarean delivery. *Obstetrics & Gynecology: Original Research, 102*(4), 791–800. Retrieved March 7, 2004, from http://www.acog.org/from_home/publications/green_journal/wrapper.cfm?document=2003/ong14583fla.htm

Martin, J. A., Hamilton, B. E., Sutton, P. D., Ventura, S. J., Menacker, F., & Munson, M. L. (2003). Births: Final data for 2002. *National Vital Statistics Reports, 52*(10), 1–114. Retrieved March 7, 2004, from http://www.cdc.gov/nchs/data/nvsr/nvsr52/nvsr52_10.pdf

Simpson, K. R., & Atterbury, J. (2003). Trends and issues in labor induction in the United States: Implications for clinical practice. *Journal of Obstetric, Gynecologic, and Neonatal Nursing (JOGNN), 32*(6), 767–779.

Simpson, K. R., & Creehan, P. A. (2001). *Perinatal nursing* (2nd ed.). Philadelphia: Lippincott Williams & Wilkins.

Weismiller, D. G. (1998). Transcervical amnioinfusion. *American Family Physician, 57*(3), 504–512. Retrieved April 26, 2003, from http://www.aafp.org/afp/980201ap/articles.html

Wilk, P. R., & Galan, H. (2002). Postdate pregnancy. In B. D. Cowan, F. Talavera, R. S. Legro, F. B. Gaupp, & L. P. Shulman (Eds.), *eMedicine*. Retrieved April 5, 2003, from http://www.emedicine.com/med/topic3248.htm

Websites

Labor Induction

http://www.hattiesburgclinic.com/front/61801/inside/show. asp?durki=634

http://www.parents.com/articles/pregnancy/1014.jsp?page=1

Cesarean Birth

http://www.noah-health.org/english/pregnancy/pregnancy.html (Scroll down to the "Delivery" section on the page. Click on the link "Cesarean Birth." When you are done exploring that section, click on the link "Vaginal Birth After Cesarean.")

Photos

http://pregnancy.about.com/library/blsection.htm

WORKBOOK

NCLEX-STYLE REVIEW QUESTIONS

1. A woman who has an episiotomy asks the nurse, "When will I get my stitches taken out?" How should the nurse best reply?

   a. "I don't know. Ask the doctor."

   b. "It depends on the type of episiotomy. A mediolateral episiotomy requires that the stitches be removed, while a midline does not."

   c. "The doctor will remove the stitches when the perineum stops hurting."

   d. "The stitches will be absorbed on their own. They do not need to be removed."

2. A primigravida is tired of being pregnant. She asks the nurse, "Why can't my doctor just schedule a cesarean delivery? My friend had a cesarean and everything went very well." What is the best reply by the nurse?

   a. "A cesarean birth involves major surgery, which puts you and your baby at higher risk for complications. Your physician will discuss the options with you."

   b. "I will ask your doctor. Sometimes he will allow a first-time mother to have a cesarean birth if she wants to do so."

   c. "Oh no. This would not be good for the baby. Try not to think too much about it. It is always better to have a vaginal delivery."

   d. "Why do you want to do that? Don't you know a vaginal delivery is the preferred way to have a baby?"

3. A woman whose fetus is breech is scheduled for external version. She says to the nurse, "I'm really scared of the procedure. Will it hurt badly?" What is the best reply by the nurse?

   a. "Don't worry. An external version procedure is not painful."

   b. "Sometimes the procedure is uncomfortable. If it becomes too painful, let the doctor know and she will stop the procedure."

   c. "The procedure can be quite uncomfortable, but it is best for your baby. You want to do what's best for the baby, right?"

   d. "You can do it. I'll hold your hand throughout the procedure and you should be just fine."

4. A woman is dilated 9 centimeters and the fetus is in an anterior position at a +1 station. The bag of waters is ruptured. She has been in labor for several hours and is exhausted, so she asks the nurse, "My friend was tired at the end of her labor, and the doctor used forceps to help deliver the baby. Could the doctor pull the baby out with forceps so I can get this over with?" What response by the nurse is best?

   a. "I don't know. Let me ask the doctor."

   b. "The cervix must be completely dilated before forceps can be applied safely."

   c. "No. Once the water bag ruptures, the doctor cannot apply forceps."

   d. "Forceps are too dangerous. I'll get a vacuum extractor ready for your delivery."

STUDY ACTIVITIES

1. Develop a 15-minute presentation on cesarean delivery to give to a group of first-time mothers at a prenatal education class.
2. Discuss how care of the newborn during cesarean delivery is different from care of the newborn after vaginal delivery. What additional risk factors does the newborn delivered by cesarean have?
3. Using the table below, compare methods of cervical ripening.

Method	How it Works to Ripen the Cervix	Special Nursing Considerations

CRITICAL THINKING: What Would You Do?

Apply your knowledge of cesarean birth and assisted deliveries to the following situations.

1. Amy Jones is a 21-year-old gravida 1 who is attending a prenatal childbirth education class. She comments that she thinks she will not attend next week's class because cesarean delivery is going to be discussed, and she does not plan to have a cesarean. How would you reply to Amy's comment?

2. A woman who is close to term asks the nurse at a normal obstetric visit, "My doctor says I have a Bishop score of 4. What does that mean?"

   a. How would you reply?

   b. If the physician felt that the woman's labor needed to be induced, what recommendation would she likely make to the woman? Why?

3. You are going to assist the physician to perform a fetal fibronectin test. What equipment do you need?

4. Ellen Hess, a 30-year-old gravida 2, has chosen to attempt a VBAC. After 4 hours of labor, she reports to you severe pain and a "popping" sensation in her abdomen. What would you do?

Postpartum and Newborn

The Postpartum Woman

12

STUDENT OBJECTIVES

On completion of this chapter, the student will be able to

1. Describe the physiologic adaptation of the woman during the postpartum period.
2. Discuss major points related to psychological adaptation during the postpartum period.
3. Describe a postpartum assessment.
4. Discuss the responsibilities of the practical (vocational) nurse in caring for the woman in the early postpartum period.
5. Compare and contrast the nursing care of the woman who delivers vaginally with that of the one who delivers by cesarean.
6. Outline the nurse's role in preparing the woman for discharge.

KEY TERMS

attachment
boggy uterus
bonding
breakthrough pain
colostrum
diastasis recti abdominis
dyspareunia
en face
grand multiparity
involution
lochia
postpartum blues
puerperium

The processes of pregnancy and birth challenge the woman's psychological and physiologic coping mechanisms. It is during the postpartum period, sometimes referred to as the 4th trimester of pregnancy, that the woman must adjust to the reality of her new role as mother. This is also the period during which her body must return to the nonpregnant state. The postpartum period, or **puerperium**, encompasses the 6 weeks after birth. For ease of discussion, the puerperium can be subdivided into three categories: the immediate postpartum period, which covers the first 24 hours; the early postpartum period or 1st week; and late postpartum period, which refers to weeks 2 through 6. This chapter discusses the adaptations a low-risk woman makes during the puerperium and the nursing care that promotes healing and wellness.

MATERNAL ADAPTATION DURING THE POSTPARTUM PERIOD

Physiologic Adaptation

The woman's body undergoes tremendous changes to accommodate pregnancy. Every body system and organ is affected. It is during the weeks after pregnancy that the body recovers from the stress of pregnancy and returns to its normal prepregnancy state.

Reproductive System

The organs and hormones of the reproductive system must gradually return to their nonpregnant size and function. The shrinking or returning to normal size of the uterus, cervix, and vagina is called the process of **involution**.

Uterus

Uterine Contraction and Involution. Immediately after the placenta delivers, the uterus contracts inward, a process that seals off the open blood vessels at the former site of the placenta. If the uterus does not contract effectively, the woman will hemorrhage. The clotting cascade also is initiated, a process that causes clot formation to control bleeding. Large blood vessels at the former placental site degenerate and are replaced by smaller ones. Gradually the decidua is shed, new endometrial tissue forms, and the placental area heals without leaving fibrous scar tissue.

Uterine contraction also leads to uterine involution. Involution is assessed by measuring fundal height. Immediately after delivery the fundus is firm and located in the midline halfway between the umbilicus and symphysis pubis. One hour after delivery the uterus should be contracted firmly, with the fundus midline at the level of the umbilicus. The day after

delivery the fundus is found 1 cm below the umbilicus. The normal process of involution thereafter is for the uterus to descend approximately 1 fingerbreadth (1 cm) per day until it has descended below the level of the pubic bone and can no longer be palpated. This occurs by the 10th postpartum day (Fig. 12-1).

There are several factors that promote uterine contraction and involution. Breast-feeding stimulates oxytocin release from the woman's posterior pituitary gland. Oxytocin stimulates the uterus to contract. Early ambulation and proper nourishment also foster normal involution.

In addition, there are factors that can inhibit or delay uterine involution. A full bladder impedes uterine contraction by pushing upward on the uterus and displacing it. Any condition that overdistends the uterus during pregnancy can lead to ineffective uterine contraction after delivery. Examples include a multifetal pregnancy and hydramnios. Maternal exhaustion and excessive analgesia during labor and delivery also can hinder contraction of the uterus. Other factors include retained placental fragments, infection, and **grand multiparity**, five or more pregnancies. When the uterus does not contract effectively, blood and clots collect in the uterus, which makes it even more difficult for the uterus to contract. This leads to a **boggy uterus** and hemorrhage if the condition is not arrested. A boggy uterus feels soft and spongy, rather than firm and well contracted.

● **Figure 12.1** Normal uterine involution occurs at a predictable rate. One hour after childbirth the fundus is at the level of the umbilicus. On the first postpartum day the fundus is approximately 1 fingerbreadth or 1 cm below the level of the umbilicus. Thereafter, it descends downward at the rate of 1 fingerbreadth per day until it becomes a pelvic organ again on the 10th day postpartum.

Afterpains. After a multipara delivers, the uterus contracts and relaxes at intervals. This leads to afterpains, which can be quite severe. For the primipara, the uterus normally remains contracted, and afterpains are less severe than that of the multipara. However, breast-feeding, because it causes the release of oxytocin, increases the duration and intensity of afterpains for both the primipara and multipara.

Lochia. The uterine lining that helped nourish the pregnancy must be shed. Blood, mucus, tissue, and white blood cells are cast away from the uterus during the postpartum period. This discharge is called **lochia**. Lochia discharge progresses through three stages:

- Lochia rubra: Occurs during the first 3 to 4 days; is of small to moderate amount; is composed mostly of blood; is dark red in color; and has a fleshy odor.
- Lochia serosa: Occurs during days 4 to 10; decreases to a small amount; and takes on a brownish or pinkish color.
- Lochia alba: Occurs after day 10; and becomes white or pale yellow because the bleeding has stopped and the discharge is now composed mostly of white blood cells.

Lochia may persist for the entire 6 weeks after delivery but often subsides by the end of the 2nd or 3rd week. The lochia should never contain large clots. Other abnormal findings include reversal of the pattern (e.g., the lochia has been serosa, then goes back to rubra); lochia that fails to decrease in amount or actually increases versus gradually decreasing; or a malodorous lochia.

Warning! Normal lochia has a fleshy, but not offensive, odor. If the lochia is malodorous or smells rotten, infection is most likely present. This finding must be reported immediately to the RN or the practitioner.

Ovaries

Ovulation can occur as soon as 3 weeks after delivery. Menstrual periods usually begin within 6 to 8 weeks for the woman who is not breast-feeding. However, the lactating woman may not resume menses for as long 18 months after giving birth. Although lactation may suppress ovu-

Did you know? Ovulation can occur without return of the menstrual period. Conversely, the woman can have menstrual bleeding without ovulating. Explain to the woman that she may be able to conceive even if the menses does not resume immediately.

lation, it is not a dependable form of birth control. It is wise for the woman to use some type of birth control when she resumes sexual activity, unless she wishes to immediately become pregnant again.

Cervix

During labor the cervix thins and dilates. This process does not occur without some trauma. Directly after delivery the cervix is still partially open and contains soft, small tears. It may also appear bruised. Although abnormal, large tears may be an uncommon cause of postpartum hemorrhage. The internal os closes after a few days. Gradually the muscle cells regenerate, and the cervix recovers by the end of the 6-week puerperium. The external os, however, remains slightly open and has a slit-like appearance, in comparison with the dimple-like appearance of the cervix of a nulliparous woman (Fig. 12-2).

Vagina and Perineum

The vagina may have small tears that will heal without intervention. Immediately after delivery, the walls of the vagina are smooth. Rugae begin to return to the vaginal walls after approximately 3 weeks. The diameter of the introitus gradually becomes smaller by contraction but rarely returns to its prepregnant size. Muscle tone is never fully restored to the pregravid state; however, Kegel exercises may help increase the tone and enhance sexual enjoyment. Because breast-feeding suppresses ovulation, estrogen levels remain lower in the lactating woman, which can lead to vaginal dryness and **dyspareunia**, painful intercourse.

The labia and perineum may be edematous after delivery and may appear bruised, particularly after a difficult delivery. If an episiotomy was done or a perineal tear repaired, absorbable stitches will be in place. The edges of the episiotomy or repair should be well approximated. The episiotomy takes several weeks to fully heal. The labia tend to be flaccid after childbirth.

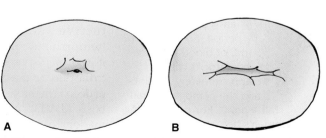

● **Figure 12.2** Appearance of the cervix in nulliparous and multiparous women. **(A)** This drawing represents the cervix of a nulliparous woman. Notice the dimple-like structure of the external os. **(B)** This is a representation of the cervix of a multiparous woman. The external os of the multiparous cervix is slit-like in appearance.

Tone may improve over time but never completely returns to the prepregnant state.

Breasts

Colostrum, the antibody-rich breast secretion that is the precursor to breast milk, is normally excreted by the breasts in the last weeks of pregnancy and continues to be excreted in the first few postpartum days. Prolactin levels rise when estrogen and progesterone levels fall after delivery of the placenta. Suckling at the breast also causes prolactin levels to rise. Prolactin stimulates milk production by the breasts, and the milk normally comes in on the 3rd day. See Chapter 14 for a detailed discussion of breast physiology, milk production, and breast-feeding.

Test Yourself

- Where is the fundus normally located on the day after delivery?

- Name three factors that can inhibit or delay uterine involution.

- Name the three stages, in order, through which lochia passes.

Cardiovascular System

The additional fluid volume that is present during the pregnancy is eliminated in the early postpartum period via the skin and urinary routes and through blood loss. The woman who experiences a normal vaginal delivery loses approximately 300 to 500 mL of blood during delivery. If she has a cesarean delivery, normal blood loss is between 500 and 1,000 mL. As the blood volume returns to normal, some hemoconcentration occurs that causes an increase in the hematocrit.

If you can remember this, you'll be able to approximately determine the amount of blood loss in the early postpartum period. For every 250 mL of blood loss, the hematocrit will fall approximately 2 points, and the hemoglobin will fall 1 point. For example, if the woman's hemoglobin and hematocrit were 12.0 and 34, respectively, before delivery, then fall to 10.0 and 30 the day after, she has lost approximately 500 mL of blood.

High plasma fibrinogen levels and other coagulation factors mark the postpartum period. This is protective against hemorrhage, but it also predisposes to the development of deep vein thrombosis (DVT), formation of blood clots in the deep veins of the legs. Dehydration, immobility, and trauma can add to the risk for DVT. Refer to Chapter 19 for discussion of DVT in the postpartum period.

The white blood cell count is elevated to approximately 15,000 to 20,000/ mL, and may reach as high as 30,000/mL. Leukocytosis helps protect the woman from infection, as there are multiple routes for infection to occur in the early postpartum period.

Immediately after delivery, the woman may experience a shaking postpartum chill. This is thought to be caused by hormonal and physiologic changes and is not harmful, unless accompanied by fever greater than 100.4°F or other signs of infection. The shivering normally resolves within minutes, especially if a prewarmed blanket is placed over the woman.

Vital Signs

The temperature may be elevated slightly during the first 24 hours because of the exertion and dehydration of labor. After the first 24 hours, a temperature of 100.4°F or greater is abnormal and may indicate infection.

Here's a tip to help you get accurate blood pressure readings. Take the woman's blood pressure with the woman in the same position each time. The preferred position is supine because orthostatic hypotension is common immediately after delivery. If you take the blood pressure immediately after the woman sits up from a lying position, the reading may be falsely low.

The blood pressure should remain at the woman's baseline level. An elevated blood pressure could be a sign of developing preeclampsia and should be reported. (See Chapter 17.) A falling blood pressure, particularly in the presence of a rising pulse is suggestive of hemorrhage. The woman should be assessed carefully for a source of blood loss if her blood pressure drops.

It is normal for the pulse to be slow in the 1st week after delivery. A heart rate as low as 50 beats per minute is considered normal. Occasionally the woman may experience tachycardia. This is more likely to occur after a difficult labor and delivery, or it may indicate excess blood loss.

Musculoskeletal System

The most pronounced changes are found in the abdominal muscles, although other muscles may be weak because of the exertion of labor. The abdomen is soft and sagging in the immediate postpartum period. Often the woman has to wear loose clothing for the first few weeks. The abdomen usually regains its tone with exercise. However, in some women the abdomen remains slack. In this situation if another pregnancy occurs, the abdomen will be pendulous and the woman will have more problems with backache. **Diastasis recti abdominis** is a condition in which the abdominal muscles separate during the pregnancy, leaving part of the abdominal wall without muscular support. Exercise can improve muscle tone, if diastasis recti abdominis occurs. A woman is predisposed for poor muscle tone and diastasis if she has poor muscle tone or is obese before the pregnancy, her abdomen is overdistended during the pregnancy, or she is a grand multipara.

Gastrointestinal System

Immediately after delivery the postpartum woman often is very hungry. The energy expended during labor uses up glucose stores, and food has generally been restricted. Restriction of fluids and loss of fluids in labor, in the urine, and via diaphoresis often lead to increased thirst.

The postpartum woman may be troubled by constipation. Intra-abdominal pressure decreases rapidly after childbirth, and peristalsis is diminished. These factors make it more difficult for feces to travel down the gastrointestinal tract. The woman may be afraid to defecate in the early postpartum period because of hemorrhoidal discomfort and perineal pain. Suppressing the urge to defecate complicates the problem of constipation and may actually cause increased pain when defecation finally occurs. Iron supplementation adds to the problem. However, by the end of the 1st postpartum week, bowel function has usually returned to normal.

Urinary System

The urinary system must handle an increased load in the early postpartum period as the body excretes excess plasma volume. Healthy kidneys are able to adjust to the increased demands. Urinary output exceeds intake. Transient glycosuria, proteinuria, and ketonuria are normal in the immediate postpartum period.

During the process of labor and delivery trauma can occur to the lower urinary system. Pressure of the descending fetal head on the ureters, bladder, and urethra can lead to transient loss of bladder tone and urethral edema. Trauma, certain medications, and anesthesia given during labor can also lead to a temporary loss of bladder sensation. The result can be urinary retention. Sometimes the woman voids small amounts but does not completely empty the bladder. Or she may not be able to void at all. If the urethra has been traumatized, voiding may be painful.

The urinary system is more susceptible to infection during the postpartum period. Hydronephrosis, dilation of the renal pelves and ureters, is a normal change that occurs during pregnancy because of hormonal influences. This condition persists for approximately 4 weeks after delivery. Hydronephrosis and urinary stasis predispose the woman to urinary tract infection (UTI).

Integumentary System

Copious diaphoresis occurs in the first few days after childbirth as the body rids itself of excess water and waste via the skin. The perspiration is noticed particularly at night. The woman may wake up and be drenched in sweat. This is a normal finding and is not a cause for concern.

Striae, stretch marks, are found on the abdomen and sometimes on the breasts. Immediately after birth they appear red or purplish. Over time they fade to a light silvery color and remain faintly visible.

Weight Loss

Immediately after delivery approximately 10 to 12 pounds are lost with expulsion of the fetus, placenta, and amniotic fluid. The woman loses an additional 5 pounds in the early postpartum period because of fluid loss from diaphoresis and urinary excretion. The average woman will have returned to her prepregnant weight 6 months after childbirth, if she was within the recommended weight gain of 25 to 30 pounds during pregnancy. Some women take longer to lose the additional pounds. In general, the breast-feeding woman tends to lose weight faster than the woman who does not breast-feed because of increased caloric demands.

Here's an assessment tip! A full bladder can push up on the uterus, which displaces it (usually to the right side) and interferes with effective uterine contraction. If you palpate the fundus and find that it is above the umbilicus, deviated to the right side, and boggy, the most likely cause is a full bladder. Assist the woman to void, and then re-evaluate the fundus.

Test Yourself

- A falling blood pressure and rising pulse in the early postpartum period is suggestive of _____.

- Name two factors that contribute to constipation in the postpartum period.

- How long does it take for the average woman to return to her prepregnant weight after delivery?

Psychological Adaptation

Role change is the most significant psychological adaptation the woman must make. This process may be especially pronounced for first-time mothers, but it occurs with each new addition to the family. Each child is a unique being with her own temperament and needs. In fact, the whole family must adapt to the addition of a new member.

Maternal role development begins during pregnancy as the expectant mother anticipates the birth of the baby. She fantasizes about and prepares for her newborn's arrival. After the birth, the woman must take on the role of mother to the baby. This is a continuous process that occurs over the months and years as the child grows and changes.

The nurse can influence the development of positive family relationships in many ways. Careful assessment of maternal psychological adaptation and anticipatory guidance regarding postpartum blues and expected psychological adjustments can go a long way toward fostering positive transition for the woman and the new family.

Maternal Role Development

The adjustment of the woman to her new role as mother occurs through a series of developmental stages. Although each woman takes on her role as mother in her own way, influenced by her culture, upbringing, and role models, there are patterns of behavior that can be noted. One nurse researcher, Reva Rubin, observed that women go through three general phases in the first few days and continuing through the first year after delivery. These phases are taking in, taking hold, and letting go.

Taking In Phase

In the early puerperium the new mother demonstrates dependent behaviors. She has difficulty making decisions and needs assistance with self-care needs. She tends to be inwardly focused and concerned about her own physical needs, such as food, rest, and elimination. She relives the delivery experience, and has a great need to talk about the details. This process is important for her to integrate the experience into her concept of self. She may remain in this dependent, reintegration phase for several hours or days. This is not an optimum time to teach detailed newborn care because the new mother is not readily receptive to instruction. Listen with an attitude of acceptance. No feeling the woman expresses is "wrong." Help her interpret the events of her birth experience.

Taking Hold Phase

Most women move quickly from the dependent stage to increasing independence in self and newborn care. After she has rested and recovered somewhat from the stress

Don't yield to temptation!

Sometimes it may seem easier to do the infant care yourself, rather than observe and support the woman as she cares for the newborn. However, it is important for you not to assume the mothering role. The new mother needs practice and praise to begin to feel confident in her new role. Otherwise she may feel incompetent to carry out her parenting role when she goes home.

of the delivery, the new mother has more energy to concentrate on her infant. At this point she becomes receptive to infant care instruction. The first-time mother in particular needs reassurance that she is capable of providing care for her newborn. She may feel that the nurse is more adept than she is at meeting the newborn's needs. Therefore, it is important to encourage her to perform care for her newborn while you provide gentle guidance and support. She responds well to praise for her early attempts at child care during this phase. This phase lasts anywhere from 2 days to several weeks.

Letting Go Phase

Most nurses do not witness the transition into the third postpartum phase of psychological adjustment because this phase occurs in the late puerperium. Letting go of previous roles and defining her new parenting role requires grief work. It is normal for the woman to experience a wide range of emotions as she gives up her fantasy child and gets to know the real child. She begins to see her infant as separate from herself. It is during this phase that family relationships are adjusted to accommodate the infant.

Development of Positive Family Relationships

The enduring emotional bond that develops between the parent and infant is called **attachment**. However, this process does not happen automatically. Attachment occurs as parents interact with and respond to their infant. In the early postpartum period, the woman may have a wide range of emotions and responses to her newborn. Humans seem to respond to gains and losses in similar ways. Disbelief and shock are often the initial reactions. You may hear the mother say over and over, "I can't believe I just had a baby." Ambivalence also is a normal response. The new parents may communicate uncertainty over their readiness to take on the parent role. Frequently the new mother may experience negative feelings about the baby in the first few days after birth. However, she may not express these feelings because of the cultural expectation that "mothers always love their babies." If she does express negativity, such as "I'm

A PERSONAL GLIMPSE

I delivered my first child after 14 hours of intense labor. I went through my labor naturally without an epidural with the help of my doula. I pushed for 2 hours, so I was pretty exhausted after delivery. The midwife had to cut an episiotomy because she said it was a tight fit. My baby weighed 9 pounds! The next day while the baby was in the room I remember that everything felt so unreal. I kept telling myself that I should feel happy. But all I really wanted to do was to cry. The nurse came in and told me what a beautiful baby I had and asked me her name. I started to cry and said that I wasn't sure that I could be a good mother. I felt scared and confused and unready to take care of a baby. The nurse told me that the feelings I was having were very normal. She said that this was a huge change for me and that it takes time to get adjusted to the new mother role. She asked me if I had someone to help me at home. I told her that my sister was going to stay with me for several weeks. The nurse gave me a card with the phone number for the hospital. She wrote her name on it and told me that she would be happy to answer any questions I had after I went home. She said that I could talk to any of the nurses, if she wasn't on duty when I called. I felt relieved. The nurse then stayed with me a while and watched while I changed the baby's diaper. She told me that I was a quick learner and that I was very gentle with the baby. I felt so much better. I knew that it was going to be ok.

Holly

LEARNING OPPORTUNITY: Why do you think this new mother felt better after her interaction with the nurse? In what ways can you in your role as a nurse support the new mother when she expresses negative feelings about her baby or her abilities as a mother?

● **Figure 12.3** A mom and dad bond with their newborn immediately after birth. At first some parents are tentative, but gradually they will bond.

not sure that I like my baby," the nurse or family members may reply in a way that denies or dismisses the emotion. "Oh, I'm sure you don't mean that," is one such dismissive response. It is important to remember that negative feelings are part of the process as mother and baby adjust to each other and become acquainted.

The initial component of healthy attachment is a process called **bonding**. This is the way the new mother and father become acquainted with their newborn (Fig. 12-3). The process begins with a predictable pattern of parental behavior. Initial inspection of the newborn begins with fingertip touching. The new mother explores her newborn's extremities, counting his fingers and toes. She then advances to using the palms of her hands to touch the newborn and begins to explore larger body

areas. Eventually she enfolds the newborn with her hands and arms and holds her close. As bonding continues she begins to spend more time holding the newborn in the **en face** position in which she interacts face-to-face with the newborn. She places the baby's face within her direct line of vision and makes full eye contact with the newborn. The new mother often will talk to the baby in high-pitched tones and smile and laugh while she continues the en face posture. Box 12-1 lists the sequence of initial attachment.

Acceptance is not as hard as you think. If the new mother makes a negative comment, you can respond in a way that is accepting and supportive. You might reply, "It is natural to have feelings of uncertainty as you adjust to having a new baby." Or, "Having a new baby can seem a bit overwhelming at first. Take your time as you get to know your baby." Be creative. I'm sure you can come up with some great supportive phrases.

One important component in the development of healthy attachment between the new parents and their baby is the amount and type of social support the new family has available to them. If supportive friends and relatives surround them, attachment is enhanced. When a new mother is isolated and without adequate social support, attachment is threatened. If you encounter this situation, it is important to assist the woman to find sources of support. Perhaps there is someone she can call who might be willing to provide

BOX 12.1	Progression of Initial Attachment Behaviors

The new mother and father both begin their interaction with the new baby in a fairly predictable sequence. Note that this process may take anywhere from hours to days.
1. Exploration begins with fingertip touching.
2. Next the new parent explores the infant's extremities.
3. Fingertip touching gives way to touching with the palmar surface of the hands.
4. Then larger body surfaces are touched and caressed.
5. Soon the infant is enfolded with the hands and arms and cuddled closely to the parent.
6. Progressively more time is spent in the en face position talking to and smiling at the new baby.

support. Discuss the situation with the RN in charge. A referral to social services may be in order.

Healthy bonding behaviors include naming the newborn and calling the newborn by name. Making eye contact and talking to the newborn are other indicators that healthy attachment is occurring. It is important to differentiate between a new parent who is nervous and anxious about her new role and one who is rejecting her parenting role. Warning signals of poor attachment include turning away from the newborn, refusing or neglecting to provide for the care of the newborn, and disengagement from the newborn.

It was once thought that the mother was the first and most important person to bond with the new baby. It is now accepted that the baby can make many bonds (Fig. 12-4). The father benefits from early contact with the newborn immediately after delivery. It is common

for the father to describe strong emotions of pride, joy, and other positive emotions when he first holds his newborn. The father may be engrossed with the newborn. He progresses through a pattern of touching similar to that of the mother.

Siblings can also bond with the new baby. There are special considerations that the parents need to make for older siblings of a new baby. The birth of a new baby requires a role change for the sibling. Sometimes the new baby does not meet the sibling's expectations. For instance, the baby might be a boy, but the sibling wanted a sister. It is common for the sibling to regress for a few days after the birth.

Postpartum Blues

Approximately 50% to 70% of postpartum women will experience the **postpartum blues**, sometimes called the "baby blues." The postpartum blues is a temporary depression that usually begins on the 3rd day and lasts for 2 or 3 days. The woman may be tearful, have difficulty sleeping and eating, and feel generally let down. It is thought that a combination of factors contributes to the baby blues. Psychological adjustment along with a physiologic decrease in estrogen and progesterone are thought to be the greatest contributors. In addition, too much activity, fatigue, disturbed sleep patterns, and discomfort also may contribute. It is important for the woman and her family to know that this is a normal reaction; however, if the depression lasts for more than several days, or if the symptoms become severe, further psychological evaluation is needed. (See Chapter 19 for a discussion of postpartum depression.)

Test Yourself
- Name two characteristics of women who are in the taking in phase of psychological adjustment after delivery.
- Define attachment.
- List the normal progression of interaction that occurs during the initial bonding experience between a new parent and the newborn.

● Nursing Process for the Early Postpartum Period

Most women who deliver vaginally go home within 24 to 48 hours after delivery. This challenges the nurse caring for the woman in the early

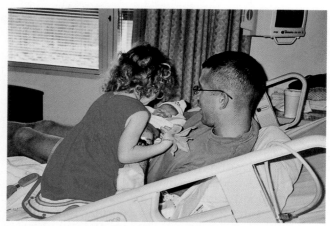

● *Figure 12.4* The proud father snuggles with his newborn son and introduces big sister to her new baby brother.

postpartum period to do thorough assessments to pick up on any complications that might be developing, and to use every available opportunity to do teaching regarding self- and newborn care.

ASSESSMENT

After the initial recovery period, the woman may be transferred to a postpartum room. If she delivered in a labor, delivery, recovery, and postpartum (LDRP) setting, she will stay in the room in which she delivered. Whatever the setting, the postpartum nurse must do a thorough initial assessment.

Data Collection

Much of the data collection is done before the woman delivers and can be found on the initial admission assessment done in the labor and delivery unit (L&D). It is important to check the initial assessment and the prenatal record as part of the initial data collection. The L&D nurse gives report when the woman is transferred to the postpartum nurse. The report should include significant medical history, pregnancy history, labor and birth history, newborn data, and initial postpartum recovery data.

The medical and pregnancy histories are important because they alert the postpartum nurse to risk factors that might lead to postpartum hemorrhage or other complications and give clues as to bonding potential. The report includes the gravida and para, the estimated date of delivery (EDD), blood type and Rh, complications experienced during the pregnancy, group B streptococcus (GBS) culture status, and any medical problems, including sexually transmitted infections (STIs).

The labor and birth history includes the length of labor, type and time of birth, type and timing of analgesia or anesthesia administered, type and timing of any IV medications given, and any complications experienced during labor. Important information regarding the newborn includes sex, Apgar scores, resuscitation efforts, congenital anomalies, current status, the mother's plans for feeding, and whether or not feeding was initiated in the delivery room. Initial postpartum recovery data that should be reported includes status of the fundus, lochia, and perineum; type of pain, if any, and success of analgesics and comfort measures to control the pain; whether or not the woman ambulated after delivery and how she tolerated it; type and amount of IV fluids infusing, if any; status of the bladder; and response of the woman and her partner to the newborn.

Physical Assessment
Initial Assessment in the First Hour After Delivery

If the woman is going to hemorrhage, she is most likely to do so within the 1st postpartum hour. For this reason, she is monitored closely during this time period. Her vital signs are monitored every 15 minutes during the 1st hour. With each vital sign check, determine the position and firmness of the uterine fundus, the amount and character of lochia, the status of the perineum, and monitor for signs of bladder distention. If the woman had a cesarean delivery, also check the incisional dressing for intactness and determine if any incisional bleeding is occurring. Measure the temperature and determine the status of the breasts once immediately after delivery and then again just before transfer to postpartum. Some institutions continue monitoring as above every 30 minutes for the 2nd hour, then every 4 hours during the first 24 hours after delivery.

Complete Postpartum Assessment

At least once per shift a complete head-to-toe assessment should be completed. A quick visual survey and speaking to the woman reveals her level of consciousness and affect. Assist her to empty her bladder, if necessary, before commencing the full assessment. First, take the vital signs. Respirations should be even and unlabored. Be sure to rule out shortness of breath and chest pain. The heart rate should be regular without murmurs and may be as slow as 50 beats per minute. The lungs should be clear in all five lobes (Fig. 12-5). After the vital signs assessment, there are 11 main areas that must be assessed and monitored in the postpartum period. These areas are

* breasts
* uterus

● **Figure 12.5** The nurse auscultates the lungs as part of a complete postpartum assessment.

- lochia
- bladder
- bowel
- perineum
- lower extremities
- pain
- laboratory studies
- maternal–newborn bonding
- maternal emotional status

Breasts. Inspect the breasts and nipples for signs of engorgement, redness, or cracks. Palpate the breasts gently to determine if they are soft, filling, or engorged with milk. Note if there are any painful areas. With a gloved hand palpate the nipples to determine if they are erect or inverted. The breasts should be soft during the 1st postpartum day, and begin filling on the 2nd and 3rd days. Engorgement may occur on the 3rd day. There should be no reddened areas on the breasts, and the nipples should be intact without cracks or fissures.

Uterus. With the woman lying supine, palpate the fundus (Nursing Procedure 12-1). Note the position of the uterus and palpate the uterus to determine consistency, tone, position, and size. It should be firm, not boggy, located in the midline, and at the appropriate height in relation to the umbilicus, depending on what hour/day it is after delivery.

Notice this difference. When a woman has had a cesarean delivery, she usually has less lochia than a woman who delivers vaginally. This occurs because the surgeon thoroughly wipes out the uterine cavity before suturing it closed, which removes much of the blood and debris. However, she should still progress through the same stages (i.e., rubra, serosa, then alba), and the flow should progressively become smaller in amount.

Lochia. Determine the amount and character of the lochia. Is it scant, small, moderate, or heavy? Is it rubra or serosa? Is there a foul smell? Be sure to check under her buttocks for pooling. Ask her how many times she has changed her sanitary napkins/pads since the previous assessment and determine if she is saturating pads. The lochia should be rubra of small to moderate amount without large clots and no foul odor.

Bladder and Bowel. The woman should be voiding adequate amounts (more than 100 mL per each voiding) regularly. Voiding frequently in amounts smaller than 100 mL with associated suprapubic distention (a rounded area just above

Nursing Procedure 12.1
Fundal Palpation and Massage

EQUIPMENT

Warm, clean hands
Clean gloves

PROCEDURE

1. Explain procedure to the woman.
2. Instruct her to empty her bladder, if necessary.
3. Wash hands thoroughly.
4. Position her supine with the head of the bed flat.
5. Locate and place one hand on the uterine fundus. It should feel hard and rounded—something like a melon.
6. Place the other hand in a cupped position just above the symphysis pubis, as in the picture. Use this hand to gently support the uterus.

7. Gently massage the fundus, if it is soft or boggy.
8. Notice the location, height, and position of the uterus.
9. Wash hands.
10. Document the tone (soft, boggy, or firm) and the location of the fundus in finger breadths above or below or at the level of the umbilicus. Note whether or not the fundus is midline or deviated to one side.

Note: Vigorous fundal massage or overstimulation can cause the uterus to become flaccid, rather than helping it to contract. Take measures to avoid over-massaging the fundus.

● **Figure 12.6** Notice that the woman is in the Sims' position. The nurse lifts the upper buttock and inspects the perineum.

the symphysis pubis) is indicative of urinary retention. Next, visually inspect the abdomen and auscultate for bowel sounds. Bowel sounds should be present in all four quadrants. Ask the woman if she has had a bowel movement after delivery.

Perineum. Assist the woman to the Sims' position. Lift the top buttock, and with a good light source (such as a penlight or flashlight) inspect the perineum for redness, edema and ecchymosis. If an episiotomy was done or a tear occurred, check the sutures and be certain the edges are well approximated. Determine if there is any drainage from the stitches. Palpate gently with a gloved hand to determine if there are any

hematomas forming in the area. Note any hemorrhoids. The perineum should be intact, with only minimal swelling and no hematomas. Figure 12-6 depicts a nurse performing an assessment of the perineum.

Lower Extremities. Inspect the extremities for edema (Fig. 12-7A), equality of pulses, and capillary refill. Check for Homans' sign (Fig. 12-7B). Feel along the calf area for any warmth or redness. The calves should be of equal size and warmth bilaterally. There should be no reddened, painful areas, and there should be no pain in the calves when the feet are dorsiflexed (negative Homans' sign), or when the woman is walking.

Pain. Determine if the woman is experiencing any pain. If so, investigate the source (e.g., afterpains, episiotomy, painful urination, pain in the calves). Determine the characteristics, quality, timing, and relief after comfort measures.

Laboratory Studies. Monitor the hemoglobin and hematocrit (H&H). Note the H&H before delivery. Most practitioners order a postpartum H&H on the morning after delivery. If the values drop significantly, the woman may have experienced postpartum hemorrhage. Note the blood type and Rh. If the woman is Rh-negative, she will need a RhoGAM workup. Determine the woman's rubella status. If she is nonimmune, she will need a rubella immunization before she is discharged home.

Maternal–Newborn Bonding and Maternal Emotional Status. Anytime the newborn is in the room, note maternal–newborn interactions.

A   B

● **Figure 12.7** Assessment of the lower extremities. **(A)** The nurse checks the right lower extremity for edema. **(B)** The nurse dorsiflexes the foot and asks the woman if she feels pain in the calf of her leg. No pain is recorded as a negative Homans' sign. If pain is present, a positive Homans' sign is recorded and the RN or physician is notified. A positive Homans' sign may indicate the presence of deep vein thrombosis. Homans' sign is recorded and the RN or physician is notified. A positive Homans' sign may indicate the presence of deep vein thrombosis.

BOX 12.2	**Warning Signs of Poor Attachment**

- Making negative statements about the baby
- Turning away from the baby
- Refusing to name the baby
- Refusing to care for the baby
- Withdrawing
- Verbalizing disappointment with the sex of the baby
- Failing to touch the baby
- Limited handling of the baby

Assess successfulness of breast-feeding attempts. Notice the quantity and quality of social support available to the woman. Monitor her mood and affect. Box 12-2 lists warning signs of poor attachment.

Test Yourself

- List five major components of the woman's history that are important for the postpartum nurse to know when assuming care of the woman after delivery.

- Describe the appropriate way to perform an assessment of the episiotomy.

- Name three important laboratory studies to which the nurse should pay attention after delivery.

SELECTED NURSING DIAGNOSES

- Risk for Injury: Postpartum hemorrhage related to uterine atony, undetected lacerations, or hematoma formation
- Acute Pain related to sore nipples, afterpains, or episiotomy discomfort
- Risk for Infection related to multiple portals of entry for pathogens, including the former site of the placenta, episiotomy, bladder, and breasts
- Risk for Injury: Falls related to postural hypotension and fainting
- Urinary Retention related to periurethral edema, injury to the bladder during birth, or lingering effects of anesthesia
- Risk for Constipation related to slowed peristalsis, inadequate fluid or fiber intake, and fear of pain during defecation
- Risk for Injury: Thrombus formation related to increased coagulation factors and inadequate fluid intake

- Disturbed Sleep Pattern related to excess fatigue, overstimulation, or adjusting to newborn's frequent feeding needs
- Risk for Impaired Parent–Newborn Attachment

OUTCOME IDENTIFICATION AND PLANNING

Appropriate goals may include that the woman will not experience injury from postpartum hemorrhage; will express adequate pain control; will not exhibit signs and symptoms of infection; will not experience injury from falls; will have adequate urinary elimination without retention; will experience adequate bowel elimination; will not experience injury from DVT; will verbalize feeling rested after sleeping; and will exhibit behaviors that indicate the beginning of a healthy attachment with the newborn. Other goals and interventions are planned according to the individual needs of the woman and her partner.

IMPLEMENTATION

Promoting Hemostasis

As discussed earlier in the chapter the postpartum woman is subject to hemorrhage from several sources. The most common type of hemorrhage is related to uterine atony. If the uterus feels boggy or soft to palpation, massage it until it tones up beneath your fingers. Monitor IV fluids and administer oxytocics, such as Pitocin, to prevent uterine atony. Teach the woman to perform periodic self-fundal massage.

Be prepared. Anytime the woman has been in bed for a length of time, the lochia will pool in the vagina. Therefore, when she gets up for the first time after delivery, or in the morning after reclining all night, it is normal for the lochia to seem heavy and to flow down her legs. Reassure her before she gets up that this is a normal occurrence and does not signify that she is hemorrhaging.

Bright red bleeding that occurs in a steady stream in the presence of a firm fundus is most likely caused by a vaginal or cervical laceration that was not repaired. Report this finding to the RN or the primary care provider immediately. Also report bleeding from or separation of the edges of the episiotomy. Monitor for and report any very painful, soft, and possibly pulsing, masses palpable in the perineal area. These are signs of hematoma formation.

Providing Pain Management

There are several possible sources of pain that can occur during the postpartum period. To manage the pain adequately, you must first determine the source of pain.

Managing Breast Pain. Breast pain should be investigated to determine if it is unilateral and associated with increased warmth and redness. This could be a sign of mastitis, a postpartum complication that is discussed in Chapter 19. If the breasts are painful bilaterally because of engorgement, interventions chosen will be dependent on whether or not the woman is breast-feeding. If she is breast-feeding, warmth seems to help the most. Have her run warm water over her breasts in the shower, or place a warm washcloth as a compress on the breasts. If the engorgement is preventing the baby from latching on, assist the woman to express some milk before attempting to breast-feed.

If the breasts are engorged and the woman is bottle-feeding her newborn, instruct her to keep a support bra on 24 hours per day. Cool compresses, or an ice pack wrapped in a towel, will usually be soothing and help to suppress milk production.

If the nipples are painful during breast-feeding attempts, examine the nipples for cracks or fissures. Observe the woman when she puts her newborn to the breast and ensure that she is positioning the newborn properly to prevent sore, cracked nipples. Encourage the use of a lanolin-based cream to keep the nipples soft and promote healing. A mild analgesic may be helpful. (See Chapter 14 for additional breast-feeding interventions.)

Managing Afterpains. If the source of pain is afterpains, ibuprofen or other nonsteroidal anti-inflammatory drugs (NSAIDs) are usually helpful. The primary care provider often will order 600 to 800 mg of ibuprofen every 6 to 8 hours as needed for pain. For multiparas, it may be appropriate to schedule the medication around the clock, rather than waiting for the woman to ask for it. Timing administration of the drug so that it is given 30 to 45 minutes before breast-feeding is also helpful because breast-feeding intensifies uterine cramping and associated afterpains. Nonpharmacologic methods that might be helpful include warm compresses to the abdomen, positioning for comfort, adequate rest and nutrition, and early ambulation.

Managing Perineal Pain. If the pain is arising from the perineum, the perineum should be visualized before taking measures to control the pain to rule out development of a hematoma and to

Nursing Procedure 12.2
Application of Perineal Ice Packs

EQUIPMENT

A commercial ice pack or a clean glove and ice
Clean gloves

PROCEDURE

1. Explain procedure to the woman.
2. Wash hands thoroughly.
3. Position her in dorsal recumbent position.
4. Activate the commercial pack as instructed in the directions for use, or fill a clean glove with crushed ice and tie a knot at the opening at the top of the glove.
5. Cover the pack or the glove with a thin covering, such as a towel.
6. Place the pack on the perineum.
7. Assist her to a position of comfort.
8. Wash hands.
9. Leave in place for 20 minutes then remove for 10 minutes. Repeat as necessary for comfort during the first 24 hours postpartum.

Note: If the ice pack is allowed to stay next to the perineum continuously for prolonged periods, tissue damage could result.

make certain the episiotomy is well approximated. Early interventions within the first 24 hours include ice packs to the perineum (Nursing Procedure 12-2). Ice will help reduce swelling and ease painful sensations. Most institutions use special perineal ice packs that incorporate the cold source into the perineal pad. The ice pack should be on for 20 minutes, then off for 20 minutes to be most effective.

Be careful. When administering combination products for pain, be certain you know the dose of each product in the combination. Be particularly watchful that you do not exceed the maximum daily-recommended dosage of acetaminophen when giving products that contain this medication.

After the first 24 hours, warm sitz baths can be especially comforting to a sore perineum (Nursing Procedure 12-3). Throughout the first few postpartum days, mild analgesics combined with a narcotic are usually most helpful for perineal pain. Examples of combination products include acetaminophen with codeine (Tylenol No. 3) and hydrocodone with

Nursing Procedure 12.3
Assisting the Postpartum Woman With a Sitz Bath

EQUIPMENT

New sitz bath in manufacturer's packaging with directions
Clean gloves

PROCEDURE

1. Explain procedure to the woman.
2. Instruct her to empty her bladder, if necessary.
3. Wash hands thoroughly.
4. Place the sitz bath in the toilet as per the manufacturer's instructions.
5. Place the tubing in the allotted slot and clamp the tubing.
6. Fill the bag with warm (102°F to 105°F) water and hang it at a level of a few feet above the toilet.
7. Unclamp the tubing and allow the warm water to fill the basin.
8. Reclamp the tubing and refill the bag with warm water. Seal the bag with the locking mechanism provided.
9. Assist the woman to sit on the basin so that her perineum is submerged in the water.
10. Ensure that she can reach the emergency call bell.
11. Instruct her to unclamp the tubing periodically to allow water to run over the perineum and into the toilet.
12. Encourage the woman to stay on the sitz bath for at least 20 minutes.
13. Provide a clean towel with which to pat dry and clean sanitary napkins to apply when she is finished.
14. With clean-gloved hands, assist her to rinse out the basin, dry it and store it for the next use.
15. Wash hands.

Note: Encourage the woman to use the sitz bath three times per day for at least 20 minutes per session, or as needed for comfort. Some women may prefer cooler water temperatures, which is an acceptable practice.

---

acetaminophen (Lortab, Vicodin). Local anesthetics, such as witch hazel pads or benzocaine sprays, may be helpful. The pain of hemorrhoids can be reduced by use of sitz baths, witch hazel pads, and/or products that contain hydrocortisone.

Preventing Infection

There are multiple portals of entry for infection in the postpartum period. However, the number one way of preventing infection continues to be handwashing. Wash your hands before and after

caring for the patient, even if you will be wearing gloves. It is also important to teach the woman to wash her hands before touching her breasts or feeding the baby; before and after using the restroom or performing perineal care; and before eating. Early ambulation, adequate fluid intake, and good nutrition strengthen the immune system and help to prevent infection.

The best way to prevent mastitis (infection in the breast), in addition to frequent handwashing, is to avoid cracked nipples. Assist the woman to properly position the infant at the breast to prevent this complication. Other measures that help prevent cracked nipples are to rub the nipples with a few drops of expressed milk after breast-feeding and allow the nipples to air dry. Lanolin cream may also be a helpful measure. The woman should breast-feed at regular, frequent intervals. Milk stasis can lead to obstruction of a duct, which can lead to inflammation and then infection.

Endometritis, or infection of the uterine lining, is another type of infection that can occur in the postpartum period. Handwashing before and after using the bathroom and performing perineal care are the best ways to prevent this infection. In addition, have the woman use a peribottle to perform perineal care and change her sanitary napkins/pads at least every 4 hours. Instruct her to fill the peribottle with warm water (a gentle soap can be added, if desired). After using the restroom, she should squeeze the bottle while aiming at the perineum so that the water flows from front to back. She can then use a washcloth or tissue to gently pat and dry the perineum from front to back. Instruct the woman to avoid touching the center part of the sanitary napkins/pads; she should handle the pads only by the ends. The part of the peripad that touches her perineum should be sterile. These measures can also help prevent infections of the episiotomy.

The postpartum woman is prone to bladder infections because of urethral trauma and perhaps from stasis related to incomplete bladder emptying. Urinary catheterization may be necessary to treat urinary retention; however, this invasive procedure increases the risk for urinary tract infection (UTI). Taking steps to avoid urinary catheterization, when possible, is helpful in decreasing the risk for UTI. Adequate fluid intake and measures to prevent retention are also helpful.

Preventing Injury from Falls

The first time the woman gets up, she is at risk for fainting and falling because of postural hypotension. When the woman is going to get out of bed for the first time after delivery, assist her to dangle her legs at the side of the bed for 5 minutes. If she is not feeling dizzy, assist her to the bathroom. Remain with her until she returns to bed. If she begins to feel dizzy at anytime, help her to sit down with her head forward for a few minutes. If she begins to black out, gently support her to the floor until she comes to. Another time she is at increased risk for fainting is the first time she is in the shower. The warm water may cause peripheral dilation of blood vessels, which leads to hypotension and fainting. Stay in the woman's room while she is showering for the first time. Have a shower chair available for her to sit on if she begins to feel faint.

Promoting Urinary Elimination

The best way to assist the woman to empty her bladder is to help her up to the restroom to void. However, sometimes this is not possible because of incomplete recovery from regional anesthesia. In this instance, assist the woman to sit up on the bedpan, a position that may promote emptying of the bladder. Be certain that the woman has privacy. If she is having difficulty voiding, running water in the sink, or using the peribottle to run warm water over the perineum may help. It also helps to give her plenty of time in which to void. If she feels rushed, this may contribute to urinary retention. If the woman cannot void on her first trip to the bathroom after delivery, it may be appropriate to allow her to wait for a while longer. If she is still unable to void and it has been longer than 6 hours, or there are signs of bladder distention, you may need to perform an in-and-out urinary catheterization to empty her bladder. Likewise, catheterization may be necessary if she is voiding small amounts (less than 100 cc) in frequent intervals.

Promoting Bowel Elimination

All of the normal measures that help prevent constipation are helpful in the postpartum period. Adequate fluid intake keeps the feces soft, facilitating passage. Early ambulation stimulates normal bowel peristalsis. Adding plenty of fruits, vegetables, and fiber to the diet also helps to prevent constipation. A bulk-forming agent, such as Metamucil, may also be helpful. Sometimes the primary care provider orders a stool softener for the first few days after birth. Encourage the woman not to suppress the urge to defecate.

Preventing Injury From Thrombus Formation

Assist the woman to ambulate as soon as possible after delivery. Early ambulation decreases the chance of thrombus formation by promoting venous return. Encourage liberal fluid intake. Dehydration contributes to the risk of thrombus formation.

Promoting Restful Sleep

Monitor the woman's sleep–wake cycle. Encourage her to continue presleep routines she normally uses at home. Promote a relaxing, low-stress environment before sleep. Dim the lights and monitor noise and traffic near the woman's room during sleep time. Medicate for pain, if needed, at bedtime. Plan care activities so that sleep is disturbed as infrequently as possible. For instance, if the postpartum recovery is going well, and vital signs have been stable, consult with the RN about waiting until the 6 a.m. laboratory draw to obtain vital signs, rather than awaking the patient at 2 a.m. Or instruct the woman to call you if she awakens in the night to use the restroom; you can perform the vital signs at this time.

Of course it is challenging for a new mother to get enough sleep because newborns may awaken to feed every 2 to 3 hours. Encourage the woman to rest when the baby is sleeping. She may also wish to get in the habit of maintaining a quiet atmosphere and keeping the lights low when feeding the baby during the night. This practice helps to develop the baby's sleep–wake pattern so that it coincides with light and dark periods of the day. If the lights are turned on, and the parents talk loudly and play with the baby in the middle of the night, he will think it is playtime and stay awake longer.

Promoting Parent–Newborn Attachment

It is important to allow as much parent–newborn contact as possible during the early postpartum period. Encourage the parents to cuddle the newborn closely. Role model attachment behavior by talking to the newborn and calling the newborn by name. Point out positive features of the baby. Encourage the parents to participate in the care of the newborn. Provide privacy for the family to interact with the newborn. Assist the parents to be attuned to the baby's cues that he is ready for interaction, that he is overstimulated, or that he is ready for sleep. Encourage the parents to interact with the newborn while she is in the alert state. Meet the woman's needs for pain relief, rest, and self-care so that she will have the energy to care for and interact with her newborn.

EVALUATION: GOALS AND EXPECTED OUTCOMES

- **Goal:** Maternal injury from postpartum hemorrhage is avoided.

Expected Outcomes:
- Fundus is firm and in the midline.
- Lochia flow is rubra (dark red in color) and small to moderate in amount.
- There is no bright red bleeding from any source.
- **Goal:** The woman's pain is manageable.
  Expected Outcomes:
  - The woman reports pain before it becomes severe.
  - The woman verbalizes a tolerable pain level and a decrease in pain level after interventions.
- **Goal:** The woman remains free from the signs and symptoms of infection.
  Expected Outcomes:
  - The woman remains afebrile (temperature less than 100.4°F).
  - There is no redness or heat in localized areas of the breast.
  - Lochia has a normal fleshy scent without a foul odor.
  - Episiotomy remains well approximated without purulent discharge.
  - There is no severe pain when voiding.
- **Goal:** No injury is experienced because of fainting/falling.
  Expected Outcomes:
  - If the woman faints, she is gently guided to the floor.
  - There is no evidence of head injury, bruises, or lacerations from a fall.
- **Goal:** Urinary retention is avoided.
  Expected Outcomes:
  - Voids spontaneously within 6 hours of delivery.
  - Urinary output is greater than 100 cc per episode every 3 to 4 hours.
- **Goal:** Normal bowel elimination occurs without constipation.
  Expected Outcome:
  - Passes a soft, formed stool within the first 3 days after birth.
- **Goal:** Deep vein thrombosis is avoided.
  Expected Outcomes:
  - Homans' sign is negative.
  - There is no unilateral swelling of the lower extremities.
  - There is no redness or heat in the calf area.
- **Goal:** Experiences adequate amounts of restful sleep.
  Expected Outcome:
  - Verbalizes feeling rested with adequate energy to care for self and infant.
- **Goal:** Demonstrates signs of healthy attachment to the newborn.

Expected Outcomes:
- Calls the newborn by name.
- Interacts with the newborn in the en face position.
- Talks to the newborn lovingly.
- Makes positive comments about the newborn.

Test Yourself

- Name two ways the nurse can promote hemostasis for the postpartum woman.
- List three nursing actions that can help a new mother avoid endometritis.
- What are three things a nurse can do to help promote rest and sleep for a new mother?

● Nursing Process for Postpartum Care After Cesarean Birth

The woman who has a cesarean birth faces the major postpartum challenges; however, she has also undergone major surgery. This section discusses how postpartum nursing care differs for the woman who has a cesarean birth. Remember that most of the nursing considerations discussed above for the postpartum woman also apply to the woman who delivers by cesarean section.

ASSESSMENT

In addition to the normal postpartum assessment, the woman who has experienced a cesarean delivery requires close monitoring. Auscultate lung sounds at least every 4 hours in the first 24 hours and at least every 8 hours thereafter. The lungs should be clear without adventitious sounds and not diminished in any lobe.

If a narcotic, such as Duramorph, was used in conjunction with the spinal or epidural anesthesia, the woman must be monitored closely for signs of respiratory depression. Many anesthesiologists have preprinted orders that include how often the respirations should be monitored after this type of anesthesia. Usually the respiratory rate is counted every 1 to 2 hours for the first 24 hours. Report respiratory rates of 12 per minute or less. Pulse oximetry, either continuous or intermittent, is often ordered. The oxygen saturation should remain above 95%.

Monitor the IV for rate of flow and correct solution. Check the IV site at least every 2 hours for redness, swelling, and pain. The IV usually remains in place for the first 24 hours after delivery. At that time, it may be removed or a saline lock may be put in place.

The sources of pain and discomfort for the woman who delivers by cesarean are similar to those of a woman who has delivered vaginally. Usually a woman who experiences cesarean birth does not have an episiotomy, although rarely this may be the case. However, she does have an abdominal incision that is an additional source of pain. The buildup of intestinal gas and referred shoulder pain are other sources of pain. Pruritus, itching, is a common side effect of narcotic administration during regional anesthesia. This can be a source of discomfort for the woman who had a cesarean birth.

The abdominal incision is a site for possible hemorrhage and infection. Monitor for drainage on the dressing in the first 24 hours. Assess the incision at least once every 8 hours after the dressing is removed. The incision should be well approximated with sutures or staples. A small amount of redness is normal. An increase in the amount of redness, edema, or drainage from the site is an abnormal finding.

Monitor bowel sounds at least every 4 hours. Check closely for abdominal distention and pain associated with gas formation. It may be difficult for the woman to pass flatus after cesarean delivery because of decreased peristalsis. Ask the woman if she is passing gas. Instruct her to report bowel movements.

Observe the Foley catheter for urinary output. The catheter usually remains in place for the first 24 hours after cesarean birth. Output should be at least 30 mL per hour. The urine should be clear yellow or a light straw color. Cloudy urine is associated with infection. After the Foley catheter is removed, observe the woman for the first few voids to make certain she is voiding adequately without retention.

Assess for signs of thrombus formation. The calves should be of equal size without redness, warmth, or pain. The woman who delivers by cesarean is at even higher risk for thrombus formation than is the woman who delivers vaginally.

SELECTED NURSING DIAGNOSES

- Ineffective Breathing Pattern related to respiratory depression from narcotics
- Risk for Injury: Hemorrhage from the normal postpartum routes and from the incision
- Risk for Infection related to postpartum status, stasis of secretions in the lungs, abdominal incision, and presence of the Foley catheter

- Acute Pain related to incision, discomfort from pruritus, or inability to pass flatus
- Risk for Injury: Thrombus formation related to postpartum status, bed rest, and lowered activity levels

OUTCOME IDENTIFICATION AND PLANNING

Appropriate goals include that the woman will maintain an adequate respiratory rate; will not experience injury from hemorrhage; will remain free from signs of infection; will verbalize a tolerable pain level; and will remain free of injury from thrombus formation.

IMPLEMENTATION

Monitoring for an Adequate Respiratory Pattern

If the woman has had narcotics administered via the spinal or epidural routes, monitor her closely for respiratory depression. The respirations should be monitored at least every 2 hours for the first 24 hours after spinal narcotics are administered. Have naloxone (Narcan) readily available. The anesthesiologist writes orders for naloxone administration if the respiratory rate falls below 10 to 12 per minute. Monitor oxygen saturation, as ordered. Report continuous levels below 95%.

Preventing Injury From Hemorrhage

Do not forget to check the fundus. It is not necessary to massage the fundus unless it is soft and the woman is bleeding vaginally. Any manipulation of the fundus increases pain. However, it is important to note the position and height of the fundus and whether or not it is well contracted.

Assess the dressing for drainage. Mark any areas of drainage so that you can tell if the area is increasing during subsequent assessments. If the dressing becomes saturated, reinforce it and apply pressure to the site. Notify the RN or primary care provider for further orders.

Preventing Infection

One major difference between care of the woman who has delivered vaginally and one who has had a cesarean is that of lung status. The lungs of a woman who has experienced cesarean birth must be assessed carefully at least every 4 hours during the first 24 hours. You must also assist the woman to turn, cough, and deep breathe at least every 2 hours. It will not be easy for her to take deep breaths or to cough. Assist her to splint her incision with a pillow while she coughs. This stabilizes the area and reduces pain. An incentive spirometer will be ordered. Assist the woman to use it hourly for the first 24 hours when she is awake.

The incision is another possible site for infection. During the first 24 hours the original dressing usually covers the incision. After the physician has removed the dressing, assess the incision for increasing redness, edema, or drainage. Proper incision care includes washing the hands thoroughly before touching the incision for any reason. Instruct the woman to wash the incision with soap and water, and then pat it dry thoroughly. Nothing wet should remain against the incision.

The continuous Foley catheter that is in place during the first 24 hours is another potential source of infection. Provide frequent perineal and Foley care. Monitor IV fluids to ensure adequate infusion of fluids. When the woman is well hydrated, her kidneys will produce enough urine to keep a steady flow going. The flow helps to wash out bacteria. When the catheter is removed, assist the woman to void within 6 hours of removal.

Providing Pain Management

Pain management for the woman after cesarean birth is an area that challenges the postpartum nurse. During the first 24 hours, the anesthesiologist usually manages the pain. Generally, if the woman had a spinal narcotic administered, she will have orders for a PRN medication for **breakthrough pain**. Breakthrough pain occurs when the basal dose of analgesia does not control the pain adequately.

Another form of pain control that may be ordered is patient-controlled analgesia (PCA). This type of analgesia allows the woman to control how often she receives pain medication. A narcotic (usually morphine) is given via a pump into the IV line. The pump is locked to prevent tampering. The pump is set per physician orders so that the patient can receive a prescribed amount of narcotic each time she pushes a button. A lockout interval is also prescribed so that the woman cannot accidentally overdose herself. Many women require reassurance that they cannot administer too much medication when PCA is used.

Infrequently, narcotics will be ordered at PRN intervals after cesarean birth. In this instance, plan to administer the narcotic around the clock for the first 24 hours. Research has shown that it is easier to control pain before it becomes severe and that adequate pain control in the first 24 hours reduces the total amount of pain medication needed by the woman. Adequate pain control is necessary for the woman to ambulate well and for her to provide self- and newborn care.

Pruritus is a common side effect of narcotics given by the spinal or epidural routes. This side effect can become quite uncomfortable for the woman and can lead to scratching and excoriation. An antipruritic, usually diphenhydramine (Benadryl), is frequently ordered to help control this side effect. If nothing is ordered, notify the anesthesiologist. Other comfort measures include applying lotion, administering a back rub, and using cool compresses or diversion to help control the itching. In some cases it becomes necessary to administer naloxone (Narcan). It is best to avoid this if possible because naloxone reverses the effect of the narcotic and can lead to increased pain sensation.

Another common source of pain for the woman who delivers by cesarean is gas pain. Because peristalsis is naturally slowed in the postpartum period and because of the lingering effects of anesthesia and analgesia, and manipulation of the intestines during surgery, the woman is at increased risk for gas formation. If it builds up and cannot be released, the woman becomes bloated and can experience severe pain.

This pain is usually not relieved by analgesics. Many surgeons order simethicone (Mylicon) prophylactically. If this is the case, simethicone will be given around the clock. It may also be ordered PRN. Frequent and early ambulation stimulates peristalsis and passing of flatus. Instruct the woman to avoid very hot or very cold beverages, carbonated beverages, and drinking through straws. All of these things can increase the formation and discomfort of gas. Other medical interventions may become necessary, such as rectal suppositories or enemas. Encourage the woman to lie on her left side. This position allows the gas to be expelled more easily.

Preventing Injury From Thrombus Formation

Many women come back from surgery with thromboembolic disease stockings (TEDS) already in place. If not, there will be an order to apply them. Pneumatic compression devices also may be ordered during the first 24 hours. These devices stimulate venous return to the heart, an action that helps prevent pooling and thrombus formation. Once the woman can get out of bed and ambulate, frequent ambulation is advised. This is the best way to prevent a thrombus from forming. Another important nursing action is to ensure adequate fluid intake.

EVALUATION: GOALS AND EXPECTED OUTCOMES

- **Goal:** The respiratory pattern is not compromised.

Expected Outcomes:
- Maintains an adequate respiratory pattern (16 to 20 breaths per minute).
- Oxygen saturation remains above 95%.
- **Goal:** Injury from hemorrhage is avoided.
  Expected Outcomes:
  - Fundus remains firm in the midline.
  - Lochia flow remains scant to small.
  - There is no drainage or bleeding from the incision.
- **Goal:** Remains free from signs and symptoms of infection.
  Expected Outcomes:
  - Temperature remains below 100.4°F.
  - Lungs remain clear to auscultation.
  - Incision is clean, dry, well-approximated without redness or drainage.
  - Lochia does not have a foul odor.
  - Urine remains clear.
- **Goal:** Pain is manageable.
  Expected Outcomes:
  - Reports pain before it becomes severe.
  - Uses PCA, as ordered.
  - Voices adequate pain relief after interventions.
  - States pruritus is at a tolerable level.
- **Goal:** Remains free from thrombus formation.
  Expected Outcomes:
  - Negative Homans' sign.
  - No unilateral swelling, redness, or warmth in the lower extremities.
  - No shortness of breath or chest pain.

● Nursing Process for Preparing the Postpartum Woman for Discharge

Discharge planning for the new mother begins upon admission and continues until she is dismissed home. Most interventions related to discharge focus on teaching the woman to care for herself and the baby when she goes home. It is also important to observe how the woman and her partner are adapting to their new role as parents and to support healthy adaptation behaviors.

ASSESSMENT

Bearing a child is a life-changing event. Observe how the parents interact with each other and with the baby. Watch for interactions between other members of the family, such as grandparents and siblings of the new baby. Determine what behaviors are helping the new family adjust and note if any actions are getting in the way of positive adjustment.

Because teaching is the focus of most nursing interventions when planning for discharge, it is important to determine the woman's knowledge base. It is important not to assume that a woman knows certain things just because she may be educated, or she is a nurse, or she has other children, and so on. The only way to know what a woman knows about self-care and baby care is to ask and to observe. This section focuses on maternal self-care at home. Newborn care is discussed in Chapter 15.

SELECTED NURSING DIAGNOSES

- Health-Seeking Behaviors
- Risk for Injury related to Rh negative blood type and/or nonimmunity to rubella
- Deficient Knowledge of self care

OUTCOME IDENTIFICATION AND PLANNING

Appropriate goals include that the woman and her partner will demonstrate positive adjustment to the parental role; no injury will occur related to Rh status or rubella nonimmunity; and the woman will verbalize danger signs that should be reported immediately. Another goal is that the woman will demonstrate the ability to perform self-care to include breast care, fundal checks and massage, care of lochia and the perineum, pain management, and prevention of constipation and fatigue.

IMPLEMENTATION

Supporting Health-Seeking Behaviors
Reinforce positive family behaviors. Take particular care to praise the woman and her partner for positive parenting skills. When assistance is needed as the parents learn new skills, provide positive verbal support. If the woman makes a mistake, don't focus on the mistake in a negative way. For instance, it is not helpful to tell the mother, "No. That's not the way to do it. Do it like this." Instead focus on the things she is doing right and use positive language to guide her when she is having difficulty with the task. Use words that convey acceptance, such as, "Some women find it helpful to do it this way." Or "the baby might find this to be soothing."

Anticipatory guidance is helpful when siblings are involved. Explain to the parents that it is normal for the older sibling to regress in the first few days after the birth of the baby. Tell them it helps if they do not focus undue attention on regressive behaviors, such as a return to bedwetting, sucking the thumb, or clinging to a favorite toy or blanket. It is particularly important for the parents not to criticize or belittle the older child for regressive behaviors. Explain that the behavior is temporary and will pass as the child adjusts to his new role in the family. Suggest that the parents set aside time every day that is just "big brother or sister" time. The sibling will find it easier to adjust if he is assured that his parents still care for and value him. Another helpful suggestion is to provide the older child with a doll and allow the child to take care of the doll, as the parent is caring for the baby. This activity helps the older child to feel included and can help to develop nurturing skills.

Preventing Injury From Rh-Negative Blood Type or Nonimmunity to Rubella

Before the woman is discharged, it is important to check to see if the woman who is Rh negative is a candidate for RhoGAM. If the woman is Rh-negative and the baby is Rh-positive, the woman will need an injection of RhoGAM to prevent the development of antibodies to Rh-positive blood. The RhoGAM must be given within 72 hours of delivery to be most effective. If the baby is Rh negative, the woman will not need RhoGAM. Box 12-3 highlights nursing considerations for administering RhoGAM.

You must also determine the woman's rubella status. If she is nonimmune to rubella, the rubella titer is less than 1:8, she will need to receive the rubella vaccine before she is discharged. It is important for her to know that she should not get pregnant for at least 3 months after receiving the vaccine. Box 12-4 discusses nursing considerations for giving the rubella vaccine.

Providing Patient Teaching

Because the postpartum stay is very short, it is important to grab every available opportunity for teaching. On the day of discharge, give the woman written self-care instructions. It is best to ask her questions regarding how she plans to care for her breasts, perineum, pain, and so on; to determine how much information she has retained; and to reinforce areas she may not have absorbed. Instruct the woman that she needs to make an appointment with her primary care provider for a 6-week postpartum checkup. It is important for the woman to know danger signs that should be reported to the primary care provider. Box 12-5 lists these danger signs.

Breast Care

Teach breast care as you are assisting the woman to breast-feed or when she takes a shower. Explain that plain water is sufficient to clean the nipples

---

BOX 12.3	Pharmacology Focus: Prevention of Antibody Development

Medication: Rh immune globulin (RhoGAM)
Method of action: Prevents development of antibodies to Rh D-positive blood, if given to the Rh-D negative woman within 72 hours of abortion, invasive procedure such as amniocentesis, or delivery of an Rh D-positive infant.
Usual dosage and administration: One vial given via the IM route
Antidote: None
Nursing interventions:
1. Ensure that the woman is a candidate for RhoGAM. She
   a. Is Rh D-negative
   b. Has never been sensitized to Rh D-positive blood
   c. Has had an abortion, ectopic pregnancy, or delivered an Rh D-positive infant within the past 72 hours
2. Explain that the woman is receiving RhoGAM to prevent her from being sensitized to Rh-positive blood. This will prevent hemolytic disease of the newborn in subsequent pregnancies.
3. Inform the woman that RhoGAM is a blood product.
4. Ensure that you are administering the correct vial to the woman. RhoGAM is cross-matched to each specific woman. The lot number should be checked by two nurses before RhoGAM is administered.
5. Explain that there may be soreness at the site.
6. Ask the woman which site she prefers for the IM injection. The deltoid and gluteal muscles are both acceptable sites.
7. Give the woman a card indicating her Rh status and the date of RhoGAM administration. Instruct her to carry the card with her at all times.

---

because soap is drying and can contribute to sore, cracked nipples. Encourage the use of lanolin cream on the nipples. After a feeding, teach the woman to express a drop of breast milk, rub it into each nipple, and allow the nipples to air dry. She should wear a good support bra at all times.

Fundal Massage

Teach self-fundal massage when you are assessing the fundus. Assist her to touch the top of the uterus and to gently massage it as she makes certain it stays firmly contracted. Explain to her that the uterus should no longer be palpable by the 10th day.

Perineum and Vaginal Care

Instruct the woman on proper perineal care the first time she gets up to use the bathroom. Help her fill the peribottle with warm water, and

BOX 12.4	Pharmacology Focus: Development of Immunity to Rubella

Medication: Live rubella vaccine
Method of action: Causes the body to produce antibodies against the rubella virus, thereby stimulating the development of immunity to rubella.
Usual dosage and administration: One vial given subcutaneously in the upper, outer aspect of the arm.
Antidote: None
Nursing interventions:
1. Determine whether there are any contraindications for administering the vaccine. The woman
   a. Is sensitive to neomycin
   b. Is immunosuppressed
   c. Has received a blood product within the past 3 months
2. Explain possible adverse reactions.
   a. Discomfort at the injection site.
   b. Development of rash, sore throat, headache, and general malaise within 2 to 4 weeks of the injection.
3. Obtain informed consent before administering the vaccine.
4. Instruct the woman on the importance of avoiding pregnancy for at least 3 months. Because the rubella vaccine is a live virus, it could be teratogenic to the fetus.
5. Inform the breast-feeding woman that the rubella vaccine crosses over into the breast milk. The newborn benefits from short-term immunity but may become flushed, fussy, or develop a slight rash. Suggest that the woman speak to the pediatrician if she has concerns.

BOX 12.5	Postpartum Danger Signs

- Fever greater than or equal to 100.4°F
- Shaking chills
- Localized reddened, painful area on one breast
- Frequency, urgency, and painful urination
- Sudden onset of shortness of breath and/or chest pain
- Severe unremitting abdominal or back pain that is unrelieved by normal pain measures
- Foul smelling lochia
- Increased or heavy lochia flow or passage of clots
- Return to lochia rubra after it has been serosa or alba
- Severe pain, redness, or swelling in the episiotomy or cesarean incision
- Swollen, reddened, painful area on the calf
- Prolonged or severe depression
- Thoughts of harming the baby or self (suicidal thoughts)

instruct her to squirt the water over her perineum to wash away lochia. Watch as she pats dry. Be certain that she pats from front to back. Explain the importance of this action to help prevent bladder and episiotomy infections. Show her how to open the sanitary napkins and how to handle them to avoid contaminating the center of the pad. Explain that she will need to continue to use sanitary napkins until the lochia stops. Tampons are not used because they contribute to uterine infection until the placental site has healed. Reinforce that she should continue perineal care after every voiding and defecation until the lochia stops. Encourage handwashing before and after performing perineal care.

Remind the woman that lochia flow should become progressively lighter. Lochia rubra generally lasts for approximately 2 to 3 days. This is followed by lochia serosa for the remainder of the 1st week after delivery. After the 1st week, the flow should be lochia alba. She shouldn't saturate peripads, and there shouldn't be any large clots.

Here's a good teaching tip. If the woman engages in vigorous exercise during the postpartum period, the amount of lochia will temporarily increase. This is a normal finding.

Teach the woman to avoid sexual intercourse, tampons, or introduction of any substance into the vagina until the placental site and episiotomy or tear have healed to prevent additional trauma and infection. Healing is indicated when the lochia flow stops and there is no discomfort when two fingers are placed inside the vaginal opening. Hormonal changes associated with breast-feeding sometimes contribute to vaginal dryness and associated dyspareunia. For this reason breast-feeding mothers may find it helpful to use a water-soluble jelly (e.g., KY jelly) for lubrication during sexual intercourse.

Pain Management
Teach the woman about pain management as you provide pain management for her. Explain that it is more effective to control pain before it becomes severe. Many women are afraid to take pain medication when they are breast-feeding. Reassure her that the analgesics the primary care provider has ordered will not harm her baby. Clarify that breast-feeding is promoted when the mother is comfortable and pain free. Tell her the name of the medication that you are giving her and briefly

describe its benefit. For instance, when the woman complains of afterpains, administer the ordered ibuprofen, and explain that ibuprofen is usually very effective in controlling the pain of cramping. If she complains of her stitches hurting, administer the ordered analgesic-narcotic combination and make clear that this medication is most effective at controlling episiotomy pain. Tell her how frequently she can have each medication and why it is important not to take pain medication more frequently or at higher dosages than what is ordered.

Explain the benefits of using nonmedicinal ways of easing pain, such as applying warmth to the abdomen to help soothe afterpains. When you assist her with the sitz bath, encourage her to continue using it at home until the episiotomy has healed. Some women worry that the stitches will have to be removed and anticipate that this will be painful. Reassure her that the stitches will be absorbed by the body and do not need to be removed.

Nutrition

Nutrition is an important aspect of self-care. Meal times are a good time to discuss nutrition with the woman. Determine what her normal pattern of intake is. Give her brochures that explain the food pyramid. Discuss with her how to use the food pyramid to plan meals. Instruct the woman who is not breast-feeding to decrease her caloric intake by approximately 300 kcal per day (i.e., she should reduce her intake to prepregnancy levels). Because the lactating woman was using 300 kcal extra per day during the pregnancy, she will need to add an additional 200 kcal, for a total of 500 kcal above prepregnancy requirements.

Constipation

As you are caring for the woman, explain how different activities contribute to or prevent constipation. Describe how activity helps the bowel to regain its tone, which helps prevent constipation. When you fill her water pitcher, explain that she needs to drink liberally of noncaffeinated fluids to help keep the stool soft. Explain that caffeine is a diuretic, so it is best to limit caffeinated fluids. Encourage her to drink fluids that she enjoys. If she does not like water, explore alternatives with her, such as noncaffeinated herbal tea, juice, and sugar-free gelatin. Explain to her the importance of heeding the urge to defecate. Ignoring the urge can contribute to constipation. Teach her about high fiber foods when you serve her a meal or bring her a snack. If the primary care provider has prescribed a stool softener, tell her the name of the medication and its intended effect when you administer it. Offer her a large glass of water when she takes the stool softener and emphasize the importance of adequate hydration when taking a stool softener.

Proper Rest

It is important for the woman to know that it is easy to over-do it in the first few days after having a baby. Explore the possibility of asking a friend or relative to help out for the first few days. Reassure her that her health and that of her baby are the most important concerns while she is recovering from childbirth. Give her hints such as, "When you are tired, rest. If you are exhausted, you will not have the energy to care for your baby." It might be helpful to suggest that she rest with her feet up when the baby is napping during the day. Reassure her that housecleaning chores can wait, if she is too tired to do them. Also, the woman should not do heavy lifting. Teach the woman the good rule of thumb not to lift anything heavier than the baby for the first 6 weeks after delivery.

When the father is present, explain to him how much energy it takes for the body to repair itself after childbirth. If he was present at the birth, he probably readily understands this concept. If appropriate, encourage him to help out with household chores and older sibling care while the woman recuperates.

EVALUATION: GOALS AND EXPECTED OUTCOMES

- **Goal:** Both parents demonstrate positive adjustment to the parental role.
  Expected Outcomes:
  - Cares for her newborn with confidence.
  - Demonstrates positive attachment behaviors with her newborn.
- **Goal:** No injury will occur related to Rh type or rubella nonimmunity.
  Expected Outcomes:
  - Receives RhoGAM within 72 hours after delivery, if eligible.
  - Receives rubella vaccine (or instructions as to where to obtain the vaccine) if nonimmune.
- **Goal:** Demonstrates adequate self-care behaviors.
  Expected Outcomes:
  - Explains danger signals that need to be reported.
  - Demonstrates the ability to perform self-care to include
    - Breast care
    - Fundal checks and massage
    - Perineal care

- Pain management
- Constipation prevention
- Avoidance of fatigue and sleep deprivation

Test Yourself

- Describe four major ways that assessment of the woman after cesarean delivery is different from that for a woman who delivers vaginally.
- Explain the proper way to perform perineal care.
- List four signs of infection that the new mother should report.

KEY POINTS

- The organs of the reproductive system gradually return to the nonpregnant size and function in the process of involution.
- Fundal height decreases at a rate of 1 fingerbreadth (1 cm) per day until the uterus is no longer palpable on the 10th postpartum day.
- Multiparas more frequently experience afterpains than do primiparas.
- Lochia progresses from rubra to serosa to alba as the uterine lining and other cells are cast away from the uterus.
- Kegel exercises can help the postpartum woman regain tone in the perineal area, although the size and tone of the introitus never fully return to the prepregnant state.
- The extra fluid volume that built up during the pregnancy is eliminated in the early postpartum period, leading to high urinary output and diaphoresis.
- The woman's temperature may be slightly elevated during the first 24 hours after delivery because of dehydration and exhaustion. After that it should be under 100.4°F. The blood pressure should remain at the level it was during labor. It is normal for bradycardia to be found in the early postpartum period.
- The woman is often very hungry and thirsty after delivering a baby. She should be allowed to eat and drink unless there are medical contraindications for doing so.
- Trauma to the lower urinary tract can lead to urinary retention in the postpartum period.
- The woman must adapt to her new role as mother. She usually does this in three stages: taking in, taking hold, and letting go.

- Bonding is the initial component of healthy attachment between a parent and the newborn. Healthy bonding generally occurs in a predictable sequence.
- Postpartum blues is a temporary mood disorder that manifests itself through tearfulness and other signs of mild depression.
- Postpartum assessment involves data collection to include pregnancy history, medical history, and labor and birth history. It also involves a thorough head-to-toe physical assessment with focus on expected postpartum changes.
- The focus of nursing interventions in the early postpartum period is on preventing and detecting hemorrhage, treating pain, preventing infection, preventing falls, detecting and treating urinary retention, preventing constipation, preventing and detecting thrombus formation, promoting sleep, and promoting healthy parental–newborn attachment.
- Additional nursing considerations for the woman who has a cesarean birth involve the surgical status of the woman. Respiratory compromise is a possible complication that requires monitoring and nursing intervention.
- The woman who delivers by cesarean has an abdominal incision that can be an additional source of pain, infection, and hemorrhage.
- Helping the woman to turn, cough, and deep breath and encouraging early and frequent ambulation after cesarean delivery are necessary measures to help prevent respiratory compromise and thrombus formation.
- The focus of nursing interventions when assisting the woman to prepare for discharge is teaching the woman to perform self- and infant care.
- Self-care includes breast care, fundal massage, assessment of lochia, perineal care, pain management, prevention of constipation, and prevention of fatigue.

REFERENCES AND SELECTED READINGS

Books and Journals
Bukowski, R., & Silver, H. (2000). The puerperium. In A. T. Evans & K. R. Niswander (Eds.), *Manual of obstetrics* (6th ed., pp. 479–495). Philadelphia: Lippincott Williams & Wilkins.
Cunningham, F. G., Gant, N. F., Leveno, K. J., Gilstrap, L. C. III, Hauth, J. C., & Wenstrom, K. D. (2001). The puerperium. In *Williams obstetrics* (21st ed., pp. 403–421). New York: McGraw-Hill Medical Publishing Division.
Franzblau, N., & Witt, K. (2002). Normal and abnormal puerperium. In R. Levine, F. Talavera, G. F. Whitman-Elia, F. B. Gaupp, & L. P. Shulman (Eds.), *eMedicine.* Retrieved

February 2, 2003, from http://www.emedicine.com/med/topic3240.htm

Ladewig, P. W., London, M. L., Moberly, S., & Olds, S. B. (2002) *Contemporary maternal–newborn nursing care* (5th ed.). Upper Saddle River, NJ: Prentice Hall.

Martell, L. K. (2003). Postpartum women's perceptions of the hospital environment. *Journal of Obstetric, Gynecologic, & Neonatal Nursing (JOGNN), 32*(4), 478–485.

Scoggin, J. (2000). Physical and psychological changes. In S. Mattson & J. E. Smith (Eds.), *Core curriculum for mater-nal–newborn nursing.* AWHONN publication (2nd ed., pp. 302–313). Philadelphia: WB Saunders.

Websites
Postpartum Resources
http://www.childbirth.org/articles/postpartum.html
http://www.sbpep.org/

Helping Dads Support the New Mom
http://www.dona.org/PDF/DadsandPostpartum-Doulas.pdf

WORKBOOK

NCLEX-STYLE REVIEW QUESTIONS

1. An 18-year-old primipara is getting ready to go home. She had a third degree episiotomy with repair. She confides in the nurse that she is afraid to go to her postpartum checkup because she is afraid to have the stitches removed. Which reply by the nurse is best?

   a. "It doesn't hurt when the midwife takes out the stitches. You will only feel a little tugging and pulling sensation."

   b. "It is very important for you to go to your checkup visit. Besides, the stitches do not have to be removed."

   c. "Many women have that fear after having an episiotomy. The stitches do not need to be removed because the suture will be gradually absorbed."

   d. "Oh, you mustn't miss your follow-up appointment. Don't worry. Your midwife will be very gentle."

2. A woman has just delivered her third baby. Everything has progressed normally up to this point. When the nurse tries to take the woman's blood pressure, she notices that the woman is shaking and that her teeth are chattering. Which action should the nurse take first?

   a. Finish taking the vital signs, and then decide what to do

   b. Notify the RN immediately

   c. Place two prewarmed blankets on the woman

   d. Put on the call bell to summon for help

3. The night shift LPN is checking on a woman who had a cesarean delivery with spinal Duramorph anesthesia several hours earlier. The nurse counts a respiratory rate of 8 in 1 minute. What should the nurse do first?

   a. Administer naloxone (Narcan), per the preprinted orders

   b. Awaken the woman and instruct her to breathe more rapidly

   c. Call the anesthesiologist from the room for orders

   d. Perform bag-to-mouth rescue breathing at a rate of 12 per minute

4. The nurse is performing the initial postpartum assessment for her shift on a woman who had a cesarean delivery the day before. The nurse notices that the woman is scratching her face and her arms. What action by the nurse is indicated?

   a. Administer naloxone (Narcan) immediately, per the preprinted orders

   b. Ask the woman if she wants something for the itching, and then call the anesthesiologist for orders

   c. Determine the severity of the itching and offer to give diphenhydramine (Benadryl), as ordered

   d. Observe and wait until the woman complains about the itching before treating it

5. A woman who has chosen to bottle-feed says that her breasts are painfully engorged. Which nursing intervention is appropriate?

   a. Assist the woman into the shower and have her run warm water over her breasts

   b. Assist the woman to place ice packs on her breasts

   c. Encourage the woman to breast-feed because she is producing so much milk

   d. Provide a breast pump and assist the woman in emptying her breasts

STUDY ACTIVITIES

1. With your clinical group, develop a one-page postpartum instruction sheet to send home with the new mother that covers all of the essential information she needs for self-care at home.
2. Explain how nursing care of a woman after cesarean birth differs from that of a woman who delivers vaginally. What additional risk factors does the woman have after cesarean?
3. Using the table below, compare the different sources of postpartum pain.

Pain Source	Possible Causes	Nursing Care to Prevent and Treat
Breast		
Afterpains		
Perineal pain		
Gas pain and distention after cesarean		
Cesarean incision		

CRITICAL THINKING: What Would You Do?

1. You enter the room of Heather, a 22-year-old primipara, and find her on the floor looking a little dazed. When you ask her what happened, she tells you that she remembers trying to get up to go the restroom and that she started feeling a bit dizzy and faint. The next thing she knew she was on the floor.

   a. What is the likely cause of Heather's fall? What nursing actions could have prevented this occurrence?

   b. Later that day, Heather reports that she feels like she just "dribbles" when she tries to urinate and she feels like she is bleeding too much. What assessments should you make first? What do you expect to find?

   c. What measures can the nurse take to help relieve Heather's urinary retention?

   d. On the 3rd postpartum day Heather says that she is experiencing chills and thinks she is coming down with a fever. In addition to taking the temperature, what other assessments should the nurse make? Why?

2. Marla delivered her fifth child yesterday after a difficult labor that lasted almost 24 hours. The baby weighed 7 pounds 6 ounces, and she is breast-feeding.

   a. What factors put Marla at risk for postpartum hemorrhage?

   b. While you are checking Marla's lochia, you notice that her lochia has saturated through two sanitary napkins/pads since you last checked on her an hour ago. What do you think is causing the bleeding? What is your first action and why? What would you do next? Justify your answer.

3. Mindy had a cesarean delivery. This is her 2nd postoperative day. She is in her bed when you come in to take vital signs. She looks miserable and she says that she just can't get comfortable.

   a. What assessments should you make first?

   b. You determine that Mindy is suffering from incisional pain and gas pain. What remedies should you offer for these two sources of pain?

   c. You perform a complete assessment and discover that Mindy has a positive Homans' sign. What action should you take?

Nursing Assessment of Newborn Transition

13

Physiologic Adaptation
  Respiratory Adaptation
  Cardiovascular Adaptation
  Thermoregulatory Adaptation
  Metabolic Adaptation
  Hepatic Adaptation
  *Behavioral and Social
    Adaptation*

Nursing Assessment of the Normal
  Newborn
  General Body Proportions and Posture
  Vital Signs
  Physical Measurements
  Head-to-Toe Assessment
  Neurologic Assessment
  Behavioral Assessment
  Gestational Age Assessment

STUDENT OBJECTIVES

On completion of this chapter, the student should be able to:

1. Identify respiratory adaptations that occur as the newborn makes the transition to life outside the womb.
2. Outline cardiovascular changes that occur immediately after birth.
3. Explain thermoregulatory capabilities of the newborn and why he has a difficult time maintaining body heat.
4. Discuss the role of the liver in the newborn's adaptation to extrauterine life.
5. Describe expected behavioral characteristics of the newborn.
6. Illustrate the major steps of the initial nursing assessment of the newborn.
7. Define expected weights and measures of the newborn.
8. Compare and contrast expected versus unexpected assessment parameters of the newborn.
9. Outline how each newborn reflex is elicited.

KEY TERMS

brown fat 305-306
caput succedaneum 312
cephalhematoma 312
epispadias 315
Epstein's pearls 314
Harlequin sign 310-312
hypospadias 315
jaundice 306, 307, 312
lanugo 310
meconium 316
molding 312
mottling 310
phimosis 315
physiologic jaundice 307
pseudomenstruation 315
simian crease 316
smegma 315
surfactant 305
thermoregulation 305
thrush 314
vernix caseosa 310

The newborn is a unique individual different than the fetus, older infant, child, and adult. The newborn's anatomy and physiology change immediately after birth and continue to change as he or she grows. It is essential for the nurse to be aware of adjustments the newborn must make as he transitions to life outside the womb. It also is important for the nurse to know the characteristics of a normal newborn in order to make accurate assessments. In addition, this knowledge will enable the nurse to appropriately answer parents' questions and concerns about their newborn. This chapter explores the immediate and ongoing adaptation of the normal newborn to life outside the womb and describes initial nursing assessments.

PHYSIOLOGIC ADAPTATION

The fetus is fully dependent upon the mother for all vital needs, such as oxygen, nutrition, and waste removal. At birth, the body systems must immediately undergo tremendous changes so that the newborn can exist outside the womb. Table 13-1 compares the anatomy and physiology of the fetus and newborn.

Respiratory Adaptation

Fetal lungs are uninflated and full of amniotic fluid because they are not needed for oxygen exchange. Immediately after birth, the newborn's lungs must inflate, the remaining fluid must be absorbed, and oxygen exchange must begin.

One factor that helps the newborn clear fluid from the lungs begins during labor. Much of the fetal lung

Think about this. An infant who is born by cesarean delivery does not have the same benefit of the vaginal squeeze as does the infant born vaginally. Closely monitor the respirations of the newborn after cesarean delivery. She usually has more fluid in her lungs that must be absorbed after birth, which makes respiratory adaptation more challenging for this newborn.

fluid is squeezed out as the fetus moves down the birth canal. This so-called vaginal squeeze is an important way nature helps to clear the airway in preparation for the first breath. The vaginal squeeze also plays a role in stimulating lung expansion. The pressure of the birth canal on the fetal chest is released immediately when the infant is born. The lowered pressure from chest expansion draws air into the lungs.

Chemical changes stimulate respiratory centers in the brain. The newborn's lifeline to oxygen is cut off when the umbilical cord is clamped. Oxygen levels fall and carbon dioxide levels rise causing the newborn's pH to fall. The resulting acidosis stimulates the respiratory centers of the brain to begin their lifelong function of regulating respiration.

It is critical for the newborn to make strong respiratory efforts during the first few moments of life. This effort is best demonstrated and stimulated by a vigorous cry because crying helps to open the small air sacs (alveoli) in the lungs. Immediate sensory and thermal changes stimulate the newborn to cry. It is warm and dark inside the uterus; sounds are muffled; and the fetus is cradled by the confines of the womb. The

TABLE 13.1	Anatomic and Physiologic Comparison of the Fetus and Newborn	
Comparison	Fetus	Newborn
Respiratory system	Fluid-filled, high-pressure system causes blood to be shunted from the lungs through the ductus arteriosus to the rest of body	Air-filled, low-pressure system encourages blood flow through the lungs for gas exchange; increased oxygen content of blood in the lungs contributes to the closing of the ductus arteriosus (becomes a ligament)
Site of gas exchange	Placenta	Lungs
Circulation through the heart	Pressures in the right atrium greater than in the left; encourages blood flow through the foreman ovale	Pressures in the left atrium greater than in the right; causes the foreman ovale to close
Hepatic portal circulation	Ductus venosus bypasses; maternal liver performs filtering functions	Ductus venosus closes (becomes a ligament); hepatic portal circulation begins
Thermoregulation	Body temperature maintained by maternal body temperature and warmth of the intrauterine environment	Body temperature maintained through a flexed posture and brown fat

environment changes drastically at the moment of birth. The temperature is colder; it is brighter and louder; the security of the uterus is lost; and the newborn is touched directly for the first time.

Another important factor in the newborn's respiratory adaptation is **surfactant**. Surfactant, a substance found in the lungs of mature fetuses, keeps the alveoli from collapsing after they first expand. The work of breathing is increased greatly when the lungs lack surfactant. The newborn without enough surfactant expends large amounts of energy to breathe and quickly becomes exhausted without medical intervention. By the end of 35 weeks' gestation, the fetus usually has enough surfactant to breathe without lung collapse. Maturity of the respiratory system can be determined prenatally by measuring the lecithin/sphingomyelin (L/S) ratio of amniotic fluid. Box 13-1 lists signs of respiratory distress in the newborn; if seen, such signs must be reported promptly.

Cardiovascular Adaptation

The cardiovascular system also must make rapid adjustments immediately after birth. Fetal circulation differs from newborn circulation in several important ways. As you will recall from Chapter 5, only a small amount of blood flows to the fetal lungs. The rest is shunted away from the lungs. Remember, fetal blood that circulates to the heart has already been oxygenated through the placenta, so only the blood that is needed to supply oxygen to the lung tissue goes to the lungs. The lungs are small and noncompliant in utero; the respiratory system is a resistant, high-pressure system; and pressures in the right atrium are higher than in the left. These pressures help route blood through the foreman ovale and ductus arteriosus, away from the nonfunctioning lungs, back into the general circulation. The ductus venosus shunts fetal blood away from the liver because the woman's liver provides most of the filtering and metabolic functions necessary for fetal life.

Newborn circulation is similar to adult circulation. Deoxygenated blood that enters the heart after birth

must go to the lungs for gas exchange; therefore, the fetal shunts must close. Several factors contribute to their closing. The lungs fill with air, causing the pressure to drop in the chest as soon as the newborn takes his first breath. This change results in a reversal of pressures in the right and left atria, causing the foreman ovale to close so that blood is redirected to the lungs. The oxygen content of blood circulating through the lungs increases with the first few breaths. This chemical change contributes to the closing of the ductus arteriosus, which eventually becomes a ligament. The ductus venosus also closes, allowing nutrient-rich blood from the gut to circulate through the newborn's liver.

Thermoregulatory Adaptation

The newborn is challenged to maintain an adequate body temperature by producing as much heat as is lost. The process by which heat production is balanced with heat loss is called **thermoregulation**. This process is developed poorly in the newborn because of two key factors. First, the newborn is prone to heat loss. The newborn's ratio of body mass to body surface area is much smaller than that of an adult. In other words, the amount of heat-producing tissue, such as muscle and adipose tissue, is small in relation to the amount of skin that is exposed to the environment. Second, the newborn is not readily able to produce heat by muscle movement and shivering.

There are four main ways that a newborn loses heat—conduction, convection, radiation, and evaporation (Fig. 13-1). Conductive heat loss occurs when the newborn is placed on a cold surface, causing body heat to be transferred to the colder object. Heat is lost by convection when air currents blow over the newborn's body. Heat can also be lost to a cold object that is close to, but not touching, the newborn. This radiation heat loss can occur if the newborn is placed close to a cold windowpane, causing body heat to radiate toward the window and be lost. Evaporative heat loss happens when the newborn's skin is wet. As the moisture evaporates from the body surface, heat is taken with the moisture.

The normal newborn is not entirely without protection from heat loss. The newborn naturally assumes a flexed, fetal position that conserves body heat by reducing the amount of skin exposed to the surface and conserving core heat. The newborn can also

---

BOX 13.1	**Signs of Respiratory Distress in the Newborn**

- Tachypnea (sustained respiratory rate greater than 60 breaths per minute)
- Nasal flaring
- Grunting (noted by stethoscope or audible to the ear)
- Intercostal or xiphoid retractions
- Unequal movements of the chest and abdomen during breathing efforts
- Central cyanosis

A word of caution is in order.

It takes oxygen to produce heat. If the newborn is allowed to become cold stressed, he will eventually develop respiratory distress. This is one important reason to protect the newborn from unnecessary heat loss.

● **Figure 13.1** Mechanisms of heat loss. (**A**) Conduction—heat is lost to a cold surface, such as a cold scale or circumcision board, touching the newborn's skin. (**B**) Convection—heat is lost to air currents that flow over the newborn (e.g., from a fan, air conditioner, or movement around the crib). (**C**) Radiation—heat moves away from the newborn's body toward a colder object that is close by, such as a cold window or the sides of the crib. (**D**) Evaporation—heat is lost along with the moisture that evaporates from the newborn's wet skin, if he is not dried immediately after birth or if damp clothes or blankets are left next to his skin.

A. Conduction

B. Convection

C. Radiation

D. Evaporation

produce heat by burning **brown fat,** a specialized form of heat-producing tissue found only in fetuses and newborns. Deposits of brown fat are located at the nape of the neck, in the armpits, between the shoulder blades, along the abdominal aorta, and around the kidneys and sternum. Unfortunately, brown fat is not renewable; once stores are depleted, the newborn can no longer use this form of heat production.

Test Yourself

- Name two ways a vaginal birth assists the newborn's respiratory adaptation.

- What is the function of surfactant?

- Describe two factors that make it difficult for a newborn to maintain his body temperature.

Metabolic Adaptation

Throughout life a steady supply of blood glucose is necessary to carry out metabolic processes and produce energy. Glucose is also an essential nutrient for brain tissue. Neonatal hypoglycemia is defined as a blood glucose level of less than 40 mg/dL. The newborn is highly susceptible to hypoglycemia if he is excessively stressed during labor or during the transition period immediately after birth. Respiratory distress and cold stress are two stressors that often lead to neonatal hypoglycemia. Early signs of hypoglycemia in the newborn include jitteriness, poor feeding, listlessness, irritability, low temperature, weak or high-pitched cry, and hypotonia. Respiratory distress, apnea, seizures, and coma are late signs.

Hepatic Adaptation

Although immature, the newborn's liver must handle a heavy task. The fetus has a high percentage of circulating red blood cells to make use of all available oxygen in a low-oxygen environment. After birth, the newborn's lungs begin to function, and more oxygen is available immediately. Therefore, the "extra" red blood cells gradually die and must be broken down by the liver.

Bilirubin (a yellow pigment) is released as the blood cells are broken down. Normally the liver conjugates bilirubin (i.e., makes it water soluble), and then bilirubin is excreted in the feces. However, in the newborn's case, the liver is immature and overwhelmed easily by the large volume of red blood cells. Unconjugated bilirubin is fat soluble. As it builds up in the bloodstream, it crosses into the cells and stains them yellow. If a large amount of unconjugated bilirubin is present (serum levels of 4 to 6 mg/dL and greater), a yellow staining of the skin occurs, which is called **jaundice**. Jaundice is first seen on the head and face; as bilirubin levels rise, it progresses to the trunk and then to the extremities in a cephalocaudal manner.

In approximately one-half of all term newborns a condition known as **physiologic jaundice** will occur. Physiologic jaundice is characterized by jaundice that occurs after the first 24 hours of life (usually on day 2 or 3 after birth); bilirubin levels that peak between days 3 and 5; and bilirubin levels that do not rise rapidly (greater than 5 mg/dL per day). Jaundice that occurs within the first 24 hours is considered pathologic. However, when jaundice is noted, it must be recorded and reported. A more in-depth discussion of jaundice and its treatment can be found in Chapter 20. Breast-feeding jaundice is covered in Chapter 14.

The liver manufactures clotting factors necessary for normal blood coagulation. Several of the factors require vitamin K in their production. Bacteria that produce vitamin K normally are found in the gastrointestinal tract. However, the newborn's gut is sterile because normal flora have not yet taken up residence. Therefore, the newborn cannot produce vitamin K, which in turn causes the liver to be unable to produce some clotting factors. This situation could lead to bleeding problems, so newborns are given vitamin K (AquaMEPHYTON) intramuscularly shortly after birth to prevent hemorrhage (see Chapter 15 for discussion of the vitamin K administration procedure).

Behavioral and Social Adaptation

Each newborn has a unique temperament and personality that becomes apparent readily. Some newborns are quiet, rarely cry, and are consoled easily. Other newborns are frequently fussy or fretful and are more difficult to console. There are as many variations and characteristics as there are newborns.

In 1973 Dr. T. Berry Brazelton developed the Neonatal Behavioral Assessment Scale based on research he had done on the newborn's personality, individuality, and ability to communicate. Dr. Brazelton's key assumptions include that the newborn is a social organism capable of communicating through behavior and controlling his or her responses to the environment.

Dr. Brazelton identified six sleep and activity patterns that are characteristic of newborns. It is important to remember that individual infants display uniqueness in their sleep–wake cycles. Brazelton's states of reactivity are as follows:

1. Deep sleep: quiet, nonrestless sleep state; newborn is hard to awaken
2. Light sleep: eyes are closed, but more activity is noted; newborn moves actively and may show sucking behavior
3. Drowsy: eyes open and close and the eyelids look heavy; body activity is present with intermittent periods of fussiness
4. Quiet alert: quiet state with little body movement, but the newborn's eyes are open and she is attentive to people and things that are in close proximity to her; this is a good time for the parents to interact with their newborn
5. Active alert: eyes are open and active body movements are present; newborn responds to stimuli with activity
6. Crying: eyes may be tightly closed, thrashing movements are made in conjunction with active crying (Adapted from Howard-Glen, 2000, p. 364).

Test Yourself
- Define neonatal hypoglycemia.
- What pigment causes jaundice?
- Describe the quiet alert state of the newborn.

NURSING ASSESSMENT OF THE NORMAL NEWBORN

The initial nursing assessment (sometimes called the admissions assessment) is usually completed within the first few hours after birth. (APGAR scoring and other newborn assessments and care performed in the delivery room are discussed in Chapter 15.) The registered nurse (RN), nurse practitioner, or pediatrician is responsible for the full assessment, but the LPN may be asked to assist with portions of the examination. Therefore, you should be familiar with the procedure and expected findings to assist the practitioner and to be able to promptly report unexpected deviations from normal.

The examination should be conducted in a warm area that is free from drafts to protect the newborn from chilling. There should be plenty of light available to facilitate visual inspection. Indirect lighting works best. All equipment should be checked for proper functioning and should be readily available to allow for economy of motion. An experienced practitioner can complete a thorough examination in a short period of time, which is ideal because newborns become easily fatigued when overstimulated by prolonged examination.

The general order of progression is from general observations to specific measurements. Least disturbing aspects of the examination should be completed before more intrusive techniques are used. It is generally advisable to proceed using a head-to-toe approach. The overall physical appearance of the newborn is evaluated first, followed by measurement of vital signs, weight, and length. Then a thorough head-to-toe assessment is done, ending with assessment of neurologic reflexes and the gestational age assessment. The behavioral assessment is integrated throughout the examination as the practitioner notes how the newborn responds to sensory stimulation.

General Body Proportions and Posture

A typical newborn has a head that is large in proportion to the rest of his body. The newborn's neck is short, and the chin rests on the chest. The newborn maintains a flexed position with tightly clenched fists. The newborn's abdomen is protuberant and his chest is rounded. Note the newborn's sloping shoulders and rounded hips. The newborn's body appears long with short extremities.

Vital Signs

Vital signs are of particular interest to the nurse because they yield clues as to how well the newborn is adapting to extrauterine life. Determine respiratory effort and character at the beginning of the examination while the newborn is quiet. Respirations are activity dependent. The respiratory rhythm is often irregular, a characteristic known as episodic breathing. Momentary cessation of breathing interspersed with rapid breathing movements is typical of an episodic breathing pattern. Extended periods of apnea are not normal. The abdomen and chest rise and fall together with breathing movements. The normal respiratory rate is 30 to 60 breaths per minute and should be counted for a full minute when the infant is quiet.

Here's an interesting way to remember normal heart rate and blood pressure for the newborn. A newborn starts with a low blood pressure (60/40 mm Hg) and a high pulse (120 to 160 bpm). By the time she grows up, the opposite is true: her blood pressure is high (120/80 mm Hg) and her pulse is low (60 to 80 bpm).

The heart rate is taken apically for a full minute. The normal heart rate is the same for the newborn as it is for the fetus, ranging between 110 and 160 beats per minute (bpm), depending upon activity level. When the newborn is sleeping the heart tends to beat in the lower range of normal, and is not considered problematic as long as it stays above 100 bpm. The newborn's heart rate increases with activity and may increase to the 180s for short periods of time with vigorous activity and crying. The rhythm should be regular.

The newborn's temperature is measured in the axilla; the axillary temperature is considered to be reflective of the newborn's core body temperature (Fig. 13-2). Normal temperature range is between 97.7°F and 98.6°F (36.5°C and 37°C). Blood pressures are not taken routinely. If they are measured, the cuff must be an appropriate size, and the pressure may be measured on an arm or leg. Table 13-2 delineates the expected vital signs of the term newborn.

Physical Measurements

Weight and length of a newborn are dependent on several factors, including ethnicity, gender, genetics, and maternal nutrition and smoking behaviors. Generally speaking, the normal weight range for a full-term newborn is between 5 pounds 8 ounces and 8 pounds 13 ounces (2500 to 4000 grams). Nursing Procedure 13-1 lists the steps for obtaining the newborn's weight and length.

It is normal for the newborn to lose 5% to 10% of his birth weight in the first few days. For the average newborn, this physiologic weight loss amounts to a total loss of 6 to 10 ounces, and the cause is a loss of excess fluid combined with a low fluid intake during the first few days of life. The newborn should regain the weight within 7 to 10 days, after which he or she begins to gain approximately 2 pounds every month until 6 months of age.

Length can be difficult to measure accurately because of the newborn's flexed posture and resistance to stretching. The newborn should be placed on his back with his legs extended completely. Experienced nurses can hold

● **Figure 13.2** The nurse measures the newborn's axillary temperature.

TABLE 13.2	Expected Vital Signs of the Term Newborn	
Vital Sign	Expected Range	Characteristics
Heart rate	110–160 beats per minute (bpm); during sleep as low as 100 bpm and as high as 180 bpm when crying	Rhythm regular; murmurs may be normal, but all murmurs require medical evaluation
Respiratory rate	30–60 breaths per minute	Episodic breathing is normal; chest and abdomen should move synchronously
Axillary temerature	97.7°F–98.6°F (36.5°C–37°C)	Temperature stabilizes within 8–10 hours after delivery
Blood pressure	60–80/40–45 mm Hg	Not normally recorded for the normal newborn

Nursing Procedure 13.1
Obtaining Initial Weight and Measuring Length

EQUIPMENT

Calibrated scale
Paper to place on the scale
Tape measure
Marker or pen
Clean gloves

PROCEDURE

Weighing the Newborn

1. Thoroughly wash your hands.
2. Don a pair of clean gloves.
3. Place a paper or other designated covering on the scale to prevent direct contact of the newborn's skin with the scale.
4. Set the scale to zero.
5. Remove the newborn's clothes, including diapers, and blankets and place the newborn on the scale.
6. Hold one hand just above the newborn's body. Avoid actually touching the newborn.
7. Note the weight, in pounds and ounces and in grams.

Measuring the Newborn

8. Use the marker to place a mark on the paper at the top of the newborn's head.
9. Use one hand to firmly hold the newborn's heels together and straighten the legs.
10. Place a second mark on the paper at the newborn's heel.
11. Measure the area between the two marks with a tape measure. This is the newborn's length.
12. Remove your gloves and thoroughly wash your hands.
13. Record the newborn's weight and length in the designated area of the chart.
14. Be sure to report your findings to the mother, her partner, and other family members, as appropriate.

Note: Gloves are only necessary when handling the newborn before the first bath because of traces of blood, mucus, vernix, and other secretions on the body. Use universal precautions to protect yourself from blood-borne pathogens. To avoid inaccurate results, do not leave clothes, including diapers, on the newborn when he is weighed.

the tape measure and extend the newborn's legs simultaneously to obtain a crown-to-heel measurement. However, it is acceptable to use a writing instrument to make a mark where the crown of the head falls on a paper placed under the newborn and another mark at the heel with the leg extended. Then the length can be measured between the two marks. The average length is 20 inches, with the range between 19 and 21 inches (48 to 53 centimeters[cm]).

Head and chest circumference are two additional important newborn measurements. The head circumference (Fig. 13-3) is obtained by placing a paper tape measure around the widest circumference of the head (i.e., from the occipital prominence around to just above the eyebrows). To measure the chest circumference, place the infant on his back with the tape measure under the lower edge of the scapulae posteriorly and then bring the tape forward over the nipple line (Fig. 13-3). The average head circumference is between 13 and 14 inches (33 and 35.5), approximately 1 to 2 inches larger than that of the chest. Normal ranges for physical measurements of the term newborn are summarized in Table 13-3.

Head-to-Toe Assessment

Skin

The normal newborn's skin is supple with good turgor, reddish at birth (turning pink within a few hours), and flaky and dry. **Vernix caseosa**, a white cheese-like substance that covers the body of the fetus during the second trimester and protects the skin from the drying effects of amniotic fluid, is normally found only in creases of the term newborn. **Lanugo** is a fine downy hair that is present in abundance on the preterm infant but is found in thinning patches on the shoulders, arms, and back of the term newborn. The hair should be silky and soft. Fingernails are present and extend to the end of the fingertips or slightly beyond.

Common newborn skin manifestations are described in Table 13-4. Milia may be noted on the face. These tiny white papules resemble pimples in appearance. Reassure parents that these are harmless and will subside spontaneously. Acrocyanosis results from poor peripheral circulation and is not a good indicator of oxygenation status. The mucous membranes should be pink, and there should be no central cyanosis. Birth-

A

B

● *Figure 13.3* (**A**) The nurse obtains the head circumference. (**B**) The nurse obtains the chest circumference.

marks and skin tags may be present. These are not a cause for concern and can generally be removed easily if the parents desire. **Mottling** is a red and white lacy pattern sometimes seen on the skin of newborns who have fair complexions. It is variable in occurrence and length, lasting from several hours to several weeks. Mottling sometimes occurs when the newborn is exposed to cool temperatures. **Harlequin sign,** also referred to as Harlequin coloring, is characterized by a clown-suit like appearance of the newborn. The newborn's skin is dark red on one side of the body while the other side of the body is pale. The dark red color is

TABLE 13.3	Average Physical Measurement Ranges of the Term Newborn	
Measurement	Average Range Metric System	Average Range US Customary System
Weight	2,500–4,000 grams	5 pounds 8 ounces–8 pounds 13 ounces
Length (head-to-heel)	48–53 centimeters	19–21 inches
Head circumference	33–35.5 centimeters	13–14 inches
Chest circumference	30.5–33 centimeters	12–13 inches

TABLE 13.4	Common Skin Manifestations of the Normal Newborn
Skin Manifestation	Family Teaching Tips
Acrocyanosis	A bluish color to the hands and feet of the newborn is normal in the first 6 to 12 hours after birth. Acrocyanosis results from slow circulation in the extremities.
Milia	Small white spots on the newborn's face, nose, and chin that resemble pimples are an expected observation. Do not attempt to pick or squeeze them. They will subside spontaneously in a few days.
Erythema toxicum	The so-called newborn rash commonly appears on the chest, abdomen, back, and buttocks of the newborn. It is harmless and will disappear.
Mongolian spot	These bluish-black areas of discoloration are commonly seen on the back, buttocks, or extremities of African-American, Hispanic, Mediterranean, or other dark-skinned newborns. These spots should not be mistaken for bruises or mistreatment and gradually fade during the first year or two of life.
Telangiectatic nevi	These pale pink or red marks ("stork bites") are sometimes found on the nape of the neck, eyelids, or nose of fair-skinned newborns. Stork bites blanch when pressed and generally fade as the child grows.

(table continues on page 312)

TABLE 13.4 (continued)	Common Skin Manifestations of the Normal Newborn
Skin Manifestation	**Family Teaching Tips**
Nevus flammeus or port-wine stain	A port-wine stain is a dark reddish purple birthmark that most commonly appears on the face. It is caused by a group of dilated blood vessels. It does not blanch with pressure or fade with time. There are cosmetics available that help cover the stain if it is disfiguring. Laser therapy has been successfully used to fade port-wine stains.

caused by dilation of blood vessels, and the pallor is caused by constriction of blood vessels. This harmless condition occurs most frequently with vigorous crying.

It is important to evaluate the newborn's skin for signs of jaundice. Natural sunlight is the best environment in which to assess for jaundice. If sunlight is not easily available inside the nursery, indirect lighting should be used. Press the newborn's skin over the forehead or nose with your finger and note if the blanched area appears yellow. It is also helpful to evaluate the sclera of the eyes, particularly in dark-skinned newborns. A yellow-tinge to the sclera indicates the presence of jaundice.

Some skin characteristics are attributable to birth trauma or operative intervention. Bruising may be noted over the presenting part or on the face if the labor or delivery was unusually short or prolonged. Forceps marks may be seen on the face. Occasionally there will be a nick or cut on the infant born by cesarean delivery, particularly if the cesarean was done rapidly under emergency conditions.

bones as the fetus moves through the birth canal (Fig. 13-4), or **caput succedaneum** (caput), swelling of the soft tissue of the scalp caused by pressure of the presenting part on a partially dilated cervix or trauma from a vacuum-assisted delivery. These conditions are often of concern to new parents. Reassure them that the molding or caput will decrease in a few days without treatment.

You may notice this relationship. Molding and caput are more common or more pronounced in first-born babies than in the newborns of multiparas. In addition, many newborns delivered by cesarean do not experience molding or caput unless the fetus is in the birth canal for a prolonged period of time before delivery.

A **cephalhematoma** may be noted. This is swelling that occurs from bleeding under the periosteum of the

Test Yourself
- Name the major nursing actions to take while weighing and measuring a newborn.
- What is the significance of acrocyanosis?
- How would you explain the presence of milia to the parents?

Head and Face
The head may be misshapen because of **molding,** an elongated shape caused by overlapping of the cranial

● **Figure 13.4** Molding.

A PERSONAL GLIMPSE

The doctor was just about to use the vacuum extractor because I had been pushing for 3 hours. I gave one additional strong push and felt the absolute relief of my baby sliding out of my body. The doctor said, "It's a girl." My husband was crying, and I couldn't wait to see our little girl. I wanted to examine her, touch her, feed her, and look into her eyes. They laid our tiny baby girl on my chest, and the first thing I noticed was her very long, pointy head. "Oh, my poor little girl," I thought, "that looks so painful and awful." I had heard and read about molding but had no idea it would be so pronounced. I must have had a look of serious concern on my face because the nurse touched my arm and said, "don't worry, her head will be back to a normal size and shape in just a day or two." The nurse then covered my sweet baby's pointy head with a soft pink cap, and my baby and I began to get to know each other.

Isabel

LEARNING OPPORTUNITY: How can nurses' knowledge of normal newborn assessment findings provide assurance to new parents?

Describe how a nurse's reaction to a common newborn finding could encourage or discourage parents.

---

skull, usually over one of the parietal bones. A cephalhematoma is caused by birth trauma, usually requires no treatment, and will spontaneously resolve. However, the newborn should be evaluated carefully for signs of anemia (pallor) or shock from acute blood loss.

It also is important to make certain the cephalhematoma does not cross over suture lines. If it does, a skull fracture is suspected. Sometimes it is difficult for the inexperienced practitioner to tell the difference between a cephalhematoma and caput. Figure 13-5 compares features of these conditions.

Sutures occur in the place where two cranial bones meet. The normal newborn's sutures are palpable with a small space between them. It may be difficult to palpate sutures in the first 24 hours if significant molding is present. However, it is important to determine that the sutures are present. Rarely sutures will fuse prematurely (craniostenosis). It is important to detect this condition because it will require surgery to allow the brain to grow.

Fontanels occur at the junction of cranial bones where two or more sutures meet. The anterior and posterior fontanels are palpable. The anterior fontanel is diamond shaped and larger than the posterior fontanel, which has a triangular shape. The posterior fontanel closes within the first 3 months of life, whereas the anterior fontanel does not close until 12 to 18 months of life. When the newborn is in a sitting position, the anterior fontanel should be flat, neither depressed nor bulging. It is normal to feel pulsations that correlate with the newborn's heart rate over the anterior fontanel. Bulging fontanels may indicate hydrocephalus or increased intracranial pressure, and sunken fontanels are a sign of severe dehydration.

Facial movements should be symmetrical. Facial paralysis can occur from a forceps delivery or from pressure on the facial nerve as the fetus travels down the birth canal. It is easiest to assess for facial paralysis when the newborn is crying. The affected side will not

● ***Figure 13.5*** Comparison of caput succedaneum and cephalhematoma. **(A)** Caput is a collection of serous fluid between the periosteum and the scalp. It is found on the area that was pressing against the cervix during labor, or the area to which the vacuum cup was attached. Caput often crosses suture lines. **(B)** Cephalhematoma is a collection of blood between the periosteum and the skull. It does not cross suture lines, unless there is a skull fracture, which is a rare occurrence.

move, and the space between the eyelids will widen. Facial paralysis is usually temporary, but occasionally the deficit is permanent.

Eyes

The eye color of a newborn with light skinned parents is usually blue-gray, whereas a darker skinned infant usually has a dark eye color. It is normal for the eyelids to be swollen from pressure during birth. A chemical conjunctivitis may develop after instillation of eye prophylaxis in the delivery room (see Chapter 15 for discussion of eye prophylaxis).

The sclera should be clear and white, not blue. The pupils should be equal and reactive to light. A red reflex should be present. The red reflex is elicited by shining an ophthalmoscope onto the retina of the eye. The normal response is to see a red reflection from the retina. Absence of the red reflex is associated with congenital cataracts. Small subconjunctival hemorrhages may be present. These usually disappear within a week or two and are not harmful.

Eye movements are usually uncoordinated, and some strabismus (crossed eyes) is expected. A "doll's eye" reflex is normal for the first few days: that is, when the newborn's head is turned, the eyes travel to the opposite side. Persistence of this reflex after the second week should be evaluated.

The newborn is able to perceive light and can track objects held close to the face. He or she likes shapes and colors and shows a definite preference for the human face. Crying is usually tearless because the lacrimal apparatus is underdeveloped.

Nose

The newborn's nose is flat, and the bridge may appear to be absent. The nostrils should be bilaterally patent because the newborn is an obligate nose breather. Nostril patency is presumed if the newborn breathes easily with a closed mouth. The newborn clears obstructions from the nose by sneezing. There should be no nasal flaring, which is a sign of respiratory distress. The sense of smell is present, as evidenced by the newborn's turning toward milk and by turning away from or blinking in the presence of strong odors.

Mouth

The mucous membranes should be moist and pink. Sucking calluses may appear on the central part of the lips shortly after birth. The uvula should be midline. Place a gloved finger in the newborn's mouth to evaluate the suck and gag reflexes and to check the palate for intactness. The suck reflex should be strong, the gag reflex present, and both the hard and soft palates should be intact. Well-developed fat pads are present bilaterally on the cheeks.

Epstein's pearls are small white cysts found on the midline portion of the hard palate of some newborns. They feel hard to the touch and are harmless. Precocious teeth may be present on the lower central portion of the gum. The teeth will need to be removed if they are loose to prevent the infant from aspirating them.

Don't forget! A cleft palate can be present even in the absence of a cleft lip. Check the roof of the mouth carefully to be sure it is intact.

A fungal infection (caused by *Candida albicans*) in the oral cavity, called **thrush,** may be seen in the newborn. The newborn can contract the infection while passing through the birth canal. The fungus causes white patches on the oral mucosa, particularly the tongue, which resemble milk curds. It is important not to remove the patches because doing so will cause bleeding in the underlying tissue. Thrush is treated with an oral solution of nystatin (Mycostatin, Nilstat).

Ears

The pinna should be flexible with quick recoil, indicating the presence of cartilage. The top of the pinna should be even with, or above, an imaginary horizontal line drawn from the inner to the outer canthus of the eye and continuing past the ear (Fig. 13-6). Low-set ears are associated with congenital defects, including those that cause mental retardation and internal organ defects.

In recent years most hospitals have developed newborn hearing screening programs in accordance with recommendations of the American Academy of Pediatrics (AAP) for universal screening. There are two main ways that a newborn's hearing can be tested satisfactorily using current technology: evoked otoacoustic emissions (EOAE) and auditory brain-stem

● **Figure 13.6** Determining placement of the ears. The top of the pinna should lie above an imaginary line drawn from the inner to the outer canthus of the eye continuing past the ear on either side. Note the line in the drawing.

response (ABR). Both methodologies are noninvasive and easy to perform. Each test takes less than 5 minutes to perform. Each method assesses hearing differently, and each has unique advantages and disadvantages. The important task for the nursery nurse is to make certain that each newborn is screened adequately before he or she is discharged from the hospital.

Neck

The newborn's neck is short and thick. The head should move freely and have full range of motion. Significant head lag is present when the newborn is pulled to a sitting position from a supine one (Fig. 13-7). Newborns can hold up their heads slightly when placed on their abdomens. There should be no masses or webbing.

The clavicles should be intact. Occasionally a clavicle is fractured during a difficult delivery. Signs of a fractured clavicle include a lump along one clavicle accompanied by crepitus (a grating sensation) at the site. An asymmetrical Moro reflex is another indication (refer to the discussion of the Moro reflex later in the chapter).

Chest

The anteroposterior and lateral diameters of the chest are equal, making the chest appear barrel-shaped. The xiphoid process is prominent. Chest movements should be equal bilaterally and synchronous with the abdomen.

Breast enlargement and breast engorgement is normal for both sexes. A thin milky secretion, sometimes called "witch's milk," may be secreted from the nipples. The breasts should not be squeezed in an attempt to express the liquid. Assess for supernumerary (accessory) nipples below and medial to the true nipples.

● **Figure 13.7** The newborn exhibits significant head lag when pulled to a sitting position from lying on his back.

Abdomen

The newborn's abdomen is dome shaped and protuberant. Respirations are typically diaphragmatic, which make them appear abdominal in nature. Peristaltic waves should not be visible. Bowel sounds should be audible within 2 hours of birth. The abdomen should be soft to palpation without palpable masses. The umbilical cord should be well formed, with three vessels present. The base of the cord should be dry without redness or drainage, and the umbilical clamp should be fastened securely.

Genitourinary

The newborn should void within the first 24 hours of life. Vigorous newborns may urinate for the first time in the delivery room minutes after birth. The stream of a male newborn should be strong enough to cause a steady arch during voiding, and the female should be able to produce a steady stream. The kidneys are not able to concentrate urine well during the first few days, so the color is light, and there is no odor. It is normal to find a small amount of pink or light orange color in the diaper for the first few voidings. This so-called brick dust in the diaper is caused by excess uric acid in the urine.

Both male and female genitalia may be swollen. **Smegma**, a cheesy white sebaceous gland secretion, is often found within the folds of the labia of the female and under the foreskin of the male. It is best to allow the secretion to gradually wear away because vigorous attempts at removal can irritate the tender mucosa. Immediately report the presence of ambiguous genitalia (i.e., it is difficult to tell if the newborn has male or female genitalia).

Female. The labia and clitoris may be edematous. In the term newborn, the labia majora cover the labia minora. A hymenal tag may be present. An imperforate hymen (a hymen that completely covers the vaginal opening) should be reported. A blood-tinged mucous secretion may be discharged from the vagina in response to the sudden withdrawal of maternal hormones. This secretion is called **pseudomenstruation**. Reassure the parents this condition is not cause for alarm.

Male. The urinary meatus should be positioned at the tip of the penis. If the opening is located abnormally on the dorsal (upper) surface of the glans penis, the condition is called **epispadias**. **Hypospadias** occurs when the opening to the urethra is on the ventral (under) surface of the glans. **Phimosis**, tightly adherent foreskin, is a normal condition in the term newborn. The tissue should not be forced over the glans penis. Monitor the adequacy of the urinary stream. If phimosis interferes with urination, intervention will be needed. Spontaneous erections are a common finding.

The male scrotum is pendulous, edematous, and covered with rugae (deep creases). Dark-skinned newborns have deeply pigmented scrotum. Both testes should be descended. Use your thumb and forefinger to gently palpate the scrotal sac while gently pressing down on the inguinal canal with the opposite hand. Repeat the procedure on the opposite side. Failure of the testes to descend (undescended testicles) is a condition called *cryptorchidism*. This condition requires medical evaluation. A hydrocele, fluid within the scrotal sac, may be present and should be noted.

You can diagnose a hydrocele quite easily. Take a penlight and hold it against the scrotal sac. If fluid is present (hydrocele), the light will transilluminate the scrotum. If there is no hydrocele, the light will not shine through solid structures.

Extremities

The term newborn maintains a posture of flexion. He has good muscle tone, and his extremities return quickly to an attitude of flexion after they are extended. The extremities are short in relation to the body and without deformities. Full range of motion is present in all joints, and movements are bilateral and equal.

Count the fingers and toes. Syndactyly refers to fusing or webbing of the toes or fingers, and polydactyly is the term used when extra digits are present. The palms of the hands should have creases. A single straight palmar crease, a **simian crease**, is an abnormal finding that is associated with Down's syndrome. Brachial pulses should be present and equal.

The legs are bowed and the feet flat because of a fatty pad in the arch of the foot. Creases should cover at least two thirds of the bottom of the feet. Palpate the femoral and brachial pulses on each side of the body. The pulses should be equal and strong. A strong brachial pulse with a weak femoral pulse is abnormal and should be reported (Fig. 13-8).

Here's a helpful hint. It takes practice to learn how to palpate the femoral pulses, but this is an important assessment skill to develop. Practice on a newborn who is resting quietly. Leave your fingers in one place long enough to adequately determine if the pulse is present. You will gain confidence as you are consistently able to find the pulses.

You may be asked to assist the RN while she attempts to elicit Ortolani's maneuver and Barlow's sign (Nursing Procedure 13-2) to evaluate the hip for signs of dislocation or subluxation (partial dislocation). A positive sign is associated with subluxation.

Other signs of a dislocated hip included uneven gluteal folds and one knee that is lower than the

A

B

● **Figure 13.8** (**A**) Palpating the femoral pulse (**B**) Palpating the brachial pulse.

other when the newborn is supine with both knees flexed.

The feet may appear to turn inward because of the way the fetus was positioned in the womb or birth canal. If the feet are easily reducible, that is they can be easily moved to a normal position, the "deformity" is positional and will resolve spontaneously. If the feet do not move to a normal position, true clubfoot may be present. A specialist should evaluate this condition.

Back and Rectum

The spine is straight and flat. The lumbar and sacral curves do not appear until the infant begins to use his back to sit and stand upright. Feel along the length of the spine. There should be no masses, openings, dimples, or tufts of hair. Any of these findings may be associated with spina bifida (an opening in the spinal column with or without herniation of the meninges).

The anus should be patent. **Meconium,** the first stool of the newborn, is a thick black tarry substance composed of dead cells, mucus, and bile that collects in the rectum of the fetus. Passage of meconium should

Nursing Procedure 13.2
Ortolani's Maneuver and Barlow's Sign

EQUIPMENT

Warm, clean hands
Flat surface

PROCEDURE

1. Wash hands thoroughly.
2. Position the newborn flat on his back on a firm surface.
3. Position the knees together and flex the knees and hips 90 degrees.
4. Place your middle fingers over the greater trochanter of the femur and your thumbs on the inner aspect of the thigh.
5. Apply upward pressure and abduct the hips. A clicking or a clunking sound is a positive Ortolani's sign and is associated with dislocation of the hip.

6. Next apply downward pressure and adduct the hips. Continue to maintain 90 degrees flexion. If you feel the head of the femur slip out of the acetabulum, the joint is unstable, and Barlow's sign is positive.

7. Position the newborn comfortably on the back or side.
8. Wash hands thoroughly.
9. Document your findings.

Note: In this instance, a positive Ortolani's or Barlow's sign is not wanted. It is not normal to hear clicking or clunking or to feel the femoral head slip out of the hip socket.

---

occur within the first 24 to 48 hours and confirms the presence of a patent anus.

Test Yourself

- Name two differences between caput succedaneum and cephalhematoma.

- What is pseudomenstruation?

- Define subluxation of the hip.

Neurologic Assessment

General Appearance and Behavior

The first part of the neurologic examination involves quiet observation of the general appearance and behavior of the newborn. The newborn should main-tain an attitude of flexion. Hypotonus (decreased tone) is an abnormal finding, as is hypertonus, distinct tremors, jitteriness, or seizure activity. Any of these states may be associated with neurologic dysfunction, hypoglycemia, hypocalcemia, or neonatal drug withdrawal. The cry should be vigorous and of medium pitch. A high-pitched, shrill cry is associated with neurologic dysfunction.

Reflexes

The normal newborn reflexes (Fig. 13-9) should be elicited at this point in the examination. Although there are other reflexes, the ones discussed here are generally the most common reflexes to be assessed. In addition, the newborn should demonstrate the protective reflexes of sneezing, coughing, blinking, and withdrawing from painful stimuli.

Rooting, sucking, and swallowing reflexes are important to the newborn's nutritional intake. The

● **Figure 13.9** Normal newborn reflexes. **(A)** The nurse elicits the suck reflex in the newborn **(B)** Palmar grasp. The newborn curls her fingers tightly around the nurse's fingers. **(C)** The nurse elicits the stepping reflex. **(D)** The newborn is exhibiting the Moro reflex. Notice the "C" shape of the arms. **(E)** Tonic neck reflex (fencer's position). Notice how the extremities on the side he is facing are extended while the opposite extremities are flexed.

rooting reflex is elicited by gently stroking the newborn's cheek. If the reflex is present she will turn toward the touch with an open mouth looking for food. The new mother can be taught to use this reflex to help the newborn begin breast-feeding (see Chapter 14). Place a gloved finger in the newborn's mouth to test the sucking reflex. The suck should be strong. Swallowing is evaluated when the infant eats. Listen and watch for coordinated swallowing efforts.

The plantar and palmar grasp reflexes are evaluated by placing a finger in the palm or parallel to the toes. The digits will wrap around the finger and hold on. The grasp should be equal and strong bilaterally. The stepping reflex is checked by supporting the newborn in a standing position on a hard surface. He will lift his legs up and down in a stepping motion. Babinski's sign is positive if the newborn's toes fan out and hyperextend and dorsiflexion of the foot occurs in response to a hard object (such as the blunt end of a writing pen) being traced from the heel along the lateral aspect of the foot up and across the ball of the foot. After the infant starts walking, this reflex should disappear and the toes will curl inward, rather than fanning outward.

The Moro reflex is also known as the *startle reflex*. When the newborn is startled, he will extend his arms and legs away from his body and to the side. Then his arms will come back toward each other with the fingers spread in a "C" shape. His arms look as if he is trying to embrace something. The Moro reflex should be symmetrical and can be elicited until approximately 6 months of age. The tonic neck reflex is another total body reflex. With the infant lying quietly on his back, turn his head to one side without moving the rest of his body. He will extend the arm and leg on the side he is facing and flex the opposite arm and leg. This position has been called the "fencer's position" because it looks as if the newborn is poised to begin fencing.

Behavioral Assessment

It is important to note how the parents react to the newborn's behavior states and how the parents talk about the newborn. Newborns who demonstrate self-quieting behaviors are usually considered to be "good" babies. Parents respond positively to newborns who are cuddly and sociable. When a newborn resists cuddling or is difficult to console, the parents may feel rejected, and bonding can be affected adversely.

Teach the parents to watch the newborn for cues as to when he wants to interact. The quiet alert state is a good time for focused interaction with the newborn. When the newborn is in the active alert stage, he likes to play. The drowsy state lets the parents know the newborn needs rest. Crying signals that the newborn has a need. Teach the parents to check for physical problems first, such as a wet diaper, hunger, or need to burp. If the newborn is still crying, the parents can try soothing actions, such as walking, rocking, or riding in the car. Reassure the parents that, contrary to popular opinion, you cannot spoil a newborn by picking him up when he is crying. Being held is reassuring and comforting to the newborn.

This is vital! Teach the parents to NEVER shake an infant. Shaking an infant can cause permanent brain damage. If the parent is frustrated because the crying does not stop no matter what has been tried, encourage the parent to take a minute to stop and count to 10 or ask a friend for help.

Gestational Age Assessment

The gestational age assessment is a critical evaluation. The RN is ultimately responsible for performing the gestational age assessment; however, the LPN should be familiar with the instruments used and be able to differentiate characteristics of the full-term newborn from those of the premature newborn. Chapter 20 details gestational age assessment and compares the preterm with the full-term newborn.

KEY POINTS

- The newborn must adapt rapidly to life outside the womb and without the placenta that supplies every need in utero.
- In order to adjust to life outside the uterus, the newborn must fill his lungs with air, absorb remaining fluid in his lungs, and begin oxygen exchange.
- All the fetal shunts (foramen ovale, ductus arteriosus, and ductus venosus) must close so that blood will travel to the lungs for gas exchange and so that blood will pass through the liver.
- The newborn exhibits poor thermoregulation because he is prone to heat loss through the skin and because he cannot produce heat through muscle movement and shivering. He loses heat through the processes of convection, conduction, radiation, and evaporation. However, the newborn conserves heat by maintaining a flexed position and produces heat by metabolizing brown fat.
- The newborn's liver is immature. Sometimes it cannot handle the heavy load from the breakdown of red blood cells, and physiologic jaundice appears. This condition is harmless if bilirubin levels do not rise dramatically and if jaundice is not present before the newborn is 24 hours old. Not all of the necessary blood coagulation factors are manufactured directly after birth and the gut is sterile, so vitamin K is given intramuscularly to stimulate appropriate clotting.
- Each infant is unique, but all infants have similar sleep and activity patterns. These include deep sleep, light sleep, drowsiness, quiet alert state, active alert state, and crying.
- The nursing assessment of newborn characteristics is an important way the nurse determines how well the newborn is adapting to life outside the womb. In general, the least disturbing aspects of the examination are done first, such as general observation regarding the newborn's posture. In addition, the respiratory rate and heart rate are taken early in the examination while the newborn is quiet. Then the examination proceeds in a head-to-toe manner, covering vital signs, physical measurements, and assessment of each body part.
- The expected weight range is 5 pounds 8 ounces to 8 pounds 13 ounces (2,500 to 4,000 grams). Length is 19 to 21 inches (48 to 53 cm). Head circumference is 13 to 14 inches (33 to 33.5 cm) and chest circumference is 12 to 13 inches (30.5 to 33 cm).
- The skin should be supple with good turgor and have a pink color to it. There are many variations that are normally present on newborn skin.

◗ Head and face: Molding may be present. The newborn is an obligate nose breather. The hard and soft palates should be intact.

◗ Neck and chest: The neck is short and thick. Webbing should not be present. Periodic breathing episodes are normal.

◗ Abdomen: The abdomen is protuberant. The cord should be clamped and drying at the base with three vessels present.

◗ Genitourinary: The newborn should void within the first 24 hours. Genitalia of both sexes may be swollen.

◗ The back should be straight and free of hairy tufts, dimples, or tumors. Meconium, the first stool, should be passed in the first 24 hours.

◗ The main reflexes elicited to determine neurologic status are rooting, sucking, swallowing, grasping, Moro, Babinski's, and tonic neck or the fencer's position.

REFERENCES AND SELECTED READINGS

Books and Journals

American Academy of Pediatrics Task Force on Newborn and Infant Hearing. (1999). Newborn and infant hearing loss: Detection and intervention (RE9846). *Pediatrics, 103*(2), 527–530. Retrieved July 14, 2002, from http://www.aap.org/policy/re9846.html.

Cunningham, F. G., Gant, N. F., Leveno, K. J., Gilstrap, L. C., III, Hauth, J. C. & Wenstrom, K. D. (2001). The newborn infant. In *Williams Obstetrics* (21st ed., pp. 385–402). New York: McGraw-Hill Medical Publishing Division.

DeMichele, A. M., & Ruth, R. A. (2003). Newborn hearing screening. In R. A. Faust, F. Talavera, P. S. Roland, C. L. Slack, & A. D. Meyers (Eds.), *eMedicine*. Retrieved January 8, 2004, from http://www.emedicine.com/ent/topic576.htm.

Hansen, R. W. R. (2002). Neonatal jaundice. In I. Oussama, R. Konop, B. S. Carter, C. L. Wagner, & N. N. Finer (Eds.), *eMedicine*. Retrieved January 15, 2004, from http://www.emedicine.com/ped/topic1061.htm..

Howard-Glen, L. (2000). Adaptation to extrauterine life and immediate nursing care. In S. Mattson & J. E. Smith (Eds.), *Core Curriculum for Maternal–ewborn Nursing* (2nd ed., pp. 346–359). AWHONN publication. Philadelphia: WB Saunders.

Howard-Glen, L. (2000). Newborn biological/behavioral characteristics and psychosocial adaptations. In S. Mattson & J. E. Smith (Eds.), *Core Curriculum for Maternal–Newborn Nursing* (2nd ed., pp. 360–373). AWHONN publication. Philadelphia: WB Saunders.

St. John, E. B. (2002). Hemorrhagic disease of newborn. In O. Itani, R. Konop, D. A. Clark, C. L. Wagner, & N. N. Finer (Eds.), *eMedicine*. Retrieved January 8, 2004, from http://www.emedicine.com/ped/topic966.htm.

Yan, A. C. (2002). Erythema toxicum. In K. P. Connelly, R. Konop, R. A. Schwartz, M. Poth, & D. M. Elston (Eds.), *eMedicine*. Retrieved January 15, 2003, from http://www.emedicine.com/ped/topic697.htm.

Websites
Newborn Appearance and Behavior
http://www.beryl.net/HTL/NewBaby/22917.htm
http://www.childrenshospitaloakland.org/health_library/pa/hhg/newbappe.htm

Newborn Guidelines
http://www.rcp.gov.bc.ca/Guidelines/Newborn

Newborn skin characteristics
http://www.umm.edu/ency/article/002301.htm

WORKBOOK

NCLEX-STYLE REVIEW QUESTIONS

1. An infant is born by cesarean delivery. In what way is respiratory adaptation more difficult for this infant than the one who is born by vaginal delivery?

    a. More fluid is present in the lungs at birth.

    b. Surfactant is missing from the lungs.

    c. The respiratory centers in the brain are not stimulated.

    d. There is less sensory stimulation to breathe.

2. A new mother says, "I think something is wrong with my baby. She has a milky fluid leaking from her nipples!" What is the nurse's best response?

    a. "I don't know. Let me have the charge nurse check the baby."

    b. "It's nothing to worry about. That's a normal finding."

    c. "This is a normal occurrence. You may clean her with a damp washcloth, but be careful not to squeeze the nipples."

    d. "This means the baby was exposed to an infection during birth. I'll notify the doctor at once!"

3. You are assessing a newborn that is 1 day old. You notice a small amount of white drainage and redness at the base of the umbilical cord. How should you respond?

    a. Call the doctor immediately to ask for intravenous antibiotics.

    b. Carefully clean the area with a damp washcloth and cover it with an absorbent dressing.

    c. Notify the charge nurse because this finding represents a possible complication.

    d. Show the mother how to clean the area with soap and water.

4. A newborn's axillary temperature is 97.4°F. His T-shirt is damp with spit-up milk. His blanket is loosely applied, and several children are in the room running around his crib. The room is comfortably warm, and the bassinet is beside the mother's bed away from the window and doors. What are the most likely mechanisms of heat loss for this newborn?

    a. Conduction and evaporation

    b. Conduction and radiation

    c. Convection and radiation

    d. Convection and evaporation

STUDY ACTIVITIES

1. Do an Internet search using the key words "newborn crying." How many Internet sites returned? List three to four that would be good references for new parents. Compare your list to that of your clinical group.

2. Use the table below to describe important newborn assessments for each body system.

Body System	Critical Parameters to Assess	Expected Findings and Deviation From Normal
Respiratory Cardiovascular Gastrointestinal Metabolic Hepatic Skin		

3. Research resources in your community designed to help first-time parents in their new role. How many sources did you find? Were you surprised? Share your findings with your clinical group. Discuss ways the community might be more supportive of new parents.

Critical Thinking: What Would You Do?

Apply your knowledge of normal newborn adaptation to the following situation.

1. Mary, a 28-year-old woman, delivered her first baby several hours ago. She and the father of the baby had joyful interaction with the baby immediately after delivery. The newborn breast-fed well with assistance from the delivery room nurse. You are coming on duty for the evening shift and have just entered the room to assess the baby.

    a. You find the baby sleeping with only a diaper on in an open bassinet. It appears the bassinet has been moved against the wall under a window. The baby's skin is mottled, and her extremities feel cool to the touch. What is your initial assessment of the situation? What actions should you take first?

b. What instructions should you give to the parents?

2. On day 3 of life, you notice that the skin of Mary's baby is a light yellow color.

   a. What is the likely cause of the yellow color?

   b. Mary asks you if the yellow color indicates illness. How do you reply?

3. Mary says she is frustrated. She has been trying to "play" with the baby, but he keeps looking away and yawning. She is worried that her baby doesn't "like" her.

   a. How should you reply to Mary?

   b. Mary expresses concern about a blue-black spot she found on the baby's back. She is worried that he received a bruise in the nursery. How do you explain this finding to Mary?

Newborn Nutrition

14

STUDENT OBJECTIVES

On completion of this chapter, the student should be able to

1. Describe factors that influence the woman's choice of feeding method.
2. Identify advantages of breast-feeding for both the woman and the newborn.
3. Discuss situations for which breast-feeding would not be recommended.
4. Discuss the physical and hormonal control of the breast during lactation.
5. Describe the role of the nurse when assisting a woman to breast-feed.
6. Outline appropriate nursing interventions for three common problems the breast-feeding woman might encounter.
7. List signs that a newborn is not breast-feeding well.
8. Differentiate between breast milk and formula.
9. Compare the various types of formulas available to feed newborns and infants.
10. Name situations in which formula feeding would be beneficial.
11. Outline appropriate teaching topics for the bottle-feeding woman.
12. List several questions the nurse should ask the parents of a newborn who is not tolerating formula.

KEY TERMS

amenorrhea
artificial nutrition
colostrum
engorgement
foremilk
hind milk
immunologic
lactation consultant
mastitis

I n utero the fetus obtains all of its nutrition in a passive manner. The nutrients cross from the maternal circulation, across the placenta, and enter the fetus' circulation. From there the nutrients are taken directly to the tissues and used at the cellular level. At birth, this passive intake of nutrition ends, and the newborn must actively consume and digest food.

The newborn has specific nutritional needs. The healthy term newborn needs 108 kcal/kg/day and 160 to 180 mL/kg/day. Breast milk, or an iron-fortified infant formula, will provide the newborn with all the calories and fluids necessary. In addition, breast milk and infant formulas are balanced to meet the carbohydrate, protein, and fat needs of the newborn. Table 14-1 summarizes some of the specific nutritional needs of the newborn.

CHOOSING A FEEDING METHOD

The healthy term newborn can be fed one of two ways. The woman can choose to either breast-feed or bottle-feed her newborn. The choice is ultimately the woman's to make. The nurse has a clear role in providing the woman with enough information for her to make an informed decision. In addition, the nurse has a supportive and teaching role after the woman has made her decision.

There are many factors that influence the woman's decision about whether to breast-feed or bottle-feed. Some of these factors are culture, age, prior experience with or exposure to breast-feeding, and her intent or need to return to work or school.

Culture

Each culture has its own viewpoint on feeding the newborn. Most cultures support breast-feeding. In some situations, such as immigration to a new country, formula feeding is seen as more desirable, and the woman may choose to formula feed, even if she previously breast-fed in her native country. In some cultures the desire is for a strong or large baby, and formula is seen as the way to achieve these desired goals (Riordan & Auerbach, 1998). In some cultures the woman will feed her newborn formula until her milk comes in and then she will breast-feed. In the United States, breast-feeding tends to be more predominant in whites, with 59.7% breast-feeding in the hospital after birth. African-American women have the lowest rate, with 27.2% breast-feeding after birth in the hospital. Hispanics have a 51.7% in-hospital breast-feeding rate (Lawrence & Lawrence, 1999).

Age and Education

Breast-feeding is highest in women older than 35 years of age. Younger women tend to choose bottle-feeding; fewer than 44% of women younger than 20 years of age breast-feed their newborns. This may be attributable to a lack of knowledge regarding the benefits of breast-feeding for the woman and the newborn; a lack of a role model for breast-feeding; or the woman's viewpoint that her breasts are only sexual in nature. Level of education also has an impact on the newborn feeding choice; 73.8% of women with a college degree breast-feed, whereas 46.8% of women with less than a high school education breast-feed (Lawrence & Lawrence, 1999).

Past Experience

A woman's past experience with or exposure to breast-feeding has a great impact on her decision whether or not to breast-feed this newborn. If the woman has previously breast-fed an infant, that experience will affect her decision on how to feed this newborn. The feeding experiences of the woman's support systems also play an important part in assisting the woman in her feeding choice. Their past or current experiences, whether positive or negative, regarding either type of feeding, will influence the woman's current choice of feeding.

Intent to Return to Work or School

The need to return to work or school soon after the newborn's birth plays an important role in the woman's feeding choice. Women who have chosen to breast-feed in the hospital can continue to breast-feed and pump while at work or school or breast-feed when the infant is present and offer formula while she is away, or she can elect to stop breast-feeding. Some women prefer not to begin breast-feeding because of

TABLE 14.1	Daily Nutritional Needs of the Newborn					
Protein	Vitamin A	Vitamin C	Vitamin D	Vitamin E	Vitamin K	Calcium
2.2 g/kg	400 µg/day	40 mg/day	5 µg/day	4 mg/day	2.0 µg/day	210 mg/day

their work or school obligations and choose to feed formula from the newborn's birth.

BREAST-FEEDING

Breast-feeding is the recommended method for feeding newborns. The American Academy of Pediatrics (AAP) advocates exclusive breast-feeding until 6 months of age and continuation of breast-feeding until at least 12 months of age. The infant does not have to be weaned at 12 months; the benefits of breast-feeding for both the woman and the infant continue as long as the woman is nursing.

Breast milk is superior nutritionally to **artificial nutrition,** that is, infant formula. Breast-feeding is recommended and encouraged by organizations such as the AAP, World Health Organization (WHO), and the Association of Women's Health, Obstetric, and Neonatal Nurses (AWHONN). Each of these organizations has a policy statement that defines their position on breast-feeding and their recommendations for infant feeding.

Advantages and Disadvantages of Breast-feeding

Advantages

The advantages for the woman include more rapid uterine involution and less bleeding in the postpartum period, a quicker return to her prepregnancy weight level, and decreased incidence of ovarian and premenopausal breast cancers (Riordan & Auerbach, 1998).

The advantages for the newborn are numerous. Breast milk provides **immunologic** properties from the woman that help protect the newborn from infections and strengthen the newborn's immune system. Breast-feeding also provides a unique experience for maternal–newborn bonding. There is a decreased risk in overfeeding of the breast-fed newborn, which results in a lower incidence of overweight infants. Breast-fed infants tend to have lower incidences of otitis media, diarrhea, and lower respiratory tract infections. Breast-feeding also provides a possible protective effect against certain conditions or diseases, such as sudden infant death syndrome, insulin dependent diabetes, and allergic diseases. Finally, there is a possible correlation between enhanced cognitive development and breast-feeding (Riordan & Auerbach, 1998).

There also are several benefits that affect not only the woman and newborn, but also the community at large. Breast-feeding is more economic. The breast-feeding woman does not need to purchase formula, bottles, or nipples. Breast milk is always available, needs no preparation or storage, and no cleanup of utensils or dishes after the feeding is required. When away from home, the woman does not need to carry extra equipment or supplies to feed her newborn. Breast-feeding reduces health care costs because breast-fed infants are healthier and have less illness than do formula-fed infants (Riordan & Auerbach, 1998).

Disadvantages

There is no disadvantage to either the woman or the newborn during breast-feeding. What can be claimed as a disadvantage is actually a circumstance or condition in which breast-feeding is deemed inappropriate. However, there are certain maternal conditions or situations that would contraindicate breast-feeding. Examples of these conditions include:

- Illegal drug use
- Active untreated tuberculosis
- Human immunodeficiency virus (HIV) infection
- Chemotherapy treatment (See Appendix E.)
- Herpetic lesions on the breast

In addition, there are certain conditions the newborn may have that would contraindicate breast-feeding. Galactosemia, an inborn error of metabolism, requires a specialty formula for the newborn because breast milk is high in lactose. With phenylketonuria, another inborn error of metabolism, the newborn may require partial to complete feedings of a specialty infant formula. There are other medical conditions that may necessitate the newborn receiving formula. In some situations, the woman may produce little to no breast milk. In these situations, the infant's diet should be supplemented with or switched over completely to formula.

In addition to reasons that would contraindicate breast-feeding, there are also perceived disadvantages to breast-feeding. Some women feel that breast-feeding would exclude others from caring for or feeding the newborn. Some fathers express an interest in wanting to feed the newborn and feel that breast-feeding would take away this opportunity. In these circumstances the woman can pump her breast milk, and the father or other caregiver could feed the newborn. This way the newborn still receives the superior nutrition that only breast milk can provide and the father or other caregiver can have the feeding time with the newborn. This also gives the woman a respite from feeding the newborn.

There are other perceived disadvantages to breast-feeding. Some women feel that they will be unable to return to work or school if they breast-feed. Others feel that breast-feeding is too difficult or uncomfortable. Breast-feeding may be perceived as sexual in nature, or some women may feel it may detract from the woman's sexuality. Some women feel restrained by breast-feeding in that it ties them to the baby, or they think it will make the baby "too clingy."

Physiology of Breast-feeding

Newborn Features That Facilitate Breast-feeding

The newborn possesses several unique characteristics that make breast-feeding physiologically possible. These characteristics are found only in the newborn and infant and disappear as the infant gets older. Specifically, the newborn is born with a uniquely shaped nose and mouth, the rooting reflex, and the innate ability to suck.

Newborn Facial Anatomy. The newborn is designed uniquely for breast-feeding. The nose, which looks flattened after birth, is designed to create air pockets when up against the breast. This allows the newborn to breathe without obscuring the nasal opening. Newborns are nose breathers, which allows them to breathe while their mouth is full, without having to release the breast to take a breath. The newborn's mouth is designed to compress the milk ducts located behind the nipple under the areola. The tongue, pharynx, and lower jaw are unique in their shape when these structures are compared with those of the older child or adult. The newborn also has fat pads on each cheek that aid in the sucking process.

Rooting and Sucking Reflex. In addition to these unique anatomical findings, the newborn has a set of reflexes that assist in breast-feeding. The rooting reflex is seen when the newborn's cheek is brushed lightly and the newborn turns toward the stimulation. When the newborn feels the woman's breast touching his face, he turns toward the breast and opens his mouth. This is a feeding cue the woman can observe and know that her newborn is ready to nurse. When the newborn's lips are lightly touched, the newborn will respond by opening his mouth.

The sucking reflex is seen when the nipple is placed into the newborn's mouth and the newborn begins to suck. The term newborn has the ability to coordinate her sucking, swallowing, and breathing in a manner that facilitates nursing and prevents choking, while giving the infant breaks during nursing to rest. The newborn sucks in a burst pattern; sucking several times and then pausing. The length of the pause should be equal to the time the newborn sucks. The type of sucking also changes during the feeding. At the beginning of the feeding, the newborn nurses with rapid, short sucks. These sucks stimulate the breast to release the milk. When the milk is freely flowing, the newborn nurses with longer, slower sucks.

The Breast

The breast is a unique organ that is designed for the purpose of providing the newborn with nourishment. The anatomy of the breast, and the way it makes milk, are unique to the female. The breast makes milk in response to several different stimuli. These include the physical emptying of the breast, hormonal stimulation, and sensory stimulation that the woman's brain receives from her newborn.

Breast Anatomy. The breast is very vascular, with a rich lymphatic and nervous supply. The breast is made up of 15 to 20 lobes containing the milk-producing alveoli. The alveoli are clustered together and empty into ducts. The alveoli produce the milk. The alveoli are surrounded by smooth muscle cells, which help to eject the milk into the ducts. The ducts lead to the nipple, where the milk is released.

Physical Control of Lactation. When the breast is emptied, either by the newborn sucking or by use of a breast pump, the breast responds by replenishing the milk supply. If the breast is not emptied completely, it will not make as much milk the next time. This is why it is important for the newborn to nurse long enough to establish a good milk supply. If the woman is pumping, she should allow sufficient time for the pump to drain both breasts and not stop pumping until the flow of milk has stopped. If the newborn completely empties the breast and then nurses again shortly after the feeding, it will cause the breast to increase its milk supply.

Hormonal Control of Lactation. The breast also is under hormonal control. When the newborn sucks on the breast, the anterior pituitary gland releases prolactin, which causes milk production and milk release in the breast. The newborn's sucking also causes the pituitary to release oxytocin. Oxytocin causes contractions of the muscles in the uterus and also in the myoepithelial cells that surround the alveoli in the breast. Figure 14-1 shows how the hormones respond to the stimulation of the newborn sucking on the breast.

During the first few days, the more often the newborn nurses, the more lactogen receptor sites in

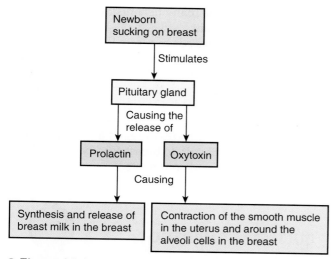

● *Figure 14.1* Diagram of the hormonal effect on lactation.

sessions. The breast starts to produce **colostrum,** a thick, and yellowish gold substance during the 2nd trimester. Colostrum is higher in antibodies than breast milk and has a lower fat and higher protein content than what is found in breast milk. There is between 2 and 20 mL of colostrum present for each feeding until the woman's milk comes in about the 3rd day.

the breast are activated to respond to lactogen, which will aid in the production of milk. If the breast is not stimulated, either by the newborn's sucking or by a breast pump, the number of sites is reduced, which can affect the quantity of the woman's milk supply. The nurse should encourage the woman to feed her newborn every 1½ to 3 hours until her milk supply is established. If she is unable to nurse her newborn, she should pump at least every 3 hours around the clock.

Sensory Stimulation. In addition to hormones and the physical emptying of the breast, the woman's body responds to the sensory information her brain picks up from her newborn. As the woman holds her newborn and the newborn touches her breast or grasps her finger with his hand, the woman's skin is stimulated. These tactile sensations are sent to her brain. As the woman sees her baby, these visual images are also sent to her brain. As the woman hears her baby cry or coo, her brain is also picking up these sounds and processing them. Finally, the olfactory sensations of the smell of a woman's baby are also sent to the woman's brain. These sensory sensations aid the woman's body in having a let-down reflex. This is why some women will report a let-down reflex when hearing another baby cry in public. The let-down reflex can be inhibited by maternal alcohol consumption, so the breast-feeding woman should avoid drinking alcoholic beverages.

Composition of Breast Milk

Breast milk is a unique substance that is unable to be duplicated because of the immunologic factors present. Breast milk is not produced until approximately 3 days after birth. Until this time, the newborn receives a substance called colostrum during the nursing

The woman's milk usually comes in between 3 and 5 days. Breast milk has 20 calories per ounce on the average. Breast milk has two different compositions: foremilk and hind milk. **Foremilk** is very watery and thin and may have a bluish tint. This is what the infant first receives during the nursing session. As the session progresses, the milk changes to hind milk. **Hind milk** is thicker and whiter. It contains a higher quantity of fat than foremilk and therefore has a higher caloric content than foremilk. The hind milk will satiate the infant longer between feedings. If the infant is thirsty and not very hungry, he or she will not nurse very long and will receive only the foremilk. The hungry infant nurses longer to get the hind milk.

It's OK to reassure the woman. Until her milk comes in, the woman may feel that her newborn is not getting enough to eat. Assure the woman that her newborn is getting enough calories and that the frequent nursing will aid in establishing an ample milk supply.

When the woman's milk comes in, she will notice her breasts feel fuller and heavier. A quality nursing bra will help her with supporting her breasts during this time. Many women experience leaking of breast milk or engorgement at this time (see "Teaching About Breast-feeding Special Concerns").

Nutritional Needs of the Breast-feeding Woman

The breast-feeding woman does not need to consume a large diet to produce milk for her infant. A well-balanced nutritious diet and drinking enough fluids to satisfy her thirst will provide her with the nutrition needed to lactate. A woman does not have to consume milk to make milk, but she does need fluids. If the woman does not consume enough fluids to satisfy her thirst or does not rest and eat a balanced diet, she may notice that she stops producing breast milk or that the quantity of her breast milk is diminished. A multivitamin will not make her breast milk more nutritious but will help ensure she obtains her daily required vitamins and minerals for her own body.

Nursing Care of the Breast-feeding Woman

The nurse has several roles when assisting a woman who is breast-feeding. These roles include assessing breast-feeding readiness, assisting with breast-feeding technique, assessing newborn fluid intake, and providing teaching about special breast-feeding topics.

Assessing Breast-feeding Readiness

Ideally, during the prenatal period the caregiver has introduced the question of whether or not the woman wants to breast-feed. At this time the woman should have been given information regarding the benefits of breast-feeding for both her and her newborn. In addition, the caregiver should have assessed the woman's breasts for any problems that might affect breast-feeding. If the woman has flat or inverted nipples, she still can breast-feed. A woman who has these types of nipples needs extra support in the beginning of breast-feeding, until she and the newborn become comfortable with nursing. A woman with flat or inverted nipples may need to use a breast pump for a few minutes before nursing the newborn to help pull out and harden the nipples so the newborn can make a good latch. She may also need to use a nipple shield to assist the newborn in latching on. The sooner women with problematic nipples are identified, the sooner the nurse can assist the woman with interventions and support from a **lactation consultant** (a nurse or layperson who has received special training to assist and support the breast-feeding woman). It is hoped this will minimize any discouragement and/or discomfort the woman may experience during the breast-feeding session and maximize the positive experience of the session.

Women who have had breast augmentation or reduction surgery can still breast-feed, as long as the surgeon left the milk ducts intact. Discuss with the woman who has had breast surgery what her surgeon told her regarding breast-feeding.

Some women are opposed to or repulsed by the thought of the newborn sucking on her breast. Women who are opposed to the newborn nursing on the breast may be willing to pump their breast milk and feed their newborn expressed breast milk from a bottle after

being informed of the many benefits of breast milk for the newborn and infant.

Lastly, the nurse needs to assess the woman's support systems. If the woman has family members or friends who have breast-fed before or are supportive of her decision to breast-feed, the woman is more likely to continue to breast-feed. On the other hand, if the woman's support systems are against breast-feeding, the woman may become discouraged and stop breast-feeding or not even begin to breast-feed because of the negative influences and comments.

CULTURAL SNAPSHOT

There are many culturally specific practices associated with breast-feeding. It is important to know the woman's cultural practices regarding modesty, breast-feeding in public or in front of others, the uses of a breast pump, or rituals for the purpose of bringing in good milk or a bountiful supply.

Assisting With Breast-feeding Technique

While assisting the woman, provide support and encouragement; many breast-feeding women are unsure of their ability to nurse their newborn. If the newborn will not nurse after you have provided assistance, contact the registered nurse in charge and take steps to contact the hospital lactation consultant for additional help.

Beginning the Breast-feeding Session. The first breast-feeding ideally should be in the delivery room within an hour after birth, unless the newborn's or woman's condition prevents this. Thereafter, the newborn should be nursed on demand at least every 1½ to 3 hours. If the newborn does not wake up by 3 hours, the woman should wake the newborn and encourage him or her to feed. Supplemental bottles

Here are some breast-feeding hints. Some women may become discouraged if their newborn is sleepy, will not latch immediately, or is crying vigorously and will not latch. Reassure the woman that the newborn will nurse. Take steps to rouse a sleepy newborn: changing the diaper, gentle rubbing of the back or head, and washing the newborn's face with a wet washcloth. If the newborn is crying and not exhibiting signs of hunger, check for other causes of crying, such as a wet or dirty diaper or constricting clothing. Try to calm the newborn before attempting to put the newborn to the breast.

of sterilized water or glucose solutions are discouraged because these will give the new-born a feeling of fullness and space out the feedings longer, which may in turn decrease the woman's milk supply.

CULTURAL SNAPSHOT

Some cultures place a high importance on privacy and/or modesty. The breast-feeding woman may not want to expose herself completely to breast-feed or may not want to breast-feed in the presence of the nurse. Some women may be uncomfortable breast-feeding in front of a male nurse.

When the nurse brings the newborn to the woman in the hospital for feedings, the first step is to check the newborn's and the woman's identification (ID) bands and make sure they match. After identity is confirmed, the nurse should provide the woman privacy by pulling a curtain around the bed or closing the door. Then assist the woman into a comfortable position. The woman should sit up in bed or a chair or lie on her side in bed. Use pillows as needed to support the woman's back and arms. Make sure there is nothing constricting or obstructing the breast, such as a too-tight bra or a cumbersome hospital gown that is in the woman's line of sight or falling between her and the newborn.

Positioning the Newborn. There are three basic positions for a woman to hold her newborn in while nursing. These are the cradle hold, football hold, and side-lying position (Fig. 14-2). Women who have breast-fed before may already know these three basic holds. However, a woman who has not breast-fed before or who has just had surgery needs more help with positioning her baby correctly. Correct positioning and latching on of the newborn will avoid nipple tissue trauma and sore nipples.

Cradle Hold. In the cradle hold, the newborn's abdomen is facing and touching the woman's abdomen. Make sure the newborn is not being held on his back and turning his head over his shoulder to reach the breast. In this position, the newborn's lower arm should be tucked between the woman's arm and breast and not between the newborn and the breast. The woman supports the breast being offered to the newborn with her free hand (see Fig. 14-2*A*).

Football Hold. In the football hold, the newborn is held with her head under the woman's breast. The newborn's head is supported under the woman's breast by the palm of the woman's hand while a pillow underneath the newborn supports her body. The woman's arm rests along the side of the newborn's body resting on the pillow. This is a good position for

A PERSONAL GLIMPSE

Todd is my second baby. My husband and I hadn't been planning for another child when I found out that I was pregnant. The pregnancy was completely normal with a few more aches and pains than I remembered with my first child, Richard. Right after the delivery I felt completely exhausted and ravenous. The nurse was insisting that I breast-feed and kept giving me a lot of information. I just couldn't deal with it. It seems like such a blur. I feel guilty that I didn't listen more. They whisked the baby away an hour after he was born. I was kind of relieved because I was so tired. But then when they brought him back to my room the nurse said, "They told me that you breast-fed in the delivery room. And since this is your second child, I'm sure you remember how to do it. He should feed for 5 to 10 minutes on each breast." I just looked at her. She handed me the baby and told me to call if I needed anything. Todd was fussy. I kept trying to get him to latch on but couldn't seem to figure out how to do it. I was sitting up in bed and having trouble getting comfortable. My stitches were hurting. But I didn't want to ask the nurse for help because I was afraid she would think I was dumb for not remembering how to get started with breast-feeding. The truth is I was very sick with my first child, so I only breast-fed for a couple of weeks, and it seemed so long ago. I finally gave up and called the nursery for a bottle. Todd immediately gulped down an ounce and a half. After that he didn't seem interested in breast-feeding. Now that he is a year old, I sometimes wish I had tried a little harder to breast-feed. I feel that somehow I missed out on a very special experience.

Rowena

LEARNING OPPORTUNITY: What assumptions did the nurse make that discouraged the mother from asking for help? How could the nurse have approached this situation to give the new mother the help that she needed?

women who have undergone surgery or women with large breasts. It also facilitates the newborn and woman being able to see each other with an unobstructed view (see Fig. 14-2*B*).

Side-Lying Position. The side-lying position is with both the woman and the newborn on their sides facing each other while lying in bed. This position facilitates maternal rest and is good for a woman who has undergone surgery. The newborn should be supported with a blanket roll behind his back so he does not roll backward during the feeding. As with the cradle hold, the woman's and newborn's abdomens should be touching and the newborn should not be resting

A

B

C

● *Figure 14.2* (**A**). The nurse is teaching the woman to use the cradle hold to breast-feed her newborn (photo © B. Proud). (**B**). The nurse is teaching the woman to use the football hold to breast-feed her newborn. Note how the woman's arm supports the newborn's body while the newborn's head rests in the palm of the woman's hand. (**C**). In the side-lying position, the woman can rest while feeding her newborn.

on his back during the nursing session or stretching his head over his shoulder to reach the breast (see Fig. 14-2*C*).

Latching On. After correct positioning, the next step is for the newborn to latch onto the breast. The newborn's mouth needs to be wide open with the tongue down at the floor of the mouth. When the newborn latches onto the breast he or she must take the entire nipple and part of the areola into the mouth. If the newborn takes only the nipple, the milk ducts will not be compressed sufficiently to empty the breast. It will also cause the woman's nipple to become sore and/or cracked and bleeding.

Have the woman make a "c" shape with her free hand and grasp the breast. Make sure that the woman's hand that is supporting the breast being offered does not bump into the newborn's jaw or prevent the jaw from making a good latch. The woman may need to reposition her hand so that it is closer to the chest wall and further from the newborn's jaw. Figure 14-3*A* shows the newborn positioned correctly on the breast, and Figure 14-3*B* shows how the newborn's mouth compresses the milk ducts.

When the newborn is latched onto the breast, make sure the woman does not dimple the breast near the newborn's mouth and nose. Many women will do this thinking they are providing breathing space for the newborn. This action can cause the nipple to be pulled out of the mouth completely, or it can cause the nipple to be pulled to the front of the mouth. If the nipple is toward the front of the newborn's mouth, the newborn's gums will compress it and cause sore nipples. This action can put pressure on the milk ducts, thereby reducing the flow of milk to the newborn, and also can prevent the breast from emptying completely.

Assessing the Breast-feeding Session. After the newborn has latched on and is nursing, the nurse needs to evaluate the effectiveness of the latch and sucking. A newborn who is correctly latched onto the breast will resist being pulled off of the breast. Audible swallowing, rhythmic jaw gliding, and seeing the areola dimple slightly near the newborn's mouth with sucking are positive signs that the newborn is latched on properly and sucking effectively.

In the postpartum period after the newborn has been nursing for a few minutes, many women report an increase in the flow of lochia or uterine cramping. This is a good indication that the newborn is nursing well. With effective sucking at the breast, the hormone

● *Figure 14.3* (**A**). Newborn with all of nipple and areola in mouth. (**B**). Diagram of newborn on breast correctly compressing milk ducts.

oxytocin is released, which causes uterine contractions. After her milk has come in, the woman may report leaking from the opposite breast or a let-down reflex. This is another good indication that the newborn is latched on and sucking well at the breast.

Ending the Breast-feeding Session. The nursing session should last approximately 10 to 20 minutes per breast. When the newborn is finished, the woman should remove the newborn from the breast. To do so, she should place her finger in the newborn's mouth, between the gums and cheek, to break the suction, and then gently pull the newborn away from the breast. It is important for her to break the suction first if the newborn is still latched on, or it might cause tissue damage to the breast.

After the feeding session, the woman may wish to burp her newborn. Because the newborn swallows less air during a breast-feeding session than in a bottle-feeding one, the newborn may not always burp. Three ways the woman may hold the newborn to burp is over the shoulder, sitting upright, or lying across her lap with the newborn's head elevated slightly above the level of its stomach.

After nursing, the woman should leave the flaps of her nursing bra open to allow her nipples to air dry. Some women express a few drops of colostrum or breast milk onto their nipples before letting them air dry to help with soreness or cracking of the nipples. If the woman has sore nipples, she can apply a purified lanolin ointment (Lansinoh) to her nipples after the nursing session.

Assessing Newborn Fluid Intake

The nurse should assess the newborn's fluid intake. A small bit of milk left in the mouth after the feeding is a good indication the newborn is sucking well. The newborn should be satiated between feedings and after nursing appear to be drowsy or asleep. By the end of the 3rd day of life, the newborn should have at least six very wet diapers and about three bowel movements per day. Newborns who are breast-fed exclusively will have a yellow or mustard colored seedy type of bowel movement that is very loose and not formed. The nurse should explain to the woman that this is normal for the breast-fed newborn. Many breast-fed newborns will have a bowel movement during the nursing session.

The newborn's weight should be monitored daily. The breast-feeding newborn should lose no more than 10% of his birth weight and should return to birth weight by 7 to 14 days of age. The nurse should evaluate the newborn's weight with regards to his feeding status and notify the registered nurse and the primary care provider if problems exist.

Teaching About Breast-feeding Special Concerns

The nurse has a very large role in teaching the breast-feeding woman. Items to be covered include tips on relieving common maternal breast-feeding problems; signs that the newborn is not feeding well; normal increases in the newborn's feeding schedule to accommodate for growth spurts; available resources for the breast-feeding woman; using supplements; breast-feeding amenorrhea; contraception while breast-feeding; and pumping and storing breast milk.

Relieving Common Maternal Breast-feeding Problems. The breast-feeding woman needs information regarding problems she may encounter at home. Some of the most commonly reported problems include sore nipples, engorgement, a plugged milk duct, or mastitis.

Sore Nipples. The newborn latching onto the breast incorrectly generally causes sore nipples. If the woman reports sore nipples or cracked and bleeding nipples, observe how the newborn latches on. The newborn's mouth must open wide, and she must take all of the nipple and part of the areola into the mouth. Other reasons for sore nipples are that the newborn may be a vigorous breast-feeder or the woman may have sensitive or tender skin.

Some women find rubbing a few drops of expressed breast milk onto their nipples after the nursing session helpful. A purified lanolin ointment (Lansinoh) may help other women. Contact the lactation consultant if the woman continues to have sore nipples and the newborn is latched on and positioned correctly.

Engorgement. **Engorgement** occurs when the milk comes in and the woman's body responds with increasing the blood supply to the breast tissues. The woman may have pain in her breasts because of swelling. Cold packs to the breast or warm showers; pumping a small amount of milk; and taking acetaminophen (Tylenol) will help alleviate the discomfort. Reassure the woman that this is temporary and will go away within a few days. Tell the woman not to completely empty her breasts between feedings, as this will increase her milk supply beyond the newborn's needs.

This is helpful advice. Many women with engorgement experience milk leaking from the breasts. Breast pads in the bra will help to absorb the leaking milk. Encourage the woman to change the bra pads as they become damp to avoid maceration or possible infection of the nipple and/or areola.

Plugged Milk Ducts. A common problem encountered during the nursing period is a plugged duct. This happens when one of the milk ducts becomes obstructed, causing a backup of the milk. The woman usually notices a sore, reddened, hard lump in one area of her breast. The woman should be taught to continue nursing; take acetaminophen (Tylenol); apply warm compresses and massage the site; nurse in different positions, including on her hands and knees to facilitate drainage of the breast; and to avoid constricting clothing or bras, including underwire bras. If the site does not improve within a few days, she should contact her health care provider.

Mastitis. Another common problem associated with breast-feeding is **mastitis.** Mastitis is an infection of the breast tissue. Women with mastitis usually describe having a run-down feeling or flu-like symptoms and a low-grade fever. Tell the woman not to ignore these signs and symptoms but to immediately report to her health care provider that she feels these symptoms and is breast-feeding. Treatment consists of antibiotics, analgesics, bed rest, and fluids. The woman needs to know that she can continue to breast-feed during this time. Mastitis will not affect her milk quality, and the antibiotics prescribed usually do not affect the newborn or infant. If the health care provider does prescribe medication that is contraindicated for breast-feeding and there is no alternative medication, the woman can pump and dump her breast milk and resume breast-feeding when the medication course is completed.

Signs the Newborn Is Not Feeding Well. The woman also needs to be taught to evaluate how well her newborn is nursing and when to call for help. Dry mouth, not enough wet diapers per day, difficulty rousing the newborn for a feeding, not enough feedings per day, or difficulty with latching on or sucking are signs that the newborn is not receiving enough breast milk. Explain to the woman that if she notices any of these signs, she should immediately contact the newborn's health care provider and a lactation consultant. Newborns can become dehydrated and suffer from a lack of nutrition very quickly and may need to be hospitalized.

Growth Spurts. Another important teaching topic for the breast-feeding woman is information on how the newborn increases the milk supply. Newborns have growth spurts in which they will nurse longer and more frequently for a few days and then space out their feedings after those few days. This causes the woman's breasts to increase their milk volume to match the growing newborn's needs. A woman who does not understand that the newborn increases the frequency and duration of feedings over a period of days to increase the milk supply may misinterpret this as she does not have enough milk to feed her newborn. This may cause the woman to stop breast-feeding.

Available Resources for the Breast-feeding Woman. The breast-feeding woman needs to be made aware of the many resources available to assist her and her newborn with breast-feeding. Lactation consultants, the La Leche League, and breast-feeding support groups in the community can give both practical and emotional support to the breast-feeding woman.

Lactation consultants are found in the hospital, in the community, and sometimes in the primary care provider's office. In the hospital, lactation consultants can help the woman with positioning and getting the newborn latched on and sucking. After discharge, the hospital may provide follow-up visits or telephone calls to the woman to help ensure that the newborn is breast-feeding as expected. The newborn's pediatrician may have an agreement with a lactation consultant who can provide assistance to the breast-feeding woman.

The La Leche League is a national organization that provides support, education, and literature to the breast-feeding woman. The woman can find the League listed in the telephone book, or the hospital may provide the woman with the telephone number of the local chapter. In addition, the hospital may have a list of breast-feeding support groups the woman can join; these groups can provide both breast-feeding support and socialization.

Using Supplements. Many women have questions about supplements for their nursing newborn. The newborn who is being breast-fed does not need supplemental bottles of water. The foremilk is watery, and the newborn will nurse only a little if thirsty. This will provide the newborn with all fluid needs. In the hospital, newborns are not started on any vitamin or iron supplements. The follow-up health care provider will instruct the woman on when and what types, if any, of supplements the newborn may need.

The woman should be informed that her breast milk is nutritionally superior to any other newborn food and that the newborn should not be started on any solids, including rice cereal, until at least 6 months of age. If there is a family history of allergies, solids should be delayed even longer. Breast milk will exclusively provide the newborn with all of her nutritional needs for the first 12 months.

Breast-feeding Amenorrhea. A very important topic of which the breast-feeding woman should be aware is breast-feeding amenorrhea. The return of the woman's menstrual cycle occurs between 6 to 10 weeks after delivery. The first postpartum menstrual cycle is anovulatory in 75% of women. The woman who is breast-feeding exclusively (i.e., without providing any supplemental bottles or solids) may experience breast-feeding **amenorrhea.** Some women who exclusively breast-feed may not have a return of their menstrual cycle for several months. The woman needs to know that ovulation can happen in the absence of a menstrual period, and she can become pregnant. It is important for her to use contraception during this time.

Contraception While Breast-feeding. The breast-feeding woman needs information about her choices in contraception. Contraception that contains hormones, especially estrogen, can lead to a decrease in the milk supply in the breast-feeding woman. The woman should be informed of this and make alternative contraceptive choices if breast-feeding is to continue. The first choice of contraception for the breast-feeding woman should be nonhormonal. If she chooses a hormonal type of contraception, a nonestrogen type, such as the mini-pill, should be offered before one that contains estrogen. Table 14-2 summarizes different contraceptive choices for the breast-feeding woman.

Pumping and Storing Breast Milk. The breast-feeding woman should be taught about pumping and storing her expressed breast milk. The woman who will be returning to work or school after giving birth can still breast-feed exclusively. The woman should breast-feed exclusively for at least 6 weeks before introducing the bottle. After 6 weeks, she should introduce one feeding per day of expressed breast milk. She also should pump her breasts during this bottle-feeding so her milk supply is not reduced. The bottle should be introduced only after she has

TABLE 14.2	Contraceptive Choices for the Breast-feeding Woman			
Nonhormonal		**Hormonal**		
Permanent	Temporary	Nonestrogen	Estrogen	
Tubal ligation Vasectomy	Abstinence Condom Diaphragm Spermicide	Mini-pill Depo-Provera	Birth control pill	

established a good milk supply and the newborn is nursing well.

Pumping. The woman should wash her hands before pumping her breasts and should use clean equipment. It is recommended the woman use a hospital-grade, dual electric breast pump, which pumps both breasts at the same time (Fig. 14-4). It may be necessary for the woman to use techniques to aid the let-down reflex. Bilaterally massaging the breasts and applying warm packs aids in the let-down of the milk. The woman may also find that looking at a picture of her infant and mentally thinking about her infant's smell, texture, and sounds aids in having a let-down reflex. At home, the woman may want to pump one breast while having the infant nurse on the opposite breast because this will aid her in having a let-down reflex and allow her to collect more breast milk.

Pumping of both breasts at the same time has been shown to increase the quantity of milk expressed at one sitting. The woman should be encouraged to pump until the flow of milk has stopped, usually about 15 to 20 minutes. When she is done pumping, she can refrigerate, freeze, or feed her infant the expressed

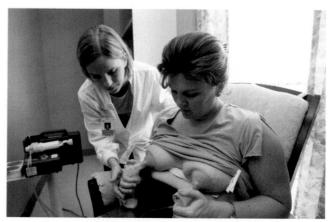

● *Figure 14.4* The nurse is assisting the woman to use a hospital pump to pump milk from both breasts at the same time.

breast milk immediately. She also needs to clean her equipment right after pumping. Tap water and a small amount of dish soap are usually sufficient to clean the equipment.

After pumping, she may want to rub a small amount of breast milk onto her nipples and allow them to air dry before covering them with a bra. If the woman experiences soreness with the breast pump, check to make sure she is using it properly and starting the pumping session at the lowest suction necessary.

Storing Breast Milk. Breast milk should be stored in hard plastic bottles or breast milk bags but not in glass containers. There are bags made especially for breast milk storage, and these should be used and not plastic bottle liners. The leukocytes in breast milk adhere to the glass, and this decreases the bacteriostatic properties of the milk. Breast milk should be reheated by placing the bottle/bag into a pan of hot water. It should not be heated in the microwave because this kills the antibodies in breast milk. In addition, milk reheated in the microwave may have hot spots that could burn the newborn's mouth and esophagus. See Table 14-3 provides a timetable for breast milk storage.

Test Yourself

- In what three positions can a woman hold her newborn to breast-feed?

- How can the nurse assess the effectiveness of the newborn's breast-feeding?

- What common problems might a breast-feeding woman encounter?

TABLE 14.3	Breast Milk Storage	
Location of Storage	**Duration of Storage**
Room temperature (19°C–22°C)	Up to 10 hours
Refrigerator (0°C–4°C)	Up to 8 days
Freezer with door opening frequently	2 weeks
Separate freezer compartment with door opening frequently	4 months
Separate deep freeze	6 months
Thawed after being frozen	24 hours

FORMULA FEEDING

Artificial nutrition, that is infant formula or another type of animal milk, has been given to infants since ancient times. In the United States, commercially prepared infant formula has been around since the early 1900s. Today there are several brands available to women who choose not to breast-feed or who need a supplemental formula. There are differences in the composition of formulas available in the hospital. There are also alternative formulas to meet specific infant needs.

Advantages and Disadvantages of Formula Feeding

Infant formulas are helpful in certain circumstances. Many women choose to forgo breast-feeding and feed their infant only formula. The woman who chooses to do so should not be made to feel guilty regarding her decision. However, the nurse should make sure that the woman has made an informed decision and has heard the advantages of breast-feeding before feeding her infant formula.

Advantages

There are specific circumstances in which formula feeding is necessary. These include infants who are adopted or cases in which breast-feeding would be harmful to the infant. In some cases the woman may need to temporarily stop breast-feeding, such as for surgery or while taking a medication that can pass to the infant through the breast milk. For many women, it is easier to quantify how much the infant has consumed with formula feeding than with breast-feeding, which reduces their worries about the infant getting enough to eat. Some women feel it is easier to formula feed than to breast-feed their infant. Formula feeding also allows others to be involved in the infant's care by feeding the infant and preparing the formula and bottles for feeding.

There are certain maternal circumstances in which breast-feeding is discouraged and the newborn should be fed formula. These include maternal illicit drug use, the woman who is receiving chemotherapy, the woman who has HIV or one who has herpetic lesions on her breast.

If the newborn has an inborn error of metabolism, such as phenylketonuria, maple sugar urine disease, or galactosemia, the newborn needs a specific formula that the newborn can digest to avoid or minimize the problems associated with such diseases.

There are women who are opposed to or repulsed by the thought of breast-feeding. For these women, formula feeding gives them an alternative to nursing their newborn. For some women, the breast milk supply dries up sooner than expected. These women may need to formula feed until their newborn is old enough to wean. Some women do not make enough milk to supply the newborn's needs. These women may need to offer supplemental formula.

Disadvantages

Formula feeding has several disadvantages. It is inferior nutrition and has none of the immunologic properties provided by breast milk. Formula is harder for the newborn to digest than breast milk. There is a higher correlation between infants who are formula fed and some illnesses, such as otitis media and allergies.

Make sure the woman is informed! If the woman is on the Women, Infants, and Children's (WIC) program, the woman will need to purchase 25% of the formula because WIC is only a supplemental program.

Infant formula also is expensive. If the family is on a limited budget, formula feeding will create additional financial needs. In addition to buying the formula, the family will need to purchase bottles, nipples, and the equipment needed to clean these items.

There are more steps involved in formula feeding the newborn than in breast-feeding. With formula feeding, the woman or caregiver must mix the right amount of powder or formula concentrate to water; store the mixed preparation; warm it when the newborn is ready to eat; and then wash all of the utensils afterward. Formula can be purchased in three forms: ready to feed, concentrate, and powder. Because of the differences in formulation, there can be errors with the proper dilution of the formula. Errors in preparation can lead to under- and overnutrition in the newborn. These errors can result in serious illness and even death.

Composition of Formula

There are three main types of formula: milk-based, soy-based, and hypoallergenic formulas. Most term newborn formulas are derived from cow's milk and the main carbohydrate source is lactose or corn syrup solids. The protein used is a whey-casein blend to simulate what is found in breast milk. The iron composition in infant formula is defined as either high or low. Iron-fortified formulas contain 1.2 mg of iron per 100 mL. Iron-fortified, or high-iron formula, is the preferred formula to give to the healthy term newborn. Some women are reluctant to feed their newborn iron-fortified formula, thinking it will cause constipation. Studies have shown that there is no significant difference in

Warn the woman that the newborn may be injured if formula is not properly mixed. Some women may be unable to afford formula and try to make the formula last longer by adding more water than the directions specify. This will cause malnutrition in the newborn. If too much powder is added to the water, the newborn will receive more calories per ounce. This can lead to an overweight infant or formula intolerance, with resulting diarrhea or emesis.

constipation rates between infants fed iron-fortified and low-iron formulas.

Alternative formulas are available for newborns with special medical needs. Soy-based infant formulas are for newborns who are allergic to cow's milk or when there is a strong family history of cow's milk allergies. Hypoallergenic formulas are for newborns with allergy or malabsorption problems. These formulas have the proteins partially or completely broken down in them. There are also a variety of formulas specially designed for specific medical conditions the newborn may have, including carbohydrate intolerance, impaired fat absorption, cystic fibrosis, congestive heart failure, and intestinal resection or short gut problems. These formulas should be given to the newborn only under a primary care provider's order. Some pediatricians will treat esophageal reflux with a formula thickened with some rice cereal or a specialized formula that already has rice cereal added to it.

There are many different compositions of formulas in the hospital. Formulas vary based on the needs of the newborn. Preterm formulas differ from term formulas in the amounts of vitamins and minerals and caloric and iron content. Preterm formulas have higher levels of sodium, potassium, calcium, and iron than do term infant formulas. Term formula, like breast milk, has 20 calories per ounce, whereas preterm formulas have 22 or 24 calories per ounce. See Table 14-4 for a comparison of different brands of formulas.

Nursing Care of the Formula Feeding Woman

The nurse in the hospital has three major roles when assisting the bottle-feeding woman. These are assisting with formula-feeding technique, assessing the formula-feeding woman and newborn, and teaching about special concerns of formula feeding.

Assisting With Formula-Feeding Technique

In the hospital, standard infant formula comes ready to feed. This means that the nurse does not need to mix or add any additives to the formula before feeding the newborn. The first step in feeding the formula-fed newborn

TABLE 14.4	Comparison of Common Formulas	
Category	Formulas (Manufacturer's Name)	Newborn Population/Medical Condition for which Formula Designed
Milk-based formulas	Enfamil (Mead-Johnson), Good Start (Nestle), Similac (Ross)	For full-term healthy newborns
Soy-based formulas	Isomil (Ross), ProSobee (Mead Johnson), Soyalac (Loma Linda)	Milk protein allergy, lactose intolerance, lactase deficiency, or galactosemia
	Lactofree (Mead Johnson)	Lactose intolerance, lactase deficiency
Specific medical conditions	RCF (Ross Carbohydrate Free) (Ross)	Carbohydrate intolerance
	Portagen (Mead Johnson)	Impaired fat absorption, intestinal resection, lymphatic anomalies
	Nutramigen (Mead Johnson)	Protein sensitivity, galactosemia, malabsorption problems
	Pregestimil (Mead Johnson)	Malabsorption syndromes, cystic fibrosis, intestinal resection, short gut syndrome
	Alimentum (Ross)	Food protein sensitivity, cystic fibrosis
	Lonalac (Mead Johnson)	Congestive heart failure, reduced sodium intake
	Similac PM 60/40 (Ross)	Infants predisposed to hypocalcemia and infants with impaired renal, digestive, and cardiovascular functions
	Lofenalac (Mead Johnson), Phenyl-free (Mead Johnson), Phenex-1 (Ross), Phenex-2 (Ross), Pro-Phree (Ross)	Phenylketonuria
	Similac Special Care (Ross), Premature Enfamil (Mead Johnson), Neosure (Ross)	Premature infants

Note: This is not an exhaustive list of all of the types of formulas available or conditions for which formulas may be used.

is to check the primary care provider's order. Many primary care providers have a preference regarding which formula the woman should feed her newborn. Check the label on the formula bottle before taking it to the woman to feed her newborn. Make sure the brand, caloric content, and iron composition matches that of the primary care provider's order.

Compare the newborn's and woman's ID bands to ensure a match. Use pillows as needed to ensure the woman is in a comfortable position and can hold and see her newborn easily. Make sure the woman is in a comfortable position sitting upright. The formula-feeding woman should not feed her newborn in a lying down position. The newborn should be in a semireclined position in the woman's arms. An angle of at least 45 degrees is preferred (Fig. 14-5).

Teach the woman to assess her newborn's hunger cues and her newborn's ability to suck, swallow, and breathe during the feeding. The woman should also observe her newborn's color while eating. Instruct the woman on what to do if the newborn starts to choke during the feeding. Make sure the nasal aspirator and a burp cloth are within the woman's reach.

Gently shake the bottle of formula because some settling of contents may occur. Attach a sterile nipple and ring unit to the

This tip could save a life! It is easier for the newborn to aspirate while sucking from a bottle. Instruct the woman to keep the light on in the room so that she can observe her newborn during the whole feeding.

Teach the woman not to prop! Sometimes the woman will prop the bottle against a surface so that she does not have to hold the bottle while the newborn sucks. This practice increases the newborn's risk of aspiration and can lead to overfeeding and baby bottle syndrome. Propping the bottle also decreases opportunities for positive bonding with the baby.

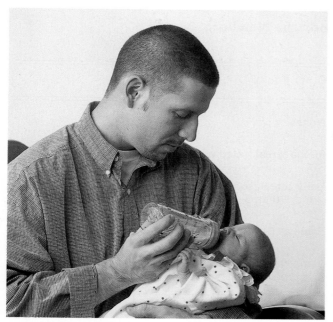

● *Figure 14.5* A newborn receives a formula feeding from her father. Notice the correct positioning.

bottle. The woman should feed 1 to 2 ounces at a feeding in the immediate newborn period. She should burp her newborn after every ½ ounce is consumed. As the newborn grows, she should advance the feeding amount slowly, no more than ½ to 1 ounce per feeding. Instruct the woman regarding cues that the newborn is satiated and finished eating. If the newborn consumes too much formula at one time, emesis or diarrhea may result.

The nurse can assist the bottle-feeding woman by feeding the newborn if the woman is unable to (e.g., she is having surgery) or if she is sleeping and requests her newborn to be fed in the nursery during the night.

Assessing the Formula-Feeding Woman and Newborn

The nurse should assess the newborn's feeding ability, amount of formula consumed at each feeding, tolerance of the infant formula, and the woman's comfort level with formula feeding her newborn. Any signs that the newborn is not sucking well, has difficulty swallowing and breathing, or is not tolerating the formula should be reported to the nurse in charge immediately. Signs the newborn is not tolerating the formula include emesis and diarrhea. These assessments should be reported to the nurse in charge. Also assess the newborn's bowel movements. Explain to the woman that her newborn's stool should progress from meconium to transitional and then to a pasty yellow solid consistency (see Chapter 15).

Teaching About Formula Feeding
Special Concerns

The nurse has a large role in teaching the formula-feeding woman. Teaching topics include how to prepare bottles of formula, adding supplements to the bottle, maternal breast care, and managing common problems in the formula-fed newborn.

Preparing Bottles of Formula. Teach the woman about the different forms of formula and how to mix each type. Powder formula is the least expensive and requires the addition of water. Concentrate also requires the addition of water but is more costly than the powder form. Ready-to-feed formula is the most expensive but does not require the addition of any water to the formula before feeding. Explain the importance of preparing the formula according to the package directions because malnutrition or dehydration can result from adding too much or too little water to the formula.

The woman will need to know what type of water to add to the powder or concentrate type of formula. This depends on what type of water she has available (e.g., city tap, well, or purified bottled water). She should be taught to mix only as much formula as the newborn needs in 24 hours. After mixing, the formula needs to be refrigerated. After 24 hours, unused formula should be discarded.

Teach the woman how to warm cold formula. The bottle containing the formula should be placed in a pan of hot water until the formula is warm. The bottle should be shaken before feeding the newborn. The microwave should never be used to warm the formula because it can create hot spots that could burn the newborn. When the newborn has finished eating, any remaining formula should be discarded. This is because as the newborn sucks, saliva mixes with the formula and remains in the bottle, and then digestive enzymes in the saliva begin to break down the remaining formula.

Teach the woman to wash the feeding utensils in hot soapy water or in the dishwasher after every feeding. Sterilizing the bottles and nipples is not necessary after each feeding.

Adding Supplements. The newborn's primary care provider will determine if and when the newborn needs any type of supplementation, such as multivitamins or fluoride. Teach the woman that the newborn does not need any other type of nutrition.

Contradict a wives' tale! Some women add rice cereal to the formula because they have heard that doing so will make the newborn sleep longer. This should not be done unless recommended by a primary care provider for a specific reason, such as reflux.

TABLE 14.5	Amount of Formula and Other Foods the Newborn and Infant Should Be Receiving	
Age	Amount of Formula	Other Foods
Birth to 4 months	2–6 ounces per feeding 20–24 ounces per day	None
4–6 months	4–6 ounces per feeding 24–32 ounces per day	Infant cereal mixed with formula
6–8 months	6–8 ounces per feeding 24–32 ounces per day	Baby cereal, soft mashed fruits and vegetables, no more than 3–4 ounces of fruit juice
8–10 months	7–8 ounces per feeding 21–32 ounces per day	Same as 6–8 months and begin to add pureed meats
10–12 months	16–32 ounces per day	Same as 8–10 months but consistency may be firmer and portions may be slightly bigger

Instruct her not to add anything to the formula. Some pediatricians tell parents to offer infant cereal mixed with formula, but not juice, around 4 to 6 months. The woman should not begin to feed solid foods until the infant's primary care provider has recommended it, usually around 6 to 8 months of age. Around 12 months of age, the infant's primary care provider will discuss weaning the infant from the formula.

Maternal Breast Care. Women who choose to formula feed exclusively need to know how to care for their breasts in the immediate postpartum period. Explain to the woman that she will produce milk, even though she is not nursing, and that this is a normal physiologic process in response to giving birth. The woman will experience engorgement when her milk comes in. She should be taught not to express any milk because this will continue the milk production process. She should wear a tight bra; the constriction will help prevent leaking and aid in the drying up of the milk supply. In addition, a tight bra will help lessen discomfort from the full breasts. Some women benefit from having their breasts bound tightly with an elastic-type bandage. In the past, some primary care providers prescribed medications that would aid in the drying up of the woman's milk supply. However, it was determined that the benefit of their use did not outweigh the associated risks.

Common Problems in the Formula-Fed Newborn. The woman needs to be taught to monitor for problems in the formula-fed newborn. These include the newborn not wanting to eat, not tolerating the formula, and dental caries.

The woman who is formula feeding is able to accurately determine how many ounces per feeding and per day the newborn is receiving. Table 14-5 lists the amount of formula and other foods the newborn and infant should be receiving at different ages. If the newborn or infant is not taking in enough formula for his age and weight, dehydration may result, and the infant may not gain sufficient weight to develop appropriately and be healthy. If a newborn or infant is refusing to eat, the woman should contact the pediatrician because there may be an underlying medical condition.

Some newborns take in the recommended amount of formula and then have large amounts of emesis after or during feedings. This also needs to be brought to the attention of the newborn's primary care provider because this is not an acceptable situation for growth and nutrition. This may be a symptom of overfeeding, gastroesophageal reflux, formula intolerance, or an underlying medical condition. The nurse should ask the woman the following questions: How much formula is the newborn taking per feeding and per day? When does emesis occur (during or after the feeding, with burps, or with repositioning)? How much emesis does the newborn have per episode? What is the consistency of the emesis? Which formula is being fed, and how is it prepared? What other foods are being fed? The answers to these questions will assist the nurse and the primary care provider to determine the probable cause of the emesis.

If the newborn has diarrhea, this also needs to be investigated. Again, the nurse needs to ask specific questions: How much and what type of formula is the newborn being fed, and how is it prepared? How many episodes of diarrhea has the newborn had in the past 24 hours? What is the consistency of the bowel movement, and is there blood present in the stool? It is important to assess the newborn's intake and output to check for dehydration, as well as to physically examine the child. Possible causes are overfeeding, illness, formula intolerance, or an underlying medical condition.

Inform the parents that newborns and infants can become dehydrated much more quickly than adults can, and that any cases of emesis or diarrhea should be quickly reported to the nurse in the hospital or the primary care provider if the newborn or infant is at home.

Infants can develop dental caries from frequent sucking on a bottle that is filled with milk or juice. This situation has been referred to as "baby bottle syndrome" or "bottle-mouth caries." Often this happens when parents give the infant a bottle at bedtime and the infant sucks on the bottle throughout the night. The frequent exposure of the immature teeth to high levels of sugars found in the milk or juice leads to dental caries. The parents should be informed not to give the infant a bottle when he or she is in the crib. They also should not allow the toddler to carry a bottle around; this practice of continual drinking of formula increases the risk of damage to the infant's teeth and is associated with a higher incidence of aspiration and otitis media.

Test Yourself

- What different types of formula are there?
- When is formula feeding an advantage?
- What topics should the nurse cover when teaching a woman to formula feed?

KEY POINTS

- The woman's decision to breast-feed is influenced by several factors. Some of these factors include culture, age, education, past experience with breast-feeding, and the woman's intent to return to work or school.
- Maternal advantages of breast-feeding include more rapid uterine involution, less bleeding in the postpartum period, and less ovarian and pre-menopausal breast cancers. Newborn advantages to breast-feeding include a strengthened immune system, fewer overweight infants, and lower incidences of certain infections, such as otitis media, diarrhea, and lower respiratory tract infections.
- There are certain situations in which breast-feeding is not recommended. Maternal situations include a woman actively using illegal drugs, one who has

untreated tuberculosis, one with HIV, or a woman receiving chemotherapy medications. Newborn conditions that would exclude breast-feeding include the newborn with galactosemia.

- The breast is under both physical and chemical control to stimulate lactation. The hormones prolactin and oxytocin stimulate milk production and release from the breast. The newborn sucking on and emptying the breast also leads to milk production.
- When assisting a woman to breast-feed, the nurse should provide for privacy, help the woman into a comfortable position, help the woman to hold her newborn correctly, and assess the newborn for a correct latching on and positioning on the breast. The nurse should assess the woman's breasts and nipples, her comfort level with breast-feeding, her support systems, and the newborn's feeding ability.
- When caring for a woman with sore nipples, the nurse should observe the latching on and the positioning of the newborn during nursing. A few drops of expressed breast milk or a purified lanolin treatment applied to the nipples after breast-feeding may help with the soreness.
- When caring for a woman with a plugged milk duct, the nurse should advise the breast-feeding woman to apply warm packs to the site, take a warm shower, take acetaminophen (Tylenol), nurse in different positions, avoid constrictive clothing or bras, and massage the site.
- When caring for a woman with mastitis, the nurse should advise the breast-feeding woman to contact her health care provider, take the antibiotics as prescribed, and continue to breast-feed even on the affected side. If breast-feeding is too uncomfortable on the affected side, she should pump the milk at each feeding so her milk supply does not diminish.
- Signs that a newborn is not breast-feeding well include dry mouth, fewer than expected wet or dirty diapers, difficulty rousing the newborn for feedings, and not enough feedings per day.
- Breast milk is superior to formula because it is easier to digest and has immunologic, bacteriocidal, and fungicidal properties that cannot be duplicated in artificial nutrition. Breast milk is economical and ready to feed and requires no special preparation or storage.
- There are many types of formulas available. The type of formula offered depends upon the newborn's gestational age and medical needs. The formulas for healthy term infants differ from the formula made for specific medical conditions. The formulas vary in types of protein sources, caloric content, and mineral and electrolyte concentrations.
- The formula-feeding woman needs education in the areas of preparation and storage of formula,

care of feeding utensils, how formula is available in the store, and the WIC program.

▶ Formula feeding would be beneficial in cases in which the woman is unavailable to breast-feed, such as adoption, surgery, or taking a medication that passes through the breast milk and would be harmful to the newborn. Formula feeding also is beneficial when the newborn has a specific medical condition, such as galactosemia.

▶ The formula-feeding woman should be taught how to feed her newborn and how much and when to increase feedings, how to prepare and store the formula and care for the equipment, how to care for her breasts after delivery, and when to notify the nurse or pediatrician.

▶ For the formula-fed newborn who is having emesis or diarrhea, the nurse should ask: What type of formula is the newborn on and how is it prepared? How much is the newborn eating per session and per day? What does the emesis/bowel movement look like? What other foods are being consumed by the newborn? How much emesis is there per episode? How many episodes has the newborn had in the last 24 hours?

REFERENCES AND SELECTED READINGS

Books and Journals

Blackburn, S. T., & Loper, D. L. (1992). *Maternal, fetal, and neonatal physiology*. Philadelphia: WB Saunders.

Conkin, C., Campbell, J., Montgomery, C. E., & Phillips, S. (Eds.). (2002). *Pediatric nutrition reference guide*. Houston, TX: Texas Children's Hospital.

Lawrence, R. A., & Lawrence, R. M. (1999). *Breastfeeding: A guide for the medical profession* (5th ed.). St. Louis: Mosby.

Riordan, J., & Auerbach, K. G. (1998). *Breastfeeding and human lactation* (2nd ed.). Sudbury: Jones and Bartlett Publishers.

Websites

American Academy of Pediatrics
http://aappolicy.aappublications.org

National Guideline Clearinghouse
http://www.guideline.gov

La Leche League International
http://www.lalecheleague.org

World Health Organization
http://www.who.int/nut/inf.htm

WORKBOOK

NCLEX-STYLE REVIEW QUESTIONS

1. A woman tells the nurse, "I don't need to use any contraception because I plan on breast-feeding exclusively." Upon which fact should the nurse base her response?

   a. Women who exclusively breast-feed do not ovulate.

   b. Ovulation can occur even in the absence of menstruation.

   c. The birth control pill is the best form of contraception for breast-feeding women.

   d. Breast-feeding women should not use contraception because it will decrease their milk supply.

2. During a prenatal visit an 18-year-old G 1 P 0 in her 36th week says to the nurse, "I don't know if I should breast-feed or not. Isn't formula just as good for the baby?" Upon what information should the nurse base her response?

   a. The benefits of breast-feeding are equal to those of formula feeding.

   b. It is ultimately the woman's choice whether she wants to breast-feed or not.

   c. The immunologic properties in breast milk cannot be duplicated in formula.

   d. The economic status of the woman is an important breast-feeding consideration.

3. The nurse is assessing the breast-feeding woman during a feeding session. What assessment has priority during the feeding session?

   a. Assess the position, latching on, and sucking of the newborn.

   b. Assess the woman's visitors and their opinions regarding breast-feeding.

   c. Check the woman's perineal pad for increased lochia flow.

   d. Determine if the woman needs a visit from the lactation consultant.

STUDY ACTIVITIES

1. Use the following table to compare information contained in your nursing pharmacology reference with information the hospital lactation specialist has on medications and their use during breast-feeding. If the two references disagree, from where did the lactation specialist get her information? Which information do you think is more accurate? Why?

Medication	Pharmacology Reference	Lactation Specialist
Magnesium sulfate		
Phenobarbital		
Depo-Provera		
Vicodin		
Coumadin		

2. Call your local WIC clinic. Interview the nurse to determine what she does to encourage the woman to breast-feed the newborn.

3. Interview the lactation consultant at the local hospital. What foods does she tell the woman to avoid when she is breast-feeding, and why? How many calories should the woman consume? How much liquid should she drink? Share your findings with your clinical group.

CRITICAL THINKING: What Would You Do?

Apply your knowledge of newborn nutrition to the following situations.

1. You are working in the prenatal clinic. Here is a list of several of the patients you encounter and the questions they ask you.

   a. Sally is a 20-year-old G 1 P 0. She tells you she is unsure about feeding her baby and asks you if she should breast-feed or bottle-feed. How would you respond?

   b. Betsy, a G 3 P 1, states she needs to return to work 6 weeks after the baby is born. "I don't know if it's even worth it to begin to breast-feed when I know I'll just have to stop in 6 weeks. It seems like a lot of work." How would you respond?

   c. Elizabeth is a 15-year-old G 1 P 0. She asks you, "I don't want to breast-feed, but I heard you still make milk after the baby is born. How do you stop it from happening?" How would you respond to Elizabeth's question?

2. You are working the mother–baby unit at the hospital. Here are some of your patients for the day and the questions they ask you.

   a. Susan is a 24-year-old G 3 P 1. She delivered 1 day ago and wants to breast-feed. When you examine her newborn, she tells you that she thinks she doesn't have enough milk to feed her baby and asks you to give her baby a bottle so he doesn't starve. How would you respond?

   b. It has been 3 days since Alicia's cesarean delivery, and she is formula feeding her new-born a milk-based formula. She tells you her baby spits up with every feeding. What questions would you ask her and why?

   c. Lanya is a 30-year-old G 2 P 2 who had a postpartum tubal ligation earlier today. It is time to breast-feed her baby, but her abdomen is sore. How would you suggest Lanya feed her newborn and why?

   d. Tricia is a 28-year-old G 1 P 1 who is formula-feeding. She asks you how to mix formula and how she should care for the bottles and nipples. What information would you give her and why?

   e. Maria is a 24-year-old G 1 P 1. She has some questions for you about how long her breast milk is good for after she pumps it. How would you respond?

The Normal Newborn

STUDENT OBJECTIVES

On completion of this chapter, the student should be able to

1. Explain how to support immediate transition from fetal to extrauterine life.
2. Illustrate how to assign an Apgar score to a newborn.
3. Outline principles of thermoregulation for the newborn.
4. Describe immediate care of the newborn to include eye prophylaxis and administration of vitamin K.
5. Explain the nurse's role in protecting the infant from misidentification in the hospital.
6. Intervene appropriately with the newborn who has hypoglycemia.
7. Institute effective infection control procedures in the nursery.
8. Protect the newborn from abduction.
9. Recognize signs of pain in the newborn.
10. Compare and contrast the care of the newborn male who is uncircumcised with that of one who is circumcised.
11. Explain what immunizations should be given and what newborn screening tests should be done before the newborn is discharged home.
12. Teach the parents normal newborn care.

KEY TERMS

circumcision 356 – 358
cold stress 344
kangaroo care 348
ophthalmia neonatorum 349
thermoneutral environment 348

As you learned in Chapter 13, the newborn must make rapid adjustments to successfully adapt to life outside of the womb. The nurse's role is to support the newborn as he adapts to these changes and quickly recognize the development of complications so that intervention can be initiated immediately. Teaching the parents the skills needed to care for their newborn is another critical role of the nurse. This chapter discusses the basic care that must be given when caring for newborns and their families.

● The Nursing Process in Immediate Stabilization and Transition of the Newborn

The current standard of care for resuscitation of the newborn immediately after birth is outlined in the Neonatal Resuscitation Program (NRP) (American Academy of Pediatrics NRP Steering Committee, 2000).[1] The basic principles of newborn resuscitation are reviewed here. Refer to an NRP textbook for detailed guidelines on newborn resuscitation. The licensed practical nurse (LPN) normally is not responsible for a complete resuscitation; however, an ability to initiate resuscitation and assist throughout the process is essential.

The first 6 to 12 hours after birth are a critical transition period for the newborn. The healthy newborn may stay with the mother immediately after delivery and be cared for by the same nurse who is overseeing the mother's recovery. In some facilities the newborn is taken to a transition nursery after a short initial bonding period with his parents. In either case, the nurse caring for the newborn during the transition period must be alert to early signs of distress and be ready to intervene quickly to prevent complications and poor outcomes.

ASSESSMENT

Immediate assessments of the newborn are concerned with the success of cardiopulmonary adaptation. A strong, healthy cry is usually the first response of the neonate to external stimuli, as discussed in Chapter 13. A vigorous or lusty cry, heart rate greater than 100 beats per minute (bpm), and pink color are associated with effective cardiopulmonary adaptation. These assessments are made rapidly during the first seconds

after birth. If the newborn does not immediately cry, the cry is weak, or he does not meet the heart rate or color criteria, it is critical for the nurse to act quickly during the first minute after birth (see interventions in the following text).

A traditional immediate assessment of cardiopulmonary adaptation is the Apgar score. The Apgar score was developed by Dr. Virginia Apgar as a means of quickly assessing the success of the newborn's transition to extrauterine life. The score is no longer used as a guide to resuscitation, but it continues to be used to evaluate the effectiveness of resuscitation efforts and to help determine the intensity of care the newborn will require in the first few days of life.

Five parameters are used to determine the total Apgar score: heart rate, respiratory effort, muscle tone, reflex irritability, and color. Each factor receives a score of 0 to 2 points, for a maximum total score of 10 (Table 15-1). Apgar scoring is performed by the nurse and recorded in the delivery room record at 1 and 5 minutes after birth. If the newborn receives a score of less than 7 at 5 minutes, scoring is continued every 5 minutes until the score is 7 or above, the newborn is intubated, or until the newborn is transferred to the nursery.

Scores of 7 to 10 at 5 minutes are indicative of a healthy baby who is adapting well to the extrauterine environment. These newborns typically do well and can be cared for in the regular newborn nursery or can room-in with their mothers. Scores between 4 and 6 at 5 minutes after birth indicate that the newborn is having some difficulty in adjusting to life outside the womb and needs close observation. These newborns are usually taken to a special nursery where they may receive oxygen and other special monitoring until their condition improves. Newborns who receive a score of 0 to 3 at 5 minutes are experiencing severe difficulty in making the transition to extrauterine life. These infants usually require observation and care in a neonatal intensive care unit (NICU).

During the transition period, continue to observe the newborn for signs of respiratory distress or cardiovascular compromise. As you will recall from Chapter 13, signs of respiratory distress include nasal flaring, tachypnea, grunting, sternal retractions, and seesaw respirations. Observe for excess mucus, which could obstruct the airway. Measure the heart and respiratory rates at least every 30 minutes during the first 2 hours of transition.

Observe the newborn closely for **cold stress**, which is a body temperature of less than 97.6°F

---

[1] Developed and maintained by the American Heart Association (AHA) and the American Academy of Pediatrics (AAP).

TABLE 15.1	**Apgar Scoring**				

Apgar scoring is done at 1 and 5 minutes after birth. The newborn is considered to be "vigorous" if the initial scores are 7 and above. If the 5-minute score is less than 7, scoring is done every 5 minutes thereafter until the score reaches 7. The numbers in the left-hand column represent the number of points that are assigned to each parameter when the criteria in the corresponding column are met.

	Heart Rate	Respiratory Effort	Muscle Tone	Reflex Irritability	Color
2	Heart rate above 100 beats per minutes (bpm)	Strong, vigorous cry	Maintains a position of flexion with brisk movements	Cries or sneezes when stimulated*	Body and extremities pink
1	Heart rate present, but less than 100 bpm	Weak cry, slow or difficult respirations	Minimal flexion of extremities	Grimaces when stimulated	Body pink, extremities blue (acrocyanosis)
0	No heart rate	No respiratory effort	Limp and flaccid	No response to stimulation	Body and extremities blue (cyanosis) or completely pale (pallor)

* Stimulation is provided by suctioning the infant or by gently flicking the sole of the foot.

(36.5°C). Use a thermal skin probe for continuous temperature assessment while the newborn is under the radiant warmer. Measure the axillary temperature at least every 30 minutes until the temperature stabilizes. Then check the temperature again at 4 hours and at 8 hours. If the temperature remains stable, it may be assessed every 8 hours until discharge.

Hypoglycemia is a potential problem that can, if prolonged, have devastating effects on the newborn. Therefore, it is critical for the nurse to know signs and symptoms of hypoglycemia in the newborn, which include:

- Jitteriness or tremors
- Exaggerated Moro reflex
- Irritability
- Lethargy
- Poor feeding
- Listlessness
- Apnea or respiratory distress
- High-pitched cry

The main sign of hypoglycemia is jitteriness, which can be exhibited as an exaggerated Moro reflex. Conversely, the hypoglycemic newborn may have no symptoms. If hypoglycemia is prolonged without treatment, the newborn may have seizures or lapse into a coma. Permanent brain damage can result, leading to lifelong disability.

The nurse must be familiar with factors that increase the risk for hypoglycemia in the newborn (Box 15-1). Any condition that adversely affects blood flow to the placenta during preg-

nancy puts the newborn at risk for hypoglycemia. If the mother's blood sugar was elevated during the latter part of the pregnancy, such as in maternal diabetes, or if she received medications that elevate her blood sugar, the newborn also is at risk for hypoglycemia. Any condition that puts physiologic stress on the fetus, such as prolonged labor or maternal infection, may deplete glycogen stores, putting the newborn at risk for low blood sugar.

BOX 15.1	**Risk Factors for Hypoglycemia**

History of any of the following during the pregnancy increases the risk that the newborn will develop hypoglycemia.
- Gestational hypertension
- Maternal diabetes (pre-existing or gestational)
- Prolonged labor
- Fetal distress during labor
- Ritodrine or terbutaline administered to mother

Newborn characteristics that increase the risk for hypoglycemia. Note that many of these conditions result from an at-risk pregnancy.
- Intrauterine growth restriction (IUGR)
- Macrosomia (a very large baby)
- Large-for-gestational age
- Small-for-gestational age
- Prematurity
- Postmaturity
- Respiratory or cardiovascular depression requiring resuscitation

This is a critical point. Never mistake jitteriness in the newborn for "shivering." If the newborn has shaky movements or startles easily, the first thing you should check is the blood sugar. This is particularly important because newborns can develop hypoglycemia even though there are no recognizable risk factors for its development.

If a newborn is exhibiting signs of, or is at risk for, hypoglycemia, check the glucose level using a heel stick to obtain a blood sample for testing (Nursing Procedure 15-1). Blood levels between 40 and 60 mg/dL during the first 24 hours of life are considered normal. Levels less than 40 mg/dL are indicative of hypoglycemia in the newborn.

A full physical assessment, including gestational age assessment as discussed in Chapter 13, is completed within the first few hours of life.

SELECTED NURSING DIAGNOSES

- Impaired spontaneous ventilation related to ineffective transition to newborn life
- Risk for injury: hypoglycemia related to immature metabolism and/or presence of risk factors
- Ineffective thermoregulation related to immature heat-regulating mechanisms
- Risk for infection related to immature immune system, possible exposure to pathogens in the birth canal or in the nursery, and umbilical cord wound
- Risk for imbalanced fluid volume related to immature blood clotting mechanisms
- Risk for injury: misidentification related to failure of delivery room personnel to adequately identify the newborn before separation from the parents

PLANNING AND GOALS

Maintaining the safety of the newborn during transition from intrauterine to extrauterine life is the primary goal when planning care immediately after delivery and in the first 6 to 12 hours of life. Appropriate patient goals include that the newborn will experience adequate cardiovascular, respiratory, thermoregulatory, and metabolic transitions to extrauterine life, and that he will remain free from signs and symptoms of infection, maintain hemostasis, and will be adequately identified before separation from the parents.

IMPLEMENTATION

Supporting Cardiovascular and Respiratory Transition

Nursing interventions to support newborn vital functions begin before the birth occurs. If you will be assisting in the immediate care of the newborn, ensure that adequate supplies are present for a full resuscitation and that all equipment is functioning properly. Most delivery settings have a newborn resuscitation board that is stocked with needed supplies. Check that oxygen is readily available and that there is a functioning suction source. Ensure that a warmer is in the delivery area, and turn it on several minutes before the delivery is expected.

Observe the newborn carefully at birth. The delivery attendant will usually suction the mouth and nose with a bulb syringe and clamp and cut the umbilical cord. If the newborn cries vigorously, you may drape a blanket over the mother's abdomen and support the infant there when the birth attendant hands the newborn to you. Quickly palpate the base of the umbilical cord and count the pulse for 6 seconds. Multiply that number by 10 to calculate the heart rate. A pulse above 100 bpm and a vigorous cry are reassuring signs that indicate the newborn is making a successful transition.

If the newborn does not cry immediately, he must be transported to a preheated radiant warmer for prompt resuscitation. He should be dried quickly to prevent heat loss from evaporation and to provide stimulation to encourage a first breath. If the newborn still does not make adequate breathing efforts, a bag and mask connected to 100% oxygen are used to provide respiratory support until spontaneous breathing occurs.

Most newborns do not need to be resuscitated, and the ones who do generally respond well to a short period of positive-pressure ventilation with a bag and mask. However, a very small number of infants also require chest compressions, intubation, and medications. Refer to the NRP for complete resuscitation guidelines.

Give constant attention to the airway. Newborns often have abundant secretions. The initial intervention is to position the newborn on the side or with the head in a slightly lower position than the body to help prevent aspiration

Nursing Procedure 15.1
Performing a Heel Stick

EQUIPMENT

Alcohol wipe
2 × 2 square gauze
Tape
Adhesive bandage
Warm pack
Lancet or other puncturing device
Device to read the glucose level and all supplies needed for its use
Clean gloves

PROCEDURE

1. Thoroughly wash your hands.
2. Place a warm pack on the newborn's heel for several minutes before attempting to obtain specimen.

3. Don a pair of clean gloves.
4. Hold the foot so that it is well supported with your thumb or finger covering the flat surfaces of the foot to avoid puncturing this area and causing damage to nerves or blood vessels. The highlighted areas on the lateral aspects of the foot in the illustration are appropriate areas from which to perform a heel stick.

Lateral plantar artery
Lateral plantar nerve
Calcaneous
Safe areas for puncture
Medial plantar artery
Medial plantar nerve
Medial calcaneal nerve

5. Locate a fat pad on either side of the foot. Palpate the chosen site to ensure there is enough padding to avoid puncturing the bone, which could lead to infection.

6. Clean the site with alcohol and allow to air dry.
7. Using the lancet, puncture the site to a depth of no greater than 2 mm. If using a commercial puncturing device, follow the manufacturer's guidelines for use. Place the lancet in a sharps container.

8. Wipe away the first drop of blood. Do not squeeze the tissue close to the puncture site or the reading may not be accurate.
9. Collect the specimen from the second drop of blood. Follow the manufacturer's instructions regarding processing the specimen.

10. Make a pressure dressing from the gauze and tape it over the puncture site. An alternative is to hold pressure for a few moments and then apply an adhesive bandage when the bleeding stops.
11. Remove the gloves and thoroughly wash your hands.
12. Record the glucose level in the designated area of the chart.

Note: Warmth causes vasodilation and draws blood to the surface, making it easier to obtain a specimen. Many facilities have commercial warm packs available for this purpose, such as the one used in the photograph. If a commercial pack is not available, a washcloth dampened with warm (not hot) water may be placed on the heel and covered with a towel or blue pad, or a diaper dampened with warm water may be used. Always check the temperature of the washcloth or diaper with the inside of your wrist before placing it on the newborn's heel. Burns can easily result if the temperature is too hot.

● *Figure 15.1* The nurse uses a bulb syringe to suction the mouth of the newborn before suctioning the nares. The bulb is depressed first and then placed in the newborn's oral cavity. Secretions are suctioned into the bulb of the syringe when pressure is released from the bulb. The bulb is then squeezed several times to empty it of secretions before subsequent attempts to suction the newborn.

of secretions. A bulb syringe is used to suction the mouth first and then the nose (Fig. 15-1).

Did you know? It is important to suction the mouth of a newborn before the nose. If the nose is suctioned first, the newborn may gasp or cry and aspirate secretions in the mouth.

Keep the bulb syringe with the newborn and teach the parents how and when to suction the baby. If copious secretions are present that do not resolve with a bulb syringe, a small suction catheter connected to a suction source may be used. Be careful not to apply suction for longer than 5 seconds at a time and to minimize suction pressures to avoid damaging the delicate respiratory structures.

Maintaining Thermoregulation

It is critical to protect the newborn from chilling. Cold stress increases the amount of oxygen and glucose needed by the newborn. She can quickly deplete glucose stores and develop hypoglycemia. She can also develop respiratory distress and metabolic acidosis if chilling is prolonged. As stated in the previous section, if the newborn cries vigorously and has an adequate heart rate, he may stay with his mother. Quickly dry the newborn on the mother's abdomen, swaddle him snugly, and apply a cap to prevent heat loss. Another way to maintain the newborn's temperature and promote early bonding is to dry the newborn quickly, place a diaper or blanket over the genital area and a cap on the head, then place the newborn skin-to-skin with

the mother or father and cover them both with blankets. This method of keeping the newborn warm is called **kangaroo care** (Fig. 15-2). Kangaroo care is an excellent way to meet the needs of the newborn and provide family-centered care.

It is important to support thermoregulation in the newborn, particularly in the first 24 hours of life. The environmental temperature necessary to maintain a **thermoneutral environment**, an environment in which heat is neither lost nor gained, is slightly higher for the newborn than that required for an older child or adult. Take care to prevent unnecessary heat loss in the nursery. For example, drafts of air can cause convective heat loss, and placing a newborn on a cold surface can lead to conductive heat loss. Conversely, do not allow the newborn to become overheated. Hyperthermia can be just as harmful as hypothermia. A skin temperature probe should be in place on the skin anytime the newborn is under the radiant warmer, and alarms should be set to signal if the skin temperature becomes too hot.

Preventing Injury from Hypoglycemia

The best way to prevent injury from hypoglycemia is to prevent the condition altogether. If the mother is breast-feeding, encourage early

● *Figure 15.2* Kangaroo care. A new father keeps his newborn warm using skin-to-skin contact. This method of warming a newborn is called kangaroo care. It is also an excellent way for parents to bond with their newborn.

and frequent feedings. If she is experiencing difficulty, it may be necessary to have a lactation consultant assist the mother. Refer to Chapter 14 for detailed information on breast-feeding and nutrition. If the newborn is to be bottle-fed, early feedings should be initiated.

Asymptomatic newborns at risk for hypoglycemia should be tested at 2, 4, 6, 12, 24, and 48 hours after delivery (Kauffman & Word, 1997). When a newborn displays signs of hypoglycemia, she should be tested. If a heel stick specimen reveals a glucose level of less than 40 mg/dL, it is important to have the results confirmed by laboratory analysis before treatment is initiated. It is common for bedside glucose analyzers to under-read glucose results.

Most facilities have protocols to guide the nurse in the treatment of hypoglycemia. Many pediatricians have preprinted orders that can be initiated if the glucose level falls below a predetermined level (usually 40 mg/dL). In the past, glucose water was used to treat low blood glucose levels, but most authorities now recommend feeding breast milk or formula to the alert newborn. If the infant's symptoms are severe enough to interfere with regular feeding, intravenous dextrose solutions are administered.

Preventing Infection
Within the first hour after birth, an antibiotic ointment must be placed in the newborn's eyes (Fig. 15-3) to prevent **opthalmia neonatorum**, a severe eye infection contracted in the birth canal of a woman with gonorrhea or chlamydia. There are three ophthalmic agents that have been approved for eye prophylaxis: 1% silver nitrate, 0.5% erythromycin, and 1% tetracycline. Silver

● **Figure 15.3** The nurse administers antibiotic ointment to the eyes of the newborn to prevent opthalmia neonatorum.

nitrate is used infrequently because it is irritating to the eyes. In some facilities it is the practice to instill the eye drops in the delivery area immediately after birth, but it is recommended that the instillation be delayed up to 1 hour to allow the newborn and parents to bond while the infant is in a quiet alert state.

Another possible infection site is the umbilical cord stump. Careful handwashing and strict aseptic technique should be used when caring for the cord. Often an antiseptic solution such as triple dye, bacitracin ointment, or povidone-iodine is used initially to paint the cord to help prevent the development of infection.

Preventing Imbalanced Fluid Volume
One possible cause of hemorrhage and fluid volume loss is an immature clotting mechanism. Vitamin K is necessary in the formation of certain clotting factors. In the adult, vitamin K is manufactured in the gut by normal flora, but the gut of the newborn is sterile; it has not yet been colonized with symbiotic bacteria. Therefore, it is necessary to supply the newborn with vitamin K to prevent possible bleeding episodes. Within the first hour after birth 0.5 to 1 mg of vitamin K (AquaMEPHYTON) is given intramuscularly (IM). Refer to Nursing Procedure 15-2.

One potential source of hemorrhage is the clamped umbilical cord. An unusually large cord may have large amounts of Wharton's jelly, which may disintegrate faster than the cord vessels and cause the clamp to become loose. This situation could lead to blood loss from the cord. Another cause could be an improperly applied or defective cord clamp. Inspect the umbilical cord for signs of bleeding.

Preventing Misidentification of a Newborn
Fortunately it is a rare occurrence for newborns to be switched in the hospital and go home with the wrong parents, but it has happened. When the mistake is uncovered years later, the situation often results in heartache and heart-wrenching choices for all parties involved. Because of the serious consequences of mistaken identity, the delivery room nurse must take the utmost care to positively identify the newborn before he is separated from his parents.

Many facilities footprint the newborn and fingerprint the mother, but this practice is in decline because footprints are not considered a valid way to identify someone. Most hospitals use some form of bracelet system. Three to four bracelets with identical numbers on the bands are prepared immediately after delivery and before the newborn is separated from his parents. Information

Nursing Procedure 15.2
Administering an Intramuscular Injection to the Newborn

EQUIPMENT

Warm, clean hands
Clean (nonsterile) exam gloves
Syringe
0.5-inch 23- to 25-gauge safety needle
Alcohol pad
Flat surface

PROCEDURE

1. Wash hands thoroughly.
2. Check physician order for medication and dose.
3. Follow normal nursing procedure for drawing medications from a vial or ampule. Do not draw more than 0.5 mL for intramuscular (IM) injection to a newborn.
4. Identify the newborn by identity band. Place the newborn on a flat surface with good lighting.
5. Select an injection site on the vastus lateralis (anterior lateral aspect of the thigh) or rectus femoris (midanterior aspect of the thigh) muscle.

6. Apply clean gloves.
7. Clean the site with an alcohol pad. Use a circular motion from the center of the chosen site outward in ever-widening circles. Hold the alcohol pad between two of your fingers.
8. With your nondominant hand, hold the leg in place.
9. Using your dominant hand, insert the needle at a 90-degree angle with a quick darting motion.
10. Stabilize the needle with your nondominant hand and pull back gently on the plunger to aspirate for blood.
11. If no blood is noted, slowly inject the medication.
12. Use the alcohol pad to stabilize the skin as you withdraw the needle.
13. Discard the syringe and needle in a sharps container. Discard the gloves in a trash receptacle.
14. Wash hands thoroughly.
15. Document on the medication administration record.

Note: If blood is aspirated in step 10, withdraw the needle to avoid intravenous (IV) injection. Discard the syringe, needle, and medication in a sharps container. Go back to step 1 and begin again.

Rectus femoris muscle

Vastus lateralis muscle

included on the bands is the mother's name, hospital number, and physician, and the newborn's sex, and date and time of birth. Two bands are placed on the newborn, one on the arm and one on the leg. A matching band is placed on the mother and another band may be placed on the father or other designated adult. Instruct the parents to always check the bands when the newborn is brought to them to ensure they are receiving their newborn.

EVALUATION: GOALS AND EXPECTED OUTCOMES

- **Goal:** The newborn will experience adequate cardiovascular and respiratory transition.
  Expected Outcomes: The newborn sustains a heart rate above 100 bpm, maintains a respiratory rate between 30 and 60 breaths per minute without signs of distress, and retains a patent airway.
- **Goal:** The newborn will experience thermoregulatory transition.
  Expected Outcome: The newborn's body temperature stays between 36.5°C and 37.5°C (97.7°F and 99.5°F).
- **Goal:** The newborn will experience adequate metabolic transition.
  Expected Outcome: The newborn's blood glucose level is between 40 and 60 mg/dL.
- **Goal:** The newborn remains free from the signs and symptoms of infection.
  Expected Outcomes: The newborn does not experience purulent conjunctivitis, purulent drainage from the umbilical cord, and has no other signs of sepsis, such as poor suck reflex and lethargy.
- **Goal:** The newborn maintains adequate hemostasis.
  Expected Outcomes: The newborn has no bleeding episodes.
- **Goal:** The newborn will be adequately identified before separation from the parents.
  Expected Outcomes: The newborn possesses a permanent form of identification before he is separated from his parents and can be positively identified by his parents.

Test Yourself

- List the five parameters measured by the Apgar score.
- What is cold stress?
- Describe kangaroo care. List two purposes that it serves.

● The Nursing Process in Providing Care to the Normal Newborn

ASSESSMENT

Nursing care of the normal, stabilized newborn is directed toward controlling risk and early detection of developing complications. The nurse who is responsible for the care of newborns must be familiar with signs that indicate the newborn needs special care.

One common problem is the potential for aspiration from secretions and mucus that are present in the airways during the first few days of life. Monitor the newborn closely for excessive secretions. Gagging and frequent regurgitation are normal in the first few hours of birth. Signs of respiratory distress or central cyanosis should not be present.

Another potential problem is that of infection. Carefully monitor the newborn for signs of infection. An infected umbilical cord will show signs of redness and edema at the base and may have purulent discharge. Early signs of sepsis in the newborn include poor feeding, irritability, lethargy, apnea, and temperature instability. Late signs are an enlarged spleen and liver, jaundice, and petechiae.

Perform a thorough skin assessment. Turgor should be present, and the skin should be intact. Inspect the diaper area for signs of rash or breakdown. Assess for signs of jaundice. As you will recall from Chapter 13, jaundice that occurs within the first 24 hours of life is associated with abnormal lysis of red blood cells and is pathologic in nature.

Between 1983 and 2002, 217 cases of infant abduction by a nonfamily member were reported in the United States (Burgess & Lanning, 2003). Although infant abduction is a rare event, it has devastating effects on hospital personnel and family members of the victim. Studies of the problem have led to a "typical abductor" profile, which is outlined in Box 15-2. When taking care of newborns, be especially alert to any suspicious activity by visitors or persons unknown to you.

The newborn is subjected to numerous startling and noxious stimuli at birth. The womb is dark, confined, and warm. Sounds are muffled through the abdominal and uterine walls. During labor and delivery this situation is reversed. Suddenly the newborn is exposed to a world that is bright, cold, and loud. His extremities flail out when he is startled with seemingly nothing to

BOX 15.2	Profile of a Typical Infant Abductor

- Overweight female of childbearing age
- Has no prior criminal record
- Suffers from low self-esteem and is emotionally immature
- Uses manipulation and deceit within interpersonal relationships
- May be cohabitating or married, but the relationship is often strained
- Often indicates that she has lost a baby or cannot have one
- May announce a false pregnancy and prepare for the arrival of a newborn
- Usually plans the abduction by visiting several hospitals and asking detailed questions regarding nursery routines and exit routes
- Although the abduction is planned, a specific infant is not usually targeted; the abductor strikes when opportunity presents itself
- Frequently poses as a nurse or other health care personnel during the abduction
- Usually demonstrates the ability to take good care of the infant
- Often stays in the community from which the infant was taken

Note: The typical abductor profile was developed from an analysis of 119 cases occurring between 1983 and 1992 (Burgess & Lanning, 2003).

stop them. He does not know his boundaries. In addition the newborn is exposed to invasive and sometimes painful procedures. These early experiences have the potential to cause the newborn to respond to the environment in a disorganized way.

SELECTED NURSING DIAGNOSES

- Ineffective airway clearance related to mucus and secretions
- Risk for infection related to cross-contamination of equipment, poor handwashing, poor hygienic practices, transmission from mother to baby
- Risk for impaired skin integrity
- Risk for injury: newborn abduction
- Risk for disorganized infant behavior related to pain, invasive procedures, or environmental overstimulation

PLANNING AND GOALS

Most continuing newborn care is aimed at monitoring for and preventing complications. After the newborn has had a successful transition, appropriate goals include that the newborn will maintain a clear airway; be free of infection; have

clean intact skin; not be abducted from the hospital; and respond to the environment in an organized way. The goal of maintaining an adequate body temperature continues to be addressed throughout the hospital stay. Interventions to meet that goal are interwoven throughout the following implementation section. The goal of maintaining adequate nutrition and hydration is covered in detail in Chapter 14.

IMPLEMENTATION

Keeping the Airway Clear
Keep the bulb syringe in the bassinet with the newborn at all times. Turn the newborn on the side and suction frequently as secretions and mucus accumulate. Teach both parents how to use the bulb syringe. Position the newborn on the side or back to sleep, as recommended by the American Academy of Pediatrics (2003), to decrease the risk of sudden infant death syndrome (SIDS).

Preventing Transmission of Infection
A newborn may contract infection from his mother, visitors, nursery personnel, or the environment. Infection can be particularly devastating for a newborn because the immune system is immature and the newborn has not yet developed effective defenses against invading pathogens. Therefore, it is essential to practice good infection control techniques when caring for newborns.

Handwashing remains the mainstay of infection control, even in newborn nurseries. Many nurseries require a 3-minute surgical-type scrub at the beginning of the shift. Follow the protocol of the facility in which you are working. Of course the hands should be washed thoroughly before and after caring for a newborn. In no instance should a nurse care for a newborn and then proceed to handle or give care to another newborn without washing hands in between. Many newborn nurseries have waterless hand sanitizer available. Hand sanitizer is acceptable to use between newborns when visible soiling of the hands has not occurred.

Other methods for reducing the transmission of infection include keeping all of the newborn's belongings together in the bassinet and not sharing items between newborns. This practice reduces the possibility of cross-contamination. Equipment that is used on multiple newborns, such as a stethoscope, is usually wiped down with alcohol between uses. Rooming-in also reduces the likelihood of cross-contamination. It is no longer considered necessary for nursery personnel to have special scrub suits laundered by the hospital, or for them to wear cover gowns when leaving the nursery. This traditional practice was not found to reduce the incidence of infection in nurseries and has been abandoned.

It is necessary, for the nurse's protection, to use universal precautions. A newborn should not be handled without gloves until after the bath. After this time the newborn may be cared for without gloves unless contact with bodily fluids is likely, such as during diaper changes and when drawing blood for testing.

Providing Skin Care

The first bath (Nursing Procedure 15-3) is delayed until the newborn's temperature is stable. Warm water is usually sufficient for bathing; however, a mild soap can be used. The sponge bath is given under a radiant warmer to minimize heat loss. If a radiant warmer is not used, it is important to keep the infant wrapped and expose only the body part being washed.

Be careful to wash off all traces of blood to minimize transmission of infection from maternal blood-borne pathogens to the newborn or to health care providers. A mild shampoo may be

Nursing Procedure 15.3
Giving the First Bath

EQUIPMENT

Clean exam gloves
Basin of warm water (98°F to 100°F)
Mild soap and shampoo
Washcloth
Towel
Comb
Cap
Clean diaper
Shirt
Two receiving blankets

PROCEDURE

1. Assemble equipment.
2. Wash hands.

3. Use only clear water (no soap) on the eyes first (proceeding from inner canthus to outer canthus), then the rest of the face.
4. Hold the newborn with your nondominant arm using the football hold. Use the washcloth with the other hand to wipe off visible blood.
5. Lather the hair with shampoo and rinse thoroughly.

6. Comb through the hair to remove dried blood and to facilitate drying.
7. Place the infant back in the crib or under the radiant warmer (per the facility policy).
8. Bathe and rinse the neck and chest. Be sure to remove blood from the creases of the neck and armpits.

(procedure box continues on page 354)

Nursing Procedure 15.3 (continued)
Giving the First Bath

9. Proceed to the abdomen. Take care not to soak the cord in water (a wet cord increases the risk for infection).
10. Wash the extremities, then the back.

11. Next bathe the genital region. For boys, do not force the foreskin over the glans. For girls, wash from front to back, avoiding contamination of the urethral and vaginal areas with bacteria from the rectum.
12. Last, bathe the anal region.
13. Apply a clean cap, t-shirt, and diaper.
14. Double wrap the newborn with two receiving blankets.
15. Rinse and dry the basin. Store unused soap and shampoo containers and comb in the basin in the storage area of the bassinet.
16. Place the towel and washcloth in the dirty linen hamper.
17. Remove gloves.
18. Wash hands.

Note: The room should be warm, approximately 75°F (24°C) to prevent chilling. In many facilities the first bath is given under the radiant warmer. Bathing should proceed from the cleanest part of the body (face) and end with the dirtiest areas (diaper area). Each body area should be washed, rinsed, and then dried before proceeding to the next area to prevent heat loss from evaporation.

used on the head. Combing the hair helps to remove dried blood. Vernix serves as a lubricant and is protective against infections; therefore, it is best to gently massage the vernix into the skin and allow it to wear off naturally. However, in many facilities vernix is wiped away completely at the first bath to make the baby more presentable.

Be careful. It is important that harsh soaps not be used when bathing newborns. These soaps can irritate the skin. Hexachlorophene in particular is not recommended for bathing because it can be absorbed through the skin and cause central nervous system damage.

Encourage the parents to participate in the bath (Fig. 15-4). This is an excellent time to allow them to interact with their baby and help them gain confidence in parenting skills. When the bath is finished, check the axillary temperature. If it is

● *Figure 15.4* The new father dries his newborn son after giving him his first bath.

within the expected range (see Chapter 13), dress the newborn in a shirt, diaper, and cap. Swaddle the newborn in a blanket and place him in an open crib. If the temperature is below 36.4°C (97.5°F), return the newborn to the radiant warmer.

Warm water can be used to clean the perineal area and buttocks at diaper changes. Frequent diaper changes will help prevent diaper rash and skin breakdown. No special oils or ointments are necessary on clean, intact skin. Talc powders are not recommended because they can cause respiratory irritation when particles are inhaled. Fold the diaper down in the front so that the cord is left open to air (Fig. 15-5). This action protects the cord area from irritation when the diaper is wet and promotes drying of the cord.

Providing Safety

Education and watchful vigilance are the keys to preventing infant abductions. Each facility that cares for newborns should have specific policies and procedures in place that address this problem. Review these policies and know the protocols for the facility in which you will be working.

Most nurseries and mother–baby units are in a part of the hospital that has some security features to discourage abductions. Most nurseries are locked from the outside, and a security code is necessary to gain entrance. Security cameras are usually placed strategically near entrances and exits. Some facilities use security bracelets that set off an alarm if someone attempts to remove it, or it may trip an alarm when a person exits the unit with a newborn. The matching identification bands for newborns and parents also are part of the security plan. In many facilities, identification photos are taken of each newborn. Cooperation of the parents is essential to

● *Figure 15.5* The diaper is folded down so that it does not cover the drying cord.

FAMILY TEACHING TIPS

Keeping the Newborn Safe

Review the following points with parents of newborns frequently throughout their hospital stay. Instruct the parents to:
- Never leave their newborn unattended.
- Not remove the identification bands on the newborn until he is discharged from the hospital and to alert the nurses if an identification band falls off or becomes illegible for any reason.
- Not release their newborn to anyone who does not have a hospital picture ID that matches the specific security color or code chosen by the facility to identify personnel authorized to transport and handle newborns.
- Question anyone who does not have the proper identification, or whose picture does not match the identification tag she is wearing, even if she is dressed in hospital attire.
- Alert the nurses immediately if they are suspicious of any person or activity.
- Know the nurses caring for them and their newborn.
- Know when the newborn will be taken for tests, what health care provider authorized the test, and how long the procedure is expected to last.

the effectiveness of any security plan, especially because most infants who are abducted are taken from the mother's room. Family Teaching Tips: Keeping the Newborn Safe lists key points to discuss with parents regarding the safety and security of their newborn while in the hospital.

Enhancing Organized Infant Behavioral Responses

Newborns respond to the environment in more predictable and organized ways when their needs are anticipated. The psychosocial task of infants is developing a sense of trust. Newborns begin to develop trust when the adults around them consistently meet their needs. Feeding the newborn, keeping him dry and comfortable, and holding him are actions that promote trust. Kangaroo care with either parent provides comfort and encourages attachment. Swaddling a newborn snugly is comforting and promotes sleep. Nonnutritive sucking on a gloved finger or pacifier can also be comforting.

EVALUATION: GOALS AND EXPECTED OUTCOMES

- **Goal:** The newborn will maintain a patent airway.

  Expected Outcomes: The newborn's respiratory rate remains between 30 and 60 breaths per minute while at rest, and there are no signs of respiratory distress.

- **Goal:** The newborn will maintain a normal body temperature.
  Expected outcomes: The newborn maintains axillary temperature above 36.4°C (97.5°F) and below 37.5°C (99.5°F)
- **Goal:** The newborn will remain free of the signs and symptoms of infection.
  Expected Outcomes: The newborn has strong, coordinated suck and swallow reflexes, vigorous feeding behaviors, and a drying umbilical cord without purulent drainage or foul odor.
- **Goal:** The newborn will maintain skin integrity.
  Expected Outcomes: The newborn has clean, intact skin.
- **Goal:** The newborn will not be abducted from the hospital.
  Expected Outcomes: The newborn remains safely in the company of family members and/or nursery personnel at all times.
- **Goal:** The newborn will respond to the environment in an organized way.
  Expected Outcomes: The newborn begins to develop predictable sleep/wake patterns, and interacts with caregivers with sustained alertness during interaction.

Test Yourself

- Name three characteristics of a "typical" infant abductor.
- List four things the nurse can do to decrease the spread of infection to newborns.
- Describe three steps parents can take to reduce the risk of infant abduction while in the hospital.

● The Nursing Process in Preparing the Newborn for Discharge

ASSESSMENT

Risk management and promoting healthy adaptation to newborn life continue to guide the nurse when planning for discharge of a healthy newborn. Continue to assess respiratory, cardiovascular, thermoregulatory, nutritional, and hydration status. Monitor for signs of infection. Check vigilantly for developing jaundice.

Watch for signs of pain in the newborn, particularly if he is scheduled for a painful procedure such as circumcision. Until recently, it was not clearly understood how newborns perceive pain and what, if any, long-term effects there might be if pain is prolonged or untreated. Many research studies now support the real physiologic pain responses experienced by the newborn. It appears that untreated pain in the newborn can lead to increased sensitivity to painful experiences later or result in more immediate consequences, such as illness during the neonatal period.

The newborn may experience pain and discomfort from any number of routine procedures carried out in a newborn nursery. Injections and heel sticks are two such sources of painful stimuli. One common procedure that causes pain is **circumcision**, surgical removal of the foreskin of the penis. Because the newborn cannot express pain verbally, other measures must be used to evaluate pain. Pain can be assessed in the newborn by paying attention to behavior, such as crying, sleeplessness, facial expression, and body movements. Changes in heart and respiratory rates, blood pressure, and oxygen saturation can also be used to determine physiologic responses to pain.

It also is important to assess the adaptation of the mother and father to the parenting role. Experienced parents may feel very comfortable in their role and carry out newborn care without difficulty. New parents may ask lots of questions, or may appear afraid to handle the newborn. Assess for signs of positive bonding with the newborn. Refer to Chapter 12 for an in-depth discussion of bonding.

SELECTED NURSING DIAGNOSES

- Pain related to painful procedures such as injections, heel sticks, and circumcision
- Risk for infection related to inadequate immunity in the neonatal period
- Risk for injury from undetected metabolic and hearing disorders
- Deficient knowledge (parental) related to normal newborn care

PLANNING AND GOALS

Prevention of, and relief from, pain are applicable goals throughout the newborn's stay in the hospital; however, these goals become particularly important when the newborn is scheduled for an invasive procedure such as circumcision. Protection from infection and injury from preventable diseases by immunizing against and screening for hepatitis B, phenylketonuria, and other metabolic disorders is a critical goal during this time period. It also is important to evaluate parental knowledge and ability to care for the newborn throughout the hospital stay, but as the time draws near for discharge, this task becomes particularly important.

IMPLEMENTATION

Preventing and Treating Pain

It is the ethical responsibility of the nurse to prevent and treat pain. Enough research exists to document the adverse effects of unnecessary and untreated pain in the neonate. The best treatment is prevention. When possible, avoid situations that may be painful or distressing to the newborn. If there is a choice between an invasive versus noninvasive procedure, choose the noninvasive procedure whenever practical. Use common sense and make suggestions to the charge nurse or physician as appropriate. For instance, it may be less painful to insert an intravenous device than to give multiple intramuscular injections. Or it might be more tolerable for the newborn to have laboratory specimens drawn by venipuncture than to undergo numerous heel sticks.

Provide for a quiet, soothing environment as often as possible. Simple comfort measures can be initiated that decrease the amount of pain perceived by the newborn. Swaddling and holding the infant securely are soothing measures. Non-nutritive sucking on a pacifier can be comforting. Placing sucrose on the pacifier, if allowed by hospital policy, adds the benefit of analgesia suitable for minor pain stimulus.

Assisting With Circumcision

There has been much debate concerning whether or not circumcision should be routinely performed. In the 1970s and 1980s, the American Academy of Pediatrics (AAP) held to a strict policy of strongly discouraging circumcisions based on the rationale that there were no valid medical indications for the procedure. Since that time, the AAP has softened its stance, currently stating, "Existing scientific evidence demonstrates potential medical benefits of newborn male circumcision; however, these data are not sufficient to recommend routine neonatal circumcision." The procedure is contraindicated in newborns who:

- Are still in the transition period
- Are preterm or sick
- Have a family history of bleeding disorder until the disorder is ruled out in the newborn
- Have received a diagnosis of a bleeding disorder

- Have a congenital genitourinary disorder, such as epispadias or hypospadias

The AAP advises that parents should be given enough information to make an informed choice and that pain relief measures should be provided if the procedure is done. Refer to Box 15-3 for a comparison of the advantages and disadvantages of male circumcision. Whatever the parents decide, the nurse must be supportive of their decision.

If the parents decide to have their male newborn circumcised, informed consent is necessary. It is the physician's responsibility to obtain informed consent, although the nurse is usually responsible for witnessing the parents' signatures to a written documentation of that consent. If the parents have unanswered questions, the physician must be notified before the procedure is done. Because of the overwhelming evidence regarding the adverse effects of pain on the newborn, many physicians recommend that language be put into the written consents informing the parents that anesthesia will not be used (if the physician does not use anesthesia) and listing the possible harmful effects of doing the procedure without anesthesia.

After the written consent is signed, prepare for the procedure by gathering all necessary supplies and equipment. Check the physician preference card to determine what procedure the physician

---

BOX 15.3 | Advantages and Disadvantages of Male Circumcision

Advantages
- There is a possible reduction in sexually transmitted infections and urinary tract infections.
- Risk of penile cancer is reduced (it is thought that careful attention to hygiene in uncircumcised males can mitigate the slight increase in risk).
- Neonatal circumcision has fewer complications than adult circumcision (medical necessity for adult circumcision is rare).

Disadvantages
- Neonates experience pain during circumcision.
- All anesthetic methods to block or reduce the pain of circumcision have side effects and possible complications.
- Circumcision can lead to the complications of hemorrhage and infection (infrequent occurrences, but potentially life-threatening), and genital mutilation (extremely rare).

Note: The religious and cultural values of the parents may play a large role in the decision on whether or not to circumcise. These values must be respected.

A PERSONAL GLIMPSE

The nurse walked into my room and found me crying and holding my newborn son. She asked me if I was in pain or if something was wrong with the baby. I said, No. She asked if I needed to talk and I nodded my head. I blurted out, "I just don't know if I should circumcise my son or not. My husband thinks we should, but I don't want my baby to be in pain. I just don't know that it is a necessary procedure."

She sat down on the side of my bed and calmly explained that there was no right or wrong decision. She assured me that she and the other nurses and doctors would support us in any decision that we made for our son. Then she gave me several pamphlets to read explaining the pros and cons of circumcision, the pros and cons of choosing not to circumcise, and the latest recommendations from the American Academy of Pediatrics. I felt much better after our talk, and my husband and I were able to make an informed decision about whether or not our son would have this procedure.

Heather

LEARNING OPPORTUNITY: What things can the nurse tell parents about pain control for painful procedures?

In what ways can the nurse act as an advocate for parents when they are trying to decide on whether or not to allow procedures on their newborn?

---

uses and what special materials are required. The newborn will usually be strapped to a padded circumcision board. If the board is not padded, add blankets or other soft material to the board. Swaddle the infant's upper body during the circumcision.

Check the orders for preprocedure pain relief methods. Acetaminophen may be given within 1 hour before the procedure and then every 4 to 6 hours afterward during the first 24 hours per physician orders or facility protocol. If an anesthetic cream, such as EMLA, is to be used for the procedure, it must be applied approximately 1 hour before the procedure to adequately numb the area. The type of anesthesia that provides the best pain relief appears to be a dorsal penile nerve block. The physician performs the nerve block with buffered lidocaine at least 5 minutes before the circumcision to allow for complete anesthesia in the area. Other methods that can decrease the pain sensation include dimming

the lights during circumcision, playing soft music or prerecorded intrauterine sounds for the newborn, and offering a sucrose-dipped pacifier to the infant before and throughout the procedure.

There are several acceptable methods for performing circumcision. Two of the most common are the Gomco (Yellen) clamp (Fig. 15-6) and the Plastibell procedures. Both methods require that the prepuce (foreskin) be separated from the glans penis and incised before the clamp is applied.

Care immediately after the procedure involves holding and comforting the newborn. If the parents are not readily available or cannot perform this action, the nurse must step in to soothe the newborn. Position the newborn on the back or side to avoid excess pressure and pain on the circumcision site. Administer analgesics as ordered on a schedule for pain. Monitor the newborn for signs of unrelieved pain.

Assess the newborn every hour for the first 12 hours after circumcision for evidence of bleeding. If bleeding occurs, apply gentle pressure as needed. Carefully observe for return of voiding and observe the urine stream. Failure to void indicates a complication of circumcision and must be reported to the charge nurse and physician. If a Plastibell was not used, A&D ointment or petroleum jelly must be applied to the site to prevent it from sticking to the diaper. Refer to Family Teaching Tips: Uncircumcised and Circumcised Penis Care for important teaching points to discuss with parents after circumcision or, if circumcision was not done, how to care for the uncircumcised penis.

Preventing Infection Through Neonatal Immunization

Hepatitis B vaccination is recommended by the Centers for Disease Control (CDC) for all newborns before they leave the hospital, regardless of the mother's HBsAg status (all pregnant women who receive prenatal care are tested for hepatitis B surface antigen [HBsAg]). Hepatitis B vaccine requires parental consent. Be sure the parents' written consent is obtained before injecting the vaccine. Instruct the parents to follow up with the recommended vaccination schedule for all immunizations, starting at 2 months and continuing throughout infancy.

The hepatitis B vaccination is especially important in newborns of mothers who are infected with hepatitis B or in whom infection is suspected. Many newborns who contract hepatitis B virus (HBV) from their mothers become chronic carriers of the disease. In some cases the

● *Figure 15.6* Circumcision using the Gomco (Yellen) clamp. (**A**) The newborn's upper body is swaddled, and his legs are strapped to the circumcision board. (**B**) The nurse injects a small amount of sucrose into the newborn's mouth and allows the newborn to suck on her gloved finger as a method of nonpharmacologic pain relief. (**C**) The physician injects a local anesthetic to numb the area in preparation for the procedure. (**D**) The penis and scrotum are prepped with povidone-iodine and the area draped with sterile towels. Forceps are used to pull the foreskin (prepuce) forward, and an incision is made into the prepuce. (**E**) The prepuce is drawn over the cone. (**F**) The clamp is applied.

G

H

● *Figure 15.6* (continued) (**G**) Pressure is maintained for 3 to 4 minutes, then a scalpel is used to cut away excess foreskin. (**H**) The clamp is removed and a petrolatum gauze dressing applied.

newborn develops an acute case of hepatitis B and dies of the infection. In other cases the newborn has no symptoms but has an increased risk for developing cirrhosis or hepatocellular carcinoma later in life. If the woman is HBsAg positive, the newborn is bathed thoroughly after birth (to remove traces of blood and decrease the risk of transmission from the mother's blood on his skin when he receives his vaccination). In addition, the newborn is given the hepatitis vaccination and one dose of hepatitis B immune globulin (HBIG) within 12 hours of birth. This dosing schedule is 98% to 99% effective in preventing transmission of HBV from an infected mother to her newborn. If the mother's HBsAg status is unknown, the HBV vaccine is given, and the HBIG dose can be postponed as long as 1 week while awaiting the mother's results.

Preventing Injury Through Neonatal Screening

It is crucial that newborns be screened for several disorders that have the potential to cause lifelong disability if diagnosis and treatment are delayed (Box 15-4). The laws in most states require this initial screening, which is done within 72 hours of birth. The ideal time to collect the specimen is after the newborn is 36 hours old and 24 hours after he has his first protein feeding. Use a heel stick to draw blood from the newborn and collect a specimen on a special collection card. The card has five rings, and each ring must be filled with the newborn's blood (Fig. 15-7). The specimen is then labeled and sent to a special laboratory for testing. A second test is performed at 1 to 2 weeks of age. The mother must be instructed on where and when to take her newborn for the follow-up screening test.

A hearing screen is now encouraged for all newborns before they are discharged home. There are two tests that are used to screen a newborn's hearing: the Auditory Brainstem Response (ABR) and Otoacoustic Emissions (OAE). Both tests use clicks or tones played into the newborn's ear. The ABR measures how the brain responds to sound through electrodes placed on the newborn's head. OAE measures sound waves produced in the inner ear. A probe is placed inside the newborn's ear canal, and the response or echo is measured. Both tests are effective screening devices. An abnormal screening result is followed-up with more extensive testing.

Because significant costs are involved for equipment and follow-up, it is mandated that insurance companies pay for this service. Early diagnosis and treatment results in better outcomes, including better chances for healthy attachment with parents, for newborns who have hearing disorders.

BOX 15.4	Newborn Screening

Disorders for which newborn screening is commonly done:
- Phenylketonuria (PKU)
- Congenital hypothyroidism
- Galactosemia
- Maple syrup urine disease
- Homocystinuria
- Biotinidase
- Sickle cell disease
- Congenital adrenal hypoplasia
- Cystic fibrosis

Note: According to the National Newborn Screening and Genetics Resource Center, all 50 states mandate screening for PKU, congenital hypothyroidism, and galactosemia.

Uncircumcised and Circumcised Penis Care

Review the following points with parents of newborn boys before discharge.

For the uncircumcised newborn, instruct the parents to:

- Wash the penis with each diaper change.
- Not force the foreskin to retract. Bleeding, infection, and scarring can result.
- Teach the child, when he is old enough, to wash under the foreskin daily by gently retracting the foreskin as far as it will go (without using forcible retraction).

For the circumcised newborn, instruct the parents to:

- Inspect the circumcision site each time the diaper is changed. Call the doctor if more than a few drops of blood are present in the diaper.
- Wash the penis with warm water dribbled gently from a washcloth at each diaper change.
- Reapply petroleum jelly at each diaper change for the first 24 to 48 hours unless a Plastibell was used.
- Fasten the diaper loosely to prevent unnecessary friction and irritation.
- Remember that yellow crusting over the area indicates normal healing. The crust should not be removed.
- Hold and comfort your baby frequently while the site is healing. Nonnutritive sucking with a pacifier may be soothing.
- Call the physician if a Plastibell does not fall off within 5 to 8 days.
- Report the following warning signs after circumcision:
  - Bleeding spot larger than a quarter in the diaper.
  - No wet diapers within 6 to 8 hours after circumcision.
  - Fever, low-grade temperature, bad smell to the drainage, pus at the site.
  - Plastibell falls off before 5 days or is displaced.
  - Scarring after the area has healed.

Supporting the Parent's Role through Discharge Teaching

Parent education is an essential part of normal newborn care. There are many things the parents need to know to effectively meet the needs of their infant. Because hospital stays are short, it is difficult to adequately teach parents everything they need to know and to give them time to absorb the information and ask questions. At the very least, instructions should be written so that the parents can refer to them as needed. Family Teaching Tips: General Tips for Newborn Care at Home provides helpful information for new parents.

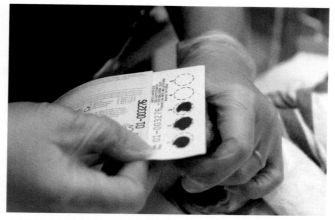

● *Figure 15.7* The nurse collects a blood specimen on a special card to screen the newborn for treatable disorders that otherwise might cause mental retardation, disability, or even death.

Some hospitals have newborn teaching videos that can be sent home with the parents. Newborn care classes often are available that can be started before discharge and continued for several weeks or months afterward. Some hospitals have home visitation programs in which a nurse or clinical nurse specialist follows up with the new family at home. All of these are ways to extend the teaching time and allow for parents to absorb the material and formulate questions.

Pay close attention. It is important that teaching be individualized to the needs of the parents. If the parents are inexperienced, it is important that they feel confident in their ability to care for their child. Tactfully role model care of the newborn, then give them the chance to develop their skills while you are available to assist. Sincerely compliment them when they do well.

Return demonstrations and home visits allow for direct observation of the parents' ability to care for their child. Several important topics that need to be discussed with parents are covered in this section.

Handling the Newborn. New parents are often anxious about picking up their newborn for the first time. Assist them to slide one hand under the neck and shoulders and place the other hand under the buttocks or between the legs before gently lifting the newborn. Because newborns cannot support their head for the first few months, it is necessary for parents to provide this support when holding the baby.

Demonstrate different ways to hold the newborn (Fig. 15-8). The football hold is one position that allows the parent to support the head and

FAMILY TEACHING TIPS

General Tips for Newborn Care at Home

FEEDING

- Most newborns eat every 2 to 4 hours. Feeding patterns become fairly regular in approximately 2 weeks.
- Regurgitation ("spitting up") is expected. Vomiting should be reported to the pediatrician. Frequent vomiting can quickly lead to dehydration. Projectile vomiting may indicate an obstruction.

SLEEPING

- Newborns sleep approximately 16 to 20 hours per day.
- It is a good idea for the caregiver to rest frequently throughout the day and sleep when the baby sleeps.
- For the first 3 to 4 months, it is difficult for infants to fall asleep by themselves. It is helpful for the parent to rock, walk, cuddle, or otherwise comfort the infant as he tries to fall asleep. After 4 months of age, the parent can help the baby learn to fall asleep at predictable times.
- There are wide variations of "normal" as to when babies sleep through the night. Some are able to do so by 6 to 7 weeks of age. Others may not until they are 3 or 4 months old.
- It does not help a baby sleep through the night to introduce solid foods too soon. A newborn's digestive system is immature and not ready to handle large protein molecules until approximately 4 months of age.

CRYING

- It is normal for a newborn to cry approximately 2 hours per day for the first 6 to 7 weeks of life.
- A "fussy period" during the day is to be expected.
- Crying is the way a baby communicates. First check the baby for physical causes of discomfort, such as a wet or dirty diaper or hunger. Then try all or some of the following suggestions to help quiet the baby.
  - Rock the baby.
  - Carry the baby and walk.
  - Take the baby for a stroll in the stroller.
  - Put the baby in a baby swing or a rocking cradle.
  - Gently pat or stroke the baby's back.
  - Swaddle the baby.
  - Take the baby for a ride in the car.
  - Turn on some white noise—washing machine, vacuum cleaner, air conditioner, radio not tuned to a station, etc.
- Never shake a baby for any reason. If you have tried everything and the baby continues to cry, put the baby down in a safe place and take a time-out. It won't hurt him to cry for a short time by himself. Also, you could ask someone else to take over for awhile.

SENSORY INPUT

- Babies' brains need stimulation to develop. Use the five senses to communicate with the baby.
- Visual stimulation can be as simple as making faces with your baby during periods of alertness. Mobiles are another means of visual enrichment.
- Talking, singing, and reading give the baby auditory stimulation.
- Holding and cuddling the baby and letting him touch different textures and shapes develops the sense of touch.
- Pay attention to your baby's cues. She will let you know when she has had enough stimulation and needs rest.

HEALTH MAINTENANCE

- Be sure to make an appointment with the pediatrician within the time frame given to you at discharge; usually at 2 weeks of age.
- Be sure to take the baby for follow-up screening and for immunizations at the appropriate times.
- Recognize signs of illness and follow up with the physician if these signs are present.
  - Fever
  - Vomiting
  - Unusually fussy
  - Diarrhea (frequent, watery stools)
  - Yellow or blue color to the skin
  - Breathing that appears stressed
  - Refuses to eat or has a poor suck
  - Appears listless.

A

B

C

● *Figure 15.8* (**A**) The nurse teaches the new mother to support the newborn using the football hold. (**B**) The grandfather is using the familiar cradle hold. (**C**) The new father demonstrates the shoulder hold.

body with one hand because the body is tucked under the arm. This leaves one hand free for other tasks. Instruct the parents to use the football hold judiciously while walking because the head is largely unprotected with this hold. Cradling the baby is familiar to most parents, as is the shoulder hold, which is sometimes comforting for a colicky baby. Newborns should always be placed on their backs to sleep to reduce the risk for SIDS.

Teach the parents to swaddle the newborn. Swaddling gives the newborn a sense of security and is comforting. Demonstrate and then let the parents give a return demonstration. Place the blanket in such a way that the newborn is positioned diagonally on the blanket. Fold down the top corner of the blanket under the

infant's head. Pull the left corner around the front of the infant and tuck it under his arm. Pull up the bottom corner and tuck it in the front. Pull the right corner around the front of the infant and tuck it under the left arm (Fig. 15-9).

Handwashing before and after handling the baby is the best way parents can protect their newborn from infection. They should also encourage visitors to wash their hands before touching the baby. Anyone with obvious illness should not visit until he or she is well again.

Clearing the Airway. Teach the parents how to use the bulb syringe. Depress the bulb first and then place it in the newborn's mouth, if excess secretions are noted. The nose is suctioned last. Clean the bulb with warm water and a mild soap. Sneezing is a normal response to particles in the

● *Figure 15.9* The nurse shows the new mother how to swaddle her newborn.

air and is not indicative of a cold. Yellow or green nasal drainage are signs of illness that should be reported to the physician. If the baby turns blue or stops breathing for longer than a few seconds, the parents should seek immediate emergency care (call 911).

Maintaining Adequate Temperature. Parents should be taught to protect their newborn from drafts and to adequately dress the infant. However, sometimes the temptation is to overdress the newborn. The best advice is to instruct the parents to dress the newborn in the amount and quality of clothes that would keep the parents comfortable in the environment. Check the baby's temperature if he seems ill. Temperatures of less than 97.7°F or greater than 100° F should be reported to the physician.

Monitoring Stool and Urine Patterns. It is normal for the newborn to have 6 to 10 wet diapers per day after the first day of life. Instruct the parents to report if the newborn does not void at all within a 12-hour period. Frequent, regular voiding indicates the newborn is getting enough milk.

Newborn stools initially are dark greenish-black and tarry. These stools are referred to as meconium. Transitional stools are lighter green or light green-yellow and are looser in character than is meconium. Most babies are having transitional stools by the time they are discharged home. In general, breast-fed babies have softer, less formed stools that have a sweetish odor to them. Bottle-fed babies tend to have more well-formed stools that are a little darker in color with a more unpleasant odor.

Signs of constipation are infrequent hard, dry stools. Babies normally turn red in the face and strain when passing stools. These signs do not indicate constipation. Diarrhea is defined as fre-

quent stools with high water content. Because newborns dehydrate quickly, it is important for parents to notify the physician if the newborn has more than two episodes of diarrhea in one day.

Providing Skin Care. Teach new parents about normal, expected skin changes such as Mongolian spots and newborn rash (refer to Chapter 13 to review this material). A sponge bath should be given until the cord falls off, approximately 10 to 12 days after birth. Newborns need protection from chilling when they are bathed. It also is important for parents to monitor the water temperature to prevent scalding the newborn's tender skin. Daily tub baths are not necessary and may dry the skin. Some physicians want the parents to cleanse the cord site with alcohol several times daily.

Maintaining Safety. Newborns quickly learn to roll over and can move around on surfaces, even if unintentionally. For this reason, newborns and infants should never be left unattended on high surfaces, such as on dressing tables or beds. They also should not be left unattended around any amount of water to avoid the possibility of drowning. Plastic should not be used to cover infant mattresses or on any object to which the newborn has contact to protect from suffocation. Pillows are not needed and may be dangerous for the young infant.

Parents need to be taught to differentiate normal from abnormal newborn observations and behaviors. A yellow tint to the skin is indicative of jaundice and should be reported to the physician promptly. Untreated jaundice can lead to permanent brain damage. Listlessness and poor feeding behaviors are signs of illness that should be reported. Teach the parents normal behavior states of newborns and help them learn to read the special cues their baby gives regarding when and how much interaction he can tolerate (refer to Chapter 13).

Proper use of car seats is a critical skill for new parents to learn. Car seats save lives, and infants should never be transported in a car without one. Most states have laws regarding their use, and parents must be familiar with these laws. Newborns are safest in rear-facing seats placed in the middle of the back seat of the car. Parents should never place car seats in the front seat of cars equipped with air bags because death and injury have occurred when air bags deploy and infants are strapped into the front seat. If it is absolutely necessary to place the infant in a car seat in the front seat, there must be no air bag or the air bag must be professionally disabled. Parents should be thoroughly familiar with the operation of the car seat they choose.

EVALUATION: GOALS AND EXPECTED OUTCOMES

- **Goal:** The newborn will maintain an adequate level of comfort during the hospital stay.
  Expected Outcomes: The newborn shows signs of contentment, is not overly fussy, and does not show other signs of pain, particularly during and after painful procedures.

- **Goal:** The newborn remains free from signs and symptoms of preventable diseases.
  Expected Outcomes: The newborn is immunized against Hepatitis B, the parents describe when to take the newborn for repeat vaccinations for all childhood diseases, the newborn receives mandatory screening for metabolic and hearing disorders, and the parents explain what follow-up is necessary and what to do if the screens are abnormal.

- **Goal:** The parents will be able to adequately care for their newborn at home.
  Expected Outcomes: The parents demonstrate the skills needed to adequately care for their newborn; verbalize signs that should initiate a call to the physician when follow-up is needed, and how to find answers to questions that come up during the care of their newborn.

Test Yourself

- Name one advantage and one disadvantage of circumcision.

- What substance, in addition to the vaccination, is given to a newborn whose mother is positive for the hepatitis B surface antigen?

- List three ways parents can deal with newborn crying?

KEY POINTS

- The delivery room should be prepared for resuscitation of the newborn before birth. Resuscitation supplies should be checked and the warmer turned on in anticipation of the birth. If resuscitation is needed, Neonatal Resuscitation Program guidelines should be followed.

- The Apgar score is a way of determining how well the newborn is transitioning to life outside the womb. Five parameters (respiratory effort, heart rate, muscle tone, reflex irritability, and color) are all used to assign a score at 1 and 5 minutes of life. A healthy, vigorous newborn has a 5-minute score of 7 or greater.

- Steps should be taken to prevent the newborn from becoming overly cold or overly hot. A thermoneutral environment is ideal in which the temperature is maintained at a level so that heat is neither gained nor lost.

- Eye prophylaxis to prevent eye infection from gonorrhea should be instituted within the first hour after birth. Vitamin K is given IM to prevent bleeding problems.

- Identification bands are placed immediately in the delivery room before newborn and parents are separated.

- Hypoglycemia is a blood glucose level less than 40 mg/dL. Newborns can have no symptoms or may demonstrate multiple signs. The most common sign is shakiness or jitteriness. Hypoglycemia is best prevented and treated with early and regular feedings.

- Maintaining the newborn with his own crib and supplies, using excellent handwashing technique, and minimizing exposure to sick people are all measures nurses take to decrease the risk for cross-contamination and infection in the newborn.

- Nurses must be vigilantly on guard for suspicious activity in and around a nursery. The risk for abduction is a real threat. The nurse should teach the parents to ask to see identification before releasing their newborn to anyone.

- Newborns show behavioral and physiologic responses, such as crying, grimacing (or making other faces), and increased heart and respiratory rates, to painful procedures.

- Circumcision remains a controversial procedure. The AAP strongly recommends the use of analgesia and anesthesia for the procedure. If the parents choose not to circumcise, they must be taught proper hygiene for the uncircumcised penis.

- All newborns should receive a hepatitis B vaccination and screening for metabolic diseases such as phenylketonuria and congenital hypothyroidism that can lead to profound mental retardation and disability if left untreated.

- Parents need to learn how to hold and position their infant, how to clear the airway, maintain adequate body temperature, monitor stool and urine patterns, provide skin care, and maintain safety of their newborn.

REFERENCES AND SELECTED READINGS

Books and Journals

American Academy of Pediatrics. (2003). Campaign launched to avoid sudden death in child care settings. News release. Retrieved June 25, 2004, from http://www.aap.org/advocacy/archives/jansids.htm

American Academy of Pediatrics. (2002). Hearing: Newborn screening. Medical Library article. Retrieved August 29, 2002, from http://www.medem.com/MedLB/article_detaillb.cfm?article_ID = ZZZS5I9Y65D&sub_cat = 108

American Academy of Pediatrics NRP Steering Committee. (2000). *Neonatal Resuscitation Program: Textbook of Neonatal Resuscitation* (4th ed.). Elk Grave Village, IL: American Academy of Pediatrics.

American Academy of Pediatrics Policy Statement. (2000). Prevention and management of pain and stress in the neonate. *Pediatrics, 105*(2), 454–461. Retrieved August 29, 2002, from http://www.aap.org/policy/re9945.html

American Academy of Pediatrics Policy Statements. (1971, 1975, 1977, 1989). *Circumcision*. Found on the CIRP Circumcision Information and Resource Pages website. Retrieved August 29, 2002, from http://www.cirp.org/library/statements/aap/

Anand, K. J. S., & Hickey, P. R. (1987). Pain and its effects in the human neonate and fetus. *New England Journal of Medicine, 317*(21), 1321–1329. Retrieved August 29, 2002, from http://www.cirtl.org/pain.htm

Brooks, C. (1997). Neonatal hypoglycemia. *Neonatal Network, 16*(2), 15–21.

Burgess, A. W., & Lanning, K. V. (Eds.). (2003). *An analysis of infant abductions*. Developed from a study by the National Center for Missing and Exploited Children, the US Department of Justice, and the University of Pennsylvania's School of Nursing. 2nd ed. Retrieved January 20, 2004, from http://www.missingkids.com/en_US/publications/NC66.pdf

Cranmer, H., & Shannon, M. (2001). Pediatrics, hypoglycemia. D. Slapper, R. Konop, W. Wolfram, J. Halamka, & W. K. Mallon, (Eds.), *eMedicine*. Retrieved August 31, 2002, from http://www.emedicine.com/emerg/topic384.htm

Cunningham, F. G., Gant, N. F., Leveno, K. J., Gilstrap, L. C. III, Hauth, J. C., & Wenstrom, K. D. (2001). The newborn infant. *Williams obstetrics* (21st ed., pp. 385–402). New York: McGraw Hill Medical Publishing Division.

Evans, N. (1998). Hypoglycaemia. *Department of neonatal medicine protocol book, Royal Prince Alfred Hospital*. Retrieved August 30, 2002, from http://www.cs.nsw.gov.au/rpa/neonatal/html/newprot/hypogly.htm

Fletcher, M. A. (1999). Physical assessment and classification. In G. B. Avery, M. A. Fletcher, & M. G. MacDonald (Eds.), *Neonatology: Pathophysiology & management of the newborn* (5th ed., pp. 301–320). Philadelphia: Lippincott Williams & Wilkins.

Freij, B. J., & McCracken, G. H. (1999). Acute infections. In G. B. Avery, M. A. Fletcher, & M. G. MacDonald (Eds.), *Neonatology: Pathophysiology & management of the newborn* (5th ed., pp. 1189–1207). Philadelphia: Lippincott Williams & Wilkins.

Geyer, J., Ellsbury, D., Kleiber, C., Litwiller, D., Hinton, A., & Yankowitz, J. (2002). An evidence-based multidisciplinary protocol for neonatal circumcision pain management. *JOGNN, 31*(4), 403–410.

Kauffman, G. R., & Word, T. M. (1997). Neonatal hypoglycemia (medical negligence). *Trial, 33*(5), 42–46.

Kelly, J. M. (1999). General care. In G. B. Avery, M. A. Fletcher, & M. G. MacDonald (Eds.), *Neonatology: Pathophysiology & management of the newborn* (5th ed., pp. 333–343). Philadelphia: Lippincott Williams & Wilkins.

North American Nursing Diagnosis Association (NANDA). (2001). *NANDA nursing diagnoses: Definitions & classification 2001–2002*. Philadelphia: Author.

Owens, A. M. (2003). Researchers spend hours studying newborns' pain at being circumcised. *National Post*, Toronto, December 30, 2003. Retrieved January 20, 2004, from http://www.cirp.org/news/nationalpost 12-30-03/

Richardson, H. (1997). Kangaroo care: Why does it work? *Midwifery Today, 44*(Winter):50–51. Retrieved August 28, 2002, from http://www.midwiferytoday.com/articles/kangaroocare.asp

Websites
Newborn Care
http://www.nlm.nih.gov/medlineplus/infantandnewborncare.html

Cord Care
http://www.rcp.gov.bc.ca/Guidelines/Newborn/Master.NB10.CordCare.February.pdf

Vitamin K
http://www.rcp.gov.bc.ca/Guidelines/Newborn/Master.NB12.VitK.pdf

WORKBOOK

NCLEX-STYLE REVIEW QUESTIONS

1. Baby Boy Alvarez is 5 minutes old. The nurse performs a quick assessment and determines that the newborn has a heart rate of 110 bpm, a weak cry, and acrocyanosis. His extremities are held in partial flexion, and he grimaces when a catheter is placed in his nose. What Apgar score does the nurse record?

   a. 5–The newborn is having extreme difficulty transitioning.

   b. 5–The newborn is having moderate difficulty transitioning.

   c. 6–The newborn is having moderate difficulty transitioning.

   d. 6–The newborn is vigorous and transitioning with minimal effort.

2. The delivery room nurse has just brought a 10-pound newborn to the nursery. You will be monitoring the newborn during the transition period. Which assessment parameter will *most* likely inhibit this newborn's transition?

   a. Apgar score

   b. Blood sugar

   c. Heart rate

   d. Temperature

3. The newborn has just been delivered. He is placed in skin-to-skin contact with his mother. A blanket covers all of his body except his head. His hair is still wet with amniotic fluid, etc. What is the most likely type of heat loss this baby may experience?

   a. Conductive

   b. Convective

   c. Evaporative

   d. Radiating

4. A woman dressed in hospital scrub attire without a name badge presents to the nursery and says that Mrs. Smith is ready for her baby. She offers to take the baby back to Mrs. Smith. What response by the nurse is best in this situation?

   a. "I don't know you. Are you trying to take a baby?"

   b. "Leave immediately! I'm calling security."

   c. "May I see your identification, please?"

   d. "You must be Mrs. Smith's sister. She said her sister is a nurse."

STUDY ACTIVITIES

1. Develop a poster that shows nurses ways to prevent transmitting infections in the nursery.
2. Develop a handout for nurses with helpful tips on preventing infant abductions. Use an Internet search to help you find material for the handout.
3. Make a discharge teaching handout for parents of a newborn.

CRITICAL THINKING: What Would You Do?

Apply your knowledge of the nurse's role in newborn care to the following situations.

1. A neighbor calls to tell you that his wife just delivered her newborn in the living room. The ambulance is on the way but is not yet there. You run to the house and find the baby loosely wrapped in a blanket. The neighbor says the baby was born approximately 2 minutes before you arrived.

   a. What actions do you take first and why?

   b. The newborn becomes jittery and irritable. What do you suspect may be the problem?

   c. What two interventions will need to be carried out as soon as the newborn and mother can be safely transported to a health care facility?

2. Mrs. Mathias just delivered a baby boy. He cries immediately and is pink. The newborn's cry sounds "wet" and "gurgly."

   a. What action should the nurse take first?

   b. If the respirations continue to sound wet, what step would the nurse take next?

3. Newborn Boy Hinojosa is crying and thrashing about after a circumcision.

   a. What is the likely cause of his crying?

   b. What should the nurse do in this situation?

4. A new mother calls the nursery from home. She and her newborn were discharged 2 days ago. She is worried about a small amount of yellow crust she notes at the circumcision site. She is also worried because the baby has been crying and fussy for the last hour.

   a. How would you advise the mother regarding the yellow crusting?

   b. What suggestions could you give her for the crying?

Childbearing at Risk

Pregnancy at Risk: Conditions That Complicate Pregnancy

16

STUDENT OBJECTIVES

On completion of this chapter, the student should be able to

1. List the advantages of tight glycemic control for the pregnant woman with diabetes.
2. Differentiate between the care of the pregnant woman with pregestational diabetes and one with gestational diabetes.
3. Describe typical nursing concerns for the pregnant woman with diabetes.
4. Explain the goals of treatment and nursing care for the pregnant woman with heart disease.
5. Differentiate between pregnancy concerns for the woman with iron-deficiency anemia and one with sickle cell anemia.
6. List treatment considerations for the pregnant woman with asthma.
7. Detail the risk to pregnancy from epilepsy.
8. Describe the impact on pregnancy from the TORCH infections.
9. Differentiate between common sexually transmitted infections according to cause, treatment, and impact on pregnancy.
10. Outline treatment for the pregnant woman with human immunodeficiency virus/acquired immunodeficiency syndrome (HIV/AIDS).
11. Describe nursing considerations for the pregnant woman with a sexually transmitted infection.
12. Outline components of a treatment plan for the pregnant woman who is the victim of intimate partner violence.
13. Delineate special concerns associated with adolescent pregnancy.
14. Describe the impact of delayed childbearing on pregnancy.

KEY TERMS

dermatome
diabetogenic effect of pregnancy
gestational diabetes
hyperglycemia
hyperinsulinemia
hypoglycemia
macrosomia
perinatologist
pregestational diabetes
status asthmaticus
status epilepticus
TORCH

In the very recent past, many women with chronic conditions were unable to successfully accomplish pregnancy and/or childbirth. Now that there are effective treatments available for many of these conditions, more women are entering pregnancy with chronic medical conditions. Consequently, the obstetric nurse is challenged to stay abreast of current research findings to intervene appropriately and to educate the woman carrying an at-risk pregnancy. The licensed vocational/practical nurse (LPN) assists the registered nurse (RN) to provide care for the pregnant woman at risk.

Highly specialized knowledge is needed to successfully manage the at-risk pregnancy. Maternal–fetal medicine is a branch of medical science that focuses on the perinatal period. A maternal–fetal medicine specialist is also referred to as a **perinatologist**. This physician specialist is an obstetrician who has received advanced training and specializes in the care of at-risk pregnancies. The perinatologist is competent in the diagnosis and treatment of the pregnant woman who presents with a pre-existing medical condition or who experiences a complication of pregnancy. The perinatologist sometimes provides consultations for the obstetrician who is managing the pregnancy. Alternatively, he or she may co-manage the woman's pregnancy with the obstetrician or be the primary care provider.

PREGNANCY COMPLICATED BY MEDICAL CONDITIONS

Chronic medical conditions and acute infections are risk factors for the pregnant woman. There are several ways in which pregnancy and medical conditions are interrelated. Pregnancy can affect the underlying medical disorder. The normal physiologic changes of pregnancy sometimes alleviate and at other times intensify the symptoms of illness. On the other hand, medical conditions can affect the progress and outcome of pregnancy. Frequently, the fetus is affected adversely by chronic medical conditions of the pregnant woman.

Diabetes Mellitus

Diabetes mellitus (DM) is a chronic disease in which glucose metabolism is impaired by lack of insulin in the body or by ineffective insulin utilization. DM, particularly if it is controlled poorly, can adversely affect pregnancy outcomes. Conversely, pregnancy affects glucose metabolism, which makes the disease challenging to manage. Approximately 4% of pregnancies are complicated by DM (Moore, 2002).

It is recommended that specialists be involved in the care of the pregnant woman with DM. Sometimes the obstetrician consults with an endocrinologist, who then manages the woman's DM throughout her pregnancy. At other times the obstetrician consults with the perinatologist or the perinatologist manages the woman with DM during her pregnancy. A team approach to the management of DM during pregnancy results in the best outcomes. It is recommended that the team be composed of the primary care physician, a registered nurse, a certified diabetic educator, a registered dietitian, and a social worker (Moore, 2002).

Classification of Diabetes Mellitus

There are two overall categories of DM: type 1 and type 2. These two diseases are very different in nature. They both affect glucose metabolism, but type 1 is characterized by a lack of insulin in the body, whereas type 2 is most often associated with insulin resistance. A woman who enters pregnancy with either type 1 or type 2 DM is said to have **pregestational diabetes**. According to the March of Dimes (2003), approximately 1 in 100 women of childbearing age has pregestational DM. Most women of childbearing age do not have full-blown type 2 DM. More often, a woman who is at risk for type 2 DM will develop **gestational diabetes** (GDM), a type of DM that is unique to pregnancy but in many respects mimics type 2 DM. The large majority (90%) of women whose pregnancies are complicated by DM have GDM (Moore, 2002).

Pregestational Diabetes Mellitus

Historically, the woman with pregestational type 1 DM had a higher incidence of spontaneous abortions (miscarriages). If the woman was able to carry the pregnancy to term, the fetus was at high risk for congenital anomalies and/or stillbirth. Fortunately, outcomes have been improved greatly with early monitoring and strict control of blood glucose levels. However, if DM is controlled poorly, particularly in the early weeks of pregnancy, the woman is two to four times more likely to experience a poor outcome, such as a child with a serious birth defect or stillbirth. Other pregnancy-related complications associated with pre-existing DM include pregnancy-induced hypertension, polyhydramnios (excess levels of amniotic fluid), preterm delivery, and shoulder dystocia (Cunningham et al., 2001c). The diabetic woman is three times as likely to experience a cesarean birth as a woman who does not have DM (Moore, 2002).

Some women who have had DM since childhood have damage to the blood vessels. Pregnancy has a tendency to speed up this damage. For example, if a woman has diabetic retinopathy (damage to the retina that can cause blindness), her vision may deteriorate during pregnancy. Fortunately, by approximately 6 months after delivery, vision returns to the prepregnant state. The most serious sequelae (consequences) of circulatory insufficiency occur in the kidneys, which can lead to renal damage and hypertension.

The placenta tends to be smaller, and maternal–fetal circulation is often decreased in longstanding DM, which may lead to chronic fetal hypoxemia and growth retardation, although, as with GDM (see discussion below), the fetus may be exceptionally large because of elevated maternal blood glucose levels. (Refer to Chapter 20 for a more detailed description of the newborn of the woman with diabetes.)

Gestational Diabetes Mellitus

The woman who develops GDM is at increased risk for developing type 2 DM. In fact, more than half of these women will go on to develop type 2 DM within 20 years. It may be that the pancreas of the woman with GDM has sufficient resources to sustain normal blood sugars when she is not pregnant; however, the stress of pregnancy may be enough to bring on GDM. She then experiences sustained periods of hyperglycemia and hyperinsulinemia, which puts her and the unborn child at risk.

The underlying pathophysiology of GDM is insulin resistance. Normal pregnancy is marked by insulin resistance. Tissues become resistant to insulin to provide sufficient levels of glucose for the growing fetus. Although the exact cause of insulin resistance in pregnancy is not known, it is thought that the hormones estrogen, progesterone, and human placental lactogen (HPL) are at least partially responsible. As these pregnancy hormones rise, insulin resistance increases. The result in a normal pregnancy is threefold:

1. Blood glucose levels are lower than normal (mild hypoglycemia) when fasting.
2. Blood glucose levels are higher than normal (mild hyperglycemia) after meals.
3. Insulin levels are increased (**hyperinsulinemia**) after meals.

Together these changes are referred to as the **diabetogenic effect of pregnancy**. GDM develops when the woman cannot tolerate this normal pregnancy change. Risk factors for GDM are listed in Box 16-1.

The greatest risk for the fetus of the woman with GDM is excessive growth, resulting in macrosomia and birth trauma (shoulder dystocia). Insulin does not cross the placenta; however, blood sugar does. Large amounts of glucose cross the placenta when the woman's blood sugar levels are elevated. The fetus does not have insulin resistance, so her pancreas produces increased levels of insulin to handle the high sugar load. As with any disproportionate intake of sugar, the excess calories are stored in the fetus' body in the form of fat. The fetus is also at risk for delayed lung maturity and other complications seen in the newborn of the woman with DM (refer to Chapter 20). Research indicates that long-range complications for the infant include risk for obesity and type 2 DM.

BOX 16.1 | **Risk Factors for Gestational Diabetes Mellitus (GDM)**

- History of a large-for-gestational age infant
- History of GDM
- Previous unexplained fetal demise
- Advanced maternal age (greater than 35 years)
- Family history of type 2 DM or GDM
- Obesity (greater than 200 pounds)
- Non-Caucasian ethnicity
- Fasting blood glucose of greater than 140 mg/dL
- Random blood glucose of greater than 200 mg/dL

Most women who develop GDM do not experience symptoms, although they may notice increased thirst, urinary frequency, hunger, or fatigue. Therefore, screening for GDM is a standard of obstetric care. Most obstetricians screen for GDM at approximately 24 to 28 weeks of pregnancy, although screening may be done as early as 20 weeks in states that have high rates (greater than 5%) of insulin resistance. If the woman has a history of GDM, she is usually screened at the first prenatal visit. The diagnosis of GDM is based on the results of the oral glucose tolerance test (OGTT). The OGTT is also referred to as a glucose challenge test. Box 16-2 outlines normal and diagnostic values of the OGTT.

Treatment

Prepregnancy Care

The woman who has type 1 DM is advised to consult with her physician before she becomes pregnant. Persistent maternal **hyperglycemia** (elevated blood glucose levels) is harmful to the growing fetus, particularly during the first 8 weeks of pregnancy, when organogenesis is occurring. Therefore, it is important for the woman to attain a state of euglycemia (normal blood glucose levels) in the months before becoming pregnant. It is also recommended that, several months before becoming pregnant, the woman with diabetes start taking a daily multivitamin supplement that contains at least 400

BOX 16.2 | **Diagnostic Values for the Oral Glucose Tolerance Test (OGTT)**

Normal values are
- Fasting—less than 95 mg/dL
- 1 hour—less than 180 mg/dL
- 2 hours—less than 155 mg/dL
- 3 hours—less than 140 mg/dL
GDM is diagnosed if two or more values meet or exceed the levels listed above.

micrograms of folic acid. Adequate folic acid intake is the best way to prevent neural tube defects, for which the woman's fetus is particularly susceptible.

Monitoring Glycemic Control

It is important to track the pattern of glycemic control. Average blood sugar levels during the past 4 to 8 weeks are determined by measuring glycosylated hemoglobin (HbA$_1$C). HbA$_1$C is a blood test that determines the percentage of red blood cells (RBCs) that have glucose incorporated in the hemoglobin. Sustained periods of hyperglycemia result in higher HbA$_1$C levels. Because elevated glucose levels are the most damaging to the fetus during the 1st trimester, the goal is for the HbA$_1$C to be less than 7% for 2 to 3 months before pregnancy is achieved. At this level, the risk of congenital anomalies is equal to that of the general population (1% to 2%). As a comparison, when the HbA$_1$C is greater than 8.5%, the risk of fetal deformity increases to 22.4% (Moore, 2002). HbA$_1$C levels are monitored throughout the pregnancy.

Monitoring Renal Function

In addition to glucose assessments, the physician monitors renal function in the woman with long-standing (greater than 10 years) type 1 DM, or if vascular disease is present. Renal function is the best indicator of pregnancy success for the woman with DM (Moore, 2002). Plasma creatinine and blood urea nitrogen (BUN) along with a 24-hour urine for protein and creatinine clearance are measured in each trimester.

Maintaining Glycemic Control

The most important goal of treatment is for the woman to maintain tight glycemic (blood sugar) control before and throughout pregnancy. Because of the increased challenge of managing blood sugar during pregnancy, the woman must monitor her blood sugar many times during the day. Frequently she will need to check her glucose levels seven times per day: upon awakening, after breakfast, before and after lunch, before and after dinner, and before bedtime. The goal is to maintain fasting blood glucose levels of less than 90 mg/dL. Glucose levels should not exceed 120 mg/dL 2 hours after meals, and should generally measure 80 to 110 mg/dL between meals. There are three main facets to glycemic control for the woman with type 1 DM: insulin, diet, and exercise (Fig. 16-1). Glycemic control for the woman with GDM focuses heavily on diet therapy and exercise. Insulin therapy is used if these modalities fail to control the diabetes.

Insulin Therapy. Blood glucose levels vary with advancing gestation. In the first few months of pregnancy, the woman's insulin requirements fluctuate widely, and she is at risk for episodes of **hypoglycemia**, low blood glucose levels, particularly between meals.

This phenomenon occurs because the rapidly growing embryo requires a constant supply of glucose, which may deplete maternal blood sugar levels. At the beginning of the 2nd trimester, insulin requirements stabilize, then begin to increase at approximately 24 weeks' gestation, continuing to increase until term. During labor, insulin needs are variable, and in the first 24 hours after delivery, insulin requirements fall dramatically. Because the pancreas of a woman with type 1 DM does not produce insulin, she must be on an insulin regimen. Twice-daily baseline doses of insulin may be ordered to be self-administered subcutaneously. Often a combination of regular and intermediate and/or long-acting insulin is ordered. The baseline doses are supplemented by regular insulin on a sliding scale basis, depending on glucose levels obtained throughout the day.

Insulin may be administered in low doses throughout the day with the use of an insulin pump. An insulin pump is a small device, approximately the size of a pager, that can be worn with a belt or placed in a pocket. A flexible tube placed in the subcutaneous tissue of the abdomen delivers the insulin. The pump has several advantages. Its action mimics that of a healthy pancreas. The woman gets a continuous basal flow of insulin, which helps keep her blood sugar stable throughout the day. She can give herself an insulin bolus by pushing a button before eating or if her glucose level is elevated above a predetermined level. Some women find the pumps more comfortable and less intrusive than self-administering insulin several times per day.

Insulin therapy is recommended for women with GDM when, despite diet and exercise, fasting blood sugar levels cannot be maintained lower than 95 mg/dL or 2 hour postprandial (after meals) sugars below 120 mg/dL. When insulin becomes necessary, the woman is usually hospitalized to titrate the dose and to provide education on self-administration.

Caution is in order! Although gestational diabetes (GDM) is similar to type 2 DM, oral hypoglycemic agents are not used because they are considered to be teratogenic (damaging to the fetus).

Diet Therapy. Another important part of diabetes management during pregnancy is diet therapy. In fact, the cornerstone of treatment for GDM is diet therapy, although insulin may be required, depending upon the severity of glucose intolerance. The goals of dietary intervention for any type of DM during pregnancy, in addition to supplying the nutritional needs of the woman and her fetus, are to maintain blood sugar levels in the normal range and to prevent

Goals:
Tight glycemic control
with a healthy mother and baby

● *Figure 16.1* Treatment overview for diabetes in pregnancy. For women with pregestational type 1 DM, the foundation of glycemic management is insulin therapy along with dietary management, exercise, and fetal surveillance. For the woman who develops gestational diabetes (GDM), dietary modification is generally the foundation of treatment. Some women with GDM require insulin therapy, and others do not. Exercise and fetal surveillance are also important facets of care.

ketoacidosis. Consultation with a registered dietitian, preferably one who is also a certified diabetic educator, is recommended because diet requirements are individualized.

The objective is to eat so as to avoid surges and dips in blood sugar. The recommended diet includes a total caloric intake of 30 to 35 kcal/kg of ideal body weight per day. The nutrients are divided so that approximately 55% of dietary intake is composed of carbohydrates, 20% is protein, and 25% is fat (less than 10% should be saturated fat). Ideally the woman spreads her food intake over the day by eating three regular meals interspersed with three snacks.

Exercise. Exercise is another way to help control blood sugar for the woman with DM. However, the pregnant woman should always consult with her physician before exercising, particularly if her diabetes is poorly controlled or she has diabetes complications, such as vascular damage, hypertension, or renal insufficiency. It is generally recommended that exercises should put minimum stress on the trunk region to avoid fetal injury (Cunningham et al., 2001c). Exercise that involves the upper arm muscles, such as swimming, is ideal.

Fetal Surveillance

Fetal surveillance is critical for the woman with DM. An initial sonogram is done during the 1st trimester to determine gestational age and fetal viability. A more detailed, high-level sonogram is usually repeated at 18 to 20 weeks to look closely for structural defects in the fetus. Fetal anatomy is carefully assessed for abnormalities, and amniotic fluid volume is measured. Maternal serum alpha-fetoprotein levels are measured at 16 to 20 weeks to screen for neural tube defects. If HbA_1C levels were elevated in early pregnancy, a fetal echocardiogram is recommended in the 2nd trimester. Serial sonograms in the 3rd trimester (from approximately 26 weeks) are done every 4 to 6 weeks to measure fetal growth. The fetus of the woman with DM may grow to be unusually large, a condition known as **macrosomia**, which is diagnosed if the birth weight exceeds 4,500 grams (9.9 pounds) or the birth weight is greater than the 90th percentile for gestational age. Macrosomia occurs more commonly in women with gestational DM. Conversely, if the woman has longstanding DM or vascular disease, the fetus may be predisposed to intrauterine growth restriction (IUGR).

Third trimester fetal surveillance is vital to help detect signs of fetal stress that precede fetal death. Fetal activity counts are initiated daily at 28 weeks' gestation. At 28 to 34 weeks' gestation, twice-weekly nonstress testing (NST) is begun. A weekly biophysical profile (BPP) is generally recommended, and contraction stress tests (CSTs) are done if the NST is nonreactive or the BPP is nonreassuring. (Refer to Chapter 7 to review prenatal fetal testing.)

Determining Timing of Delivery

Determining the optimum time and method of delivery is a consideration in the care of the pregnant woman with DM. The challenge for the obstetrician is to schedule the delivery to avoid fetal death, while giving the fetus time to mature fully. Fetal lung maturation is often delayed, which predisposes the newborn to respiratory distress. Therefore, 3rd trimester amniocentesis may be done to document fetal lung maturity (a lecithin-to-sphingomyelin ratio of at least 2:1). Many women with DM have labor induced at 39 weeks' gestation if the cervix is favorable and the fetal lungs are mature. If the pregnancy is allowed to progress too long, there is an increased chance for delivery complications, such as shoulder dystocia and fetal demise.

● Nursing Process for the Pregnant Woman With DM

ASSESSMENT

The woman with type 1 DM usually has the disease diagnosed during childhood or adolescence. Therefore, she may be accustomed to monitoring her blood glucose levels and self-administering insulin. However, it is likely that she will need to increase the number of times she monitors daily. Have her do a return demonstration of self-glucose monitoring and recording of results. Be sure that she has a log and understands the importance of recording each blood sugar level.

Once GDM has been diagnosed, assess for understanding of therapeutic regimen management. Instruct the woman to bring her blood sugar log to every prenatal visit. Review the log with her and discuss blood sugar patterns noted. Assess her ability to self-manage her condition. Inquire regarding signs and symptoms of urinary tract infection and/or candidiasis. In the 3rd trimester, institute fetal surveillance as ordered by the physician.

During labor, frequent monitoring of blood glucose levels is required, sometimes as frequently as every hour. If the woman is unable to maintain normal glucose levels, an intravenous insulin drip may be initiated, with the insulin dose titrated to maintain glucose levels within a predetermined range. Chapter 20 covers care of the infant of the woman with diabetes.

SELECTED NURSING DIAGNOSES

- Ineffective Therapeutic Regimen Management
- Risk for Injury (maternal) related to unstable glucose levels: hypoglycemia or hyperglycemia and increased risk for obstetric complications
- Risk for Infection: vaginal candidiasis and/or urinary tract infection (UTI) related to elevated blood glucose levels
- Risk for Injury (fetal): fetal demise or birth trauma related to unstable maternal blood sugars or maternal hyperinsulinemia
- Risk for Disproportionate Growth: fetal macrosomia related to maternal hyperglycemia

OUTCOME IDENTIFICATION AND PLANNING

Appropriate goals may include that the woman will manage the therapeutic regimen successfully; maternal injury from hypoglycemia, hyperglycemia, and obstetric complications will be avoided; and the woman will remain free from infection. Fetal goals may include that the fetus will maintain health status, will be appropriate size for gestational age at birth, and will avoid birth trauma. Other goals and interventions are planned according to the individualized needs of the woman throughout pregnancy, birth, and the postpartum period.

IMPLEMENTATION

Monitoring Management of Therapeutic Regimen

With the assistance of the primary health care provider, information obtained regularly by self-monitoring or blood testing at home with a portable glucose monitor gives immediate feedback on effect of diet, activity, and medications on glucose levels. At every office visit carefully review the woman's blood sugar log. If she is having difficulty maintaining her blood glucose levels within the expected parameters, explore with her possible reasons.

Dietary recall for the past 3 days may be helpful for identifying patterns of food intake that interfere with blood sugar control. Refer the woman for a consult with a registered dietitian, if she is having difficulty following the prescribed dietary regimen. Review with the woman her exercise patterns to determine if improved blood sugar control might result from implementation of an exercise regimen

Carefully explore the woman's compliance with insulin administration. If she is having difficulty controlling her blood glucose levels, ask her to do a return demonstration by having her check her blood sugar levels. If possible, request that she do a return demonstration of insulin preparation and/or administration. Assist her to correct her technique, if necessary.

Frequent episodes of hypoglycemia may be caused by too much insulin or too little food. Explore her pattern of food intake in conjunction with insulin administration. Be certain she is eating three regular meals and three snacks daily. Food intake should follow insulin administration. A pattern of regular exercise may decrease insulin needs. Notify the physician of frequent episodes of hypoglycemia, particularly if the woman began a regular exercise program 3 to 4 weeks previously.

Preventing Maternal Injury

The woman with DM is at risk for unstable blood sugar levels and the associated risks. Take particular care to review the signs and symptoms of hypoglycemia (Box 16-3) with the woman and her family. The woman with pregestational DM is often aware of her hypoglycemic symptoms because she has been dealing with diabetes for some time. Explain that it is important to pay attention to the warning signals because she is more prone to hypoglycemia during pregnancy.

Pay close attention! One of the disadvantages of maintaining a euglycemic state is increased risk for hypoglycemia. Teach the woman the signs of hypoglycemia. Instruct her to keep a ready source of glucose (e.g., a candy bar or glass of orange juice) close by. Family members should know how to administer glucagon intramuscularly in the event of hypoglycemic coma.

Although any woman with DM is at risk for developing diabetic ketoacidosis (DKA), the woman with type 1 DM during pregnancy is at highest risk. She should know the signs of developing hyperglycemia and avoid triggers for DKA. Box 16-4 details these signs and triggers.

The woman with DM is at increased risk for pregnancy-induced hypertension (PIH). In the 3rd trimester the physician will likely recommend weekly blood pressure and urinary protein measurements. At every office visit carefully screen the woman for signs of PIH, such as headache, visual disturbances, epigastric pain, generalized edema, urinary protein, and elevated

blood pressure. Inform the woman to immediately call the physician if she should experience any of the symptoms of PIH.

Monitoring for and Preventing Infection

The woman with diabetes is at increased risk for urinary tract infections (UTI) because of elevated blood sugar levels. Review with the woman the

---

BOX 16.3	**Signs of Hypoglycemia**

It is particularly important for the pregnant woman and her family to be familiar with the signs and symptoms of hypoglycemia because she is more vulnerable to the condition during pregnancy. Sometimes it helps to remember that the symptoms of hypoglycemia mimic those of the fight-or-flight response. The woman may experience any of the following symptoms.
- Anxiety
- Shakiness
- Confusion
- Headache
- Tingling sensations around the mouth
- Hunger
- Sudden behavior change
- Pale skin
- Cold, clammy skin
- Increased pulse
- Seizure
- Unresponsiveness

BOX 16.4	**Diabetic Ketoacidosis (DKA) and Pregnancy**

The onset of DKA is marked by the classic symptoms of hyperglycemia, which include
- Polydipsia (excessive thirst)
- Polyuria (increased frequency and amount of urine)
- Polyphagia (excessive hunger)

As DKA develops, the following symptoms appear
- Glucose >300 mg/dL
- Ketonuria
- Kussmaul respirations
- Acetone (like alcohol) breath
- Sleepiness
- Language slurring
- Decreased consciousness

Triggers for DKA include (but are not limited to) the following
- Too little insulin or too much food
- Infection
- Tocolytic therapy (to prevent preterm labor)
- Corticosteroid use
- Insulin pump failure

signs of a UTI, which include increased frequency, voiding small amounts, burning with urination, and cloudy urine. Teach her to drink 8 to 10 glasses of noncaffeinated beverages every day to help prevent UTI, and to wipe from front to back after using the restroom. Frequent hand-washing (before and after meals and using the restroom) continues to be the best way to prevent infection. Remind the woman that if a UTI occurs, prompt treatment is essential because UTI can cause premature labor.

Candidiasis is another problem for which the woman with diabetes is prone. Signs of vaginal candidiasis include white, cheesy-type vaginal discharge, severe itching, and discomfort. The discharge does not have a foul odor but is highly irritating to tender vaginal tissue. Fluconazole (Diflucan) is an oral tablet that is sometimes prescribed for woman with vaginal candidiasis. However, normally the use of fluconazole during pregnancy is not recommended. Occasionally the benefits of treatment with this medication outweigh the possible risks to the fetus. The physician will discuss these risks with the woman. Most frequently the physician recommends treatment with over-the-counter vaginal creams and suppositories to control the symptoms of vaginal candidiasis during pregnancy. Verify that the woman understands treatment advice and that her questions have been adequately answered.

Monitoring Fetal Status

It is very important for the pregnant woman with DM to understand the risk of fetal demise, particularly if blood sugar levels are difficult to control and/or the woman requires insulin to manage her diabetes. The 3rd trimester is generally the time of greatest danger. Institute fetal surveillance per the physician's orders. It is always appropriate to teach the woman to monitor fetal activity and kick counts, starting at approximately 26 to 28 weeks' gestation. Perform twice-weekly NSTs in the physician office or as ordered. Give the fetal monitor tracing to the RN to assess and report results to the physician. Nonreactive NSTs usually are followed up with a CST and/or a BPP.

Estimating Fetal Weight

The fetus of the woman with DM is at risk for disproportionate growth resulting in fetal macrosomia (fetal weight greater than 4,000 grams). Assist the physician or RN to measure fundal height at each prenatal visit. Report findings that do not correlate with gestational age (refer to Chapter 7 to review fundal height assessment). Larger-than-expected size may be related to a large fetus or polyhydramnios.

Instruct the woman on the importance of serial sonograms to estimate the fetal weight. The macrosomic infant is much more likely to experience the delivery complication of shoulder dystocia (difficulty delivering fetal shoulders after delivery of the head), leading to birth trauma. Many physicians induce labor in the woman as soon as fetal lung maturity can be established in an attempt to prevent shoulder dystocia. Alternatively, the physician may elect to perform a cesarean delivery if macrosomia is suspected.

EVALUATION: GOALS AND EXPECTED OUTCOMES

- **Goal:** The woman will successfully manage the therapeutic regimen.
  Expected Outcomes:
  - Monitors and records blood sugar levels as ordered.
  - Adjusts her diet to recommendations by the physician and dietitian.
  - Exercises at least three times per week using recommended exercises.
  - Self-administers insulin, if ordered.
- **Goal:** Maternal injury from hypoglycemia and hyperglycemia will be avoided.
  Expected Outcomes:
  - Recognizes and treats hypoglycemia promptly.
  - Recognizes hyperglycemia and takes measures to prevent DKA.
- **Goal:** The woman will remain free from infection.
  Expected Outcomes:
  - Does not experience a UTI (or if she does, seeks prompt treatment).
  - Seeks prompt treatment for vaginal candidiasis.
- **Goal:** The fetus will maintain health status.
  Expected Outcomes:
  - Fetal activity counts are within normal limits.
  - NST is reactive.
  - BPP score is greater than 7.
  - CST is negative.
- **Goal:** The fetus will avoid birth trauma.
  Expected Outcomes:
  - Fetal weight is estimated to be appropriate for gestational age.
  - No birth injury results from shoulder dystocia.

Test Yourself

- What test is used to monitor long-term glucose control during pregnancy for the woman with diabetes?

- What term is used to describe the fetus whose weight exceeds 4,500 grams?

- What are the three cornerstones of therapy for the pregnant woman with diabetes?

Cardiovascular Disease

Heart disease is the third leading cause of death in women of childbearing age and complicates approximately 1% of all pregnancies (Cunningham et al., 2001a). In the past, most cases of heart disease during pregnancy were caused by rheumatic heart disease. Now, however, congenital heart disease is the underlying problem in at least 50% of pregnancies complicated by heart disease.

Significant cardiovascular changes occur in a normal pregnancy. Blood volume and cardiac output increase. Systemic vascular resistance drops. In a normal healthy woman, these cardiovascular changes are tolerated with minor notice. In the woman with heart or vessel disease, whose heart is already compromised, the increased demands of pregnancy can lead to cardiac failure. Heretofore undiagnosed heart disease can be unmasked or cardiac symptoms can worsen in the woman with pre-existing disease. The periods of greatest risk for the pregnant woman with cardiac disease are at the end of the 2nd trimester (when blood volume peaks), during labor, and in the early postpartum period secondary to fluid shifts.

The New York Heart Association's (NYHA) classification system (Table 16-1) is used to rate the severity of heart disease in the pregnant woman. Generally, women with Class I or II heart disease have a good prognosis for pregnancy. However, women with Class III or IV are at much higher risk for poor pregnancy outcomes and require more extensive monitoring and treatment throughout the pregnancy. In addition, the risk of maternal and fetal complications increases if the woman has any of the following conditions: cyanosis, erythrocytosis, stenotic lesions, or right-to-left shunt.

Clinical Manifestations and Diagnosis

Signs and symptoms (Box 16-5) vary depending on the underlying cause of heart disease. Tachycardia that lasts for more than several minutes accompanied by dizziness or light-headedness suggests a tachyarrhythmia and requires further investigation. The woman with an existing stenotic valve tends to have an increase in symptoms during pregnancy, whereas the woman with incompetent valves tends to experience fewer symptoms during pregnancy. Pregnancy is particularly dangerous for the woman with severe (greater than 80 mm Hg systolic) pulmonary hypertension.

The earliest warning sign of cardiac decompensation is persistent rales in the bases of the lungs. The woman will probably notice a nocturnal cough. Serious heart failure is marked by a sudden decrease in the ability to perform normal duties, exertional dyspnea, and attacks of coughing with a smothering feeling.

TABLE 16.1	NYHA's Clinical Classification of Heart Disease			
Class	Amount of Compromise	Symptoms	Physical Limitations	Pregnancy Prognosis
I	Uncompromised	Asymptomatic	None	Good
II	Slightly compromised	• Asymptomatic at rest • Symptomatic with normal physical exertion	Slight	Good
III	Markedly compromised	Symptoms occur with minimal activity	Marked	Moderate; may need hemodynamic monitoring and special anesthetic management during labor
IV	Severely compromised	Symptoms occur at rest	Unable to perform any physical activity without discomfort	Poor, will need hemodynamic monitoring and special anesthetic, management during labor

BOX 16.5 Signs and Symptoms of Heart Disease

The woman may complain of
- Dyspnea
- Orthopnea
- Nocturnal cough
- Dizziness
- Fainting
- Chest pain

Physical examination may reveal
- Cyanosis
- Clubbing of the fingers
- Neck vein distention
- Tachycardia
- Heart murmurs
- Edema

Upon physical examination tachycardia, edema, and hemoptysis may be noted.

Treatment

A team approach is indicated to manage pregnancy complicated by heart disease. The obstetrician, cardiologist, perinatologist, and other specialists often collaborate in the care of the pregnant woman with heart disease. Treatment varies depending on the etiology of the heart condition; however, there are general principles for management. These principles involve activity levels, stress management, diet, and medication. No matter what the underlying cause of the condition, the main goal is prevention, early detection, and early treatment of cardiac decompensation.

Activity Levels

Activity is allowed as tolerated. The woman is cautioned to rest frequently and not allow herself to become overly fatigued. Because pregnancy greatly increases the workload of the heart, complete bed rest is sometimes necessary, particularly for the woman who is severely compromised (see Table 16-1).

Stress Management

Heart failure can be precipitated by any unusual stress that increases demands upon the cardiovascular system. Examples include infection, anemia, underlying medical disorders, and excessive emotional or physical stress. The physician carefully screens for any condition that might precipitate the stress response. Pneumococcal and influenza vaccines are recommended because infection is particularly harmful for the pregnant woman with heart disease. Antibiotic prophylaxis to prevent endocarditis is necessary before some high-risk procedures (e.g., some dental work and other invasive procedures) for the woman with moderate to severe heart disease.

Diet and Medications

The woman is advised to limit salt intake and weight gain during pregnancy. Most cardiac medications are continued during pregnancy, with the exception of warfarin (Coumadin) and angiotensin-converting enzyme (ACE) inhibitors. Warfarin crosses the placenta and increases the risk of congenital anomalies. An alternative is treatment with heparin. The large molecules of this anticoagulant do not cross the placental barrier. ACE inhibitors increase the risk of fetal mortality and can lead to intractable renal failure in the newborn.

Management During Labor and the Postpartum Period

Special precautions must be taken during labor. The supine position is contraindicated for any pregnant woman, but avoidance of supine hypotensive syndrome during labor for the woman with heart disease is imperative. Supine hypotensive syndrome can lead to decreased placental perfusion with resultant fetal compromise. The condition can also increase maternal cardiac output and quickly lead to maternal compromise.

Here's a helpful reminder. The signs of supine hypotensive syndrome include decreased blood pressure, dizziness, pallor, and clammy skin. It is imperative that you prevent this condition by positioning the woman in a semirecumbent position with a pillow or wedge under one hip. The pregnant woman with heart disease should never be flat on her back.

The stress and pain of labor greatly increases the demand on the heart, making pain relief a crucial part of labor management for the woman with heart disease. Epidural analgesia with narcotics and/or epidural anesthesia is the pain relief option of choice during labor. During the second stage of labor, vigorous pushing using Valsalva maneuver can lead to cardiac decompensation. Cesarean section is reserved for usual obstetric complications. Vaginal birth is preferred, if possible. It is no longer recommended that the woman with heart disease be given prophylactic antibiotics during labor and delivery, including cesarean delivery.

The woman remains at risk for heart failure in the postpartum period. She is monitored closely for signs of postpartum hemorrhage, anemia, infection, and thromboembolism. All of these complications greatly increase the risk of cardiac decompensation.

Nursing Care

The most important nursing action is to monitor for and teach the woman to recognize signs of cardiac decompensation. Listen to breath sounds at each office visit and during labor. Report rales in the bases of the lungs and complaints of nocturnal coughing. Elevated blood pressure and tachycardia are other warning signs that should be reported immediately. Increased respiration, shortness of breath and productive coughing may indicate the development of pulmonary edema or pulmonary emboli, either of which is life threatening.

It is especially important for the pregnant woman with heart disease to protect herself from infection. Instruct her to avoid crowds and anyone with signs of respiratory infection, even the common cold. Explain that cigarette smoking increases the risk of contracting an upper respiratory infection. Advise her of the importance of frequent handwashing. Administer pneumococcal and influenza vaccines, as ordered. Remind the woman of the importance of reporting her heart condition to all health care providers, including the dentist, so that prophylactic antibiotics can be administered, if necessary.

Inquire regarding illicit drug use and cigarette smoking in a nonjudgmental way. Explain that many illicit drugs and cigarette smoking adversely affect the heart and increase the risk for decompensation. Make clear that intravenous drug use increases the risk for infective endocarditis, a potentially lethal complication.

Assist the woman with tests for fetal well-being. Explain that serial ultrasound measurements allow the physician to monitor growth of the fetus. Instruct the woman to do fetal kick counts in the 2nd and 3rd trimesters. Decreased fetal movement should be reported immediately. Assist with amniocentesis, as indicated. Amniocentesis may be done to determine fetal lung maturity in anticipation of early delivery if the woman's cardiac status begins to deteriorate in the 3rd trimester.

Monitor the woman particularly closely during labor. Position her so that the gravid uterus does not compress the major blood vessels. Assess pain levels frequently. Administer intravenous analgesia as ordered. Assist with epidural anesthesia administration. Monitor vital signs as recommended for the at-risk pregnancy (see Chapter 10). Continue to observe for signs of cardiac decompensation in the postpartum period. Immediately report fever, increased bleeding, and any signs of decompensation.

Anemia

Anemia is a condition in which the blood is deficient in red blood cells (RBCs), hemoglobin, or in total volume. Anemia is not itself a disease. Rather, it is a symptom of an underlying disorder. There are three main causes of anemia: blood loss, hemolysis (increased RBC destruction), and decreased production of RBCs. There

are multiple etiologies associated with each category. Iron-deficiency anemia is the most common anemia experienced during pregnancy. Other anemias that could complicate pregnancy include megaloblastic anemia from folate deficiency, pernicious anemia from vitamin B_{12} deficiency, sickle cell anemia, and thalassemia. This section focuses on iron-deficiency and sickle cell anemia.

Iron-Deficiency Anemia

Iron-deficiency anemia is characterized by reduced production of RBCs because the body does not have enough iron to manufacture the hemoglobin molecule. The RBCs that are produced are smaller in size (microcytic) and are pale in color (hypochromic). Because the pregnant woman has increased iron requirements, she is particularly vulnerable to iron-deficiency anemia.

Clinical Manifestations and Diagnosis

Common signs and symptoms of iron-deficiency anemia in the pregnant woman are tachycardia, tachypnea, dyspnea, pale skin, low blood pressure, heart murmur, headache, fatigue, weakness, and dizziness. Pica (ingestion of nonfood substances such as clay and laundry starch) and pagophagia (frequent chewing or sucking on ice) are both associated with iron-deficiency anemia.

Treatment

Treatment for iron-deficiency anemia is directed toward a diet rich in iron and folate in addition to iron and folate supplementation. Recent studies have shown that folate supplementation increases the effectiveness of iron therapy. Rarely does the pregnant woman with anemia require a blood transfusion.

Sickle Cell Anemia

Sickle cell anemia is a hemolytic anemia that is caused by an abnormal hemoglobin molecule called hemoglobin S (Hgb S). Individuals who have sickle cell anemia inherit two copies of the genetic mutation for Hgb S, one from the father and one from the mother. Some people are carriers of the trait because they inherit only one copy of the mutation. Individuals who are carriers are said to have sickle cell trait. In the United States, sickle cell anemia most commonly occurs in African-American individuals. Every year 1 in 400 African-American newborns is born with sickle cell anemia, and approximately 1 in 12 African-Americans has sickle cell trait (Mayfield, 1996).

Sickle cell anemia is a chronic condition characterized by acute exacerbations of the disease called "crises." Stress typically triggers a crisis, in which the abnormal hemoglobin causes RBCs to "sickle" when oxygen is released from the hemoglobin. The abnormal cells are sticky and clump together in such a way that they cannot flow easily through the capillaries. If enough of the cells clump, blood flow to the area is blocked, causing tissue ischemia and pain at the site of blockage. The reticuloendothelial system fights to rid the body of the abnormal hemoglobin by breaking down the sickled cells. Unfortunately, the bone marrow cannot produce enough RBCs to replace the damaged ones, so anemia results. The pregnant woman with sickle cell anemia is at higher risk for hypertension, particularly preeclampsia-eclampsia and preterm delivery. Newborns of the woman with sickle cell anemia are more likely to be small for gestational age.

Clinical Manifestations and Diagnosis

The woman with sickle cell trait rarely experiences symptoms, and when she does, the symptoms are generally mild. The woman with sickle cell anemia, however, is at risk for a sickle cell crisis at any time during the pregnancy. Dehydration and infection are two examples of conditions that predispose the woman to a crisis. Depending upon which area of the body is affected, the woman may experience recurrent bouts of pain in the joints, bones, chest, and abdomen. She also may experience nonspecific symptoms of anemia, such as fatigue, tachycardia, and dyspnea. Physical examination may reveal enlarged lymph nodes, enlarged spleen (splenomegaly), hematuria (bloody urine), or jaundice.

Treatment

Treatment between crises is directed at preventing a crisis, if possible. Maintaining adequate hydration, avoiding infection, getting adequate rest, and eating a balanced diet are all common sense strategies that decrease the risk of a crisis. Hydroxyurea (Hydrea), a medication that decreases the frequency and severity of crises, is not recommended during pregnancy because it is teratogenic in animals.

The initial prenatal visit requires additional laboratory work for the woman with sickle cell anemia to include hemoglobin electrophoresis, serum iron, total iron binding capacity, ferritin levels, liver function tests, electrolyte analysis, kidney function tests, urinalysis, and urine culture. Hepatitis B vaccine may be administered if the woman does not have hepatitis B. Asymptomatic bacteriuria is treated with antibiotics to prevent a full-blown urinary tract infection. The woman may be instructed to return for more frequent than normal prenatal visits. Prenatal visits are scheduled every 2 weeks in the 2nd trimester and every week throughout the 3rd trimester.

When the woman experiences a painful crisis, the physician orders a CBC, type and cross match, and sometimes arterial blood gas (ABG) measurements.

Intravenous (IV) fluids are started to hydrate the patient and decrease blood viscosity. Narcotics are generally required to control the pain of an attack. Fetal monitoring is indicated, if the fetus is viable, and supplemental oxygen by face mask may be necessary. Antibiotics are given to treat infection, if it is present. Occasionally an exchange transfusion[1] may be indicated to reduce the amount of sickled RBCs in the circulation.

Nursing Care

At each visit do a 1- to 3-day diet recall to help identify patterns of food intake for the pregnant woman with any type of anemia. She may be embarrassed to give an accurate recall. In these instances, it may be helpful for a family member to assist with the dietary recall. Draw blood as ordered to monitor hemoglobin and hematocrit.

The woman with iron-deficiency anemia needs counseling regarding foods that are high in iron. These include animal protein, dried beans, fortified grains and cereals, dried fruits, and any food cooked in cast iron cookware. Instruct her that iron absorption will be enhanced if she includes foods high in vitamin C along with iron-rich foods. Absorption of her iron supplement will be enhanced if she drinks orange juice when she takes her supplement. Her diet should also contain adequate amounts of folate. Foods high in folic acid include fortified grains, dried beans, and leafy green vegetables.

Iron supplements predispose to constipation. The pregnant woman may be tempted to stop taking iron supplements because of constipation. Instruct her regarding the importance to her and her baby of continuing iron supplementation. All of the normal measures that help prevent constipation, such as maintaining adequate fluid intake, getting enough exercise, and establishing regular bowel habits are helpful for the pregnant woman taking iron supplements.

The woman with sickle cell anemia needs support and teaching throughout her pregnancy. Emphasize the importance of using common sense approaches to prevent crises. Instruct the woman to wash her hands frequently and to avoid highly crowded areas to decrease her risk of contracting an infection. Adequate fluid intake and rest are important for maintaining health in the pregnant woman with sickle cell anemia. Assist her to make and keep her prenatal appointments.

---

[1] For an exchange transfusion, a predetermined amount of blood is withdrawn from the patient (typically 500 cc) and 2 units of packed red blood cells are transfused.

Test Yourself

- What is the earliest sign of cardiac decompensation.

- Which are signs of supine hypotensive syndrome?

- Describe two conditions or situations that might trigger a crisis for the woman with sickle cell anemia.

Asthma

Asthma is a chronic, inflammatory disease of the airways characterized by acute exacerbations of reversible airway obstruction. As many as 4% of all pregnancies are complicated by asthma. This condition, also known as reactive airway disease (RAD), can be a severe threat to the health of the woman and her fetus, if the disease is not controlled properly. Pregnant women with poorly controlled asthma experience a higher incidence of preeclampsia-eclampsia, antepartum and postpartum hemorrhage, premature labor, respiratory failure, and death. Fetal complications include intrauterine growth restriction, fetal demise, and preterm birth. Perinatal outcomes are similar to those of the general population if the condition is well controlled throughout pregnancy.

Clinical Manifestations and Diagnosis

The course of the disease varies during pregnancy. Physical examination during remission may be completely normal. During an acute asthma episode the respiratory rate increases and the woman feels short of breath and anxious. An expiratory wheeze is characteristic. Other auscultation findings may include diffuse rhonchi, bronchovesicular sounds, or bronchial sounds throughout the lung fields. Retractions of the respiratory muscles may be noted. Complaint of nocturnal awakening is a classic symptom. Other symptoms frequently include a cough and chest tightness. Pulsus paradoxus, a pulse that weakens during inspiration, is often noted.

Treatment

The goals of antepartum asthma management are prevention of acute episodes, control of symptoms, maintenance of normal pulmonary function, and avoidance of emergency department visits and hospitalization.

The initial prenatal visit includes a thorough history of the course of the woman's asthma before pregnancy and in prior pregnancies, if applicable. The health care provider inquires as to the frequency of acute episodes, the severity of the disease, history of hospitalizations, and any known environmental stimuli that are asthma triggers for the woman. Medication history is carefully elicited. Baseline spirometry measurement is done to determine pulmonary function (Robinson & Norwitz, 2000). Other tests include allergen skin testing, pulse oximetry, ABG measurement, and chest x-ray (Miller & Greenberger, 1999).

Management of an Acute Exacerbation

Management of an acute attack often requires hospitalization for the pregnant woman. She may be treated on a 23-hour observation status, or her condition may necessitate a full admission. Oxygen is given by face mask to maintain the PO_2 above 60 mm Hg and the oxygen saturation greater than 95%. Fluids are given intravenously for hydration to loosen mucus in the airways. Epinephrine injected subcutaneously is often beneficial for relieving severe dyspnea. Frequent nebulizer treatments with a beta-agonist such as albuterol are done to bring the attack under control. Corticosteroids and/or theophylline may be started intravenously. Fetal well-being is generally assessed by external fetal monitoring methods after 20 weeks' gestation, although other measures of fetal well-being, such as ultrasound or biophysical profile, may also be ordered.

Status asthmaticus is a potentially fatal complication of an acute asthma attack. Severe asthma symptoms that do not respond after 30 to 60 minutes of treatment are diagnosed as status asthmaticus. This condition can lead to pneumothorax, pneumomediastinum, acute cor pulmonale, cardiac arrhythmias, and respiratory failure (Cunningham et al., 2001b). Status asthmaticus in the pregnant woman is treated aggressively, with early intubation and mechanical ventilation in the intensive care setting.

Labor and Birth Management

There are several important points to remember about managing the woman with asthma during labor. The woman may fear that asthma symptoms will be exacerbated by the stress of labor. This is not generally the case. In fact, symptoms tend to diminish during labor. Regularly scheduled asthma medications should continue to be administered throughout labor. Adequate hydration and analgesia minimize the risk of bronchospasm. Fentanyl is the narcotic of choice because it does not cause histamine release, which could lead to bronchospasm. Epidural analgesia is the ideal method of pain control for the laboring woman with asthma.

Vaginal delivery is attempted, if at all possible. If there are indications for a surgical delivery, epidural or spinal anesthesia is preferred over general anesthesia. If a general must be administered, atropine and glycopyrrolate (Robinul) may be ordered preoperatively to induce bronchodilation.

Nursing Care

Teaching is a major role when providing nursing care for the pregnant woman with asthma. Be sure that the woman does a return demonstration on the use of her inhaler. Do not assume that she knows how to use it. She should also do a return demonstration for use of the peak flow meter. Remind her of the importance of monitoring fetal activity and kick counts during the 2nd and 3rd trimesters. Family Teaching Tips: Managing Asthma During Pregnancy outlines the major points to make when educating the pregnant woman with asthma.

Epilepsy

Epilepsy is a group of neurologic disorders that involve a long-term tendency to have recurrent unprovoked seizures (Morrell, 2002). Approximately 1 in 200 pregnancies is complicated by epilepsy, making this disorder the most commonly encountered neurologic condition in pregnant women.

Clinical Manifestations

Several difficulties are encountered during pregnancy that relate to the condition of epilepsy. Drug metabolism is changed during pregnancy, making it more difficult to establish therapeutic antiepileptic drug (AED) levels. Thirty percent to 50% of women with epilepsy experience an increase in seizure frequency during pregnancy, whereas others experience a decrease or no change in seizure frequency. The major risk to the pregnancy during a seizure results from blunt trauma. Trauma can lead to miscarriage, premature rupture of membranes, and placental abruption.

The fetus of the woman with epilepsy is at almost two times greater risk of experiencing congenital malformations than is the fetus of a woman in the normal population. In the past it was thought that epilepsy itself increased the risk for birth defects. However, the latest research indicates that AEDs used to treat epilepsy are the major cause of fetal defects. Cleft lip and palate, cardiac defects, and neural tube defects comprise the majority of malformations noted in the fetus.

Treatment

Preconceptual care is highly recommended for the woman with epilepsy who wishes to become pregnant. A thorough history and physical examination establishes the diagnosis of epilepsy and the efficacy of the current treatment regimen in controlling seizures. If the woman has been seizure free for several years while receiving low-dose therapy, the physician may try to wean the woman from the AED. The woman with epilepsy should be followed by her obstetrician in consultation with a neurologist.

FAMILY TEACHING TIPS

Managing Asthma During Pregnancy

- Do not stop taking your asthma medications. The risk to you and your baby is much higher from uncontrolled asthma than it is from taking your medications. Remember, you are "breathing for two."
- Check with your doctor before taking any over-the-counter medications. Some of these medications have been shown to cause harm to your developing baby.
- Protect yourself from asthma triggers.
  - Keep a symptom diary to identify your unique triggers.
  - Avoid cigarette smoke, exposure to animals, and dusty, damp environments.
  - Stay inside in air-conditioned surroundings during pollen seasons and when the pollution or mold index is high.
  - Wear a mask or scarf over your mouth on excessively cold days to help warm the air.
  - Protect yourself from colds and flu because respiratory infections can trigger acute asthma attacks.
    - Avoid crowds where viruses may be prevalent.
    - Wash your hands frequently.
    - Take the flu shot if you have moderate or severe asthma. The flu shot is based on a killed virus, so it is safe to use during pregnancy.
  - Avoid foods or chemicals that might have caused a reaction in the past, such as sulfites or MSG.
- Continue your allergy shots as long as you are not having reactions to the shots. If you are not currently taking allergy shots, it is usually not advised to begin doing so during pregnancy because of the risk of reactions.
- Monitor your peak expiratory flow rate (PEFR) regularly, as recommended by your doctor. If you have severe asthma, you will need to measure your PEFR at least twice daily. A decrease in the PEFR usually precedes an acute asthma attack hours to days before physical symptoms begin.
- Develop a crisis management plan in consultation with your physician. The plan should include how to recognize warning signs and what to do when early signs of worsening status occur. Go immediately to the nearest emergency department if any of the following occur after rescue drugs are taken.
  - Rapid improvement does not result.
  - Improvement is not sustained.
  - Condition worsens.
  - The episode is severe.
  - Fetal movement decreases.

At the very first sign of breathing difficulties use your peak flow meter to measure your PEFR. If it is low or has decreased from your last reading, call the doctor immediately. Other warning signs of an impending attack may include a headache, itchy throat, sneezing, coughing, or feeling tired.

High-dose (4 to 5 mg daily) folate supplementation is recommended in the months preceding and throughout pregnancy because AEDs increase the risk for neural tube defects. At 14 to 18 weeks' gestation, it is recommended that maternal serum alpha-fetoprotein levels be drawn and a high-resolution sonogram be performed to screen for neural tube defects. Beginning at 36 weeks, many physicians prescribe additional vitamin K supplementation because AED therapy can lead to vitamin K-deficient hemorrhage of the newborn.

Although there is an increased risk for cesarean delivery, epilepsy is not an indication for induction of labor or for cesarean delivery. Most women can expect a normal vaginal delivery. One percent to 2% of women experience seizures either during labor or after delivery. If the seizure is severe, a cesarean delivery may be indicated.

Status epilepticus is an emergency complication of epilepsy whereby seizure activity continues for 30 minutes or more after treatment is initiated or when three or more seizures occur without full recovery between seizures. Immediate measures are taken to protect the woman from injury while protecting the airway. Emergency intubation with mechanical ventilation is sometimes required. Blood work is drawn for glucose, electrolytes, CBC, AED levels, and blood and urine toxicology screens. An IV line is started to allow for IV administration of benzodiazepines, such as diazepam or lorazepam. Once seizures are under control, fosphenytoin is given via the IV route.

Nursing Care

Teach the woman the importance of carefully following her treatment regimen and of maintaining regular prenatal care. Emphasize the importance of eating a diet high in folic acid and of taking folic acid supplementation. Advise the woman to get plenty of rest and sleep and to exercise regularly. Assist her to schedule lab work at regular intervals. Provide support when prenatal testing is done to screen for fetal anomalies.

Infectious Diseases

There are a number of infectious disease categories that present increased morbidity and mortality to the infant whose mother is victim of one or more of these infections. Some type of infective process is seen in approximately 15% of all pregnancies.

TORCH

TORCH (Box 16-6) is an acronym for a special group of infections that can be acquired during pregnancy and transmitted through the placenta to the fetus. The "T" stands for toxoplasmosis, the "O" for other infections

---

BOX 16.6 | TORCH Infections

TORCH (an acronym for the infections)
Toxoplasmosis
Other: hepatitis B, syphilis, varicella and herpes zoster
Rubella
Cytomegalovirus (CMV)
Herpes simplex virus (HSV)
All are teratogenic. All cross the placenta. Fetal effect is determined by gestational age at exposure. TORCH syndrome is characterized by IUGR, microcephaly, hepatosplenomegaly, rash, thrombocytopenia, and CNS findings, such as ventricular calcifications and hydrocephaly.

Assessment
1. History: flu-like symptoms, fatigue, cat exposure, genital lesions, rash, exposure to sick children
2. Physical exam: lymphadenopathy, headache, malaise, jaundice, N/V, low-grade temperature, rash, ulcerated and painful lesions of the genitals
3. Psychosocial: fear, anxiety, apprehension

Diagnostics
1. Serologic tests
   • TORCH screen
   • CBC
   • HBsAg and HBeAg
   • Liver function tests
2. Cultures
   • CMV
   • HSV
3. Pap smear
4. Serial ultrasounds (monitor for IUGR and other defects throughout pregnancy)

Interventions
1. Instruct the woman regarding specifics of
   a. the infection
   b. transmission
   c. medication and medical management
2. Reinforce importance of handwashing
3. Encourage questions
4. Suggest a multidisciplinary conference with family members, if anxiety and fear levels are high
5. Encourage breast-feeding. These mothers may be afraid to breast-feed their babies.

(hepatitis B, syphilis, varicella and herpes zoster), the "R" is for rubella, the "C" is for cytomegalovirus (CMV), and the "H" stands for herpes simplex virus (HSV).

Each infection is teratogenic, and the effects are different, depending upon when during the pregnancy infection occurs. Fetal infection may lead to TORCH syndrome characterized by central nervous system (CNS) dysfunction. Mental retardation, microcephaly, hydrocephalus, CNS lesions, jaundice, hepatosplenomegaly, hearing deficits, and chorioretinitis are examples of sequelae for the newborn that is infected with one of the TORCH agents. Fetal infection may also lead to spontaneous abortion, intrauterine growth restriction (IUGR), stillbirth, and premature delivery. Prevention is the focus of interventions because many of the TORCH infections do not have effective treatment regimens.

A TORCH screen can be performed if the physician has reason to believe the woman might have one of the TORCH infections. Diagnosis is made by serial antibody titers. If the woman is seronegative (no antibodies in the blood) after two titers (taken 10 to 20 days apart), infection is ruled out. If the woman is seropositive (antibodies in the blood) for the first titer, but the titers do not rise by the second draw, she is considered to have a latent ("old") infection. This is important because it is very rare that a latent infection is passed to the fetus. However, if the woman's antibody titers have risen by the second draw, she is considered to be acutely infected.

Toxoplasmosis

Toxoplasmosis is an infection caused by the protozoan *Toxoplasma gondii*, also referred to as *"T. gondii."* It is transmitted via undercooked meat and through cat feces. Toxoplasmosis is a fairly common infection in humans and usually produces no symptoms. However, when the infection is transmitted from the woman through the placenta, a condition called congenital toxoplasmosis can occur. Approximately 400 to 4,000 cases of congenital toxoplasmosis occur per year in the United States (Jones, Lopez, & Wilson, 2003). The classic triad of symptoms for congenital toxoplasmosis is chorioretinitis, intracranial calcification, and hydrocephalus in the newborn.

Toxoplasmosis is difficult to diagnose because it rarely produces symptoms in the woman. This infection is particularly harmful to the fetus if it is contracted between 10 and 24 weeks of pregnancy. Treatment is with one or all of the following: spiramycin (Rovamycine, an investigational drug in the United States), pyrimethamine (Daraprim), and folinic acid. The newborn is also treated with antibiotics.

Infection can be prevented through several common sense approaches. Advise the pregnant woman to have someone else clean the cat litter box. If there is no one else to perform this duty, she should wear gloves and wash her hands thoroughly before and after cleaning the box. The box should be cleaned daily. She should wear gloves when working in the garden or when doing yard work. She should wash her hands thoroughly before and after handling raw meat, and she should eat only meats that have been completely cooked (i.e., no rare or medium rare meats). Any surface or item that is touched by raw meat should be thoroughly cleaned in hot, soapy water after contact.

All fruits and vegetables need to be washed carefully before being served.

Other Infections: Hepatitis B, Syphilis, Varicella and Herpes Zoster

Hepatitis B. Hepatitis B virus (HBV) is transmitted sexually or through contact with blood or body fluids. It can also be transmitted to the fetus by contact with vaginal secretions and blood during delivery. In adults who become acutely infected, approximately 1% die of liver disease caused by the virus. Eighty-five percent to 90% completely recover and develop immunity to hepatitis B; 10% to 15% become chronic carriers and are at higher risk for developing cirrhosis and liver cancer.

Obstetricians screen their pregnant patients for hepatitis B surface antigen (HBsAg). A woman who has an acute HBV infection has elevated HBsAG titers. If the newborn is not treated, there is an increased risk that the infant will develop HBV infection. Approximately 25% of infants who become infected develop significant liver disease, and 50% develop chronic HBV infection.

As many as 90% of these neonatal infections can be prevented by neonatal immunoprophylaxis. If the mother is HBsAG positive, the neonate should receive hepatitis B immunoglobulin (HBIg) and the hepatitis B vaccine within 12 hours of birth. The immunoglobulin provides immediate protection, and the vaccine provides long-term protection from infection. Regardless of the woman's HBV status, all infants should be vaccinated against hepatitis B at birth, 1 to 2 months after birth, and again at 12 months of age.

Syphilis. Syphilis is a sexually transmitted infection (STI) with the bacterium (spirochete) *Treponema pallidum* (*T. pallidum*). The bacteria are transmitted via sexual contact or through broken skin. The main symptom of primary syphilis is a painless red pustule, which usually appears within 2 to 6 weeks after exposure. The pustule quickly erodes and develops a painless, bloodless ulcer called a chancre. Because it is painless, the newly infected person may not notice the chancre. The chancre, which sheds infectious fluid, usually appears on the body part that served as the portal of entry for the bacteria.

If the pregnant woman becomes infected with syphilis, the bacteria can cross the placenta, causing infection in the developing fetus. Spontaneous abortion occurs in 25% to 50% of women who develop acute syphilis early in the pregnancy. Preterm birth and fetal demise are other sequelae of active syphilis infection. If the woman carries the pregnancy to the age of viability, there is a 40% to 70% chance that the infant will be born infected with syphilis.

The infected infant may be born with birth defects, such as blindness, deafness, or other deformities.

Hutchinson's triad is characteristic and includes inflammation of the cornea, deafness, and notched teeth. Another characteristic of early congenital syphilis is snuffles, a nasal discharge that can be bloody. The newborn may have a vesicular or bullous rash that is contagious. On the other hand, the syphilis-infected infant may not immediately exhibit symptoms at birth. Symptoms can develop as long as weeks to months later. Swollen lymph glands, spleen and liver enlargement, jaundice, anemia, bone deformities, and vesicular rash may occur.

Screening for syphilis with the RPR or VDRL is one of the routine blood tests performed for every pregnant woman in the early part of pregnancy and repeated when she goes into labor. A positive screen requires further testing that is more specific to *T. pallidum*. Syphilis is curable, if properly treated. The treatment of choice for syphilis is benzathine penicillin B (Bicillin) administered intramuscularly as a single dose. Penicillin may be given during pregnancy and is safe to use while breast-feeding. Erythromycin is given to individuals who are sensitive to penicillin. Newborns with congenital syphilis are also treated with penicillin.

Varicella and Herpes Zoster. Varicella zoster is the virus that causes chickenpox. Herpes zoster is the recurrent form of the virus that lies dormant in the dorsal root ganglia of the spinal cord. Reactivation of herpes zoster results in shingles. Contact with shingles by persons who are nonimmune to chickenpox leads to the development of chickenpox in that individual. Varicella zoster and herpes zoster are members of the herpesvirus family.

Varicella zoster is transmitted by respiratory droplets and is highly contagious. The virus incubates for approximately 2 weeks and is contagious 2 days before onset of the skin lesions until the lesions crust over, generally 5 days after the initial onset. Herpes zoster (shingles) is characterized by a localized rash within a **dermatome**, an area on the body surface supplied by a particular sensory nerve. The rash is very painful. Occasionally pain precedes the rash. Anyone who has had chickenpox is at risk for developing shingles.

The incidence of varicella zoster during pregnancy is low, occurring in 1 to 5 of 10,000 pregnancies (Lie, 2003). Transmission of varicella zoster by the pregnant woman to her unborn child is very rare, occurring in 1 to 2 percent of cases (Van Earden & Bernstein, 2003). The highest risk (2%) occurs if the woman contracts varicella in the 2nd trimester, between 13 and 20 weeks' gestation. Transmission of herpes zoster is even more unlikely. However, the severity of fetal varicella syndrome, if it is contracted, gives cause to treat this infection during pregnancy with great care.

Fetal varicella syndrome is associated with low birth weight, scar-producing skin lesions, limb hypoplasia, and contractures. The syndrome can also result in damage to the ears, eyes, and CNS, leading to mental retardation, paralysis, and seizures. Prognosis for the neonate is poor. The newborn is at risk for neonatal varicella, a severe form of chickenpox with a 20% to 30% mortality rate, if the woman contracts varicella from 5 days before to 2 days after delivery. Another danger of varicella during pregnancy is the risk to the woman of developing varicella pneumonitis. This is a form of pneumonia that can be very severe, with a mortality rate as great as 40%. Even if the woman survives, the severity of the pneumonia could result in death of the fetus.

Any pregnant woman who reports a possible exposure to chickenpox or shingles should have a serologic test performed to detect varicella antibodies. Varicella zoster immune globulin (VZIG) may be given within 96 hours of exposure to help prevent the development of chickenpox. VZIG may also be given to the neonate (within 96 hours of exposure), if the woman develops chickenpox 5 days before, or within 48 hours after, delivery.

The best treatment is prevention. A woman of childbearing age who has not had chickenpox should be vaccinated. She should be instructed to avoid pregnancy for at least 1 month after vaccination. Pregnant women should not be vaccinated; however, susceptible individuals in the household of a pregnant woman who is susceptible to chickenpox should be vaccinated. This is the most effective way to prevent transmission to the pregnant woman. The nonimmune woman should receive one dose of varicella vaccine immediately after delivering her baby and a second dose at the 6-week postpartum visit.

Rubella

Rubella is a highly contagious disease caused by a virus. Rubella is usually a mild illness when it occurs in adults and children. Twenty percent to 50% of rubella infections are "silent," that is there are no symptoms. When symptoms occur, they are generally mild and include low-grade fever, rash, lymphadenopathy, general malaise, and conjunctivitis. Complications are rare.

The problem occurs when a woman contracts rubella while she is pregnant. Congenital rubella infection can result, which is anything but mild. Consequences of congenital rubella include spontaneous abortion, stillbirth, and congenital anomalies of varying severity. Hearing impairment is the single most common defect associated with congenital rubella infection. The greatest risk occurs if the woman develops rubella in the 1st trimester. Rubella contracted during the period of organogenesis (in the first 11 weeks of pregnancy) can result in multiple anomalies. Maternal rubella infection contracted after 20 weeks of pregnancy rarely results in birth defects. There is no cure for congenital rubella infection. Treatments are supportive and directed toward control of symptoms and complications.

The best treatment for congenital rubella infection is prevention. Ideally, all women of childbearing age would be tested for immunity to rubella before they become pregnant. Nonimmune women should be vaccinated before becoming pregnant and are advised to wait at least 28 days after vaccination to achieve pregnancy. Women are routinely tested for immunity to rubella in early pregnancy and again before delivery. The nonimmune woman is not vaccinated during pregnancy. She should be careful to avoid anyone with flu-like symptoms or rash during the pregnancy. Vaccination is administered in the early postpartum period before discharge from the hospital or birthing center. Breast-feeding is not a contraindication to receiving the rubella vaccine. Currently the Centers for Disease Control and Prevention (CDC, 2004) recommends that the combination measles, mumps, and rubella (MMR) vaccine be given to children at 12 to 15 months of age and a second dose at age 4 to 6 years before starting school. Routine vaccination of all children decreases spread of rubella and decreases the risk that a nonimmune pregnant woman will contract the infection.

Cytomegalovirus

Cytomegalovirus (CMV) is the silent menace. CMV is the most common cause of congenital viral infection, occurring in 0.2% to 2.2% percent of live births. A virus in the herpes family causes CMV. It is transmitted by contact with infected bodily fluids, such as saliva, blood, breast milk, urine, and semen. A common source of infection is young children.

Most individuals infected with CMV do not experience symptoms. If they do have symptoms, the symptoms mimic those of mononucleosis: sore throat, low-grade fever, swollen lymph glands, body aches, and fatigue. CMV is diagnosed by two or more antibody titers. If the antibody titers are rising, acute CMV infection is presumed.

A woman who contracts CMV for the first time while she is pregnant has a 30% to 40% risk of passing the infection to the fetus. The risk to the fetus from CMV infection is greatest during the first 20 weeks of pregnancy. Most affected newborns (approximately 90%) do not demonstrate symptoms at birth. However, as many as 15% of these infants develop one or more neurologic abnormalities, such as blindness, deafness, learning disabilities, and mental retardation. Signs that are more likely to be present at birth include hydrocephaly, microcephaly, IUGR, hepatosplenomegaly, jaundice, and rash. About 20% of newborns who have symptoms at birth will die. Ninety percent of the newborns who survive will develop serious neurologic deficits, such as mental retardation. The antiviral drug ganciclovir (Cytovene), which is used to treat adult AIDS patients with CMV-related eye infections, is currently being investigated for its efficacy in treating newborns with congenital CMV infection.

Because there is no cure for congenital CMV, prevention is strongly recommended. Pregnant women who have contact with small children should practice meticulous handwashing, particularly after contact with saliva and urine. Diapers, tissues, and other potentially infected items should be carefully disposed. Drinking glasses and eating utensils should not be shared. Pregnant health care workers should practice universal precautions. Although CMV is passed through breast milk, breast-feeding is not contraindicated because CMV infection contracted during birth or from breast-feeding rarely causes serious problems.

Herpes Simplex Virus

Herpes simplex virus (HSV) is a sexually transmitted infection caused by herpes simplex virus 1 (HSV-1) and herpes simplex virus 2 (HSV-2). The virus is spread by direct contact. In general, HSV-1 causes oral herpes, also known as cold sores, and HSV-2 causes genital herpes. However, both types can be transmitted to the mouth and/or genital region through kissing, oral-genital sex, and other sexual contact, and both types can cause serious illness in a newborn. Fortunately, neonatal herpes is rare, occurring in less than 0.1% of newborns.

Symptoms of genital herpes usually develop within 2 to 14 days after exposure to the virus. Without antiviral treatment, the lesions may last for as long as 20 days. The first attack is generally the most severe, although more than 75% of individuals with primary HSV infections have no symptoms. Painful lesions develop in the area that was exposed to the virus, usually the genital or anal regions. The lesions eventually completely heal and do not cause scarring. However, the virus lies dormant in the nervous system and can cause recurrent attacks. Flu-like symptoms, such as lymphadenopathy, headache, muscle aches, and low-grade fever, sometimes occur a day or two before an outbreak.

The majority of cases of neonatal herpes are contracted by contact with active virus in the birth canal, although a small percentage (5%) of fetuses are infected in utero. Most infants of women who have longstanding herpes do not develop neonatal herpes. This is thought to occur because maternal antibodies to herpes virus cross the placenta and protect the fetus. Preterm infants are more likely to contract herpes because antibodies do not begin to cross the placenta until approximately 28 weeks of gestation, so preterm infants do not have the same protection as full-term infants. The highest risk for neonatal herpes occurs in infants of women who develop herpes for the first time during the last trimester of pregnancy and who have active lesions in the birth canal at the time of delivery. In fact, the risk can be as high as 50%.

If the woman has a lesion at delivery, the safest alternative is cesarean delivery to prevent the baby from coming in contact with the virus in the birth canal. It is also recommended that no vaginal examinations be done, if there are active lesions. If there are no lesions present when the woman goes into labor, the American College of Obstetricians and Gynecologists recommends a vaginal delivery. It is recommended that internal monitoring with a fetal scalp electrode not be used during labor in women who have a history of genital herpes because the small break in the fetal scalp made by the electrode can serve as a portal of entry for the virus.

Sexually Transmitted Infections

A sexually transmitted infection (STI) is one that is transmitted primarily by sexual contact or through contact with blood or bodily fluids.[2] Many of the TORCH infections are STIs, including hepatitis B, syphilis, and herpes simplex. Other STIs of importance to the pregnant woman include trichomoniasis, gonorrhea, chlamydia, genital warts, and human immunodeficiency virus/acquired immunodeficiency syndrome (HIV/AIDS).

Many STIs are reportable diseases tracked by the CDC. Reportable infections include syphilis, chlamydia, gonorrhea, and AIDS. Some states require other STIs (in addition to those aforementioned) to be reported. One increasing concern is that many STIs increase the risk for the individual to contract HIV/AIDS. If symptoms of the infection include a break in the integrity of the skin or mucous membranes, these sites can provide a portal of entry for HIV.

Chlamydia

Chlamydia is the most prevalent reportable STI, occurring at a rate of 278.3 cases per 100,000 population in the year 2001. This represents a 10.4% increase over rates for the year 2000. Chlamydia is caused by infection with the bacterium *Chlamydia trachomatis* and is transmitted during oral, vaginal, and anal sex.

Approximately 75% of women who have chlamydia have no symptoms, which makes identification of the infection problematic. It also underscores that fact, that although this is the most prevalent STI, it is most likely grossly underreported. If the woman experiences symptoms, these may include vaginal discharge, abnormal vaginal bleeding, and abdominal or pelvic pain. Of

several methods of diagnostic testing that are available, amplified DNA tests are the most sensitive. Acceptable specimens include urine and cervical secretions.

Fortunately, chlamydia is easily curable with antibiotics. Treatment is with one dose of azithromycin (Zithromax) or twice-daily dosing for 7 days with erythromycin. As with other STIs, the sexual partners of the individual also require treatment.

Untreated chlamydia increases the risk of contracting HIV/AIDS. The most frequent sequela of untreated chlamydia is pelvic inflammatory disease (PID), a serious infection of the reproductive tract that can lead to infertility and chronic pelvic pain. Inflammation of the fallopian tubes that occurs with PID often results in scarring, which increases the risk of ectopic pregnancy. A pregnant woman who contracts chlamydia is at increased risk for going into preterm labor. The fetus can come into contact with bacteria in the vagina during the birth process. If this happens, the newborn can develop pneumonia or conjunctivitis that can lead to blindness.

Gonorrhea

Gonorrhea is an STI caused by the bacterium *Neisseria gonorrhoeae* (*N. gonorrhoeae*). The years between 1975 and 1997 realized a 73.8% decline in cases of gonorrhea. In 1998, the rates increased by almost 8% and have remained steady through 2001 (CDC, 2001). Gonorrhea is second in prevalence only to chlamydia, with 361,705 cases reported for the year 2001. The highest percentage (approximately 75%) of cases occurs in adolescents and young adults (National Institute of Allergy and Infectious Diseases [NIAID], May 2002). The bacteria are transmitted during sexual contact. The primary site of infection for the woman is the cervix, although infection can occur anywhere along the genital tract, in the urethra and rectum, and in the oro- and nasopharynx (throat).

Initial symptoms, which usually develop within 2 to 10 days of exposure to the bacteria, are mild and may go unnoticed. The woman who contracts gonorrhea may have vaginal bleeding during sexual intercourse, pain and burning while urinating, and a yellow or bloody vaginal discharge. A discharge from the rectum, itching around the anus, and painful bowel movements with fresh blood on the feces are signs of rectal infection. Infrequently the infection is asymptomatic.

There are several methods used to diagnose gonorrhea. A culture taken from the cervix, rectum, or throat is the diagnostic method of choice because it positively identifies *N. gonorrhea*. However, a culture takes several days to grow, so results are not immediately available. Other tests are sometimes used that produce rapid, although less accurate, results. These tests include gram staining, oxidase testing, and acid

---

[2] Many references, including government resources, refer to STIs as sexually transmitted diseases (STDs). Because of the stigma associated with these diseases, this text uses sexually transmitted infection (STI).

production testing. A presumptive diagnosis of gonorrhea is made when the rapid tests yield positive results, so that treatment can begin before the culture results are available.

Treatment is usually with a combination of two antibiotics that treat both gonorrhea and chlamydia because these infections often occur together. Some antibiotics commonly prescribed to treat gonorrhea are not used during pregnancy. One problem that has arisen recently is strains of *N. gonorrhoeae* that are resistant to antibiotics. The CDC publishes guidelines for physicians to help prevent and treat antimicrobial resistance. Efforts are under way to develop a vaccine against gonorrhea.

Untreated gonorrhea can lead to PID, which can leave the woman infertile or susceptible to ectopic pregnancy because of scarring in the reproductive tract. The bacteria can also spread through the bloodstream and infect joints, heart valves, or the brain. Infection with gonorrhea greatly increases the risk of acquiring HIV infection.

Risk to pregnancy from gonococcal infection includes increased risk for abortion and preterm delivery. Risk to the fetus occurs if the fetal eyes become infected during birth, a condition known as ophthalmia neonatorum. Blindness can result from this infection; however, cases are rare because all newborns receive prophylactic treatment with ocular antibiotic ointment within the hour after birth.

Human Papillomavirus

Human papillomavirus (HPV) is spread by skin-to-skin contact, usually during sexual activity. This virus can cause condylomata acuminata (genital warts) and cervical cancer. An individual with asymptomatic HPV infection can unknowingly pass the virus on to sexual partners.

Condylomata acuminata develop in clusters on the vulva, within the vagina, on the cervix, or around the anus. The lesions may remain small, or they can develop into large clusters of warts that resemble cauliflower. An abnormal Papanicolaou (Pap) smear may be the first indication of HPV infection and should lead to further inspection for the virus. The diagnosis is made by visualization of the warts or by applying a solution of acetic acid to areas of suspected infection. Acetic acid causes infected areas to turn white. A biopsy of tissue can be taken and examined microscopically for evidence of infection.

Genital warts can disappear without treatment. The type of treatment chosen depends on many factors, including age of the patient; duration, location, extent, and type of warts; the patient's immune status; risk of scarring; and pregnancy status. Several medical treatments are available, most of which consist of topical applications. Many of these treatments involve the use of substances that are teratogenic and thus are contraindicated during pregnancy. Surgical removal of the warts through a variety of techniques, including blunt dissection, laser, and cryosurgery, is another treatment option.

Genital warts have a tendency to increase in size during pregnancy. This may result in heavy bleeding during vaginal delivery. The pregnant woman can pass HPV to her fetus during the birth process. In rare instances, neonatal HPV infection can result in life-threatening laryngeal papillomas. HPV infection can be transmitted to the infant but may not appear for as long as 3 years after birth.

Trichomoniasis

Trichomoniasis, or infection with Trichomonas, is an STI caused by one-celled protozoa. It can infect the urethra, vagina, cervix, and structures of the vulva. Trichomoniasis is transmitted during unprotected sexual contact with someone who has the infection. It is possible for the woman to transmit trichomoniasis to the fetus during vaginal delivery, although this is a rare occurrence.

Symptoms of trichomoniasis include large amounts of foamy, yellow-green vaginal discharge, vaginal itching, unusual vaginal odor, painful sex, and dysuria. As many as half of all women with trichomoniasis have no symptoms. The most common diagnostic test is called a "wet mount." The practitioner takes a swab of vaginal secretions and examines the sample under the microscope. Unique movements of the organism allow for accurate diagnosis in 40% to 60% of cases. A culture can also be done, which is more sensitive than a wet mount, but results are not available for several days.

Treatment is with metronidazole (Flagyl). Although metronidazole is available in vaginal suppository and cream formats, oral dosing is recommended by the CDC, even during pregnancy, because of its increased effectiveness in treating Trichomonas infection. Oral metronidazole is given as a 2-gram single dose or as a 500-mg, twice-daily dose for a period of 7 days. The cure rate is 90% to 95%. In rare cases in which symptoms persist despite adequate treatment, further treatment with high doses of metronidazole is recommended. There are a few documented cases of metronidazole-resistant strains of Trichomonas. Expected side effects of treatment with oral metronidazole are metallic taste and dark urine. Nausea and vomiting can occur with high doses or when alcohol is taken during treatment.

HIV/AIDS

In 1981, health care providers were first confronted with the STI acquired immunodeficiency syndrome (AIDS), which is caused by the human immunodeficiency virus (HIV). HIV attacks the protective cells of the immune system, leaving the body unprotected against pathogens that normally do not cause illness in humans. Individuals who die of AIDS usually succumb to these opportunistic infections.

Since 1981 there have been more than 816,000 cases of AIDS in the United States. Women are at a higher risk than men for heterosexual transmission of the virus because the vaginal rugae are perfect for harboring the virus over time. African-American and Latino women are becoming infected in greater proportion than nonminority women. Washington, DC; Texas; California; New York; New Jersey; and Florida have the highest AIDS rates among women.

HIV is most often transmitted during unprotected sexual activity with an infected partner. The virus can enter the body through the mucous membranes of the genitals, rectum, or mouth. People infected with HIV often do not look or feel sick and may transmit the virus to others before they know they are infected.

HIV can also be transmitted through contact with infected blood. The risk of contracting HIV infection through receiving a blood transmission is very small because of screening and treatment of donated blood. However, an individual can be exposed to HIV-infected blood by sharing needles for IV drug use, intramuscular injections of anabolic steroids, or tattooing.

A woman who has HIV during pregnancy is at risk for transmitting the infection to the fetus during pregnancy or childbirth and to the newborn while breast-feeding. This risk can be substantially decreased if the woman receives appropriate antiretroviral treatment during pregnancy and childbirth and if she refrains from breast-feeding.

Clinical Manifestations. There are several ways to stage HIV disease. This text describes three stages of HIV infection: early, intermediate, and advanced. These stages correspond to CD4-positive T-cell (CD4 cell) counts. In the early stage, CD4 counts remain above 500/mL of blood (normal). In the intermediate stage, the CD4 counts measure between 200/mL and 500/mL (below normal). The advanced stage, which is also known as AIDS, is characterized by CD4 counts below 200/mL. CD4 cells are specialized T-cells and key infection fighters of the immune system.

The early (initial) stage of infection may be characterized by flu-like symptoms, such as fever, headache, sore throat, aching joints, malaise, and lymphadenopathy, which last for several weeks. Conversely, approximately one-half of individuals do not experience symptoms at all during the early stage.

After the initial infection, the individual moves into the intermediate stage. This stage can be divided into two phases: latent and acute HIV disease. The latent stage is "silent" in that no symptoms occur. This phase lasts for an average of 8 to 10 years. Although the person has no symptoms, the virus is replicating

rapidly and destroying CD4 cells. Unfortunately, unless the person is tested for HIV during the latent stage, he does not know that he is infected and may pass the virus on to others.

It is unknown why some HIV-positive individuals move rapidly into acute HIV disease in as little as 1 year, whereas others do not develop symptoms for 20 years or more. As stated previously, the average length of time before the onset of symptoms is 8 to 10 years. Once symptoms appear, the individual may seek treatment. Typical symptoms of acute HIV disease (Box 16-7) include swollen lymph nodes, feeling tired, weight loss, night sweats, fever, persistent oral or vaginal yeast infections, severe oral or genital herpes infections, shingles, skin rashes or scaly skin, and short-term memory loss. Women may develop severe PID that is not responsive to treatment.

The diagnosis of AIDS is made in the advanced stage of HIV infection. The CDC defines AIDS as an HIV-positive individual who has less than 200 CD4-positive T cells (CD4 cells) per milliliter of blood. It is at this stage that the person is immunosuppressed and becomes susceptible to opportunistic infections. Symptoms of opportunistic infections vary depending on the causative organism (bacteria, viruses, fungi, parasites, etc.). Symptoms may include extreme fatigue, dysphagia, coughing, dyspnea, nausea, vomiting, persistent diarrhea, severe weight loss, fever, confusion, ataxia,

---

BOX 16.7	Typical Symptoms of Acute HIV disease

Acute HIV disease describes the symptoms that appear during the latter part of the intermediate phase of HIV infection. CD4 cell counts remain above 200/mL of blood during this phase. Typical symptoms include:
- Persistent generalized lymphadenopathy
- Generalized malaise
- Weight loss
- Night sweats
- Fever
- Thrush (oral yeast infection)
- Candidiasis (vaginal yeast infection)
- Oral hairy leukoplakia (lesion characterized by white plaque on the lateral aspects of the tongue)
- Aphthous ulcers (painful, shallow ulcers of the oral mucosa)
- Herpes simplex virus (outbreaks are often severe)
- Shingles (herpes zoster)
- Anemia with associated pallor
- Thrombocytopenia
- Aseptic meningitis
- Peripheral neuropathies
- Short-term memory loss

seizures, blindness, and even coma. The individual is also susceptible to various rare cancers that are difficult to treat.

Diagnosis. A pregnant woman may become infected with HIV during pregnancy, or she may enter pregnancy with HIV. It is very important that the pregnant woman's HIV status is known. The CDC recommends that practitioners offer confidential HIV testing at the beginning of pregnancy and again during labor. The woman may refuse testing, but the practitioner is encouraged to counsel with the woman and explore reasons for refusal.

At present there are two methods to test for HIV infection: the enzyme-linked immunosorbent assay (ELISA) and the Western blot analysis. Both test for antibodies to the virus versus the virus itself. Antibodies to HIV usually develop within 6 to 12 weeks after exposure; however, it can take as long as 6 months for antibodies to appear. Researchers are trying to develop tests that can detect the HIV virus so that infection can be diagnosed much earlier and more reliably than is currently possible.

Unfortunately, all infants born to HIV-infected women have antibodies to HIV because the woman's antibodies cross the placenta. Therefore, an infant cannot be diagnosed with HIV infection using traditional testing methods until she is 18 months of age. Diagnosis in infants younger than 18 months of age requires viral culture on two separate specimens, both of which must be positive to make the diagnosis. This testing should be accomplished as soon as possible after birth so that therapy can be implemented quickly.

Treatment. The two main goals of treatment for the pregnant woman infected with HIV are to prevent progression of the disease in the woman and to prevent perinatal transmission of the virus to the fetus.[3] The best way to prevent perinatal transmission is to prevent HIV infection in the woman or to identify HIV infection before pregnancy or as early as possible during pregnancy. Therefore, early prenatal care for all women, regardless of risk, is imperative.

For the pregnant woman with HIV, therapy is composed of oral zidovudine (ZDV) prophylaxis, beginning as early as 14 weeks' gestation and continuing throughout pregnancy. Some studies have shown that adding a protease-inhibitor to the drug regimen may further reduce the risk of perinatal transmission of HIV. ZDV may be withheld in the 1st trimester of pregnancy to avoid possible teratogenic effects, although to date adverse fetal effects of ZDV administration in early pregnancy have not been demonstrated.

It is recommended that the HIV-positive woman be given the choice of cesarean delivery scheduled at 38 weeks' gestation to further reduce the risk of perinatal transmission. Several studies have shown that women who take antiretroviral medication during pregnancy and experience vaginal delivery have a 7% chance of transmitting the virus to their babies; whereas, women who take ZDV throughout pregnancy and have a cesarean delivery before the membranes rupture have as low as a 1% chance of perinatal transmission. If the woman elects for a vaginal delivery, IV ZDV is recommended to be given during labor and birth. Oral ZDV should be administered to the infant for the first 6 weeks of life. Breast-feeding is contraindicated. If these recommendations for prophylaxis are followed, the risk for perinatal transmission decreases from 25% to 35% for the untreated woman to as low as 2% for the treated woman.

If the woman is in an advanced stage of HIV disease during pregnancy, she should continue to receive treatment even in the 1st trimester. There have been no studies that show definite teratogenic properties of antiretroviral therapy. The risk to the woman and to her pregnancy from withholding treatment must be weighed against the potential risk to the fetus from drug therapy.

Nursing Care. Reassure the client that her confidentiality will be protected. Provide information concerning HIV infection and AIDS in an open, nonjudgmental manner. Explain the benefits of knowing HIV status early in pregnancy. Encourage the woman to be tested. Be certain that the woman knows how to protect herself from HIV infection by avoidance of high-risk behaviors.

If the woman is HIV positive, ensure that she understands the risk to her sexual partners and the importance of condom use. Counsel her regarding expected treatments. Explain the risks of perinatal transmission of HIV and the benefits of therapy. Explore her understanding of the treatment regimen.

● Nursing Process for the Pregnant Woman With an STI

Although different organisms cause STIs, avoiding high-risk behaviors can prevent them all. The nurse is in an excellent position to work with the pregnant woman who is diagnosed with an STI.

ASSESSMENT

Begin the assessment with a thorough history. Inquire regarding risk factors for STIs in a way that makes the woman feel safe to answer honestly. It is usually best to try to elicit the following

---

[3] Discussion of treatment for HIV for nonpregnant individuals is outside the scope of this textbook.

information with open-ended questions, if possible. Is there a previous history of STI? Has she or her partner ever been treated for an STI? Has she had multiple sexual partners? Is she in a new sexual relationship? Does her partner always use a condom, or does she use the female condom for every sexual act including oral sex? Does she engage in anal sex with her partner? Does she or her sexual partner engage in IV drug use? Does she or her partner share needles for IV drug use?

The history should include questions regarding symptoms of STI. Does she have a vaginal discharge? If so, have her describe the discharge. Is sex painful? Does she bleed during or after sex? Has she noticed swollen lymph nodes? Has she been running low-grade fevers? Has she noticed any rashes or skin lesions? Has she experienced night sweats or lost weight without trying to do so?

Perform a physical assessment. Measure her weight. Compare her current weight to her previous or normal weight. Note any recent weight loss. Record her temperature and other vital signs. Some STIs cause a low-grade fever. Palpate the lymph nodes in the neck and groin regions. Report any swollen or nonmobile nodes. Inspect the oral mucosa and tongue for lesions. Inspect the skin thoroughly for rashes or lesions.

Take note of signs of emotional distress, anxiety, or low self-esteem. Does she practice good personal hygiene? Self-esteem issues can express themselves by self-neglect and poor grooming. Does she make appropriate eye contact? Inquire regarding her social support. Does she have friends? Does she live with anyone? Does she have a partner? Is he or she supportive of her? Notice nonverbal behaviors such as fidgeting, hand wringing, or inattention.

SELECTED NURSING DIAGNOSES

- Risk for Infection (STI) related to unsafe sexual practices, IV drug use, or needle sharing.
- Ineffective Protection related to altered immune status or broken skin barrier.
- Deficient Knowledge of STI and treatment regimen.
- Risk for Situational Low Self-Esteem related to the stigma associated with STIs.
- Anxiety related to pregnancy outcome and fetal safety.

OUTCOME IDENTIFICATION AND PLANNING

Goals for a pregnant woman with an STI include risk control, prevention of the spread of infection,

adequate knowledge, maintaining positive self-esteem, anxiety control, and safe delivery of a healthy, infection-free infant. Goals and interventions are planned according to the individualized needs of the woman and her fetus throughout pregnancy, birth, and the postpartum period.

IMPLEMENTATION

Controlling Risks for STIs
Explain the risks of contact with infected bodily fluids and blood. Clarify that women are at higher risk than are men for contracting an STI during heterosexual intercourse. Make clear that the highest risk of STI transmission during sexual activity is engaging in anal intercourse without a condom. Emphasize the importance of using a latex condom for every act of sexual intercourse and a latex barrier for oral sex. Inform the woman to avoid sexual intercourse when there are open lesions or discharge on the genitals. Oral sex should also be avoided when lesions or discharge are present on the mouth or genitals.

Instruct the woman regarding proper handwashing techniques and the importance of frequent handwashing. If the woman is an IV drug user, assist her to find a needle exchange program, if one is available in the area. Help her devise a plan to avoid needle sharing. Assist her to enter a treatment program, if this is feasible and acceptable to the woman.

Maintaining Immune Status and Protection From Additional Infections
Teach the woman that infection with one STI puts her at higher risk for contracting another STI. This is particularly true for STIs that cause lesions or skin breakdown. Explain the importance of having all sexual partners treated for the infection. She should take her medication as directed.

Give instructions specific to the STI. If the woman is HIV positive, ensure that she understands the importance of diligently taking her antiretroviral medications daily. Explain that these medications control the viral load (amount of virus in the blood) and help maintain CD4 counts in the protective range.

Ensuring Knowledge of STI and Treatment Regimen
Teach the woman the specifics of the STI she is experiencing. Be sure that she can explain how the infection is transmitted, what the symptoms of infection are, how to avoid spreading the infection to her sexual partners, how to decrease the risk of transmitting the infection to her fetus, and what the treatment plan and goals are.

Verify understanding of the treatment regimen by asking the woman to describe the medications she is taking and when and how she is to take them. Have her explain the expected action of each medication, as well as expected side effects. Teach her to immediately report side effects she may find intolerable so that the physician can adjust her medications without jeopardizing her treatment. Explain the importance of completing the full course of treatment, even after symptoms subside, to prevent the development of resistant strains of the organism.

Enhancing Self-esteem

Maintain an open, accepting demeanor when interacting with the woman. Ensure she is in a comfortable, private place before interviewing her. Avoid asking potentially embarrassing questions in the presence of others.

Avoid negative criticisms and judgmental questions such as "Why didn't you?" or "You should have . . ." Encourage the woman to identify personal strengths. Convey confidence in the woman's ability to take care of her unborn child.

Reducing Anxiety

Use a calm, reassuring approach. Seek to understand the woman's perception of the risk to herself and to her fetus. Encourage the woman to verbalize her feelings. Use active listening. Ask for clarification when you do not understand.

Give factual information. Correct any misperceptions or misinformation the woman may have. Reassure the woman regarding the probable outcome of her pregnancy. Use up-to-date facts from reliable sources to avoid false reassurances. Help her understand the risks without causing unnecessary fear. For instance, you can explain that with treatment the risk of an HIV-positive woman transmitting HIV to her unborn child is less than 8%. Put another way, more than 90% of babies born to women with HIV disease who receive appropriate treatment will be born free of infection and will remain so.

EVALUATION: GOALS AND EXPECTED OUTCOMES

- **Goal:** The woman will control risks for STIs.
  Expected Outcomes:
  - Verbalizes ways she will reduce her risk for contracting or transmitting STIs.
  - Maintains a monogamous sexual relationship with one partner who is also monogamous or partner uses a latex condom for every act of sexual intercourse.

- Avoids anal sex.
- Avoids intravenous drug use or participates in a needle exchange program.
- **Goal:** The woman will not spread infection.
  Expected Outcomes:
  - Remains free of additional infections.
  - Maintains a plasma CD4 cell count above 200/mL (if HIV positive).
- **Goal:** The woman will have adequate knowledge of the STI and its treatment.
  Expected Outcomes:
  - Explains how the STI is transmitted.
  - Describes how to prevent transmission to sexual partners and decrease the risk of transmission to the fetus.
  - Explains her treatment regimen.
  - Verbalizes the goals of her treatment plan.
- **Goal:** The woman will maintain positive self-esteem.
  Expected Outcomes:
  - Demonstrates positive self-regard.
  - Makes positive statements about the self.
  - Maintains adequate personal hygiene.
  - Voices confidence in her ability to take care of her unborn child.
- **Goal:** The woman will have decreased anxiety.
  Expected Outcomes:
  - Expresses reasonable expectations regarding the outcome of the pregnancy.
  - Verbalizes decreased anxiety.

Test Yourself

- Which infection is best prevented by instructing the pregnant woman to avoid changing the cat litter box?

- Which sexually transmitted infection is most frequently diagnosed with a "wet mount?"

- What is the purpose of antiretroviral medications for the pregnant woman who is HIV positive?

PREGNANCY COMPLICATED BY INTIMATE PARTNER VIOLENCE

Intimate partner violence (IPV) is defined as abuse perpetrated by an individual against an intimate partner. The goal of the abusive behavior is to exert and maintain power and control over the partner. Abuse refers to any type of injury committed against a person, including physical, emotional, psychological, and

| BOX 16.8 | **Examples of Abusive Acts** |

The terms "abuse" or "abused" are often misunderstood to refer only to egregious acts of violence that result in serious physical injury. Therefore, it is important for the health care professional to give specific examples of abuse when screening for intimate partner violence (IPV).

Physical Acts of Abuse
• Punching
• Hitting
• Kicking
• Slapping
• Shoving
• Biting
• Scratching
• Grabbing
• Choking
• Poking
• Shaking
• Hair pulling
• Burning

Emotional Acts of Abuse
• Threats of harm to self, the intimate partner, or others
• Refusing to interact with the intimate partner without explanation ("silent treatment")
• Name calling
• Put downs
• Derogatory comments
• Any act of control
  • Financial (controlling all the money)
  • Decision making (without consulting the partner)
  • Isolation from family or friends
  • Prohibiting access to transportation or telephone
• Threatening or completing acts of violence against pets or children
• Destroying property the intimate partner cares about
• Blaming the intimate partner for his or her violent outbursts

Sexual Acts of Abuse
• Forcing the partner to watch or perform any sexual act against the partner's will.

sexual maltreatment (Box 16-8). An intimate partner is any person who is now or who ever has been in an intimate relationship with the victim. This definition includes present and former spouses, boyfriends, girlfriends, and dating partners. IPV occurs in relationships without regard to sexual preference. In other words, IPV occurs between same sex partners, as well as between heterosexual partners. IPV crosses social, cultural, religious, and economic boundaries. Other terms used to describe IPV are domestic violence, spouse abuse, domestic abuse, and battering (CDC, 2003).

It is difficult to determine the extent of IPV, partly because it is unknown how many cases of IPV go unreported. Some of the difficulty is related to the varied definitions that are used to collect and report these data. The CDC is attempting to correct this problem through the use of standardized terminology and definitions. Although IPV can be directed against men, more women report being abused. Anywhere from 25% to 31% of American women have experienced physical or sexual assault at the hands of an intimate partner; whereas, only 7% of men report being victims of this type of abuse. Yearly, approximately 1.5 million women report criminal acts of violence from an intimate partner. Of these women, approximately 324,000 are pregnant at the time the violence occurs (CDC, 2003).

Pregnancy is a vulnerable time for a woman. IPV may begin or escalate during pregnancy, particularly if the pregnancy is unplanned (Gazmararian et al., 2000). According to the American College of Obstetricians and Gynecologists (ACOG) and the CDC (2004), 4% to 8% of all pregnant women experience abuse during the pregnancy. In a Maryland study of pregnancy-associated deaths, it was discovered that a pregnant, or recently pregnant, woman is more likely to die of homicide than any other cause, including cardiovascular causes, such as pregnancy-induced hypertension (Horon & Cheng, 2001).

The pregnant woman is at risk for certain complications associated with abuse. According to Cunningham et al. (2001b), a woman's risk of developing intrauterine infection or experiencing preterm labor is doubled if she is a victim of domestic violence. She is also at increased risk for abruptio placenta and delivering by cesarean section, and her infant is more likely to have a low birth weight (Anderson, 2002).

Clinical Manifestations and Diagnosis

Abuse may begin slowly and escalate with time, or abusive episodes may begin early in a relationship. There is a generally accepted model, the Cycle of Violence (Fig. 16-2), that explains the pathophysiology of IPV. Abusive episodes usually progress in three identifiable phases:

1. Tension building phase
2. Explosion phase
3. Absence of tension or the "honeymoon" phase

Although it is not always possible to identify IPV during interactions with the victim or abuser, there are warning signs. The perpetrator of IPV often exhibits an overly protective attitude toward the victim. The abuser may accompany the victim to all office visits and may answer questions for the victim. It is important to remember that he may seem pleasant and congenial. Conversely, he may make degrading remarks about the victim in front of health care providers or others.

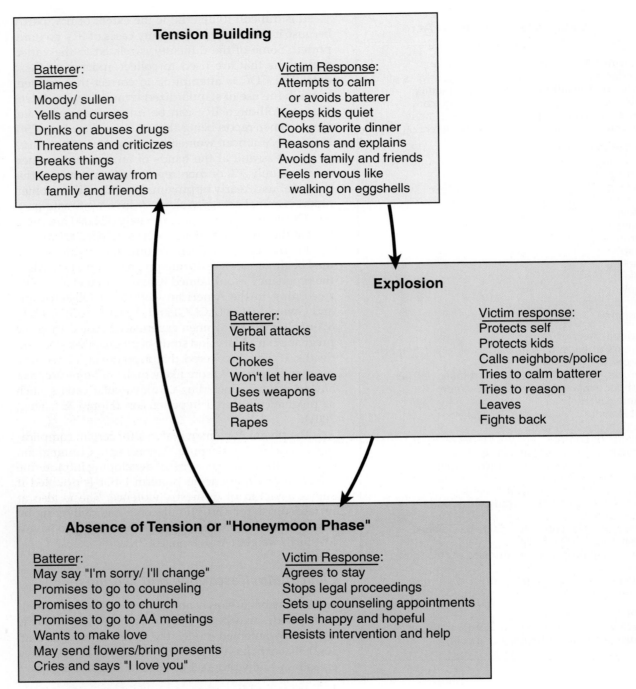

● **Figure 16.2** The cycle of violence.

The victim may appear quiet and passive. She may avoid eye contact. She may have an unkempt appearance and may appear depressed. She may exhibit anxiety, nervousness, and suicidal tendencies. She may abuse alcohol or drugs in response to the abuse. Common medical complaints include headache or neck pain, chest pain, palpitations, numbness and tingling, pelvic pain, dyspareunia, and urinary tract infection

(Wadman & Foral, 2003). Clues that should raise suspicion of abuse are listed in Box 16-9.

Treatment

Because every woman is at risk for IPV, routine screening of all women is the key to assisting those who are ready to report abuse and receive help. In particular,

BOX 16.9	**Clues That May Indicate the Woman Is Being Abused**

Any of the following signs should raise the suspicion of possible intimate partner violence (IPV). It is important to remember that a woman who is being abused may not show obvious signs of abuse.
- History of
  - Repeated assaults
  - Drug or alcohol abuse
  - Depression
  - Suicide attempts
- Injury* to the head, face, or neck
- Loose or broken teeth
- Injury to the breasts or abdomen
- Types of injury to include
  - Injury inflicted by a weapon
  - Cigarette and rope burns
  - Bite marks
  - Bruises and welts
- Pattern and distribution of injury to include
  - Areas normally covered by clothes
  - Occurring on both sides of the body (often on extremities)
  - Defensive posture injuries (such as to the hands or feet that occur when the victim tries to ward off the attacker)
- Injuries in various stages of healing
- Injuries that do not match the cause of trauma described by the woman or her partner

Signs unique to the pregnant woman may include
- Presents for late prenatal care or has no prenatal care
- Attends prenatal visits sporadically
- High gravidity and parity rates
- Poor weight gain during pregnancy
- History of
  - Spontaneous abortion(s)
  - STIs
  - Previous fetal death

* Injury can be evidenced by bruises, scrapes, scratches, or cuts, as well as burns, broken bones, etc.

Adapted from Anderson (2002), Wadman & Foral (2003), and others.

the prenatal period presents an excellent opportunity for screening for IPV. Prenatal visits offer opportunities for the health care provider to develop rapport and trust with the woman. The perinatal period is also a unique time of opportunity because the woman may be motivated to think about the future and the safety of her unborn child.

Although screening is a powerful tool, common barriers may get in the way (Williams, Dou, & Leal, 2003). The health care provider may feel the she does not have enough time to ask about IPV. Often providers feel uncomfortable addressing the issue. The provider may be afraid that he will embarrass or offend the woman. Many times screening is avoided because the

provider feels helpless to do anything to change the situation. Because screening is a critical intervention for the victim of IPV, ACOG and the CDC recommend provider training to overcome these barriers.

Once IPV is identified, interventions are directed toward safety assessment and planning. Danger signals include statements from the woman that she or her children are in danger, that the violence has recently escalated, the partner has threatened to kill, or that there are lethal weapons (particularly guns) in the home. If the likelihood of danger exists, the health care provider assists the woman to develop a safety plan (Box 16-10).

Trained health care providers discuss options with the woman. Basically, the woman has three options:

- Stay with the abuser.
- Remove the abuser through arrest or with protective orders.
- Leave the relationship temporarily or permanently.

It is important for the provider to keep in mind that the woman is the only one who can truly determine which option is best for her.

Nursing Care

There are many reasons that it is difficult to discuss domestic violence with patients. Myths abound, such

BOX 16.10	**Components of a Safety Plan**

Whether or not the woman elects to stay in the abusive relationship, she should have a safety plan. The health care provider instructs her to
- Memorize the National Domestic Violence Hotline: 1-800-799-SAFE (7233) or 1-800-787-3224 (for hearing-impaired or deaf victims).
- Pack a bag in advance with cash, credit cards, and clothes for herself and children. The bag should remain at a trusted friend or family member's house.
- Have important personal documents readily accessible. These include
  - Birth certificates
  - Driver's license
  - Bank account information
  - Important telephone numbers
  - Insurance information and cards
  - Court documents or orders
  - Copies of utility bills
- Establish a code word with family and friends to indicate when violence is escalating and help is needed.
- Identify a safe place to go. This may be a women's shelter or other safe place. Each community has unique resources that should be identified for the woman.

as IPV happens in only certain socioeconomic or ethnic groups or the woman could just leave if she were not so weak or codependent. Often it is the nurse's own discomfort with the subject of abuse that keeps the silence. The nurse may feel powerless to do anything about the situation, and therefore does not bring up the subject. There may be a lack of knowledge about how to screen for abuse. Whatever the barrier, the nurse can learn to screen pregnant women for IPV.

Assist the RN to assess for abuse. Always screen the woman alone, away from children and the abuser (Cockey, 2003). Provide privacy. Ask simple, direct, open-ended questions in a nonjudgmental way to show the victim that you are a safe person when she is ready to disclose. Avoid questions that imply that the woman is responsible for the violence or that it is easy to walk away from a violent relationship. Questions to avoid include, "Why do you not just leave? What did you do to make your partner so angry? Why do you go back to your partner?" Remember, determining whether or not a woman should leave an abusive relationship is always only her decision to make.

Sometimes it is better to err on the side of caution! You may not be the best person to screen for IPV. If you haven't been trained, it is better to report your suspicions of abuse to an RN or other health care provider who has been trained to deal with victims of abuse. However, do not allow your discomfort with the subject to hinder you from learning how to screen for violence.

Always document the woman's responses to questioning about IPV. If the woman denies being in an abusive relationship, document her denial. It is important to quote the woman directly. Do not use terms such as "alleges" when you are documenting the woman's replies. This terminology may cast doubt on the veracity of the woman's answers if the medical record is ever used as evidence in a court of law.

If the woman discloses IPV, be careful to respond with supportive statements. One of the most important things you can communicate to the victim of abuse is the fact that the abuse is not her fault! You can say, "This is not your fault. No one deserves to be treated this way." Examples of other helpful statements include, "I'm sorry that you've been hurt. Do you want to talk about it? I am concerned for your safety. You have options. Help is available."

Document your assessment objectively. If there are physical indications of abuse, draw these on a body map, then use measurable terminology to describe each lesion or observation. Photographs can be invaluable aids in a courtroom. You must get the woman's written consent before photographing her, however.

Be knowledgeable about local resources that are available for the victim of IPV. Resources include office and hospital personnel with specialized training, IPV advocacy groups, women's shelters, hotlines, child protective services, and law enforcement resources. Many cities have city-wide plans to respond to IPV. Be familiar with your city's plan.

The compassionate nurse who develops the trust of the abused woman can help turn the tide of abuse. Recovery from IPV does not happen in only one or two interventions; rather, it is a consistent atmosphere of encouragement and esteem building that may assist the victim to become a survivor.

PREGNANCY COMPLICATED BY AGE-RELATED CONCERNS

The typical childbearing years envelop the ages of 15 through 44 years; however, females can, and sometimes do, become pregnant anywhere from ages 9 through 56 years of age. At either end of the age spectrum pregnancy carries higher risk for morbidity and mortality for the woman and her fetus. Although age-related concerns warrant special "at-risk" considerations, they are not in the pathophysiologic category, as are the medical conditions heretofore discussed. Instead, they are a natural part of the reproductive process requiring additional accommodations throughout the perinatal period.

Adolescent Pregnancy

Adolescent, or teen, pregnancy is defined as pregnancy occurring at 19 years of age or younger. The consequences of teenage pregnancy are well documented. According to the United States Department of Health and Human Services (2000), teenage mothers are "less likely to get or stay married, less likely to complete high school or college, and more likely to require public assistance and to live in poverty than their peers who are not mothers." There are also considerable consequences for the infants of adolescent mothers, particularly for those whose mothers are younger than 15 years. Infants of teen mothers are more likely to be below normal birth weight, experience higher neonatal mortality rate, and have a higher incidence of sudden infant death syndrome.

The good news is that the adolescent pregnancy rate has decreased steadily since 1990. Teen birth rates were at an all time low in 2001. The birth rate for teens younger than 15 years fell from 1.4 per 1,000 in 1991 to 0.8 per 1,000 in 2001. The 2001 rate for the youngest teens is the lowest it has been since 1966. The rate also fell for adolescents 15 through 19 years of age, from 38.6 in 1991 to 24.7 in 2001, which is a record low

(Hamilton, Sutton, & Ventura, 2003). The two foremost explanations for this decline are the number of female adolescents engaging in sexual intercourse has leveled off after increasing during the 1980s and condom use among sexually active teens has significantly increased (Anderson, Smiley, Flick, & Lewis, 2000).

Clinical Manifestations

Many pregnant teens seek late prenatal care, often in the 3rd trimester, or they return sporadically for prenatal visits. Sometimes they get no prenatal care. There are many factors that contribute to poor prenatal care and subsequent complications of pregnancy. Recent research points to the social situation of the adolescent as the root cause of increased pregnancy risk, rather than age itself. The pregnant teen is more likely than her older counterpart to be unmarried, have less education, be a member of an ethnic minority, and to live in poverty (Anderson et al., 2000).

The adolescent faces many barriers to receiving adequate prenatal care. The pregnant teen may be fearful of disclosing her pregnancy to her parents or caregivers, so she may attempt to hide the pregnancy by wearing loose clothing and avoiding prolonged interaction with adults. Or she may lack family support or transportation to regularly attend prenatal visits. Because body image is extremely important to the adolescent, she may use behaviors associated with eating disorders, such as purging or self-starvation, to avoid weight gain during the pregnancy. The pregnant adolescent may not get adequate nutrition secondary to poor food choices. There is increasing evidence that pregnant teens are at increased risk for domestic violence. This situation can also lead to sporadic attendance to prenatal visits. Whatever the reason for not receiving good prenatal care, the pregnant adolescent is at increased risk for complications, such as inadequate weight gain, anemia, and preeclampsia-eclampsia. All of these conditions can result in fetal complications, such as intrauterine growth restriction, low birth weight, and preterm birth.

Diagnosis of adolescent pregnancy is made with the same tests used for older women. However, the diagnosis can be easily missed if the practitioner does not keep in mind the prospect of pregnancy when performing a history and physical. Adolescents often deny the possibility of pregnancy (even to themselves), making diagnosis even more challenging. The adolescent should be screened for pregnancy if she reports irregular periods, nausea and vomiting, or fatigue.

Treatment

The best treatment for teenage pregnancy is prevention. Many physicians and advanced practice nurses are actively involved in programs designed to prevent adolescent pregnancy. Others are involved in research studies attempting to discover which methods work and which do not. Much of the literature on adolescent pregnancy concentrates on prevention.

The challenge of managing an adolescent pregnancy is considerable. Although obtaining information about the woman's physical and psychological response to pregnancy and social support available to her is notable for any pregnant woman's care, this part of the history is particularly valuable for the pregnant teen. If the adolescent does not have adequate social support, she is more likely to experience adverse outcomes. Other areas of the history to which the practitioner pays close attention include determining the teen's perception of options available to her, HIV and other STI risk factors, and school status. Because IPV is associated with adolescent pregnancy, it is particularly important for the practitioner to screen for domestic violence.

The informed practitioner does several things to assist the pregnant teen. Advocacy for the pregnant adolescent includes giving information in an open, nonjudgmental way and supporting the adolescent's choices. This approach requires that the practitioner treat the adolescent with dignity and respect by providing and protecting the right to privacy and confidentiality. Advocacy includes assisting the teen to freely make choices without coercion.

> **CULTURAL SNAPSHOT 16-1**
>
> Remember that each adolescent is an individual. Her beliefs and values are influenced by her culture. Plan interventions based on the unique needs of each teen.

One crucial part of management includes helping the teen to develop an adequate support network. Parents, teachers, friends, and the father of the baby are all potential resources for the pregnant adolescent. These individuals may benefit from guidance on ways they can effectively help.

Nursing Care

Caring for Developmental Needs

Keep in mind the developmental needs of the pregnant adolescent. Pregnancy does not change the developmental tasks, although it may complicate the issues. According to Erickson (Cramer, Flynn, & LaFave, 1997), developing an identity is an essential developmental task of the adolescent. It is important to help the pregnant teen to work on identity issues while she also begins to adopt the role of motherhood.

As with other teens, the pregnant adolescent's normal priorities include acceptance by her peer group and focusing on appearance. In addition, the adolescent, particularly the very young adolescent, is typically self-centered, a characteristic that can make it difficult for her to consider the needs of others. Take into account these priorities and characteristics as you plan your nursing care.

Caring for Physical Needs

Adequate nutrition is essential to the health of the pregnant teen. However, nutritional considerations may not have a high priority from the adolescent's viewpoint. Assist the teen to identify healthful foods that are appealing and easy to prepare. It may help to determine what foods the teen normally eats and then suggest more healthful alternatives. For instance, rather than forbidding desserts, help the teen to choose desserts that have nutritional value, such as fresh fruits or frozen yogurt. You might suggest that the teen try low-salt tortilla chips, baked potato chips, or whole grain crackers, rather than regular potato chips.

Cultural sensitivity is in order. Do not forget that food choices are influenced culturally. Be sure that you understand the teen's cultural context when you counsel her regarding prenatal nutrition.

Pregnant teens are at higher risk for delivering prematurely, particularly if they experience a repeat pregnancy during their teen years. One way to help decrease the risk of a repeat pregnancy is to counsel the teen regarding birth control methods. STIs are another potential problem. Encourage the use of barrier methods of birth control (particularly male use of latex condoms) that supply protection from STIs.

Caring for Emotional and Psychological Needs

The emotional and psychological needs of the adolescent are complex. When the emotional demands of pregnancy are added, the strain can be tremendous. It is frequently helpful to include significant support persons in the care planning. It is easier for them to provide meaningful support if they know how pregnancy might affect emotional functioning.

Be knowledgeable regarding community resources for the pregnant teen. If you or the primary practitioner refers the teen to another entity, follow up to make certain the adolescent receives the services for which she was referred. If not, try to determine the barriers that prevent her from following through with treatment. Assist her to work through the barriers to obtain needed services.

Remain nonjudgmental and open minded when dealing with pregnant teens. There are many factors working against the teen. Scolding and punishment are not helpful interventions. They tend to push the adolescent away and do little to resolve the real issues with which the teen must contend.

Pregnancy in Later Life

While adolescent birth rates have been steadily declining, births for women in their late 30s and early 40s have risen. In 1990, the birth rate for women 35 through 39 years of age was 31.7 per 1,000. The rate increased by 28% to 40.6 per 1,000 in 2001. For women ages 40 to 44 years, the birth rate increased by 47%, from 5.5 in 1990 to 8.1 per 1,000 in 2001. The rate for women aged 45 to 49 years has more than doubled from 0.2 in 1990 to 0.5 in 2001 (Hamilton et al., 2003).

There are risk factors that are associated with delayed childbearing. For women, fertility declines with age. Although assisted reproductive technology is much more effective than it was in the past, there is a higher incidence of multiple fetal pregnancies (i.e., twins, triplets) when these technologies are used to help a woman get pregnant. A woman older than 35 years is more likely to conceive a child with chromosomal abnormalities, such as Down's syndrome. She is also at higher risk for spontaneous abortion (miscarriage), pregnancy-induced hypertension, gestational diabetes, preterm delivery, and bleeding and placental abnormalities. She has almost twice the risk of a younger woman of having a fetal demise; she is more likely to have cesarean delivery; and she is more likely to deliver a low birth-weight baby. As ominous as these statistics sound, it is helpful to remember that the majority of pregnancies to women older than 35 years end with healthy babies and healthy moms.

Clinical Manifestations

In general the woman who waits to have her first baby until she is in her late 30s or early 40s has more education than her younger counterparts. Frequently she has chosen to postpone childbearing to pursue career choices. She is most likely to be married, to have financial resources, and to have planned the pregnancy. She is also more likely to have a chronic condition, such as diabetes or hypertension. It is of note that the older pregnant woman may be more likely to use alcohol during pregnancy, particularly if she is unmarried (CDC, 2002).

Some older women report more aches and pains during pregnancy, whereas others do not. If the older woman is physically fit, it is less likely that pregnancy will cause excessive tiredness and distress. The hormonal changes of pregnancy are often a cause of facial skin breakouts, even for the older woman.

Treatment

A preconceptual visit is recommended for any woman who wishes to become pregnant. For the older woman it is especially important that she have a complete physical before becoming pregnant, particularly if she has a chronic medical condition. Because it may be more difficult for the older woman to conceive, fertility experts recommend that she seek medical help if she is not pregnant within 6 months of trying.

Once pregnancy is achieved, genetic testing and counseling is offered to the woman older than 35 years. The miscarriage rate is higher as the woman ages, most likely because of chromosomal abnormalities of the conceptus. Trisomy 21 (Down's syndrome), trisomy 18 (Edward's syndrome), and trisomy 13 (Patau's syndrome) all occur with greater frequency as the woman ages. Therefore, chorionic villus sampling or early amniocentesis is offered.

Nursing Care

It is helpful to approach the older pregnant woman with an open mind. Be ready to answer questions and to suggest pregnancy and parenting resources. A woman that chooses to delay childbearing until she is past 35 years of age does not want to be constantly reminded that she is an "older" pregnant woman. Neither does she want to be reminded of the increased risks associated with late childbearing. If the woman complains of receiving "rude" remarks from strangers about her age, suggest that it is OK to ignore such remarks. If she has a good sense of humor, she may be able to make a joke out of the situation. For example, one woman who was asked if she had planned to have a child at her age replied that she was "certainly old enough to know better."

Suggest a good skin care routine to combat facial breakouts. The older pregnant woman may benefit from a trip to a spa for a facial. It will give her a chance to relax, and she can obtain advice from a skin expert. Caution her not to begin a vigorous exercise routine during pregnancy. If she enters pregnancy already physically fit, she may continue her exercise pattern as long as she does not experience a complication of pregnancy.

A PERSONAL GLIMPSE

My husband and I married in our late 20s. We decided to wait until we were both in our 30s to have children because we had lots of school loans to pay off and wanted to be financially secure before raising a family. I got pregnant with my daughter when I was 33. It was a normal pregnancy; I felt great, and the baby and I were completely healthy throughout. When Libby was 3 years old, we decided to try and have another baby. I conceived easily and eagerly made my first doctor appointment to officially confirm the pregnancy. I assumed that this pregnancy would be as uncomplicated as my first. Imagine my surprise when I sat down with the nurse and she started grilling me about the potential for genetic problems and health problems in my baby because I was over 35 years old. She started talking about the need for me to have special blood tests and an amniocentesis. It was all rather overwhelming and scary. I was shocked. How could 3 years make such a difference in the way that my pregnancies would be managed?

Julia

LEARNING OPPORTUNITY: How can the nurse present information to the woman at risk without increasing her anxiety level? Does the risk level dramatically increase at the age of 35? Why or why not?

Test Yourself

- True or false: Intimate partner violence (IPV) occurs only in heterosexual relationships.
- List three components of a safety plan for a victim of IPV.
- Name two dysfunctional behaviors the pregnant adolescent might use to keep from gaining weight during pregnancy.

KEY POINTS

- Tight glycemic control for the pregnant woman with diabetes dramatically decreases the incidence of complications. Glucose levels over time are determined by measuring glycosylated hemoglobin (HbA1C).
- The pancreas of the woman with type 1 diabetes does not produce insulin, so it must be administered subcutaneously. Insulin can be self-injected or administered via an insulin pump. The cornerstone of therapy for gestational diabetes is diet therapy.
- Fetal surveillance is critical for the pregnant woman with diabetes. Fetal activity counts and nonstress testing is done to determine fetal well-being. Amniocentesis to determine fetal lung maturity may be done in the 3rd trimester to help determine the optimum time for delivery.
- Typical nursing concerns for the pregnant woman with DM include management of the therapeutic regimen, risk for maternal and fetal injury, risk for infection, and fetal macrosomia.

▶ The main goal of treatment for the pregnant woman with heart disease is prevention and early detection of cardiac decompensation. This goal is met by monitoring activity levels, managing stress, diet modification, and medication therapy.

▶ Iron-deficiency anemia requires iron supplementation and a diet high in iron-rich foods. Because iron supplements predispose to constipation, the nurse teaches the woman to maintain adequate hydration, exercise regularly, and get plenty of fiber in the diet.

▶ Preventing a crisis is the goal of treatment for the woman with sickle cell anemia. Interventions involve maintaining adequate hydration, avoiding infection, getting adequate rest, and eating a well-balanced diet.

▶ Teaching is an important part of asthma management. The woman should be advised to continue taking her asthma medications during pregnancy. She should avoid over-the-counter medications and protect herself from asthma triggers and infection.

▶ Because antiepileptic drugs (AEDs) are a major cause of fetal defects, preconceptual care is recommended. High-dose folic acid supplements are given before and throughout pregnancy to help prevent neural tube defects, and vitamin K supplementation is often given during the last weeks of pregnancy to prevent neonatal hemorrhage.

▶ TORCH stands for toxoplasmosis, other (hepatitis B, syphilis, varicella, and herpes zoster), rubella, cytomegalovirus, and herpes simplex virus. These infections can lead to serious fetal anomalies and other complications. Prevention of infection is the best treatment strategy because many of the TORCH infections do not have effective treatment.

▶ Chlamydia is caused by sexual transmission of the bacterium *Chlamydia trachomatis*. It is frequently asymptomatic but easily treated with antibiotics.

▶ Gonorrhea is caused by the bacterium *Neisseria gonorrhoeae* and is treated with antibiotics. Gonorrhea increases the risk of PID, spontaneous abortion, and preterm delivery.

▶ Human papillomavirus (HPV) is a virus that causes genital warts. The warts have a tendency to increase in size during pregnancy and can lead to heavy bleeding during delivery. HPV can be transmitted to the fetus during birth.

▶ Trichomoniasis is caused by a protozoan. It is treated with metronidazole (Flagyl) given orally.

▶ A pregnant woman with HIV/AIDS can pass the infection to her unborn child during pregnancy or childbirth or while breast-feeding. Disease progression and response to treatment are determined by measuring CD4 counts. Therapy during pregnancy is prophylactic administration of oral zidovudine (ZDV) throughout pregnancy. Breast-feeding is contraindicated.

▶ Nursing considerations for the pregnant woman with a sexually transmitted infection (STI) include risk for additional infection, ineffective protection, deficient knowledge, risk for low self-esteem, and anxiety. Education regarding STI prevention and treatment are important nursing functions.

▶ The Cycle of Violence describes the typical pathophysiology of IPV. Tension building is followed by the explosion phase, which leads to the honeymoon phase.

▶ Treatment of IPV includes the screening of all pregnant women. Once IPV is identified, interventions are directed toward safety assessment and planning. The victim should be assisted to develop a safety plan.

▶ A pregnant teen is at high risk for poor prenatal care. Body image is an important consideration that may lead to attempts to limit weight gain during pregnancy. She is also at risk for domestic violence, inadequate weight gain, anemia, and preeclampsia-eclampsia. Nutrition and social support are important areas of intervention for the pregnant adolescent.

▶ The woman who delays childbearing past 35 years of age is at increased risk for complications of pregnancy. However, she is frequently mature, has a career, is financially stable, and married. Most pregnancies to older women end successfully with a healthy mother and a healthy baby. Preconceptual care is ideal.

REFERENCES AND SELECTED READINGS

Books and Journals

American College of Obstetricians and Gynecologists (ACOG) & Centers for Disease Control (CDC). (2001). *Intimate partner violence during pregnancy: A guide for clinicians.* PowerPoint Training Slide Lecture. Released May 29, 2001. Retrieved September 14, 2003, from http://www.cdc.gov/reproductivehealth/violence/ipvdp.htm

American Diabetes Association. (2003). Gestational diabetes: Position statement. *Diabetes Care, 26*(Suppl 1), S103–S105.

Anderson, C. (2002). Battered and pregnant: A nursing challenge. *AWHONN Lifelines, 6*(2), 95–99.

Anderson, N. E., Smiley, D. V., Flick, L. H., & Lewis, C. Y. (2000). Missouri rural adolescent pregnancy project (MORAPP). *Public Health Nursing, 17*(5), 355–362.

Burnett, L. B., & Adler, J. (2001). Domestic violence. In S. A. Conrad, F. Talavera, R. C. Harwood, J. Halamka, & B. Brenner (Eds.), *eMedicine.* Last updated July 20, 2001. Retrieved September 14, 2003, from http://www.emedicine.com/emerg/topic153.htm

Burton, J., & Reyes, M. (2001). Breathe in breathe out: Controlling asthma during pregnancy. *AWHONN Lifelines, 5*(1), 24–30.

Caughey, A. B., & Sandberg, P. (2002). Seizure disorders in pregnancy. S. R. Trupin, F. Talavera, D. Chelmow, F. B. Gaupp, & L. P. Shulman (Eds.), *eMedicine*. Last updated June 28, 2002. Retrieved August 10, 2003, from http://www.emedicine.com/med/topic3433.htm

Centers for Disease Control and Prevention (CDC). (2000). National and state-specific pregnancy rates among adolescents—United States, 1995–1997. *MMWR, 49*(27). Retrieved September 20, 2003, from http://www.cdc.gov/mmwr/preview/mmwrhtml/mm4927a1.htm

Centers for Disease Control and Prevention (CDC). (2001). *STD surveillance 2001*. Prepared by the Division of Sexually Transmitted Diseases of the National Center for HIV, STD and TB Prevention. Retrieved September 6, 2003, from http://www.cdc.gov/std/stats/TOC2001.htm

Centers for Disease Control and Prevention (CDC). (2002). Alcohol use among women of childbearing age—United States, 1991–1999. *MMWR, 51*(43), 273–276. Retrieved September 28, 2003, from http://www.cdc.gov/mmwr/preview/mmwrhtml/mm5113a2.htm

Centers for Disease Control and Prevention (CDC). (2003*). Intimate partner violence fact sheet*. Prepared by the Centers for Disease Control and Prevention and the National Center for Injury Preventions and Control. Last reviewed August 21, 2003. Retrieved September 13, 2003, from http://www.cdc.gov/ncipc/factsheets/ipvfacts.htm

Centers for Disease Control and Prevention (CDC). (2004). Recommended childhood and adolescent immunization schedule—United States, January—June 2004. Approved by the Advisory Committee on Immunization Practices, the American Academy of Pediatrics, and the American Academy of Family Physicians. Retrieved August 5, 2004, from http://www.cdc.gov/nip/recs/child-schedule.pdf

Cockey, C. D. (2003). Screening for violence in pregnancy: Nurses should ask about violence in private—but not all do. *AWHONN Lifelines, 7*(6), 495–497.

Cramer, C., Flynn, B., & LaFave, A. (1997). *Erick Erickson's 8 stages of psychosocial development summary chart*. Retrieved August 6, 2004, from http://web.cortland.edu/andersmd/ERIK/sum.HTML

Cunningham, F. G., Gant, N. F., Leveno, K. J., Gilstrap, L. C. III, Hauth, J. C., & Wenstrom, K. D. (2001a). Cardiovascular disease. In *Williams obstetrics* (21st ed., pp. 1181–1207). New York: McGraw-Hill Medical Publishing Division.

Cunningham, F. G., Gant, N. F., Leveno, K. J., Gilstrap, L. C. III, Hauth, J. C., & Wenstrom, K. D. (2001b). Critical care and trauma. In *Williams obstetrics* (21st ed., pp. 1159–1180). New York: McGraw-Hill Medical Publishing Division.

Cunningham, F. G., Gant, N. F., Leveno, K. J., Gilstrap, L. C. III, Hauth, J. C., & Wenstrom, K. D. (2001c). Diabetes. In *Williams obstetrics* (21st ed., pp. 1359–1381). New York: McGraw-Hill Medical Publishing Division.

Fischer, R. (2003). Genital herpes in pregnancy. In A. Witlin, F. Talavera, R. S. Legro, F. B. Gaupp, & L. P. Shulman (Eds.), *eMedicine*. Last updated March 20, 2003. Retrieved September 1, 2003, from http://www.emedicine.com/med/topic3554.htm

Gazmararian, J. A., Petersen, R., Spitz, A. M., Goodwin, M. M., Saltzman, L. E., & Marks, J. S. (2000). Violence and reproductive health: Current knowledge and future research directions [abstract]. *Maternal and Child Health Journal (special issue): Violence and Reproductive Health, 4*(2). Retrieved September 14, 2003, from http://www.cdc.gov/reproductivehealth/wh_viol_mchjv4n2.htm

Hamilton, B. E., Sutton, P. D., & Ventura, S. J. (2003). Revised birth and fertility rates for the 1990s and new rates for Hispanic populations, 2000 and 2001: United States. *National Vital Statistics Reports NVSS, 51*(12). Retrieved September 20, 2003, from http://www.cdc.gov/nchs/data/nvsr/nvsr51/nvsr51_12.pdf

Hicks, P. (2000). Gestational diabetes in primary care. *Medscape General Medicine, 2*(1). Retrieved August 3, 2003, from http://www.medscape.com/viewarticle/408910

Horon, I. L., & Cheng, D. (2001). Enhanced surveillance for pregnancy-associated mortality: Maryland, 1993–1998 [abstract]. *JAMA, 285*(11), 1455–1459. Retrieved September 14, 2003, from the JAMA&Archives website http://pubs.ama-assn.org/

Jones, J., Lopez, A., & Wilson, M. (2003). Congenital toxoplasmosis. *American Family Physician, 67*(10), 2131–2147. Retrieved August 31, 2003, from http://www.aafp.org/afp/20030515/2131.html

Kazzi, A. A., & Marachelian, A. (2001). Pregnancy, asthma. In A. J. Sayah, F. Talavera, M. Zwanger, J. Halamka, & S. H. Plantz (Eds.), *eMedicine*. Last updated June 6, 2001. Retrieved August 10, 2003, from http://www.emedicine.com/emerg/topic476.htm

Laino, C. (2003). Gestational diabetes raises risk of metabolic syndrome. In D. Flapan (Ed.), *Medscape Medical News*. Retrieved July 26, 2003, from http://www.medscape.com/viewarticle/457507

Lie, D. A. (2003). Varicella zoster in first trimester of pregnancy. *Medscape Primary Care, 5*(1). Posted March 21, 2003. Retrieved September 1, 2003, from http://www.medscape.com/viewarticle/450603

Liu, P., & Euerle, B. (2002). Syphilis. In D. R. Lucey, F. Talavera, J. L. Brusch, E. Mylonakis, & B. A. Cunha (Eds.), *eMedicine*. Last updated August 16, 2002. Retrieved September 1, 2003, from http://www.emedicine.com/med/topic2224.htm

March of Dimes. (Undated). Cytomegalovirus infection in pregnancy. *Quick reference: Infections and diseases*. Retrieved September 1, 2003, from http://www.marchofdimes.com/professionals/681_1195.asp

March of Dimes. (2003). *Diabetes in pregnancy*. Retrieved July 19, 2003, from http://www.marchofdimes.com/professionals/681_1197.asp

Mayfield, E. (1996). *New hope for people with sickle cell anemia*. U.S. Food and Drug Administration. (Last updated February 1999). Publication No. (FDA) 99-1251. Retrieved August 17, 2003, from http://www.fda.gov/fdac/features/496_sick.html

Metcalf-Wilson, K. (2002). Confidentiality, communication and compliance: The three 'C's' of female adolescent care. *AWHONN Lifelines, 6*(4), 344–348.

Miller, M. M., & Greenberger, P. A. (1999). Asthma and pregnancy: A review. *Medscape General Medicine, 1*(3). Retrieved August 3, 2003, from http://www.medscape.com/viewarticle/408736

Montgomery, K. S. (2003). Health promotion for pregnant adolescents. *AWHONN Lifelines, 7*(5), 432–444.

Moore, T. (2002). Diabetes mellitus and pregnancy. In R. K. Zurawin, F. Talavera, C. V. Smith, M. Cooper, & L. P. Shulman (Eds.), *eMedicine*. Last updated October 3, 2002. Retrieved July 17, 2003, from http://www.emedicine.com/med/topic3249.htm

Morrell, M. J. (2002). Epilepsy in women. *American Family Physician, 66*(8). Retrieved August 10, 2003, from http://www.aafp.org/afp/20021015/1489.html

National Institute of Allergy and Infectious Diseases (NIAID). (2002, May). *Gonorrhea*. Health matters fact sheet prepared by the NIAID. Retrieved September 6, 2003, http://www.niaid.nih.gov/factsheets/stdgon.htm

National Institute of Allergy and Infectious Diseases (NIAID). (2002, November). *Syphilis*. Health matters fact sheet prepared by the NIAID. Retrieved September 6, 2003, from http://www.niaid.nih.gov/factsheets/stdsyph.htm

National Institute of Allergy and Infectious Diseases (NIAID). (2003, June). *HIV infection and AIDS: An overview*. Fact sheet prepared by the Office of Communications and Public Liaison, National Institute of Allergy and Infectious Diseases, and National Institutes of Health, Bethesda, MD. Retrieved September 7, 2003, from http://www.niaid.nih.gov/factsheets/hivinf.htm

National Institutes of Health. (1993). *Report of the working group on asthma and pregnancy* (NIH Publication No. 93-3279). Retrieved August 9, 2003, from http://www.nhlbi.nih.gov/health/prof/lung/asthma/astpreg.txt

National Institutes of Health. (2002). Contraception and pregnancy. In *The management of sickle cell disease*, 4th ed. NIH publication No. 02-2117. Retrieved August 16, 2003, from http://www.nhlbi.nih.gov/health/prof/blood/sickle/sc_mngt.pdf

Ostlund, I., et al. (2003). Maternal and fetal outcomes if gestational impaired glucose tolerance is not treated. *Diabetes Care, 26*(7), 2107–2111.

Robinson, J. N., & Norwitz, E. R. (2000). Respiratory complications. In A. T. Evans & K. R. Niswander (Eds.), *Manual of obstetrics* (6th ed., pp. 82–89). Philadelphia: Lippincott, Williams & Wilkins.

Rochester, J. A., & Kirchner, J. T. (1997). Epilepsy in pregnancy. *American Family Physician, 56*(6). Retrieved August 10, 2003, from http://www.aafp.org/afp/971015ap/rochest.html

Rogers, M. F., Fowler, M. G., & Lindegren, M. L. (2001). Revised recommendations for HIV screening of pregnant women. *MMWR, 50*(RR19), 59–86. A CDC Report. Retrieved September 7, 2003, from http://www.cdc.gov/mmwr/preview/mmwrhtml/rr5019a2.htm

Schleiss, M. R. (2003). Cytomegalovirus infection. In D. Jaimovich, R. Konop, L. L. Barton, R. W. Tolan, & R. Steele (Eds.), *eMedicine*. Last updated April 1, 2003.

Retrieved September 1, 2003, from http://www.emedicine.com/ped/topic544.htm

Silver, H. (2000). Cardiovascular complications. In A. T. Evans & K. R. Niswander (Eds.), *Manual of obstetrics* (6th ed., pp. 40–50). Philadelphia: Lippincott, Williams & Wilkins.

Smith, J. E., & Mattson, S. D. (2000). Domestic violence. In J. E. Smith & S. D. Mattson (Eds.), *Core curriculum for maternal–newborn nursing* (2nd ed.). Philadelphia: WB Saunders.

Spencer, D. (2002). Women's health and epilepsy. In A. S. Blum, F. Talavera, J. E. Cavazos, M. J. Baker, & N. Lorenzo (Eds.), *eMedicine*. Retrieved August 10, 2003, from http://www.emedicine.com/neuro/topic613.htm

United States Department of Health and Human Services. (2000). Family planning. *Tracking Healthy People 2010, Part B: Operational definitions*. Retrieved September 20, 2000, from http://www.healthypeople.gov/Document/html/tracking/od09.htm

Van Earden, P., & Bernstein, P. (2003). Varicella zoster infections in pregnancy. *Medscape Ob/Gyn and Women's Health, 8*(1). Posted June 10, 2003. Retrieved September 1, 2003, from http://www.medscape.com/viewarticle/455972

Wadman, M. C., & Foral, J. (2003). Domestic violence. In J. A. Salomone, F. Talavera, D. E. Houry, J. Adler, & J. S. Cohen (Eds.), *eMedicine*. Last updated March 18, 2003. Retrieved September 14, 2003, from http://www.emedicine.com/aaem/topic538.htm

Williams, G. B., Dou, M., & Leal, C. C. (2003). Violence against pregnant women. *AWHONN Lifelines, 7*(4), 348–354.

Winter, W. E., & Schatz, D. A. (2003). Current role of the oral glucose tolerance test. *Medscape Diabetes and Endocrinology, 5*(1). Retrieved July 26, 2003, from http://www.medscape.com/viewarticle/448038

Websites

Asthma and Pregnancy

http://allergy.mcg.edu/advice/preg.html

http://nationaljewish.org/medfacts/medfacts.html#AsthmaMedFacts

http://www.nhlbi.nih.gov/health/prof/lung/asthma/astpreg.txt

TORCH Infections and STIs

http://health.discovery.com/diseasesandcond/encyclopedia/1509.html

http://www.niaid.nih.gov/factsheets/stdsyph.htm

http://www.cdc.gov/nip/vaccine/varicella/faqs-clinic-vac-preg.htm

http://www.bcm.tmc.edu/pedi/infect/cmv/

Intimate Partner Violence

http://www.ndvh.org/

WORKBOOK

NCLEX-STYLE REVIEW QUESTIONS

1. A woman presents to the prenatal clinic for her 28-week prenatal visit. She has pregestational diabetes. Which type of diabetes does she *most* likely have?

   a. Type 1

   b. Type 2

   c. Undetermined

   d. Uncontrolled

2. A woman with Class III heart disease is in for a prenatal visit. If she is in early heart failure, which sign is *most* likely to be discovered during physical assessment?

   a. Audible wheezes

   b. Persistent rales in the bases of the lungs

   c. Elevated blood pressure

   d. Low blood pressure

3. A 30-year-old gravida 1 has sickle cell anemia. She is not currently in crisis. Which nursing intervention has the highest priority? Instructions on

   a. avoidance of infection

   b. constipation prevention

   c. control of pain

   d. iron-rich foods

4. A 25-year-old woman is in for her first prenatal visit at 28 weeks' gestation. Which assessment finding would most lead you to believe that she may be a victim of intimate partner violence?

   a. A calm demeanor

   b. Bilateral pedal edema

   c. A small bruise on her upper thigh

   d. Multiple bruises in varying stages of healing

STUDY ACTIVITIES

1. Use the following table to list and compare differences between gestational diabetes and type 1 diabetes during pregnancy.

	Gestational DM	Type I DM
Clinical presentation		
Treatment		
Nursing care		

2. Research the Internet to find at least five reliable websites that give patient education information regarding sickle cell anemia.

3. Investigate your community for resources to help adolescents during pregnancy and parenting. Share your findings with your clinical group.

CRITICAL THINKING: What Would You Do?

Apply your knowledge of medical conditions during pregnancy to the following situation.

1. Elizabeth, a 32-year-old gravida 2, has just received a diagnosis of gestational diabetes.

   a. What test was done to diagnose the condition? What were the results of the test?

   b. What risk factors for gestational diabetes may be present in Elizabeth's history?

   c. Explain the priorities of care for Elizabeth during her pregnancy.

2. Tanya is 29 years old and has asthma. She is pregnant with her first child.

   a. What will pregnancy likely do to Tanya's asthma severity?

   b. Outline a teaching plan for Tanya.

3. Rachel is pregnant with her third child. Her HIV test just came back positive. Rachel says she does not know how she contracted HIV. She thinks it could have been from a blood transfusion she received after her last delivery.

   a. What are the most common methods of HIV transmission? Name three risk factors for HIV.

   b. What are the priorities of care for Rachel?

   c. What medication will the physician likely prescribe for her?

   d. Rachel wants to know how best to protect her unborn child from the infection. How will you respond?

   e. Rachel asks if her other children should be tested. How do you respond? Why or why not?

Pregnancy at Risk: Pregnancy-Related Complications

17

STUDENT OBJECTIVES

On completion of this chapter, the student should be able to

1. Choose appropriate nursing interventions for the woman with hyperemesis gravidarum.
2. Describe clinical manifestations of ectopic pregnancy.
3. Compare and contrast the six types of spontaneous abortion.
4. Discuss the treatment for incompetent cervix.
5. Provide patient teaching (e.g., pathology, treatment, and follow-up care) to a woman experiencing a hydatidiform mole.
6. Compare and contrast placenta previa and abruptio placenta according to characteristics of bleeding and other clinical manifestations.
7. Apply the nursing process to the care of a pregnant woman with a bleeding disorder.
8. Differentiate four categories of hypertensive disorders in pregnancy.
9. Discuss interventions that the nurse uses to care for the woman with preeclampsia-eclampsia.
10. Relate ways the management of a multiple gestation pregnancy is different from that of a singleton gestation.
11. Explain the threat to pregnancy posed by ABO and Rh incompatibilities.

KEY TERMS

abruptio placentae
cerclage
choriocarcinoma
eclampsia
ectopic pregnancy
gestational hypertension
hydatidiform mole
hyperemesis gravidarum
incompetent cervix
placenta previa
preeclampsia
proteinuria
salpingectomy
salpingitis
spontaneous abortion
vasospasm

In Chapter 16 the effect of pre-existing and acquired medical conditions on pregnancy was examined. This chapter focuses on conditions unique to pregnancy that place the woman and/or fetus at risk. Although an uneventful pregnancy is hoped for and often expected, complications can develop. Prenatal care is essential for early risk identification and early detection of developing complications.

The licensed practical or vocational nurse's (LPN's) role includes identification of risk factors for pregnancy-related complications through patient interview and data collection. Although the LPN does not independently provide care for a woman with a complicated pregnancy, he must be able to identify signs of complications and know what problems need prompt intervention. An understanding of the basic pathology and clinical manifestations of these conditions allows the nurse to intervene appropriately, to teach the patient about her condition and care, and to answer questions confidently.

The psychological and emotional impact a complication of pregnancy has on the woman and her family should not be forgotten or ignored. A complication that results in loss of the fetus can be devastating. The woman and her family will need support and guidance to help them cope with the loss. Sometimes the complication of pregnancy puts the woman's life in danger and difficult treatment choices must be made, such as the risk to the mother of continuing the pregnancy versus the risk to the fetus if he is delivered early. This chapter highlights information the nurse will need to provide basic physiologic and emotional care for the woman with a pregnancy at risk because of obstetric risk factors or complications.

HYPEREMESIS GRAVIDARUM

Hyperemesis gravidarum is a disorder of early pregnancy that is characterized by severe nausea and vomiting. Hyperemesis occurs in 0.5 to 10 cases per 1,000 pregnancies, with a higher incidence among white and younger women. The disorder most often appears between 8 and 12 weeks' gestation and usually resolves by week 16. The exact cause is unclear, although there is an association between hyperemesis and high levels of human chorionic gonadotropin (hCG) or estrogen. Some researchers have identified a connection between pyridoxine deficiency and hyperemesis. The risk of hyperemesis is increased with a multiple gestation (pregnancy with more than one fetus), molar pregnancy, or when there is a history of hyperemesis gravidarum. Stress and psychological factors can contribute to the condition.

Clinical Presentation

This disorder is distinguished from "morning sickness" because the nausea and vomiting are severe and result in dehydration, weight loss, and electrolyte imbalances, particularly hypokalemia. Acid-base imbalances may occur. Before a diagnosis of hyperemesis gravidarum is made, other causes of nausea and vomiting, such as hepatitis, hyperthyroidism, and disorders of the liver, gallbladder, and pancreas should be excluded. An ultrasound examination is helpful to rule out a molar pregnancy.

Clinical features of the disorder include symptoms of dehydration, such as poor skin turgor, postural hypotension, and elevated hematocrit. Although rare, esophageal tears or perforation can occur with unremitting vomiting. Prolonged starvation from severe or untreated hyperemesis can lead to thiamine deficiency and Wernicke's encephalopathy, a severe neurologic disorder marked by inflammation and hemorrhage in the brain.

Treatment

Emergency treatment is directed toward correcting fluid, electrolyte, and acid-base imbalances. Hospitalization becomes necessary when severe dehydration is present. Intravenous (IV) solutions that contain dextrose are frequently used to give the woman an energy source so that the body does not break down protein and fat for energy. Potassium is added to IV fluids because untreated hypokalemia can lead to cardiac disturbances. Other electrolytes or multivitamins may be added to the intravenous fluids as indicated to correct imbalances.

The woman is given nothing by mouth (NPO) for the first 24 hours or until the vomiting stops. Although vomiting sometimes ceases after rehydration, antiemetics are frequently required to control it. None of the antiemetics are approved by the United States Food and Drug Administration (FDA) for treatment of nausea and vomiting during pregnancy. Because many of these medications are in pregnancy Category C,[1] the physician must carefully weigh the benefit of using the drug against the possible harmful effects to the fetus.

When antiemetics are prescribed, they are usually more effective when ordered on a regular, around-the-clock schedule versus as-needed (PRN) dosing. Until vomiting is controlled, these medications are given by parenteral injection or via rectal suppository. Once the vomiting has subsided, antiemetics are given by mouth. Recent research has highlighted the benefits of several alternative therapies. In severe cases that do not respond to conventional treatment, additional measures may be taken. Steroid therapy is sometimes helpful, or the woman may require enteral feeding or parenteral nutrition.

---

[1]Pregnancy Drug Categories are described in Chapter 7 (Box 7-6).

CULTURAL SNAPSHOT

- Ginger is an herbal remedy commonly used to treat nausea. Some cultures consider ginger to be a "hot" herb that treats "cold" conditions. Although there is no information regarding possible adverse fetal effects during pregnancy, recent research demonstrates that ginger can reduce nausea significantly.
- Acupuncture/acupressure, specifically stimulation of the "P6 Neiguan point," located on the palmar aspect of the forearm above the wrist, has been shown to reduce nausea and vomiting by at least 50%. Some researchers recommend this traditional therapy as a first-line treatment before prescribing antiemetic medications.

Nutritional issues are addressed once the vomiting has stopped. A clear liquid diet is given and then advanced, as tolerated, to a bland diet. A dietitian is consulted to assist in determining caloric requirements. Pyridoxine supplementation may be ordered because deficiency of this B vitamin is associated with hyperemesis. Many physicians order thiamine supplements to prevent Wernicke's encephalopathy.

Nursing Care

Assess the woman for nausea and administer antiemetics, as ordered. It also is important to assess the amount and character of emesis. Record intake and output and weigh the woman daily. Assess for signs of dehydration, such as poor skin turgor and weight loss. Monitor laboratory values. An elevated hematocrit is associated with dehydration. Observe potassium levels, as ordered. Hypokalemia may result from severe vomiting, or hyperkalemia can occur with potassium supplementation. Monitor the fetal heart rate at least once per shift.

Did you know? A small amount of food taken at frequent intervals is easier to tolerate than one large meal, particularly for someone who is experiencing nausea.

After the vomiting has stopped, implement measures to promote intake. A relaxed, pleasant atmosphere is conducive to eating. The area for eating should be well ventilated and free of unpleasant odors. In addition, eating with others can promote intake. Every effort should be made to provide foods that the woman enjoys. Carbohydrates, such as breads, cereals, and grains, are sometimes easier to tolerate than other food types. Foods high in fat should be avoided because such foods may exacerbate nausea.

Provide mouth care before and after meals. This reduces unpleasant tastes in the mouth, thereby encouraging intake and retention of food. In addition, it is a good idea to restrict oral fluids at mealtime to avoid early satisfaction of hunger before sufficient nutrients are consumed.

Observe family dynamics. Because psychological factors can contribute to this disorder, a psychiatric or social worker consult might be indicated. Consult with the RN regarding this possibility. It may be therapeutic to allow the woman to ventilate her feelings regarding the pregnancy, her condition, and the hospitalization.

BLEEDING DISORDERS

Bleeding disorders can occur during early or late pregnancy. Bleeding disorders that occur during early pregnancy include ectopic pregnancy and spontaneous abortion. Although incompetent cervix is not technically a bleeding disorder, it is discussed in this section because it is a cause of early pregnancy loss. Molar pregnancy is most often found in early pregnancy but occasionally may not be diagnosed until midpregnancy. Placenta previa and abruptio placentae are bleeding disorders that become apparent during late pregnancy. These disorders can lead to hemorrhage during pregnancy and the birth process. The nurse must be alert to signs and symptoms of a bleeding disorder and must notify the physician if one is suspected. When the diagnosis is made promptly, hypovolemic shock from a bleeding episode may be avoided.

Ectopic Pregnancy

The term "ectopic" refers to an object that is located away from the expected site or position. An **ectopic pregnancy** is a pregnancy that occurs outside of the uterus. The fertilized ovum does not find its way to the uterus, so it implants in another location. In approximately 97.7% of all ectopic pregnancies, the pregnancy is found in a fallopian tube (Braun, 2003). This condition is referred to as a "tubal" pregnancy. Other sites, such as the abdomen, ovary, or cervix, can serve as implantation sites (Fig. 17-1), although this occurs rarely. The estimated incidence is 25 cases per 1,000 pregnancies, or 1 in 40 pregnancies (Braun, 2003). Ectopic pregnancy is the leading cause of pregnancy-related death in the first trimester.

Ectopic pregnancy occurs because some factor or condition prevents the fertilized egg from traveling down the fallopian tube, so it implants before it reaches the uterus. Adhesions, scarring, and narrowing of the tubal lumen may block the zygote's progress

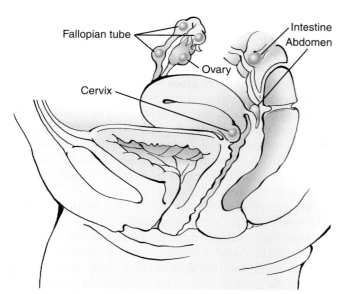

Figure 17.1 Possible implantation sites for an ectopic pregnancy.

to the uterus. Any condition or surgical procedure that can injure a fallopian tube increases the risk. Examples include **salpingitis**, infection of the fallopian tube, endometriosis, history of prior ectopic pregnancy, any type of tubal surgery, congenital malformation of the tube, or multiple elective abortions. Conditions that inhibit peristalsis of the tube can result in tubal pregnancy. Hormonal factors are thought to play a role because tubal pregnancy occurs more frequently in women who take fertility drugs or who use progesterone intrauterine contraceptive devices (IUDs).

Clinical Presentation

Symptoms usually appear 4 to 8 weeks after the last menstrual period (LMP), although the woman may not seek medical treatment until 8 to 12 weeks. The most commonly reported symptoms are pelvic pain and/or vaginal spotting. Other symptoms of early pregnancy, such as nausea and vomiting, also may be present.

Rarely, a woman may present with late signs, such as shoulder pain or hypovolemic shock. These signs are associated with tubal rupture, which occurs when the pregnancy expands beyond the tube's ability to stretch. The risk of tubal rupture increases with advancing gestation. Therefore, prompt diagnosis is critical to preventing rupture. If the tube ruptures, hemorrhage occurs into the abdominal cavity, which can lead to hypovolemic shock. Manifestations of shock include rapid, thready pulse; rising respiratory rate; shallow, irregular respirations; falling blood pressure; decreased or absent urine output; pale, cold, clammy skin; faintness; and thirst.

The diagnosis is not always immediately apparent because many women present with complaints of diffuse abdominal pain and minimal to no vaginal bleeding. Steps are taken to diagnose the disorder and to rule out other causes of abdominal pain. A serum or urine pregnancy test is done to detect the presence of hCG. Transvaginal ultrasound is used to locate the gestational sac and is often diagnostic. Culdocentesis (a procedure in which fluid is drawn from the cul-de-sac behind the vagina) may be done to identify the type of fluid located in the cul-de-sac. The presence of blood is associated with a ruptured tube. Laparoscopy may be required to confirm the diagnosis.

Treatment

Management depends on the condition of the woman. If she presents in shock with abdominal bleeding from a ruptured tube, she will be transported to surgery immediately for exploratory laparotomy, control of hemorrhage, and removal of the damaged tube. The ovaries and uterus are left intact. Volume expanders and blood transfusions may be used for massive hemorrhage.

In nonemergent diagnosed cases of tubal pregnancy, the physician must decide how best to remove the pregnancy. Laparoscopic surgery is the most common method of removing an ectopic pregnancy. If the woman desires to have children in the future, the physician makes every attempt to save the tube through the use of microsurgical techniques and minimally invasive surgery. When the tube cannot be saved or if the woman has finished childbearing, a **salpingectomy**, removal of the fallopian tube, is done.

A newer method of treating a small, unruptured ectopic pregnancy is the use of methotrexate, a drug that is also used in the treatment of cancer. The medication works by interfering with DNA synthesis, which disrupts cell multiplication. Because the cells of the zygote are rapidly multiplying, methotrexate targets the pregnancy for destruction. The medication is given intramuscularly. Sometimes a single dose is sufficient; at other times the physician may order multiple injections. The advantage to this approach is that surgery on the tube is avoided. Whatever treatment method is chosen, anti-D immunoglobulin (RhoGam) is given to the Rh-negative nonsensitized woman.

Think about this. Because surgery on a fallopian tube is a risk factor for ectopic pregnancy, treatment with the anticancer drug methotrexate can actually help prevent future ectopic pregnancies because surgery on the tube is avoided.

Nursing Care

Suspect ectopic pregnancy if the woman presents to the emergency department with abdominal pain and absence of menstrual periods for 1 to 2 months. Record vital signs and the amount and appearance of vaginal bleeding. Immediately report heavy bleeding or signs and symptoms of shock to the physician or registered nurse (RN).

If the physician decides surgery is necessary, assist the RN to prepare the patient. An IV line is started and laboratory testing done. At a minimum, a complete blood count (CBC) and blood type and cross-match are ordered. Check to see that written surgical consent is obtained and that the surgical preparatory checklist is completed.

Once the patient is in stable condition, emotional issues become the focus of nursing care. Be available for emotional support of the woman and her family. It is important to remember that the woman is grieving a loss, and each individual has her own way of expressing grief. Suggest outside sources of support, such as pastoral care or grief counseling.

Before discharge, instruct the woman regarding danger signs that should be reported, including fever, severe abdominal pain, or a vaginal discharge with bad odor. Explain that weekly follow-up care with her physician is necessary to measure hCG levels. Discuss contraceptive options and advise the woman that she should not attempt pregnancy until her hCG levels have returned to nonpregnant levels. If the woman desires more children, explain the possibility of another ectopic pregnancy and review the symptoms of ectopic pregnancy. Encourage her to seek grief counseling or attend a support group after discharge.

Early Pregnancy Loss

Early pregnancy loss is the most common complication of pregnancy and occurs in approximately 75% of women who are trying to conceive (Petrozza & O'Brien, 2002). A more specific term used to describe early pregnancy loss is **spontaneous abortion**, loss of a pregnancy before the age of viability (less than 20 weeks of gestation or fetal size of less than 500 grams). The common name for early pregnancy loss is *miscarriage*.

Here's a tip for you. It is best to use the term "miscarriage" when talking to patients about spontaneous abortion because the term "abortion" carries negative connotations for many people.

The rate of early pregnancy loss is difficult to determine because as many as 50% of losses occur before the woman realizes she is pregnant. The rate of recognized early pregnancy loss is 15% to 20%; therefore, the overall rate may be as high as 60% to 70%. Approximately 80% of spontaneous abortions occur during the first trimester (Puscheck & Pradhan, 2002).

It is difficult to determine the exact cause of miscarriage. Frequently, multiple factors contribute, and in many instances the cause cannot be determined. There are three overall categories: fetal, maternal, and environmental. Fetal factors are usually genetic in nature. In fact, the most common cause of spontaneous abortion in the first trimester is chromosomal defects in the fetus. Faulty implantation and defects in the sperm or ovum are other fetal-related causes. Maternal causes are varied and include advanced maternal age, autoimmune diseases, uterine anatomic abnormalities and fibroids, cervical incompetence, infection, endocrine dysfunction, and coagulation disorders. Environmental factors include poor nutrition; exposure to tobacco, chemicals, or radiation; and use of alcohol, street drugs, or certain prescription drugs.

Some authorities classify spontaneous abortion according to the timing of the loss. Early abortion occurs before 12 weeks and late abortion occurs between 12 and 20 weeks. Early abortion is most frequently caused by fetal factors, whereas maternal factors tend to cause late abortions.

Clinical Presentation

Typical symptoms of spontaneous abortion include cramping and spotting or frank bleeding, which can be severe. Blood clots or tissue may be expelled. Abdominal and suprapubic pain are common and may radiate to the lower back, buttocks, and perineum. Fever and chills are associated with sepsis.

There are several different types of spontaneous abortion: threatened, inevitable, incomplete, complete, and missed (Table 17-1). The definition of each type is related to whether or not the uterus is emptied, or for how long the products of conception are retained.

This is a good rule of thumb. Always consider any woman of childbearing age with vaginal bleeding to be pregnant until proven otherwise.

To make the diagnosis of spontaneous abortion the physician often orders laboratory and imaging studies. An hCG level is drawn to confirm that the woman is pregnant. A CBC can identify anemia associated with blood loss and can provide evidence of infection. Blood typing is important to determine if the woman is $Rh_o(D)$ negative. Blood cross-matching and coagulation studies may be ordered in cases of severe blood loss. Urinalysis is done to rule out a

TABLE 17.1	Comparison of Abortion Types	
Abortion Type	**Clinical Presentation**	**Treatment**
Threatened abortion	Vaginal bleeding or spotting occurs. Cramping is often present, but the cervix does not dilate. The symptoms may resolve and the pregnancy may be maintained, or threatened abortion can progress to one of the other types.	Vaginal rest is indicated (e.g., no sexual intercourse or douches). Sometimes bed rest is prescribed. The woman is instructed to report bleeding heavier than a normal menstrual period, cramping, or fever. If tissue is passed, she is to save it for examination by the physician.
Inevitable abortion	Cramping and spotting or vaginal bleeding with cervical dilation. Amniotic fluid may leak.	Surgical removal of the pregnancy is the treatment of choice. The type of procedure performed depends largely on the gestational age. Pregnancies less than 14 weeks are usually evacuated by dilatation and curettage (D&C). (Refer to "Induced Abortion" in Chapter 4 for a discussion of specific techniques.)
Incomplete abortion	Some of the products of conception are expelled and others are retained. Usually, the fetus delivers and the placenta and membranes are retained.	Treatment is similar to that used for inevitable abortion.
Complete abortion	All of the products of conception (fetus, membranes, placenta) are expelled.	Usually no surgical procedures are recommended. The woman is dismissed home with instructions to monitor for complications such as heavy or increased bleeding or fever.
Missed abortion	The fetus dies, but remains in utero. Signs of pregnancy are present, but the fundus does not grow as expected in a normal pregnancy and may regress (get smaller). No fetal heart tones are present.	Ultrasound is used to confirm the diagnosis. If a dead fetus is carried for longer than 4 weeks, the risk of a hemorrhagic disorder is high; therefore, a coagulation profile is drawn. The uterus is then evacuated by D&C, or oxytocin or prostaglandin is used to induce labor, which results in passing of the products of conception.
Habitual (recurrent) abortion	The loss of three or more consecutive pregnancies before the fetus is viable.	Attempts are made to determine and treat the cause. For example, an incompetent cervix is often a cause of habitual abortion.

urinary tract infection. Transvaginal ultrasound is the diagnostic procedure of choice. The uterine cavity is visualized to determine if any products of conception are present and whether or not the embryo or fetus is alive.

Treatment

Treatment depends on which type of early pregnancy loss is occurring (see Table 17-1). Treatment for a threatened abortion is conservative because currently there is no specific therapy that can reliably prevent threatened abortion from progressing to spontaneous abortion. The physician develops a "wait-and-see" attitude. Usually she orders bed rest and pelvic rest, which includes no sexual intercourse, douches, or tampons. The woman is instructed to report heavy bleeding, cramping, or fever. Most other types of spontaneous abortion require some type of surgical intervention, unless all

the products of conception are expelled (complete abortion). Vacuum aspiration or dilatation and curettage (D&C) are the most common methods used to clear the uterus of the products of conception (see Chapter 4 for discussion of the various procedures). Intravenous oxytocin (Pitocin) or oral Methergine may be ordered after uterine evacuation to help prevent bleeding. Ibuprofen may be ordered to control uterine cramping.

Nursing Care

Assess the woman's vital signs, amount and appearance of vaginal bleeding, and pain level. Count the number of perineal pads used or weigh perineal pads to assess the amount of bleeding. Document whether or not the pad is saturated and note if clots are present. Report a falling blood pressure and rising pulse, or other symptoms of shock, and an elevated temperature, which is associated with infection. If the pregnancy is greater than 10 to12 weeks, evaluate the fetal heart rate with a Doppler device. Save all expelled tissue for evaluation by the physician. Administer anti-D immunoglobulin (RhoGam) if the woman is $Rh_o(D)$ negative.

After the pregnancy has been expelled, either spontaneously or through surgical intervention, continue to monitor vital signs and bleeding. Administer oxytocin or Methergine as ordered to control bleeding. Provide analgesics as ordered and comfort measures to treat pain. Usually the woman is dismissed home a few hours after vacuum aspiration or D&C, if she is in stable condition. Family Teaching Tips: Instructions for Self-Care After Spontaneous Abortion explains self-care at home.

This is important! If a woman is $Rh_o(D)$ negative, she should receive $Rh_o(D)$ immune globulin (RhoGAM) any time a pregnancy is terminated for any reason. The length or type of pregnancy does not change this need.

Grief reactions are to be expected. Allow the woman and her partner or support person privacy to discuss their feelings with each other. Offer parents the opportunity to view the fetus. It is important to acknowledge the loss and resist the temptation to reassure the woman that she "can always have more babies." The woman must work through her feelings and come to terms with the current loss before it is helpful or appropriate to focus on future pregnancies.

FAMILY TEACHING TIPS

Instructions for Self-Care After Spontaneous Abortion

- Return for follow-up care if you experience any of the following danger symptoms.
  - Large amount of vaginal bleeding
  - Foul-smelling discharge
  - Severe pelvic pain
  - Temperature above 38°C (100.4°F)
- Do not use tampons or douche and refrain from sexual intercourse for approximately 2 weeks.
- Return for weekly physician visits to monitor hCG levels, if ordered. Avoid sexual intercourse or use contraception until hCG levels become negative.
- You will likely experience intermittent menstrual-like flow and cramps during the week after miscarriage. Ibuprofen is recommended to control painful cramping. Resume regular activities when you feel well.
- Grief counseling is beneficial.

A PERSONAL GLIMPSE

I was shocked when I found out I was pregnant with our fourth child. I was almost 40 years old and had a teenager and two school-age kids. At first, my husband and I were not eager to return to the days of sleepless nights and changing diapers. However, the idea of a sweet, new baby in our family grew on my husband and me, and our three kids were thrilled and excited. During the 10th week of my pregnancy, I started to have cramping and slight bleeding. I called my OB's office and the nurse said to come to the office immediately. I called my husband at work and asked him to come home and take me to the doctor. While I was waiting for him to arrive, the cramping grew stronger and the bleeding grew heavier. I started to cry because I knew I was losing my baby. After examining me, my doctor confirmed my fear; I had experienced a miscarriage. I was told that the miscarriage wasn't complete and that they would have to do a procedure to remove what remained in my uterus. No one really explained the procedure to us, and I felt so lonely lying on the table. After the procedure, the nurse gave me some medicine for pain and made sure I was comfortable; she told me that I could probably go home in a few hours. Before leaving the room, the nurse turned to my husband and me and said, "I know this has been difficult for you, but you and your husband are very fortunate to have three children at home." Although she may have meant no harm, this nurse made me feel guilty for grieving the loss of this unexpected, but wanted pregnancy.

Elisabeth

▶**LEARNING OPPORTUNITY:** In what ways can the nurse acknowledge that the loss of a pregnancy is a unique and deeply personal experience for the woman and her family?
Describe helpful things the nurse can say when a woman loses a pregnancy. Describe unhelpful responses.

The intensity and range of emotional responses of the woman experiencing a spontaneous abortion will vary greatly. The woman may feel overwhelmed by grief. She may feel guilty that she might have done something to cause the pregnancy loss. She may express anger with a divine power for allowing her to lose the baby. Accept and support the woman's emotions. The woman needs ongoing grief support after discharge; make sure the woman is referred for this service.

CULTURAL SNAPSHOT

Expressions of grief are influenced culturally. Some cultures discourage displays of emotion, whereas others encourage dramatic expression of grief. The degree of grief cannot be determined by the presence or absence of emotional expression.

Incompetent Cervix

When a woman has an **incompetent cervix**, painless cervical dilatation occurs with bulging of fetal membranes and parts through the external os. Usually loss of the pregnancy cannot be prevented. Therefore, although incompetent cervix is not technically a bleeding disorder, it often is a cause of habitual or recurrent abortion.

The exact cause of incompetent cervix is unknown, but there are factors that increase the risk. Any type of trauma to the cervix, such as surgical trauma (e.g., dilatation and curettage, conization or cauterization of the cervix) or exposure to diethylstilbestrol (DES) while in utero increases the likelihood that incompetent cervix will occur.

Treatment of incompetent cervix involves placing a purse-string type suture in the cervix to keep it from dilating. This procedure, known as **cerclage** is done between 14 and 26 weeks of gestation, generally after incompetent cervix has been diagnosed in a previous pregnancy. The suture is then removed when the pregnancy is at term or the woman goes into labor.

Test Yourself

- An elevation in what hormone is associated with hyperemesis gravidarum?

- List two conditions that increase the risk for ectopic pregnancy.

- Name two types of abortion in which the cervix dilates.

Hydatidiform Mole

A **hydatidiform mole**, also referred to as a molar pregnancy and gestational trophoblastic disease, is characterized by benign growth of placental tissue. There are two types of molar pregnancies: partial and complete. In both cases errors in chromosomal duplication occur during fertilization. The consequence is grapelike (hydatidiform) swelling of the chorionic villi and trophoblastic hyperplasia. Chromosomal abnormalities are present when there is a fetus; however, fetal tissue is found only in partial molar pregnancies. A molar pregnancy has some features of a malignancy in that the trophoblastic tissue proliferates (multiplies) out of control. In fact, 20% of women who experience a complete molar pregnancy develop **choriocarcinoma**, malignancy of the uterine lining, within 6 months to 1 year after molar pregnancy.

Fortunately, molar pregnancy occurs rarely. In Western countries, the rate is 1 per 1,000 to 1,500 pregnancies. The rate is uniform among ethnic groups living in the United States; however, in Asian countries the rate is much higher. Risk factors for a complete mole include extremes of age. Young women in their early teens and older women who are near the end of their reproductive lives are at highest risk. Women older than 40 years have a sevenfold increase in risk compared with younger women (Moore & Ware, 2002).

Clinical Presentation

Before the widespread use of ultrasound, molar pregnancy was most often diagnosed in the second trimester. Now the condition is diagnosed frequently in the first trimester before classic symptoms are evident. Thus, the most common presenting sign for both partial and complete moles is vaginal bleeding. Typically the woman presents between 8 and 16 weeks' gestation with complaints of painless (usually) brown to bright red vaginal bleeding. The bleeding may be intermittent or continuous and can be severe. An hCG level is obtained, the results of which is more often than not higher than expected for gestational age. Transvaginal ultrasound reveals the characteristic snowstorm pattern caused by grapelike vesicles that fill the uterus.

If a complete molar pregnancy continues into the second trimester undetected, other signs and symptoms appear. The woman often presents with complaints of dark to bright red vaginal bleeding and pelvic pain. Infrequently, she will report passage of grapelike vesicles. The physical examination may reveal a uterus that measures larger than expected for dates. Fetal heart tones are absent, and fetal parts cannot be detected. The snowstorm pattern is seen with abdominal ultrasound, and in 50% of the cases giant ovarian cysts are detected, which are the source of pelvic pain. Other less common findings include gestational hypertension (sometimes referred to as pregnancy-induced hypertension or PIH) before the 24th week (27%), hyperemesis gravidarum (26%), and hyperthyroidism (7%) (Kurowski & Yakoub, 2003).

Treatment

If the woman is hemorrhaging when she presents, the clinical team must move quickly to stabilize her condition. She requires IV volume expanders and blood transfusions. Clotting studies are ordered because coagulation disorders can develop as a complication of hemorrhage. Antihypertensives are administered if the blood pressure is elevated.

Once the woman is in stable condition, preparation for surgery begins. A chest x-ray is ordered to assess for vesicle emboli or lung metastasis. Blood samples are drawn to establish the baseline hCG level and to type and cross-match the blood, if this has not been previously accomplished.

Surgical treatment options include evacuation of the uterus by suction curettage, if the woman wishes to have children in the future. Abdominal hysterectomy is the treatment of choice when continued fertility is not desired. Labor induction techniques are not used because of the danger of hemorrhage. After the uterus is evacuated, RhoGAM is given to the woman who is $Rh_o(D)$ negative.

Continued follow-up for 1 year is extremely important. The woman returns to the doctor's office every 1 to 2 weeks to have hCG levels drawn. This monitoring is done to detect the development of choriocarcinoma, which is highly treatable if caught early. The woman is instructed not to become pregnant during the year after a molar pregnancy and is usually placed on a regimen of oral contraceptives. Although the practice is controversial, some physicians recommend prophylactic chemotherapy because one in five women with a complete molar pregnancy will experience choriocarcinoma.

Nursing Care

The woman is at risk for several complications; therefore, it is important to watch her closely during the postpartum period. Vaginal bleeding and the condition of the uterine fundus must be monitored frequently. Observe vital signs and the woman's level of consciousness because shock can result from hemorrhage caused by uterine atony or accidental perforation of the uterus during surgery. Administer oxytocin as ordered to control uterine atony. Methergine or Hemabate are other medications that may be ordered to stimulate the uterine muscle to contract.

Disseminated intravascular coagulation (DIC), a bleeding disorder related to lack of clotting factors, is another possible complication. Molar tissue releases substances that break down clotting factors, increasing the woman's risk for DIC. Review clotting studies for abnormal values and monitor IV and injection sites for bleeding. Continual oozing from these sites should be reported immediately.

Trophoblastic embolus or pulmonary edema as a consequence of fluid overload is a possibly fatal condition; therefore, every nursing assessment should

include a thorough evaluation of respiratory status and auscultation of the lung fields. Respiratory distress or crackles in the lungs must be reported to the RN or physician immediately. Continuous or intermittent pulse oximetry may be ordered. If oxygen saturation levels fall below 95%, supplemental oxygen is indicated.

In addition to nursing measures directed at preventing hemorrhage (see "Nursing Process for Caring of the Woman With a Bleeding Disorder") and detecting respiratory distress, emotional support is an important nursing function. The woman has to cope with a complication of pregnancy that can cause severe illness, but a baby will not result from her ordeal. Family Teaching Tips: Follow-up Care After Molar Pregnancy lists important aspects of patient education for a woman being discharged after treatment for a molar pregnancy.

Test Yourself

- What procedure is used to treat an incompetent cervix?

- How is hydatidiform mole diagnosed?

- Name three important discharge teaching points for the woman who has experienced a molar pregnancy.

FAMILY TEACHING TIPS

Follow-up Care After Molar Pregnancy

- Frequent physician visits will be necessary for 1 year after termination of a molar pregnancy to evaluate for the development of choriocarcinoma, a type of malignancy associated with molar pregnancy.
- Serum hCG levels are monitored at each visit to detect rising hCG levels, which may indicate the presence of choriocarcinoma.
- Avoid pregnancy for at least 1 year after treatment because hCG levels rise during pregnancy, making it difficult to differentiate between pregnancy and choriocarcinoma.
- Immediately report unexpected vaginal bleeding after evacuation of a molar pregnancy. Irregular vaginal bleeding is associated with choriocarcinoma.
- Report severe persistent headaches, cough, or bloody sputum. These are symptoms of metastasis, which requires immediate, aggressive treatment.

Placenta Previa

Placenta previa is a condition in which the placenta is implanted close to or covers the cervical os. Normally, the placenta implants in the upper uterine segment. In placenta previa, the placenta implants in the lower part of the uterus. As the pregnancy progresses, the part of the placenta that lies over the cervix bleeds because of rupture of blood vessels in the placenta.

The cause is not known. It may be that the site of normal implantation is scarred or damaged so that the embryo implants in a site that is more favorable for placental development. Conditions that increase the risk for placenta previa include history of elective abortions, multiparity, advanced maternal age (older than 35 years), previous cesarean birth or uterine incisions, maternal smoking, and prior placenta previa. The condition occurs approximately once for every 200 pregnancies (Queenan, 2000). The actual incidence of placenta previa at delivery is approximately one-tenth that diagnosed by ultrasound in the second trimester. However, this is true only for partial and marginal previas (see discussion in next paragraph). A complete placenta previa diagnosed in the second trimester rarely resolves to a normal implantation at delivery.

Placenta previa is classified according to the degree to which the placenta covers the cervix. Total placenta previa occurs when the placenta completely covers the cervix. If the placenta covers part of the cervix, the term partial placenta previa is used. Sometimes the placenta does not cover the cervix but is located on the border of the cervix. This condition is called marginal placenta previa. Figure 17-2 compares three classifications of placenta previa.

Clinical Presentation

Painless, bright red bleeding that begins with no warning is a strong indicator of placenta previa. Bleeding may be light to severe and usually stops spontaneously. However, bleeding will recur, and each subsequent episode usually produces heavier bleeding than the previous one. The first bleeding occurs on average between 27 and 32 weeks' gestation.

For any woman who presents with painless bleeding, a digital examination of the cervix should not be done until placenta previa has been excluded. This precaution is necessary because digital manipulation of placental tissue through the cervical os can cause uncontrollable bleeding. The diagnostic test of choice is transvaginal ultrasound because it is 100% predictive of placenta previa. Abdominal ultrasound is sometimes ordered. This method is 95% accurate in making the diagnosis.

Usually the first bleeding episode does not harm the fetus, unless it is unusually severe. The fetal heart rate should be within normal limits. Total placenta previa is associated with atypical fetal presentations, such as breech and transverse lie. It is thought that the abnormally located placenta prevents the fetus from assuming the expected head-down presentation. In severe bleeding episodes the fetus can become anemic, hypoxic, or develop hypovolemic shock because of loss of fetal blood and decreased oxygen transport across the placenta.

NEVER assist with a vaginal examination on a pregnant woman who is bleeding until the physician is sure that there is no placenta previa. During a vaginal examination, the fingers could penetrate the placenta, causing massive hemorrhage.

Treatment

If the initial bleeding episode does not stop or is massive, an immediate cesarean delivery is done to save the life of the woman and her fetus. If the initial bleeding episode stops and the fetus is still immature,

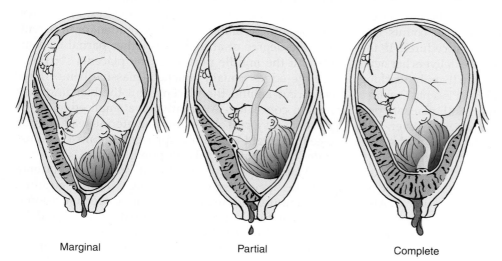

Marginal   Partial   Complete

● *Figure 17.2* Three classifications of placenta previa.

hospitalization with bed rest is indicated. IV access is maintained, and at least two units of blood are placed on hold for immediate transfusion, if necessary.

If the woman is Rh$_o$(D) negative, a Kleihauer-Betke test is performed to determine if fetal blood cells are in the maternal circulation, which indicates fetal–maternal hemorrhage. This test helps to determine the appropriate dosage of anti-D immunoglobulin (RhoGam) to be given. Rh$_o$Gam is injected for each bleeding episode to prevent isoimmunization, development of antibodies against Rho(D) positive blood in the pregnant woman. (See discussion later in this chapter.)

Serial nonstress tests (NSTs) are done to monitor fetal well-being. Continuous electronic fetal monitoring (EFM) is required during acute bleeding episodes. In some instances the woman is allowed to go home after the bleeding stops, but she must have someone with her at all times who can transport her immediately to the hospital if bleeding begins again.

A cesarean delivery is necessary in almost all cases of placenta previa. If the woman with a total previa were allowed to labor, massive hemorrhage could occur because placental blood vessels would break open and bleed as the cervix dilated. The physician often schedules the delivery as soon as it is reasonably certain that the fetal lungs are mature. The woman and fetus fare better when the delivery is accomplished in a planned fashion, as opposed to rushing to the operating room during an acute bleeding episode. Occasionally, a woman with a marginal placenta previa can deliver vaginally, as long as heavy bleeding does not occur during labor.

Nursing Care

The woman who has been diagnosed with placenta previa requires careful nursing observation. Maintain IV access at all times while the woman is hospitalized. Institute a perineal pad count so that bleeding can be quantified. Monitor the vital signs at regular intervals, and assess for signs of shock. Perform NSTs as ordered, and listen to the fetal heart rate at least every 4 hours. Instruct the woman to perform and record kick counts (see Chapter 7 for description of this procedure). If the woman is discharged home before she delivers her newborn, give her instructions for self-care (Family Teaching Tips: Home Care for the Woman With Placenta Previa).

Postpartum care of the woman with placenta previa is the same as for other women. However, it is important to observe her closely for signs and symptoms of infection and postpartum hemorrhage. She is at higher risk for both of these complications because of the proximity of the open, bleeding vessels at the former placenta site to the opening of the uterus. Also, the lower segment of the uterus cannot contract as effectively as can the upper segment; therefore, sometimes not enough pressure is exerted on the blood vessels to stop the bleeding.

FAMILY TEACHING TIPS

Home Care for the Woman With Placenta Previa

- Arrange for a dependable person with transportation to be available immediately to transport you to the hospital should a bleeding episode occur.
- Perform fetal kick counts at least daily. Decreased fetal activity is a sign of fetal stress. Kick counts are designed to measure fetal activity.
- Remain on bed rest (usually with bathroom privileges) while at home. Do no housework or lifting. Moderate-to-vigorous activity could bring about a bleeding episode.
- Vaginal rest is essential. Do not insert anything into the vagina (e.g., no sexual intercourse, no douching, no tampons). These activities could stimulate bleeding, and subsequent bleeding episodes tend to be more severe than the first.

Abruptio Placentae

Abruptio placentae, or placental abruption, is the premature separation of a normally implanted placenta. The incidence of abruptio placenta is 1% (Deering & Satin, 2002). Although the placenta is located in the normal place, it pulls away from the uterine wall before the end of labor. The cause of abruptio placentae is unknown; however, there are associated risk factors. Any condition that is characterized by elevated blood pressure puts the woman at risk for abruption. Preeclampsia and pre-existing chronic hypertension fall into this category. Maternal age greater than 35 years and multiparity increase the risk for placental abruption. Trauma (e.g., motor vehicle collisions or domestic violence), cigarette smoking, use of cocaine, and preterm premature rupture of the membranes are additional risk factors for abruption.

A placental abruption is classified in several ways. The bleeding is either concealed (hidden) or apparent, and the degree of abruption is either partial or complete. If the middle portion of the placenta separates but the edges remain attached, massive hemorrhage can occur behind the placenta but the bleeding may remain concealed. Alternatively, a small edge of the placenta may pull away from the uterine wall and the bleeding might be readily apparent. Figure 17-3 illustrates types of placental abruption.

Maternal complications of abruptio placenta include hemorrhagic shock, DIC, uterine rupture, renal failure, and death. If a classic cesarean incision is done, all future pregnancies must be delivered by cesarean birth. Fetal complications are related to the degree of placental separation and maturity of the fetus. Hypoxia, anemia, growth retardation, and even

● *Figure 17.3* Types of placental abruption.

Partial abruption, concealed hemorrhage

Partial abruption, apparent hemorrhage

Complete abruption, concealed hemorrhage

fetal death may occur. When preterm delivery is indicated, the neonate is at risk because of prematurity.

Clinical Presentation

The physician often makes the preliminary diagnosis based on signs and symptoms of the patient. The diagnosis is confirmed after delivery upon manual inspection of the placenta. The classic signs are pain, dark red vaginal bleeding, a tender abdomen that is rigid to palpation, and hypertonic labor. Pain has a sudden onset and is constant. Bleeding is apparent in most (approximately 80%) cases. The uterus may not relax well between contractions, the amniotic fluid often is bloody, and signs of maternal shock and fetal distress may be present. The fundal height may increase with severe intrauterine bleeding.

Ultrasound may assist with the diagnosis, but a negative sonogram does not rule out the possibility of abruption. As with other bleeding disorders, DIC is a potential complication of placental abruption. The physician carefully monitors fibrinogen levels and other clotting studies to detect the development of DIC.

Treatment

For cases in which there is severe bleeding, a large-bore IV is started and IV fluids are infused until cryo-precipitate, fresh frozen plasma, or whole blood is available for transfusion. Four units of packed red blood cells are cross-matched and are readily available from the laboratory. Oxygen is administered via face mask. The physician may perform an amniotomy to decrease intrauterine pressure. Immediate cesarean birth is done if the condition of either the woman or her fetus becomes unstable. After delivery of the fetus, if the physician is unable to control the bleeding, a hysterectomy may be done to save the woman's life.

Vaginal delivery is preferred to cesarean birth for small abruptions in which the woman and fetus remain hemodynamically stable or when the fetus has died. Contraindications for a vaginal birth include fetal dis-

tress, bleeding severe enough to threaten the life of the mother and fetus, or unsatisfactory progress of labor. The physician may rupture the membranes artificially to induce or augment labor, and oxytocin may be used. Although placental abruption is characterized by failure of the uterus to relax effectively, the benefits of vaginal delivery outweigh the risk of oxytocin induction in most cases (Cunningham et al., 2001b, pp. 629-630; Queenan, 2000, p. 301).

Maybe this will jog your memory on the exam! The classic way to tell the difference between placenta previa and abruptio placenta is that the bleeding with previa is bright red and *painless*, whereas the bleeding with an abruption is usually darker red (the blood may even be old) and *painful*. No pain = previa. Lots of pain = abruption.

Nursing Care

The woman with a suspected or diagnosed placental abruption requires careful monitoring. She is allowed nothing by mouth until her condition is stable. Assess for signs of shock. Watch for bleeding from the gums, nose, and venipuncture sites, which may indicate DIC. Insert a large-bore IV line and infuse IV fluid and blood products as ordered. Continuous EFM is necessary. The RN should evaluate the strip frequently. Immediately notify the RN if any signs of fetal distress become evident. Be prepared to quickly prepare the woman for an emergency cesarean birth if ordered.

After delivery, the woman requires close monitoring for postpartum hemorrhage because she is at risk for uterine atony. Continue to observe for signs of DIC. This complication may develop after delivery. Place the woman on strict monitoring of intake and output. Pay particular attention to the urinary output. Acute renal failure can occur.

● Nursing Process for the Woman With a Bleeding Disorder

ASSESSMENT

Take a thorough obstetric history, unless the severity of the bleeding necessitates immediate intervention. It is important to evaluate the chief complaint and history of the current condition and to note any risk factors for antepartum hemorrhage (e.g., grand multiparity, advanced maternal age, or previous history of a bleeding disorder).

During an acute bleeding episode it is critical to determine the characteristics of bleeding. How much is the woman bleeding? What is the color and consistency? Is pain present? If so, where and to what degree? In some conditions, bleeding can be hidden, such as a ruptured ectopic pregnancy and some placental abruptions. Ask yourself, "Is the fundal height increasing?" Take vital signs to determine if shock is present. Initial symptoms of shock include cool, clammy skin, restlessness, apprehension, and confusion. Late signs of shock include tachycardia and, when blood loss is severe, hypotension.

Obtain the fetal heart rate (FHR) and apply the EFM if the fetus is more than 20 weeks' gestation. It is important to assess and record the baseline FHR and to review the monitor strip for indications of fetal distress. Fetal tachycardia that progresses to bradycardia or decreased variability with late decelerations are ominous signs that must be reported to the charge RN or physician at once. Absence of the FHR is associated with fetal death or hydatidiform mole.

Palpate the uterus to determine if the resting tone is soft and to evaluate the characteristics of contractions, if present. Measure fundal height and compare it to previous measurements; concealed bleeding can cause increasing uterine distention.

Evaluate the woman's pain. Pelvic or shoulder pain in very early pregnancy is associated with ectopic pregnancy. Pain is generally not associated with placenta previa, unless the woman is also experiencing labor, in which case the pain will subside with each contraction. Cramping and abdominal pain may accompany spontaneous abortion and abruptio placentae.

SELECTED NURSING DIAGNOSES

- Ineffective Tissue Perfusion: placental related to hypovolemia from excessive blood loss
- Deficient Fluid Volume related to fluid volume loss from bleeding
- Risk for Injury (fetal) related to hypoxia and complications of prematurity
- Risk for Injury (maternal) related to fetal/maternal blood incompatibilities and complications of the bleeding disorder
- Risk for Infection related to open, bleeding vessels
- Acute Pain related to separation of placenta from the uterine wall or contractions associated with pregnancy loss
- Anxiety related to threat of harm and/or death to self and fetus

OUTCOME IDENTIFICATION AND PLANNING

Maintaining the safety of the pregnant woman and her fetus is the primary goal when planning care. Goals and interventions are planned according to the individual needs and situation of the woman. Appropriate goals may include that the woman's placental perfusion and fluid volume will be maintained; fetal injury from chronic or acute hypoxia will be avoided; maternal injury and Rh isoimmunization will be avoided; the woman will remain free of signs and symptoms of infection; she will express the ability to cope with her pain; and her anxiety will be reduced.

IMPLEMENTATION

Maintaining Placental Perfusion and Fluid Volume

The priority of care for any woman who is bleeding is to prevent and treat shock. For acute bleeding episodes, or when the potential for hemorrhage exists, start an IV line with a large-bore catheter per physician order. Infuse fluids, as ordered, to maintain blood volume. Collect blood specimens for type and cross-matching, and make certain that blood is available at all times for possible transfusion (2 to 4 units). If there is severe bleeding, administer blood and blood products as ordered.

It is important to monitor vital signs closely for signs of shock. Maintain strict intake and output monitoring with special attention to the urine output, which should remain above 30 milliliters (mL) per hour. In addition, maintain the woman in a lateral position to promote placental perfusion. Give oxygen by face mask if bleeding is heavy or if there are signs of fetal distress.

Sometimes the nurse will need to prepare the woman for surgery, either emergently to control the bleeding, or on a planned basis to prevent hemorrhage. In a planned situation, obtain informed consent, carry out preoperative orders, and complete the preoperative checklist. When the woman must be prepared for surgery emergently, move quickly and efficiently to get her ready.

If active bleeding is not occurring, but the potential for hemorrhage exists (e.g., placenta previa), assist the woman to remain on bed rest with bathroom privileges, as ordered. It is important to maintain an ongoing perineal pad count to monitor for increased bleeding. Evaluate fundal height for sudden size increase, a condition that may occur when there is concealed hemorrhage.

Avoiding Fetal Injury

When the pregnancy has reached the point of viability (usually considered 20 weeks and greater), the fetus should be monitored continuously during bleeding episodes until the woman is in stable condition. Watch the fetal monitoring tracing closely for signs of fetal distress, such as loss of variability, a gradually increasing or decreasing baseline, and late decelerations. If any of these signs are present, administer oxygen to the mother, reposition her to a side-lying position, and increase the rate of IV fluids. Notify the RN or physician immediately.

If the woman's condition has been stabilized and there are no signs of fetal distress, the woman may remain hospitalized for observation. Assist her to maintain bed rest, as ordered, and institute preterm labor precautions (refer to Chapter 18). Administer betamethasone as ordered to increase fetal lung maturity in the event delivery must occur before term.

Preventing Maternal Injury

Maternal injury can occur from complications, such as DIC, which are sometimes the sequelae of a bleeding disorder. Obtain specimens for laboratory studies as ordered. Typical blood work includes a complete blood count (CBC) to detect the presence of anemia and infection. Often coagulation studies are necessary because some disorders (such as abruptio placentae) are associated with a high risk of clotting dysfunction. Coagulation studies include platelet and fibrinogen levels, fibrin/fibrinogen degradation products, and prothrombin time/activated partial thromboplastin time.

In addition to close monitoring of laboratory results, observe for and report signs of DIC (e.g., bleeding from the nose, gums, and venipuncture sites). Watch for cough, dyspnea, fever, confusion and disorientation, symptoms that are also associated with DIC. Monitor the blood urea nitrogen and creatinine levels. Levels may be elevated secondary to renal failure. Assess the skin carefully for petechiae and purpura.

Injury can also result if bleeding causes fetal blood to come in contact with maternal blood. For this reason, blood typing is always done with any bleeding disorder of pregnancy. The woman who is Rh$_o$(D) negative may need a Kleihauer-Betke test to determine if any fetal blood has entered her cir-

culation. This test can help the physician determine how much anti-D immunoglobulin (RhoGam) is needed. Every woman who is Rh$_o$(D) negative should receive anti-D immunoglobulin (RhoGam) if there is risk of fetal–maternal hemorrhage. All bleeding episodes and evacuation of the products of conception from the uterus increase this risk.

Preventing Infection

Take measures to prevent infection. It is important to use aseptic technique as indicated. In addition, teach the woman to wash her hands before and after eating, using the restroom, and performing perineal care. Monitor the temperature and white blood cell count. Report elevations in either parameter. Instruct the woman to report any vaginal discharge with a foul odor.

Managing Pain

Assess carefully regarding the woman's pain. It is important to ask the following questions regarding pain. Where is it? What is it like? When did it start? How often does it occur? What makes it worse? What makes it better? Intensity is best evaluated using a pain scale. Many nurses ask the woman to rate the pain on a scale of 0 to 10. Zero represents no pain at all and 10 represents the worst pain imaginable. If you use a pain scale, you can more effectively evaluate the success of your interventions.

Give the woman information about what is causing the pain (if you have that information) and how long she can expect it to last. Explain to her the medications the physician has ordered to help decrease her pain and tell her how frequently she can have them. For acute pain it is often better to schedule the pain medications, rather than waiting for the woman to ask for them. Explain that it is easier to treat pain before it becomes severe. Be sure that the room temperature, lighting, and noise level are at a comfortable level for the woman. It is also helpful to try to eliminate any factors that might be interfering with her ability to cope with the pain (e.g., if the woman is overly fatigued or bored, it will be more difficult for her to deal with the pain sensation). Consult with the RN regarding nonpharmacologic methods of pain relief, such as warm or cold applications, massage, or relaxation techniques. Be sure to inform the RN or the physician right away if measures to reduce pain are ineffective.

Reducing Anxiety

Care should be taken to attend to the woman's emotional needs. It can be frightening when there is active bleeding and health care providers are moving quickly to intervene. Use a calm and confident manner. It is a good idea to offer explanations for all procedures and treatments as they are being performed using language the woman and her family can understand. Promote expression of feelings and encourage the presence of supportive family members and friends, as appropriate. If the fetus dies because of complications of the bleeding disorder, or if the woman requires an unplanned, emergency hysterectomy, she will need additional support to deal with these losses. Request a social service consult if support is inadequate.

EVALUATION: GOALS AND EXPECTED OUTCOMES

- **Goal:** Placental perfusion and fluid volume are maintained
  Expected Outcomes: Skin and mucous membranes remain hydrated.
  - Hematocrit, serum electrolytes, and urine specific gravity remain within normal limits.
- **Goal:** Fetal injury is avoided.
  Expected Outcomes: Fetal monitor tracing shows presence of variability and reactivity without late decelerations.
- **Goal:** The woman remains injury free.
  Expected Outcomes: Coagulation studies remain within expected limits.
  - If DIC develops, the condition is caught early and treated immediately.
  - The woman who is $Rh_o(D)$ negative does not become isoimmunized to $Rh_o(D)$-positive blood.
- **Goal:** The woman shows no signs of infection.
  Expected Outcomes: Vital signs remain within expected limits.
  - Fever is absent, and the white blood cell count remains within the normal range.
- **Goal:** The woman expresses the ability to cope with her pain.
  Expected Outcomes: She reports reduced pain (measured on a pain scale) after interventions.
  - She reports she is able to carry on with the activities of daily living and get enough sleep and rest despite the pain.
- **Goal:** The woman's anxiety is reduced.
  Expected Outcomes: Available social supports are used.
  - Effective coping strategies are used.
  - Decreased levels of anxiety are reported.

Test Yourself

- Name two characteristics that are different between abruptio placentae and placenta previa.

- Name three early symptoms of shock.

- Name one way to evaluate the extent of concealed hemorrhage.

HYPERTENSIVE DISORDERS IN PREGNANCY

Hypertension during pregnancy is the second leading cause of maternal morbidity and mortality in the United States, complicating 6% to 8% of all pregnancies (most of these are first-time pregnancies) and being responsible for almost 15% of maternal deaths. These disorders are not only dangerous for the pregnant woman, but also significantly increase the risk for the fetus (Lenfant, 2001). There are four basic categories of elevated blood pressure during pregnancy:

1. Gestational hypertension
2. Preeclampsia/eclampsia
3. Chronic hypertension
4. Preeclampsia superimposed on chronic hypertension

Gestational Hypertension

Gestational hypertension (formerly called pregnancy-induced hypertension or PIH) is the current term used to describe elevated blood pressure (greater than or equal to 140/90 mm Hg) that develops for the first time during pregnancy without the presence of protein in the urine. Gestational hypertension may resolve spontaneously after the baby is born, in which case the condition is referred to as transient hypertension. If the blood pressure remains elevated after delivery, the diagnosis becomes chronic hypertension. The concern is that gestational hypertension may develop into the more serious preeclampsia-eclampsia syndrome; therefore, urine checks for protein are done and blood pressure is monitored closely at each physician visit. If the blood pressure increases to a level that might endanger the woman or her fetus, the physician will prescribe antihypertensives.

Preeclampsia-Eclampsia

Preeclampsia is a serious condition of pregnancy in which the blood pressure rises to 140/90 mm Hg or higher accompanied by **proteinuria,** the presence of protein in the urine. Preeclampsia usually occurs after the 20th week of gestation and resolves when the pregnancy terminates. The syndrome may develop gradually, or it may appear suddenly without warning. The underlying cause of this disorder is unknown. It appears that exposure to trophoblastic tissue is the triggering factor, but it is not known what causes some pregnant women to develop sensitivity to the tissue while others do not. Risk factors for preeclampsia are listed in Box 17-1.

Medical researchers have been attempting to discover ways to prevent and predict preeclampsia-eclampsia

BOX 17.1	Risk Factors for Preeclampsia-Eclampsia

- Family history of preeclampsia-eclampsia
- African-American descent
- Nulliparity
- Pre-existing medical conditions such as
  - Chronic hypertension
  - Systemic lupus erythematosus
  - Renal disease
  - Diabetes
- Obstetric complications including
  - Multiple gestation
  - Hydatidiform mole (molar pregnancy)
  - Carrying a fetus that develops erythroblastosis fetalis
- Extremes of age
  - Younger than 20 years (increased risk probably due in large part to nulliparity)
  - Older than 35 years (increased risk most likely related to presence of chronic diseases)

because of the severe effects this condition can have on the woman and her fetus (Table 17-2). Various methods have been tried to prevent the condition, including high-protein, low-salt diets; low-dose aspirin therapy; and calcium supplementation. None of these therapies has been found to be effective in preventing preeclampsia.

Because there are no diagnostic tests available that can predict which woman will develop preeclampsia, early detection through regular prenatal care is the best alternative. Early prenatal care reduces morbidity and mortality associated with preeclampsia-eclampsia. However, a recent study indicates that there are differences in outcomes between ethnic groups.

Women who receive no prenatal care are more than seven times as likely to die of complications of preeclampsia and eclampsia as women who receive any prenatal care, according to a study in the April 2001 issue of *Obstetrics and Gynecology*. African-American women are 3.1 times more likely to die of preeclampsia or eclampsia than are white women. Although black and white women who received prenatal care had a lower risk of death, there is a far greater reduction for white women than for black women. This suggests that the quality of prenatal care may play a role, say researchers (ACOG News Release, 2001).

In a normal pregnancy a woman's blood pressure does not rise significantly above her baseline. In fact, during the second trimester the blood pressure decreases. However, in a pregnancy complicated by preeclampsia, the blood pressure rises. The elevated blood pressure occurs because the woman's blood vessels become more sensitive to substances that cause vasoconstriction, a condition that increases peripheral resistance and blood pressure. The rise in pressure is reinforced when the kidneys respond to decreased blood flow by releasing substances that raise the blood pressure.

The primary problem underlying the development of preeclampsia is generalized **vasospasm**, spasm of the arteries, which affects every organ in the body. Vasospasm causes generalized vasoconstriction, which leads to hypertension. The elevated blood pressure adversely affects the central nervous system and decreases blood flow to the kidneys, liver, and placenta. Vasospasm also leads to endothelial damage, which causes abnormal clotting. Tiny clots (microemboli) cause damage to internal organs, especially the liver and kidneys. Edema of the tissues, body organs, or both may result from this process (Fig. 17-4).

TABLE 17.2	Complications of Preeclampsia-Eclampsia That Can Cause Maternal and/or Fetal Injury or Death

Effects of Preeclampsia-Eclampsia	Potential Complications
Maternal Effects of Preeclampsia-Eclampsia	
Seizure activity	Bodily injury (especially the tongue), aspiration, placental abruption, or cerebral hemorrhage
Endothelial damage to pulmonary capillaries	Pulmonary edema
Severely elevated blood pressure and cerebral edema	Cerebral bleeding and complications associated with cerebral vascular accident (CVA or stroke). This complication is rare.
Edema and reduced blood flow to the liver	HELLP syndrome and/or rupture of the liver
Platelet aggregation and consumption of clotting factors	Thrombocytopenia and disseminated intravascular coagulopathy (DIC)
Fetal Effects of Preeclampsia-Eclampsia	
Reduced blood flow to the placenta	Intrauterine growth restriction (IUGR), oligohydramnios, and placental abruption
Preterm delivery to save mother or baby	Respiratory distress syndrome and other complications of prematurity

● **Figure 17.4** Pathophysiology of preeclampsia. Every body organ is affected.

Clinical Presentation

Preeclampsia is diagnosed when blood pressures of greater than 140 mm Hg systolic or 90 mm Hg diastolic develop after the 20th week of gestation. The hypertension must be documented on at least two different occasions and be accompanied by proteinuria (measured initially by dipstick of a clean-catch or catheterized urine specimen followed by a 24-hour urine collection). The presence of edema or weight gain is no longer considered a criterion for diagnosis of this disorder because edema occurs commonly in pregnancy and is not specific to preeclampsia. However, edema is significant if it is nondependent or if it involves the face and hands.

Depending on symptoms, preeclampsia is categorized as mild or severe (Table 17-3). Symptoms of mild preeclampsia are limited to slightly elevated blood pressure and limited protein in the urine. Severe preeclampsia is manifested by blood pressure above 160/110 mm Hg, greater than 2+ of protein in the urine, and symptoms related to edema of body organs and decreased blood flow to tissues. The central nervous system (CNS), especially the brain, is sensitive to small changes in fluid volume. Nervous system irritability occurs, resulting in hyperactive deep tendon reflexes and clonus (Fig. 17-5). A severe headache may indicate the presence of cerebral

edema. If the retina of the eye becomes edematous, the woman will report blurred or double vision and spots before her eyes. Visual changes and a severe headache indicate that a seizure is likely to occur. Liver involvement results in elevation of liver enzymes. Severe edema of the liver causes nausea and pain in the epigastric region. In addition, a low platelet count may result in prolonged bleeding time, and pulmonary edema may occur when the disease process affects the lungs.

If the woman with severe preeclampsia experiences a convulsion or a coma, she has progressed from preeclampsia to **eclampsia**, the presence of seizure activity or coma in a woman with preeclampsia. Seizures are typically generalized tonic-clonic in nature and only rarely progress to status epilepticus. Potential complications of eclamptic seizure activity include cerebral hemorrhage, stroke,

Be careful! Don't let the term "mild" (when applied to preeclampsia) fool you. Mild preeclampsia can progress rapidly to severe preeclampsia or full-blown eclampsia with seizures. This is a serious disorder. Any woman with signs of preeclampsia should be monitored closely.

TABLE 17.3	Comparison of Mild and Severe Preeclampsia and Eclampsia		
	Mild Preeclampsia	Severe Preeclampsia	Eclampsia
Blood pressure	140/90 mm Hg or higher; diastolic pressure remains below 100 mm Hg	160/110 mm Hg or higher	Same as for severe preeclampsia
Proteinuria	Trace to 1+ in a random specimen; 300 mg or greater in 24-hour specimen	Persistent 2+ or more; 500 mg or greater in 24-hour specimen	Same as for severe preeclampsia
Serum creatinine	Normal	Elevated	Elevated
Platelet count	Normal	Low (thrombocytopenia)	Same as for severe preeclampsia; may develop HELLP syndrome
Liver enzymes	Normal to minimally elevated	Markedly elevated	Same as for severe preeclampsia
Headache, visual disturbances, epigastric (abdominal) pain	Absent	Present	Present; epigastric pain is an important warning of an impending seizure
Fetal growth	Normal (not restricted)	May be restricted, unless there is a sudden onset near term and the baby is delivered promptly	Same as for severe preeclampsia
Edema	Trace to 1+ pedal, if present	May or may not be present; edema of the face or hands is significant	May or may not be present
Pulmonary edema	Absent	May be present	May be present
Seizure activity or coma	Absent	Absent	Present

B

● *Figure 17.5* (**A**) Patellar reflexes are best checked with the woman in a sitting position and the legs hanging freely. Absent reflexes are graded as "0," hypoactive reflexes are "1+," normal reflexes are "2+," brisk reflexes are "3+" and "4+." (**B**) The nurse checks for clonus by dorsiflexing the foot, then quickly letting go. Normally the foot rebounds smoothly against the nurse's hand. If clonus is present, the foot jerks rapidly. Clonus is recorded in "beats." One beat means the foot made one jerky movement against the hand, and so on.

A

hepatic rupture, abruptio placentae, fetal compromise, and death of the woman or fetus. The woman with preeclampsia remains at risk for seizure activity throughout pregnancy, labor, and in the first few days of the postpartum period. In fact, the signs of preeclampsia-eclampsia may occur suddenly in the postpartum period even if they were not noticeable before delivery.

HELLP syndrome is a severe form of preeclampsia-eclampsia. HELLP is an acronym for *h*emolysis, *el*evated *l*iver enzymes, and *l*ow *p*latelets, which are the laboratory findings in a woman with this complication of preeclampsia-eclampsia. The presence of HELLP syndrome or eclampsia greatly increases the mortality associated with preeclampsia.

Treatment

The primary goals of therapy are to deliver a healthy baby and restore the woman to a healthy state. To accomplish these goals the physician must consider several issues.

The most important decision regarding management of preeclampsia involves the timing of delivery because the only cure for preeclampsia is to end the pregnancy. If the fetus is at term (>37 weeks), the physician will usually induce labor because a vaginal birth is preferred to a cesarean delivery. If the fetus is preterm, management depends upon the severity of the disease and determination of fetal lung maturity. The benefits and risks of conservative management (bed rest and observation) are weighed against the benefits and risks of a preterm delivery. If the woman's condition deteriorates rapidly or the intrauterine environment becomes hostile, the physician delivers the baby promptly to save the life of the woman, the baby, or both.

Conservative management may be chosen for the woman with mild preeclampsia. If she is compliant with the treatment plan and understands the danger signals, she may receive care at home. Otherwise, hospitalization is required. Activity restriction is implemented, which usually involves bed rest on the left side with bathroom privileges. The woman should stay in a minimally stimulating environment; therefore, visitors are usually restricted to one or two support persons. The blood pressure is monitored at least every 4 hours and the weight is measured daily. Urine protein is determined via a 24-hour urine collection, or a protein dipstick is used to check each voiding. Deep tendon reflexes are assessed, and the presence of clonus is determined at lease once per shift. The woman is asked to report signs of worsening condition, such as headache, visual disturbances, or epigastric pain.

If conservative management is attempted to allow a preterm fetus to mature, close observation of the fetus is indicated. Fetal kick counts are done after every meal, and NSTs are done at least twice weekly. A biophysical profile (see Chapter 7) and serial sono-grams may be done to monitor fetal status and growth. In addition, amniocentesis may be done to determine lung maturity using the lecithin/sphingomyelin (L/S) ratio. A ratio of 2:1 is indicative of lung maturity. If imminent delivery seems necessary and the baby is preterm, glucocorticoids (usually betamethasone) may be administered to the woman in an attempt to hasten maturity of the fetal lungs.

Preventing maternal seizures is another important goal of therapy. If severe preeclampsia ensues, bed rest in a darkened, quiet room is implemented and visitors are restricted. The most effective medication to prevent and treat eclamptic seizures is magnesium sulfate, which is usually administered via the IV route (Box 17-2). This medication is reserved for the woman with severe disease. The drug works by directly relaxing skeletal muscles and raising the seizure threshold. IV MgSO$_4$ is the drug of choice to treat eclamptic seizures, although other anticonvulsants such as phenytoin (Dilantin) or diazepam (Valium) are sometimes ordered.

BOX 17.2 | **Pharmacology Focus: Magnesium Sulfate**

Method of Action:
Prevents seizures by relaxing muscles and through direct action on the central nervous system (CNS).

Usual Dosage and Administration
IV route: Loading dose of 4 to 6 grams diluted in 100 mL fluid infused over 15 to 20 minutes, followed by maintenance dose of 2 grams per hour
Antidote: Calcium gluconate 1 gram IV push over 2 minutes

Nursing Interventions
1. Carefully prepare and administer magnesium sulfate exactly as ordered.
2. Use a pump to regulate flow when administering via IV route.
3. Monitor vital signs per agency protocol every 15 to 30 minutes.
4. Perform hourly assessments of the following parameters
   a. Urinary output and protein levels
   b. Deep tendon reflexes
   c. Edema
5. Request serum magnesium levels every 4 to 6 hours, as ordered.
6. Discontinue magnesium sulfate and notify the physician if deep tendon reflexes are absent, respirations are less than 14 per minute, or urinary output is less than 30 mL/hour.
7. Therapeutic levels of magnesium sulfate are between 4 and 7 mEq/L. Patellar reflexes disappear at 10 mEq/L; respiratory arrest occurs at 12 mEq/L.

Note: The RN administers this medication. However, the LPN may assist with monitoring of the patient who is receiving IV magnesium.

Administration of magnesium sulfate requires careful management. If the medication is given intravenously, an IV pump must be used to control the rate of the infusion. Fluid overload could lead to pulmonary edema, a complication for which the woman with preeclampsia is at risk.

Magnesium sulfate is eliminated via the kidneys, and preeclampsia can cause kidney damage. Therefore, close attention must be given to urinary output, which is measured hourly. An hourly output of less than 30 mL must be reported because a low urinary output can lead to high serum levels of magnesium. The therapeutic level of magnesium sulfate is 4 to 8 mg/dL. This level is effective to in preventing seizures without causing toxicity. Magnesium toxicity begins when serum magnesium levels approach 9 mg/dL. First the reflexes disappear, then as the levels increase, respiratory depression and cardiac arrest can occur. For this reason, the reflexes and respiratory rate of the woman receiving magnesium sulfate are monitored at frequent intervals. Serum magnesium levels are drawn at prescribed intervals. Calcium gluconate is the antidote to magnesium sulfate. The RN gives this medication by IV push to treat magnesium overdose.

Because magnesium sulfate causes muscular relaxation, uterine contractions are inhibited. If delivery is indicated, the woman usually requires oxytocin induction of labor. She is at risk for postpartum hemorrhage because the uterine muscle may be unable to contract effectively. Careful monitoring for this complication is indicated after delivery.

The treatment of hypertension is controversial. Antihypertensives are only given to treat severely elevated blood pressure (greater than 160/105 mm Hg) because a rapid drop in the blood pressure can lead to decreased placental perfusion, resulting in fetal distress. Hydralazine (Apresoline) is the drug of choice for severely elevated blood pressure. Nifedipine (Procardia) is another antihypertensive that might be administered.

Nursing Care

Care of the woman with preeclampsia or eclampsia is challenging. The woman and fetus require frequent monitoring for symptoms of worsening condition. The experienced RN is responsible for assessment and care of the woman with preeclampsia, although the practical nurse may assist.

In the hospital, monitor blood pressure at least every 4 hours for mild preeclampsia and more frequently for severe disease (Nursing Procedure 17-1). In addition, it is important to auscultate the lungs every 2 hours. Adventitious sounds may indicate developing pulmonary edema. Weigh the woman daily on the same scale at the same time of day while she is wearing

Nursing Procedure 17.1
Measuring Blood Pressure in Preeclampsia

EQUIPMENT

Blood pressure cuff appropriate to the size of the woman*
Sphygmomanometer
Stethoscope

PROCEDURE

1. Wash hands.
2. Assist the woman to the same position for each reading; preferably she should be sitting.
3. Apply the blood pressure cuff to the arm in the usual fashion and support the arm.
4. Auscultate carefully. Note the systolic pressure; use phase 1 Korotkoff (the reading where the first clear, rhythmic sound becomes audible).
5. Diastolic pressure is noted at phase 5 Korotkoff (the number at which the sound completely disappears).
6. If the pressure is greater than 140/90 mm Hg, reposition the woman to her left side, wait 5 minutes and repeat the reading.

7. If the pressure continues to be elevated, determine if the woman is experiencing headache, blurred vision, or epigastric pain.
8. Reposition the woman comfortably on her left side, supported by pillows.
9. Replace equipment appropriately and wash hands.
10. Report immediately to the RN blood pressures greater than 140/90 mm Hg and/or abnormal symptoms.
11. Record the blood pressure per agency protocol. If the pressure was taken twice, record each reading, noting the time of each and maternal position.

Note: Most facilities use automated blood pressure equipment such as a Dinamap blood pressure device. These devices can be set to automatically take and record the blood pressure at preset intervals. There is also a manual override feature. Many fetal monitoring systems include automated blood pressure monitoring capabilities. With these systems the blood pressures are automatically taken and recorded on the fetal monitor strip.

* Care should be taken to choose a cuff that fits the woman correctly. If a small cuff is used to measure the blood pressure for a large woman, the reading may be elevated falsely. Conversely, if a large cuff is used on a small woman, the reading may be lowered falsely.

the same amount of clothing. Report any sudden increase in weight.

Teach the woman to report headache, visual changes, and epigastric pain, which are warning signs of an impending seizure. It is important to keep the environment quiet and nonstimulating because bright lights and loud noises could precipitate a seizure. Institution of seizure precautions is a must. Seizure precautions include padding the side rails and keeping suction equipment, an oral airway, supplemental oxygen, and medications readily available for use at the bedside. If a seizure does occur, follow proper procedure (Nursing Procedure 17-2).

The woman should remain on bed rest in the left lateral position, although some women with mild preeclampsia are allowed bathroom privileges. Maintain strict monitoring of intake and output. IV fluids may be ordered. It is important to control the infusion carefully with an IV pump to maintain adequate hydration without causing overload. Report urinary output of less than 30 mL/hour.

Adequate nutrition is important to promote fetal growth and maternal well-being. There is no special diet for preeclampsia, but careful attention is needed so that nutrients are consumed in adequate amounts (see Chapter 7). Salt does not need to be restricted below normal levels, but care should be taken to avoid excessive intake. See Nursing Care Plan 17-1.

The nurse also cares for the psychosocial needs of the woman hospitalized for preeclampsia. Boredom may be an issue because of prolonged bed rest. Encourage the woman to read, keep a journal, or do crafts. The woman may be anxious about the well-being of her fetus or because she had to leave older children at home. Keep the woman informed of the results of NSTs and other tests of fetal well-being. Reassure her that she can monitor fetal well-being by doing kick counts regularly. Allow her to ventilate her feelings of fear or frustration. Short daily visits by older children or telephone calls may also help alleviate anxiety.

Postpartum care of the woman varies depending on whether magnesium sulfate was used during the intrapartum period. If it was, the woman receives care in the labor and delivery unit or a high-risk antepartum unit for the first 24 to 48 hours after delivery. During that time magnesium sulfate administration is continued, and close monitoring of respirations, deep tendon reflexes, clonus, and urinary output is continued as before delivery. Close observation for postpartum hemorrhage is indicated.

If the medication was not used, the woman may be transferred to a postpartum unit. In addition to normal

---

Nursing Procedure 17.2
What to Do in the Event of an Eclamptic Seizure

EQUIPMENT

Suction equipment
Equipment to deliver oxygen
Magnesium sulfate
IV access materials
Fetal monitor

PROCEDURE

When the seizure begins:
1. If you are in the room when a seizure begins, summon help with the call bell and note the time the seizure began.
2. Gently attempt to place the woman on her side, if possible. Do not force her to this position if injury will result.
3. Provide oxygen by face mask.

During the seizure:
4. The RN will prepare and administer IV magnesium sulfate loading dose per orders or standing protocol to stop the seizure.
5. If IV access is not in place, establish access as soon as it is safe to do so.
6. Suction PRN, if it is safe to do so, because aspiration is a real threat. Do not force the suction catheter into the mouth, particularly if you are using a hard plastic suction tip.
7. Watch for signs of spontaneous birth of the baby. Sometimes a seizure will precipitate birth.
8. Note the characteristics of the seizure so that you may accurately record a description after the emergency is over.

After the seizure:
9. Continue to suction PRN.
10. Continue administering oxygen to prevent/treat maternal–fetal hypoxia.
11. Begin continuous monitoring of the fetal heart rate, if a continuous monitor is not already in place.
12. Notify the physician of the seizure, if another nurse has not already completed this task.
13. Document the following parameters.
    a. Time the seizure began
    b. Characteristics of the seizure: tonic-clonic activity, fecal or urinary incontinence, cyanosis, etc.
    c. All nursing actions completed and medications administered
    d. Response of the woman to interventions
    e. Evaluation of the electronic fetal monitor tracing

NURSING CARE PLAN 17-1

The Woman With Preeclampsia

CASE SCENARIO

Hilda Rodriguez is a 35-year-old Gravida 1, Para 0 at 33 weeks' gestation. She was admitted to the hospital with the diagnosis of mild preeclampsia. Admitting vital signs are BP 150/98 mm Hg, T 98.7°F, P 70 bpm, R 20/min. She denies contractions, headache, blurred vision, or epigastric pain. Her deep tendon reflexes are 2+ (normal), and she does not have clonus (also a normal finding). Proteinuria of 1+ is found in a random voided specimen. Fetal heart rate is in the 150s, and a nonstress test at the physician's office today was reactive.

NURSING DIAGNOSIS

Ineffective Tissue Perfusion (maternal vital organs, peripheral tissues and placenta) related to constriction of blood vessels (vasospasms).

GOAL

Maintenance of adequate arterial blood supply to major organs, peripheral tissues, and placenta.

EXPECTED OUTCOMES

- The woman remains alert, awake, and responsive
- Blood pressure remains 140/90 mm/Hg or lower
- Urinary output is at least 30 mL/hour
- Extremities remain warm to touch
- Peripheral edema +1 or less
- No facial edema or ascites
- Weight remains stable without sudden increases

NURSING INTERVENTIONS	*RATIONALE*
Maintain bed rest in side-lying position, as ordered (strict or with bathroom privileges).	Bed rest in a side-lying position improves blood flow to the kidneys and other vital organs.
Monitor neurologic status (level of responsiveness) as per facility protocol.	Lowered levels of consciousness may indicate the presence of cerebral edema.
Monitor vital signs q 4 hours or more frequently as ordered; report blood pressure >140/90 mm Hg or as ordered.	A highly elevated blood pressure can interfere with blood flow to major body organs and extremities.
Perform strict intake and output measurements.	Vasospasms associated with preeclampsia can lead to hypovolemia, a condition that decreases blood flow to vital organs.
Monitor urinary output q 4 hours or as ordered; report outputs totaling less than 30 mL/hour, or 120 mL per 4-hour time period.	Reduced urinary output can indicate decreased blood flow to the kidneys, which should be treated promptly to prevent kidney damage.
Measure daily weights. a. Use the same scale at the same time each day with the same amount of clothing. b. Report sudden weight gain. c. Monitor for edema.	Sudden weight gain and edema indicates that fluid is being retained. Although the woman has more overall body water, the fluid is trapped in tissues so that less fluid is in the blood, a condition that leads to decreased perfusion.

NURSING DIAGNOSIS:

Risk for Injury (maternal) related to cerebral irritability and possible progression of preeclampsia to eclampsia.

GOAL

Freedom from injury related to seizure activity.

EXPECTED OUTCOMES

The woman will
- Not experience injury from seizure activity
- Maintain a clear airway

(nursing care plan continues on page 428)

NURSING CARE PLAN 17-1 continued

The Woman With Preeclampsia

NURSING INTERVENTIONS	RATIONALE
Monitor vital signs as ordered; assess for increasing blood pressure.	Increasing blood pressure indicates a worsening of status. The woman is then at risk for seizure activity.
Institute seizure precautions 　a. Side rails up and padded 　b. Airway, suction, and oxygen equipment set up at bedside. 　c. Quiet, minimally stimulating environment (low lights, sound, etc.)	A noisy, stimulating environment increases the risk for a seizure. If the woman does have a seizure, padded side rails, airway, suction equipment and oxygen will all be needed to prevent serious injury from the seizure (e.g., aspiration)
Monitor for signs of impending seizure. 　d. Headache 　e. Blurred vision 　f. Epigastric pain 　g. Hyperactive reflexes: 4+ 　h. Presence of clonus	All listed signs are indicators that seizure activity will likely occur unless there is intervention.
Assist the RN to administer magnesium sulfate, as ordered.	Magnesium sulfate is a muscle relaxant and a central nervous system depressant that can prevent eclamptic seizures.

NURSING DIAGNOSIS
Risk for Injury (fetal) related to chronic hypoxia secondary to ineffective tissue perfusion of the placenta and episodes of acute hypoxia during maternal seizure activity.

GOAL
Maintenance of adequate fetal oxygenation.

EXPECTED OUTCOMES
The fetus will
- Maintain a heart rate between 120 and 160 bpm
- Remain active with normal kick counts
- Demonstrate well-being with reactive nonstress tests
- No injury occurs and fetus remains reactive if a maternal seizure occurs.

NURSING INTERVENTIONS	RATIONALE
Maintain in side-lying position, or with a wedge under one hip.	A side-lying position increases perfusion to the placenta.
Monitor fetal heart tones and reactivity, as ordered.	Monitoring is done to determine fetal status.
Instruct the client to monitor fetal kick counts after each meal. (Chapter 7 outlines the procedure for performing fetal kick counts.)	If the fetus is moving as often as expected, there is reassurance the fetus is doing well. A decrease in fetal movement is an ominous sign.
Assist the RN to perform nonstress tests (NST), as ordered.	Serial NSTs will be ordered to closely monitor fetal status. A nonreactive NST indicates the fetus may be in distress.

postpartum care, closely observe the blood pressure and monitor for other signs of worsening preeclampsia because a seizure can occur as long as several days after delivery. Observe the woman closely because she is at increased risk for postpartum hemorrhage. Monitor the platelet count, as ordered, and watch for development of complications, such as bleeding from the mouth, gums, nose, or injection sites. If the neonate is in the neonatal intensive care unit (NICU), assist the woman to visit as soon as she is able. If she cannot visit, provide pictures of the infant and provide a daily update on the baby's condition.

Chronic Hypertension and Preeclampsia Superimposed on Chronic Hypertension

Chronic hypertension is high blood pressure that is present and diagnosed before the woman becomes pregnant. When a woman with preexisting hypertension becomes pregnant, the pregnancy is already at risk. Sustained high blood pressure can be damaging to blood vessels and eventually can decrease placental perfusion, leading to fetal growth restriction. In addition, the woman with chronic hypertension is at a much higher risk of developing superimposed preeclampsia. Box 17-3 lists the complications associated with chronic hypertension in the pregnant woman.

Clinical Presentation

Chronic hypertension is said to exist if the blood pressure has been elevated consistently above 140/90 mm/Hg when the woman is not pregnant. If hypertension develops before the 20th week of gestation, the diagnosis is suspected but is not confirmed until after pregnancy. If the elevation continues after the end of the pregnancy, the diagnosis of chronic hypertension is made. Some women with preexisting hypertension may begin the pregnancy with mild disease, but then experience severe disease after the 24th week.

The diagnosis of superimposed preeclampsia is made when a woman who has chronic hypertension experiences proteinuria. The presence of preeclampsia superimposed on chronic hypertension is a particularly lethal one. In these cases, the preeclampsia tends to develop earlier in the pregnancy and runs a more severe course. The risk of placental abruption and incidence of fetal growth restriction is increased significantly.

Treatment and Nursing Care

Ideally, the woman with chronic hypertension meets with the physician before becoming pregnant to modify her treatment regimen. If she is taking a hypertensive medication that may be teratogenic, the physician changes her medication to one that is recommended for use during pregnancy. The physician often recommends a sodium-restricted diet, explains work and exercise limitations, and recommends weight loss, if the woman is overweight. Once pregnancy is achieved,

prenatal visits are done more frequently, usually every 2 weeks during the first half of pregnancy, and weekly thereafter. Fetal surveillance is intensified with serial ultrasound tests, frequent NSTs, and biophysical profiles.

Mild, uncomplicated cases of chronic hypertension tend to fare well without significant increases in perinatal mortality. In fact, pharmacologic therapy may not be needed in women with mild disease. However, in cases of severe hypertension (i.e., if the diastolic blood pressure exceeds 110 mm/Hg) antihypertensive therapy is almost always indicated.

Certain antihypertensive agents are typically used to control the blood pressure. Methyldopa (Aldomet), beta blockers, and calcium channel blockers may be prescribed. The benefit of treatment with one of these agents generally outweighs the risk of fetal effects when hypertension is severe. Angiotensin-converting enzyme (ACE) inhibitors and angiotensin II receptor antagonists/blockers are contraindicated, and thiazide diuretics are not recommended for use during pregnancy because of adverse fetal effects.

Test Yourself

- List four categories of high blood pressure during pregnancy.

- What is the underlying process that causes most of the problems associated with preeclampsia?

- HELLP is an acronym for _____.

MULTIPLE GESTATION

A multiple gestation refers to a pregnancy in which the woman is carrying more than one fetus.[2] Twins are the most common manifestation of multiple gestation. In the general population twins (two fetuses) occur once in 83 deliveries, triplets (three fetuses) occur once in 6,900 deliveries, and quadruplets (four fetuses) occur once in 575,000 pregnancies (Elliot, 2003). Most pregnancies resulting in more than two fetuses are the result of fertility treatments. The incidence of twins is also increased with fertility techniques.

Twins can be identical (monozygotic), resulting from one ovum fertilized by one sperm, or fraternal (dizygotic), the result of two ova fertilized by two sperm (see Chapter 5 for review). A woman has an

---

BOX 17.3	**Complications Associated With Chronic Hypertension in Pregnancy**

Medical Complications
- Ventricular hypertrophy
- Cardiac decompensation
- Cerebrovascular accident (CVA)
- Chronic renal damage

Complications of Pregnancy
- Superimposed preeclampsia
- Placental abruption
- Fetal growth restriction

Source: Cunningham, F. G., et al. (2001b). Hypertensive disorders in pregnancy. In *Williams Obstetrics* (21st ed., pg. 571). New York: McGraw-Hill.

---

[2]Singleton gestation is the term used when the woman is carrying one fetus.

increased chance of conceiving dizygotic twins if she has one or more of the following risk factors: older maternal age, multiparity, or family history of dizygotic twins. Monozygotic twins may have one or two placentas and one or two amniotic sacs. The best situation occurs when monozygotic twins each have their own placenta and amniotic sac.

When twins share a placenta, a serious condition called twin-to-twin transfusion syndrome (TTTS) can occur. In this situation, one twin receives more blood from the placenta than his sibling. This twin is called the recipient. The recipient twin gets too much blood, which can overload the cardiovascular system and result in polycythemia and heart failure. The other twin, called the donor twin, does not get enough blood from the placenta. This twin can become severely anemic and experience intrauterine growth restriction.

A multifetal pregnancy is considered to be at risk. The woman with multifetal pregnancy is at increased risk for hyperemesis gravidarum, pyelonephritis, preterm labor, placenta previa, and pregnancy-induced hypertension. The fetuses are at risk to be conjoined, to experience growth restriction, or to be born prematurely. During labor there is a higher risk for umbilical cord prolapse. During the postpartum period the woman is at risk for postpartum hemorrhage.

There also is increased fetal demand for nutrients in a multifetal pregnancy. This situation can easily lead to maternal anemia. Insufficient iron leads to iron-deficiency anemia, whereas insufficient folic acid may result in megaloblastic anemia.

Clinical Presentation

The woman carrying multiple fetuses usually presents with a uterus that is large for dates. She is more likely than a woman carrying one fetus to experience anemia, fatigue, severe nausea and vomiting, and hyperemesis gravidarum. The practitioner will perform an ultrasound examination to date the pregnancy and to rule out polyhydramnios, fibroid tumors, and molar pregnancy.

Treatment

Management of a multifetal pregnancy often includes consultation with a perinatologist. There is increased emphasis on the woman's diet, multivitamin and iron supplements, and rest. Obstetric ultrasounds are done every 4 to 6 weeks after diagnosis to assess fetal growth and presentation, and placental location. After 24 weeks' gestation, the woman is asked to schedule prenatal visits every 2 weeks, which include a cervical evaluation at every visit. Weekly NSTs are scheduled after 32 weeks.

The practitioner must choose (or recommend) a mode of delivery. In general, a cesarean delivery is indicated if twin A (the first twin) is not in a vertex presentation. If twin A is vertex, the practitioner may opt to try a vaginal delivery. Success for this method is increased if both twins are vertex. If twin B (the second twin) is breech, the practitioner may schedule a cesarean delivery, or attempt a vaginal delivery but only if twin B is not larger than twin A. If a vaginal delivery is attempted, the practitioner may perform podalic version to turn twin B after twin A is delivered. Or the practitioner may attempt a breech delivery for twin B. If twin B experiences fetal distress, or the practitioner experiences difficulty delivering twin B vaginally, a cesarean delivery may be performed for twin B.

Nursing Care

Assist the physician to perform assessments to detect complications throughout the pregnancy. Instruct the woman regarding symptoms of preterm labor (Chapter 18). Teach the woman to perform fetal movement counts daily after 32' weeks gestation. Encourage the woman to get adequate rest and a well-balanced diet.

BLOOD INCOMPATIBILITIES

There are several situations that can cause problems for the fetus related to blood incompatibilities between the woman's blood and the fetus' blood. Normally the two bloodstreams never meet. But occasionally some type of trauma occurs that allows intermingling of the two bloodstreams. This situation is more likely to occur during invasive procedures such as amniocentesis or active labor, after spontaneous abortion, or when the placenta separates at birth. Two types of blood incompatibilities are discussed: Rh incompatibility and ABO incompatibility.

Rh Incompatibility

The $Rh_o(D)$ factor is an antigen (protein) that is found on the surface of blood cells. When this factor is present on the blood cells, the individual is Rh positive, and when the factor is lacking, the person is Rh negative. If a woman who is Rh negative is exposed to Rh-positive blood, such as through an incorrectly cross-matched blood transfusion, her immune system produces antibodies to fight the $Rh_o(D)$ antigen. Once her body has produced antibodies to the $Rh_o(D)$ factor, she is sensitized to Rh-positive blood, a condition referred to as *isoimmunization*.

The problem arises when a woman who is Rh negative carries a fetus with Rh-positive blood. If the pregnant woman has been sensitized, the antibodies to the $Rh_o(D)$ factor readily cross the placenta and attack the fetus' blood cells. The fetus develops hemolytic anemia and often requires exchange transfusions in utero or shortly after birth. In years past, a woman who was Rh negative often became sensitized while carrying her first child. Sensitization most often occurred during childbirth, when fetal blood can leak into the woman's bloodstream during delivery. Thereafter, with each subsequent pregnancy, the fetus with Rh-positive blood would develop hemolytic anemia, with the disease becoming increasingly severe with each pregnancy. Now sensitization rarely occurs because the Rh-negative woman is given Anti-D immunoglobulin (RhoGam) within 72 hours of delivering an Rh-positive baby.

Clinical Presentation

The goal is to identify the woman at risk for Rh incompatibility and to prevent sensitization from occurring. The routine blood and Rh typing that are done during the first prenatal visit serve this function. Antibody screening is done to determine if the woman is sensitized. A positive antibody screen indicates that sensitization has occurred. In this instance the woman will have no symptoms at all; however, the fetus may be severely affected. The physician often performs amniocentesis or cordocentesis to diagnose and assess hemolytic disease in the fetus. If sensitization has not occurred (i.e., the antibody screen is negative), the woman will be instructed that she needs RhoGam after any invasive procedure, trauma of any kind (e.g., motor vehicle collision or physical trauma), and delivery, whether it be by abortion, miscarriage, removal of ectopic pregnancy, or vaginal or cesarean birth.

Treatment

RhoGam is a product derived from blood that prevents the Rh-negative woman from developing antibodies to the $Rh_o(D)$ factor. It is critical for a woman who is Rh-negative to receive RhoGam after childbirth, miscarriage or abortion, ectopic pregnancy, or any invasive procedure, such as amniocentesis or chorionic villus sampling. It is during these times that fetal blood is most likely to come into contact with maternal blood. Most physicians also administer a prophylactic minidose of RhoGam at 28 weeks of pregnancy.

CULTURAL SNAPSHOT

Some religions ban the use of blood products. Inform the woman that Anti-D immunoglobulin (RhoGam) is derived from blood and obtain her consent before administering the treatment. If a woman refuses RhoGam, alert the RN or physician immediately. The woman must be fully informed of the risks and consequences of refusing the treatment.

If the woman is sensitized, she is not a candidate for RhoGam, and the fetus requires close observation. As the pregnancy progresses, fetal well-being is assessed with amniocentesis, cordocentesis, biophysical profiles, NSTs, or contraction stress tests. If hemolytic disease is severe, the fetus may require exchange transfusions, or the physician may opt to deliver the fetus prematurely (refer to Chapter 20 for discussion of hemolytic disease of the newborn).

It is important to note that Rh incompatibility does not occur if the woman is Rh positive. It doesn't matter what the fetus' Rh factor is, if the woman is Rh positive, she is not a candidate for RhoGam. An Rh-negative woman who delivers an Rh-negative child is also not a candidate for RhoGam. Because the gene for Rh-negative blood is autosomal recessive, if the woman's partner is Rh negative and she is Rh negative, the fetus will be Rh negative, and RhoGam will be unnecessary. RhoGam is never to be administered to the newborn.

Think of it this way. A problem with Rh incompatibility can only exist if the woman is Rh negative. So first determine the blood type of the woman. If she is Rh positive, then there isn't a problem. If she is Rh negative, a problem exists only if the fetus is Rh positive.

Nursing Care

The nurse's responsibility in cases of Rh incompatibility is to always check the woman's blood type on laboratory reports and the prenatal record. If there is a discrepancy, notify the physician. Before discharging a woman after any invasive procedure, abdominal trauma, abortion, ectopic pregnancy, or childbirth, check her blood type. If she is Rh negative, it is important to follow up to see if she is a candidate for RhoGam. If she is a candidate, obtain orders and administer the RhoGam. Instruct the woman regarding the purpose and importance of RhoGam to subsequent pregnancies. Make certain that she understands under what circumstances she is to receive RhoGam.

ABO Incompatibility

ABO incompatibility is another cause of hemolytic disease of the newborn. The problem most frequently arises when the woman's blood type is O and the fetus' blood type is A, B, or AB. Type O blood has naturally occurring antibodies against types A, B, and AB. However, these antibodies are large and generally do not cross the placenta. Occasionally during pregnancy fetal blood may leak into the maternal circulation, causing the woman's immune system to produce antibodies to fetal blood. These antibodies are smaller than the naturally occurring antibodies and readily cross the placenta, where they work to destroy fetal blood. Fortunately, this type of blood incompatibility usually results in a much less severe form of hemolytic disease than does Rh incompatibility. The neonate rarely requires exchange transfusions, although she will likely require treatment for jaundice.

Test Yourself

- List three complications for which a multiple gestation is at risk.

- Name two situations that place the fetus at increased risk for blood incompatibilities.

- What product is administered to an Rh-negative woman after she has delivered an Rh-positive fetus?

KEY POINTS

- Nursing care of hyperemesis gravidarum focuses on assisting the woman to regain fluid balance and to obtain nutrition needed for healthy fetal development.

- Signs and symptoms of ectopic pregnancy include missed menstrual period, nausea and vomiting, abdominal pain, shoulder pain, and vaginal spotting or bleeding. If the tube ruptures, the woman will experience hemorrhage into the abdominal cavity and hypovolemic shock.

- Spontaneous abortion is loss of a pregnancy before the fetus is able to survive outside the uterus on his own (before viability). Abortions are classified according to whether or not the uterus is emptied, or for how long the products of conception are retained. The six types of spontaneous abortion are threatened, inevitable, incomplete, complete, missed, and habitual (recurrent).

- Cerclage is the surgical procedure used to treat incompetent cervix. A suture is used to close the cervix so that the pregnancy can be carried to term.

- The nurse provides patient education regarding follow-up care to the woman who experiences molar pregnancy, including the importance of frequent physician visits, monitoring of serum hCG levels, avoiding pregnancy for at least 1 year, and reporting any symptoms of metastasis (e.g., severe persistent headache, cough or bloody sputum, or unexpected vaginal bleeding).

- Placenta previa causes painless, bright red bleeding during pregnancy because the placenta is implanted abnormally, either close to or covering the cervix. Abruptio placentae is associated with

dark red, painful bleeding caused by separation of the placenta from the wall of the uterus at any time before the end of labor.

- The nursing process is used to develop the plan of care for a woman with a bleeding disorder. The focus of the care plan is maintaining placental perfusion and fluid volume, avoiding fetal injury (dealing with hypoxia), preventing maternal injury (dealing with isoimmunization), preventing infection, and reducing anxiety and pain.

- Hypertensive disorders are classified according to when in relation to the pregnancy the high blood pressure is first diagnosed, the presence or absence of proteinuria, and whether or not the condition resolves spontaneously after delivery. The four categories of hypertension are gestational hypertension, preeclampsia/eclampsia, chronic hypertension, and preeclampsia superimposed on chronic hypertension.

- Priority nursing interventions for the woman with preeclampsia-eclampsia include maintaining bed rest in a side-lying position; monitoring neurologic status, blood pressure, urinary output, and daily weights; instituting seizure precautions; observing for signs of an impending seizure (headache, blurred vision, epigastric pain, hyperactive reflexes, presence of clonus); assisting the RN to administer magnesium sulfate; and monitoring the fetus (fetal kick counts, fetal heart rate, NSTs).

- A multiple gestation, also known as multifetal pregnancy, is at risk. The woman is more likely to experience hyperemesis gravidarum, pyelonephritis, preterm labor, placenta previa, preeclampsia-eclampsia, and postpartum hemorrhage. Close observation of the pregnancy with special attention to diet and fetal well-being is recommended. Frequently, a perinatologist manages the pregnancy. The mode of delivery is dependent on several factors, the most important of which is the presentation of each twin.

- Rh and ABO incompatibilities can cause hemolytic disease of the fetus/newborn. Prevention of Rh incompatibilities through the use of RhoGam for the Rh-negative woman is the goal of therapy. If sensitization (isoimmunization) has occurred, the focus of assessment and care becomes the fetus, who may require exchange transfusions.

REFERENCES AND SELECTED READINGS

Books and Journals

ACOG News Release. (2001). Pregnancy-related mortality from preeclampsia and eclampsia. Retrieved February 15, 2003, from http://www.acog.com/from_home/ publications/press_releases/nr03-31-01-4.cfm

Braun, R. D. (2003). Surgical management of ectopic pregnancy. *eMedicine.* J. J. Kavanagh, F. Talavera, G. F.

Whitman-Elia, F. B. Gaupp, & L. P. Shulman (Eds.). Retrieved January 28, 2003, from http://www.emedicine.com/med/topic3316.htm

Chamberlain, G., & Steer, P. (Eds.). (1999). Obstetric emergencies. *British Medical Journal, 318,* 1342.

Chudacoff, R. (2000). *Hyperemesis gravidarum.* The American Surrogacy Center, Inc. Retrieved January 17, 2003, from http://www.surrogacy.com/medres/article/hyperem.html

Cunningham, F. G., Gant, N. F., Leveno, K. J., Gilstrap, L. C. III, Hauth, J. C., & Wenstrom, K. D. (2001a). Gastrointestinal disorders. In *Williams obstetrics* (21st ed., pp. 1275–1276). New York: McGraw Hill Medical Publishing Division.

Cunningham, F. G., Gant, N. F., Leveno, K. J., Gilstrap, L. C. III, Hauth, J. C., & Wenstrom, K. D. (2001b). Section VII. Common complications of pregnancy. In *Williams obstetrics* (21st ed., pp. 565–810). New York: McGraw Hill Medical Publishing Division.

Deering, S. H., & Satin, A. (2002). Abruptio placentae. *eMedicine.* B. A. Meyer, F. Talavera, A. V. Sison, F. B. Gaupp, & L. P. Shulman (Eds.). Retrieved February 9, 2003, from http://www.emedicine.com/med/topic6.htm

Edelman, A., & Logan, J. R. (2001). Pregnancy, hyperemesis gravidarum. *eMedicine.* A. J. Saya, F. Talavera, M. Zwanger, J. Halamks, & R. O'Conner (Eds.). Retrieved January 17, 2003, from http://www.emedicine.com/emerg/topic479.htm

Elliot, J. P. (2003). *Multiple gestation.* Condition summary from Best Doctors website. Retrieved November 15, 2003, from http://www.bestdoctors.com/en/conditions/g/gestation/gestation_100200.htm

Ernst, E., & Pittle, M. H. (2000). Efficacy of ginger for nausea and vomiting: A systematic review of randomized clinical trials. *British Journal of Anaesthesia, 84*(3), 367–371. Abstract retrieved January 19, 2003, from http://www.jr2.ox.ac.uk/bandolier/booth/alternat/AT128.html

Gaufberg, S. V. (2001). Threatened abortion. *eMedicine.* R. Alson, F. Talavera, M. Zwanger, J. Halamka, & J. Adler (Eds.). Retrieved February 8, 2003, from http://www.emedicine.com/emerg/topic11.htm

Kurowski, K., & Yakoub, N. (2003). Staying alert for gestational trophoblastic disease: Implications for primary care clinicians. *Women's Health in Primary Care, 6*(1), 39–47.

Lenfant, C. (2001). Management of hypertension in pregnancy. *Journal of Clinical Hypertension, 3*(2), 71–72. Retrieved August 10, 2001, from Medscape database. http://www.medscape.com

Magee, L. A. (1998). The safety and effectiveness of antiemetic therapy for NVP. Presented at the 1st International Conference on Nausea and Vomiting of Pregnancy. Retrieved January 19, 2003, from http://www.nvpvolumes.org/index.htm

Mattson, S., & Smith, J. E. (Eds.). (2000). *Core curriculum for maternal–newborn nursing. AWHONN publication* (2nd ed.). Philadelphia: WB Saunders Company.

Moore, L. E., & Ware, D. (2002). Hydatidiform mole. *eMedicine.* J. G. Pritzker, F. Talavera, A. D. Barnes, F. B. Gaupp, & L. P. Shulman (Eds.). Retrieved January 17, 2003, from http://www.emedicine.com/med/topic1047.htm

National High Blood Pressure Education Program Working Group Report on High Blood Pressure in Pregnancy. (2001). Working Group Report on high blood pressure in pregnancy. *Journal of Clinical Hypertension, 3*(2), 75–88. Retrieved August 10, 2001, from http://www.medscape.com/LeJacq/JCH/2001/v03.n02/jch0302.02/pnt-jch0302.02.html

Nettina, S. M. (2001). Complications of the childbearing experience. In *The Lippincott manual of nursing practice* (7th ed., pp. 1179–1219). Philadelphia: Lippincott Williams & Wilkins.

Petrozza, J. C., & O'Brien, B. (2002). Early pregnancy loss. *eMedicine.* B. D. Cowan, F. Talavera, C. V. Smit, F. B. Gaupp, & L. P. Shulman (Eds.). Retrieved February 8, 2003, from http://www.emedicine.com/med/topic3241.htm

Puscheck, E., & Pradhan, A. (2002). Complete abortion. *eMedicine.* S. R. Trupin, F. Talavera, R. S. Legro, F. B. Gaupp, & L. P. Shulman (Eds.). Retrieved February 8, 2003, from http://www.emedicine.com/med/topic3310.htm

Queenan, R. A. (2000). Third trimester bleeding. In A. T. Evans & K. R. Niswander (Eds.), *Manual of obstetrics* (6th ed., pp. 298–305). Philadelphia: Lippincott Williams & Wilkins.

Saju, J., & Lyons, D. L. (2002). Placenta previa. *eMedicine.* R. Levine, F. Talavera, R. S. Legro, F. B. Gaupp, & L. P. Shulman (Eds.). Retrieved February 9, 2003, from http://www.emedicine.com/med/topic3271.htm

Sepilian, V., & Wood, E. (2002). Ectopic pregnancy. *eMedicine.* R. K. Zurawin, F. Talavera, A. D. Barnes, F. B. Gaupp, & L. P. Shulman (Eds.). Retrieved February 8, 2003, from http://www.emedicine.com/med/topic3212.htm

Williams, M. C. (2000). Hepatic, biliary, and gastrointestinal complications. In A. T. Evans & K. R. Niswander (Eds.), *Manual of obstetrics* (6th ed., pp. 90–126). Philadelphia: Lippincott Williams & Wilkins.

Yoon, Y., & Ko, P. (2001). Placenta previa. *eMedicine.* J. J. Sachter, F. Talavera, M. Zwanger, J. Halamka, & S. H. Plantz (Eds.). Retrieved February 9, 2003, from http://www.emedicine.com/emerg/topic427.htm

Websites

Hyperemesis Gravidarum
http://www.am-i-pregnant.com/hg.shtml

Early Pregnancy Loss
http://www.miscarriageassociation.org.uk/
http://www.babycenter.com/refcap/252.html

Cervical Incompetence
http://www.dyspareunia.org/html/cervical_cerclage.htm

Ectopic and Molar Pregnancy
http://www.modimes.org/professionals/681_1189.asp

Bleeding During Pregnancy
http://www.perinatalmed.com/articles/vaginalbleeding.html
http://www.smartmoms.org/health-safety/health1.html

Preeclampsia
http://www.preeclampsia.org/index.asp

Rh Incompatibility and RhoGam
http://folsomobgyn.com/rh_testing_and_rhogam.htm

Package Insert for RhoGam
http://www.babycenter.com/rhogam/info.pdf

WORKBOOK

NCLEX-STYLE REVIEW QUESTIONS

1. A 28-year-old gravida 4 para 0 is seen at the prenatal clinic for complaints of lower abdominal cramping and spotting at 12 weeks' gestation. The nurse midwife performs a pelvic examination and finds that the cervix is closed. What does the nurse suspect is the cause of the cramps and spotting?

   a. Ectopic pregnancy

   b. Habitual abortion

   c. Incompetent cervix

   d. Threatened abortion

2. A 32-year-old gravida 1 para 0 at 36 weeks' gestation is brought to the obstetric department reporting abdominal pain. Her blood pressure is 164/90 mm Hg, her pulse is 100 beats per minute, and her respirations are 24 per minute. She is restless and slightly diaphoretic with a small amount of dark red vaginal bleeding. What assessment should the nurse make next?

   a. Check deep tendon reflexes.

   b. Measure fundal height.

   c. Palpate the fundus and check fetal heart rate.

   d. Obtain a voided urine specimen and determine blood type.

3. Which assessment finding best correlates with a diagnosis of hydatidiform mole?

   a. Bright red painless vaginal bleeding

   b. Brisk deep tendon reflexes and shoulder pain

   c. Dark red, "clumpy" vaginal discharge

   d. Painful uterine contractions and nausea

4. Which instruction is appropriate to give to a woman with hyperemesis gravidarum?

   a. Eat mainly high-fat foods to supply sufficient calories.

   b. Limit fluids with meals to increase retention of food.

   c. Do all your own cooking so you will build up a tolerance for food odors.

   d. Take your antinausea medicine after meals to help control the nausea.

STUDY ACTIVITIES

1. Fill in the table to indicate how ectopic pregnancy, threatened abortion, inevitable abortion, and incompetent cervix are alike and how they are different according to the signs and symptoms listed.

	Pain	Bleeding	Nauses and Vomiting	Cervical Dilation
Ectopic pregnancy				
Threatened abortion				
Inevitable abortion				
Incompetent cervix				

2. Go to the following Internet site: http://www-medlib.med.utah.edu/WebPath/webpath.html

   a. Click on "Systemic Pathology."

   b. Click on "Female Genital Tract Pathology."

   c. Choose images of the ectopic pregnancy (number 51 in the "Fallopian Tube" section), and of a molar pregnancy (numbers 84 to 86 in the "Placenta" section).

3. Think of an experience you, a relative, or a friend has had that involved a miscarriage. Be ready to share your story with your clinical group. Discuss interventions the nurse can use to help the parents to cope after a miscarriage.

CRITICAL THINKING: What Would You Do?

Apply your knowledge of hypertensive disorders of pregnancy to the following situation.

1. Maria, a 38-year-old primigravida, presents to the doctor's office for a scheduled prenatal visit at 28 weeks' gestation. During the assessment, Maria comments that she must be eating more than she thought because she gained 5 pounds during the course of 2 days. Her blood pressure is 150/92 mm Hg while sitting.

   a. What should the nurse ask next? Why?

   b. What additional assessments should be done?

c. Based on these data, what management plan is the physician likely to implement?

2. Maria is admitted to the hospital to rule out preeclampsia. The doctor's orders include bed rest with bathroom privileges, regular diet, private room, limit visitors, 24-hour urine specimen for protein and creatinine clearance, complete blood count, blood urea nitrogen and creatinine levels, liver profile, and coagulation studies.

a. How should the nurse prepare the room for Maria? What supplies are needed? Why?

b. If Maria has preeclampsia, what results does the nurse anticipate to see on the laboratory report for each test?

c. Why did the doctor write an order for a private room and to limit visitors?

3. Maria receives a diagnosis of mild preeclampsia. She is to remain in the hospital on bed rest.

a. What fetal assessment tests should be done? How frequently?

b. What special instructions and recurring assessments should be included on the care plan?

c. Maria asks the nurse, "Since my condition is mild, why can't I just go home? I could stay in bed there and I'd be so much more comfortable." How should the nurse reply?

4. The nurse is doing the a.m. assessment. Maria says, "I woke up with a terrible headache, and I can't seem to wake up enough to see well this morning. Everything looks blurry." Maria's blood pressure is 164/110 mm Hg.

a. How is Maria's condition classified now?

b. What other assessments should the nurse make? What should be done next after the assessment is completed?

c. How does the nurse expect the treatment plan will change?

Labor at Risk

18

STUDENT OBJECTIVES

On completion of this chapter, the student should be able to

1. Choose appropriate nursing interventions for the client with labor dystocia.
2. Compare and contrast PROM with preterm PROM.
3. Describe clinical manifestations of preterm labor.
4. Discuss treatment options for preterm labor.
5. Apply the nursing process to the care of a woman in preterm labor.
6. Develop a patient teaching plan for the woman with a post-term pregnancy.
7. Describe nursing interventions for the woman experiencing fetal demise.
8. Compare and contrast obstetric emergencies according to clinical manifestations, treatment, and nursing care.

KEY TERMS

chorioamnionitis
labor dystocia
pelvic rest
precipitous labor
tocolytic

There are situations that sometimes arise that put the laboring woman and her fetus at risk. It is for this reason that many women prefer to deliver in a hospital setting. However, a well-trained practitioner who monitors the laboring woman closely can often catch signs of developing complications so that intervention can prevent harm no matter what the treatment setting. The following discussion describes complications that might be encountered during labor. Although the licensed practical nurse/licensed vocational nurse (LPN/LVN) may not be directly responsible for the laboring woman, it is helpful to know the signs of labor complications to be able to summon help when needed.

DYSFUNCTIONAL LABOR (DYSTOCIA)

4-I's (?)

Labor dystocia is an abnormal progression of labor. Dystocia occurs as a result of a malfunction in one or more of the "four Ps" of labor that were discussed in Chapter 8: passageway, passenger, powers, or psyche. The pelvis may be small or contracted because of disease or injury. The fetus may be malpositioned, excessively large (macrosomic), or have an anomaly, such as hydrocephalus or omphalocele, which may not allow him to fit through the birth canal. Uterine contractions may be of insufficient quality or quantity. The woman may be unable to push effectively during the second stage of labor because of exhaustion. The woman may "fight" the contractions because of fear or pain. Frequently it is a combination of factors that results in dysfunctional labor.

Complications

Difficult labor is associated with increased maternal and fetal morbidity and mortality. The risk for infection is increased when labor is prolonged, particularly in association with ruptured membranes. Bacteria can ascend the birth canal, resulting in fetal or maternal bacteremia and sepsis. Neonatal pneumonia can result from the fetus aspirating infected amniotic fluid. Uterine rupture can result from obstructed labor. This complication can be lethal for the woman and her fetus. Labor dystocia is the most common reason cited for performing a primary cesarean delivery, which carries increased risk for mother and baby.

Some complications of labor dystocia relate only to the woman. Fistula formation is more common in prolonged labor because the presenting part exerts pressure for prolonged periods on maternal soft tissue, a situation that can result in tissue necrosis and subsequent fistula development. Pelvic floor injury is more common for the woman who experiences a difficult labor or delivery.

TABLE 18.1	Expected Labor Progress	
	Primipara	**Multipara**
Expected length of the latent phase of labor	<20 hours	<14 hours
Expected rate of dilation during active labor	At least 1.2 centimeters per hour	At least 1.5 centimeters per hour
Expected rate of fetal descent during active labor	At least 1 centimeter per hour	At least 2 centimeters per hour

Clinical Manifestations and Diagnosis

Before abnormal labor can be diagnosed, the clinician must be aware of what constitutes normal labor. Table 18-1 compares expected rates of labor progress for the primipara and multipara. For additional review of normal labor, refer to Chapters 8 and 10.

Labor dystocia can occur in any stage of labor, although it is diagnosed most commonly once the woman is in active labor or when she reaches the second stage of labor. Dystocia is characterized by disorders of protraction and arrest. A protraction disorder occurs when there is abnormally slow progression of labor. An arrest disorder refers to total lack of progress. A primipara in active labor receives a diagnosis of protraction of dilation if cervical dilation progresses at less than 1.2 centimeters/hour. She has a diagnosis of protraction of descent if the fetal head descends at less than 1 centimeter/hour. If a multipara in active labor experiences less than 1.5 centimeters/hour cervical dilation or fetal descent of less than 2 centimeters/hour, she is diagnosed with protraction disorder. Arrest disorders occur when there is no change in cervical dilation or fetal descent for a period of 2 hours provided adequate labor has been established.

Causes of Labor Dysfunction

Labor dysfunction can occur as a result of problems with the uterus or problems with the fetus.

Uterine Dysfunction

There are two types of uterine dysfunction: hypotonic and hypertonic. The most common is hypotonic dysfunction. This labor pattern is manifested by uterine contractions that may or may not be regular, but the quantity or strength is insufficient to dilate the cervix.

Hypertonic dysfunction presents in two ways. The most common is frequent ineffective contractions. Some clinicians refer to this syndrome as uterine "irritability." The underlying problem with this disorder is that the uterine muscle cells do not contract in a coordinated fashion. The end result is an elevated resting uterine tone with small, short, but frequent contractions.

The other type of hypertonic dysfunction manifests as increased frequency and intensity of uterine contractions. This type of hypertonic dysfunction often results in **precipitous labor**—labor that lasts less than 3 hours from the start of uterine contractions to birth. The complication that most frequently results from a precipitous labor is maternal soft tissue damage, such as lacerations of the cervix, vaginal wall, and perineum; and bruising or other trauma to the infant from rapid descent through the birth canal.

Be careful! Don't confuse precipitous labor with precipitous delivery, although precipitous labor may result in a precipitous birth. Precipitous labor is an abnormally fast labor (lasting less than 3 hours); whereas, a precipitous delivery refers to a delivery that is unattended by the physician or nurse midwife. A precipitous delivery may be totally unattended or it may be nurse controlled. This type of delivery may occur outside or inside of the health care facility.

Cephalopelvic Disproportion (CPD)

Labor arrest is sometimes referred to as "failure to progress." If hypotonic labor is ruled out as the cause of failure to progress, the practitioner may suspect CPD. In this situation the diameters of the fetal head are too large to pass through the birth canal. CPD can be due to a condition that causes an enlarged fetal head, such as fetal macrosomia or hydrocephalus. CPD can also result from a small maternal pelvis. In the past, maternal rickets frequently was the cause of a contracted pelvis. Improved nutrition has decreased the incidence of rickets, so today most cases of CPD are due to other causes. Nongynecoid pelvic types, such as android, anthropoid, or platypelloid, may result in CPD.

Fetal Malposition

Fetal malposition can cause prolonged labor. When the back of the fetal head is positioned toward the posterior portion of the maternal pelvis, the position is referred to as occiput posterior (see Chapter 8 for a review of fetal positions). A labor complicated by occiput posterior position is usually prolonged and characterized by maternal perception of increased intensity of back discomfort. The lay term for this type of labor is "back labor." Face presentation is another cause of prolonged labor. When the fetal face presents, the largest diameters of the fetal head are presented to the maternal pelvis, and labor is generally prolonged. Breech presentation, transverse lie, and compound presentations may also cause labor dystocia. Any of these fetal positions may result in the need for cesarean delivery, although vaginal delivery may be possible.

Treatment

Treatment depends on the cause of labor dystocia. However, because the cause is not always known, clinicians usually give what is called a "trial of labor." If uterine hypofunction is the cause of inadequate progress, augmentation of labor with artificial rupture of membranes or intravenous (IV) oxytocin infusion or both is usually the treatment of choice. Augmentation is carried out using the same process as that for labor induction. (See Chapter 11 for discussion of labor induction.) Oxytocin augmentation is the treatment of choice for uterine irritability in the absence of placental abruption. In this situation, oxytocin assists the uterus to contract more effectively so that the pattern spaces out, but individual contractions are stronger and more effective.

Hypertonic labor may result from an increased sensitivity of uterine muscle to oxytocin induction or augmentation. Treatment for this iatrogenic cause of hypertonic labor is to decrease or shut off the oxytocin infusion. If the hypertonic pattern causes the fetal heart rate to drop precipitously, the practitioner may order administration of a **tocolytic**, a substance that relaxes the uterine muscle, to slow the labor.

If the cause of labor dystocia is fetal malposition, the practitioner may attempt to manipulate the fetus to a more favorable position. For occiput posterior position, the fetus may rotate unaided to an anterior position, although the labor is generally prolonged because the fetus must rotate 180 degrees, as compared with 90 degrees if the fetal head begins descent in a transverse position. If the woman completes the first stage of labor and the fetal head has not rotated, the practitioner may use the vacuum extractor or forceps to attempt to rotate the head to an anterior position. This requires that the fetal head be at +2 station, or lower. It is possible for the fetus to deliver from an occiput posterior position. In this situation, the fetus is born face up.

There are three basic options for a breech presentation. The practitioner may use a version procedure (see Chapter 11) in an attempt to turn the fetus to a cephalic presentation. Frequently this procedure is effective; however, sometimes the fetus turns back to a breech presentation before labor ensues. Some practitioners will allow the woman to labor with the fetus in a breech presentation and attempt a vaginal delivery, although this practice has become less common because of successful version techniques and malpractice concerns.

A cesarean delivery is the third option for delivering a breech presentation.

For a transverse lie (shoulder presentation), there are two options. Either the practitioner will use external version to try to turn the fetus to a cephalic presentation, or she will deliver by cesarean. If the fetus remains in a transverse lie, he cannot deliver vaginally.

Nursing Care

Carefully assess fetal lie, presentation, and position when the woman presents to the labor and delivery area. During the active phase, assess the contraction pattern every 30 minutes. Check for uterine contractions of adequate frequency and intensity. Assess fetal response to uterine contractions. Perform a thorough pain assessment every hour to include a pain scale to rate intensity. Ask the woman to describe her pain. Inquire regarding the presence of intense back pain.

Plot cervical changes and fetal descent on a labor graph. Observe for slow progression or arrest of labor. Identify slow progression if a primipara in active labor dilates more slowly than 1.2 centimeters/hour or the fetal head descends at less than 1 centimeter/hour; or if a multipara in active labor dilates more slowly than 1.5 centimeters/hour or the fetal head descends at less than 1.5 centimeters/hour over a period of several hours. Identify arrest of dilation if no cervical change occurs during a period of 2 hours, and arrest of descent if no descent occurs during a 2-hour period.

If a disorder of dilation or descent is noted, the physician must be notified. However, there are several assessments that must first be made. Check to see if the woman has a full bladder. Remember that a full bladder can interfere with the progress of labor. Next, determine if the contraction pattern is adequate. Contractions should occur every 2 to 3 minutes apart, last 60 to 90 seconds, and be of moderate to strong intensity during the active phase of labor.

If the bladder is empty and the contraction pattern is adequate, try to determine if the fetus is in an occiput posterior position. Inquire regarding the character of the woman's pain. Suspect occiput posterior position if the woman complains of severe lower back pain. Remember, counterpressure applied to the lower back with a fisted hand sometimes helps the woman to cope with the "back labor" that is characteristic of occiput posterior positioning.

Determine if the woman might benefit from pain relief measures. Intravenous sedation or epidural anesthesia might be helpful. If the woman is "fighting" the contractions, pain control might help her relax and allow the cervix to dilate.

Call a full report of your labor assessments to the physician. Carefully note any orders for sedation, anesthesia, or oxytocin augmentation. After carrying out the ordered interventions, continue to evaluate for adequate labor progress. Notify the physician if interventions do not result in progression of labor or if signs of fetal distress occur.

Test Yourself

- Name four complications that are associated with labor dystocia.

- What is the usual medical treatment for uterine hypofunction?

- List three nursing assessments that must be made before notifying the physician of a disorder of dilation or descent?

PREMATURE RUPTURE OF MEMBRANES

Premature rupture of membranes (PROM) refers to spontaneous rupture of the amniotic sac before the onset of labor. PROM occurs in approximately 10% of pregnancies at term (Wilkes & Galan, 2002b). This condition is to be differentiated from preterm labor, which is the onset of labor before the end of 37 weeks' gestation, and preterm PROM, which refers to rupture of the amniotic sac before the onset of labor in a woman who is less than 37 weeks' gestation. Complications associated with PROM include abruptio placentae, umbilical cord compression or prolapse, and infection.

Preterm PROM is the leading known cause of preterm delivery and occurs in approximately 2% of all pregnancies. Risk factors for preterm PROM include cigarette smoking, previous preterm delivery, vaginal bleeding, low socioeconomic conditions, sexually transmitted infections, and unknown causes. The farther along in the pregnancy that PROM occurs, the better the chance for a healthy outcome. Most women with preterm PROM deliver within 1 week after the amniotic sac ruptures. PROM before the age of viability rarely results in a good outcome.

Clinical Manifestations and Diagnosis

The woman with PROM usually presents to the delivery suite with reports of a large gush or continuous, uncontrollable leaking of fluid from the vagina. She may report vaginal discharge or bleeding and pelvic pressure. However, she does not present with regular uterine contractions because she is not in labor.

Sometimes the diagnosis is obvious when large amounts of amniotic fluid are visible. A definitive diagnosis of PROM is made by speculum examination. The practitioner looks for pooling of amniotic fluid and then tests the fluid with Nitrazine paper, which turns blue in the presence of amniotic fluid. If the Nitrazine test is equivocal (uncertain), the practitioner may elect to perform a fern test. For this test, the practitioner collects a specimen of fluid from the vagina on a sterile cotton swab and then smears the specimen on a slide. When the specimen is viewed under the microscope, a ferning pattern indicates that amniotic fluid is present.

Treatment

The major problem for the woman with PROM at term is the increased risk for infection, specifically **chorioamnionitis**, bacterial or viral infection of the amniotic fluid and membranes. With each hour that passes after PROM that delivery has not occurred, the risk for infection increases. Fortunately, most women go into spontaneous labor within 24 hours of PROM. However, many practitioners prefer to induce labor with oxytocin rather than wait for nature to take its course. Both treatment options, expectant management (wait and see) and induction of labor, should be carried out in the hospital. Research has shown that the neonate born to the woman who stays at home with PROM and waits for labor to ensue before presenting to the hospital or birthing clinic for care has a much higher risk of being admitted to the neonatal intensive care unit (NICU) with neonatal sepsis (Wilkes & Galan, 2002b).

Management of preterm PROM is more complicated. If there are signs of infection, such as elevated maternal temperature; maternal tachycardia; cloudy, foul-smelling amniotic fluid; and uterine tenderness, cultures are obtained, antibiotics started, and delivery facilitated, regardless of gestational age. However, if there is no infection, expectant management may be chosen. The goal is to allow the fetus time to mature and achieve delivery before the woman or her fetus becomes infected.

The usual practice is to administer 7 days of antibiotic therapy. The practitioner often orders a course of IV antibiotics (usually ampicillin and erythromycin) for 48 hours, followed by oral antibiotics for 5 days. Antibiotic therapy for longer than 7 days is not recommended because of the risk that resistant strains of bacteria might emerge.

The woman may be put on strict bed rest or bed rest with bathroom privileges. **Pelvic rest**, a situation in which nothing is placed in the vagina (including tampons and the practitioner's fingers to perform a cervical examination), is instituted because the risk for infection increases whenever the cervix is manipulated. The practitioner may elect to perform periodic sterile speculum examinations to check for cervical changes. A digital examination is not necessary unless signs of labor, such as pelvic pressure, cramping, regular contractions, or bloody show, are present.

Fetal surveillance is performed at least daily. Generally, the woman is instructed to perform kick counts after every meal. Daily nonstress tests (NSTs) may also be ordered. If the woman is less than 32 weeks' gestation, intramuscular injections of a corticosteroid (e.g., Betamethasone and Dexamethasone) are given to hasten fetal lung maturity. Some practitioners administer a tocolytic to prolong the pregnancy long enough for the steroid injections to work. Tocolytics are not administered in the presence of infection.

Nursing Care

Assess the woman who presents with reports of PROM. Ask the woman to describe the sequence of events that occurred in association with the rupture of the amniotic sac. Check for visible signs of PROM—pooling of fluid and positive Nitrazine or fern test.

Once the diagnosis has been established, follow the practitioner's orders for management of PROM. If the woman is at term, expect continuous fetal heart rate monitoring. Watch for the sudden onset of deep variable decelerations, which may indicate umbilical cord prolapse. Take the temperature at least every 2 hours. Promptly report temperature elevation, prolonged maternal or fetal tachycardia, and cloudy or foul-smelling amniotic fluid. Watch for the

Here's a tip for you. Always give a thorough report! The length of time the membranes were ruptured before delivery is an important part of the report to the pediatrician and to the nurse assuming care of the infant. This information will alert them to monitor the newborn closely for signs of sepsis in the event of prolonged rupture of membranes.

natural onset of labor, or administer oxytocin induction, if ordered.

PRETERM LABOR

Preterm labor is labor that occurs after 19 weeks' and before the end of 37 weeks' gestation. Preterm labor often leads to preterm birth, which accounts for 70% of neonatal morbidity and mortality. Despite years of research, the incidence of preterm birth has actually increased from approximately 8% to 9% in the 1980s to 11.9% in 2001 (Bernhardt & Dorman, 2004). The current rate is much higher than the Healthy People 2010 goal of 7.6% (Church-Balin & Damus, 2003). It is widely accepted that the development of effective treatments for preterm labor would greatly reduce the health care burden of sick neonates.

Often the cause of preterm labor is not readily apparent. In fact, there is no associated risk factor in one-half of woman presenting with preterm labor (Moos, 2004). The top three risk factors associated with preterm labor are current multiple gestation pregnancy (twins, triplets, or more), history of previous preterm birth, and uterine or cervical abnormalities. Although history of previous preterm labor is one of the better predictors, this association is not helpful for predicting preterm labor for the primigravida. Other risk factors are listed in Box 18-1.

Clinical Manifestations and Diagnosis

It is not always easy to diagnose preterm labor. The presence of painful uterine contractions does not by itself indicate that the woman is in preterm labor because pain is a subjective phenomenon that can be affected by many variables. The definitive diagnosis is made when uterine contractions result in cervical change. The earlier the diagnosis is made, the greater the likelihood that treatment will be effective. If the diagnosis is made after the woman has progressed to greater than 3 centimeters, it is unlikely that preterm birth will be avoided.

The woman in preterm labor often presents with signs that include uterine contractions, which may be painless; pelvic pressure; menstrual-like cramps; vaginal pain; and low, dull backache accompanied by vaginal discharge and bleeding. The membranes may or may not be ruptured. The most frequent examinations used to diagnose preterm labor include assessment of contraction frequency, fetal fibronectin test (Box 18-2), and measurement of cervical length. No change in cervical length in the presence of a negative fetal fibronectin test indicates that the woman has less than 10% chance of delivering prematurely.

BOX 18.1	Risk Factors for Preterm Labor and Birth

Obstetric and Gynecologic Risk Factors
- Multiple gestation (twins, triplets)
- History of preterm birth
- Uterine or cervical abnormalities
  - Fibroid tumors
  - Bicornuate uterus
  - Incompetent cervix
- Preterm premature rupture of membranes
- Placenta previa
- Retained intrauterine device
- Short time period (less than 6 to 9 months) between pregnancies

Demographic and Lifestyle Risk Factors
- Extremes of maternal age (<17 years of age or >35 years of age)
- Member of an ethnic minority
- Low socioeconomic status
- Late or no prenatal care
- Smoking
- Alcohol use
- Illicit drug use
- Intimate partner violence
- Lack of social support
- High levels of stress
- Long working hours with long periods of standing

Medical Risk Factors
- Infection
  - Chorioamnionitis
  - Bacterial vaginosis
  - Bacteriuria
  - Acute pyelonephritis
  - Sexually transmitted infections
- High blood pressure
- Diabetes
- Clotting disorders
- Entering the pregnancy underweight
- Obesity

Fetal-Related Risk Factors
- Fetal demise
- Intrauterine growth restriction (IUGR)
- Congenital anomalies

Treatment

Standard obstetric care includes evaluation of risk factors for preterm delivery as early as the first office visit. If risk factors are identified, the cervix is examined for evidence of injury. A workup is done to detect asymptomatic bacteriuria, sexually transmitted infections, and bacterial vaginosis. These infections are treated, if present. At 20 and 26 weeks' gestation a transvaginal ultrasound may be done to measure the length of the cervix. A cervical length of less than 2.5 centimeters is considered abnormal. Education is given regarding the

BOX 18.2	Fetal Fibronectin Test

Fetal fibronectin is a protein that serves as an adhesive between the amniotic sac and the uterine lining. This protein is normally found in cervical secretions up to approximately 22 weeks' gestation, after which it is normally absent. The test is performed during a speculum examination of the cervix. A cotton swab is used to collect a sample of cervical secretions, which is sent to a laboratory for analysis. It takes anywhere from 6 to 36 hours to get the results of the test.

The presence of fetal fibronectin in cervical secretions (a positive test) in association with signs of preterm labor may indicate that the adhesive is coming apart too early and that preterm birth is imminent. The absence of fetal fibronectin (a negative test) is a more reliable indicator than is a positive test. A negative test indicates that the woman will not likely deliver for at least 2 weeks.

signs and symptoms of preterm labor. Weekly telephone contact with a nurse and regular prenatal visits are encouraged.

Once active preterm labor is diagnosed, the practitioner must determine how best to treat it. Often bed rest and hydration with either oral or IV fluids is enough to stop uterine irritability and prolong the pregnancy. The decision must be made as to whether or not tocolytics (Table 18-2) should be used. A fetus less than 23 weeks' gestation has almost no chance of surviving outside of the womb, so tocolytics generally are not used below this gestational age. Likewise, tocolytics are not often prescribed after 34 weeks' gestation because neonatal morbidity and mortality are very low at this point in the pregnancy. Tocolytics are administered most frequently between 24 and 33 weeks' gestation. Although the medication may not prevent preterm birth, it often allows the practitioner to buy enough time to allow corticosteroid injections to help mature the fetal lungs or to allow transfer to a facility with a higher level of neonatal intensive care.

TABLE 18.2	Tocolytic Agents		
Medication	Route of Administration	Maternal Side Effects	Fetal/Neonatal Side Effects
Magnesium sulfate	IV	*At therapeutic levels*: Pulmonary edema *At toxic levels*: Respiratory depression, tetany, paralysis, profound hypotension, cardiac arrest	*At therapeutic levels*: Nonreactive nonstress test; decreased to no fetal breathing movements
Ritodrine (Yutopar)	IV	Hypokalemia, hyperglycemia, tachycardia, hypotension, palpitations, anxiety, shortness of breath, headache, nausea or vomiting, pulmonary edema, cardiac ischemia, cardiac insufficiency, maternal death	Tachycardia, elevated serum glucose
Terbutaline (Bricanyl)	Subcutaneously	Same as ritodrine	Same as ritodrine
Indomethacin	*Loading dose*: Rectal suppository *Maintenance dose*: Orally	Renal failure, hepatitis, gastrointestinal bleeding	Premature closure of the ductus arteriosus, oligohydramnios, neonatal necrotizing enterocolitis, intraventricular hemorrhage
Nifedipine (Procardia)	Sublingually	Transient hypotension	Unknown

● Nursing Process for the Woman With Preterm Labor

ASSESSMENT

Collect a thorough history, including previous preterm births, multiple gestation pregnancies, infections, cigarette smoking, and other risk factors for preterm labor (see Box 18-1). Inquire if the woman is experiencing symptoms of preterm labor, such as uterine contractions; uncontrollable leaking of fluid from the vagina; backache; menstrual-like cramps; or vaginal pain, discharge, or bleeding.

The physical assessment includes Nitrazine testing. If the Nitrazine test results are uncertain, prepare to assist the RN or practitioner to perform a speculum exam to check for pooling of fluid and to obtain a fern test. Place the woman on the fetal monitor. Observe for uterine irritability or contractions. Palpate the uterus carefully. A hard, board-like uterine rigidity and pain that does not relent may indicate placental abruption.

Assess the woman's emotional response. The threat of preterm labor may cause apprehension, fear, and anxiety. The woman and her partner may be concerned for the well-being of the fetus. Once the diagnosis is established, the woman may be concerned about the side effects of tocolytic therapy.

SELECTED NURSING DIAGNOSES

- Risk for Imbalanced Fluid Volume related to dehydration, infusion of high volumes of IV fluid, and/or side effects of tocolytic therapy
- Risk for Injury related to side effects of tocolytic therapy
- Acute Pain related to labor contractions
- Anxiety related to threat of harm to or death of self and fetus

PLANNING AND GOALS

Maintaining the safety of the pregnant woman and her fetus is the primary goal when planning care. Appropriate goals may include that the woman will maintain a balanced fluid volume with clear lung fields; she will not experience injury from tocolytic therapy; she will report a tolerable pain level; and she will report a reduction in anxiety. Additional goals and interventions are planned according to the individual needs and situation of the woman.

IMPLEMENTATION

Maintaining a Balanced Fluid Volume

Monitoring fluid status is an important nursing function for the woman in preterm labor. Sometimes hydration with IV fluids is all that is needed to stop the premature contractions. Monitor the IV site and the rate of infusion. Administer a fluid bolus of 500 to 1,000 mL as ordered and then reduce to the ordered maintenance rate.

Monitor vital signs. A normal blood pressure in conjunction with a rising pulse upon moving from a recumbent to a sitting or standing position is associated with low fluid volume. Hypotension is associated with severe dehydration. Monitor urinary output. Record urine characteristics. Concentrated urine with a high specific gravity may indicate dehydration.

Watch for signs of fluid overload. Normally a healthy pregnant woman can withstand high fluid volumes; however, if she is receiving tocolytics, watch closely for signs of developing pulmonary edema, such as dyspnea, tachycardia, productive cough, and adventitious breath sounds.

Preventing Injury

If the woman is receiving magnesium sulfate therapy to stop preterm labor, assess her at least once per hour. Report dyspnea, tachycardia, productive cough, or adventitious breath sounds to the RN or primary care provider. Monitor respiratory rate. Report bradypnea or periods of apnea. Check the deep tendon reflexes at least hourly. Report decreased or absent reflexes immediately. Refer to Chapter 17 for other nursing actions necessary for magnesium infusion.

If the woman is receiving a Beta$_2$-adrenergic receptor agonist, such as ritodrine or terbutaline, monitor serum potassium and glucose levels, as ordered. Report low potassium or elevated glucose to the RN or primary care provider. Monitor for and report any significant changes in the vital signs, in particular tachycardia or hypotension. The primary care provider usually leaves orders detailing the pulse and blood pressure levels that should be reported. Assess for shortness of breath, anxiety, and palpitations. Immediately report any complaints of chest pain. Monitor for signs of pulmonary edema.

Managing Pain

Assess the woman's pain using a pain scale at the frequency ordered by the RN. Ask the woman at what level the pain is tolerable. Be sure to assess and record location, characteristics, and intensity. Administer pain medication as ordered by the primary care provider. Keep in mind that a sudden increase in pain intensity or pain that does not relent may be the sign of a developing complication. Report any changes in the character or intensity of pain.

Reducing Anxiety

Encourage the woman and her partner to verbalize their fears and concerns. Answer questions honestly and to the best of your ability. If you do not know the answer, say so, and explain that you will find the answer as soon as possible. Make certain that the woman and her partner know the treatment plan. Explain procedures before performing them. Allow the woman to ventilate regarding her feelings. Explore with the RN coping strategies that the woman is using. Assist the woman to use positive coping strategies whenever possible. If she is alone without a support system, ask for a social services or pastoral care consult.

EVALUATION: GOALS AND EXPECTED OUTCOMES

- **Goal:** Fluid volume balance is maintained.
  Expected Outcomes:
  - Skin and mucous membranes remain hydrated.
  - Lung fields remain clear to auscultation.
  - Hematocrit, serum electrolytes, and urine specific gravity remain within normal limits.
- **Goal:** The woman remains injury free.
  Expected Outcomes:
  - The woman reports onset of respiratory distress immediately, such as
    - Dyspnea.
    - Productive cough.
  - The woman reports cardiac signs immediately, such as
    - Chest pain.
    - Heart palpitations.
    - Racing pulse
- **Goal:** The woman expresses the ability to cope with her pain.
  Expected Outcomes:
  - Reports reduced pain (measured on a pain scale) after interventions.
  - Reports she is able to get sufficient sleep and rest despite the pain.
- **Goal:** The woman verbalizes that she is coping with her anxiety.
  Expected Outcomes:
  - Available social supports are used.
  - Effective coping strategies are used.
  - Decreased levels of anxiety are reported.

POST-TERM PREGNANCY AND LABOR

A post-term pregnancy is one that lasts longer than 2 weeks after the due date (i.e., 42 weeks). The incidence of post-term pregnancy is 3% to 12% (Wilkes & Galan, 2002a). Some pregnancies are erroneously diagnosed as post-term because of miscalculation of gestational age. Certainty of pregnancy dating is diminished when the woman seeks late prenatal care and is unsure of her last menstrual period. This is true because early sonograms are the most accurate at determining gestational age.

A post-term pregnancy is at risk for increased perinatal mortality, particularly during labor. The post-term pregnancy is more likely to be complicated by oligohydramnios and meconium staining of the amniotic fluid. Oligohydramnios increases the incidence of cord compression, with subsequent development of fetal distress during labor. Thick meconium-stained fluid increases the risk for meconium aspiration syndrome (discussed in Chapter 20). The risk for birth of an unusually large infant increases as the gestation advances. The woman in labor with a large infant is at higher risk for shoulder dystocia. A post-term pregnancy that is also complicated by intrauterine fetal growth restriction (IUGR) is particularly at risk for perinatal mortality. The theory that a post-term pregnancy is at risk for decreased placental functioning has not been verified by clinical studies (Cunningham et al., 2001a).

Clinical Manifestations and Diagnosis

The woman presents with an intrauterine pregnancy that has been determined to be at or past 42 completed weeks. Usually the primary care provider will attempt to use several methods to determine fetal age, such as when the fetal heart rate could first be heard by Doppler and by fetoscope, early ultrasound measurements, and recorded fundal height measurements. Amniotic fluid volume may be decreased, as measured by ultrasound. Fetal macrosomia may be suspected.

When an amniotomy is done, meconium staining frequently is noted.

Treatment

There are two basic treatment plans for the woman who is carrying a post-term pregnancy. One is called expectant management. This treatment protocol involves frequent testing for fetal well-being (Searing, 2001). The woman is instructed to report decreased fetal movement immediately. NSTs are performed at least twice weekly. Ultrasound to measure amniotic fluid volume and biophysical profiles (BPPs) are frequently performed. The second strategy for managing a post-term pregnancy is induction of labor at 42 weeks' gestation. (Chapter 11 discusses labor induction.) Clinical research has shown that similar outcomes occur using either strategy.

Nursing Care

Teach the woman who is post-term to monitor fetal movements daily. (Refer to Chapter 7 for description of fetal kick counts.) Explain the importance of reporting decreased fetal movement to her primary care provider immediately. She may be anxious regarding the well-being of her fetus. Provide realistic reassurances. Be certain that the primary care provider has answered all her questions and concerns adequately. If you identify a knowledge deficit, instruct her appropriately or refer her to the RN or primary care provider for clarification.

During labor, observe the fetal monitor strip closely for signs of fetal distress. Report these immediately to the RN in charge. Carefully note and record the color and amount of amniotic fluid that is released when the water bag breaks. No fluid is worrisome because it may indicate oligohydramnios with thick meconium staining. If you assisted with the amniotomy, be sure to inform the RN of this finding.

INTRAUTERINE FETAL DEATH

Fetal death is defined as death of the fetus in utero (lack of cardiac activity) at 20 weeks' or greater gestation or a weight of 500 grams or more. This definition distinguishes fetal death from early pregnancy loss, such as occurs with spontaneous abortion.

Causes of fetal death can be categorized into four general types: fetal, placental, maternal, and unknown. Approximately 25% to 40% of fetal deaths can be attributed to fetal causes, 25% to 35% placental causes, 25% to 35% unknown causes, and 5% to 10% maternal causes (Cunningham et al., 2001c). Examples of fetal causes include genetic or congenital abnormalities and infection. The most common cause of fetal demise is placental abruption. This is usually categorized under placental causes; however, preeclampsia and other disorders can increase the risk for placental abruption. Cord accidents (such as prolapse or true knot), premature rupture of the membranes, and twin-to-twin transfusion syndrome are other placental causes. Maternal causes include advanced maternal age; medical disorders, such as diabetes mellitus and hypertension; and pregnancy-related complications, such as preeclampsia-eclampsia, Rh disease, uterine rupture, and infection.

Clinical Manifestations and Diagnosis

It is when the woman no longer detects fetal movement that she often presents for treatment. Inability to find the fetal heart rate leads the primary care provider to suspect fetal death. Confirmation of death is made by sonogram. The fetal heart is visualized. Lack of cardiac activity is diagnostic.

Treatment

In the past, the woman was advised to wait until labor spontaneously ensued; however, the longer a woman carries a dead fetus, the greater her risk for developing disseminated intravascular coagulopathy (DIC). Currently the recommendation is to induce labor within the next few days.

Induction is carried out as described in Chapter 11 for fetal demise at or near term. When the gestational age is less than 28 weeks, the cervix is rarely favorable for induction. In these cases, the woman may be induced with prostaglandin E_2 vaginal suppositories or oral or intravaginal misoprostol.

Nursing Care

Physical care of the woman is carried out as for other women having labor induced. Careful attention to the history is warranted because the woman with a uterine scar from previous surgery is at risk for rupture. For the woman at term, the tocodynamometer is used to monitor uterine contractions during labor. Postpartum care is the same as for other women.

Emotional care of the woman is more complex. She may experience shock, denial, anger, and depression. Remember that grief responses vary from individual to individual. Allow the woman and her family space to comfort one another, but do not avoid her. Offer to call a pastor or other spiritual leader she may desire. Be sure to determine if the woman wishes any religious sacraments or rituals to be done. Most institutions provide postpartum care in a unit or room away from the nursery.

Don't forget the golden rule!

A woman who has just received a diagnosis of fetal demise is experiencing a terrific loss. Be available to her without intruding. Answer her questions honestly. Encourage her to hold and name her baby, if she is able.

Be sure that mementos are collected. Take pictures as dictated by institutional policy. Pictures are usually taken even if the woman refuses them. The pictures are kept on file for a year or more. The woman is told that she can change her mind and come get the pictures at any time. Collect a lock of hair, footprints, and other reminders of the baby. Refer to Chapter 19 for further discussion of how to care for the grieving woman.

Test Yourself

- Name five complications for which the postterm pregnancy is at risk.

- What condition is the woman at greater risk of developing if a fetal demise is not delivered within a few days of fetal death?

- Describe at least three ways the nurse can provide support for the woman with a fetal demise?

EMERGENCIES ASSOCIATED WITH LABOR AND BIRTH

Amniotic Fluid Embolism

Amniotic fluid embolism is a rare obstetric emergency that frequently results in death or severe neurologic impairment of the woman and her fetus. Recently a new name has been proposed for the disorder: anaphylactoid syndrome of pregnancy. The proposed new name resulted from research that indicates that amniotic fluid embolism more resembles anaphylaxis and septic shock than it does pulmonary embolism.

Amniotic fluid embolism occurs in 1 in 20,000 to 1 in 80,000 pregnancies. Maternal mortality ranges from 26% to 61%; however, very few (approximately 15%) survive without neurologic damage (De Jong & Fausett, 2003). Amniotic fluid embolism is often divided into two major phases: respiratory distress, followed by hemodynamic instability, which includes pulmonary edema and hemorrhage. The woman may become comatose, and if she survives, may remain in a vegetative state.

Clinical Manifestations and Diagnosis

In most cases, symptoms of amniotic fluid embolism occur suddenly during or immediately after labor. The woman usually develops symptoms of acute respiratory distress, cyanosis, and hypotension. If she is in labor, the fetus typically demonstrates signs of fetal distress, with bradycardia occurring in most cases.

Diagnosis is made based on the clinical symptoms and laboratory studies. Arterial blood gases (ABGs) demonstrate acidosis and hypoxemia. Bleeding times are usually prolonged. Evidence of pulmonary edema may be seen on a chest x-ray (Moore & Ware, 2002).

Treatment

Because amniotic fluid embolism is still poorly understood, varied clinical approaches have been tried in an effort to increase survival rates. Unfortunately, there is currently no curative therapy; therefore, treatment is aimed at supporting vital functions. An immediate response to the woman's initial complaint of respiratory distress is necessary to increase the woman's chances of survival. The woman often progresses quickly to full cardiopulmonary arrest and requires advanced cardiac life support, including mechanical intubation and ventilation. Delivery of the infant by cesarean within 5 minutes after the start of cardiopulmonary resuscitation (CPR) is recommended (Curran, 2003). Typically, disseminated intravascular coagulopathy is treated with massive fluid resuscitation and blood product replacement therapy. Once the woman is in stable condition, she requires care in an adult intensive care unit (ICU).

Nursing Care

Respond promptly and summon for immediate assistance if a laboring or postpartum woman reports dyspnea. Administer oxygen via face mask. Measure the vital signs, particularly the blood pressure and pulse. Hypotension, tachycardia, and other signs of shock are usually evident. Initiate CPR, if needed, and be prepared to assist with a cesarean delivery at the bedside, if needed. Be prepared to assist the RN during fluid resuscitation and blood product administration. Anticipate transfer to the ICU as soon as the woman is stable enough to transfer.

Shoulder Dystocia

Shoulder dystocia is an obstetric emergency that is dreaded by all obstetric practitioners. The fetal head delivers, but the shoulders become stuck in the bony pelvis, preventing delivery of the body. Unless the condition is remedied within a few minutes, the fetus can suffer permanent brain damage because his chest cannot expand, and he cannot take his first breath. Although macrosomia (fetal weight greater than 4,000 grams) and

A PERSONAL GLIMPSE

My wife, Sally, had just delivered our daughter. We had waited to have a child until we were in our 30s, and then it had taken us 2 years to get pregnant. I was so awed by the whole birth experience. I was taking pictures of my daughter when I heard Sally say to the nurse, "I can't breathe!" I looked over and saw that she was very pale, almost gray. In the blink of an eye she stopped breathing and one of the nurses started helping her breathe. The other nurse took the baby and me to the nursery. The nursery nurse was very kind. She let me stay with the baby as long as I wanted; however, I couldn't concentrate on the baby because I was so worried about my wife. I went to the waiting room and I was pacing up and down. After what seemed like an eternity the doctor came to talk to me. He said that he thought Sally had an embolism. He told me that she had a breathing tube and was connected to a machine that was helping her breathe. The nurse came out and took me to the ICU. I felt so frightened by all the tubes and machines that were connected to my wife. I felt very helpless. I also felt guilty for putting my wife through this. I didn't know if I could forgive myself if she didn't make it. Slowly, over the next week Sally started to get better. I have never felt more thankful in my life than on the day I was able to take Sally home. She was very weak, but she was alive. It was such a joy to see her finally able to hold our little Jessica.

Bill

LEARNING OPPORTUNITY: What could the nurses in this situation have done to help the husband cope with his wife's severe illness? What interventions could the nurse use to help promote attachment between the newborn and the woman when the woman who has been critically ill begins to get better?

maternal diabetes are the two risk factors known to be associated with shoulder dystocia, many cases occur in fetuses of normal weight. Therefore, this complication should be anticipated at every delivery.

Shoulder dystocia puts the woman and the fetus at risk. Even if correct maneuvers are used, injury can still result. The woman is at increased risk for uterine rupture and/or bladder rupture. The fetus is at increased risk for brachial plexus injuries and fractures of the humerus and clavicle (Rose, 1998).

Clinical Manifestations and Diagnosis

The "turtle sign" is the classic sign that alerts the practitioner to the probability of shoulder dystocia. The fetal head delivers, but then retracts similar to a turtle. The practitioner tries gentle downward pressure on the fetal head in an attempt to deliver the anterior shoulder, but is unable to do so using normal maneuvers.

Treatment

There are several maneuvers the practitioner can attempt to relieve shoulder dystocia. Two of them require the direct assistance of the nurse (Fig. 18-1).

- McRoberts maneuver (see Fig. 18-1*A*) is often tried first and is frequently successful. Two nurses are needed to assist with this maneuver. With the woman in lithotomy position, each nurse holds one leg and sharply flexes the leg toward the woman's shoulders. This opens the pelvis to its widest diameters and allows the anterior shoulder to deliver in almost half of the cases.
- In addition to McRoberts maneuver, one nurse can use a fist to apply suprapubic pressure (see Fig. 18-1*B*). This will sometimes dislodge the impacted shoulder.

The birth attendant can try other maneuvers, such as placing a hand in the vagina and attempting to push one of the shoulders in a clockwise or counterclockwise motion. The birth attendant may intentionally fracture a clavicle in an attempt to dislodge the fetus. In some cases the birth attendant has placed the head back in the birth canal and done an emergency cesarean delivery. This maneuver, called Zavanelli maneuver, has been successful, but is associated with increased risk of trauma.

Nursing Care

Assist the birth attendant with maneuvers, as described above. Be prepared to go for a stat cesarean delivery if the body cannot be delivered. If maneuvers are successful and a vaginal delivery is accomplished, perform a careful assessment of the newborn. Check for crepitus in the area of the clavicle, which might indicate the bone is broken. Check for spontaneous movements of both arms. Sometimes the newborn will move only one arm, which may indicate Erb's palsy. This injury is characterized by (usually temporary) nerve damage and inability to move the arm. When edema subsides, full function normally returns, although injury can persist.

This is important! Don't EVER apply pressure to the fundus (fundal pressure). This action has been linked to increased incidence of birth trauma. The shoulder can actually become more impacted, and the woman has an increased chance of uterine or bladder rupture when this maneuver is used in instances of shoulder dystocia.

● *Figure 18.1* Techniques to relieve shoulder dystocia. (**A**) McRoberts maneuver. Two nurses (or the nurse and the woman's coach) each take one of the woman's legs and sharply flex them onto the woman's abdomen. This position maximally opens the pelvis, which sometimes dislodges the impacted shoulder. (**B**) Suprapubic pressure. The nurse puts pressure just above the pubic bone. Sometimes this maneuver in conjunction with McRoberts maneuver is successful in dislodging the impacted shoulder.

A   B

Umbilical Cord Prolapse

Umbilical cord prolapse occurs when the umbilical cord slips down in front of the presenting part. It occurs rarely in vertex presentations. Factors that increase the risk include fetal malpresentation, multiple gestation, intrauterine fetal growth restriction, prematurity, and rupture of the membranes with the fetus at a high station (Curran, 2003).

Clinical Manifestations and Diagnosis

Prolapse of the umbilical cord can occur at any time. Infrequently the condition may be detected before the membranes rupture. The woman may report feeling "something coming out" when the membranes rupture. Sometimes she presents with a cord prolapse. The cord may be visible at the introitus, or it may be palpable in the vaginal vault. An occult prolapse results in cord compression, but the cord is not easily palpable. Frequently a prolapse is detected immediately after spontaneous or artificial rupture of the membranes. The fetal heart rate usually drops precipitously. Vaginal examination typically confirms the diagnosis.

Treatment

When the cord is compressed against the bony pelvis, it can compromise fetal circulation and result in fetal death unless interventions are carried out quickly. The examiner who discovers the condition should push upward on the presenting part with the fingers to move the fetus away from the cord. Immediate cesarean delivery should be accomplished to save the fetus' life.

Nursing Care

Always check fetal heart tones after spontaneous or artificial rupture of the membranes. If the fetal heart rate drops, perform a vaginal examination (or call the RN to do one), and palpate for the umbilical cord. If the woman presents with a visible prolapse, quickly place her in bed and gently palpate the cord for pulsations to verify fetal viability. Then use your fingers to press upward on the presenting part. Continue to hold the presenting part off of the cord until the infant is delivered by cesarean delivery. (You will be transported with the woman to the operating room. The sterile drapes will be placed over you.) If you discover the condition and are unable to call for help, place the patient in knee–chest position, call for help, and then continue to intervene as previously described (Curran, 2003). If another nurse is holding the presenting part off of the cord, move quickly to prepare the woman for emergency cesarean delivery.

Uterine Rupture

Uterine rupture occurs when the uterus tears open, leaving the fetus and other uterine contents exposed to the peritoneal cavity. Rarely is this a spontaneous occurrence. It is usually associated with a uterine scar

TABLE 18.3	**Placental Abnormalities**		
Condition	Description	Risk Factors	Maternal and Fetal Implications
Placenta accreta	Abnormal adherence of the placenta to the uterine wall. Variations of penetration occur, including • Placenta increta—the placenta invades the uterine muscle. • Placenta percreta—the placenta penetrates through the uterine muscle, sometimes invading the bladder and other pelvic structures.	History of previous uterine surgery; such as • Cesarean delivery (risk increases with each subsequent C section) • Myomectomy • Dilation and curettage • Induced abortion Other risk factors include • Age older than 35 • Placenta previa	*Maternal implications*: Interferes with normal placental separation in the 3rd stage of labor, resulting in hemorrhage, which may require hysterectomy to control. May also cause uterine rupture during pregnancy or labor. *Fetal implications*: Fetal death may occur if the condition results in uterine rupture.
Velamentous insertion of the umbilical cord	The umbilical cord is attached to the side (versus the center) of the placenta, and the fetal vessels separate in the membranes before reaching the placenta. Vasa previa is a variation in which the fetal vessels are in the part of the membrane that is in front of the presenting part.	Low-lying placenta, antepartum hemorrhage, in vitro fertilization (IVF) pregnancy	*Fetal implications*: Exsanguination (the fetus may bleed out) resulting in fetal death may occur when the membranes rupture.
Succenturiate placenta	An "accessory" placenta that develops at a distance from the main placenta. Vasa previa can occur in this situation when the fetal vessels traverse the membranes between the two placentas.	Same as for velamentous placenta	*Maternal implications*: May result in hemorrhage when the accessory placenta is retained. Hemorrhage may require blood transfusions and/or hysterectomy to control. *Fetal implications*: The same as for vasa previa.
Nuchal cord	The umbilical cord is wrapped once (or more) around the fetus' neck.	This condition occurs frequently in normal pregnancies with no identifiable risk factors.	*Fetal implications*: Moderate-to-deep variable decelerations may occur during labor. Rarely, a tight nuchal cord can lead to fetal death.
True knot	A true knot occurs when the umbilical cord is tied in a knot.	This condition can occur in an active fetus with a long cord.	*Fetal implications*: A true knot sometimes results in fetal death.

from previous uterine surgery. Often the scar results from a prior cesarean delivery; however, any surgery that requires an incision into the uterus can place the woman at risk for uterine rupture. Traumatic rupture can occur in connection with blunt trauma, such as occurs in an automobile collision or intimate partner violence. Incidence of uterine rupture is 0.1% to 1.5% when the previous incision type was a low cervical transverse incision, and 4% to 9% when the incision type is classical or T-shaped (Curran, 2003).

Clinical Manifestations and Diagnosis

Abrupt change in the fetal heart rate pattern is often the most significant sign associated with uterine rupture (Dauphinee, 2004). Another sign is pain in the abdomen, shoulder, or back that is not masked by epidural anesthesia. Sometimes the woman will begin to report intense pain when the epidural has been giving relief until that point. Falling blood pressure and rising pulse may be associated with hypovolemia caused by occult bleeding. A vaginal examination may demonstrate a higher fetal station than was present previously. There may or may not be changes in the contraction pattern.

Treatment

As soon as uterine rupture is recognized, the treatment is immediate cesarean delivery. This action is necessary to save the woman's life and, it is hoped, that of the fetus, as well, although uterine rupture is associated with a high incidence of fetal death. This is true because the fetus can withstand only approximately 20 minutes in utero after uterine rupture. This time period can be even shorter if the cord prolapses through the tear in the uterine wall and becomes compressed.

Nursing Care

Recognizing the signs of uterine rupture is critical for the obstetric nurse because the complication requires quick recognition and action to avoid fetal and maternal death. In cases of trial-of-labor-after-cesarean (TOLAC), the RN should monitor the woman during labor, particularly if oxytocin is used to induce or augment the labor. If signs of rupture occur, the woman is immediately prepared for cesarean delivery, and other interventions are instituted to treat hypovolemic shock.

Placental and Umbilical Cord Abnormalities

Although technically abnormalities of the placenta and umbilical cord are not obstetric emergencies, they can lead to emergency situations and can have dire outcomes for the woman and her fetus. Selected conditions that can result in maternal and fetal complications are listed in Table 18-3.

Test Yourself

- Describe three clinical manifestations of amniotic fluid embolism.
- Describe two maneuvers for which the nurse can assist when shoulder dystocia complicates delivery.
- Define vasa previa.

KEY POINTS

- Nursing interventions for labor dystocia include carefully assessing the fetal lie, presentation, and position and the woman's labor pattern throughout labor. Compare the woman's progress with expected norms and notify the practitioner when progress deviates from the expected. Assist the woman to keep her bladder empty, frequently assess adequacy of the contraction pattern, and administer pain relief interventions.

- PROM is spontaneous rupture of the amniotic sac before the onset of labor in a full-term fetus; preterm PROM is PROM in a pregnancy that is less than 37 weeks' gestation. In both cases, the woman presents to the delivery suite with uncontrollable leaking of fluid from the vagina. The woman's temperature must be monitored frequently to detect early signs of infection.

- Clinical manifestations of preterm labor include uterine contractions, with or without pain; pelvic pressure; cramping; backache; and vaginal discharge and bleeding.

- Bed rest and hydration with oral or IV fluids often is the first way the practitioner attempts to stop symptoms of preterm labor. Urinalysis and other lab work are also done to detect infection. If the membranes are not ruptured, the practitioner may prescribe tocolytics and injectable steroids to stop the labor long enough to allow the fetal lungs to mature.

- Nursing interventions for the woman in preterm labor include maintaining a balanced fluid volume, preventing injury, managing the woman's pain, and reducing anxiety.

- Patient teaching for the woman carrying a post-term pregnancy includes discussing the plan of care, whether it be expectant management or labor induction. Expectant management involves frequent fetal kick counts and NSTs to monitor fetal well-being. Instruct the woman to report decreased fetal movement immediately.

- During labor induction of a woman with fetal demise, monitor the contraction pattern to avoid uterine rupture. Monitor the woman for signs of DIC. Provide emotional care for the woman and her family.

- Amniotic fluid embolism occurs suddenly during labor or in the immediate postpartum period. The woman becomes acutely dyspneic, apprehensive, hypotensive, and cyanotic. Treatment is supportive, and the woman requires care in the ICU.

- Shoulder dystocia occurs when the fetal head is born but the shoulders fail to deliver. McRoberts maneuver and suprapubic pressure are two interventions that require the active involvement of the nurse. Carefully observe the newborn for signs of birth injury.

♦ Umbilical cord prolapse occurs when the umbilical cord slips down in front of the presenting part. Unless pressure is immediately relieved, the fetus will die or will experience permanent brain damage from lack of oxygen. An immediate cesarean delivery is required.

♦ History of a previous uterine scar increases the risk of uterine rupture during labor. Ominous fetal heart rate patterns on the fetal monitor are usually the most significant sign of rupture. Prompt cesarean delivery is necessary to save the fetus and the woman.

REFERENCES AND SELECTED READINGS

Books and Journals

Bernhardt, J., & Dorman, K. (2004). Pre-term birth risk assessment tools: Exploring fetal fibronectin and cervical length for validating risk. *AWHONN Lifelines, 8*(1), 38–44.

Church-Balin, C., & Damus, K. (2003). Commentary: Preventing prematurity. *AWHONN Lifelines, 7*(2), 97–101.

Crowley, P. (2003). Antenatal corticosteroids—current thinking. *BJOG: An International Journal of Obstetrics and Gynaecology, 110*(Suppl 20), 77–78. Retrieved December 2, 2003, from http://www.womenshealth-elsevier.com/doc/journals/pdf/bjog%20sup%2015.pdf

Cunningham, F. G., Gant, N. F., Leveno, K. J., Gilstrap L. C. III, Hauth, J. C., & Wenstrom, K. D. (2001a). Postterm pregnancy. In *Williams obstetrics* (21st ed., pp. 729–742). New York: McGraw-Hill Medical Publishing Division.

Cunningham, F. G., Gant, N. F., Leveno, K. J., Gilstrap, L. C. III, Hauth, J. C., & Wenstrom, K. D. (2001b). Preterm birth. In *Williams obstetrics* (21st ed., pp. 689–727). New York: McGraw-Hill Medical Publishing Division.

Cunningham, F. G., Gant, N. F., Leveno, K. J., Gilstrap, L. C. III, Hauth, J. C., & Wenstrom, K. D. (2001c). Section V: Abnormal labor. In *Williams obstetrics* (21st ed., pp. 423–482). New York: McGraw-Hill Medical Publishing Division.

Curran, C. A. (2003). Intrapartum emergencies. *JOGNN, 32*(6), 802–813.

Dauphinee, J. D. (2004). VBAC: Safety for the patient and the nurse. *JOGNN, 33*(1), 105–115.

Davis, D. (2003). Amniotic fluid embolism: Exploring this rare but typically fatal condition. *AWHONN Lifelines, 7*(2), 126–131.

De Jong, M. J., & Fausett, M. B. (2003). Anaphylactoid syndrome of pregnancy: A devastating complication requiring intensive care. *Critical Care Nurse, 23*(6), 42–48.

Divon, M. Y., Haglund, B., Nisell, H., Otterblad, P. O., & Westgren, M. (1998). Fetal and neonatal mortality in the postterm pregnancy: The impact of gestational age and fetal growth restriction. *American Journal of Obstetrics and Gynecology, 178*(4), 726–731.

Fisk, N. M., & Chan, J. (2003). The case for tocolysis in threatened preterm labour. *BJOG: An International Journal of Obstetrics and Gynaecology, 110*(Suppl 20), 98–102. Retrieved December 2, 2003, from http://www.womenshealth elsevier.com/doc/journals/pdf/bjog%20sup%2020.pdf

Freda, M. C. (2003). Nursing's contribution to the literature on preterm labor and birth. *JOGNN, 32*(5), 659–667.

Glimore, D. A., Wakim, J., Secrest, J., & Rawson, R. (2003). Anaphylactoid syndrome of pregnancy: A review of the literature with latest management and outcome data. *AANA Journal, 71*(2), 120–126.

Lindsey, J. L. (2002). Evaluation of fetal death. *eMedicine.* Witlin, A., Talavera, F., Smith, C. V., Gaupp, F. B., & Shulman, L. P. (Eds.). Retrieved January 11, 2004, from http://www.emedicine.com/med/topic3235.htm

Moore, L. E., & Ware, D. (2002). Amniotic fluid embolism. *eMedicine.* Kavanagh, J. J., Talavera, F., Barnes, A. D., Gaupp, F. B., & Shulman, L. P. (Eds.). Retrieved April 30, 2004, from http://www.emedicine.com/med/topic122.htm

Moore, M. L. (2003). Preterm labor and birth: What have we learned in the past two decades? *JOGNN, 32*(5), 638–649.

Moos, M. (2004). Understanding prematurity. *AWHONN Lifelines, 8*(1), 32–37.

Newton, E. R. (2002). Preterm labor. *eMedicine.* Trupin, S. R., Talavera, F., Legro, R. S., Gaupp, F. B., & Shulman, L. P. (Eds.). Retrieved November 30, 2003, from http://www.emedicine.com/med/topic3245.htm

Oyelese, K. O., Schwarzler, P., Coates, S., Sanusi, F. A., Hamid, R., & Campbell, S. (1998). A strategy for reducing the mortality rate from vasa previa using transvaginal sonography with color doppler. *Ultrasound Obstetrics and Gynecology, 12*(6), 434–438.

Rose, V. L. (1998). ACOG releases practice pattern on shoulder dystocia. *American Family Physician, 57*(10), 2546–2547.

Saju, J., & Lyon, D. (2003). Diagnosis of abnormal labor. *eMedicine.* Zurawin, R. K., Talavera, F., Legro, R. S., Gaupp, F. B., & Shulman, L. P. (Eds.). Retrieved November 3, 2003, from http://www.emedicine.com/med/topic3488.htm

Searing, K. A. (2001). Induction versus post-date pregnancies: Exploring the controversy and who's really at risk. *AWHONN Lifelines, 5*(2), 44–48.

Walling, A. D. (1999). Risk of hemorrhage and scarring in placenta accreta. *American Family Physician, 60*(2), 636.

Weismiller, D. G. (1999). Preterm labor. *American Family Physician, 59*, 593–604. Retrieved December 2, 2003, from http://www.aafp.org/afp/990201ap/593.html

Wilkes, P. T., & Galan, H. (2002a). Postdate pregnancy. *eMedicine.* Cowan, B. D., Talavera, F., Legro, R. S., Gaupp, F. B., & Shulman, L. P. (Eds.). Retrieved January 11, 2004, from http://www.emedicine.com/med/topic3248.htm

Wilkes, P. T., & Galan, H. (2002b). Premature rupture of membranes. *eMedicine.* Trupin, S. R., Talavera, F., Whitman-Elia, G. F., Gaupp, F. B., & Shulman, L. P. (Eds.). Retrieved November 23, 2003, from http://www.emedicine.com/med/topic3246.htm

Websites.

http://www.moonlily.com/obc/complications.html

Post-term Pregnancy

http://www.aafp.org/afp/080196/960801c.html

Shoulder Dystocia

http://pregnancy.about.com/cs/laborbirth/a/aa081801a.htm
http://www.obgyn.net/pb/pb.asp?page=/pb/articles/dystocia-casereport

WORKBOOK

NCLEX-STYLE REVIEW QUESTIONS

1. A 35-year-old Gravida 1 delivered after 24 hours of labor. Her membranes ruptured 4 hours after she started labor. Two hours before she delivered, she spiked a temperature of 101°F. For which of the following complications is her newborn most at risk?

   a. ABO incompatibility

   b. Fistula formation

   c. Pelvic floor injury

   d. Pneumonia

2. A 26-year-old primigravida is attempting natural childbirth. Her doula has been supporting her through the past 16 hours of labor. The laboring woman is now 6 centimeters dilated. She continues to report severe pain in her back with each contraction. She finds it comforting when her doula uses the ball of her hand to put counterpressure on her lower back. What do you think is the likely cause of the woman's back pain?

   a. Breech presentation

   b. Fetal macrosomia

   c. Occiput posterior position

   d. Nongynecoid pelvis

3. A 31-year-old Gravida 3 Para 1 calls the clinic. She is at 29 weeks' gestation. She says that she has been having uterine contractions every 10 minutes for the past 2 hours. She also feels "heaviness" in her vaginal area. Her first baby was born prematurely at 28 weeks' gestation. What advice by the nurse is best for this woman?

   a. "Come into the hospital immediately. These signs strongly indicate that you may be in premature labor."

   b. "Drink two large glasses of water. Lie down on your left side. If the contractions don't stop in an hour, come in to the hospital."

   c. "Monitor your contractions for 1 more hour. If they increase in frequency, or get stronger, come in right away."

   d. "It is not likely that you will deliver a second baby prematurely. Don't panic. If you continue to have contractions, come in to be checked."

4. You are assisting in a delivery that is complicated by shoulder dystocia. Which nursing action is indicated?

   a. Give fundal pressure.

   b. Start rescue breathing.

   c. Assist the RN to flex the woman's thighs.

   d. Watch the fetal monitor for signs of fetal distress.

STUDY ACTIVITIES

1. Use the table provided to compare fetal and maternal causes of labor arrest.

Fetal Causes of Labor Arrest	Maternal Causes of Labor Arrest

2. Interview your local March of Dimes representative to see what is being done in your community to learn more about and prevent preterm labor. Share your findings with your clinical group.

3. Develop a teaching plan for a woman with a post-term pregnancy that is being managed expectantly.

CRITICAL THINKING: What Would You Do?

Apply your knowledge of labor at risk to the following situations.

1. Julia, a Gravida 2 Para 0, just found out that her fetus is in a breech position at 36 weeks' gestation. Julia is afraid that she will have to have a cesarean delivery. What options does Julia have in this situation?

2. Julia's pregnancy proceeds to 39 weeks' gestation. She presents to labor and delivery because her "water bag broke." After the midwife confirms that the membranes have ruptured, she explains to Julia that the plan is for Julia and her husband to wait in the hospital until labor begins. Julia wants to know why she and her husband can't just go home to wait for contractions to begin.

a. How do you reply to Julia?

b. What nursing interventions will you plan for Julia during the wait before labor begins?

c. How would your care be different if Julia were at 30 weeks' gestation with ruptured membranes versus 39 weeks?

3. Kimberly has been receiving the tocolytic terbutaline for the past 12 hours. You are taking Kimberly's vital signs at the beginning of your shift. You notice that Kimberly's pulse is 130 and her blood pressure is 88/50 mm Hg. When you ask her how she is feeling, she replies, "I feel out of breath, and I have a feeling of pressure in my chest." What should you do?

Postpartum Woman at Risk

19

STUDENT OBJECTIVES

On completion of this chapter, the student should be able to

1. Identify major conditions that place a woman at risk during the postpartal period.
2. Differentiate between early and late postpartum hemorrhage
3. Describe appropriate nursing interventions for the woman with postpartum hemorrhage, regardless of the cause.
4. Compare and contrast four types of infection that may occur in the postpartum period.
5. Identify factors that place a postpartum woman at risk for a thromboembolic disorder.
6. Describe three different psychiatric problems that can complicate the postpartum period.
7. Discuss the nurse's role when caring for a postpartal woman who is grieving.
8. Identify behaviors that would suggest malattachment.

KEY TERMS

cystitis
endometritis
exudate
hematoma
hypovolemic shock
malattachment
mastitis
pyelonephritis
uterine atony
uterine subinvolution

Often considered the "fourth trimester of pregnancy," the postpartum period encompasses the first 6 weeks after childbirth. After delivery, the woman begins to experience physiologic and psychological changes that return her body to the prepregnancy state. These changes usually occur without difficulty. However, factors such as blood loss, trauma during delivery, infection, or fatigue can place the postpartum woman at risk. The nurse plays a key role in identifying the woman at risk for complications to ensure early detection and prompt intervention. Most often, the nurse is the person who identifies the problem and alerts the primary medical provider of the pressing need for intervention. Nursing interventions for the postpartum woman at risk focus on treating the complication, thereby minimizing the effects on the woman's return to her prepregnant state; promoting adaptation to her role as mother of a new infant; and supporting and enhancing maternal–infant bonding.

This chapter addresses major complications associated with the postpartum period, including hemorrhage, infection, thromboembolic disorders, and psychiatric disorders. The priority aspects of nursing care are emphasized for each complication. In addition, the chapter describes special postpartum situations, such as postpartal grieving and malattachment. The nurse's role in each situation is presented.

POSTPARTUM HEMORRHAGE

Postpartum hemorrhage is one of the leading causes of maternal deaths, accounting for approximately 30% of all pregnancy-related deaths (Roman & Rebarber, 2003). It can occur early, within the first 24 hours after delivery, or late, anytime after the first 24 hours through the 6-week postpartum period. The woman is most vulnerable to hemorrhage during the first 24 hours after delivery, with the greatest risk occurring in the first hour after delivery.

Traditionally, postpartum hemorrhage has been defined as any blood loss in an amount greater than 500 mL after a vaginal delivery or greater than 1,000 mL after a cesarean birth. However, because blood loss estimates during delivery are often inaccurate, the American College of Obstetricians and Gynecologists (ACOG) has defined postpartum hemorrhage as a decrease in the hematocrit of 10% or greater after delivery when compared with that before delivery (AGOG, 1998; Roman & Rebarber, 2003).

The causes of postpartum hemorrhage can be grouped into four major categories: **uterine atony**, inability of the uterus to contract effectively; lacerations to the uterus, cervix, vagina, or perineum; retained placenta; and disruption in maternal clotting

abilities. It is important to monitor all postpartum women for excessive bleeding because two-thirds of the women who experience postpartum hemorrhage have no risk factors. However, certain factors are known to increase the risk for postpartum hemorrhage (Box 19-1). Early detection and prompt intervention are necessary to control the hemorrhage. Otherwise the woman can progress to shock, renal failure, and ultimately death from the loss of blood.

Early Postpartum Hemorrhage

Early postpartum hemorrhage refers to blood loss (greater than 500 mL) within the first 24 hours after delivery. Early postpartum hemorrhage results from one of the three following conditions:

- Uterine atony
- Lacerations
- Hematoma

BOX 19.1 | **Risk Factors for Postpartum Hemorrhage**

Each risk factor is listed by cause.

Uterine Atony
- Multiparity
- Intrauterine infection
- Previous uterine surgery
- Prolonged or difficult labor
- History of postpartum hemorrhage
- Placenta previa or abruptio placentae
- Use of oxytocin for labor stimulation or augmentation
- Use of agents during labor that relax the uterus (tocolytics), such as
  - magnesium sulfate
  - terbutaline
  - certain anesthetics
  - nitroglycerin
- Overdistention of the uterus, such as occurs with
  - multiple gestation
  - polyhydramnios
  - fetal macrosomia

Lacerations and Hematomas
- Episiotomy
- Macrosomia
- Precipitous labor
- Traumatic delivery
- Use of forceps or vacuum extraction for delivery

Retained Placenta
- Abruptio placentae
- Placenta accreta
- Prolonged third stage of labor

Disruption in Maternal Clotting Abilities
- Fetal demise
- Thrombocytopenia
- Pregnancy-induced hypertension

Most cases of early postpartum hemorrhage result from uterine atony. With this condition, the uterus does not contract as it should. Thus, the muscles of the uterus remain relaxed and exert no compression on the open uterine blood vessels. As a result, the vessels continue to bleed. This blood loss can be extensive and rapid. Lacerations can occur as small tears or cuts in the perineal tissue, vaginal sidewall or cervix. A **hematoma** is a clot of blood that collects within tissues and leads to concealed blood loss.

Regardless of the cause, the woman is at risk for developing hypovolemia, a system-wide decrease in blood volume from too much blood loss. If the blood loss continues, the woman may develop **hypovolemic shock,** which is characterized by a weak, thready, rapid pulse; drop in blood pressure; cool, clammy skin; and changes in level of consciousness. These findings may occur abruptly and be dramatic if the blood loss is large and occurs quickly. However, with bleeding of a more gradual onset, these signs and symptoms may be extremely subtle because of the woman's ability to compensate for the blood loss over time. With continued bleeding, the woman's body eventually is overwhelmed and no longer able to compensate for the loss. At that point she exhibits the typical signs and symptoms of shock.

The woman who experiences postpartum hemorrhage is also at risk for developing anemia from the blood loss. Other complications connected with postpartum hemorrhage include complications associated with blood transfusions, further bleeding that may occur if clotting factors are used up or if disseminated intravascular coagulation (DIC) develops, need for emergency surgical intervention to include hysterectomy with loss of childbearing capability, and multiple organ failure.

Clinical Manifestations

Clinical manifestations of early postpartum hemorrhage differ according the cause of the hemorrhage.

Hemorrhage Caused by Uterine Atony. If the underlying cause of hemorrhage is uterine atony, the woman's fundus usually will be difficult to palpate. When the fundus is identified on palpation, it is soft (boggy), relaxed, and located above the level of the umbilicus. The woman's bladder may be distended, further interfering with uterine contraction. A full bladder may cause the uterus to be pushed to one side, rather than being at the midline. Vaginal bleeding (lochia) typically is moderate to heavy, possibly with numerous large clots.

Hemorrhage Caused by Lacerations. When lacerations are the cause of bleeding, the fundus is firm on palpation. However, the bleeding continues in a steady trickle. Characteristically, the bleeding is bright red in color, in contrast to the dark red color of lochia.

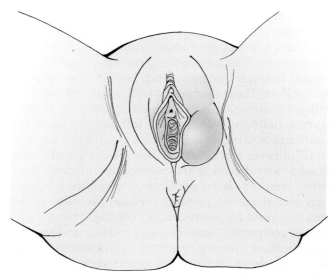

● **Figure 19.1** Perineal hematoma. Notice the localized area of swelling. A perineal hematoma usually results from trauma to the area that breaks a blood vessel, causing bleeding into the tissue. The main symptom is severe perineal pain unrelieved by normal measures, and a soft, palpable mass.

Hemorrhage Caused by Hematoma. Unlike uterine atony and lacerations, the bleeding associated with hematoma formation may not be apparent (Fig. 19-1). A blood vessel ruptures and leaks into the surrounding tissue. This causes pressure, pain, swelling (edema), and dark red or purple discoloration, most commonly on one side of the perineum. Initially, the area may feel soft. However, as leakage into the tissues continues, the area becomes firm to the touch. In addition, the area is tender on palpation.

A hematoma also can form deep in the pelvis. This is a much more difficult problem to identify. The primary symptom is deep pain unrelieved by comfort measures or medication and accompanied by vital sign instability. Regardless of where the hematoma occurs, the woman's lochia usually is within expected parameters. However, if the hematoma is large, she may experience a significant loss of blood into the tissues, leading to signs and symptoms of hypovolemic shock.

Diagnosis

Diagnosis is made on clinical signs and changes in laboratory values. Because of blood loss, the woman's hemoglobin and hematocrit levels will be decreased from her prelabor (baseline) levels, approximately 1 to 1.5 g/dL and 2% to 4%, respectively. In addition, if the woman has an underlying coagulation defect, clotting times will be increased and platelet and prothrombin levels will be decreased.

Treatment

The goal of treatment for postpartal hemorrhage is to correct the underlying cause while attempting to control the hemorrhage and reduce its effects on the woman. If the woman is exhibiting signs and symptoms of hypovolemic shock, emergency measures are instituted to support vital functions. These include rapid IV fluid replacement, blood transfusions, oxygen administration, and frequent close monitoring of all vital functions. Insertion of an indwelling urinary catheter may be necessary to monitor the woman's urine output hourly.

Treatment for Uterine Atony. If uterine atony is present, fundal massage (refer to Nursing Procedure 12-1 in Chapter 12) is initiated first. Massage attempts to help the uterus to contract, thereby compressing the blood vessels and ultimately decreasing the bleeding. Once the uterus is contracted, firm gentle pressure is applied to the uterus to help express any clots that may have collected in the uterus. The woman's bladder must be empty when fundal massage is initiated. Otherwise the uterus will not remain contracted once the massage stops.

Don't do it! Never, never, never, attempt uterine massage without first placing one hand over the symphysis pubis. Doing so could cause the uterus to turn inside out (inversion). Once this occurs, massive hemorrhage ensues and can quickly lead to death.

Drug therapy may be necessary if fundal massage fails to maintain the uterus in a contracted state. Oxytocic agents, such as oxytocin (Pitocin), ergonovine (Ergotrate), methylergonovine (Methergine), carboprost (Hemabate), and misoprostol (Cytotec) may be administered parenterally. If drug therapy is ineffective, the primary care provider may need to intervene. Bimanual compression of the uterus is frequently the first method attempted. Exploration of the uterine cavity may be the next option when other treatment measures fail. Uterine packing may be done to control hemorrhage. Another option is uterine artery embolization or ligation to control bleeding. When postpartum hemorrhage due to uterine atony continues despite all efforts to control it, a hysterectomy may be done, usually only as a last resort.

Treatment for Lacerations and Hematomas. Postpartal hemorrhage caused by lacerations is treated by surgical repair of the lacerations. Small hematomas usually require no additional treatment other than application of ice and analgesics to control pain. In most instances, small hematomas absorb spontaneously, usually during a period of 4 to 6 weeks. Surgical incision, with drainage and evacuation of clots and ligation of the bleeding vessel may be required if the hematoma is large.

● Nursing Process for the Woman With Early Postpartum Hemorrhage

The nurse plays an important role in monitoring the woman's status, assisting with measures to control bleeding, providing support to the woman and her family, and educating the woman about her condition. Maintaining the woman's safety is paramount.

ASSESSMENT

As with any patient, thorough, frequent assessment is necessary to allow for early detection and prompt intervention should hemorrhage occur. Be aware of the woman's history, labor progress, and risk factors for postpartum hemorrhage. Note the use of any analgesia or anesthesia during labor and delivery or the use of oxytocin for labor induction or augmentation. This information helps to identify potential factors that would place the woman at risk for hemorrhage.

Ask the woman about the onset of the bleeding, if appropriate. For example, "Did the bleeding seem to increase suddenly or have you noticed a constant trickling?" Ask about any associated symptoms, such as "Do you have any pain or pressure?" These types of questions help to provide information about the possible cause of the hemorrhage. Ask the woman how frequently she is changing her perineal pads, how saturated they appear, and when she changed the pad last. The bleeding of a woman who has changed her perineal pads twice in the last hour with each pad containing approximately a half-dollar sized amount of lochia is far different from that of a woman who has changed her perineal pads twice in the last hour because they were saturated. Additional evaluation of the second woman is necessary. In this case, the primary health care provider also needs to be notified.

Assess the fundus for consistency, shape, and location. Remember that the uterus should be firm, in the midline, and decrease 1 centimeter each postpartum day. Inability to locate the fundus suggests that it is not firm and contracting. Displacement to one side suggests that the woman has a distended bladder.

Observe lochia for color, amount, odor, and character, including evidence of any clots. When evaluating the lochia, turn the woman to her side and look under the buttocks for any pooling of blood that may occur while she is in bed. Note amount and characteristics of the bleeding. Dark red is the normal color of lochia in the first few postpartum days. A bright red color is associated with fresh bleeding, such as that from a laceration.

Here's an objective way to determine the quantity of blood loss!

Remember that 1 gram of weight is approximately equal to 1 milliliter (mL) of fluid. First weigh a dry, clean perineal pad. Next, weigh the used pad and then subtract the dry pad weight from this amount. The result will be the amount of blood lost. For example, a dry perineal pad weighs 5 grams. A used perineal pad weighs 34 grams. 34 − 5 = 29 grams, which is equivalent to 29 mL of blood loss.

Note whether or not bleeding decreases with fundal massage.

Determine when the woman last urinated. Remember that a full bladder can impede uterine contraction, predisposing her to hemorrhage. Inspect the woman's perineal area closely for evidence of lacerations or hematomas. Do not mistake an episiotomy for a laceration. Typically an episiotomy is approximately 1 to 2 inches in length and has clean, regular sutured edges, whereas a laceration varies in length, and its edges appear irregular and somewhat jagged. Evaluate pain and other associated symptoms. Severe pain and pressure that are unrelieved by ordinary pain control measures may indicate the presence of a hematoma.

Assess the woman's vital signs to obtain a baseline and then monitor vital signs as ordered, noting any changes suggesting hypovolemic shock. Also note the color and temperature of the woman's skin and her level of consciousness. Recall that cool, clammy skin and decreasing level of consciousness may indicate hypovolemic shock. Table 19-1 highlights assessment findings for the major causes of postpartum hemorrhage.

CULTURAL SNAPSHOT

For people of color (e.g., African American, Hispanic, and Asian), assess skin "color" (pale, red, cyanotic, jaundiced) by looking at the mucous membranes of the mouth, tongue, and gums. The unpainted nail bed also gives a clear, nonpigmented view of color.

SELECTED NURSING DIAGNOSES

- Deficient Fluid Volume related to excessive blood loss
- Risk for Injury related to hemorrhage and possible development of hypovolemic shock
- Ineffective Tissue Perfusion related to decreased circulating blood volume subsequent to postpartum hemorrhage and development of hypovolemic shock

OUTCOME IDENTIFICATION AND PLANNING

Appropriate goals for the woman experiencing postpartum hemorrhage include the following: the woman will demonstrate signs and symptoms of restored fluid balance; she will remain free of any injury; and she will exhibit signs of adequate tissue perfusion.

IMPLEMENTATION

Nursing care for the woman experiencing postpartum hemorrhage focuses on stopping the bleeding, restoring fluid balance, preventing injury, and promoting adequate tissue perfusion. As with any postpartal complication, be sure to provide emotional support to the woman and her family, explaining all events and procedures to minimize anxiety and fear. Keep the family informed of the situation, explaining laboratory tests, procedures, and signs of improvement. Allow the partner and family to discuss feelings, which may be very intense. Frustration, anger, blame, disbelief, and sorrow often are expressed. Listen, be patient, be present, and acknowledge that this is a difficult time.

Controlling and Restoring Fluid Balance

Key to restoring fluid balance is stopping the bleeding. First, try fundal massage to stop the bleeding (see Nursing Procedure 12-1 in Chapter 12). Administer oxytocics, as ordered. If an IV line with oxytocin is present, increase the rate of flow to a fast drip. Prepare the woman for surgical intervention if less drastic measures do not control bleeding. If the woman is scheduled for surgery, withhold all food and fluids, unless allowed by the physician. Be sure to explain all treatments and procedures to the woman and her family to help reduce anxiety. If the woman continues to hemorrhage, expect her to be transferred to the intensive care unit for closer, more frequent monitoring.

When a woman experiences postpartum hemorrhage, fluid is lost. If she is allowed oral intake, encourage her to increase her oral fluid intake. If

TABLE 19.1	Assessing the Source of Postpartum Hemorrhage

	Uterine Atony	Subinvolution of the Uterus	Lacerations	Retained Placental Fragments	Hematoma
Occurrence	Early	Late	Early	Early or late	Early
Condition/ placement of uterus	Fundus will be boggy and high. If the bladder is full, the fundus will also be displaced to one side.	Fundus may be firm when palpated but boggy a short time later.	Normal	Fundus will be slightly boggy when assessed but often becomes firm when massaged.	Normal
Characteristics of lochia	Moderate to heavy lochia (i.e., when a perineal pad fills up with blood in less than 1 hour)	Initially, lochia flow is normal. Then the lochia will increase over what is expected and/or will revert to an earlier type of flow (e.g., the lochia will become rubra after it has changed to serosa, etc.).	Bleeding is heavy, bright red, and continues in a steady trickle or flow.	Intermittent clots will characterize bleeding.	Normal
Characteristics of pain	May be absent.	May be absent or there may be constant cramping. Backache may be present.	May be constant.	May be characterized by intermittent or heavier than normal cramping.	Pressure and severe pain at the site (perineal hematoma). Deep pain unrelieved by comfort measures or medication (deep pelvic hematoma)
Other signs and symptoms	Tachycardia, hypotension, and other signs of hypovolemic shock if blood loss is severe.	Dizziness, light-headedness, and fatigue when changing positions or doing simple self-care tasks. Fever and other signs of infection may be present.	Bruising may be apparent.	Portions of maternal surface of placenta are missing.	Swelling (edema) and dark red or purple discoloration (perineal hematoma). Accompanied by instability of blood pressure, pulse, and hemoglobin and hematocrit (deep pelvic hematoma).

the woman is not able to drink oral fluids, or if fluid loss is significant, expect to administer fluids intravenously. Typically, isotonic IV solutions, such as normal saline or lactated Ringer's solution, are ordered for replacement. Assist with IV catheter insertion if the woman does not have one already inserted, and administer fluids as ordered. Use care in administering fluids to avoid circulatory overload from too rapid or too great an infusion.

Continue to monitor the woman's fundus and lochia frequently for changes indicating continuation or resolution of the hemorrhage. If uterine atony is causing the bleeding and the woman received IV oxytocin, fundal assessment is crucial. Although oxytocin helps to contract the uterus, and this effect is immediate, the drug has a short duration of action, placing the woman at risk for hemorrhage secondary to a recurrence of atony once the IV rate of administration is slowed or stopped.

Inspect the perineum closely for evidence and amount of bleeding. Monitor pad count and weigh pads to determine the amount of blood lost. Be sure to turn the woman on her side and inspect the area under the buttocks because blood can pool, presenting a misleading picture. Assist as necessary with fundal massage to keep the uterus in a contracted state. Be aware that the uterus may relax quickly when massage stops, placing the woman at risk for continued hemorrhage.

Monitor the woman's intake and output closely, possibly every hour if necessary, to determine the effectiveness of therapy and progression or resolution of the fluid imbalance. Urine output should be at least 30 mL/hour, indicating adequate renal function. Encourage the woman to void frequently to prevent bladder distention from interfering with uterine contraction, increasing the risk for continued hemorrhage. If the woman has difficulty voiding, try measures such as running warm water over the perineum, placing the woman's hand in a basin or sink of warm water, or having the woman hear running water at the sink. If all else fails and the woman is unable to void, anticipate the need for insertion of an indwelling urinary catheter.

Expect to assist with obtaining blood specimens for laboratory testing, such as complete blood count, electrolyte levels, coagulation studies, and type and cross-matching for blood. If ordered, administer blood component therapy to aid in replacing fluid and blood loss.

Continue to monitor the woman's vital signs frequently for changes. Be alert for a rising pulse rate, changing pulse characteristics to rapid and thready, or decreasing blood pressure, which may indicate hypovolemic shock.

Preventing Injury

A postpartum woman who is hemorrhaging is at risk for injury. Reduction in blood supply to the brain can lead to changes in the woman's level of consciousness, placing her at risk for injury from confusion, disorientation, and falls. Therefore, safety measures are necessary to ensure that the woman remains free from injury.

Keep the call light close by and urge the woman to remain in bed. Check on her frequently, and encourage a family member to stay with her, if necessary. If the woman is allowed to ambulate to the bathroom, have her sit at the side of the bed for a short time before arising to prevent orthostatic hypotension. Then assist her to ambulate and stay nearby in the event that she complains of lightheadedness or dizziness.

Continue to monitor the woman's vital signs for changes. If she reports dizziness or lightheadedness when getting up, obtain her blood pressure while lying, sitting, and standing, noting any change of 10 mm Hg or more. Should the woman's blood pressure drop with position changes, notify the primary care provider.

Promoting Adequate Tissue Perfusion

A decrease in circulating blood volume secondary to hemorrhage affects tissue perfusion because oxygen, carried by the blood, is not transported to the required areas in adequate amounts. Therefore, oxygen must be provided. Expect to administer oxygen therapy via nasal cannula as ordered. Depending on the woman's need, oxygen may be administered via mask. Institute continuous pulse oximetry to evaluate oxygen saturation levels. Notify the physician if the oxygen saturation falls below 95%.

Arterial blood gas (ABG) studies may be performed to evaluate the woman's acid-base balance and provide a more definitive evaluation of the woman's current status. Be prepared to adjust the oxygen flow rate based on the ABG findings.

Continue to assess the woman's skin color and temperature for changes. Cold, clammy skin may indicate that constriction of the peripheral vessels is occurring, suggesting that the woman is developing hypovolemic shock or that the woman's condition is worsening. Also check nail beds for color and capillary refill. Keep in mind that a capillary refill greater than 3 seconds suggests impaired blood flow.

Monitor the woman's level of consciousness for changes. A woman who is alert and oriented is exhibiting adequate cerebral perfusion. However, confusion, disorientation, or deteriorating levels of consciousness suggest diminished blood flow and inadequate cerebral perfusion.

When adequately perfused, the kidneys function to produce urine. Adequate renal function is evidenced by a urine output of at least 30 mL/hour. Therefore, monitor the woman's urine output for changes. Report any urine output less than this amount immediately.

EVALUATION: GOALS AND EXPECTED OUTCOMES

- **Goal:** The woman will demonstrate evidence of fluid balance.
- **Expected Outcomes:**
  - Intake and output are within acceptable parameters.
  - Output is at least 30 mL/hour.
  - Vital signs are within normal limits.
  - Lochia is moderate in amount, without clots.
  - Laboratory test results, including hemoglobin and hematocrit levels, have returned to acceptable levels.
- **Goal:** The woman will remain free of injury.
- **Expected Outcomes:**
  - Vital signs are maintained within acceptable parameters.
  - The woman demonstrates no signs and symptoms of hypovolemic shock.
  - The uterus remains in a contracted state.
  - The woman is alert and oriented.
  - The woman remains free of falls.
- **Goal:** The woman will exhibit signs of adequate tissue perfusion.
- **Expected Outcomes:**
  - The woman is alert and oriented to person, place, and time.
  - The woman's skin is pink, warm, and dry with quick capillary refill.
  - Vital signs are within acceptable parameters.
  - Oxygen saturation remains above 95%.
  - Urine output is at least 30 mL/hour.

Late Postpartum Hemorrhage

Late postpartum hemorrhage refers to blood loss (more than 500 mL) occurring after the first 24 hours after delivery, and at any time throughout the 6-week postpartum period. Most cases of late postpartum hemorrhage result from retained placental fragments or **uterine subinvolution**, a condition in which the uterus returns to its prepregnancy shape and size at a

rate that is slower than expected (usually the result of retained placental fragments or an infection). The woman who has had uterine surgery, including a previous cesarean birth or an abortion, is at high risk for retained placental fragments along the surgical scar.

Clinical Manifestations

As with early postpartum hemorrhage, the woman with late postpartal hemorrhage notices an increase in bleeding. This increase usually occurs abruptly several days after discharge. Along with an abrupt onset of bleeding, the woman exhibits a uterus that is not contracted firmly. On palpation, the uterus is not descending at the usual rate of 1 centimeter or fingerbreadth per postpartum day. Lochia is heavier than that which would be expected. The woman may report episodes of intermittent, irregular, or excessive vaginal bleeding. In addition, the woman may report backache, fatigue, and general malaise. She may also report pelvic pain or heaviness. Her temperature may be elevated slightly and lochia may be foul smelling if an infection is present.

Diagnosis

Similar to the findings of early postpartum hemorrhage, the woman's hemoglobin and hematocrit levels will be decreased. If retained placental fragments are the cause, the woman's serum human chorionic gonadotropin levels will be elevated. Ultrasound may reveal evidence of placental fragments. An elevated white blood cell count may be noted with an infection. However, this result may not be conclusive because a postpartal woman's white blood cell count typically is elevated in the early postpartum period.

Treatment

Treatment of late postpartum hemorrhage focuses on correcting the underlying cause of the hemorrhage. Drug therapy, similar to that used for uterine atony, may be administered to aid in contracting the uterus. Often, uterine contraction aids in removing any fragments from the uterus. If necessary, surgery, specifically dilation and curettage (D&C) may be done to remove the fragments from the myometrium. Usually, this procedure is performed only when other treatment measures have been ineffective because it can traumatize the uterus further, leading to additional bleeding. Antibiotic therapy is indicated if an infection is present.

Nursing Care

Most cases of late postpartum hemorrhage occur after the woman has been discharged from the health care or birthing facility. Therefore, patient education before discharge about expected changes and danger signs and symptoms is crucial. Instruct the woman to call her primary care provider if she experiences any signs of infection, such as fever greater than 100.4°F, chills, or foul-smelling lochia. She should also report lochia that increases (versus decreasing) in amount, or reversal of the pattern of lochia (i.e., moves from serosa back to rubra).

Test Yourself

- What is the definition of postpartum hemorrhage?
- Name the most common cause of early postpartum hemorrhage.
- Name three nursing actions that should be used for the woman who is experiencing postpartum hemorrhage secondary to uterine atony.

POSTPARTUM INFECTION

Postpartum infection, also called puerperal infection, refers to any infection that occurs after delivery. Most commonly, the infection involves the reproductive tract, but it also can involve other areas, such as the breast, wound, or urinary tract. Current research suggests that postpartum infections occur in approximately 1% to 8% of all postpartum women, with the maternal mortality rate attributable to postpartum infection ranging from 4% to 8% (Kennedy, 2003).

A postpartum infection is suspected when the woman develops a fever of 100.4°F (38°C) or greater on two consecutive occasions at least 6 hours apart during the first 10 days postpartum, but not including the first 24 hours (Simpson & Creehan, 2001). Various organisms are associated with postpartum infections, including but not limited to staphylococcus, streptococcus, *Escherichia coli*, and Chlamydia.

Specific risk factors are associated with the development of a postpartum infection, primarily involving the reproductive tract. Antepartum risk factors include: history of infection; history of chronic conditions, such as diabetes, anemia, or poor nutrition; infections of the genital tract; smoking; and obesity. Intrapartal risk factors include:

- Cesarean birth
- Urinary catheterization
- Episiotomy or lacerations
- Frequent vaginal examinations
- Retained placenta or one requiring manual removal
- Prolonged rupture of membranes (usually more than 24 hours)
- Chorioamnionitis (infection/inflammation of the fetal membranes)

- Traumatic birth, including the use of instruments such as forceps or vacuum extractor
- Use of invasive procedures, such as internal fetal monitoring, fetal scalp sampling, and amnioinfusion

Use of poor aseptic technique and inadequate handwashing are also risk factors. In addition, a woman who experiences postpartum hemorrhage has a greater risk for postpartal infection because of her weakened state and reduced ability to fight off the infection.

Although postpartal infection usually is localized, it can progress and spread to nearby structures such as the peritoneum, causing peritonitis, or to the blood, causing septicemia and posing a significant risk to the woman's well-being. Most postpartal infections occur once the woman is discharged from the health care facility. Therefore, patient teaching about possible signs and symptoms is crucial to ensure early detection and prompt intervention.

Endometritis

Endometritis refers to an infection of the uterine lining. It is the most common postpartal infection, occurring in as many as 3% of women who delivered vaginally and as many as 15% of women who had a cesarean birth (Franzblau & Witt, 2002). Bacteria, often normal vaginal flora, gain entrance to the uterus during birth or the immediate postpartum period.

Typically, endometritis is considered a polymicrobial infection. This means that anaerobic and aerobic organisms enter the uterus from the lower reproductive tract. Common causative organisms include group A streptococci (usually associated with endometritis occurring on day 1 or 2 postpartum); *E. coli* (usually associated with endometritis occurring on day 3 or 4 postpartum); *Klebsiella pneumoniae*; proteus; *Chlamydia trachomatis* (usually associated with endometritis occurring after day 7 postpartum); and Bacteroides species (usually associated with endometritis with cesarean birth).

Endometritis is a serious complication because the infection can spread to nearby organs, such as the fallopian tubes (causing salpingitis), ovaries (causing oophoritis), connective tissues and ligaments (causing parametritis), and the peritoneum (causing peritonitis).

Clinical Manifestations

The woman with endometritis typically looks ill and commonly develops a fever of 100.4°F (38°C) or higher (more commonly 101°F [38.4°C], possibly as high as 104°F [40°C]) on the 3rd to 4th postpartum day. The rise in temperature at this specific time is the most significant finding. The woman exhibits tachycardia, typically a rise in pulse rate of 10 beats per minute for each rise in temperature of 1 degree. In addition, the woman may report chills, anorexia, and general malaise. She also may report abdominal cramping and pain, including strong afterpains. Fundal assessment reveals uterine subinvolution and tenderness. Lochia commonly is increased in amount, dark, purulent, and foul smelling. However, if the woman's temperature is high, her lochia may be scant or absent.

Diagnosis

A complete blood count reveals an elevated white blood cell (WBC) count with increased eosinophiles or polymorphonuclear leukocytes. Urine culture, which may be done to rule out possible urinary tract infection, is negative. Vaginal cultures confirm the diagnosis and reveal the offending organisms. Blood cultures are positive in approximately 10% to 30% of the cases (Simmons & Bammel, 2001). Pelvic ultrasound may reveal an abscess or possible retained placental fragments that have become infected.

Pay close attention! Remember that the WBC count of a postpartal woman is elevated normally, ranging as high as 20,000 to 30,000/mm³. So use caution when interpreting this laboratory result as an indicator for infection. Do suspect infection if the woman's WBC count is near the upper range of 30,000/mm³ or higher, or if it has increased significantly above her immediate postpartum count.

Treatment

The mainstay of treatment is antibiotic therapy. Typically the woman is admitted to the health care facility for IV therapy. Until culture and sensitivity reports are available, the woman is started on broad-spectrum antibiotic therapy. Commonly used agents include combination therapy with clindamycin (Cleocin) and gentamicin. Ampicillin may be added to the treatment regimen if there is no response to the initial therapy. Cefoxitin (Mefoxin) or moxalactam are alternative agents that may be used. Oral antibiotic therapy is initiated once the woman has been afebrile for approximately 48 hours.

In addition to antibiotics, the primary care provider may prescribe oxytocic agents to aid in uterine involution and promote uterine drainage. Analgesics may be necessary if the woman is experiencing strong afterpains or abdominal discomfort. Hydration with IV and oral fluids and adequate nutrition also are important treatment measures.

Nursing Care

The woman with endometritis is visibly ill. Therefore, nursing care focuses on administering drug therapy to combat the infection, promoting physical and emotional comfort, alleviating anxiety, and teaching the woman about measures used to treat the infection and to prevent a recurrence, including proper perineal care and handwashing.

Managing Antibiotic Therapy. Administer prescribed broad-spectrum antibiotics intravenously and assess the woman for changes indicating an improvement. Monitor the woman's vital signs every 2 to 4 hours, or more often if indicated. Expect to see a reduction in temperature and a return of the pulse rate to preinfection levels as the infection resolves. Monitor for a decrease in abdominal pain and tenderness and a change in the

Keep in mind that many antibiotics can be nephrotoxic (damaging to the kidneys). Encourage an increase in fluid intake, intravenously and orally, preferably to 3,000 mL/day, and monitor the woman's intake and output. Report any decrease in urine output to less than 30 mL/hour.

woman's lochia to normal color (based on the postpartum day) and amount. Palpate the fundus to evaluate for uterine contraction. Expect to administer oxytocic agents as ordered to promote uterine involution. As with the administration of any medication, check with the primary care provider or lactation consultant to determine whether the woman can continue to breast-feed. In most cases the woman will be able to continue breast-feeding. If breast-feeding is contraindicated, encourage the woman to pump her breasts to maintain the milk supply.

In conjunction with antibiotic therapy, position the woman in the semi-Fowler's position to promote uterine drainage and prevent extension of the infection. If possible and allowed by the physician, encourage the woman to ambulate to promote drainage. Be alert for signs and symptoms of peritonitis, such as pronounced abdominal pain, and distention, a rigid, boardlike abdomen and absent bowel sounds. Also assess the woman for tachycardia, tachypnea, hypotension, changes in sensorium, and decreased urine output. These suggest septic shock, a serious, possibly fatal complication.

Encourage frequent changing of perineal pads to remove infected drainage, reminding the woman to remove the pad using a front-to-back motion to avoid contaminating the perineal area. Reinforce the need to wash her hands after each change. Offer perineal care every 2 hours or as necessary. Be sure to wear gloves when handling the woman's soiled perineal pads to prevent infection transmission.

Providing Comfort Measures. The woman needs comfort care during this time. Provide cool washcloths and frequent linen changes, especially if the woman is febrile and diaphoretic. If the woman reports chills, add extra blankets to keep her warm; however, be careful that she doesn't become overheated. Keep the room calm and quiet to ensure the woman rests.

Expect to administer analgesics for reports of abdominal pain. Encourage the woman to change positions frequently while maintaining the semi-Fowler's position. The woman probably will be fatigued because of the stress of the infection. Allow for frequent rest periods so that she does not overtax herself. In addition, assist with personal hygiene measures, including perineal care.

Alleviating Anxiety. The woman who develops endometritis typically has been discharged from the health care facility. She may become anxious and upset when readmission is necessary because now she will be separated from her newborn. Allow her to verbalize her feelings. Provide support and guidance as necessary. Enlist the aid of the woman's spouse or significant other and family to help in alleviating her anxiety.

If breast-feeding is allowed, encourage the woman to pump her breasts for feedings. Alternatively, the primary care provider may allow the baby to be brought in for feedings. If not, encourage the family to bring in pictures of the baby for the woman to keep in her room.

Providing Patient Teaching. Patient teaching is a major focus of nursing care. One key area of teaching is medication therapy, especially if the woman is to continue the therapy at home. Other areas to address include proper handwashing techniques; perineal care; expected changes in lochia; signs and symptoms of a recurrent infection; danger signs to notify the physician. Family Teaching Tips: Endometritis outlines the major discharge teaching points.

Wound Infection

Postpartal wound infections typically involve infections of the perineum that develop at the site of an episiotomy or laceration. Wound infection also can occur at the site of the abdominal incision after a cesarean birth. Perineal wound infections, although rare, commonly develop on the 3rd or 4th postpartum day. Factors increasing the risk of perineal wound infections include infected lochia, fecal contamination of the wound, and inadequate hygiene measures. In most cases, the infectious organism is normal vaginal flora.

Post-cesarean delivery incisional infections usually develop about the 4th postpartum day, often after the woman has developed endometritis. Although these infections most commonly are caused by contamination with vaginal flora, *Staphylococcus aureus* from the skin or another outside source has been identified as a cause in some cases.

FAMILY TEACHING TIPS

Endometritis

- Be sure to complete all of your antibiotics, even though you are feeling better.
- Call your care provider if you have any of the following symptoms of recurrent infection:
  - Temperature greater than 100.4°F (38°C)
  - Chills
  - Abdominal pain that does not go away with pain medication
  - Vaginal discharge that smells bad (like rotten meat)
- You should do the following things to prevent additional infection:
  - Wash your hands thoroughly before and after eating, using the restroom, or touching your vaginal area.
  - Wipe from front to back after using the restroom.
  - Remove soiled sanitary pads from front to back. Fold the pad so that the discharge is contained in the middle section of the pad, and then wrap it in toilet paper, or preferably a plastic bag. Dispose in the trash.
  - Wash hands before applying a new pad. Apply the pad from front to back. Do not touch the middle section of the pad. This part should remain very clean because it will be touching your vaginal area.
- You will heal faster and be less likely to get sick again if you do the following things:
  - Get at least 8 hours of sleep every night.
  - Rest frequently. Take a nap when the baby is napping.
  - Eat a nutritious diet.
  - Gradually increase your activity as you are able to tolerate it.
  - Drink plenty (1 to 2 liters) of fluids each day.
- Be sure to attend your scheduled follow-up visits with your primary care provider.

Risk Factors

Risk factors for the development of a postpartum wound infection include:

- History of a chronic medical disorder, such as diabetes or hypertension
- Anemia or malnutrition
- Obesity
- Chorioamnionitis
- Immunosuppression, including treatment with corticosteroids
- Development of a hematoma
- Prolonged labor, rupture of membranes, or operative time
- Hemorrhage (Franzblau & Witt, 2002; Simpson & Creehan, 2001).

Clinical Manifestations

The woman with a perineal wound infection most likely will report pain out of proportion to what is expected. Inspection of the perineum reveals redness of the area and edema of the surrounding tissue. Separation of the wound edges may be noted. Often there is a foul-smelling, possibly purulent, vaginal drainage. The area will be tender on palpation. Fever and general malaise also may be present.

The woman experiencing an incisional infection after a cesarean birth often develops endometritis before the onset of the incisional infection. In this case, the woman continues to be febrile, even with antibiotic treatment. Inspection of the abdominal wound reveals erythema and induration (area of hardened tissue). In addition, the wound edges may be separated (Fig. 19-2). **Exudate** (drainage; fluid accumulation) may or may not be present, and the drainage may or may not be purulent. A small area of fluid collection may be noted near the incision. When opened, the area may ooze serosanguinous or purulent fluid (Franzblau & Witt, 2002). The area of the wound typically is warm and tender on palpation, and the woman reports pain.

Diagnosis

A complete blood count (CBC) with differential may reveal an elevation in WBC count. A culture of the area reveals the causative organism and guides treatment. Ultrasound may be used to determine if an abscess is present (Singhal & Zammit, 2002).

Additional laboratory studies may include serum protein, albumin, pre-albumin, and transferrin. These are done to assess nutritional status, which affects wound healing. Coagulation studies and a metabolic profile may be ordered (Stillman, 2002).

● **Figure 19.2** Postcesarean wound infection. A wound infection usually has an area of induration (raised and firm to palpation) surrounded by erythema. The wound may or may not be separated, as is shown in the illustration.

Treatment

Antibiotic therapy is indicated for treatment of the infection. For the woman with a perineal infection, therapy is supportive to include analgesics, local anesthetic sprays, warm compresses, and sitz baths. If an abscess develops, surgical incision and drainage are performed.

For the woman with an incisional infection, wound care, involving opening the wound for drainage (possibly requiring a trip to the operating room), irrigation, debridement, and possibly packing may be necessary. The goal is to clean the wound and promote granulation.

Nursing Care

For the woman with a perineal infection, provide warm compresses to the wound site and sitz baths to provide comfort. These measures also aid the healing process by increasing circulation to the area. Typically these are ordered for 20 minutes several times a day. When assisting with the application of warm compresses, be sure to adhere to standard precautions and perform handwashing.

Keeping the perineal area clean also is important. Encourage the woman to change her perineal pads and to perform perineal care frequently. Urge her to use a front-to-back motion when removing perineal pads and when cleaning the perineum after voiding and moving her bowels. Also remind her to wash her hands after performing any perineal care and using the bathroom. Although always important, thorough handwashing is absolutely essential when the woman is being cared for at home. Handwashing is critical to prevent transmitting the infection to the newborn.

For the woman with an incisional infection, wound care may be ordered. This may include dressing changes, irrigations, debridement, or possibly wound packing. Always use aseptic technique when performing wound care. With each dressing change or procedure, inspect the wound for signs and symptoms indicating resolution of the infection and evidence of healing. If necessary, record measurements of the wound to aid in evaluating progress. If wound care will need to be continued after discharge or if wound care is being provided in the home, teach the woman or another family member how to perform the care. She should also be able to detect signs and symptoms of increasing infection and know the signs that indicate the wound is healing. Have the person perform a return demonstration of any procedure.

Mastitis

Mastitis refers to an infection of the mammary gland (breast). This infection is most common in women who are breast-feeding for the first time. Typically, only one breast is affected. Although the infection can occur at any time when the woman is breast-feeding, it is most common during the 2nd and 3rd weeks after delivery.

Mastitis occurs when organisms are transferred from the woman's hands, staff's hands, or newborn's mouth to the breast and enter the breast tissue through a small, often microscopic, crack, fissure, or injured area on the nipple or breast tissue. Certain risk factors have been identified as contributing to the development of mastitis. These include

- Inadequate or incomplete breast emptying during feeding or lack of frequent feeding leading to milk stasis
- Engorgement
- Clogged milk ducts
- Cracked or bleeding nipples (Simpson & Creehan, 2001)

If left untreated, mastitis can progress to an abscess, which may require surgical drainage.

Clinical Manifestations

The woman with mastitis usually develops the infection after discharge, when she is at home. Common complaints include general flu-like symptoms that occur suddenly; such as fever, malaise, and possibly chills. In addition, the woman often reports tenderness, pain, and heaviness in her breast. Inspection reveals erythema and edema in an area on one breast but not the other (Fig. 19-3). The area is hard, warm, and tender on palpation. Purulent drainage may or may not be noted.

● **Figure 19.3** Mastitis. The woman with mastitis usually has a reddened, painful area on one breast that is warm to palpation.

Diagnosis

No specific tests are used to confirm the diagnosis of mastitis. Typically, the diagnosis is made based on the woman's signs and symptoms. A sample of breast milk may be sent for analysis, but the results fail to yield accurate and reliable data (Franzblau & Witt, 2002).

Treatment

Supportive care in conjunction with antibiotic therapy is used to treat mastitis. Penicillinase-resistant agents such as dicloxacillin (Dynapen) are the drugs of choice. Therapy usually is continued for 10 days. Analgesics may be prescribed for comfort.

Nursing Care

Nursing care focuses on resolving the infection and preventing further milk stasis. Preventing milk stasis is important for relieving the discomfort and preventing extension of the infection with possible abscess formation. Encourage the woman to breast-feed (unless contraindicated) every 1½ to 2 hours. Frequent feeding enhances complete emptying of the breast. If the woman is unable to breast-feed, for example because the affected breast is too sore or antibiotic therapy contraindicates breast-feeding, encourage the woman to manually express breast milk or use a breast pump to empty her breasts.

If the woman is breast-feeding, recommend the use of warm compresses or a warm shower before feeding to promote the let-down reflex and stimulate the flow of milk. Warm compresses also are soothing and increase blood flow to the area to stimulate healing. Suggest that the woman begin breast-feeding on the affected breast first, if possible. Doing so promotes the milk ejection reflex in the affected breast, thereby making complete emptying more efficient. Massaging the affected area over the breast during feeding also helps to ensure complete emptying.

As with any woman who is breast-feeding, encourage the woman to increase her fluid intake to ensure adequate milk formation. Review proper techniques for breast-feeding and proper infant positioning (refer to Chapter 14). Provide support and encouragement for continuing breast-feeding. If necessary, a lactation consultant can be consulted for specific assistance. Nursing Care Plan 19-1 discusses the care of a woman with mastitis.

Urinary Tract Infection

Urinary tract infection (UTI) involves an infection of the bladder (**cystitis**) or the kidneys (**pyelonephritis**). Anatomically, a woman's urethra is shorter than a man's urethra, thereby increasing the woman's risk for UTI. In addition, trauma during birth and inadequate bladder emptying may lead to urinary stasis intrapartally and postpartally, increasing the woman's risk for developing a UTI. Moreover, frequent vaginal examinations during delivery, urinary catheterizations, and delivery involving instrumentation further compound the risk.

Clinical Manifestations

The signs and symptoms exhibited by a woman with cystitis differ from those of a woman with pyelonephritis. Typically, those associated with pyelonephritis are more dramatic and severe. The woman with cystitis characteristically reports burning and pain on urination. She reports urgency and frequency and voids only small amounts at a time. The woman usually has a low-grade fever and possibly suprapubic pain.

In addition to burning, pain, urgency, and frequency, the woman with pyelonephritis presents with a high, spiking fever that rises and falls abruptly. Often she has shaking chills and reports nausea and vomiting.

Flank pain and tenderness are common. In addition, tenderness at the costovertebral angle (the area on the back just above the waistline) is noted on palpation.

Diagnosis

A urinalysis and clean catch urine for culture and sensitivity are done to determine evidence of an infection. The urinalysis typically reveals white blood cells, protein, blood, and presence of bacteria. The clean catch urine specimen, considered diagnostic for UTI, reveals greater than 10^5 colony-forming units. In addition, a complete blood count may reveal an elevated white blood cell count.

Treatment

Antibiotic therapy is the treatment of choice based on the urine culture and sensitivity results. For the woman with cystitis, antibiotics are administered orally. For the woman with pyelonephritis, antibiotic therapy is ordered intravenously. Typically therapy begins with a broad-spectrum antibiotic and is later adjusted based on the urine culture and sensitivity reports.

In addition to antibiotic therapy, antipyretics and analgesics, such as acetaminophen (Tylenol); antispasmodics; urinary analgesics; such as phenazopyridine hydrochloride (Pyridium); and antiemetics may be ordered. Hydration and good perineal hygiene also are important.

Nursing Care

Nursing care focuses on promoting comfort, ensuring adequate hydration, and providing patient teaching. The woman with cystitis typically does not require admission to a health care facility for treatment. However, the woman with pyelonephritis usually is admitted for IV hydration and antibiotic therapy.

Providing Comfort. Providing comfort measures is important. The woman with a UTI typically has pain and burning on urination, which can make voiding difficult. In addition, this discomfort can prevent the woman from emptying her bladder completely, resulting in urinary stasis. Urinary stasis provides a good medium for organism growth, further compounding her risk for infection, and possibly increasing her risk for extension of the infection, for

Pay attention! If the woman is experiencing pain and burning on urination, she may be hesitant to drink the necessary amount of fluid, fearing that increasing fluid intake will increase the number of times she will need to void and thus increase her pain. Explain that a high urinary output often decreases the pain associated with UTI.

NURSING CARE PLAN 19.1

The Woman With Mastitis

CASE SCENARIO:
Jessica Thompson is a 22-year-old gravida 1 para 1, who delivered her baby vaginally 2 weeks ago. She is breast-feeding. She has just been readmitted to the postpartum ward of the hospital with a diagnosis of mastitis in the right breast. Her admitting vital signs are BP 128/70, T 101.2°F, P 106 bpm, R 22/minute. She says that she feels like she has the flu. She is very tired all the time, and her body aches all over. Assessment of her breast-feeding techniques indicates that the baby feeds better from the left breast, so Jessica usually starts with the left breast. Since her right breast began hurting 2 days ago, she has avoided using that breast to feed the baby because she says, "It just hurts too much." She also reports that sometimes the baby uses a pacifier between feedings. Jessica says that she isn't sure that she should keep breast-feeding because she is afraid that "the infection might hurt my baby." The physician has ordered clindamycin (Cleocin) 900 mg IV every 8 hours; acetaminophen (Tylenol) 1,000 mg PO every 4 to 6 hours PRN temperature greater than 100.4°F; ibuprofen (Motrin) 800 mg PO every 8 hours PRN pain.

NURSING DIAGNOSIS:
Hyperthermia related to inflammation secondary to infectious process as evidenced by T 101.2°F.

GOAL: Regulation of temperature.

EXPECTED OUTCOMES:
* Temperature will decrease to less than 100.4°F.
* Pulse rate will decrease to less than 100 bpm.
* Muscle aches will resolve.

NURSING INTERVENTIONS	RATIONALE
Monitor vital signs, including temperature every 4 hours until it has been less than 100.4°F for at least 24 hours.	Monitoring the vital signs will allow tracking of temperature spikes and overall response to therapy.
Monitor WBC, as ordered.	White blood cell count will begin decreasing as the infection resolves.
Administer the antipyretic, acetaminophen, as ordered.	Antipyretics control body temperature.
Administer antibiotic, clindamycin, as ordered.	Antibiotics will treat the infection that is causing the fever.
Place a pitcher of ice water at the bedside and refill it frequently, as needed. Offer juices, popsicles, and other liquids every 1 to 2 hours.	Temperature elevation can result in fluid loss. Also, adequate hydration is needed so that the body can effectively fight infection.

NURSING DIAGNOSIS
Ineffective Breast-feeding Pattern related to incomplete emptying of the right breast and pacifier use.

GOAL: Maintenance of effective breast-feeding.

EXPECTED OUTCOMES:
* Initiates breast-feeding on demand at least every 1.5 to 2 hours.
* Infant exhibits proper latch during breast-feeding.
* Empties both breasts regularly.

NURSING INTERVENTIONS	RATIONALE
Encourage Jessica to continue breast-feeding.	Breast-feeding with mastitis is safe for the baby. In fact, stopping breast-feeding does not help the woman recover and may cause her condition to get worse.
Request a consult with a lactation specialist.	A lactation specialist can evaluate the woman for subtle factors that may be interfering with the breast-feeding process and can help the baby to latch on well.

NURSING CARE PLAN 19.1 continued

The Woman With Mastitis

NURSING INTERVENTIONS	RATIONALE
Assist Jessica to breast-feed every 1.5 to 2 hours until symptoms begin to resolve.	Regular emptying of the breasts improves milk flow and decreases stasis, which can lead to blocked milk ducts and further infection.
Instruct Jessica to start on the right breast first, if she is able. If not, it may help to assist her to use a breast pump on the right breast while she is feeding on the left breast.	It is important that Jessica completely empty the affected breast at every feeding to increase milk flow and circulation to the area.
Instruct Jessica to gently massage the affected area (the lump that is warm and tender) as the breast is emptied (i.e., during breast-feeding or pumping).	Gentle massage is indicated to help unclog the clogged duct that is causing the problem.
Encourage rooming in with the infant, as long as someone can stay at the bedside with Jessica.	Rooming in allows for breast-feeding on demand, which is ideal. A competent adult must remain at the bedside to take responsibility for the baby, because the baby is not a patient. It is not appropriate for the patient to have responsibility for the infant until she is well enough to go home.
If the baby must go home at any time, assist Jessica to pump her breasts every 2 hours. The milk can be refrigerated for later consumption by the baby.	Pumping the breasts stimulates milk production, increased blood flow, and increased milk flow, all of which help decrease the symptoms of mastitis.
Discourage pacifier use.	Sucking on a pacifier or artificial nipple can decrease the amount that the infant suckles, thereby increasing the risk for milk stasis.

NURSING DIAGNOSIS
Acute Pain related to mastitis (particularly associated with breast-feeding).

GOAL: Tolerable pain levels

EXPECTED OUTCOMES:
• Verbalizes adequate relief from pain after interventions.
• Empties affected breast without undue pain.

NURSING INTERVENTIONS	RATIONALE
Administer ibuprofen, as ordered. In the first 24 to 48 hours, administer the medication around the clock versus PRN.	Ibuprofen usually provides excellent pain relief for the pain associated with mastitis. It also has anti-inflammatory properties, which further help reduce pain. Around-the-clock dosing prevents acute pain from becoming severe. Once pain becomes severe, it is more difficult to treat.
Assist Jessica to apply warm compresses or a heating pad to the affected breast. Alternatively, or additionally, encourage her to take warm showers.	Warmth helps to decrease pain and increases blood flow to the area, which increases milk flow.

NURSING DIAGNOSIS
Fatigue related to infectious process.

GOAL: Ability to perform self- and baby-care functions.

EXPECTED OUTCOMES:
• Verbalizes feeling rested.
• Reports increased energy levels.
• Performs self- and baby-care without complaints of fatigue.

(nursing care plan continues on page 470)

NURSING CARE PLAN 19.1 continued

The Woman With Mastitis

NURSING INTERVENTIONS	RATIONALE
Encourage frequent rest periods.	Promotes healing.
Encourage adequate nutrition.	Promotes healing and provides energy source.
Encourage wakefulness during the early evening hours. Discourage late afternoon naps.	Promotes sleep during the night, which provides the most restful sleep.
Encourage the use of bedtime rituals, preferably ones she uses at home.	Promotes sleep.
Limit visitors, as appropriate.	Reduces stimuli and allows for rest.
Reduce light and noise stimuli at bedtime.	Promotes sleep.
Encourage significant other to care for the baby (other than feedings) during the night.	Promotes periods of uninterrupted sleep.
Group nursing interventions and care activities.	Avoids unnecessary interruptions and promotes rest.

NURSING DIAGNOSIS
Deficient Knowledge: Self-care after discharge

GOAL: Demonstrates ability to care for self at home.

EXPECTED OUTCOMES:
• Washes hands before and after using the restroom, eating, touching the breasts.
• Answers questions accurately regarding self-care.
• Breast-feeds infant every 2 to 3 hours without prompting.

NURSING INTERVENTIONS	RATIONALE
Teach importance of handwashing. Encourage frequent handwashing at appropriate times.	Helps prevent the spread and recurrence of infection.
Encourage Jessica to continue breast-feeding as instructed (refer to breast-feeding guidelines above).	Proper breast-feeding techniques decrease the likelihood that mastitis will recur.
Instruct regarding early warning signs, which include	If the woman initiates intervention at the first warning sign, she may be able to prevent a recurrence of mastitis.
• Breast engorgement	
• Nipple soreness or cracking	
• A painful lump in one breast, which is a sign of a plugged duct	
If she has any of the warning symptoms, she should do the following	These measures encourage the flow of milk; help prevent milk stasis; and prevent early mastitis from becoming more severe.
• Rest in bed, if possible.	
• Breast-feed frequently from the affected breast.	
• Put a warm compress on the affected breast.	
• Gently massage lumpy areas while the infant is feeding.	
• Call her physician if she develops fever 100.4°F or above or if she does not get better within 24 hours.	

example, from the bladder to the kidneys. Therefore, assist the woman with comfort measures, such as running warm water over the perineum or using a sitz bath when voiding. In addition, administer analgesics such as acetaminophen (Tylenol) as ordered. A urinary analgesic (e.g., phenazopyridine hydrochloride [Pyridium]) is comforting, if ordered.

Promoting Adequate Hydration. Adequate hydration is necessary to dilute the bacterial concentration in the urine and aid in clearing the organisms

from the urinary tract. Encourage the woman to drink at least 3,000 mL of fluid a day. Suggest she drink one glass per hour to ensure adequate intake and to keep a record of her intake.

Advise the woman to drink fluids that make the urine acidic, deterring organism growth. Fluids such as cranberry, plum, prune, or apricot juices are examples. Tell the woman to avoid carbonated beverages because they increase the alkalinity of urine, which promotes organism growth. If the woman has pyelonephritis, expect to administer fluids intravenously in addition to oral fluid to ensure adequate hydration.

Providing Patient Teaching. Patient teaching is essential for ensuring compliance with therapy and preventing a recurrence of cystitis or pyelonephritis. Instruct the woman to complete the full drug regimen, which can range from 5 to 10 days. Although the woman with pyelonephritis will receive antibiotic therapy intravenously, she probably will be switched to an oral form that will be continued after discharge (depending on her length of stay in the health care facility). If the woman is breast-feeding, provide instruction concerning the safety of her continuing to breast-feed based on the particular antibiotic she is taking. Other important patient teaching topics include hydration measures; comfort measures; perineal care; and preventive measures, including signs and symptoms of a recurrence.

Test Yourself

- List five risk factors for postpartum infection.
- Name five signs and symptoms of endometritis.
- Describe four clinical manifestations of postpartum wound infection.

THROMBOEMBOLIC DISORDERS

Thromboembolic disorders in the postpartum period typically involve three types:

- Superficial thrombophlebitis
- Deep vein thrombophlebitis
- Pulmonary embolism

Of these three, pulmonary embolism is the most serious and possibly fatal.

Risk Factors

The postpartal woman is at risk for thromboembolic disorders for three reasons: (1) Clotting factors that increased during pregnancy are still elevated, promoting blood clotting; (2) During pregnancy and birth, the fetal head exerted pressure on the veins of the lower extremity, causing them to dilate; and (3) The woman has spent a relative amount of time during labor and delivery being inactive or with her extremities placed in stirrups, leading to venous pooling and stasis. In addition, some women may have other factors that further increase their risk for thromboembolic disorders. These may include

- Varicose veins
- Past history of thrombophlebitis
- Obesity
- Smoking
- Age greater than 35 years
- History of three or more pregnancies
- Prolonged labor
- Use of forceps or cesarean birth

Superficial and Deep Vein Thrombophlebitis

Thrombophlebitis refers to an inflammation of the lining of the vein with the formation of clots. It can be categorized as superficial or deep vein. Superficial thrombophlebitis typically involves the saphenous veins of the lower extremities, usually affecting the calf area. Deep vein thrombophlebitis (DVT) usually affects the deeper veins of the calf, thigh, or pelvis. These deep veins carry the majority of venous return from the legs to the heart, making it a more serious condition than superficial thrombophlebitis.

Clinical Manifestations

In most cases, signs and symptoms of superficial thrombophlebitis develop within the first 3 postpartum days. The woman with deep vein thrombophlebitis may develop signs and symptoms during pregnancy or at any time during the postpartum period.

Typically the postpartum woman with superficial thrombophlebitis exhibits a tender, painful area along a vein in the calf, most commonly a varicose vein. On inspection the area is reddened and the vein is enlarged and highly visible. The area is warm and cordlike to the touch (Schreiber, 2002). The affected extremity may be swollen, and the woman may report pain when walking.

The woman with deep vein thrombophlebitis may have no symptoms. If the woman does exhibit signs, these typically include increased calf pain and tenderness. The leg is swollen visibly and, when circumference of the thigh and calf is measured, is larger than the other leg. Pedal edema also may be present. The area is warm, tender, and red. Homans' sign (pain on dorsiflexion of the foot) may be positive. Historically, a positive Homans' sign was indicative of deep vein thrombophlebitis. However, this is no longer considered a reliable sign because the pain may be attributable to muscle strain or contusion. In addition, the woman may exhibit indications of an arterial spasm, causing a decrease in circulation to the affected area. As a result, the leg may appear visibly pale or white, and pedal pulses may be diminished. Other signs and symptoms include chills, low-grade fever (usually not greater than 101°F [38.3°C]), malaise, stiffness of the affected leg, and pain on ambulation (Schreiber, 2002).

Diagnosis

Confirmation of superficial thrombophlebitis is based on the woman's signs and symptoms. For the woman with deep vein thrombophlebitis, the physician may order several diagnostic tests, such as Doppler ultrasonography or venography with a contrast medium, which reveals altered blood flow confirming the inflammation and blood clots.

Treatment

The primary goals of medical therapy are to prevent further thrombus formation and to prevent pulmonary embolism, a potentially fatal complication. Treatment for superficial thrombophlebitis includes analgesics, elevation of the affected extremity, bed rest, and local application of heat. Anticoagulant therapy such as Heparin or low-molecular-weight-heparin (enoxaparin [Lovenox]) may be ordered and is usually administered subcutaneously. Heparin is administered with caution in the postpartum period and usually is not given in the immediate postpartum period because of bleeding concerns. As the woman's condition improves, ambulation is encouraged.

For the woman with deep vein thrombophlebitis, treatment is similar to that for superficial thrombophlebitis, including analgesics, heat, bed rest, application of compression stockings, and elevation of the leg. In addition, anticoagulant therapy typically is ordered. Heparin is usually given intravenously by continuous infusion pump; enoxaparin (Lovenox) is given subcutaneously. After several days of heparin or enoxaparin therapy, the woman is started on oral anticoagulant therapy with warfarin (Coumadin). Heparin therapy is decreased gradually as the warfarin therapy reaches therapeutic levels. Oral anticoagulant therapy is continued for approximately 6 weeks.

Nursing Care

Nursing care for the woman with superficial thrombophlebitis and deep vein thrombophlebitis includes instituting bed rest; applying compression stockings, as ordered; and elevating the affected extremity to promote venous return. Inspect the lower extremities for changes in color, temperature, and size. Palpate pedal pulses and measure the circumference of each lower extremity and compare the results bilaterally to determine the degree of edema. Assist the woman to remove the compression stockings for an hour every 8 to 12 hours.

Apply warm compresses as ordered. When applying the compresses, ensure that they are at the proper temperature to avoid burning the woman. Because of altered blood flow, the woman's ability to sense temperature extremes may be diminished, placing her at risk for a burn injury. Also be sure that the weight of the compresses does not rest on the leg, causing a further compromise in blood flow. In addition, check the woman's bed linens and change them as necessary because the linens may become damp or wet from the moist heat applications. If possible, use a waterproof pad to protect the linens. Warm moist compresses can cool quickly. Provide the woman with extra blankets if necessary to prevent chilling. Also use chemical heat packs or a pad such as an Aquathermia pad to help keep the compresses warm.

For the woman with deep vein thrombophlebitis, it is important to monitor the woman's vital signs closely for slight elevations in temperature, possibly to 101°F (38.3°C), and report this finding to the physician. Because the woman with deep vein thrombophlebitis has an increased risk for developing a pulmonary embolism, be alert for and immediately report any sudden onset of breathing difficulties.

Expect to administer anticoagulant therapy as ordered. When administering heparin, always have the antidote, protamine sulfate, readily available should the woman experience bleeding. Place the woman on bleeding precautions, which includes monitoring for evidence of bleeding, applying 5 to 10 minutes of pressure to injection or venipuncture sites, and avoiding unnecessary injections. Be sure to urge the woman to report any increase in vaginal bleeding, saturation of perineal pads or evidence of bruising, oozing at IV sites, or gingival bleeding.

The woman typically is discharged on oral anticoagulant therapy. Therefore, teach the woman about the drug and signs and symptoms to report immediately (Family Teaching Tips: Anticoagulant Therapy).

Pulmonary Embolism

Pulmonary embolism refers to a clot (thrombus) that breaks free from the vessel wall and travels to the heart and through the pulmonary circulation, where it becomes lodged and interrupts the blood flow to the

Consistency equals accuracy!
Use this guideline to measure swelling. Compare one extremity on the woman to the other when deciding if swelling is abnormal. Use an indelible pen to mark a line on the back of the leg at the largest part of the extremity to be measured. This line can be as small as 1 inch. At the same level, mark the other extremity. Use a paper tape to measure and record the circumference of both extremities. Compare these results to see if there is a difference. If you make this recording every 4 hours, it will be easy to see if the swelling is increasing or decreasing. The mark allows all nurses to measure at the same point.

FAMILY TEACHING TIPS

Anticoagulant Therapy

While you are on anticoagulant therapy, you are at risk for bleeding. Look for the following signs of bleeding:
- Bruising
- Bleeding gums
- Nosebleed
- Oozing from scratches and scrapes
- Blood in the urine
- Black or tarry stools
- Increased vaginal bleeding
- Notify the primary care provider of any change in level of consciousness, decreased ability to follow commands, or decreased sensation or ability to move extremities. These signs may indicate the presence of a cerebral bleed. This is an emergency that requires immediate intervention.

The following precautions will help prevent excessive bleeding:
- Use a soft toothbrush.
- Avoid use of razor blades (use an electric razor to shave).
- Avoid aspirin-containing products.
- Check with the primary care provider before taking any over-the-counter (OTC) medications.
- Notify your dentist and any other health care provider that you are on anticoagulant therapy.
- Apply pressure for 5 to 10 minutes after any injections or after blood is drawn or if you accidentally cut or scrape yourself.

Heparin and warfarin (Coumadin) are both considered safe for use in breast-feeding mothers (Anderson, 2002; Zimmerman, undated).

lungs. Thrombus formation occurs most commonly in the pelvic vein in postpartum women. If a large area of blood flow is compromised, cardiovascular collapse ultimately occurs, which can be fatal.

Pulmonary embolism is a complication that can result from deep vein thrombophlebitis. It also may result from superficial thrombophlebitis, but this is rare. Pulmonary embolism is the leading cause of maternal mortality.

Clinical Manifestations

The postpartum woman who develops a pulmonary embolism typically exhibits a sudden onset of dyspnea, pleuritic chest pain, and an impending sense of severe apprehension or doom. If the woman experiences any of these, report them immediately. In addition, the woman may be tachypneic, tachycardic, and hypotensive. She may have a cough with bloody sputum (hemoptysis) and report abdominal pain. Cyanosis and changes in level of consciousness also may occur.

Diagnosis

Arterial blood gases reveal a decrease in the partial pressure of oxygen and partial pressure of carbon dioxide. Ventilation/perfusion scan demonstrates a mismatching between lung tissue perfusion and ventilation, that is, a decrease in or absence of perfusion in lung areas that are being normally ventilated. Pulmonary angiography will reveal a defect in filling or an abrupt cessation of blood flow at the location of the embolus. A chest radiograph may show atelectasis, infiltrates, or pleural effusions, all of which suggest a pulmonary embolism.

Treatment

Development of a pulmonary embolism is considered a life-threatening emergency requiring immediate treatment. Administration of oxygen therapy via face mask and medication administration to treat the woman's symptoms are used. For example, if the woman is hypotensive, dopamine may be used to raise the woman's blood pressure. Heparin therapy is administered to prevent further clot formation. Thrombolytic agents may be administered to dissolve the existing clot.

Continuous monitoring via pulmonary artery catheterization and continuous electrocardiogram monitoring often are necessary. Because of the woman's critical status, she most likely will be transferred to the intensive care unit.

Nursing Care

Immediate action by the nurse is crucial for the woman who develops a pulmonary embolism. After assessing signs and symptoms of a pulmonary embolism, notify the physician at once and immediately raise the head of the bed to at least 45 degrees to facilitate breathing. Begin oxygen therapy at 8 to 10 liters per minute via face mask. Be prepared to assist with obtaining specimens for arterial blood gas analysis and prepare the woman for diagnostic testing. Monitor the woman's vital signs closely. Provide emotional support and explain all procedures and treatments to the woman, who is most likely apprehensive about what is happening. Prepare the woman for transfer to the intensive care unit.

Test Yourself

- What three factors put the postpartum woman at risk for thrombus formation?
- Name four nursing interventions appropriate for the woman with DVT.
- What symptoms are associated with pulmonary embolism?

POSTPARTUM PSYCHIATRIC DISORDERS

Three separate psychiatric conditions have been identified as occurring during the postpartum period. These include: postpartum blues (also known as "baby blues" or "maternity blues"); postpartum depression; and postpartum psychosis. Of these three conditions, postpartum blues is the most common and least serious. Research reveals that at least 50% of all postpartum women experience this transitory phase of sadness and crying. (See Chapter 12 for more discussion of this condition.)

Postpartum depression and postpartum psychosis are considered mood disorders involving one's view of life. Depression affects the woman's ability to function; however, her perception of reality remains intact. Conversely, the woman with postpartum psychosis experiences a severe distortion in her view of reality, often accompanied by hallucinations and delusions.

The exact cause of these disorders is unknown. Researchers believe that multiple factors are responsible for their development. These factors may include:

- Stress arising from the pregnancy and responsibilities associated with child rearing
- Sudden decrease in endorphins with labor and abrupt changes in hormonal levels (estrogen and progesterone) after delivery
- Low serum levels of free tryptophan (which are associated with the psychiatric diagnosis of major depression)
- Possible thyroid gland dysfunction

Regardless of the cause, the nurse plays a key role in teaching the woman about the signs and symptoms of each disorder and in early detection so that prompt treatment can be initiated.

Postpartum Depression

Postpartum depression is described as a mood disorder that involves a pervasive and sustained emotion in which the woman demonstrates a lack of interest or pleasure in usual activities. This disorder is believed to affect as many as 15% of new mothers. Some research provides evidence that this rate is even higher, possibly as high as 25% in women with multiple births and in those who deliver preterm newborns. In addition, as many as 50% of women with postpartum depression may go undiagnosed because of the stigma associated with mental illness (Beck, 2003).

Duration of the disorder is variable. Symptoms may begin at any time after delivery. Although the disorder may resolve within 3 to 6 months, research has revealed that approximately 25% of women will continue to experience depression after 1 year (Franzblau

BOX 19.2	Risk Factors for Postpartum Depression

The following factors increase a woman's risk for developing postpartum depression:
- Episodes of depression or anxiety during the pregnancy at any trimester
- Stressful life events, such as loss of employment, change in family situation, serious illness, or loss of family member
- Problems in relationship with partner or spouse
- Inadequate or lack of social support from family, friends, or partner
- Anger at the pregnancy or an undesired pregnancy
- Personal history of depression before pregnancy or family history of psychological problems
- History of sexual abuse or intimate partner abuse

& Witt, 2002). Certain factors have been identified as possibly increasing a woman's risk for postpartum depression. These factors are highlighted in Box 19-2.

Clinical Manifestations

The woman with postpartum depression commonly demonstrates strong feelings of sadness and irritability. She is frequently tearful. She may have a lack of interest in her surroundings and have trouble motivating herself to do normal activities. She may show disinterest in others and a lack of enjoyment with life. Often intense feelings of inadequacy, inability to cope, ambivalence, guilt, and unworthiness are noted.

In conjunction with these signs and symptoms, the woman may report problems sleeping, loss of libido, decreased appetite, inability to concentrate, overwhelming fatigue, feelings of insecurity and loss of control, and obsessive thinking. In addition, the woman may contemplate harming herself (suicide) or the infant.

Diagnosis

Diagnosis is made on the basis of signs and symptoms, which must be present on most days for at least 2 weeks for the diagnosis to apply. The primary care provider usually screens the woman for hypothyroidism because this condition can cause symptoms of depression.

Treatment

Treatment for the woman with postpartum depression is usually accomplished on an outpatient basis, although severe cases may require hospitalization in a psychiatric facility. A trained mental health professional guides the treatment plan, which includes the woman's family. Antidepressant therapy may be prescribed. Agents such as selective serotonin reuptake inhibitors (SSRIs), including paroxetine (Paxil), fluoxetine (Prozac), and sertraline (Zoloft), are first-line drugs in the treatment of postpartum depression. Research demonstrates that these agents are safe for use in women who are breast-feeding. Electroconvulsive treatment (ECT), which has been shown to be effective for women with major depression, may be used for the woman with postpartum depression.

Nursing Care

Early detection and treatment are critical because the disorder can be totally disruptive of the woman's life and frequently interferes with interpersonal relationships. Therefore, all postpartum women and their families need information regarding the warning signs and symptoms. This teaching should be done as a part of routine postpartum discharge instructions. In fact, some states have mandated that every pregnant woman be given written information about postpartum depression along with a list of local resources as a part of prenatal care and again before discharge from the hospital after giving birth.

It is normal for the postpartum woman to be reluctant to verbalize any feelings of sadness or lack of enthusiasm about motherhood or child caring and rearing because of fear of rejection or feelings of guilt. Thus, the nurse plays a key role in dispelling the myth that happiness automatically occurs after the birth of a child.

Instruct the woman and her family that postpartum depression can occur at any time after delivery. Therefore, the family needs to keep a listening ear to the woman's concerns. Instruct the family to be especially alert for complaints about problems sleeping, lack of energy or interest in daily activities, or fatigue out of proportion to the woman's status. It is especially important the woman understand that she should seek help immediately if she has thoughts of harming herself or her baby.

Once postpartum depression has been diagnosed, acknowledge any feelings that the woman expresses. Avoid statements that provide false reassurance or that discount the woman's feelings, such as, "Don't worry, you'll feel better soon," or "Your baby is so cute. You shouldn't feel so sad!" Assist the woman in obtaining support as necessary. Contact with others in a support group can help to alleviate feelings of isolation.

Postpartum Psychosis

Postpartum psychosis refers to a condition that usually occurs within the first 2 to 3 weeks after delivery, possibly as early as the 1st or 2nd day. With this disorder, the woman exhibits severe distortions of reality. This condition occurs in approximately 1 to 2 women for

A PERSONAL GLIMPSE

When I gave birth to our oldest daughter, my husband and I were living away from our families and friends. I remember bringing our daughter home from the hospital and feeling completely overwhelmed and anxious. Our daughter was fussy and didn't nurse well. I had no mother, sister, or girlfriend nearby to talk with or get advice from. My husband was calm and very supportive, but he worked full-time shift work. I remember feeling so lonely and depressed. I kept thinking that these feelings would go away after a few weeks. But they didn't. I wasn't eating or sleeping well, and I know I was miserable to be around. I felt completely inadequate as a mother. Finally, after 8 weeks of this my husband suggested we go see the doctor. Reluctantly, I made an appointment. When we first got to the doctor's office, the nurse sat down with us to ask us questions. When she asked why we were there, I started crying but managed to explain what I had been feeling since the birth of our daughter. She handed me some tissues and put her hand on my arm. She assured me that she and the doctor would work with me to help me feel better and return to my normal emotional state.

I am so glad that my husband suggested I get help. The doctor gave me a prescription for Paxil, and the nurse gave me all sorts of great suggestions, like joining a new mom support group and making sure that I got daily exercise. In just a few weeks, I felt so much better and now have much more confidence in my ability to be a mother to our daughter.

Lynne

LEARNING OPPORTUNITY: What clues did this woman give that indicate she was suffering from postpartum depression versus the "baby blues?" What specific actions can the nurse take to quickly recognize and provide support for the woman who has postpartum depression?

every 1,000 births (Beck, 2003; Simpson & Creehan, 2001). It is considered an emergency situation requiring immediate treatment. With treatment, postpartum psychosis generally spans 2 to 3 months.

Clinical Manifestations

Typically the woman with postpartum psychosis exhibits manifestations similar to those for any woman experiencing psychosis. Symptoms often associated with schizophrenia, bipolar disorder, or major depression may be noted. The woman with postpartum psychosis may demonstrate the following:

- Delusions that may cause her to believe that the infant is dead or defective

- Hallucinations, which may involve voices telling the woman to kill herself or her child
- Severe agitation, restlessness, or irritability
- Hyperactivity, euphoria, or little concern for self or infant (manic phase of bipolar disorder)
- Depression including preoccupation with guilt, feelings of worthlessness and isolation, extreme overconcern for the infant's health, and sleep disturbances
- Poor judgment and confusion

Because of the woman's misperception of reality, suicide and infanticide are possible.

Treatment

Postpartum psychosis is a psychiatric emergency requiring immediate treatment. Typically the woman requires hospitalization with treatment focusing on her specific symptoms. Medications such as antipsychotic agents and antidepressants are used. In addition, suicide precautions may be necessary. The woman's family should be involved in the treatment plan.

Nursing Care

The care of the woman with postpartum psychosis requires specialized psychiatric training beyond the scope of practice for the obstetric nurse. However, all nurses need to be aware of the signs and symptoms of postpartum psychosis so that early detection and prompt intervention can occur.

SPECIAL POSTPARTUM SITUATIONS

In addition to complications that can occur in the postpartum period, two other situations may require nursing intervention. These include grief and malattachment.

Grief in the Postpartal Period

Typically, the postpartum period is thought of as a happy time of celebrating the birth of a newborn. However, not all pregnancies conclude in a happy family taking home a healthy newborn. These situations may include the woman who is placing her newborn for adoption; the family faced with a newborn with congenital anomalies; and the family whose newborn (fetus) dies.

Grief is a universal process that is experienced uniquely by each individual. Grief is a natural response to a loss; whether the loss is the result of a choice, such as occurs with adoption; or when the situation is completely out of the individual's control, such

as occurs when the newborn has a congenital anomaly or dies. Shock and disbelief are most frequently the first feelings experienced. The feeling of numbness or unreality may last hours, days, or weeks. Anger, even to the point of rage, bargaining, and depression are natural stages of the grieving process. It is normal for individuals to pass in and out of the stages several times as they work through their feelings. When the individual reaches the acceptance stage, healing has usually occurred.

Frequently men and women differ in their responses to grief. These differences can cause a rift between the woman and her spouse unless the couple receives intervention to help them work through the differences. Sometimes the woman will respond to feelings of sadness and guilt with tearfulness and isolation. The man may respond to these same feelings by throwing himself into his work. The woman may misperceive that her spouse "doesn't care" or isn't grieving. Counseling is frequently beneficial.

The Woman Placing the Newborn for Adoption

Giving the newborn up for adoption is a complicated and difficult choice facing some women. The woman often enters into a very somber period of grief and detachment. Each case is unique and must be handled as the circumstances develop. Sometimes she is emotional and needs to discuss the dreams and hopes that she is releasing with this decision. Sometimes circumstances are beyond her control, leading her to this decision. In all cases, the woman requires support, personal care, and comfort through the early postpartum period.

The woman who is placing her newborn for adoption requires nonjudgmental support. It is critical for you to be aware of your own attitudes about the situation to avoid the temptation to influence the outcome toward your beliefs. Be very aware that your role is to be an advocate for the woman, which involves keeping her informed of her rights and options and supporting her in whatever decision that she makes. It is also important for you to recognize that each state has laws that govern the rights of each party in the adoption process. Be knowledgeable of your institution's policies regarding handling of the adoption process.

The Family Whose Newborn Has Congenital Anomalies

Helping parents adjust to a newborn with congenital anomalies is a challenge for the postpartum nurse. Involving a newborn specialist very early in this situation is important because many anomalies can be corrected with early interventions and neonatal surgery. Despite early positive interventions, the family still experiences a measure of loss and grief for the normal newborn, the perfect son or daughter.

For the family with a newborn who has a congenital anomaly, encourage frequent interaction. Point out positive features of the newborn. Role model healthy behaviors by talking and playing with the baby as you would with any newborn. Give the parents information about the disorder or point them in the direction of resources that can assist them as they make treatment decisions, etc. When the family goes home, they may benefit by participation in a parent support group.

The Family Whose Newborn (Fetus) Has Died

Death often forces individuals to face core issues and personal values; it leaves emotions raw while people struggle for meaning. When a newborn or fetus dies, the parents are often totally unprepared to deal with their new reality. They frequently voice questions to which there are no good answers. Each person and family will respond to the situation in their own way.

Coping with death of the fetus or newborn can be stressful for the nurse, as well as the family. You may feel inadequate to help and be tempted to withdraw from the situation. In planning care for the family whose newborn or fetus has died, it is important to recognize your feelings so that you don't let your feelings interfere with your ability to care for the woman and her family. It may be helpful to talk through your feelings with a friend or co-worker. Do not let personal beliefs and values overshadow the family's beliefs and values. Allow the family to experience their own grief process; provide assistance and support to the family in ways that are meaningful and helpful to them.

Several measures can help provide meaning to the family during this difficult time. Grief is not a process of forgetting sad occasions. Rather, it is a process of remembering good things about the person who died. The baby who died is a part of a family and has a place with them. The family can name their newborn, even if it was stillborn. Memory items such as footprints and hand prints, a name record, blessing, and souvenir birth record identify this baby as a member of a particular family. Parents have identified photos of the newborn as a precious memory. Keep in mind that the photos must be comforting photos, that is, ones with the baby clothed, washed, and positioned comfortably. Allow the family or mother to assist with clothes, bathing, animal toys, or blankets. The more the family is involved, the more memories they will have when they recall this difficult time. Each family is unique in their beliefs regarding death and burial. For some, this will be a very quiet process; for others it will be emotional and surrounded by many friends and family. Follow the cues set by the family.

Malattachment in the Postpartal Period

The relationship of attachment begins when a women first finds out that she is pregnant. Through the prenatal visits, the information about the well-being of her baby reinforces this attachment. As she hears the heart beat, sees the baby's movements on ultrasound, and feels the movement inside her uterus, the woman begins to perceive this something inside her body as a "someone" other than herself. Preparations of the nursery and choosing names continue this bonding process.

Many things influence the degree of attachment. A stable relationship, good prenatal course, and positive anticipation of a healthy infant help a woman to begin an internal relationship with her baby before he or she is born. This enduring emotional bond between the baby and a primary caregiver is called attachment. Difficulties during the pregnancy, immaturity of the woman, or an unreliable support system puts the family at risk for **malattachment** or emotional distancing in the maternal–infant relationship. Pregnancies after a miscarriage or infant death often give rise to fears that interfere with normal attachment. Pregnancy complications or difficult relationships with the father of the baby can also adversely affect attachment. In addition, alcohol and drug abuse can contribute to malattachment and infant neglect.

Key signs of malattachment include lack of eye contact, lack of verbal stimulation, and a lack of response to the newborn's cries or cues. Other direct observations that show evidence of malattachment are listed in Table 19-2. If you observe any of these signs, report them to the RN. Lack of bonding between the mother and her newborn can be very serious if the woman is allowed to go home without proper support. Therefore, interventions include involving the whole family in the bonding and care of the infant. Discharge planning includes a predischarge consult with a clinical psychologist or clinical social worker to assess

CULTURAL SNAPSHOT

In the United States, fathers take a more active role in the direct care of their newborns shortly after birth. Families from different cultures may incorporate other relatives in newborn care. Be careful not to misinterpret lack of the father's involvement as malattachment. Family cultural beliefs may prescribe that only female members, such as the woman's sisters, mother, or mother-in-law, are allowed to handle the baby until the child is older. In some cultures, the woman is expected to remain secluded at home for approximately 4 to 6 weeks after delivery. Ask the family directly about who will be attending to the needs of the woman and infant once they go home.

TABLE 19.2	Comparing Attachment and Malattachment	
Attachment	**Malattachment**	
Uses endearments and pet names	Speaks of the newborn as an object; "it"	
Speaks softly and uses "baby talk"	Makes no eye contact with the newborn	
Calls newborn by name, often	Does not use the newborn's name	
Becomes involved in routine care of diapering, bathing, and feeding	Shows disinterest in daily care and feeding of the newborn	
Holds newborn close to body or in direct face-to-face contact	Places newborn in crib or lays newborn on lap facing away from mother	
Responds to crying, smiling, feeding, and elimination with positive reinforcement	Ignores crying and newborn cue behaviors; reacts negatively to elimination needs	
Easily calms upset newborn	Does not perceive newborn's needs; newborn is frustrated and nervous	

support systems available for the mother. A referral for home care may be appropriate.

Test Yourself

- What signs indicate that the woman may be experiencing postpartum depression versus the "baby blues?"

- Name five stages of grief that individuals normally experience when faced with a loss.

- List three things the nurse can do to help a family cope with the birth of a newborn with a congenital anomaly.

KEY POINTS

- Hemorrhage, infection, thromboembolic disorders, and psychiatric disorders are conditions that put the postpartum woman at risk.
- Early postpartum hemorrhage occurs in the first 24 hours after birth and is most frequently caused by uterine atony. Late postpartum hemorrhage can occur anytime after the first 24 hours. Frequent causes are infection, subinvolution, and retained placental fragments.

- Nursing interventions for the woman with postpartum hemorrhage are focused on identifying the cause and stopping the bleeding. Establishing an IV line and frequent monitoring of vital signs and urinary output are critical actions. To determine the cause, assess the condition of the uterine fundus and characteristics of the lochia, and observe for shock and pain out of proportion with the observed blood loss, which may indicate concealed bleeding.

- Endometritis, infection of the uterine lining, is the most common postpartal infection. IV antibiotics are necessary for serious infections.

- Wound infection can involve the episiotomy or laceration or cesarean incision. Risk factors include chronic medical conditions, obesity, and any factor that decreases a woman's resistance. Antibiotic therapy and drainage of the wound may be required.

- Mastitis is a localized infection of breast tissue that is caused by milk stasis in a milk duct and infection with organisms that enter the breast through a crack or fissure in the nipple. Treatment involves antibiotics, emptying the breasts (preferably by breast-feeding), and warm compresses.

- Urinary tract infection (UTI) is the fourth type of infection that can complicate the postpartum period. Symptoms include frequency, urgency, and burning upon urination. Pyelonephritis is a more serious infection than cystitis because it involves the kidneys. Pyelonephritis is accompanied by high, intermittent fever with flank tenderness. Antibiotics are the therapy of choice.

- All postpartum women are at risk for thromboembolic disorders because of increased clotting factors that remain elevated after birth, exertion of the fetal head on the veins of the lower extremities during pregnancy, and the length of time in labor and delivery of being inactive or placed in stirrups, which can lead to stasis and pooling of blood in the extremities.

- The three psychiatric disorders that can affect the woman in the postpartum period include the postpartum blues, postpartum depression, and postpartum psychosis. Postpartum blues is temporary and self-limited tearfulness and blue mood. Depression is diagnosed if symptoms are interfering with the woman's ability to function in daily life for a period of 2 weeks or more. Psychosis occurs when the woman's perception of reality is distorted. Depression and psychosis require treatment by a mental health professional.

- The nurse's role is to support the woman who is grieving. Listen and be accepting of her feelings. Encourage the use of a support group and counseling for the couple. If the newborn dies, help the family make memories by encouraging them to hold the baby and say goodbye, by taking pictures, and by giving them a memento box with clothes the baby wore or blankets, etc.

▶ Malattachment may be occurring if the woman does not interact with or hold her baby. If she turns away or doesn't talk to the baby or call him by name, she may be having problems with attachment. Notify the RN if you notice any of these symptoms.

REFERENCES AND SELECTED READINGS

Books and Journals

American College of Obstetricians and Gynecologists (ACOG). (1998). *Postpartum hemorrhage*. ACOG Technical Bulletin, 243. Washington, DC. Author.

Anderson, P. O. (2002). *Safety of commonly used drugs in nursing mothers*. UCSD Medical Center Department of Pharmacy. Retrieved April 25, 2004, from http://health.ucsd.edu/pharmacy/resources/breastfeeding.htm

Beck, C. T. (2003). Recognizing and screening for postpartum depression in mothers of NICU infants. *Advances in Neonatal Care, 3*(1), 37–46. Retrieved April 25, 2004, from http://www.medscape.com/viewarticle/450938

Chandran, L. (2003). Endometritis. In E. Alderman, R. Konop, W. Wolfram, P. D. Petry, & M. Strafford (Eds.), *eMedicine*. Retrieved April 23, 2004, from http://www.emedicine.com/ped/topic678.htm

Cheng, D. (2003). *Postpartum depression*. Focus on Women's Health Article: U.S. Department of Health and Human Services, Office on Women's Health. Retrieved April 24, 2004, from http://www.4woman.gov/HealthPro/healtharticle/

Cheng, D., & D'Agnati, D. D. (2002). *About postpartum depression*. State of Maryland, Department of Health and Mental Hygiene. Retrieved September 27, 2002, from http://mdpublichealth.org/womenshealth/pdf/postpartum_booklet.pdf

Cockey, C. D. (2003). Low-dose warfarin prevents clot recurrence. *AWHONN Lifelines, 7*(2), 106–108.

Cunningham, F. G., Gant, N. F., Leveno, K. J., Gilstrap, L. C. III, Hauth, J. C., & Wenstrom, K. D. (2001). *Williams obstetrics* (21st ed.). New York: McGraw-Hill Medical Publishing Division.

Depression After Delivery, Inc. (2001). *Postpartum psychosis*. Retrieved September 27, 2002, from http://www.depressionafterdelivery.com

Franzblau, N., & Witt, K. (2002). Normal and abnormal puerperium. In R. Levine, F. Talavera, G. F. Whitman-Elia, G. B. Gaupp, & L. P. Shulman (Eds.), *eMedicine*. Retrieved April 23, 2004, from http://emedicine.com/med/topic3240.htm

Hanna, B., Jarman, H., Savage, S., & Layton, K. (2004). The early detection of postpartum depression: Midwives and nurses trial a checklist. *JOGNN, 33*(2), 191–197.

Kennedy, E. (2003). Pregnancy, postpartum infections. In A. J. Sayah, F. Talavera, M. Zwanger, J. Halamka, &

R. O'Connor (Eds.), *eMedicine*. Retrieved April 23, 2004, from http://www.emedicine.com/emerg/topic482.htm

Mandeville, L. K., & Troiano, N. H. (Eds.). (1999). *High-risk and critical care intrapartum nursing*. AWHONN publication (2nd ed.). Philadelphia: Lippincott Williams & Wilkins.

Maternal & Neonatal Health. (Undated). Preventing postpartum hemorrhage: Active management of the third stage of labor. *Maternal & Neonatal Health: Best Practices*. Retrieved September 1, 2002, from http://www.mnh.jhpiego.org/best/pphactmng.pdf

Mattson, S., & Smith, J. E. (Eds.). (2000). *Core curriculum for maternal–newborn nursing*. AWHONN publication (2nd ed.). Philadelphia: WB Saunders.

Roman, A. S., & Rebarber, A. (2003). Seven ways to control postpartum hemorrhage. *Contemporary OB/GYN, 48*(3), 34–53. Retrieved April 23, 2004, from http://www.medscape.com/viewarticle/451545

Schreiber, D. (2002). Deep vein thrombosis and thrombophlebitis. In F. Counselman, F. Talavera, G. Setnik, J. Halamka, & B. Brenner (Eds.), *eMedicine*. Retrieved April 24, 2004, from http://www.emedicine.com/emerg/topic122.htm

Simmons, G. T., & Bammel, B. (2001). Endometritis. In A. C. Sciscione, F. Talavera, A. V. Sison, F. B. Gaupp, & L. P. Shulman (Eds.), *eMedicine*. Retrieved April 23, 2004, from http://www.emedicine.com/med/topic676.htm

Simpson, K. R., & Creehan, P. A. (2001). *AWHONN Association of Women's Health, Obstetric and Neonatal Nurses: Perinatal Nursing*. Philadelphia: Lippincott Williams & Wilkins.

Singhal, H., & Zammit, C. (2002). Wound infection. In B. J. Daley, F. Talavera, A. L. Friedman, M. E. Zevitz, & J. Geibel (Eds.), *eMedicine*. Retrieved April 24, 2004, from http://www.emedicine.com/med/topic2422.htm

Stillman, R. M. (2002). Wound care. In B. J. Daley, F. Talavera, A. L. Friedman, M. E. Zevitz, & J. Geibel (Eds.), *eMedicine*. Retrieved April 24, 2004, from http://www.emedicine.com/med/topic2754.htm

Wainscott, M. P. (2003). Pregnancy, postpartum hemorrhage. In A. J. Sayah, F. Talavera, M. Zwanger, J. Halamka, & S. H. Plantz (Eds.), *eMedicine*. Retrieved April 23, 2004, from http://www.emedicine.com/emerg/topic481.htm

Yokoe, D. S., Christiansen, C. L., Johnson, R., Sands, K. E., Livingston, J., Shtatland, E. S., & Platt, R. (2001). Epidemiology of and surveillance for postpartum infections. *Emerging Infectious Diseases, 7*, 837–841. Retrieved April 23, 2004, from www.cdc.gov/ncidod/eid/vol7no5/pdf/yokoe.pdf

Zimmerman, D. (undated). *Medical care of the breastfeeding mother*. Retrieved April 24, 2004, from http://www.terem.com/abstracts40.htm

Websites
Postpartum Hemorrhage
http://www.babycenter.com/refcap/baby/physrecovery/1152328.html
http://pregnancy.about.com/cs/postpartumrecover/a/pph.htm

Postpartum Depression
http://www.nimh.nih.gov/publicat/depwomenknows.cfm
http://www.4woman.gov/faq/postpartum.pdf

WORKBOOK

NCLEX-STYLE REVIEW QUESTIONS

1. A woman is in for her postpartum checkup. She has a fever of 101°F and reports abdominal pain and a "bad smell" to her lochia. What diagnosis do you suspect?

   a. Mastitis

   b. Endometritis

   c. Subinvolution

   d. Episiotomy infection

2. The nurse enters the room of a woman who delivered 12 hours ago. The woman is leaning forward in bed and is obviously having difficulty breathing. The area around her mouth is blue. What should the nurse do first?

   a. Administer oxygen by nasal cannula.

   b. Obtain arterial blood for blood gas analysis.

   c. Raise the head of the bed.

   d. Tell the woman that she doesn't need to worry.

3. A woman delivered a healthy baby girl 2 days ago. Which observation by the nurse indicates the need for additional assessment and follow-up? The woman

   a. actively participates in the care of her baby.

   b. comments that her baby has red hair like her grandmother.

   c. reports that she will be happy to get home because she doesn't like hospital food.

   d. tells a friend, referring to her baby, "it just cries all the time."

4. When caring for a postpartum woman who exhibits a large amount of bleeding, which areas would the nurse need to assess before the woman ambulates?

   a. Attachment, lochia color, complete blood cell count

   b. Blood pressure, pulse, complaints of dizziness

   c. Degree of responsiveness, respiratory rate, fundus location

   d. Height, level of orientation, support systems

STUDY ACTIVITIES

1. Use the following table to compare superficial and deep vein thrombophlebitis.

	Superficial Thrombophlebitis	Deep Vein Thrombophlebitis
Clinical manifestations		
Diagnosis		
Treatment		
Nursing care		

2. Research the resources in your community for postpartum depression. How many of these are available at no charge to the woman? How can the woman find out about these resources? Share your findings with your clinical group.

3. Develop a teaching plan for young teenage mothers to help them decrease their chances for developing a postpartum infection.

CRITICAL THINKING: What Would You Do?

Apply your knowledge of postpartum complications to the following situation.

1. Josie is an outgoing 15-year-old girl who delivered a baby girl 24 hours ago. You walk in because you hear the newborn crying. Josie is talking to a friend on the telephone about the football game next week. When you check on the baby in the crib beside Josie's bed, the baby is jittery and red in the face.

   a. What is your impression of this situation? What ongoing assessments will you do to evaluate this situation?

   b. What do you need to do for the baby? Which individuals do you need to involve in the discharge planning process?

2. You just received Tiffany from the labor and delivery (L&D) unit after a normal delivery of a little girl. Her fundus is slightly firm, above the umbilicus, and positioned to the right. Her sanitary pad is full, but the L&D nurse reported that she received perineal care just before transport.

a. What is the likely source of the heavy lochia? What nursing interventions should be done?

b. If the fundus remains firm and in the midline, but a steady flow of lochia is noted despite fundal massage, what do you suspect is causing the problem? What nursing interventions should be done in this instance?

3. A woman who had a cesarean birth 3 days ago asks you to look at her incision, which is red and warm to touch with a small amount of yellow drainage along the edges.

a. What conclusions do you reach as a result of your assessment? What additional assessments should be made? What interventions are appropriate in this situation?

b. What if the woman reported hardness in an area of one of her breasts? How would you assess her breasts? What instructions would you give her?

The Newborn at Risk: Gestational and Acquired Disorders

20

STUDENT OBJECTIVES

On completion of this chapter, the student will be able to

1. Explain the various components of the gestational age assessment.
2. Classify the high-risk newborn by birth weight and gestational age while anticipating related problems.
3. Differentiate symmetric and asymmetric growth retardation in SGA infants.
4. Compare and contrast the characteristics of premature, full-term, and post-term newborns.
5. List possible contributing factors for preterm birth.
6. Identify five complications associated with preterm newborns.
7. List the characteristics of a post-term newborn.
8. Identify the major acquired disorders associated with newborns.
9. Describe the signs and symptoms commonly assessed in newborns with an acquired disorder, such as meconium aspiration syndrome.
10. Discuss the care needed for a newborn of a chemically dependent mother and one with a congenitally acquired infection.

KEY TERMS

apnea
appropriate for gestational age (AGA)
asphyxia
aspiration
Erb palsy
erythroblastosis fetalis
gestational age
hemolysis
hydramnios
hyperbilirubinemia
hypoglycemia
intrauterine growth restriction (IUGR)
intraventricular hemorrhage
kernicterus
large for gestational age (LGA)
lecithin
low birth weight (LBW)
macroglossia
macrosomia
meconium aspiration
necrotizing enterocolitis (NEC)
polycythemia
post-term
preterm
respiratory distress syndrome (RDS)
retinopathy of prematurity (ROP)
ruddy
small for gestational age (SGA)
surfactant
term
very low birth weight (VLBW) 1500 gm

The majority of newborns are born around 40 weeks' gestation weighing from 5.5 to 10 lb (2.5 to 4.6 kg) and measuring 18 inches to 23 inches (45 to 55 cm) in length. However, variations in **gestational age** (the length of time between fertilization of the egg and birth of the infant) and variations in birth weight occur. These variations increase the newborn's risk for perinatal problems. In addition, newborns also may develop problems at birth or soon after birth. These problems may be the result of conditions present in the woman during pregnancy or at the time of delivery, events occurring or factors present with delivery, or possibly the result of an unknown cause. Regardless, these acquired disorders also place the newborn at risk for serious health problems.

VARIATIONS IN SIZE AND GESTATIONAL AGE

Newborns may be classified based on their size or gestational age. When using size, the newborn's weight, length, and head circumference are considered. Size classifications include:

- **small for gestational age (SGA),** which is a newborn whose weight, length, and/or head circumference falls below the 10th percentile for gestational age;
- **appropriate for gestational age (AGA),** which is a newborn whose weight, length, and/or head circumference falls between the 10th and 90th percentiles for gestational age; and
- **large for gestational age (LGA),** which is an infant whose weight, length, and/or head circumference is above the 90th percentile for gestational age.

Two other classifications, based on weight, may be used to classify newborns by size. **Low birth-weight (LBW)** newborns are those who weigh less than 2,500 g. **Very low–birth-weight (VLBW)** newborns weigh less than 1,500 g.

Newborn classification based on gestational age includes:

- **preterm,** or premature, a newborn born at 37 weeks' gestation or less; commonly called premature
- **post-term,** or postmature, a newborn born at 42 weeks' or more gestation
- **term,** a newborn who is born between the beginning of week 38 and the end of week 41 of gestation.

A gestational age assessment is key to determining a newborn's classification.

GESTATIONAL AGE ASSESSMENT

Assessment of gestational age is a critical evaluation. The registered nurse (RN) is ultimately responsible for performing the gestational age assessment. However, the licensed vocational/practical nurse (LPN) should be familiar with the instruments used and be able to differentiate characteristics of the full-term newborn from those of the premature or post-term newborn. Although prenatal estimates, particularly the sonogram, are fairly accurate in determining gestational age, the most precise way to assess gestational age is through direct evaluation of the newborn. Several tools are available to assist the nurse in determining gestational age. The Newborn Maturity Rating and Classification developed by Ballard (Fig. 20-1) is a common gestational age assessment tool used in newborn nurseries. This tool is used as a basis for the discussion below.

Gestational age assessment typically involves the evaluation of two main categories of maturity: physical and neuromuscular maturity. Physical maturity can be assessed immediately after birth. Generally, the physical characteristics remain fairly constant and do not change rapidly with time. However, neuromuscular maturity, as evidenced by neuromuscular characteristics, can be influenced by several factors, such as medications given to the mother during labor and the time that has elapsed since birth. Therefore, it is best to do a gestational age assessment within the first few hours after birth. If the newborn is premature or postmature, it is important to have that information early on because his needs will differ from those of the term newborn.

Physical Maturity

Six categories are rated to determine physical maturity. These include:

1. Skin
2. Lanugo
3. Plantar creases
4. Breast buds
5. Ears
6. Genitals

Each category is rated on a scale of 0 to 5, with 5 being the highest or most completed development. Table 20-1 summarizes the gestational assessment findings in a term, premature, and postmature newborn.

Neuromuscular Maturity

Like physical maturity, six categories are rated. These categories are:

	0	1	2	3	4	5
SKIN	gelatinous red, trans-parent	smooth pink, visible veins	superficial peeling &/or rash, few veins	cracking pale area, rare veins	parchment, deep cracking, no vessels	leathery, cracked, wrinkled
LANUGO	none	abundant	thinning	bald areas	mostly bald	
PLANTAR CREASES	no crease	faint red marks	anterior transverse crease only	creases ant. 2/3	creases cover entire sole	
BREAST	barely percept.	flat areola, no bud	stippled areola, 1–2 mm bud	raised areola, 3–4 mm bud	full areola, 5–10 mm bud	
EAR	pinna flat, stays folded	sl. curved pinna, soft with slow recoil	well-curv. pinna, soft but ready recoil	formed & firm with instant recoil	thick cartilage, ear stiff	
GENITALS Male	scrotum empty, no rugae		testes descend-ing, few rugae	testes down, good rugae	testes pendulous, deep rugae	
GENITALS Female	prominent clitoris & labia minora		majora & minora equally prominent	majora large, minora small	clitoris & minora completely covered	

A

B

Score	Wks
5	26
10	28
15	30
20	32
25	34
30	36
35	38
40	40
45	42
50	44

C

● **Figure 20.1** Ballard's assessment of gestational age criteria. (**A**) Physical maturity assessment criteria. (**B**) Neuromuscular maturity assessment criteria. *Posture*: With infant supine and quiet, score as follows: arms and legs extended = 0; slight or moderate flexion of hips and knees = 2; legs flexed and abducted, arms slightly flexed = 3; full flexion of arms and legs = 4. *Square Window*: Flex hand at the wrist. Exert pressure sufficient to get as much flexion as possible. The angle between hypothenar eminence and anterior aspect of forearm is measured and scored. Do not rotate wrist. *Arm Recoil*: With infant supine, fully flex forearm for 5 sec, then fully extend by pulling the hands and release. Score as follows: remain extended or random movements = 0; incomplete or partial flexion = 2; brisk return to full flexion = 4. *Popliteal Angle*: With infant supine and pelvis flat on examining surface, flex leg on thigh and fully flex thigh with one hand. With the other hand, extend leg and score the angle attained according to the chart. *Scarf Sign*: With infant supine, draw infant's hand across the neck and as far across the opposite shoulder as possible. Assistance to elbow is permissible by lifting it across the body. Score according to location of the elbow: elbow reaches opposite anterior axillary line = 0; elbow between opposite anterior axillary line and midline of the thorax = 1; elbow at midline of thorax = 2; elbow does not reach midline of thorax = 3; elbow at proximal axillary line = 4. *Heel to Ear*: With infant supine, hold infant's foot with one hand and move it as near to the head as possible without forcing it. Keep pelvis flat on examining surface. (**C**) Scoring for a Ballard assessment scale. The point total from assessment is compared to the left column. The matching number in the right column reveals the infant's age in gestation weeks. (From: Ballard, J. L. [1991]. New Ballard score expanded to include extremely premature infants. *Journal of Pediatrics, 119,* 417–423.)

1. Posture
2. Square window (measurement of wrist angle with flexion toward forearm until resistance is met)
3. Arm recoil (extension and release of arm after arm is completely flexed and held in position for approximately 5 seconds)
4. Popliteal angle (measurement of knee angle on flexion of thigh with extension of lower leg until resistance is met)
5. Scarf sign (arm pulled gently in front of and across top portion of body until resistance is met)
6. Heel to ear (movement of foot to near the head as possible)

Each category is rated on a scale of 0 to 5. See Table 20-1 for a summary of the findings associated with term, premature, and postmature newborns.

THE SMALL-FOR-GESTATIONAL-AGE NEWBORN

Small for gestational age (SGA) is a term used to describe a baby who is born smaller than the average size in weight for the number of weeks' gestation at the time of delivery. The criterion is that the SGA newborn's weight falls below the 10th percentile of that

TABLE 20.1	Comparing Gestational Age Assessment Findings		
Assessment Parameter	**Term Newborn**	**Preterm Newborn**	**Post-term Newborn**
Physical Maturity			
Skin	Cracking of the skin and few visible veins	Very thin with little subcutaneous fat and easily visible veins	Leathery, cracked, and wrinkled
Lanugo	Thinning of lanugo with balding areas	Abundance of fine downy hair up to 34 weeks	Almost absent lanugo with many balding areas
Plantar creases	Creases covering at least the anterior 2/3 of foot	Smooth feet with few creases	Creases covering entire foot
Breast buds	Raised areola with 3- to 4-mm breast bud	Flat areola with little to no breast bud	Full areola with 5- to 10-mm breast bud
Ear	Cartilage present within pinna with ability for natural recoil when folded	Little cartilage, allowing shape to be maintained when folded	Cartilage thick; pinna stiff
Genitals	Male with pendulous scrotum covered with rugae; testicles descended	Male with smooth scrotum and undescended testicles	Male with pendulous scrotum with deep rugae
	Female with large labia major covering minora	Female with prominent clitoris; labia minora not covered by majora	Female with clitoris and labia minora completely covered by labia majora
Neuromuscular Maturity			
Posture	Flexed position with good muscle tone	Hypotonic with extension of the extremities	Full flexion of arms and legs
Square window	Flexible wrists with a small angle, usually ranging from 0 to 30 degrees	Angle greater than 45 degrees	Similar to that for term newborn
Arm recoil	Quick recoil with angle at elbow less than 90 degrees	Slowed recoil time with angle greater than 90 degrees	Similar to that for term newborn
Popliteal angle	Resistance to extension with knee angle 90 degrees or less	Decreased resistance to extension with large angle at knee	Similar to that for term newborn
Scarf sign	Increased resistance to movement with elbow unable to reach midline	Increased flexibility with elbow extending past midline	Similar to that for term newborn
Heel to ear	Moderate resistance to movement	Little to no resistance to movement	Similar to that for term newborn

which is expected. Gestationally, the newborn may be preterm, term, or post-term. It is preferred that the SGA baby is identified before birth, typically using the ultrasound method, allowing the health care team to determine anticipated treatment.

The SGA newborn usually appears physically and neurologically mature but is smaller in size than other infants of the same gestational age. These infants are often weak, unable to tolerate large feedings, and experience difficulty staying warm.

Although some SGA babies are small because their parents are small (genetics), most are small because of circumstances that occurred during the pregnancy, causing limited fetal growth. This condition is known as **intrauterine growth restriction (IUGR)**. It occurs when the fetus does not receive adequate amounts of oxygen and nutrients necessary for the proper growth and development of organs and tissues. IUGR can begin at any time during the pregnancy.

Contributing Factors

IUGR, the most common underlying condition leading to SGA newborns, results from interference in the supply of nutrients to the fetus. Lack of adequate maternal nutrition may be a contributing factor. As a result, the mother is unable to meet the increased nutritional demands of pregnancy. Thus, the fetus does not receive the necessary nutrients for growth. Another factor may involve an abnormality in the placenta or its function.

If a mother smokes during pregnancy, the newborn's birth weight can be reduced by 200 grams. Maternal tobacco use is the most common preventable cause of IUGR.

The placenta may have become damaged, such as when the placenta separates prematurely, or a decrease in blood flow to the placenta reduces its ability to transport nutrients. Maternal conditions that interfere with adequate blood flow to the placenta, such as pregnancy-induced hypertension or uncontrolled diabetes, contribute to placental malfunction. In some situations, placental functioning may be normal, but the fetus is unable to use the nutrients being supplied, such as when the fetus develops an intrauterine infection.

Common factors leading to a restriction in growth rate associated with SGA newborns include:

- Chromosomal abnormalities
- Congenital defects
- Congenital infections
- Multiple gestations in which each fetus competes for supplied nutrients in the blood
- Maternal history of long-term problems, such as chronic kidney disease, high blood pressure, severe malnutrition or anemia, intrauterine infection, substance abuse, and cigarette smoking
- Fetal nutritional deficiencies
- Maternal complications during pregnancy, such as gestational diabetes, placental abruption or placenta previa, preeclampsia, or pregnancy-induced hypertension (PIH)

Characteristics of the SGA Newborn

Typically, SGA newborns experiencing IUGR are classified as symmetrically growth restricted or asymmetrically growth restricted, based on appearance.

Symmetrically Growth-Restricted Newborns

The symmetrically growth-restricted newborn accounts for 90% of IUGR newborns. These newborns have not grown at the expected rate for gestational age on standard growth charts. Generally, all three growth measurements (weight, length, and head circumference), when plotted on a standard growth chart, fall below the 10th percentile. Because there is prolonged limited growth in the size of organs affecting body growth, both head and body parts are in proportion but are below normal size for gestational age.

The newborn may appear active on inspection and demonstrate more developed neurologic responses because of a more advanced age in comparison to size. However, the newborn typically appears wasted with poor skin turgor. Sutures in the skull may be separated widely, and the abdomen may be sunken.

If the fetus experienced hypoxia early on in gestation and this hypoxia continued throughout the pregnancy, the newborn is at an increased risk for central nervous system (CNS) abnormalities and developmental delays.

Asymmetrically Growth-Restricted Newborns

The asymmetrically growth-restricted newborn has not grown at the expected rate for gestational age based on standard growth charts. When the three growth measurements (weight, length, and head circumference) are plotted on a standard growth chart, one of the measurements falls below the 10th percentile. Accounting for 10% of IUGR, these newborns typically are those with normal measurements for head circumference and length but demonstrate a comparatively low birth weight.

Asymmetrically growth-restricted newborns typically appear thin and pale with loose dry skin. They have a wasted, wide-eyed look, with a head that is disproportionately large when compared with body size. The umbilical cord appears thin and dull looking, compared with the shiny, plump cord of an AGA or LGA newborn.

Typically, these newborns demonstrate more developed organ systems, resulting in fewer neurologic complications and an improved survival rate when compared with newborns with symmetrical growth restriction. However, the newborn still may encounter many other risks and complications.

Potential Complications

Harsh conditions in utero can lead to a decrease in the amount of oxygen available to the fetus (hypoxia), causing the fetus to experience chronic fetal distress. Unable to meet the demands of normal labor and birth because of intrauterine fetal distress, the fetus will gasp in utero or with the first breaths at delivery, resulting in **aspiration** (when the baby breaths fluid into the lungs) of amniotic fluid or fluid containing the first stool called meconium.

The growth-restricted fetus is at increased risk for cesarean delivery because of fetal distress. Birth by cesarean predisposes the newborn to a respiratory distress condition called transient tachypnea of the newborn (TTN), which is caused by retained fetal lung fluid.

Because of the high demand for metabolic fuel and loss of brown fat used to survive in utero, coupled with the large ratio of body surface area to weight, the SGA newborn may experience thermoregulation problems (difficulty maintaining body temperature). As a result, the newborn may develop hypothermia. In addition, the newborn typically experiences **hypoglycemia** (low blood sugar) because of a high metabolic rate in response to heat loss and low glycogen stores. Hypoglycemia is the most common complication.

In response to chronic hypoxia in utero, red blood cell production increases, leading to **polycythemia** (excess number of red blood cells). Polycythemia also is caused by endocrine, metabolic, or chromosomal disorders of the SGA newborn and can occur with placental transfusion at the time of delivery.

Nursing Care

The care provider or RN is responsible for assessing gestational age and identifying potential complications. The LPN aids in carrying out the measures as identified in the plan of care for the SGA newborn at risk. Expect to perform routine newborn care with a focus on breathing and blood glucose patterns, thermoregulation, and parental interaction.

Review the maternal history and note any factors that might contribute to SGA. Estimate gestational age to determine SGA status and establish if IUGR is symmetric or asymmetric. Be alert for potential complications and risk factors of the newborn related to respiratory distress, hypothermia, hypoglycemia, polycythemia, and altered parental interaction with the newborn. Conduct and document routine nursing care with special emphasis on the following:

- Monitor respiratory status, including respiratory rate and pattern and observe for signs and symptoms of respiratory distress, such as cyanosis, nasal flaring, and expiratory grunting
- Provide measures to maintain skin temperature between 36.5°C and 37.0°C (97.7°F to 98.6°F)
- Monitor blood glucose levels to maintain levels >40 mg/dL
- Monitor results of other blood studies, such as hematocrit (<65%), hemoglobin (<22 g/dL), and bilirubin (<12 mg/dL)

- Observe feeding tolerance, including amounts taken and any difficulties or problems encountered, such as inability to suck at breast, fatigue, excessive spitting up, or diarrhea
- Monitor intake and output and daily weights
- Observe for jaundice
- Encourage parents to visit frequently and care for their infant

THE LARGE-FOR-GESTATIONAL AGE NEWBORN

A large-for-gestational age (LGA) newborn is one who is larger than the average baby. More precisely, an LGA newborn is one whose weight when plotted on a standard growth chart is above the 90th percentile. Typically the newborn weighs more than 4,000 grams. Generally, the newborn's overall body size is proportional, but both head and weight fall in the upper limits of intrauterine growth charts. Most LGA infants are genetically or nutritionally adequate. However, their size is misleading because development often is immature because of gestational age.

Some newborns are categorized as LGA incorrectly due to miscalculation of the date of conception. Therefore a thorough assessment of gestational age is essential to identify potential problems and requirements of these newborns.

Contributing Factors

In the majority of cases, the underlying cause of the large size of the LGA newborn is unknown. However, certain factors have been identified. Genetic factors may contribute to the development of large size in the newborn. For example, parents who are large have an increased tendency for a LGA newborn. Male newborns also are typically larger than female newborns. In addition, multiparous women have two to three times the number of LGA newborns than do primiparous women. The belief is that with each succeeding pregnancy, the fetus grows larger.

Congenital disorders also have been implicated. Beckwith's syndrome, a rare genetic disorder is associated with excessive intrauterine growth, causing hormonally induced excessive weight gain and **macroglossia** (abnormally large tongue), which can cause feeding difficulties. Transposition of the great vessels, a congenital heart disease, also is associated with LGA newborns. Other factors include umbilical abnormalities, such as omphalocele, hypoglycemia, and hyperinsulinemia of the newborn.

Maternal diabetes is the most widely known contributing factor. LGA newborns are frequently born to diabetic women with poor glucose control. Continued high blood glucose levels in the women lead to an increase in insulin production in the fetus. Increased insulin levels act as a fetal growth hormone, causing **macrosomia**, an unusually large newborn with a birth weight of greater than 4,500 grams (9 lbs 14 oz). After birth, the pancreas of the LGA newborn continues to produce high levels of insulin. However, the newborn is no longer exposed to the elevated glucose levels of the mother; therefore, the newborn's blood sugar falls leading to hypoglycemia.

Characteristics of the LGA Newborn

A newborn who is LGA typically demonstrates less motor skills ability and difficulty in regulating behavioral states (more difficult to arouse and maintain a quiet alert state). Commonly, a LGA newborn exhibits immaturity with reflex testing and possibly signs and symptoms of birth trauma, such as bruising or a broken clavicle. In addition, the newborn's skull may show evidence of molding, cephalohematoma, or caput succedaneum.

Potential Complications

Most commonly, LGA newborns develop complications associated with the increase in body size. This increased size is a leading cause of breech position and shoulder dystocia, which results in an increased incidence of birth injuries and trauma from a difficult extraction. Subsequent problems include fractured skull or clavicles; cervical or brachial plexus injury from peripheral nerve damage; and **Erb palsy** (a facial paralysis resulting from injury to the cervical nerves).

Trauma to the central nervous system can occur during birth. As a result, perfusion to the fetus is decreased. Oxygen and carbon dioxide exchange is diminished, ultimately resulting in **asphyxia** (severe hypoxia). CNS trauma also can interfere with the newborn's ability to maintain thermoregulation.

Frequently the LGA infant's head size diameter is disproportionately larger than the mother's pelvic outlet, creating cephalopelvic disproportion (CPD). As a result, cesarean delivery may be necessary. Subsequently, the LGA newborn is at risk for additional complications, such as those associated with effects of anesthesia. Other complications may include respiratory distress syndrome and transient tachypnea of the newborn.

Nursing Care

Identifying the newborn at risk for LGA is important for anticipating the plan of care. Carefully review the maternal history for any risk factors that would con-

tribute to an LGA newborn. Note any prenatal ultrasound reports, such as fetal skull size measurement. Estimate gestational age to determine LGA status. Conduct and document routine nursing care with a special emphasis on the following:

- Monitor vital signs frequently, especially respiratory status for changes indicating respiratory distress
- Observe for signs and symptoms of hypoglycemia, including monitoring results of blood glucose levels
- Note any signs of birth trauma or injury
- Help parents verbalize feelings about any bruising or trauma they notice, including their fears of causing their newborn more pain
- Encourage parent–newborn bonding by providing interaction and support, such as showing how to arouse a sleepy newborn, console a fussy newborn, and offer feedings

Test Yourself

- What two major areas are evaluated with a gestational age assessment?
- What is the underlying factor commonly associated with most SGA newborns?
- LGA newborns are at an increased risk for what complications associated with their size?

THE PRETERM NEWBORN

At one time, prematurity was defined only on the basis of birth weight: any live infant weighing 2,500 g (5 lb 8 oz) or less at birth. Time proved this definition inadequate because some term infants weigh less than 2,500 g, and some premature infants weigh more than 2,500 g. The American Academy of Pediatrics advocates the use of the term "preterm": (premature) infant to mean any infant of less than 37 weeks' gestation.

Determining the gestational age of the preterm newborn is crucial. The Dubowitz scoring system was devised as an assessment tool based on external and neurologic development. Variations of the system are currently in use in many hospitals (see discussion of gestational age assessment and Figure 20-1 earlier in this chapter). The newborn is evaluated by the criteria on the chart, and the gestational age of the infant is calculated from the score. This assessment usually is performed within the first 24 hours of life and at least by the time the newborn is 42 hours old.

The preterm infant's untimely departure from the uterus may mean that various organs and systems are not sufficiently mature to adjust to extrauterine life. Often, small community hospitals or birthing centers are not equipped to care adequately for the preterm infant. When preterm delivery is expected, the woman often is taken to a facility with a neonatal intensive care unit (NICU) before delivery. However, if delivery occurs before the woman can be transported, transportation of the newborn may be necessary. Teams of specially trained personnel may come from the NICU to transport the neonate by ambulance, van, or helicopter. The newborn is transported in a self-contained, battery-powered unit that provides warmth and oxygen. Intravenous (IV) fluids, monitors, and other emergency equipment also may be used during the transport of the newborn.

Contributing Factors

The underlying cause of preterm birth, in most cases, is unknown. Despite development of medication to control preterm uterine activity, controlling preterm labor to prevent preterm delivery remains a problem.

Most often, preterm births result from a combination of factors, such as poor health habits and diet, inadequate living conditions, and overwork of the pregnant woman. Other contributing factors include low income, frequent pregnancies occurring in close succession, and maternal age extremes (younger than 20 years and older than 40 years).

One of the most common factors contributing to preterm delivery is premature rupture of membranes (PROM). This may be due to various underlying conditions, such as acute or chronic maternal infection or disease.

Multiple births are often preterm because of **hydramnios** (excessive amniotic fluid), a larger than average intrauterine mass, and/or early cervical dilation. Other factors related to the birth of preterm newborns involve the need for earlier delivery to ensure maternal or fetal well-being. These include eclampsia from pregnancy-induced hypertension, placenta previa, and abruptio placenta.

Preterm births also may result from emotional or physical trauma to the woman, such as when the woman requires nonobstetric-related surgery; habitual abortion or habitual premature birth; fetal infection, such as syphilis; and fetal malformations.

Characteristics of the Preterm Newborn

Compared with the term infant, the preterm infant is tiny, scrawny, and red. The extremities are thin, with little muscle or subcutaneous fat. The head and abdomen are disproportionately large, and the skin is thin, relatively translucent, and usually wrinkled. Veins of the abdomen and scalp are more visible. Lanugo is plentiful over the extremities, back, and shoulders. The ears have soft, minimal cartilage and thus are extremely pliable. The soft bones of the skull tend to flatten on the sides, and the ribs yield with each labored breath. Testes are undescended in the male; the labia and clitoris are prominent in the female. The soles of the feet and the palms of the hands have few creases (Fig. 20-2). Many of the typical newborn reflexes are weak or absent.

Complications of the Preterm Newborn

The preterm newborn's physiologic immaturity causes many difficulties involving virtually all body systems, the most critical of which is respiratory. Typically, respirations are shallow, rapid, and irregular, with periods of apnea (temporary interruption of the breathing impulse). Respirations may become so labored that the chest wall, perhaps even the sternum, is retracted.

Pediatricians and nursery staff should be alerted to the impending birth of a preterm infant so that equipment for resuscitation and emergency care is ready. If the birth occurs in a facility without a NICU, plans should be made to transport the newborn immediately after birth.

A

B

● *Figure 20.2* Sole creases in a preterm newborn (**A**) and a term newborn (**B**).

Respiratory Distress Syndrome

Respiratory distress syndrome (RDS), also known as hyaline membrane disease, occurs in about 50,000 of the 250,000 premature infants born in the United States each year. It occurs because the lungs are too immature to function properly. Normally, the lungs remain partially expanded after each breath because of a substance called **surfactant**, a biochemical compound that reduces surface tension inside the air sacs. The premature infant's lungs are deficient in surfactant and thus collapse after each breath, greatly reducing the infant's vital supply of oxygen. This damages the lung cells, and these damaged cells combine with other substances present in the lungs to form a fibrous substance called hyaline membrane. This membrane lines the alveoli and blocks gas exchange in the alveoli.

The preterm newborn with RDS may exhibit problems breathing immediately or a few hours after birth. Typically, respirations will be increased, usually greater than 60 breaths per minute. Nasal flaring and retractions may be noted. Mucous membranes may appear cyanotic. As respiratory distress progresses, the newborn exhibits see-saw like respirations in which the chest wall retracts and the abdomen protrudes on inspiration and then the sternum rises on expiration. Breathing becomes noticeably labored, the respiratory rate continues to increase, and expiratory grunting occurs. Breath sounds usually are diminished, and the newborn may develop periods of apnea.

If premature delivery is expected, an attempt may be made to prevent RDS. Through amniocentesis, the amount of **lecithin**, the major component of surfactant, may be measured to determine lung maturity. If insufficient lecithin is present 24 to 48 hours before delivery, the mother may be given a glucocorticosteroid drug (betamethasone) that crosses the placenta and causes the infant's lungs to produce surfactant. The infant begins to produce surfactant about 72 hours after birth; therefore, the critical time comes within these first several days. Infants who survive the first 4 days have a much improved chance of recovery unless other problems are overwhelming.

After birth, surfactant replacement therapy with synthetic or naturally occurring surfactant, obtained from animal sources or extracted from human amniotic fluid, has proved successful in the treatment of RDS. Surfactant is administered as an inhalant through a catheter inserted into an endotracheal tube, at or soon after birth. The therapy may be used as preventive treatment ("rescue") to avoid the development of RDS in the newborn at risk. Newborns with RDS usually receive additional oxygen through continuous positive airway pressure, using intubation or a plastic hood. This helps the lungs to remain partially expanded until they begin producing surfactant, usually within the first 5 days of life. The preterm newborn who develops RDS requires supportive care that focuses on measures to promote adequate oxygenation.

Intraventricular Hemorrhage

Intraventricular hemorrhage (IVH) is a complication of preterm birth that occurs more often in the newborn of less than 32 weeks' gestation. In addition to early gestational age, other factors commonly associated with IVH include birth asphyxia, low birth weight, respiratory distress, and hypotension. Ultrasonography, computed tomography, and magnetic resonance imaging can be used to determine if bleeding has occurred.

Signs of possible IVH include hypotonia, apnea, bradycardia, a full (or bulging) fontanelle, cyanosis, and increased head circumference. Neurologic signs such as twitching, convulsions, and stupor are also possible warning signs. However, mild bleeding can occur without these symptoms.

Preventing IVH focuses on avoiding situations that increase or cause fluctuations in the cerebral blood pressure. Appropriate measures include keeping the head and body in alignment when moving and turning the newborn (avoiding twisting the head at the neck), reducing procedures that cause crying (as a result of pain), and minimizing endotracheal suctioning. Any unnecessary disturbances of the newborn are to be avoided. In addition, analgesics may be administered to relieve or reduce discomfort and lessen the danger of increased intracranial blood pressure.

Cold Stress

All newborns are subject to heat loss, and maintaining thermoregulation is crucial. For the preterm newborn, thermoregulation is a major problem. The preterm newborn has a large body surface area when compared to the body weight, allowing for greater heat loss through evaporation, radiation, conduction, and convection. In addition, the preterm newborn has little subcutaneous fat to act as insulation. This in conjunction with the preterm newborn's immature muscular development interfering with the newborn's ability to keep his body flexed and to actively move about to generate heat. Moreover, the preterm newborn cannot shiver or sweat, mechanisms useful for generating and dissipating heat, respectively. Immaturity of the central nervous system and the lack of integrated reflex control of peripheral blood vessels (to cause vasodilation or vasoconstriction) also affect the preterm newborn's ability to maintain body temperature. Therefore, cold stress is a greater threat to the preterm newborn than it is to the term newborn. Cold stress may result in hypoxia, metabolic acidosis, and hypoglycemia. To prevent heat loss and to control other aspects of the premature infant's environment, an isolette or a radiant warmer is used (Fig. 20-3). The isolette has a clear Plexiglas top that allows a full view of the newborn from all aspects. The isolette

A   **B**

● *Figure 20.3* Maintenance of thermoregulation. (**A**) Newborn under a radiant warmer.
(**B**) Newborn in an isolette.

maintains ideal temperature, humidity, and oxygen concentrations and isolates the infant from infection. Portholes at the side allow access to the newborn with minimal temperature and oxygen loss. A heat-sensing probe attached to the newborn's skin controls the temperature of the isolette or the radiant warmer. Oxygen typically is administered. If oxygen is administered through an oxygen hood, it must be warmed and moisturized before it is administered.

Retinopathy of Prematurity

Retinopathy of prematurity (ROP) refers to a complication commonly associated with the preterm newborn. It results from the growth of abnormal immature retinal blood vessels. Preterm birth may be a factor contributing to this growth. In addition, the use of high concentrations of oxygen has been identified as a major cause. The immature blood vessels constrict when high levels of oxygen are given, depriving the retinal tissues of adequate nutrition. In addition, in some newborns capillaries increase, leading to scarring and eventually retinal detachment. These events lead to varying degrees of blindness.

Remember that usually the younger the preterm infant, the higher the probability of ROP.

ROP was once thought to be irreversible, but laser therapy and cryosurgery have been effective in reducing the degree of blindness. Laser treatment has proved more effective and less damaging to surrounding eye tissues than cryosurgery. Prevention of this complication is key by monitoring the preterm newborn's blood oxygen level and keeping it within normal limits. Levels greater than 100 mm Hg greatly increase the risk of ROP.

Necrotizing Enterocolitis

Necrotizing enterocolitis (NEC) is an acute inflammatory disease of the intestine. Although it may occur in full-term neonates, it most often occurs in small preterm newborns. The cause is not clearly defined. Precipitating factors are hypoxia, causing poor tissue perfusion to the bowel; bacterial invasion of the bowel; and feedings of formula, which provide material on which bacterial enzymes can work. Clinical manifestations include distention of the abdomen, return of more than 2 mL of undigested formula when the gastric contents are aspirated before a feeding, and occult blood in the stool. The newborn feeds poorly and may experience vomiting and periods of apnea. This disorder usually occurs within the first 10 days of life. Diagnosis is confirmed by abdominal radiographs. The infant with necrotizing enterocolitis is gravely ill and must be cared for in the NICU.

Initially, oral feedings are discontinued and nasogastric suction, IV fluids, and antibiotics are given. There is a danger that a necrotic area will rupture, causing peritonitis. A temporary colostomy may be needed to relieve the obstruction, and surgical removal of the necrotic bowel may be necessary.

● *Figure 20.4* Typical resting posture of preterm newborn. Note the lax position and immature muscular development.

Other Complications

The preterm newborn desperately needs nourishment but has a digestive system that may be unprepared to receive and digest food. The stomach is small, with a capacity that may be less than 1 to 2 oz. The sphincters at either end of the stomach are immature, causing regurgitation or vomiting if feedings distend the stomach. The immature liver cannot manage all the bilirubin produced by **hemolysis** (destruction of red blood cells with the release of hemoglobin), making the infant prone to jaundice and high blood bilirubin levels **(hyperbilirubinemia)** that may result in brain damage.

The preterm infant does not receive enough antibodies from the mother and cannot produce them. This characteristic makes the infant particularly vulnerable to infection.

Muscle weakness in the premature infant contributes to nutritional and respiratory problems and to a posture distinct from that of the term infant (Fig. 20-4). The infant may not be able to change positions and is prone to fatigue and exhaustion, even from eating and breathing. Skilled, gentle intensive care is needed for the newborn to survive and develop. The parents also need supportive, intensive care.

Test Yourself

- When is a newborn classified as preterm?
- What is observed on the hands and feet of a preterm newborn?
- Which complication associated with preterm newborns is due to a surfactant deficiency?

● Nursing Process for the Preterm Newborn

The physical condition of a preterm newborn demands the skilled assessment and planning of nursing care, emphasizing maintenance of adequate oxygenation, continuous electronic cardiac and respiratory monitoring, frequent manual monitoring of vital signs, thermoregulation, infection control, hydration, provision of adequate nutrition and sensory stimulation for the newborn, and emotional support for the parents.

ASSESSMENT

Although assessment of the preterm newborn is similar to that for any newborn, the initial assessment focuses on the status of the respiratory, circulatory, and neurologic systems to determine the immediate needs of the infant. Box 20-1 highlights the assessment findings of a preterm newborn.

SELECTED NURSING DIAGNOSES

Based on the initial assessment, some of the nursing diagnoses that may be appropriate include the following:

- Ineffective Breathing Pattern related to an immature respiratory system

A PERSONAL GLIMPSE

My son was born 8.5 weeks before his expected due date. I was unable to hold him until 12 hours after his birth. I was discharged from the hospital with a Polaroid snapshot of him and the phone number of the hospital's neonatal intensive care unit.

For 2 weeks I visited him, learning new medical terms and gaining an understanding of all the obstacles he would have to overcome before being released. These days were an emotional roller coaster filled with feelings of joy over being blessed with a son; enormous concern over his condition; and a great deal of guilt. The thing I wanted most in the world was to take him home, healthy and without the IVs, equipment, monitors, and the hard hospital chairs. When I left him each day, I was leaving a part of myself, and I felt as though I would not be whole until he was home with me.

Looking back, I so appreciated that the staff was optimistic when informing me of things, but not overly so. Unmet expectations can be devastating! There is not a moment that I am not thankful for my son and his health and not a night that I don't sleep better after I have checked on him sleeping in bed.

Kerry

LEARNING OPPORTUNITY: Give specific examples of what the nurse could do to support this mother and help decrease her fears and anxieties.

BOX 20.1	Assessment Findings of a Preterm Newborn

- Skin: Usually thin, translucent to gelatinous with vessels easily seen, becoming loose and wrinkled after a few days. Generalized edema and ecchymosis (typically from birth trauma to presenting parts) are normally seen, along with a small amount of vernix caseosa and subcutaneous fat (for insulation to maintain heat) and inadequate stores of brown fat. Lanugo is characteristically present on sides of face, extremities, and back with thin and fine hair on head and eyebrows and soft and thin nails.
- Color: Ranging from pink or dark red (**ruddy**) to acrocyanosis, a bluish discoloration of the palms of the hands and soles of the feet. (This condition is considered normal immediately after birth but should not persist longer than 48 hours.) Generalized cyanosis is possible because of the preterm newborn's ill state; jaundice may be seen by day 2 to day 8.
- Behavior/activity level: Incapable of moving smoothly from one state or level of alertness to another to control his environmental input. The preterm newborn maintains a hypersensitive/hyperalertness; may have a feeble or even absent cry and show an exaggerated response to unpleasant stimuli. Typically, the preterm newborn shows less spontaneous activity than a term newborn; will become lethargic with onset of illness; agitation may be revealed by vital signs such as an increased heart rate and blood pressure, an increase or decrease in respiratory rate, or decreased oxygen saturation levels.

- Muscle tone: Characteristically weak, leaving a flaccid and open resting position and allowing for increased heat loss of body temperature, as well as an increased inability to control his behavioral state.
- Breasts: Engorgement rarely seen. Nipples and areola are usually not easily noted.
- Head: Large in proportion to body size; bones of the skull are soft, with overriding sutures and small fontanels, leaving a narrow, flattened appearance to head and face.
- Eyes: Small and sometimes fused; eyelids may become edematous after treatment.
- Ears: Soft, flat, and small with little cartilage, allowing for the pinna to bend and fold, leading to potential injury to ear.
- Nose: Small with visible milia; breathing predominately through nose; nasal flaring indicative of respiratory distress.
- Chest: Weak musculoskeletal structure; lung auscultation typically wet and noisy; heart beat rapid and difficult to hear over lung sounds. Apnea common.
- Abdomen: Full and soft with a weak muscle tone, allowing for visible bowel loops and marked abdominal distention.
- Genitalia: In female, labia minora and clitoris prominent because the labia majora are underdeveloped; in male, small scrotum and, frequently, undescended testes.

- Ineffective Thermoregulation related to immaturity and transition to extrauterine life
- Risk for Infection related to an immature immune system and environmental factors
- Risk for Imbalanced Nutrition, Less Than Body Requirements related to an inability to suck
- Risk for Impaired Skin Integrity related to urinary excretion of bilirubin and exposure to phototherapy light
- Activity Intolerance related to poor oxygenation and weakness
- Risk for Disorganized Infant Behavior related to prematurity and excess environmental stimuli
- Parental Anxiety related to a seriously ill newborn with an unpredictable prognosis
- Risk for Impaired Parenting related to separation from the newborn and difficulty accepting loss of ideal newborn
- Interrupted Family Processes related to the effect of prolonged hospitalization on the family

OUTCOME IDENTIFICATION AND PLANNING

The major goals for the preterm newborn include improving respiratory function, maintaining body temperature, preventing infection, maintaining adequate nutrition, preserving skin integrity, conserving energy, and promoting sensory stimulation. Goals for the family include reducing anxiety and improving parenting skills and family functioning. The premature newborn is cared for by highly skilled nurses in an NICU. Nursing care is planned and implemented to address each of the goals identified.

IMPLEMENTATION

Improving Respiratory Function

Not all preterm newborns need extra oxygen, but many do. Isolettes are made with oxygen inlets and humidifiers for raising the oxygen concentration inside from 20% to 21% (room air) to a higher percentage. In addition, a clear plastic hood placed over the infant's head supplies humidified oxygen at the concentration desired. Oxygen saturation of the blood may be monitored by pulse oximetry, or the oxygen and carbon dioxide levels may be measured by transcutaneous monitoring. Both of these methods help establish the desirable oxygen concentration in the newborn. In the absence of pathologic lung changes, it is safer to keep the oxygen concentration lower than 40%, unless hypoxia is documented.

Observing the preterm newborn's respirations is obviously of utmost importance. Also monitor the pulse rate and note skin color, muscle tone, alertness, and activity.

Measure the rate of respiration and identify retractions to help determine proper oxygen concentrations. Ensure that oxygen support or ventilator settings and placement of an endotracheal (ET) tube, if ordered, is as prescribed to ensure adequacy of ventilation and respiration assistance. Repositioning the newborn every 2 hours helps to reduce the risk for pneumonia and atelectasis. Frequent suctioning may be necessary to prevent airway obstruction, hypoxia, and asphyxiation. If not contraindicated, elevate the head of the bed as needed to maintain a patent airway.

Observe for changes in respiratory effort, rate, depth, breath sounds, and regularity of respirations. Note any expiratory grunting or chest retractions (substernal, suprasternal, intercostal, subcostal), including severity, and nasal flaring to determine the newborn's ability to maintain respirations.

One of the most hazardous characteristics of the preterm newborn is the tendency to stop breathing periodically (**apnea**). The hypoxia caused by this apnea and general respiratory difficulty may lead to mental retardation or other neurologic problems.

Electronic apnea alarms are used routinely. Electrodes are placed across the infant's chest with leads to the apnea monitor, providing a continuous reading of the respiratory rate. Visual and audio alarms may be set to alert the nurse when the rate goes too high or too low or if the infant waits too long to take a breath.

It is a nursing responsibility to place, check, and replace the leads on the newborn. Each day, remove electrodes and reapply them in a slightly different location to protect the infant's sensitive skin from being damaged by the electrode paste and adhesive. Cleanse the skin carefully between applications of the electrodes. Many false alarms are the result of leads that have come loose. Some of these false alarms may be prevented by using a small amount of electrode paste and being careful to keep the paste inside the circle of adhesive on the electrode.

Respiratory assistance may be used to handle apnea. Usually, gentle stimulation, such as wiggling a foot, is enough to remind the newborn to breathe. However, sometimes respirations need to be assisted by a bag and mask. Every nursery nurse should know how to "bag" an infant. The principles of this form of assisted respiration are similar to those of mouth-to-mouth rescue breathing:

1. Slightly extend the neck to open the airway.
2. Cover the infant's mouth and nose with the mask. Maintain a tight seal between the mask and the infant's face.
3. Quickly but gently squeeze the small bag filled with oxygen or air. The quantity of air needed is relatively small, and the pressure is gentle to prevent damage to the immature lungs.

Promote rest times between procedures because organized care helps to conserve the newborn's energy and reduce oxygen consumption. Supportive medications may be ordered to stimulate the central respiratory chemoreceptors, relax bronchial smooth muscle, and stimulate the CNS to increase respiratory skeletal activity.

Maintaining Body Temperature

The preterm newborn's body temperature must be monitored closely and continuously. Monitors that record temperature, pulse, respirations, and blood pressure; transcutaneous oxygen and carbon dioxide monitors; and pulse oximeters (monitors used to measure oxygen saturation) are all routinely used in the NICU. However, close observation by a nurse who is regularly assigned to the same newborn remains an essential part of the infant's care. Observe the monitoring and life-support equipment, making sure it is functioning properly, and systematically assess the infant. Time assessment and other procedures so that the infant is disturbed as little as possible to conserve energy. In addition, be sure to expose as little of the newborn's skin as possible during procedures to minimize heat loss.

Observe for signs of cold stress, such as low temperature, body cold to touch, pallor, and lethargy. The preterm newborn has weak muscle tone and activity. Therefore, leaving the newborn in an extended posture decreases heat conservation. Be aware of and avoid heat loss via the following mechanisms:

- Evaporation, such as through wet skin during bathing
- Conduction, such as when lying on a cold surface such as a scale for weighing
- Radiation, such as when the newborn is exposed to but not in contact with surfaces, for example, isolette walls near a window

- Convection, such as when the newborn is exposed to drafts

Most isolettes have a control system for temperature regulation. Attach a temperature-sensitive electrode to the infant's abdomen and connect it to the isolette thermostat. The unit may then be set to turn the heater on and off according to the infant's skin temperature. Open units with overhead radiant warmers allow maximum access to the infant when sophisticated equipment or frequent manipulation for treatment and assessment is necessary. The temperature remains more constant than in the closed unit, which is constantly having the door or portholes opened and the atmosphere breached.

The preterm newborn must not be overheated because this causes increased consumption of oxygen and calories, possibly jeopardizing the newborn's status. Use clothing, a head covering (such as a stockinette cap), and blankets when removing the newborn from the warm environment of the isolette or radiant warmer for feeding or cuddling. It is still standard practice to take and record axillary temperatures when the infant is being warmed by either of these methods.

Although monitoring equipment provides a continual reading of the heart rate, take apical pulses periodically, listening to the heart through the chest using a stethoscope for 1 full minute so as not to miss an irregularity in rhythm. Observations should include rate, rhythm, and strength. The pulse rate is normally rapid (120 to 140 beats per minute [bpm]) and unstable. Premature newborns are subject to dangerous periods of bradycardia (as low as 60 to 80 bpm) and tachycardia (as high as 160 to 200 bpm). The nurse's observations of the pulse rate, rhythm, and strength are essential to determining how the infant is tolerating treatments, activity, feedings, and the temperature and oxygen concentration of the isolette.

Preventing Infection

Infection control is an urgent concern in the care of the preterm newborn. The preterm infant cannot resist bacterial invasions, so the caregivers must provide an atmosphere that protects him or her from such attacks. The primary means of preventing infection is handwashing. All persons who come in contact with the newborn must practice good handwashing immediately before touching the newborn and when moving from one newborn to another. Handwashing is the most important aspect of infection control.

Other important aspects of good housekeeping include regular cleaning or changing of humidifier water, IV tubing, and suction, respira-

tory, and monitoring equipment. The NICU is separate from the normal newborn nursery and usually has its own staff. This separation helps eliminate sources of infection. Personnel in this area usually wear scrub suits or gowns. Personnel from other departments (radiology, respiratory therapy, or laboratory) put a cover gown over their uniforms while working with these newborns.

Observe the newborn frequently for signs and symptoms of infection including:

- Temperature instability (decrease or increase)
- Glucose instability and metabolic acidosis
- Poor sucking
- Vomiting
- Diarrhea
- Abdominal distention
- Apnea
- Respiratory distress and cyanosis
- Hepatosplenomegaly
- Jaundice
- Skin mottling
- Lethargy
- Hypotonia
- Seizures

Close observation allows for successful intervention if infection occurs. Obtain diagnostic laboratory work as ordered and report results that indicate the source and treatment of infection. Routine laboratory tests used to diagnose and treat infections include blood cultures, cerebral spinal fluid analysis, urine tests, tracheal aspirate culture, and superficial cultures. Expect antibiotics to be ordered to treat suspected or confirmed bacterial infections.

Maintaining Adequate Nutrition

When born, a preterm newborn may be too weak to suck or may not yet have developed adequate sucking and swallowing reflexes. Commonly, the preterm newborn has poorly coordinated suck, swallow, and gag reflexes, leading to possible aspiration; a limited stomach capacity, contributing to distention and inadequate intake; poor muscle tone of the cardiac sphincter, leading to regurgitation and secondary apnea and bradycardia; and finally, muscle weakness, which leads to exhaustion. In addition, preterm newborns do not tolerate carbohydrates and fats well.

For several hours or even 1 day, the preterm newborn may be able to manage without fluids, but soon IV fluids will be necessary. In many instances, an IV "life line" is established immediately after delivery. Fluids are infused through a catheter passed into the umbilical vein in the stub of the umbilical cord if it is still fresh. Intravenous fluids may be given through other veins, particularly the peripheral veins of the hands or feet. Extremely small amounts of fluid are needed, perhaps as little as 5 to 10 mL/hour or even less. They may be measured accurately and administered at a steady rate by using an infusion pump. Keep accurate, complete records of IV fluids and frequently observe for infiltration or overhydration.

Measure and record all urinary output by weighing the diapers before and after they are used. Urine volume is normally 35 to 40 mL/kg per 24 hours during the first few days, increasing to 50 to 100 mL. Also observe and record the number of urinations, the color of the urine, and edema. Edema changes the loose, wrinkled skin to tight, shiny skin.

At first, some preterm newborns receive all their fluid, electrolyte, vitamin, and calorie needs by the IV route; others can start with a nipple and bottle. Special nipples and smaller bottles may be used to prevent too much formula from flowing into the newborn's mouth.

Premature newborns are likely to have problems with aspiration because the gag reflex does not develop until about the 32nd to 34th week of gestation. As a result, gavage feedings may be necessary. The frequency and quantity of gavage feedings are individualized. Usually, feedings are given every 2 hours. Extending the feeding time too long may tire the infant (Fig. 20-5).

Typically a feeding should be completed in less than 30 minutes. If the stomach is not empty by the next feeding, allow more time between feedings or give smaller feedings. Usually, the quantity given is just as much as the infant can tolerate and is increased milliliter by milliliter as quickly as tolerated. Commonly amounts as small as 5 to 10 mL per feeding are given. Special

● **Figure 20.5** The nurse helps the caregiver administer a gavage feeding to her premature infant.

preterm newborn nursers are available. These nursers are calibrated in 1-mL markings.

The feeding is too large if the newborn's stomach becomes so distended that it causes respiratory difficulty, vomiting, or regurgitation and if there is formula left in the stomach by the next feeding.

Breast milk, the preferred source of nutrition for the preterm newborn, is thought to be higher in protein, sodium, chloride, and immunoglobulin A than is the breast milk of mothers of term infants. Mothers can pump their breast milk and freeze it to use for bottle or gavage feedings until the preterm newborn is strong enough to breastfeed. The use of her own milk to nourish her newborn is a tremendous boost to the emotional satisfaction of the mother.

The most common premature infant formula has 13 calories/oz (often called half-strength formula). A formula with 20 calories/oz (the usual strength for newborns) also may be used. If the formula is too rich (too high in carbohydrates and fats), vomiting and diarrhea may occur. If the infant does not gain weight after the initial postnatal weight loss, the formula may be too low in calories.

When a preterm newborn who is being gavage fed begins to suck vigorously on the fingers, hands, pacifier, or gavage tubing and demonstrates evidence of a gag reflex, nipple feeding should be tried. The infant who can take the same quantity of formula by nipple that was tolerated by gavage feeding without becoming too tired is ready. Alternating gavage and nipple feedings may be necessary in some cases to assist the preterm newborn in making the transition. The nipple for a preterm newborn usually is made of softer rubber than the regular nipple. It is also smaller, but no shorter, than the regular nipple.

Burp preterm newborns often during and after feedings. Sometimes simply changing the infant's position is enough assistance; at other times, it may help to gently rub or pat the infant's back. Throughout feedings, be careful to prevent aspiration. Hold the infant for the feeding, keeping oxygen available as needed. After a feeding, the best position for the preterm newborn is probably on his or her right side, with the head of the mattress slightly elevated.

Other feeding methods can be used if neither gavage nor nipple feeding is tolerated and if IV fluids are inadequate. Some preterm newborns do better if fed with a rubber-tipped medicine dropper. Others may require gastrostomy feedings. The preterm newborn who is not receiving nipple feedings should be given nonnutritive sucking opportunities, such as a pacifier.

Weigh the preterm newborn daily. These daily weights give an indication of overall health and indicate whether enough calories are being consumed. The physicians and parents probably will want to know the infant's current weight each day. Weigh the newborn with the same clothing, using the same scale at the same time each day to help ensure accurate, comparable data.

Preserving Skin Integrity

Assess skin integrity frequently but at least every shift for changes in color, turgor, texture, vascularity, and signs of irritation or infection. Pay special attention to areas in which equipment is attached or inserted. Frequent skin assessment allows for early detection and prompt intervention. A preterm newborn's skin is extremely fragile and can be injured easily. Reposition the preterm newborn every 2 to 4 hours and PRN as necessary. Handle the preterm newborn gently when repositioning. If the preterm newborn is placed on the back, make sure that aspiration does not occur. Preterm infants have a knack for wriggling into corners and cracks from which they cannot extract themselves, so close observation is necessary.

Changing the diaper as soon as possible after soiling will maintain clean and dry skin. Keep the skin clean and dry but avoid excessive bathing, which furthers dries the skin. Pad pressure prone areas by using sheep skin blankets, waterbeds, pillows, or egg crate mattresses to help prevent additional skin breakdown to these areas. In addition monitor intake and output and avoid dehydration and over hydration.

Apply creams and ointments and medication as prescribed for relief of itching, infections, and to prevent breakdown. Be sure to record the use of any special equipment or procedures.

Promoting Energy Conservation and Sensory Stimulation

The preterm newborn uses the most energy to breathe and pump blood. Plan the newborn's day to avoid exhaustion from constant handling and movement. In addition, help conserve the preterm newborn's energy by eliminating regular bathing and giving only "face and fanny" care as needed. Preterm newborns usually are dressed in only a diaper, if anything, to conserve energy, provide more freedom of movement, and allow a better opportunity to observe the infant. However, do not be misled into ignoring or avoiding the newborn or discouraging the contact essential to establishing a normal relationship.

The environment of the NICU, with its lights, noises, frequent handling, and invasive procedures can be overwhelming to the preterm newborn's immature central nervous system. Overstimulation can be as much of a problem as lack of stimulation. Therefore, assist with measures to balance the amount of stimulation the newborn receives. Speak gently and softly and minimize the amount of handling. If the preterm newborn is in an isolette, avoid tapping on the sides and opening and closing the portholes too frequently to reduce the amount of noise in the newborn's environment.

Older preterm infants have a special need for sensory stimulation. Mobiles hung over the isolette and toys placed in or on the infant unit may provide visual stimulation. A radio with the volume turned low, a music box, or a wind-up toy in the isolette may provide auditory stimulation. An excellent form of auditory stimulation comes from the voices of the infant's family, physicians, and nurses talking and singing. Being bathed, held, cuddled, and fondled provides needed tactile stimulation. Contact is essential to the infant and the family. Some NICUs have "foster grandparents" who regularly visit long-term NICU infants and provide them with sensory stimulation, cuddling, loving, crooning, and talking. These programs have proven beneficial to both the infants and the volunteer grandparents.

Reducing Parental Anxiety

Birth of a preterm newborn creates a crisis for the family caregivers. Often their long-awaited baby is whisked away from them, sometimes to a distant neonatal center, and hooked up to a maze of machines. Parents feel anxiety, guilt, fear, depression, and perhaps anger. They cannot share the early, sensitive attachment period. It may take weeks to establish touch and eye contact, ordinarily achieved in 10 minutes with a term infant. Parents often leave the hospital empty-handed, without the perfect, healthy infant of their dreams. How can they learn to know and love the strange, scrawny creature that now lives in that plastic box? These feelings are normal, but studies have shown that if these feelings are not expressed and resolved, they can damage the long-term relationship of parents and child, even resulting in child neglect or abuse.

The mother's condition also must be considered. If the infant was delivered by cesarean birth, or if the labor was difficult or prolonged, she may feel abandoned or too weak to become involved with the baby.

Nurses who work with high-risk infants can do much to help families cope with the crisis of prematurity and early separation. To ease some of the apprehension of the family caregivers, transport teams prepare the newborn for transportation, then take the newborn in the transport incubator into the mother's room so that the parents may see (and touch, if possible) the newborn before the child is whisked away. In many cases, instant photos provide the family some concrete reminder of the newborn until they can visit in person.

Explain what is happening to the newborn in the NICU and periodically report on his or her condition (by phone if the NICU is not in the same hospital) to reassure the family that the child is receiving excellent care and that they are being kept informed. Listen to the family and encourage them to express their feelings and support one another. As soon as possible, the family should see, touch, and help care for the newborn. Most NICUs do not restrict visiting hours for parents or support persons, and they encourage families to visit often, whenever it is convenient for them. Many hospitals offer 24-hour phone privileges to families so that they are never out of touch with their newborn's caregivers.

Improving Parenting Skills and Family Functioning

Before the mother is discharged from the hospital, plans are made for both parents and other support persons to visit the preterm newborn and to participate in the care. They need to feel that the newborn belongs to them, not to the hospital. To help foster this feeling and strengthen the attachment, work closely with families to help them progress toward successful parenthood. Siblings should be included in the visits to see the preterm newborn (Fig. 20-6). The monitors, warmers, ventilators, and other equipment may be frightening to siblings and family caregivers. Make the family feel welcome and comfortable when they visit. A primary nurse assigned to care for the infant gives the family a constant person to contact, increasing their feelings of confidence in the care the newborn is receiving.

Support groups of families who have experienced the crisis that a preterm newborn causes are of great value to the families. Members of these support groups can visit the families in the hospital and at home, helping the parents and other family members to deal with their feelings and solve the problems that may arise when the infant is ready to come home or if the infant does not survive.

As the time for discharge of the infant nears, the family is understandably apprehensive. The NICU nurses must teach the parents and support persons the skills they need to care for the infant. This knowledge gives them confidence that they can take care of the infant. Some hospitals allow caregivers to stay overnight before the infant's discharge so that they can participate in around-the-clock care. The knowledge that they can telephone the physician and nurse at any time after discharge to have questions answered is reassuring.

Before discharge, most preterm newborns will have successfully made the transition from isolette to open crib, thriving without artificial support systems. In addition to feeding, bathing, and general care of the infant, many families of premature newborns need to learn infant cardiopulmonary resuscitation and the use of an apnea monitor before the infant is discharged (Fig. 20-7). Some preterm infants are being sent home with oxygen, gastrostomy feeding tubes, and many other kinds of sophisticated equipment. This helps place the infant in the home much earlier, but it requires intensive training and support of the family members who care for the infant.

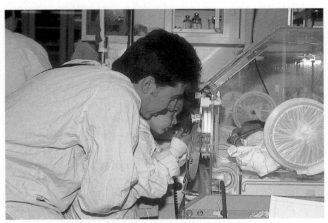

● **Figure 20.6** Encouraging sibling interaction with the preterm newborn.

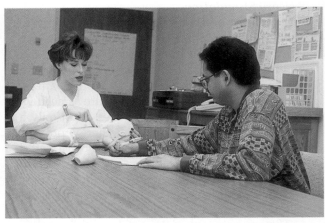

● **Figure 20.7** Teaching a parent how to perform CPR before discharge.

After the baby goes home, a nurse, usually a community health nurse, visits the family to check on the health of the mother and the baby. The nurse provides additional support and teaching about the infant's care, if necessary, and answers any questions the family might have.

EVALUATION: GOALS AND EXPECTED OUTCOMES

Evaluation of the preterm newborn is an ongoing process that demands continual readjustment of the nursing diagnoses, planning, and implementation. Goals and expected outcomes include:

- **Goal:** The preterm newborn's respiratory function will improve.
  Expected Outcomes: Respiratory rate remains less than 60 bpm; no grunting or retractions evidenced; breath sounds clear; oxygen saturation level greater than 95%; symmetrical chest expansion; no episodes of apnea.
- **Goal:** The preterm newborn's temperature will remain stable.
  Expected Outcome: Temperature is maintained at 97.7°F to 98.6°F (36.5°C to 37.0°C).
- **Goal:** The infant will remain free of infection.
  Expected Outcome: Signs of infection are not noted, as evidenced by vital signs within normal limits; breath sounds clear; and skin intact.
- **Goal:** The preterm newborn's nutritional status will remain adequate.
  Expected Outcomes: The infant ingests increased amounts of oral nutrition and gains weight daily; skin turgor improves.
- **Goal:** The preterm newborn will remain free of skin breakdown.
  Expected Outcome: The newborn's skin is intact and free of redness, rashes, and irritation.
- **Goal:** The preterm newborn will show improved tolerance to activity.
  Expected Outcomes: Vital signs remain stable and skin color remains pink during activity; supplemental oxygen is required in decreasing amounts until no longer necessary.
- **Goal:** The preterm newborn demonstrates appropriate behavior in response to stimulation.
  Expected Outcome: The newborn responds appropriately to stimuli cues.
- **Goal:** The parents demonstrate a reduction in anxiety level.
  Expected Outcome: Parents and family caregivers express feelings and anxieties concerning the newborn's condition, visit and establish a relationship; demonstrate interaction with the newborn, holding and helping to provide care.
- **Goal:** Parents demonstrate appropriate parenting skills.

Expected Outcomes: Parents and family caregivers learn how to care for the newborn in the hospital and at home; parents hold, cuddle, talk to, and feed the preterm newborn; family caregivers demonstrate knowledge of appropriate infant care.
- **Goal:** The family adapts to the crisis and begins functioning at an appropriate level.
  Expected Outcome: Family has an adequate support system and uses it; contacts a support group for families of high-risk infants.

THE POST-TERM NEWBORN

When pregnancy lasts longer than 42 weeks, the infant is considered to be post-term (postmature), regardless of birth weight.

Contributing Factors

About 12% of all infants are post-term. The causes of delayed birth are unknown. However, some predisposing factors include first pregnancies between the ages of 15 and 19 years, the woman older than 35 years with multiple pregnancies, and certain fetal anomalies, such as anencephaly.

Characteristics of the Post-term Newborn

Some post-term newborns have an appearance similar to term infants, but others look like infants 1 to 3 weeks old. Little lanugo or vernix remains, scalp hair is abundant, and fingernails are long. The skin is dry, cracked, wrinkled, peeling, and whiter than that of the normal newborn. These infants have little subcutaneous fat and appear long and thin. This lack of subcutaneous fat may lead to cold stress. These infants are threatened by failing placental function and are at risk for intrauterine hypoxia during labor and delivery. Thus, it is customary for the physician or nurse–midwife to induce labor or perform a cesarean delivery when the baby is markedly overdue. Many physicians believe that pregnancy should be terminated by the end of 42 weeks.

Potential Complications

Often, the post-term infant has expelled meconium in utero. At birth, the meconium may be aspirated into the lungs, obstructing the respiratory passages and irritating the lungs. This may lead to pneumonia. Whenever meconium-stained amniotic fluid is detected in any delivery, oral and nasopharyngeal suctioning often is performed as soon as the head is born. After delivery, gastric lavage also may be performed to remove any meconium swallowed and to prevent aspiration of vomitus.

In the last weeks of gestation, the infant relies on glycogen for nutrition. This depletes the liver glycogen stores and may result in hypoglycemia. Another complication of the post-term infant may be polycythemia in response to intrauterine hypoxia. Polycythemia puts the infant at risk for cerebral ischemia, hypoglycemia, thrombus formation, and respiratory distress as a result of hyperviscosity of the blood.

Nursing Care

Special care can be taken when knowledge of a post-term newborn is evident. Early in the pregnancy, typically before 20 weeks, ultrasound examinations are performed to help establish more accurate dating by measurements taken of the fetus. Later in the pregnancy (after 42 weeks), ultrasound is used to evaluate fetal development, weight, the amount of amniotic fluid, and the placenta for signs of aging. This information allows the physician to make an informed decision regarding the safest form of delivery.

To reduce the chances of meconium aspiration, upon delivery of the post-term newborn's head and just before the baby takes his first breath, the physician or clinical nurse will suction the infant's mouth and nose and also check for respiratory problems related to meconium aspiration.

Typically, postmature newborns are ravenous eaters at birth. With this in mind, if the newborn is free from respiratory distress, the practical nurse can offer feedings at 1 or 2 hours of age, being observant for potential aspiration and possible asphyxia. Serial blood glucose levels will be monitored because the post-term newborn is at risk for hypoglycemia because of the increased use of glucose stores. Intravenous glucose infusions may be ordered to stabilize the newborn's glucose level.

Provide a thermoregulated environment, such as a radiant heat warmer or isolette, and use measures to minimize heat loss, such as reducing drafts and drying the skin thoroughly after bathing. With an increased production in red blood cells in response to hypoxia, venous and arterial hematocrit levels may be drawn to evaluate for polycythemia. If polycythemia is suspected, a partial exchange transfusion may be done to prevent hyperviscosity.

Anticipate that the stressed post-term newborn will not tolerate the labor and delivery process too well. Therefore, expect to observe and monitor the newborn's cardiopulmonary status closely. Administer supplemental oxygen therapy as ordered for respiratory distress.

Post-term newborns can appear very different from what parents had expected to see. Help facilitate a positive parent–newborn bond by explaining the newborn's condition and reasons for treatments and procedures. Encourage them to express their feelings and to participate in their newborn's care, if possible, to alleviate their stresses and fears about the newborn's condition.

Test Yourself
- What should be provided to a preterm newborn who is not receiving nipple feedings?
- What are three potential complications associated with post-term newborns?

ACQUIRED DISORDERS

RESPIRATORY DISORDERS

A newborn is at risk for developing respiratory disorders after birth as the newborn adapts to the extrauterine environment. The risk for these disorders increases when the newborn experiences a gestational age variation.

Transient Tachypnea of the Newborn

Transient tachypnea of the newborn (TTN) involves the development of mild respiratory distress in a newborn. It typically occurs after birth, with the greatest degree of distress occurring approximately 36 hours after birth. TTN commonly disappears spontaneously around the 3rd day.

TTN results from a delay in absorption of fetal lung fluid after birth. Before birth, the fetus receives nutrients, including oxygen, via the placenta. Thus, the fetus does not breathe, and the lungs are filled with fluid. As the fetus passes through the birth canal during delivery, some of the fluid is expelled as the thoracic area is compressed. After birth, the newborn breathes and fills the lungs with air, thus expelling additional lung fluid. Any fluid that remains is later expelled by coughing or absorbed into the bloodstream.

Contributing Factors

TTN is commonly seen in newborns born by cesarean delivery. Here, the newborn does not experience the compression of the thoracic cavity that occurs with passage through the birth canal. Newborns who are preterm or SGA or whose mothers smoked during pregnancy or have diabetes also are at risk for TTN.

Clinical Manifestations

A newborn who develops TTN typically exhibits mild respiratory distress, with a respiratory rate greater than 60 breaths per minute. Mild retractions, nasal flaring, and some expiratory grunting may be noted. However, cyanosis usually does not occur. Often the newborn has difficulty feeding because he or she is breathing at such a rapid rate and is unable to suck and breathe at the same time.

Diagnosis and Treatment

Arterial blood gases may reveal hypoxemia and decreased carbon dioxide levels. A chest x-ray usually indicates some fluid in the central portion of the lungs with adequate aeration. Treatment depends on the newborn's gestational age, overall status, history, and extent of respiratory distress. Unless an infection is suspected, medication therapy usually is not given. IV fluids and gavage feedings may be used to meet the newborn's fluid and nutritional requirements. Oral feedings typically are difficult because of the newborn's increased respiratory rate. Supplemental oxygen often is ordered, and oxygen saturation levels are monitored via pulse oximetry.

Nursing Care

Caring for the newborn with TTN requires close observation and monitoring and providing supportive care. Monitor the newborn's vital signs and oxygen saturation levels closely, being alert for changes that would indicate that the newborn is becoming fatigued from the rapid breathing. Administer IV fluids and supplemental oxygen as ordered. Assist the parents in understanding what their newborn is experiencing to help allay any fears or anxieties that they may have.

Meconium Aspiration Syndrome

Meconium aspiration syndrome (MAS) refers to a condition in which the fetus or newborn develops respiratory distress after inhaling meconium mixed with amniotic fluid. Meconium is a thick, pasty, greenish-black substance that is present in the fetal bowel as early as 10 weeks' gestation. **Meconium aspiration** occurs when the fetus inhales meconium along with amniotic fluid. Meconium staining of amniotic fluid usually occurs as a reflex response that allows the rectal sphincter to relax. Subsequently, meconium is released into the amniotic fluid. The fetus may aspirate meconium while in utero or with his or her first breath after birth. The meconium can block the airway partially or completely and can irritate the newborn's airway, causing respiratory distress.

Contributing Factors

Typically, meconium aspiration syndrome is associated with fetal distress during labor. Most commonly, the fetus experiences hypoxia, causing peristalsis to increase and the anal sphincter to relax. The fetus then gasps or inhales the meconium-stained amniotic fluid.

Additional factors that contribute to the development of MAS include a maternal history of diabetes or hypertension, difficult delivery, advanced gestational age, and poor intrauterine growth.

Clinical Manifestations

MAS is suspected whenever amniotic fluid is stained green to greenish black. Other manifestations include:

- Difficulty initiating respirations after birth
- Low Apgar score
- Tachypnea or apnea
- Retractions
- Hypothermia
- Hypoglycemia
- Cyanosis

Diagnosis and Treatment

Typically, diagnosis is confirmed with a chest x-ray that shows patches or streaks of meconium in the lungs. Air trapping or hyperinflation also may be seen. Treatment begins with suctioning the newborn during delivery, before the shoulders are delivered. Tracheal and bronchial suctioning may be indicated to remove any meconium plugs that may be lower in the respiratory tract. Oxygen therapy and assisted ventilation may be necessary to support the newborn's respiratory status. In some case, extracorporeal membrane oxygenation (ECMO) may be used to support the newborn's need for oxygen. Antibiotic therapy may be ordered to prevent the possible development of pneumonia. The physician may order chest physiotherapy with clapping and vibration to help in removing any remaining meconium from the lungs.

Nursing Care

Newborns with MAS are extremely ill and often require care in the NICU. Nursing care focuses on observing the neonate's respiratory status closely and ensuring adequate oxygenation. Measures to maintain thermoregulation are key to reducing the body's metabolic demands for oxygen. Be prepared to administer respiratory support and medication therapy as ordered.

Sudden Infant Death Syndrome

Sudden infant death syndrome (SIDS) has caused much grief and anxiety among families for centuries. One of the leading causes of infant mortality worldwide, SIDS claims an estimated 2,500 lives annually in the United States alone. Although there has been a dramatic drop in the incidence of deaths during the past 20 years, SIDS is still the leading cause of death in infants between 7 and 365 days of age (Carroll & Laughlin, 1999).

Commonly called "crib death," SIDS is the sudden and unexpected death of an apparently healthy infant in whom the postmortem examination fails to reveal an adequate cause. The term SIDS is not a diagnosis but rather a description of the syndrome.

Varying theories have been suggested about the cause of SIDS. Over the years, much research has been done, but no single cause has been identified.

Contributing Factors

Infants who die of SIDS are usually 2 to 4 months old, although some deaths have occurred during the 1st and 2nd week of life. Few infants older than 6 months of age die of SIDS. It is a greater threat to low birthweight infants than to term infants. It occurs more often in winter and affects more male infants than female infants, as well as more infants from minority and lower socioeconomic groups. Infants born to mothers younger than 20 years of age, infants who are not first born, and infants whose mothers smoked during pregnancy also have been found to be at greater risk. Research has revealed that a greater number of infants with SIDS have been sleeping in a prone (face down) position than in a supine (lying on the back with the face up) position. As a result of these studies, the American Academy of Pediatrics recommends that infants must not be placed in a prone position to sleep until they are 6 months old.

Clinical Manifestations

SIDS is rapid and silent and occurs at any time of the day. The history reveals that no cry has been heard, and there is no evidence of a struggle. People who have been sleeping nearby claim to have heard nothing unusual before the death was discovered. It is not uncommon for the infant to have been recently examined by a physician and found to be in excellent health. The autopsy often reveals a mild respiratory disorder but nothing considered serious enough to have caused the death.

A closely related syndrome is apparent life-threatening event (ALTE). This is an episode in which the infant is found in distress but when quickly stimulated, recovers with no lasting problems. These were formerly called "near-miss SIDS." These infants are placed on home apnea monitors (Fig. 20-8). The apnea monitor is set to sound an alarm if the infant has not taken a breath within a given number of seconds. Family caregivers are taught infant cardiopulmonary resuscitation (CPR) so that they can respond quickly if the alarm sounds. Infants who have had an episode of

● **Figure 20.8** An apnea monitor for home monitoring.

ALTE are at risk for additional episodes and may be at risk for SIDS. Infants are usually kept on home apnea monitoring until they are 1 year old. This is a stressful time for the family because someone who is trained in infant CPR must be with the infant at all times.

Nursing Care

The effects of SIDS on caregivers and families are devastating. Grief is coupled with guilt, even though SIDS cannot be prevented or predicted. Disbelief, hostility, and anger are common reactions. An autopsy must be done and the results promptly made known to the family. Even though the family caregivers are told that they are not to blame, it is difficult for most not to keep searching for evidence of some possible neglect on their part. Prolonged depression usually follows the initial shock and anguish over the infant's death.

The immediate response of the emergency department staff should be to allow the family to express their grief, encouraging them to say good-by to their infant and providing a quiet, private place for them to do so. Compassionate care of the family caregivers includes helping to find someone to accompany them home or to meet them there. Referrals should be made to the local chapter of the National SIDS Foundation immediately. Sudden Infant Death Alliance is another resource for help. In some states, specially trained community health nurses who are knowledgeable about SIDS are available. These nurses are prepared to help families and can provide written materials, as well as information, guidance, and support in the family's home. They maintain contact with the family as long as necessary and provide support in a subsequent pregnancy.

One concern of the caregivers is how to tell other children in the family what has happened and how to help them deal with their grief and anger. Many books and booklets are available.

Caregivers are particularly concerned about subsequent infants. Recent studies have indicated that the risk for these infants is no greater than that for the general population. Many care providers, however, continue to recommend monitoring these infants for the first few months of life to help reduce the family's stress. Monitoring is usually maintained until the new infant is past the age of the SIDS infant's death.

HEMOLYTIC DISEASE OF THE NEWBORN

Hemolytic disease of the newborn is another name for **erythroblastosis fetalis**, a condition in which the infant's red blood cells are broken down (hemolyzed) and destroyed, producing severe anemia and hyperbilirubinemia. This rapid destruction of red blood cells may produce heart failure, brain damage, and death.

Before the mid-1960s, hemolytic disease was largely the result of Rh incompatibility between the blood of the mother and the blood of the fetus. The introduction of immune globulin, or RhoGAM, in the mid-1960s has markedly reduced the incidence of this disorder. Hemolytic disease occurring today is principally the result of ABO incompatibility and is generally much less severe than the Rh-induced disorder.

Rh Incompatibility

Rh factor, a protein substance (antigen), is found on the surface of red blood cells. The antigen is named "Rh" because it was first identified in the blood of rhesus monkeys. Persons who have the factor are $Rh_0(D)$ positive; those lacking the factor are $Rh_0(D)$ negative. A person's blood type is inherited and follows the rules of hereditary dominance and recession. $Rh_0(D)$ positive trait is dominant. Therefore, if both members of a couple are $Rh_0(D)$ negative, the couple's children will also be $Rh_0(D)$ negative, and there will be no hemolytic disorder. However, if the woman is $Rh_0(D)$ negative and the man is $Rh_0(D)$ positive, the child may inherit $Rh_0(D)$ positive blood and the disorder may occur.

If the man is homozygous positive for the trait, then both of his genes carry the $Rh_0(D)$ positive (dominant) trait. In this case, if the woman is $Rh_0(D)$ negative, then all of the couple's children will be $Rh_0(D)$ positive and are vulnerable to hemolytic disease. However, if the man is heterozygous positive for the trait, then one of his genes carries the antigen and the other does not. In this case, if the woman is $Rh_0(D)$ negative,

then there is a 50-50 probability that the child will be $Rh_0(D)$ positive and therefore vulnerable to hemolytic disease.

The $Rh_0(D)$ positive fetus is only vulnerable to hemolytic disease if his mother is $Rh_0(D)$ negative and has been sensitized to $Rh_0(D)$ positive blood. The woman may only become sensitized (develop antibodies) against the $Rh_0(D)$ antigen if she is exposed to the antigen. This situation may occur if the $Rh_0(D)$ negative woman receives a transfusion with $Rh_0(D)$ positive blood or it may occur during abortion or miscarriage, amniocentesis or other traumatic procedure, placental abruption, or during birth when the placenta separates and fetal blood cells escape into the woman's circulation. Because sensitization normally occurs only during birth, the first-born child is not usually affected by hemolytic disease.

With the next pregnancy, the maternal antibodies enter the fetal circulation and begin to hemolyze the baby's red blood cells. Rapid destruction of red blood cells causes excretion of bilirubin into the amniotic fluid. The fetus makes a valiant attempt to replace the red blood cells being destroyed by sending out large amounts of immature red blood cells (erythroblasts) into the bloodstream (thus the name erythroblastosis fetalis). As the process of rapid destruction of red blood cells continues, anemia develops. If the anemia is severe enough, heart failure and death of the fetus in utero may result.

ABO Incompatibility

The major blood groups are A, B, AB, and O, and each has antigens that may be incompatible with those of another group. The most common incompatibility in the newborn occurs between an infant with type O blood and a mother with type A or B blood. The reactions are usually less severe than in Rh incompatibility.

Prevention

The dramatic reduction in the incidence of erythroblastosis fetalis is due largely to the introduction of RhoGAM. It is effective only in mothers who do not have Rh antibodies, and it must be administered by injection within 72 hours after delivery of an Rh-positive infant or after abortion. Most obstetricians also give the mother an injection of RhoGAM in the 28th week of pregnancy to prevent any sensitization occurring during the pregnancy. RhoGAM essentially neutralizes any $Rh_0(D)$ positive cells that may have escaped into the mother's system, preventing isoimmunization. As mentioned, RhoGAM also must be given to the $Rh_0(D)$ negative mother after an abortion. It is never given to an infant or to a father. The use of RhoGAM on all patients who are candidates for it offers the hope of eliminating hemolytic disease caused by Rh incompatibility. The criteria for giving RhoGAM are:

- The woman must be $Rh_o(D)$ negative.
- The woman must not be sensitized.
- The infant must be $Rh_o(D)$ positive.
- The direct Coombs' test (a test for antibodies performed on cord blood at delivery) must be weakly reactive or negative.

All expectant women should have their blood tested for blood group and Rh type at the initial prenatal visit. If the woman is found to be $Rh_o(D)$ negative, she should then be followed closely throughout her pregnancy. The woman should have blood titers performed periodically as a screening method to detect the presence of antibodies. This allows the physician to evaluate the health of the fetus and plan for the infant's delivery and care.

No preventative measures exist for ABO incompatibility.

Diagnosis

When titers show the presence of antibodies, the physician tries to determine to what degree the fetus is affected. Because there is no direct way to sample fetal blood to determine the degree of anemia, indirect means must be used.

Diagnosis may be made through the use of amniocentesis. Through a needle inserted into the amniotic sac, 10 to 15 mL of amniotic fluid is removed. The fluid is sent to the laboratory for spectrophotometric analysis, which shows the amount of bile pigments (bilirubin) in the amniotic fluid. Thus, it can be determined if the fetus is mildly, moderately, or severely affected.

If analysis of the amniotic fluid shows that the fetus is severely affected, the obstetrician will either perform an intrauterine transfusion of $Rh_o(D)$ negative blood or, if the fetus is beyond 32 weeks' gestation, induce labor or perform a cesarean delivery. After delivery, the baby is turned over to a pediatrician or neonatologist, who will arrange for exchange transfusions.

Clinical Manifestations

Infants with known incompatibility (either Rh or ABO) to the mother's blood are examined carefully at birth for pallor, edema, jaundice, and an enlarged spleen and liver. If prenatal care was inadequate or absent, a severely affected infant may be stillborn or have hydrops fetalis, a condition marked by extensive edema, marked anemia and jaundice, and enlargement of the liver and spleen. These babies are in critical condition and need exchange transfusions at the earliest possible moment. If untreated, severely affected infants are at risk for severe brain damage or **kernicterus** from excess bilirubin levels. Death occurs in about 75% of infants with kernicterus; those who survive may be mentally retarded or develop spastic paralysis or nerve deafness. Exchange transfusions are given at once to infants who have signs of neurologic damage when first seen, although there is no proof that the damage is reversible. Fortunately, our current ability to detect and treat hemolytic disease has reduced the number of infants who become permanently damaged to just a few.

Treatment and Nursing Care

A severely affected newborn usually is transfused without waiting for laboratory confirmation. All other suspected infants have a sample of cord blood sent to the laboratory for a Coombs' test for the presence of damaging antibodies, Rh and ABO typing, hemoglobin and red blood cell levels, and measurement of plasma bilirubin. A positive direct Coombs' test indicates the presence of antibodies on the surface of the infant's red blood cells. A negative direct Coombs' test indicates that there are no antibodies on the infant's red blood cells.

A positive Coombs' test indicates the presence of the disease but not the degree of severity. If bilirubin and hemoglobin levels are within normal limits, the infant is watched carefully and frequent laboratory blood tests are performed. Bilirubin levels may be measured noninvasively with transcutaneous bilirubinometry or by a heel stick, results of which may be interpreted by the nursery nurse with specialized equipment. Exchange transfusions are performed at the discretion of the physician. The infant is cared for in the NICU.

Any infant admitted to the newborn nursery should be examined for jaundice during the first 36 hours or more. Early development of jaundice (within the first 24 to 48 hours) is a probable indication of hemolytic disease.

Phototherapy

Phototherapy refers to the use of special lights to help reduce bilirubin levels. These specially designed fluorescent lights help to prevent bilirubin levels from reaching the danger point of 20 mg/dL, beyond which kernicterus is a threat.

The criteria for treatment with phototherapy vary with the infant's size and age. The lights are placed above and outside the isolette (Fig. 20-9). The infant is nude (except for possibly a diaper under the perineal area to collect urine and feces), with the eyes shielded from the ultraviolet light. The eye patches may promote infection if they are not clean and changed frequently, or they may cause eye damage if they are not applied so that they stay in place. The light may cause the infant to have skin rashes; "sunburn" or tanning;

● *Figure 20.9* A newborn receiving phototherapy.

loose, greenish stools; hyperthermia; an increased metabolic rate; increased evaporative loss of water; and priapism (a perpetual abnormal erection of the penis). Infants undergoing phototherapy need as much as 25% more fluids to prevent dehydration. Monitor the serum bilirubin levels routinely when the infant is receiving phototherapy.

A fiberoptic blanket consisting of a pad attached to a halogen light source with illuminating plastic fibers also can be used. The blanket is covered with a disposable protective cover and can be wrapped about the infant to disperse therapeutic light. These blankets can be used at home, cutting hospitalization costs for the infant with hyperbilirubinemia and reducing the separation time for the infant and family. The neonate's eyes do not need to be covered when the fiberoptic blanket is used. The light can stay on all the time, and the neonate is available for care as needed.

Infants whose bilirubin has been restored to normal levels may be discharged to routine home care like any well newborn. The nurse should be sensitive to the parents' feelings of guilt and anxiety. They may feel that they caused the condition and need to ventilate their feelings. They must never be made to feel that they are responsible for the condition.

NEWBORN OF A DIABETIC MOTHER

The severity of the mother's diabetes has a direct relation to the risk for the infant. The diabetic woman who can closely control her blood glucose level before conception and throughout pregnancy, particularly in the early months, can avoid having an infant with the congenital anomalies commonly associated with diabetes. Infants of mothers with poorly controlled type 2 or gestational diabetes have a distinctive appearance.

They are large for gestational age, plump and full-faced, and coated with vernix caseosa. Both the placenta and the umbilical cord are oversized. In contrast, infants of mothers with poorly controlled, long-term, or severe type 1 diabetes actually may suffer from intrauterine growth retardation.

Newborns of diabetic mothers often are at risk for hypoglycemia in the first few hours after birth (Box 20-2). The woman's high blood glucose levels increase the blood glucose level of the fetus before birth and cause the fetal pancreas to secrete increased amounts of insulin. This process leads to the increased intrauterine growth of the fetus. After birth, however, the high levels of glucose are suddenly cut off when the umbilical cord is cut, but the newborn's pancreas cannot readjust quickly enough and it continues to produce insulin. Thus, hypoglycemia (or hyperinsulinism) occurs. This condition may be fatal if not detected quickly and treated with oral or IV glucose to raise the level of the infant's blood glucose. Hypoglycemia, if untreated, may cause severe, irreversible damage to the central nervous system.

The usual range of blood glucose levels for newborns is 45 to 90 mg/dL. If the newborn's blood glucose level is 40 mg/dL or lower, the infant is treated with IV fluids, early feedings, and IV or oral glucose. The newborn's blood glucose level is checked by heel stick on a frequent schedule for the first 24 hours of life.

These infants are subject to many other hazards, including congenital anomalies, hypocalcemia, hyperbilirubinemia, and respiratory distress syndrome. Newborns of diabetic mothers require especially careful observation.

BOX 20.2	**Signs and Symptoms of Hypoglycemia in the Newborn**

Central Nervous System Signs
• Jitteriness
• Tremors
• Twitching
• Limpness
• Lethargy
• Weak or high-pitched cry
• Apathy
• Seizures
• Coma

Other Signs
• Cyanosis
• Apnea
• Irregular, rapid respirations
• Poor feeding
• Sweating

NEWBORN OF A CHEMICALLY DEPENDENT MOTHER

Alcohol and illicit drug use by the mother during pregnancy can lead to many problems in the newborn. Newborns of mothers who use alcohol are at risk for fetal alcohol syndrome (FAS). Typically, newborns of chemically dependent mothers are SGA and experience withdrawal symptoms.

Unfortunately, identifying the pregnant woman who abuses alcohol or drugs may be difficult. Many of these women have no prenatal care or only infrequent care. They may not keep appointments because of apathy or simply because they are not awake during the day. As a result, many of these infants have suffered prenatal insults that result in intrauterine growth retardation, congenital abnormalities, and premature birth.

Fetal Alcohol Syndrome

Alcohol is one of the many teratogenic substances that cross the placenta to the fetus. Fetal alcohol syndrome (FAS) is often apparent in newborns of mothers with chronic alcoholism and sometimes appears in newborns whose mothers are low to moderate consumers of alcohol. No amount of alcohol is believed to be safe, and women should stop drinking at least 3 months before they plan to become pregnant. The ability of the mother's liver to detoxify the alcohol is apparently of greater importance than the actual amount consumed.

Clinical Manifestations

FAS is characterized by low birth weight, smaller height and head circumference, short palpebral fissures (eyelid folds), reduced ocular growth, and a flattened nasal bridge. These newborns are prone to respiratory difficulties, hypoglycemia, hypocalcemia, and hyperbilirubinemia. Their growth continues to be slow, and their mental development is retarded, despite expert care and nutrition.

Nursing Care

FAS can be prevented by increasing the public's awareness of the detrimental effects of alcohol use during pregnancy. Other helpful interventions include screening women of reproductive age for alcohol problems and encouraging women to obtain adequate prenatal care and use appropriate resources for decreasing alcohol use.

Nursing care for the newborn with FAS is supportive and focuses on preventing complications such as seizures. Sedatives or anticonvulsants may be ordered to prevent stimulation that may lead to seizure activity. Providing adequate nutrition is key to supporting weight gain. The newborn's sucking reflex may be weak, and he or she may be too irritable to feed. Monitor the newborn's daily weights and intake and output. Encourage the parents to feed the newborn. This measure also helps to promote bonding.

Newborn With Withdrawal Symptoms

Newborns of mothers addicted to cocaine, heroin, methadone, or other drugs are born addicted, and many of these infants suffer withdrawal symptoms during the early neonatal period. However, the time of onset varies widely. For example, newborns experiencing withdrawal from opiates typically experience withdrawal symptoms within 24 to 48 hours after birth. However, it may take up to 10 days before the newborn exhibits any symptoms. For the newborn withdrawing from heroin, some may develop symptoms within 72 hours after birth, whereas others may not experience symptoms for as long as 2 weeks.

Clinical Manifestations

Withdrawal symptoms commonly include tremors, restlessness, hyperactivity, disorganized or hyperactive reflexes, increased muscle tone, sneezing, tachypnea, vomiting, diarrhea, disturbed sleep patterns, and a shrill high-pitched cry (Fig. 20-10). Ineffective sucking and swallowing reflexes create feeding problems, and regurgitation and vomiting occur often after feeding.

Nursing Care

Care of the newborn experiencing drug withdrawal focuses on providing physical and emotional support. Medications, such as chlorpromazine, clonidine, diazepam, methadone, morphine, paregoric, or phenobarbital, may be ordered to aid in withdrawal and prevent complications such as seizures.

Because of neuromuscular irritability, many of these newborns respond favorably to movement and close body contact with their caregivers. Therefore, some nurseries place the newborns in special carriers that hold them close to the nurse's chest while the nurse moves about the nursery. Swaddling the infant

Irritability

Disturbed sleep patterns

Frequent sneezing

Shrill, high-pitched cry

Vomiting

Tachypnea

Constant movement

Diarrhea

Tremors

Hyperreflexia, clonus

● *Figure 20.10* Manifestations of a newborn with withdrawal.

(wrapping securely in a small blanket) with arms across the chest also is recommended as a method of quieting the agitated newborn. Keep the newborn's environment dimly lit to minimize stimulation. Maintain the newborn's airway and monitor the newborn's respiratory status closely for changes. Provide small frequent feedings, keeping the newborn's head elevated to promote effective sucking and reduce the risk of aspiration. Vomiting and diarrhea may lead to fluid and electrolyte imbalances. Monitor intake and output closely and give supplemental fluids as ordered. Use a nonjudgmental approach when interacting with the newborn and his or her mother.

NEWBORN WITH A CONGENITALLY ACQUIRED INFECTION

Newborns are at increased risk for infections because their immune systems are immature and they cannot localize infections. High-risk newborns are even more susceptible than normal newborns. Infections may be acquired prenatally from the mother (through the placenta), during the intrapartum period (during labor and delivery) from maternal vaginal infection or inhalation of contaminated amniotic fluid, and after birth from cross-contamination with other infants, health care personnel, or contaminated equipment.

Infections in the newborn can be caused by a variety of organisms. The major cause is group B beta-hemolytic streptococcal infection. The newborn can acquire this infection from the mother because this organism is naturally found in the female reproductive tract. Another means of transmission is from one newborn to another if good handwashing is not used.

The rubella virus may be transmitted to the fetus if the mother becomes infected during the 1st trimester of pregnancy. The newborn is at risk for numerous congenital anomalies, such as cataracts, heart disease, deafness, microcephaly, and motor and cognitive impairments.

Infection with *Chlamydia trachomatis* or *Neisseria gonorrhoeae* may lead to ophthalmia neonatorum, a very serious form of conjunctivitis. The organisms may be transmitted to the newborn during vaginal birth. The routine administration of erythromycin ointment to the eyes of a newborn after birth aids in preventing this infection.

A mother infected with hepatitis B can transmit the virus to the newborn via contact with infected blood at the time of delivery. To prevent the complications associated with infection, newborns of mothers who are positive for the virus are given hepatitis B immune globulin within 12 hours after birth.

Infection with herpes virus type 2 can occur in newborns in one of two ways. The virus may be transmitted via the placenta to the fetus when the mother has an active infection during pregnancy. However, the most common method of transmission is via contact with the vaginal secretions of a mother who has active herpes lesions in the vaginal area at the time of delivery.

Human immunodeficiency virus (HIV) may be transmitted to the fetus across the placenta, from the mother's body fluids during birth, or through breast milk. If the mother is known to be positive for HIV, she should not breast-feed her newborn. The infant's test results are positive for HIV antibodies for as long as 15 months because he or she has passively acquired antibodies from the mother. Only 20% to 40% of infants born to known HIV-infected mothers are infected themselves (Ahuwalia, Merritt, Beck, & Rogers, 2001). To help prevent transmission to the fetus, antiretroviral therapy is ordered for HIV-positive women during the 2nd and 3rd trimesters of pregnancy and during labor and delivery. The newborns also may receive therapy during the first 6 weeks of life.

The newborn often does not have any specific signs of illness. The clue that alerts the nurse to a possible problem may be signs such as cyanosis, pallor, thermal instability (difficulty keeping temperature within normal range), convulsions, lethargy, apnea, jaundice, or just "not looking right." Diagnosis is made through blood, urine, and cerebrospinal fluid cultures and other laboratory and radiographic tests necessary to isolate the specific organism. Treatment consists of intensive antibiotic therapy, IV fluids, respiratory therapy, and other supportive measures.

The newborn of an HIV-positive mother may not show any signs of infection at birth and appears much the same as any other newborn. Signs of HIV infection usually are not seen in infants younger than 4 to 6 months of age. By 1 year of age, about half of those who are infected have symptoms, and by 2 years of age, most HIV-infected infants have symptoms. The prognosis is poor for infants who have symptoms before 1 year of age and those who develop *Pneumocystis carinii* pneumonia. Bacterial infections, such as pneumonia, meningitis, and bacteremia, are common in infected newborns. These infants also commonly have thrush, mouth sores, and severe diaper rash. Gloves must be worn by personnel when they are performing the first bath on every newborn. Gloves also must be worn by the nurse when performing any procedure in which the nurse could be exposed to blood or body fluids that may contain blood.

KEY POINTS

▶ Newborns are classified by size as small for gestational age (SGA), appropriate for gestational age (AGA), and large for gestational age (LGA).

▶ Newborns are classified by gestational age as preterm, post-term, or term.

▶ A gestational age assessment usually evaluates two major categories of maturity: physical maturity and neuromuscular maturity.

▶ Intrauterine growth restriction (IUGR) is the most common underlying condition leading to SGA newborns; the underlying cause for LGA newborns is not known.

▶ A preterm newborn is any newborn of less than 37 weeks' gestation. This newborn typically is tiny, scrawny, and red with little muscle or subcutaneous fat. The skin appears translucent and thin.

▶ Common complications associated with preterm newborns include respiratory distress syndrome, intraventricular hemorrhage, cold stress, retinopathy of prematurity, and necrotizing enterocolitis.

▶ Care of the preterm newborn focuses on improving respiratory function, maintaining body temperature, preventing infection, maintaining adequate nutrition, preserving skin integrity, promoting energy conservation and sensory stimulation, reducing parental anxiety, and

improving parenting skills and family functioning.

▶ A postterm newborn is any newborn of greater than 42 weeks' gestation. This newborn is at high risk for meconium aspiration and hypoglycemia.

▶ Common acquired respiratory disorders of the newborn include transient tachypnea of the newborn (TTN), meconium aspiration syndrome (MAS), and sudden infant death syndrome (SIDS).

▶ Hemolytic disease of the newborn, a condition in which the infant's red blood cells are broken down and destroyed, may be the result of Rh or ABO incompatibility. Hyperbilirubinemia occurs and may be treated by exchange transfusions or phototherapy.

▶ Newborns of diabetic mothers typically are LGA, plump and full-faced, and coated with vernix caseosa and are at high risk for hypoglycemia during the first few hours after birth.

▶ The newborn of a mother who is chemically dependent on alcohol may develop fetal alcohol syndrome (FAS); the newborn of a mother who is chemically dependent on illicit drugs may experience withdrawal symptoms.

▶ Group B beta hemolytic streptococcus is the major cause of infection in the newborn. Other causes include rubella virus; *Chlamydia trachomatis* or *Neisseria gonorrhoeae* (leading to ophthalmia neonatorum); hepatitis B; herpes virus type 2; and human immunodeficiency virus (HIV).

REFERENCES AND SELECTED READINGS

Books and Journals

Ahuwalia, I. B., Merritt, R., Beck, L. F., & Rogers, M. (2001). Multiple lifestyle and psychosocial risks and delivery of small for gestational age infants. *Obstetrics and Gynecology, 97*(5 Pt 1):649–656. PMID: 11339910 [PubMed - indexed for MEDLINE]

Ballard, J. L. Khoury, J. C., Wedig, K., Wang, L., Eilers-Walsman, B. L., & Lipp, R. (1991). New Ballard score expanded to include extremely premature infants. *Journal of Pediatrics, 119*(3), 417–423.

Carroll, J. L., & Laughlin, G. M. (1999). Sudden infant death syndrome. In *Oski's pediatrics: Principles and practices* (3rd ed.). Philadelphia: Lippincott Williams & Wilkins.

Farrell, M. (2003). Gestational diabetes. *The American Journal of Maternal/Child Nursing, 28*(5), 301–305.

Hockenberry, M. J., Wilson, D., Winkelstein, M. L., & Kline, N. E. (2003). *Wong's nursing care of infants and children* (7th ed.). St. Louis: Mosby.

Johnson, T. (2003). Hypoglycemia and the full-term newborn: How well does birth weight for gestational age predict risk? *Journal of Obstetric, Gynecologic, and Neonatal Nursing (JOGNN), 32*(1), 48–57.

Pillitteri, A. (2003). *Maternal and child health nursing* (4th ed.). Philadelphia: Lippincott Williams & Wilkins.

Thomas, K. (2003). Infant weight and gestational age effects on thermoneutrality in the home environment. *Journal of Obstetric, Gynecologic, & Neonatal Nursing (JOGNN), 32*(6), 745–752.

White, R. C., et al. (2004). Developmental patterns of physiological response to a multisensory intervention in extremely premature and high-risk infants. *Journal of Obstetric, Gynecologic, & Neonatal Nursing (JOGNN), 33*(2), 266–275.

Web Addresses

Fetal Alcohol Syndrome

http://www.niaaa.nih.gov/publications/brochure.htm

Prematurity

http://kidshealth.org/parent/system/ill/nicu_diagnoses.html

http://www.marchofdimes.com/prematurity

http://premature-infant.com/index.cfm

WORKBOOK

NCLEX-STYLE REVIEW QUESTIONS

1. The nurse is assisting in a newborn assessment of gestational age using the Newborn Maturity Rating and Classification (Ballard) scoring system. Of the following characteristics, which would be noted in a newborn with the oldest gestational age? The newborn has

   a. abundant lanugo, flat areola, and pinna flat.

   b. anterior transverse plantar crease, ear recoil, and few scrotal rugae.

   c. transparent skin, no lanugo, and prominent clitoris.

   d. bald areas, plantar creases cover sole, and 3- to 4-mm breast bud.

2. A newborn is considered large for gestational age (LGA) when the newborn is larger than the average baby. Which of the following is *most* likely to be a contributing factor in a newborn that is LGA? The mother of the newborn has

   a. no other children.

   b. gained little weight during pregnancy.

   c. a diagnosis of diabetes.

   d. a history of smoking during pregnancy.

3. The nurse is caring for a preterm newborn. When developing a plan of care for the preterm newborn, which of the following nursing interventions would be the *most* important intervention to include?

   a. Repositioning at least every 2 hours

   b. Monitoring body temperature

   c. Promoting rest periods between procedures

   d. Recording urinary output

4. The nurse is caring for the newborn of a mother who abused cocaine during her pregnancy. Which of the following characteristics would the nurse likely see in this newborn? The newborn

   a. weighs above average when born.

   b. sleeps for long periods of time.

   c. cries when touched.

   d. has facial deformities.

5. The preterm newborn has specific characteristics, which differ from those of the term newborn. Identify characteristics that may be seen in the preterm newborn.
   Select all that apply:

   a. Extremities are thin, with little muscle or subcutaneous fat.

   b. Skin is thickened and without wrinkles.

   c. Head and abdomen are disproportionately large.

   d. Veins of the abdomen and scalp are visible.

   e. Lanugo is not evident on the back and shoulders.

   f. Ears have soft, minimal cartilage and are pliable.

STUDY ACTIVITIES

1. Research your community to find sources of help for families who have lost children to sudden infant death syndrome (SIDS). What support groups and organizations are available that you might recommend to families who have lost a child because of SIDS? Discuss with your peers what you found and make a list of resources to share.

2. Go to the following Internet site: http://kidshealth.org.
   Click on "Enter Parents." Type "premature" in the search box.
   Click on "A Primer on Preemies."

   a. What are the two basic needs of a premature infant discussed on this site?

   b. What are the common health problems often seen in premature infants?

   c. What suggestions does this site offer to families of children who have a premature infant?

CRITICAL THINKING: What Would You Do?

1. Andrea, the mother of Andrew, a newborn, has just been told that her son's bilirubin level is elevated and he is going to be given phototherapy. Andrea appears concerned and anxious and looks as if she is about to cry.

   a. What is the first thing you would do and say to Andrea?

   b. What would you explain to Andrea regarding the purpose of the phototherapy for Andrew?

c. What will you teach this mother in regards to what she might expect while Andrew is under the light?

2. You are teaching a nutrition class to a group of pregnant women. One of the women says that she heard it was not a problem to drink a little alcohol while she was pregnant. Another member of the group says she has heard about something called fetal alcohol syndrome.

a. What will you teach this group regarding the use of alcohol during pregnancy?

b. What is fetal alcohol syndrome?

c. What are the characteristics of infants with fetal alcohol syndrome?

d. What are the possible long-term complications of fetal alcohol syndrome?

The Newborn at Risk: Congenital Disorders

STUDENT OBJECTIVES

On completion of this chapter, the student should be able to

1. Differentiate between cleft lip and cleft palate.
2. Identify the early signs that indicate the presence of an esophageal fistula.
3. Name the greatest preoperative danger for newborns with tracheoesophageal atresia.
4. List and describe the five types of hernias that newborns may have.
5. Differentiate the three types of spina bifida that may occur.
6. Name the type of spina bifida that is most difficult to treat and state why.
7. Describe the two types of hydrocephalus that may occur.
8. State the most obvious symptoms of hydrocephalus.
9. Describe two types of shunting performed for hydrocephalus.
10. List five common types of congenital heart defects and trace the blood flow of each defect.
11. State the two most common skeletal deformities in the newborn.

KEY TERMS

atresia
bilateral
brachycephaly
chordee
congestive heart failure (CHF)
cyanotic heart disease
ductus arteriosus
ductus venosus
foramen ovale
galactosemia
hernia
hip dysplasia

12. List three signs and symptoms of congenital dislocation of the hip.
13. Describe the treatment for congenital dislocation of the hip.
14. Identify the test to detect phenylketonuria in the newborn.
15. Describe the treatment for phenylketonuria.
16. Name the tests performed on newborns to detect congenital hypothyroidism.
17. State the one serious outcome that is common to untreated phenylketonuria, congenital hypothyroidism, and galactosemia.
18. Discuss the reason Down syndrome is also called trisomy 21.
19. List 10 signs and symptoms of Down syndrome.

hypothermia
imperforate anus
overriding aorta
phenylketonuria
pulmonary stenosis
right ventricular hypertrophy
spina bifida
supernumerary
talipes equinovarus
unilateral
ventricular septal defect
ventriculoatrial shunting
ventriculoperitoneal shunting

Malformations that occur during the prenatal period and are present at birth are termed *congenital anomalies*. Many times these can be corrected during the first months or years of life. Some congenital conditions are termed inborn errors of metabolism, which are hereditary disorders that affect metabolism. Other congenital defects are caused by chromosomal abnormalities. These types of congenital malformations and disorders are discussed within this chapter. Gestational and acquired disorders of the newborn are present at birth and are caused by prenatal and perinatal damage due to maternal infection, substance use, maternal disorders or disease, birth trauma, or abnormalities specific to pregnancy. These disorders are discussed in Chapter 20.

The birth of a newborn with a congenital defect (anomaly) is a crisis for parents and caregivers. Depending on the defect, immediate or early surgery may be necessary. Early, continuous, skilled observation and highly skilled nursing care are required. Rehabilitation of the newborn and education of the family caregivers in the newborn's care are essential. The emotional needs of the newborn and the family must be integrated into the plans for nursing care. Many of these newborns have a brighter future today as a result of increased diagnostic and medical knowledge and advances in surgical techniques.

Family caregivers experience a grief response whether the newborn's defect is a result of abnormal intrauterine development or a chromosomal abnormality. They mourn the loss of the perfect child of their dreams, question why it happened, and may wonder how they will show the newborn to family and friends without shame or embarrassment. This grief may interfere with the process of parent–newborn attachment. Parents need to understand that their response is normal and that they are entitled to honest answers to their questions about the newborn's condition. Other children in the family should be informed gently but honestly about the newborn and should be allowed to visit the newborn when accompanied by adult family members. Sufficient time and attention must be devoted to the older siblings to avoid jealousy toward the newborn.

CONGENITAL MALFORMATIONS

Congenital anomalies or malformations may be caused by genetic or environmental factors. Approximately 2% to 3% of all infants born have a major malformation (Holmes, 1999). These anomalies include defects of the gastrointestinal, central nervous, cardiovascular, skeletal, and genitourinary systems. Defects such as cleft lip and severe neural tube defects are apparent at birth, but others may be discovered only after a complete physical examination. Congenital anomalies account for a large percentage of the health problems seen in newborns and children.

Gastrointestinal System Defects

Most gastrointestinal system anomalies are apparent at birth or shortly thereafter. The anomalies are often the result of embryonic growth interrupted at a crucial stage. Many of these anomalies interfere with the normal nutrition and digestion essential to the newborn's normal growth and development. Many anomalies require immediate surgical intervention.

Cleft Lip and Cleft Palate

The birth of a newborn with a facial deformity may change the atmosphere of the delivery from one of joyous anticipation to one of awkward tension. Parents and family are naturally eager to see and hold their newborn and must be prepared for the shock of seeing the facial disfigurement of a cleft lip. Their emotional reaction to such an obvious malformation is usually much stronger than to a "hidden" defect, such as congenital heart defect. They need encouragement and support, as well as considerable instruction about the newborn's feeding and care.

The most common facial malformations, cleft lip and cleft palate, occur either alone or in combination. Cleft lip occurs in about one in 1,000 live births and is more common in males. Cleft palate occurs in one newborn in 2,500, more often in females. Their cause is not entirely clear; they appear to be influenced genetically but sometimes occur in isolated instances with no genetic history. Although a cleft lip and a cleft palate often appear together, either defect may appear alone. In embryonic development, the palate closes later than the lip, and the failure to close occurs for different reasons.

The cleft lip and palate defects result from failure of the maxillary and premaxillary processes to fuse during the 5th to 8th week of intrauterine life. The cleft may be a simple notch in the vermilion line, or it may extend up into the floor of the nose (Fig. 21-1). It may be either **unilateral** (one side of the lip) or **bilateral** (both sides). Cleft palate occurs with a cleft lip about 50% of the time, most often with bilateral cleft lip. The child born with a cleft palate, but with an intact lip, does not have the external disfigurement that may be so distressing to the new parent. However, the prob-

lems are more serious. Cleft palate, which develops sometime between the 7th and 12th weeks of gestation, is often accompanied by nasal deformity and dental disorders, such as deformed, missing, or **supernumerary** (excessive in number) teeth.

In an 8-week-old embryo, there is still no roof to the mouth; the tissues that are to become the palate are two shelves running from the front to the back of the mouth and projecting vertically downward on either side of the tongue. The shelves move from a vertical position to a horizontal position; their free edges meet and fuse in midline. Later, bone forms within this tissue to form the hard palate.

Normally the palate is intact by the 10th week of fetal life. Exactly what happens to prevent this closure is not known for sure. The incidence of cleft palates is higher in the close relatives of people with the defect than it is in the general population, and some evidence indicates that environmental and hereditary factors play a part in this defect.

Clinical Presentation

The physical appearance of the newborn confirms the diagnosis of cleft lip. Diagnosis of cleft palate is made at birth with the close inspection of the newborn's palate. To be certain that a cleft palate is not missed, the examiner must insert a gloved finger into the newborn's mouth to feel the palate to determine that it is intact. If a cleft is found, consultation is set up with a clinic specializing in cleft palate repair.

Treatment

Surgery, usually performed by a plastic surgeon, is a major part of the treatment of a newborn with a cleft lip, palate, or both (Fig. 21-2). Total care involves many other specialists, including pediatricians, nurses, orthodontists, prosthodontists, otolaryngologists, speech therapists, and occasionally psychiatrists. Long-term, intensive, multidisciplinary care is needed for newborns with major defects.

Plastic surgeons' opinions differ as to the best time for repair of the cleft lip. Some surgeons favor early repair, before the newborn is discharged from the hospital. They believe early repair can alleviate some of the family's feelings of rejection of the newborn. Other surgeons prefer to wait until the newborn is 1 or 2 months old, weighs about 10 lb, and is gaining weight steadily. Newborns who are not born in large medical centers with specialists on the staff are discharged from the birth hospital and referred to a center or physician specializing in cleft lip and palate repair.

If early surgery is contemplated, the newborn should be healthy and of average or above-average weight. The newborn must be observed constantly because a newborn has a higher likelihood of aspiration than does an older infant. These newborns must

● *Figure 21.1* A cleft lip may extend up into the floor of the nose.

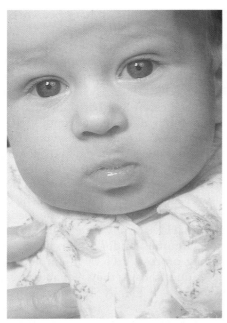

● **Figure 21.2** Infant with a surgical repair of a cleft lip.

be cared for by competent plastic surgeons and experienced nurses.

The goal in repairing the cleft palate is to give the child a union of the cleft parts to allow intelligible and pleasant speech and to avoid injury to the maxillary development. The timing of cleft palate repair is individualized according to the size, placement, and degree of deformity. The surgery may need to be done in stages over a period of several years to achieve the best results. The optimal time for surgical repair of the cleft palate is considered to be between 6 months and 5 years of age. Because the child cannot make certain sounds when starting to talk, undesirable speech habits are formed that are difficult to correct. If surgery must be delayed beyond the 3rd year, a dental speech appliance may help the child develop intelligible speech.

● Nursing Process in Caring for the Newborn With Cleft Lip and Cleft Palate

ASSESSMENT

One primary concern in the nursing care of the newborn with a cleft lip with or without a cleft palate is the emotional care of the newborn's family. In interviewing the family and collecting data, the nurse must include exploration of the family's acceptance of the newborn. Practice active listening with reflective responses, accept the family's emotional responses, and demonstrate complete acceptance of the newborn.

The family caregivers who return to the hospital with their infant for the beginning repair of a cleft palate have already faced the challenges of feeding their infant. Conduct a thorough interview with the caregiver that includes a question about the methods they found to be most effective in feeding the infant.

Physical examination of the infant includes temperature, apical pulse, and respirations. Listen to breath sounds to detect any pulmonary congestion. Observe skin turgor and color, noting any deviations from normal. In addition, observe the infant's neurologic status, noting alertness and responsiveness. Document a complete description of the cleft.

SELECTED NURSING DIAGNOSIS

Nursing diagnoses for the newborn before surgery may include:
- Imbalanced Nutrition: Less than Body Requirements related to inability to suck secondary to cleft lip
- Compromised Family Coping related to visible physical defect
- Anxiety of family caregivers related to the child's condition and surgical outcome
- Deficient Knowledge of family caregivers related to care of child before surgery and the surgical procedure

Nursing diagnoses applicable to the newborn after the surgical repairs are:
- Risk for Aspiration related to a reduced level of consciousness after surgery
- Ineffective Breathing Pattern related to anatomic changes
- Risk for Deficient Fluid Volume related to NPO status after surgery
- Imbalanced Nutrition: Less than Body Requirements related to difficulty in feeding after surgery
- Acute Pain related to surgical procedure
- Risk of Injury to the operative site related to newborn's desire to suck thumb or fingers and anatomic changes
- Risk for Infection related to surgical incision
- Risk for Delayed Growth and Development related to hospitalizations and surgery
- Deficient Knowledge of family caregivers related to long-term aspects of cleft palate

OUTCOME IDENTIFICATION AND PLANNING: PREOPERATIVE CARE

Goal setting and planning must be modified to adapt to the surgical plans. If the newborn is to be discharged from the birth hospital to have surgery a month or two later, the nurse may focus on preparing the family to care for the newborn at home and helping them cope with their emotions. The major goals include maintaining adequate nutrition, increasing family coping, reducing the parents' anxiety and guilt regarding the newborn's physical defect, and preparing parents for the future repair of the cleft lip and palate.

IMPLEMENTATION

Maintaining Adequate Nutrition. The newborn's nutritional condition is important to the planning of surgery because the newborn must be in good condition before surgery can be scheduled. However, feeding the newborn with a cleft lip or palate before repair is a challenge. The procedure may be time consuming and tedious because the newborn's ability to suck is inadequate. Breastfeeding may be successful because the breast tissue may mold to close the gap. If the newborn cannot breast-feed, the mother's breast milk may be expressed and used instead of formula until after the surgical repair heals. Various nipples may be tried to find the method that works best. A soft nipple with a crosscut made to promote easy flow of milk or formula may work well. A large nipple with holes that allow the milk to drip freely makes sucking easier. If the cleft lip is unilateral, the nipple should be aimed at the unaffected side. The infant should be kept in a upright position during feeding.

If the infant does not have a cleft lip or if the lip has had an early repair, sucking may be learned more easily, even though the suction generated is not as good as in the infant with an intact palate. Lamb's nipples (extra-long nipples) and special cleft palate nipples molded to fit into the open

palate area to close the gap have been used with success.

One of the simplest and most effective methods may be the use of an eyedropper or an Asepto syringe with a short piece of rubber tubing on the tip (Breck feeder) (Fig. 21-3). The dropper or syringe is used carefully to drip formula into the newborn's mouth at a rate slow enough to allow the newborn to swallow. As the newborn learns to eat, much coughing, sputtering, and choking may occur. The nurse or family caregiver feeding the newborn must be alert for signs of aspiration.

Whatever feeding method is used, the experience may be frustrating for both the feeder and the newborn. Have family caregivers practice the feeding techniques under supervision. During the teaching process, give them ample opportunity to ask questions so they feel able to care for the newborn (see Family Teaching Tips: Cleft Lip/Cleft Palate).

Promoting Family Coping. Encourage family members to verbalize their feelings regarding the defect and their disappointment. Convey to the family that their feelings are acceptable and normal. While caring for the newborn, demonstrate behavior that clearly displays acceptance of the newborn. Serve as a model for the family caregivers' attitudes toward the child.

Reducing Family Anxiety. Give the family caregivers information about cleft repairs. Pamphlets are available that present photographs of before and after corrections that will answer some of their questions. Encourage them to ask questions and reassure them that any question is valid.

Providing Family Teaching. By the time the infant is actually admitted for the repair, the family will have received a great amount of information, but all families need additional support

A

B

● *Figure 21.3* Specialty feeding devices used for the newborn with a cleft lip or palate include **(A)** special nipples and devices and **(B)** a special feeder.

Cleft Lip/Cleft Palate

- Sucking is important to speech development.
- Holding the baby upright while feeding helps avoid choking.
- Burp the baby frequently because a large amount of air is swallowed during feeding.
- Don't tire the baby. Limit feeding times to 20 to 30 minutes maximum. If necessary, feed the baby more often.
- Feed strained foods slowly from the side of the spoon in small amounts.
- Don't be alarmed if food seeps through the cleft and out the nose.
- Have baby's ears checked any time he or she has a cold or upper respiratory infection.
- Talk normally to baby (no "baby talk"). Talk often; repeat baby's babbling and cooing. This helps in speech development.
- Try to understand early talking without trying to correct baby.
- Good mouth care is very important.
- Early dental care is essential to observe teething and prevent caries.

throughout the procedure. Explain the usual routine of preoperative, intraoperative, and postoperative care. Written information is helpful, but be certain the parents understand the information. Simple things are important; show families where they may wait during surgery, inform them how long the surgery should last, tell them about the postanesthesia care unit procedure, and let them know where the surgeon will expect to find them to report on the surgery.

OUTCOME IDENTIFICATION AND PLANNING: POSTOPERATIVE CARE

Major goals for the postoperative care of the infant who is hospitalized for surgical repair of cleft lip or palate include preventing aspiration, improving respiration, maintaining adequate fluid volume

CULTURAL SNAPSHOT

In some cultures genetic defects are blamed on the mother—something she did or ate; stress or trauma that occurred during pregnancy; viewing a child with a defect caused her child to have the same defect. The mother may have feelings of guilt or fears of being an unacceptable mother and needs to be supported by the nurse.

and nutritional requirements, relieving pain, preventing injury and infection to the surgical site, promoting normal growth and development, and increasing the family caregivers' knowledge about the child's long-term care.

IMPLEMENTATION

Preventing Aspiration. To facilitate drainage of mucus and secretions, position the infant on the side, never on the abdomen, after a cleft lip repair. The infant may be placed on the side after a cleft palate repair. Watch the infant closely in the immediate postoperative period. Do not put anything in the infant's mouth to clear mucus because of the danger of damaging the surgical site, particularly with a palate repair.

Changing Breathing Pattern. Immediately after a palate repair, the infant must change from a mouth-breathing pattern to nasal breathing. This change may frustrate the infant, but the infant positioned to ease breathing and given encouragement should be able to adjust quickly.

Monitoring Fluid Volume. In the immediate postoperative period, the infant needs parenteral fluids. Follow all the usual precautions: check placement, discoloration of the site, swelling, and flow rate every 2 hours. Document intake and output accurately. Parenteral fluids are continued until the infant can take oral fluids without vomiting.

Maintaining Adequate Nutrition. As soon as the infant is no longer nauseated (vomiting should be avoided if possible), the surgeon usually permits clear liquids. After the cleft lip repair, no tension should be placed on the suture line, to prevent the sutures from pulling apart and leaving a scar. A specialized feeder may need to be used because bottle- or breast-feeding may increase the tension on the suture line.

For an infant who has had a palate repair, no nipples, spoons, or straws are permitted; only a drinking glass or a cup is recommended. A favorite cup from home may be reassuring to the older infant. Offer clear liquids such as flavored gelatin water, apple juice, and synthetic fruit-flavored drinks. Red juices should not be given because they may conceal bleeding. Infants do not usually like broth. The diet is increased to full liquid, and the infant is usually discharged on a soft diet. When permitted, foods such as cooked infant cereals, ice cream, and flavored gelatin are often favorites. The surgeon determines the progression of the diet. Nothing hard or sharp should be placed in the infant's mouth. After each feeding, clear water is used to rinse the mouth and suture line.

Relieving Pain. Observe the infant for signs of pain or discomfort from the surgery. Administer ordered analgesics as needed. Relieving pain not only comforts the infant, but may also prevent crying, which is important because of the danger of disrupting the suture line. Make every effort to prevent the infant with a lip repair from crying to prevent excessive tension on the suture line.

Preventing Postoperative Injury. Continuous, skilled observation is essential. Swollen mouth tissues cause excessive secretion of mucus that is handled poorly by a small infant. For the first few postoperative hours, never leave the infant alone because aspiration of mucus occurs quickly and easily. Because nothing is permitted in the infant's mouth, particularly the thumb or finger, elbow restraints are necessary. The thumb, although comforting, may quickly undo the repair or cause undesirable scarring along the suture line. The infant's ultimate happiness and well-being must take precedence over immediate satisfaction. Accustoming the infant to elbow restraints gradually before admission is helpful.

Elbow restraints must be applied properly and checked frequently (see Figure 30-1). Place the restraints firmly around the arm and pinned to the infant's shirt or gown to prevent them from sliding down below the elbow. The infant's arms can move freely but cannot bend at the elbows to reach the face. Apply the restraint snugly but do not allow the circulation to be hindered. The older infant may need to be placed in a jacket restraint. The use of restraints must be documented.

Some nurses find this approach helpful. For the infant in restraints, playing "Peek-a-Boo" and other infant games will help to comfort and entertain the baby; however "Patty Cake" does not work well with an infant in elbow restraints.

Remove restraints at least every 2 hours, but remove them only one at a time and control the released arm so that the thumb or fingers do not pop into the mouth. Comfort the infant and explore various means of comforting. Talk to the infant continuously while providing care. Inspect and massage the skin, apply lotion, and perform range-of-motion exercises. Replace restraints when they become soiled.

Preventing Infection. Gentle mouth care with tepid water or clear liquid may be recommended to follow feeding. This care helps clean the suture area of any food or liquids to promote a cleaner incision for optimal healing.

Care of Lip Suture Line. The lip suture line is left uncovered after surgery and must be kept clean and dry to prevent infection and subsequent

● *Figure 21.4* Logan bar for easing strain on sutures.

scarring. A wire bow called a Logan bar or a butterfly closure is applied across the upper lip and attached to the cheeks with adhesive tape to prevent tension on the sutures caused by crying or other facial movement (Fig. 21-4). Carefully clean the sutures after feeding and as often as necessary to prevent collection of dried formula or serum. Frequent cleaning is essential as long as the sutures are in place. Clean the sutures gently with sterile cotton swabs and saline or the solution of the surgeon's choice. Application of an ointment such as bacitracin may also be ordered. Care of the suture line is extremely important because it has a direct effect on the cosmetic appearance of the repair. Teach the family how to care for the suture line because the infant will probably be discharged before the sutures are removed (7 to 10 days after surgery). The infant probably will be allowed to suck on a soft nipple at this time.

Aseptic technique is important while caring for the infant undergoing lip or palate repair. Good handwashing technique is essential. Instruct the family caregivers about the importance of preventing anyone with an upper respiratory infection from visiting the infant. Observe for signs of otitis media that may occur from drainage into the eustachian tube.

Promoting Sensory Stimulation. The infant needs stimulating, safe toys in the crib. The nurse and family caregivers must use every opportunity to provide sensory stimulation. Talking to the infant, cuddling and holding him or her, and responding to cries are important interventions. Provide freedom from restraints within the limitations of safety as much as possible. One caregiver should be assigned to provide stability and consistency of care. Family caregivers and health care personnel must encourage the older child to use speech and help enhance the child's self-esteem. A baby experiences emotional frustration because of restraints, so satisfaction must be provided in other ways. Rocking, cuddling, and other soothing techniques are an important part of nursing care. Family members and other caregivers are the best people to supply this loving care.

Providing Family Teaching. After effective surgery and skilled, careful nursing care, the appearance of the baby's face should be improved greatly. The scar fades in time. Family caregivers need to know that the baby will probably need a slight adjustment of the vermilion line in later childhood, but they can expect a repair that is barely, if at all, noticeable (see Fig. 21-2).

Cleft lip and cleft palate centers have teams of specialists who can provide the services that these children and their families need through infancy, preschool, and the school years. Explain to the caregivers the services offered by the pediatrician, plastic surgeon, orthodontist, speech therapist, nutritionist, and public or home health nurse. These professionals can give explanations and counseling about the child's diet, speech training, immunizations, and general health. Encourage family caregivers to ask them any questions they may have. Be alert for any evidence that the caregivers need additional information and arrange appropriate meetings.

Dental care for the deciduous teeth is even more important than usual. The incidence of dental caries is high in children with a cleft palate, but preservation of the deciduous teeth is important for the best results in speech and appearance.

EVALUATION: GOALS AND EXPECTED OUTCOMES

Preoperative

- **Goal:** The newborn will show appropriate weight gain.
  Expected Outcomes: The newborn's weight increases at a predetermined goal of 1 oz or more per day.
- **Goal:** The family will demonstrate acceptance of the newborn.
  Expected Outcomes: Family caregivers verbalize their feelings about the newborn and cuddle and talk to the newborn.
- **Goal:** The family caregiver's anxiety will be reduced.
  Expected Outcomes: Family caregivers ask appropriate questions about surgery, openly discuss their concerns, and voice reasonable expectations.
- **Goal:** The family will learn how to care for the newborn and will have an understanding of surgical procedures.
  Expected Outcomes: Family caregivers ask appropriate questions, demonstrate how to

feed the newborn before surgery, and describe the surgical procedures.

Postoperative

- **Goal:** The infant's respiratory tract will remain clear, the infant will breathe easily, and the respiratory rate will be within normal limits.
  Expected Outcomes: The infant has clear lung sounds with no aspiration, and the respiratory rate stays within normal range.
- **Goal:** The infant will adjust his or her breathing pattern.
  Expected Outcomes: The infant breathes nasally with little stress and maintains normal respirations.
- **Goal:** The infant will show signs of adequate hydration during NPO period.
  Expected Outcomes: The newborn's skin turgor is good, mucous membranes are moist, and urine output is adequate; there is no evidence of parenteral fluid infiltration.
- **Goal:** The infant will have adequate caloric intake and retain and tolerate oral nutrition.
  Expected Outcomes: The infant gains 0.75 to 1 oz (22 to 30 g) per day if younger than 6 months of age or 0.5 to 0.75 oz (13 to 22 g) per day if older than 6 months and does not experience nausea or vomiting.
- **Goal:** The infant's pain and discomfort will be minimized.
  Expected Outcomes: The infant rests quietly, does not cry, and is not fretful.
- **Goal:** The surgical site will remain free of injury.
  Expected Outcomes: The surgical site is intact; the infant puts nothing into the mouth such as straws, sharp objects, thumb, or fingers.
- **Goal:** The infant's incision site will remain free of signs and symptoms of infection.
  Expected Outcomes: The incisional site is clean with no redness or drainage. The infant's temperature is within normal limits. The caregivers and family members practice good handwashing and aseptic technique.
- **Goal:** The infant will show evidence of normal growth and development.
  Expected Outcomes: The infant is content most of the time and responds appropriately to the caregiver and family. The infant engages in age- and development-appropriate activities within the limits of restraints.
- **Goal:** The family will learn how to care for the infant's long-term needs.
  Expected Outcomes: The family caregivers ask appropriate questions, respond appropriately to staff queries, and describe services available for the child's long-term care.

Esophageal Atresia

Atresia is the absence of a normal body opening or the abnormal closure of a body passage. Esophageal atresia with or without fistula into the trachea is a serious congenital anomaly and is among the most common anomalies causing respiratory distress. This condition occurs in about 1 in 2,500 live births. Several types of esophageal atresia occur; in more than 90% of affected newborns, the upper, or proximal, end of the esopha-

gus ends in a blind pouch and the lower, or distal, segment from the stomach is connected to the trachea by a fistulous tract (Fig. 21-5).

Clinical Presentation

Any mucus or fluid that a newborn swallows enters the blind pouch of the esophagus. This pouch soon fills and overflows, usually resulting in aspiration into the trachea. Few other conditions depend so greatly on careful

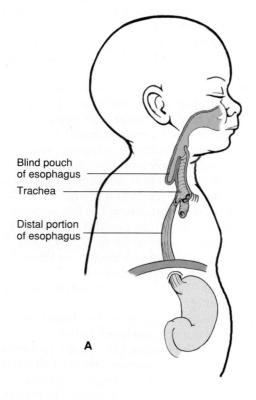

Blind pouch of esophagus
Trachea
Distal portion of esophagus

A

B   **C**   **D**

● *Figure 21.5* (**A**) The most common form of esophageal atresia. (**B**) Both segments of the esophagus are blind pouches. (**C**) Esophagus is continuous but with narrowed segment. (**D**) Upper segment of esophagus opens into trachea.

nursing observation for early diagnosis and, therefore, improved chances of survival. The newborn with this disorder has frothing and excessive drooling and periods of respiratory distress with choking and cyanosis. Many newborns have difficulty with mucus, but the nurse should be alert to the possibility of an anomaly and report such difficulties immediately. No feeding should be given until the newborn has been examined.

If early signs are overlooked and feeding is attempted, the newborn chokes, coughs, and regurgitates as the food enters the blind pouch. The newborn becomes deeply cyanotic and appears to be in severe respiratory distress. During this process, some of the formula may be aspirated, resulting in pneumonitis and increasing the risk of surgery. This newborn's life may depend on the careful observations of the nurse. If there is a fistula of the distal portion of the esophagus into the trachea, the gastric contents may reflux into the lungs and cause a chemical pneumonitis.

Treatment and Nursing Care

Surgical intervention is necessary to correct the defect. Timing of the surgery depends on the surgeon's preference, the anomaly, and the newborn's condition. Aspiration of mucus must be prevented, and continuous, gentle suction may be used. The newborn needs intravenous fluids to maintain optimal hydration. The first stage of surgery may involve a gastrostomy and a method of draining the proximal esophageal pouch. A chest tube is inserted to drain chest fluids. An end-to-end anastomosis is sometimes possible. If the repair is complex, surgery may need to be done in stages.

Often these defects occur in premature newborns, so additional factors may complicate the surgical repair and prognosis (Fig. 21-6). If there are no other major problems, the long-term outcome should be good. Regular follow-up is necessary to observe for and dilate esophageal strictures that may be caused by scar tissue.

● **Figure 21.6** Repair of tracheal esophageal atresia in premature newborns may be complicated by other factors.

Imperforate Anus

Early in intrauterine life, the membrane between the rectum and the anus should be absorbed, and a clear passage from the rectum to the anus should exist. If the membrane remains and blocks the union between the rectum and the anus, an **imperforate anus** results. In a newborn with imperforate anus, the rectal pouch ends blindly at a distance above the anus; there is no anal orifice. A fistula may exist between the rectum and the vagina in females or between the rectum and the urinary tract in males.

Clinical Presentation

In some newborns, only a dimple indicates the site of the anus (Fig. 21-7A). When the initial rectal temperature is attempted, it is apparent that there is no anal opening. However, a shallow opening may occur in the anus, with the rectum ending in a blind pouch some distance higher (Fig. 21-7B). Thus, being able to pass a thermometer into the rectum does not guarantee that the rectoanal canal is normal. More reliable presumptive evidence is obtained by watching carefully for the first meconium stool. If the newborn does not pass a stool within the first 24 hours, the physician should be notified. Abdominal distention also occurs. Definitive diagnosis is made by radiographic studies.

Treatment

If the rectal pouch is separated from the anus by only a thin membrane, the surgeon may repair the defect from below. For a high defect, abdominoperineal resection is indicated. In these newborns, a colostomy is performed, and extensive abdominoperineal resection is delayed until 3 to 5 months of age or later.

Nursing Care

When the newborn goes home with a colostomy, the family must learn how to give colostomy care. Teach caregivers to keep the area around the colostomy clean with soap and water and to diaper the baby in the usual way. A protective ointment is useful to protect the skin around the colostomy.

Hernias

A **hernia** is the abnormal protrusion of a part of an organ through a weak spot or other abnormal opening in a body wall. Complications occur depending on the amount of circulatory impairment involved and how much the herniated organ impairs the functioning of another organ. Most hernias can be repaired surgically.

Diaphragmatic Hernia

In a congenital hernia of the diaphragm, some of the abdominal organs are displaced into the left chest

A   **B**

● *Figure 21.7* Imperforate anus (anal atresia). (**A**) Membrane between anus and rectum. (**B**) Rectum ending in a blind pouch at a distance above the perineum.

through an opening in the diaphragm. The heart is pushed toward the right, and the left lung is compressed. Rapid, labored respirations and cyanosis are present on the first day of life, and breathing becomes increasingly difficult. Surgery is essential and may be performed as an emergency procedure. During surgery, the abdominal viscera are withdrawn from the chest and the diaphragmatic defect is closed.

This defect may be minimal and repaired easily or so extensive that pulmonary tissue has failed to develop normally. The outcome of surgical repair depends on the degree of pulmonary development. The prognosis in severe cases is guarded.

Hiatal Hernia

More common in adults than in newborns, hiatal hernia is caused when the cardiac portion of the stomach slides through the normal esophageal hiatus into the area above the diaphragm. This action causes reflux of gastric contents into the esophagus and subsequent regurgitation. If upright posture and modified feeding techniques do not correct the problem, surgery is necessary to repair the defect.

Omphalocele

Omphalocele is a relatively rare congenital anomaly. Some of the abdominal contents protrude through into the root of the umbilical cord and form a sac lying on the abdomen. This sac may be small, with only a loop of bowel, or large and containing much of the intestine and the liver (Fig. 21-8). The sac is covered with peritoneal membrane instead of skin. These defects may be detected during prenatal ultrasonography so that prompt repair may be anticipated. At birth, the defect should be covered immediately with gauze moistened in sterile saline, which then may be covered with plastic wrap to prevent heat loss. Surgical replacement of the organs into the abdomen may be difficult with a large omphalocele because there may not be enough

space in the abdominal cavity. Other congenital defects often are present.

With large omphaloceles, surgery may be postponed and the surgeon will suture skin over the defect, creating a large hernia. As the child grows, the abdomen may enlarge enough to allow replacement.

Umbilical Hernia

Normally the ring that encircled the fetal end of the umbilical cord closes gradually and spontaneously after birth. When this closure is incomplete, portions of omentum and intestine protrude through the opening. More common in preterm and African-American newborns, umbilical hernia is largely a cosmetic problem (Fig. 21-9). Although upsetting to

Did you know? Some people believe that taping a coin on an umbilical hernia will help reduce the hernia. This can actually result in a serious problem for the newborn and should not be done.

● *Figure 21.8* Large omphalocele with liver and intestine.

● *Figure 21.9* Small umbilical hernia in newborn.

parents, umbilical hernia is associated with little or no morbidity. In rare instances, the bowel may strangulate in the sac and require immediate surgery. Almost all these hernias close spontaneously by the age of 3 years; hernias that do not close should be corrected surgically before the child enters school.

Inguinal Hernia

Primarily common in males, inguinal hernias occur when the small sac of peritoneum surrounding the testes fails to close off after the testes descend from the abdominal sac into the scrotum. This failure allows the intestine to slip into the inguinal canal, with resultant swelling. If the intestine becomes trapped (incarcerated) and the circulation to the trapped intestine is impaired (strangulated), surgery is necessary to prevent intestinal obstruction and gangrene of the bowel.

As a preventive measure, inguinal hernias normally are repaired as soon as they are diagnosed.

Test Yourself

- What are two major concerns for the newborn with a cleft lip or cleft palate?
- What is a potential complication for the newborn who has esophageal atresia?
- How are hernias most often treated?

Central Nervous System Defects

Central nervous system defects include disorders caused by an imbalance of cerebrospinal fluid (as in hydrocephalus) and a range of disorders resulting from malformations of the neural tube during embryonic development (often called "neural tube defects"). These defects vary from mild to severely disabling.

Spina Bifida

Caused by a defect in the neural arch generally in the lumbosacral region, **spina bifida** is a failure of the posterior laminae of the vertebrae to close; this leaves an opening through which the spinal meninges and spinal cord may protrude (Fig. 21-10).

Clinical Presentation

Signs and Symptoms. A bony defect that occurs without soft-tissue involvement is called *spina bifida occulta.* In most instances, it is asymptomatic and presents no problems. A dimple in the skin or a tuft of hair over the site may cause one to suspect its presence, or it may be overlooked entirely.

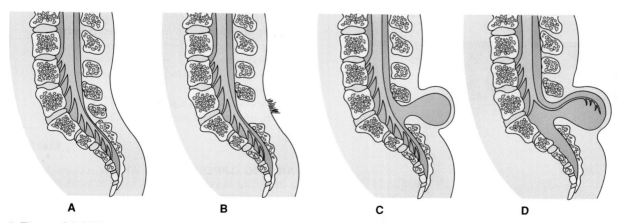

A   B   C   D

● *Figure 21.10* Degrees of spinal cord anomalies. (**A**) The normal spinal closure. (**B**) Occulta defect. (**C**) Meningocele defect. (**D**) Myelomeningocele defect clearly shows the spinal cord involvement.

When part of the spinal meninges protrudes through the bony defect and forms a cystic sac, the condition is termed *spina bifida with meningocele*. No nerve roots are involved, so no paralysis or sensory loss below the lesion appears. However, the sac may rupture or perforate, introducing infection into the spinal fluid and causing meningitis. For this reason, as well as for cosmetic purposes, surgical removal of the sac with closure of the skin is indicated.

In *spina bifida with myelomeningocele,* there is a protrusion of the spinal cord and the meninges, with nerve roots embedded in the wall of the cyst (Fig. 21-11). The effects of this defect vary in severity from sensory loss or partial paralysis below the lesion to complete flaccid paralysis of all muscles below the lesion. Complete paralysis involves the lower trunk and legs, as well as bowel and bladder sphincters.

Making a clear-cut differentiation in diagnosis between a meningocele and a myelomeningocele on the basis of symptoms alone is not always possible. Myelomeningocele may also be termed *meningomyelocele;* the associated "spina bifida" is always implied but not necessarily named. *Spina bifida cystica* is the term used to designate either of these protrusions.

Laboratory and Diagnostic Test Results. Elevated maternal alpha-fetoprotein (AFP) levels followed by ultrasonographic examination of the fetus may show an incomplete neural tube. An elevated AFP level in the maternal serum or amniotic fluid indicates the probability of central nervous system abnormalities. Additional examination may confirm this and allow the pregnant woman the opportunity to consider terminating the pregnancy. The best time to perform these tests is between 13 and 15 weeks' gestation, when peak levels are reached. Most obstetricians perform AFP testing.

Diagnosis of the newborn with spina bifida is made from clinical observation and examination. Additional evaluation of the defect may include magnetic resonance imaging (MRI), ultrasonography, computed tomography (CT) scanning, and myelography. The newborn needs to be examined carefully for other associated defects, particularly hydrocephalus, genitourinary defects, and orthopedic anomalies.

Treatment

Many specialists are involved in the treatment of these newborns, especially in the case of myelomeningocele. These specialists may include neurologists, neurosurgeons, orthopedic specialists, pediatricians, urologists, and physical therapists. After a thorough evaluation of the newborn, a plan of surgical repair and treatment is developed.

Highly skilled nursing care is necessary in all aspects of the newborn's care. The child requires years

● *Figure 21.11* A newborn with a myelomeningocele and hydrocephalus.

A PERSONAL GLIMPSE

A child with "special needs." I never thought I would have to understand just what that really means. Courtney was our second child. A perfect pregnancy. Absolutely no problems. I didn't drink, never smoked, so I planned on a perfectly healthy baby. Until the AFP test. I will never forget that test now. I was 4 months pregnant and went in for the routine test. A few days later the results were in. A neurotube defect. . . . what in the world was that?

I have been asked many times if I was glad I knew before I had Courtney that she would have problems. I've thought a lot about it and even though it made the last several months of the pregnancy a little (well, maybe more than a little) worrisome, yes, I'm very glad we knew. Courtney was born C-section at a regional medical center that is about 60 miles from home. She was in surgery just a few hours after she was born.

Words like spina bifida, hydrocephalus, v. p. shunt, catheterizations, glasses, walkers, braces, kidney infections, all became everyday words at our home. We have learned a lot in the last 5 years. Courtney has frequent doctor visits to all her specialists. She is the only 5-year-old concerned if her urine is cloudy and making sure her mom gives her medication on time.

A little over 5 years ago a "special" child was born, and we feel very blessed she was given to us!!

Rhonda

LEARNING OPPORTUNITY: What reactions do you think the nurse might anticipate in working with a pregnant woman who finds her child will be born with "special needs?" In what ways could the nurse encourage this mother to share with other parents in similar situations?

of ongoing follow-up and therapy. Surgery is required to close the open defect but may not be performed immediately, depending on the surgeon's decision. Waiting several days does not seem to cause additional problems, and this period gives the family an opportunity to adjust to the initial shock and become involved in making the necessary decisions.

● Nursing Process in Caring for the Newborn With Myelomeningocele

ASSESSMENT

A routine newborn examination is conducted with emphasis on neurologic impairment. When collecting data during the examination, observe the movement and response to stimuli of the lower extremities. Carefully measure the head circumference and examine the fontanelles. Thoroughly document the observations made. When the newborn is handled, take great care to prevent injury to the sac.

The family needs support and understanding during the newborn's initial care and for the many years of care during the child's life. Determine the family's knowledge and understanding of the defect, as well as their attitude concerning the birth of a newborn with such serious problems.

SELECTED NURSING DIAGNOSES

- Risk for Infection related to vulnerability of the myelomeningocele sac
- Risk for Impaired Skin Integrity related to exposure to urine and feces
- Risk for Injury related to neuromuscular impairment
- Compromised Family Coping related to the perceived loss of the perfect newborn
- Deficient Knowledge of the family caregivers related to the complexities of caring for a newborn with serious neurologic and musculoskeletal defects

OUTCOME IDENTIFICATION AND PLANNING: PREOPERATIVE CARE

The preoperative goals for care of the newborn with myelomeningocele include preventing infection, maintaining skin integrity, preventing trauma related to disuse, increasing family coping skills, education about the condition, and support.

IMPLEMENTATION

Preventing Infection Monitor the newborn's vital signs, neurologic signs, and behavior frequently to observe for any deviations from normal that may indicate an infection. Prophylactic antibiotics may be ordered. Carry out routine aseptic technique with conscientious handwashing, gloving, and gowning as appropriate. Until surgery is performed, the sac must be covered with a sterile dressing moistened in a warm sterile solution (often sterile saline). Change this dressing every 2 hours; do not allow it to dry to avoid damage to the covering of the sac. The dressings may be covered with a plastic protective covering. Maintain the newborn in a prone position so that no pressure is placed on the sac. After surgery, continue this positioning until the surgical site is well healed.

Diapering is not advisable with a low defect, but the sac must be protected from contamination with fecal material. Placing a protective barrier between the anus and the sac may prevent this contamination. If the anal sphincter muscles are involved, the newborn may have continual loose stools, which adds to the challenge of keeping the sac free from infection.

Promoting Skin Integrity. The nursing interventions discussed in the previous section on infection also are necessary to promote skin integrity around the area of the defect and the diaper area. As mentioned, leakage of stool and urine may be continual. This leakage causes skin irritation and breakdown if the newborn is not kept clean and the diaper area is not free of stool and urine. Scrupulous perineal care is necessary.

Preventing Contractures of Lower Extremities. Newborns with spina bifida often have **talipes equinovarus** (clubfoot) and congenital **hip dysplasia** (dislocation of the hips), both of which are discussed later in this chapter. If there is loss of motion in the lower limbs because of the defect, conduct range-of-motion exercises to prevent contractures. Position the newborn so that the hips are abducted and the feet are in a neutral position. Massage the knees and other bony prominences with lotion regularly, then pad them, and protect them from irritation. When handling the newborn, avoid putting pressure on the sac.

Promoting Family Coping. The family of a newborn with such a major anomaly is in a state of shock on first learning of the problems. Be especially sensitive to their needs and emotions. Encourage family members to express their feelings and emotions as openly as possible. Recognize that some families express emotions much more freely than others do, and adjust your responses to the family with this in mind. Provide privacy as needed for the family to mourn together over their loss, but do not avoid the family because this only exaggerates their feelings of loss and depression. If possible, encourage the family members to cuddle or touch the newborn using proper precautions for the safety of the defect. With the permission of the physician, the newborn may be held in a chest-to-chest position to provide closer contact.

Providing Family Teaching. Give family members information about the defect and encourage them to discuss their concerns and ask questions. Provide information about the newborn's present state, the proposed surgery, and follow-up care. Remember that anxiety may block understanding and processing knowledge, so information may need to be repeated. Information should be provided in small segments to facilitate comprehension.

After surgery, the family needs to be prepared to care for the newborn at home. Teach the family to hold the newborn's head, neck, and chest slightly raised in one hand during feeding. Also teach them that stroking the newborn's cheek helps stimulate sucking. Showing the family how to care for the newborn, allowing them to participate in the care, and guiding them in performing return demonstrations are all methods to use in family teaching.

For long-term care and support, refer the family to the Spina Bifida Association of America (*http://www.sbaa.org*). Give them materials concerning spina bifida. These children need long-term care involving many aspects of medicine and surgery, as well as education and vocational training. Although children with spina bifida have many long-term problems, their intelligence is not affected; many of these children grow into productive young adults who may live independently (Fig. 21-12).

EVALUATION: GOALS AND EXPECTED OUTCOMES

- **Goal:** The newborn will be free from signs and symptoms of infection.
  Expected Outcomes: The newborn's vital signs and neurologic signs are within normal limits; the newborn shows no signs of irritability or lethargy.
- **Goal:** The newborn will have no evidence of skin breakdown.
  Expected Outcomes: The newborn's skin will remain clean, dry, and intact and will have no areas of reddening or signs of irritation.
- **Goal:** The newborn remains free from injury.
  Expected Outcomes: The newborn's lower limbs show no evidence of contractures.

● *Figure 21.12* Learning to use new braces and a crutch, this girl underwent successful surgery for repair of a myelomeningocele during infancy.

- **Goal:** The family caregivers will show positive signs of beginning coping.
  Expected Outcomes: The family members verbalize their anxieties and needs and hold, cuddle, and soothe the newborn as appropriate.
- **Goal:** The family caregivers will learn to care for the newborn.
  Expected Outcomes: The family demonstrates competence in performing care for the newborn, verbalizes understanding of the signs and symptoms that should be reported, and has information about support agencies.

Hydrocephalus

Hydrocephalus is a condition characterized by an excess of cerebrospinal fluid (CSF) within the ventricular and subarachnoid spaces of the cranial cavity. Normally a delicate balance exists between the rate of formation and absorption of CSF: the entire volume is absorbed and replaced every 12 to 24 hours. In hydrocephalus, this balance is disturbed.

Cerebrospinal fluid is formed mainly in the lateral ventricles by the choroid plexus and is absorbed into the venous system through the arachnoid villi. Cerebrospinal fluid circulates within the ventricles and the subarachnoid space. It is a colorless fluid consisting of water with traces of protein, glucose, and lymphocytes.

In the *noncommunicating* type of congenital hydrocephalus, an obstruction occurs in the free circulation

● *Figure 21.13* Ventricles of the brain and channels for the normal flow of cerebrospinal fluid.

Lateral ventricles

Foramina of Monro

Third ventricle

Aqueduct of Sylvius

Foramina of Magendie and Luschka

Fourth ventricle

Subarachnoid space

of CSF. This blockage causes increased pressure on the brain or spinal cord. The site of obstruction may be at the foramen of Monro, the aqueduct of Sylvius, the foramen of Luschka, or the foramen of Magendie (Fig. 21-13). In the *communicating* type of hydrocephalus, no obstruction of the free flow of CSF exists between the ventricles and the spinal theca; rather the condition is caused by defective absorption of CSF, thus causing increased pressure on the brain or spinal cord. Congenital hydrocephalus is most often the obstructive or noncommunicating type.

Hydrocephalus may be recognized at birth, or it may not be evident until after a few weeks or months of life. The condition may not be congenital but instead may occur during later infancy or during childhood as the result of a neoplasm, a head injury, or an infection such as meningitis.

When hydrocephalus occurs early in life before the skull sutures close, the soft, pliable bones separate to allow head expansion. This condition is manifested by a rapid increase in head circumference. The fact that the soft bones can yield to pressure in this manner may partially explain why many of these newborns fail to show the usual symptoms of brain pressure and may exhibit little or no damage in mental function until later in life. Other newborns show severe brain damage, which often has occurred before birth.

Clinical Presentation

Signs and Symptoms. An excessively large head at birth is suggestive of hydrocephalus. Rapid head growth with widening cranial sutures is also strongly suggestive and may be the first manifestation of this condition. An apparently large head in itself is not nec-essarily significant. Normally every newborn's head is measured at birth, and the rate of growth is checked at subsequent examinations. If a newborn's head appears to be abnormally large at birth or appears to be enlarging, it should be measured frequently.

As the head enlarges, the suture lines separate and the spaces may be felt through the scalp. The anterior fontanelle becomes tense and bulging, the skull enlarges in all diameters, and the scalp becomes shiny and its veins dilate (Fig. 21-14). If pressure continues to increase without intervention, the eyes appear to be pushed downward slightly with the sclera visible above the iris—the so-called "setting sun" sign.

If the condition progresses without adequate drainage of excessive fluid, the head becomes increasingly heavy, the neck muscles fail to develop sufficiently, and the newborn has difficulty raising or turn-

● *Figure 21.14* A newborn with hydrocephalus. Note the pull on the eyes giving the "setting sun" appearance.

ing the head. Unless hydrocephalus is arrested, the newborn becomes increasingly helpless, and symptoms of increased intracranial pressure (IICP) develop. These symptoms may include irritability, restlessness, personality change, high-pitched cry, ataxia, projectile vomiting, failure to thrive, seizures, severe headache, changes in level of consciousness, and papilledema.

Laboratory and Diagnostic Test Results. Positive diagnosis of hydrocephalus is made with CT and MRI. Echoencephalography and ventriculography also may be performed for further definition of the condition.

Treatment

Surgical intervention is the only effective means of relieving brain pressure and preventing additional damage to the brain tissue. If minimal brain damage has occurred, the child may be able to function within a normal mental range. Motor function is usually retarded. In some instances, surgical intervention may remove the cause of the obstruction, such as a neoplasm, a cyst, or a hematoma, but most children require placement of a shunting device that bypasses the point of obstruction, draining the excess CSF into a body cavity. This procedure arrests excessive head growth and prevents additional brain damage.

Many shunt procedures use a silicone rubber catheter that is radiopaque so that its position may be checked by radiographic examination. The silicone rubber catheter reduces the problem of tissue reaction. A valve or regulator is an essential part of each catheter that prevents excessive build-up of fluid or too-rapid decompression of the ventricle. The most common procedure, particularly for newborns and small children, is **ventriculoperitoneal shunting** (VP shunt). In this procedure, the CSF is drained from a lateral ventricle in the brain; the CSF runs through the subcutaneous catheter and empties into the peritoneal cavity. This procedure allows the insertion of some excess tubing to accommodate growth. As the child grows, the catheter needs to be revised and lengthened (Fig. 21-15).

In **ventriculoatrial shunting,** CSF drains into the right atrium of the heart. This procedure cannot be used in children with pathologic changes in the heart. The CSF drained from the ventricle is absorbed into the bloodstream.

Other pathways of drainage have been used with varying degrees of success. All types of shunts may have problems with kinking, blocking, moving, or shifting of tubing. The danger of infection in the tubing is a constant concern. Children with shunts must be observed constantly for signs of malfunction or infection.

The long-term outcome for a child with hydrocephalus depends on several factors. If untreated, the outcome is very poor, often leading to death. With shunting, the outcome depends on the initial cause of

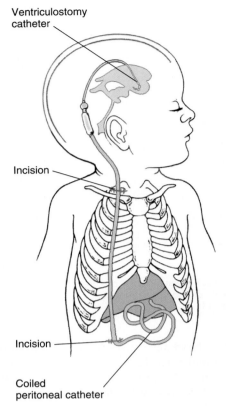

● **Figure 21.15** Ventriculoperitoneal shunt.

the increased fluid, the treatment of the cause, the brain damage sustained before shunting, complications with the shunting system, and continued long-term follow-up. Some of these children can lead relatively normal lives if they have follow-up and revisions as they grow.

● Nursing Process in Caring for the Postoperative Newborn With Hydrocephalus

ASSESSMENT

Obtaining accurate vital and neurologic signs is necessary before and after surgery. Measurement of the newborn's head is essential. If the fontanelles are not closed, carefully observe them for any signs of bulging. Observe, report, and document all signs of IICP. If the child has returned for revision of an existing shunt, obtain a complete history before surgery from the family caregiver to provide a baseline of the child's behavior.

Determine the level of knowledge family members have about the condition. For the family of the newborn or young newborn, the diagnosis will probably come as an emotional shock.

Conduct the interview and examination of the newborn with sensitivity and understanding.

SELECTED NURSING DIAGNOSES

- Risk for Injury related to increased ICP
- Risk for Impaired Skin Integrity related to pressure from physical immobility
- Risk for Infection related to the presence of a shunt
- Risk for Delayed Growth and Development related to impaired ability to achieve developmental tasks
- Anxiety related to the family caregiver's fear of the surgical outcome
- Deficient Knowledge related to the family's understanding of the child's condition and home care

OUTCOME IDENTIFICATION AND PLANNING

The goals for the postoperative care of the newborn with shunt placement for hydrocephalus include preventing injury, maintaining skin integrity, preventing infection, maintaining growth and development, and reducing family anxiety. Family goals include increasing knowledge about the condition and providing loving, supportive care to the newborn.

IMPLEMENTATION

Preventing Injury. At least every 2 to 4 hours, monitor the newborn's level of consciousness. Check the pupils for equality and reaction, monitor the neurologic status, and observe for a shrill cry, lethargy, or irritability. Measure and record the head circumference daily. Carry out appropriate procedures to care for the shunt as directed. To prevent a rapid decrease in ICP, keep the newborn flat. Observe for signs of seizure, and initiate seizure precautions. Keep suction and oxygen equipment convenient at the bedside.

Promoting Skin Integrity. After a shunting procedure, keep the newborn's head turned away from the operative site until the physician allows a change in position. If the newborn's head is enlarged, prevent pressure sores from forming on the side where the child rests. Reposition the newborn at least every 2 hours as permitted. Inspect the dressings over the shunt site immediately after the surgery, every hour for the first 3 to 4 hours, and then at least every 4 hours.

Preventing Infection. Infection is the primary threat after surgery. Closely observe for and promptly report any signs of infection, which include redness, heat, or swelling along the surgical site, fever, and signs of lethargy. Perform wound care thoroughly as ordered. Administer antibiotics as prescribed.

Promoting Growth and Development. Every newborn has the need to be picked up and held, cuddled, and comforted. An uncomfortable or painful experience increases the need for emotional support. A newborn perceives such support principally through physical contact made in a soothing, loving manner.

This is important! Always support the head of a newborn with hydrocephalus when picking up, moving, or positioning. Using egg-crate pads, lamb's wool, or a special mattress can prevent pressure and breakdown of the scalp.

The newborn needs social interaction and needs to be talked to, played with, and given the opportunity for activity. Provide toys appropriate for his or her physical and mental capacity. If the child has difficulty moving about the crib, place toys within easy reach and vision: a cradle gym, for example, may be tied close enough for the newborn to maneuver its parts.

Unless the newborn's nervous system is so impaired that all activity increases irritability, the newborn needs stimulation just as any child does. If repositioning from side-to-side means turning the newborn away from the sight of activity, the crib may be turned around so that vision is not obstructed.

A newborn who is given the contact and support that all newborns require develops a pleasing personality because he or she is nourished by emotional stimulation. Use the time spent on physical care as a time for social interaction. Talking, laughing, and playing with the newborn are important aspects of the newborn's care. Make frequent contacts, and do not limit them to the times when physical care is being performed.

Reducing Family Anxiety. Explain to the family the condition and the anatomy of the surgical procedure in terms they can understand. Discuss the overall prognosis for the child. Encourage family members to express their anxieties and ask questions. Giving accurate, nontechnical answers is extremely helpful. Give the family information about support groups such as the National Hydrocephalus Foundation (*www.nhfonline.org*) and encourage them to contact the groups.

Providing Family Teaching. Demonstrate care of the shunt to the family caregivers and have them perform a return demonstration. Provide them with a list of signs and symptoms that should be reported. Review these with the family members and make sure they understand them. Discuss appropriate growth and developmental expectations for the child, and stress realistic goals.

EVALUATION: GOALS AND EXPECTED OUTCOMES

- **Goal:** The newborn will be free from injury related to complications of excessive cerebrospinal fluid.
  Expected Outcomes: The newborn has no signs of IICP, such as lethargy, irritability, and seizure activity, and has a stable level of consciousness.
- **Goal:** The newborn's skin will remain intact.
  Expected Outcomes: The newborn's skin shows no evidence of pressure sores, redness, or other signs of skin breakdown.
- **Goal:** The newborn will remain free of infection.
  Expected Outcomes: The newborn shows no signs of infection; vital signs are stable; and there is no redness, drainage, or swelling at the surgical site.
- **Goal:** The newborn will have age-appropriate growth and development.
  Expected Outcomes: The newborn's social and developmental needs are met. The newborn interacts and plays appropriately with toys and surroundings.
- **Goal:** The family caregiver's anxiety will be reduced.
  Expected Outcomes: The family expresses fears and concerns and interacts appropriately with the newborn.
- **Goal:** The family will learn care of the child.
  Expected Outcomes: The family participates in the care of the newborn, asks appropriate questions, and lists signs and symptoms to report.

Cardiovascular System Defects: Congenital Heart Disease

Cardiovascular system defects range from mild to severe. They may be detected immediately at birth or may not be detected for several months. When a newborn is suspected of having a heart abnormality, the family is understandably upset. The heart is *the* vital organ; a person can live without a number of other organs and appendages, but life itself depends on the heart. The family caregivers will have many questions: the nurse may answer some; the physician must answer others. Many answers will not be available until after various evaluation procedures have been conducted.

Technological advances have progressed rapidly in this field, making earlier detection and successful repair much more likely. However, heart defects are still the leading cause of death from congenital anomalies in the first year of life. A brief discussion of the development and function of the embryonic heart is useful to understanding the malformations that occur.

Development of the Heart

The heart begins beating early in the 3rd to 8th week of intrauterine life. When first formed, the heart is a simple tube receiving blood from the placenta and pumping it out into its developing body. During this period, the heart rapidly develops into its normal, but complex, four-chambered structure.

Adjustments in circulation must be made at birth. During fetal life the lungs are inactive, requiring only a small amount of blood to nourish their tissues. Blood is circulated through the umbilical arteries to the placenta, where waste products and carbon dioxide are exchanged for oxygen and nutrients. The blood is then returned to the fetus through the umbilical vein.

At birth, the umbilical cord is cut, and the newborn's own independent circulatory system is established. Certain circulatory bypasses, such as the **ductus arteriosus,** the **foramen ovale,** and the **ductus venosus,** are no longer necessary. They close during the first several weeks after birth. In addition, the pressure in the heart, which has been higher on the right side during fetal life, now changes so that the left side of the heart has the higher pressure (Fig. 21-16).

During this period of complex development, any error in formation may cause serious circulatory difficulty. The incidence of cardiovascular malformations is about 8 in 1,000 live births. Some abnormalities are slight and allow the person to lead a normal life without correction. Others cause little apparent difficulty but need correction to improve the chance for a longer life and for optimal health. Some severe anomalies are incompatible with life for more than a short time; others may be helped but not cured by surgery.

Common Types of Congenital Heart Defects

Traditionally, congenital heart defects have been described as cyanotic or acyanotic conditions. **Cyanotic heart disease** implies an oxygen saturation of the peripheral arterial blood of 85% or less. This condition occurs when a heart defect allows any appreciable amount of oxygen-poor blood in the right side of the heart to mix with the oxygenated blood in the left side of the heart. Defects that permit right-to-left shunting may occur at the atrial, ventricular, or aortic level.

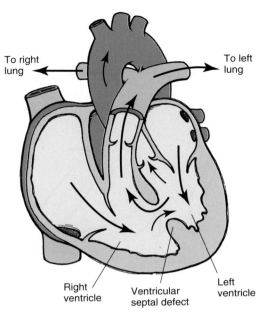

● **Figure 21.16** Normal blood circulation. Highlighted ligaments indicate pathways that should close at or soon after birth. *Arrows* indicate normal flow of blood.

● **Figure 21.17** A ventricular septal defect is an abnormal opening between the right and left ventricle. Ventricular septal defects vary in size and may occur in the membranous or muscular portion of the ventricular septum. Owing to higher pressure in the left ventricle, a shunting of blood from the left to the right ventricle occurs during systole. If pulmonary vascular resistance produces pulmonary hypertension, the shunt of blood is then reversed from the right to the left ventricle, with cyanosis resulting.

However, because defects are often complex and occur in various combinations, this is an inadequate means of classification. A more clear-cut classification system is based on blood flow characteristics. These are:

1. Increased pulmonary blood flow (e.g., ventricular septal, atrial septal, and patent ductus arteriosus)
2. Obstruction of blood flow out of the heart (e.g., coarctation of the aorta)
3. Decreased pulmonary blood flow (e.g., tetralogy of Fallot)
4. Mixed blood flow, where saturated and desaturated blood mix in the heart, aorta, and pulmonary vessels (e.g., transposition of the great arteries)

Because defects often occur in combination, they give rise to complex situations. Most nurses may never see many of the complex defects and most of the rare, isolated defects. The conditions discussed here are common enough that the pediatric nurse needs to be familiar with their diagnosis and treatment.

Ventricular Septal Defect

Ventricular septal defect is the most common intracardiac defect. It consists of an abnormal opening in the septum between the two ventricles, which allows blood to pass directly from the left to the right ventricle. No

unoxygenated blood leaks into the left ventricle, so cyanosis does not occur (Fig. 21-17).

Small, isolated defects are usually asymptomatic and often are discovered during a routine physical examination. A characteristic loud, harsh murmur associated with a systolic thrill occasionally is heard on examination. A history of frequent respiratory infections may occur during infancy, but growth and development are unaffected. The child leads a normal life.

Corrective surgery may be postponed until the age of 18 months to 2 years, when the surgical risk is less than that for newborns. However, surgical techniques have improved to the degree that the repair may be made in the first year of life with high rates of success. The child is observed closely and may be prescribed a regimen of prophylactic antibiotics to prevent frequent respiratory infections. If pulmonary involvement becomes a problem, the repair is done without further delay. Repairs in children who are at high risk are done by the use of cardiac catheterization procedures.

Atrial Septal Defects

In general, left-to-right shunting occurs in all true atrial septal defects. However, the atrial septum of many healthy people houses a patent **foramen ovale** that normally causes no problems because its valve is

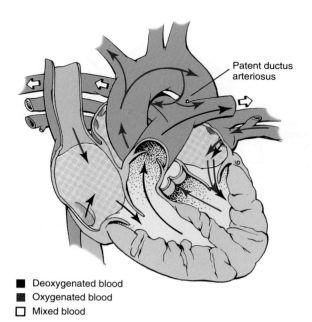

■ Deoxygenated blood
■ Oxygenated blood
☐ Mixed blood

● *Figure 21.18* An atrial septal defect is an abnormal opening between the right and left atria. Basically, three types of abnormalities result from incorrect development of the atrial septum. An incompetent foramen ovale is the most common defect. The ostium secundum defect results from abnormal development of the septum secundum and causes an opening in the middle of the septum. Improper development of the septum primum produces an opening at the lower end of the septum known as an ostium primum defect, frequently involving the atrioventricular valves. In general, left-to-right shunting of blood occurs in all atrial septal defects.

● *Figure 21.19* The patent ductus arteriosus is a vascular connection that, during fetal life, short-circuits the pulmonary vascular bed and directs blood from the pulmonary artery to the aorta. Functional closure of the ductus normally occurs soon after birth. If the ductus remains patent after birth, the higher pressure in the aorta reverses the direction of blood flow in the ductus.

anatomically structured to withstand left chamber pressure, rendering it functionally closed (Fig. 21-18).

True atrial septal defects are common heart anomalies and may occur as isolated defects or in combination with other heart anomalies. Atrial septal defects are amenable to surgery with a low surgical mortality risk. Since the advent of the heart–lung bypass machine, this repair may be performed in a dry field, replacing the older "blind" technique. The opening is closed with sutures or a Dacron patch.

Patent Ductus Arteriosus

The **ductus arteriosus** is a vascular channel between the left main pulmonary artery and the descending aorta. In fetal life it allows blood to bypass the nonfunctioning lungs and go directly into the systemic circuit. After birth the duct normally closes, eventually becoming obliterated and forming the ligamentum arteriosum. However, if the ductus arteriosus remains patent, blood continues to be shunted from the aorta into the pulmonary artery. This situation results in a flooding of the lungs and an overloading of the left heart chambers (Fig. 21-19).

Normally the ductus arteriosus is nonpatent after the 1st or 2nd week of life and should be obliterated by the 4th month. Why it fails to close is unknown. Patent ductus arteriosus is common in newborns who exhibit the rubella syndrome, but most newborns with this

anomaly have no history of exposure to rubella during fetal life. It is also common in preterm newborns weighing less than 1,200 g and in newborns with Down's syndrome.

Symptoms of patent ductus arteriosus are often absent during childhood. Growth and development may be retarded in some children with an easy fatigability and dyspnea on exertion. The diagnosis may be based on a characteristic machinery-like murmur over the pulmonary area, a wide pulse pressure, and a bounding pulse. Cardiac catheterization is diagnostic but is not required in the presence of classic clinical features.

Indomethacin (Indocin), a prostaglandin inhibitor, may be administered with some success to premature newborns to promote closure of the ductus arteriosus. If this fails to close the ductus, surgery is indicated in all diagnosed cases, even if they are asymptomatic. Some persons live a normal life span without correction, but the risks involved far outweigh the surgical ones. Surgical correction consists of closure of the defect by ligation or by division of the ductus. Division is the method of choice if the child's condition permits because the ductus occasionally reopens after ligation. The optimal age for surgery is before the age of 2 years, with earlier surgery for severely affected newborns. Prognosis is excellent after a successful repair.

Coarctation of the Aorta

This congenital cardiovascular anomaly consists of a constriction or narrowing of the aortic arch or the descending aorta usually adjacent to the ligamentum arteriosum (Fig. 21-20).

Most children with this condition have no symptoms until later childhood or young adulthood. A few newborns have severe symptoms in their first year of life; they show dyspnea, tachycardia, and cyanosis, which are all signs of developing congestive heart failure.

In older children, the condition is diagnosed easily based on hypertension in the upper extremities and hypotension in the lower extremities. The radial pulse is readily palpable, but the femoral pulses are weak or even impalpable. Blood pressure is normal or elevated in the arms and is low or undetectable in the legs. A high-pitched systolic murmur is usually present and heard over the base of the heart and over the interscapular area of the back. The diagnosis may be confirmed by aortography.

Obstruction to blood flow caused by the constricted portion of the aorta does not cause early difficulty in an average child because the blood bypasses the obstruction by way of collateral circulation. The bypass is chiefly from the branches of the subclavian and carotid arteries that arise from the arch of the aorta. Eventually the enlarged collateral arteries erode the rib margins, and the rib notching may be visualized by radiographic examination.

Uncorrected coarctation may cause hypertension and cardiac failure later in life. The optimal age for elective surgery is before the age of 2 years. Early surgery may be necessary for a gravely ill newborn who presents with severe congestive heart failure. In early infancy, the mortality rate depends on the presence of other congenital heart problems.

Surgery consists of resection of the coarcted area with an end-to-end anastomosis of the proximal and distal ends of the aorta. Occasionally a long defect may necessitate an end-to-end graft using tubes of Dacron or similar material. Prognosis is excellent for the restoration of normal function after surgery.

Tetralogy of Fallot

This is a fairly common congenital heart defect involving 50% to 70% of all cyanotic congenital heart diseases. It consists of a grouping of heart defects (tetralogy denotes four abnormal conditions): (1) **pulmonary stenosis,** (2) **ventricular septal defect,** (3) **overriding aorta,** and (4) **right ventricular hypertrophy.** The pulmonary stenosis is usually seen as a narrowing of the upper portion of the right ventricle and may include stenosis of the valve cusps. Pulmonary stenosis results, in turn, in right ventricular hypertrophy. The aorta appears to straddle the ventricular septum, overriding the ventricular septal defect. This defect allows a shunt of unsaturated blood from the right ventricle into the aorta or into the left ventricle (Fig. 21-21).

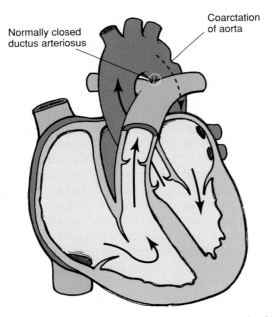

● **Figure 21.20** Coarctation of the aorta is characterized by a narrowed aortic lumen. It exists as a preductal or postductal obstruction, depending on the position of the obstruction in relation to the ductus arteriosus. Coarctations exist with great variation in anatomic features. The lesion produces an obstruction to the flow of blood through the aorta, causing an increased left ventricular pressure and workload.

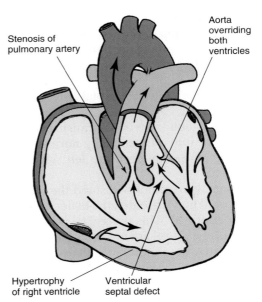

● **Figure 21.21** Tetralogy of Fallot is characterized by the combination of four defects: (1) pulmonary stenosis, (2) ventricular septal defect, (3) overriding aorta, and (4) hypertrophy of the right ventricle. It is the most common defect causing cyanosis in patients surviving beyond 2 years of age. The severity of symptoms depends on the degree of pulmonary stenosis, the size of the ventricular septal defect, and the degree to which the aorta overrides the septal defect.

The child with tetralogy of Fallot may be precyanotic in early infancy, with the cyanotic phase starting at 4 to 6 months of age. However, some severely affected newborns may show cyanosis earlier. As long as the ductus arteriosus remains open, enough blood apparently passes through the lungs to prevent cyanosis.

The infant presents with feeding difficulties and poor weight gain, resulting in retarded growth and development. Dyspnea and easy fatigability become evident. Exercise tolerance depends in part on the severity of the disease; some children become fatigued after little exertion. In the past, on experiencing fatigue, breathlessness, and increased cyanosis, the child was described as assuming a squatting posture for relief. Squatting apparently increased the systemic oxygen saturation. However, squatting rarely is seen today because these newborns' defects usually are repaired by the time they are 2 years old.

Attacks of paroxysmal dyspnea are common during infancy and early childhood. An anoxic spell is heralded by sudden restlessness, gasping respiration, and increased cyanosis that lead to a loss of consciousness and, possibly, convulsions. These attacks, called "tet spells," last from a few minutes to several hours and appear to be unpredictable, although stress does seem to trigger some episodes.

The history and clinical manifestations are usually sufficient to make a diagnosis. However, cardiac catheterization, electrocardiography, chest radiography, and laboratory tests to determine polycythemia and arterial oxygen saturation may be performed for additional definition.

The preferred repair of these defects is total surgical correction. This procedure requires the use of a cardiopulmonary bypass machine. The heart is opened, and extensive resection is done. The repair relieves the pulmonary stenosis, and the septal defect is closed by use of a patch.

Successful total correction transforms a grossly abnormal heart into a functionally normal one. However, most of these children are left without a pulmonary valve.

In infants who cannot withstand the total surgical correction until they are older, the Blalock-Taussig procedure is performed. This procedure is an end-to-end anastomosis of a vessel arising from the aorta, usually the subclavian artery, to the corresponding right or left pulmonary artery. These shunts are now seen only occasionally because total surgical repair is meeting with much greater success and lower mortality rates.

Transposition of the Great Arteries

This severe defect was at one time almost always fatal. Advancements in diagnosis and treatment have increased the success rate in treatment of this disorder. In transposition of the great arteries, the aorta arises from

the right ventricle instead of the left, and the pulmonary artery arises from the left ventricle instead of the right. These newborns are usually cyanotic from birth.

Test Yourself

- What is the difference between spina bifida with meningocele and spina bifida with myelomeningocele?

- What does the newborn have an excess of in the condition of hydrocephalus? How is hydrocephalus treated?

- List the five common types of congenital heart defects.

- In children with heart conditions what is the most common manifestation or symptom?

Risk Factors

Maternal alcoholism, maternal irradiation, ingestion of certain drugs during pregnancy, maternal diabetes, and advanced maternal age (older than 40 years) increase the incidence of heart defects in newborns. Rubella in the expectant mother during the first trimester can also cause cardiac malformations. Maternal malnutrition and heredity may be contributing factors. Recent studies have shown that the offspring of mothers who had congenital heart anomalies have a much higher risk of having congenital heart anomalies. If one child in the family has a congenital heart abnormality, later siblings have a very high risk for such a defect.

Clinical Presentation

The newborn with a severe abnormality, such as a transposition of the great vessels, is cyanotic from birth and requires oxygen and special treatment. A less seriously affected child, whose heart can compensate to some degree for the impaired circulation, may not have symptoms severe enough to call attention to the difficulty until he or she is a few months older and more active. Others may live a fairly normal life and not be aware of any heart trouble until a murmur or an enlarged heart is discovered during physical examination in later childhood.

A cardiac murmur discovered early in life necessitates frequent physical examinations. This murmur may be a functional, "innocent" murmur that may disappear as the child grows older, or it may be the chief manifestation of an abnormal heart or an abnormal circulatory system. The most common parental concern is that of feeding difficulties. Newborns with cardiac anomalies severe enough to cause circulatory difficulties have a history of being poor eaters, tiring easily from the effort to suck, and failing to grow or thrive normally. These manifestations of **congestive heart failure** (CHF) may appear during the first year of life in newborns with conditions such as large ventricular septal defects, coarctation of the aorta, and other defects that place an increased workload on the ventricles. See Chapter 36 for a full discussion of CHF.

Treatment and Nursing Care

Advances in medical technology have enabled heart repairs to be performed in newborns as young as less than 1 day old. Miniaturization of instruments, earlier diagnosis through the use of improved diagnostic techniques, pediatric intensive care facilities staffed with highly skilled nurse specialists, and more sophisticated monitoring techniques have all contributed to these advances.

Most physicians now think it is important to operate as early as possible to repair defective hearts. Inadequate circulation may prevent adequate growth and development and cause permanent, irreparable physical, mental, and emotional damage. If the child is receives a diagnosis early and correction or repair is possible, CHF may be avoided.

In cases where the child has CHF, it is important that the CHF be treated. The primary goals in the treatment of CHF are to reduce the workload of the heart and to improve the cardiac functioning, thus increasing oxygenation of the tissues. This is done by removing excess sodium and fluids, slowing the heart rate, and decreasing the demands on the heart. See Chapter 36 for a complete discussion of CHF and its treatment.

Care at Home Before Surgery

A child with congenital heart disease may show easy fatigability and retarded growth. If the child has a cyanotic type of heart disease with clubbing of the fingers or toes, periods of cyanosis and reduced exercise tolerance are evident. This young child may assume a squatting position, which reduces the return flow to the heart, thus temporarily reducing the workload of the heart.

Such a child should be allowed to lead as normal a life as possible. Families are naturally apprehensive and find it difficult not to overprotect the child. They often increase the child's anxiety and cause fear in the child about participating in normal activities. Children are rather sensible about finding their own limitations and usually limit their activities to their capacity if they are not made unduly apprehensive.

Some families can adjust well and provide guidance and security for the sick child. Others may become confused and frightened and show hostility, disinterest, or neglect; these families need guidance and counseling. The nurse has a great responsibility to support the family. The nurse's primary goal is to reduce anxiety in the child and family. This goal may be accomplished through open communication and ongoing contact.

Routine visits to a clinic or a physician's office become a way of life, and the child may come to feel different from other people. Physicians and nurses have a responsibility both to the family caregivers and the child to give clear explanations of the defect, using readily understandable terms and diagrams, pictures, or models. A child who knows what is happening can accept a great deal and can continue with the business of living.

Cardiac Catheterization

Cardiac catheterization may be performed before heart surgery to obtain more accurate information about the child's condition. The child or newborn is sedated or anesthetized for this process, and a radiopaque catheter is inserted through a vein into the right atrium. In the newborn or young child, the femoral vein often is used. Close observation of the child after the procedure is essential. Carefully monitor the site used and check the extremity for pulses, edema, skin temperature and color, and any other signs of poor circulation or infection. A pressure dressing is used over the catheterization site and left in place until the day after the procedure. The dressing should be snug and intact and monitored closely for any signs of bleeding from the site. The child is kept flat in bed with the extremity straight for as long as 6 hours after the procedure. Vital signs are monitored closely.

Preoperative Preparation

When a child enters the hospital for cardiac surgery, it is seldom a first admission; generally, it has been preceded by cardiac catheterization or perhaps other hospitalizations. The child may be admitted a few days before surgery to allow time for adequate preparation. With the current emphasis on cost containment, however, many preoperative procedures are done on an outpatient basis. Preoperative teaching should be intensive for the family and the child at an age appropriate level. They should understand that blood might be obtained for typing and crossmatching and for other determinations as ordered. Additional x-ray studies may be done.

The equipment to be used after surgery should be described with drawings and pictures. If possible, the family caregivers and the child should be taken to a cardiac recovery room and shown chest tubes and an oxygen tent. They should meet the nursing personnel and see the general appearance of the unit. Of course, nurses should use good judgment about the timing and the extent of such preparation; nothing is gained by arousing additional anxiety with premature or excessively graphic descriptions. A young child may become familiar with the surgical clothing worn by personnel and with the oxygen tent and can perhaps listen to a heartbeat. The child should be taught how to cough and should practice coughing. He or she should understand that coughing is important after surgery and must be done regularly, even though it may hurt.

Cardiac Surgery

Open-heart surgery using the heart–lung machine has made extensive heart correction possible for many children who otherwise would have been disabled throughout their limited lives. Machines have been refined for use with newborns and small children. Heart transplants may be performed when no other treatment is possible.

Hypothermia—reducing the body temperature to 68°F to 78.8°F (20°C to 26°C)—is a useful technique that helps to make early surgery possible. A reduced body temperature increases the time that the circulation may be stopped without causing brain damage. The blood temperature is reduced by the use of cooling agents in the heart–lung machine. This also provides a dry, bloodless, motionless field for the surgeon.

Postoperative Care

At the end of surgery, the child is taken to the pediatric intensive care unit for skillful nursing by specially trained personnel for as long as necessary. Children who have had closed-chest surgery need the same careful nursing as those who have had open-heart surgery.

By the time the child returns to the regular pediatric unit, chest drainage tubes usually have been removed and the child has started taking oral fluids and is ready to sit up in bed or in a chair. The child probably feels weak and helpless after such an experience and needs encouragement and reassurance. However, with recovery a child is usually ready for activity.

Family caregivers usually need to reorient themselves and to accept their child's new status. This attitude is not easy to acquire after what seemed like a long period of anxious watching. The surgeon and the surgical staff evaluate the results of the surgery and make any necessary recommendations regarding resumption of the child's activities. Plans should be made for follow-up and supervision, as well as counseling and guidance.

Skeletal System Defects

Skeletal system defects in the newborn may be noted and treatment begun soon after birth. Some skeletal system defects may not be evident until later in the child's life. Congenital talipes equinovarus (clubfoot) is usually evident at birth. Another common skeletal system defect is congenital hip dysplasia (dislocation of the hip). Children with these conditions and their parents often face long periods of exhausting, costly treatment; therefore, they need continuing support, encouragement, and education.

Congenital Talipes Equinovarus

Congenital clubfoot is a deformity in which the entire foot is inverted, the heel is drawn up, and the forefoot is adducted. The Latin *talus*, meaning ankle, and *pes*, meaning foot, make up the word *talipes*, which is used in connection with many foot deformities. Equinus, or plantar flexion, and varus, or inversion, denotes the kind of foot deformity present in this condition. The equinovarus foot has a club-like appearance, thus the term "clubfoot" (Fig. 21-22A).

Congenital talipes equinovarus is the most common congenital foot deformity, occurring in about 7 in 1,000 births. It appears as a single anomaly or in connection with other defects, such as myelomeningocele. It may be

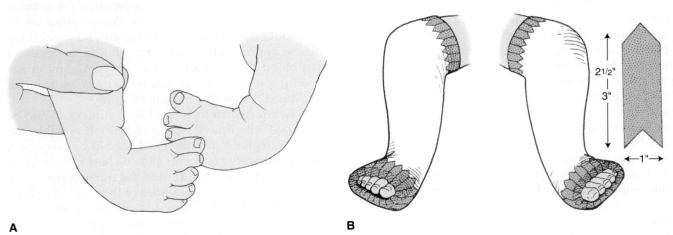

A   **B**

● *Figure 21.22* (A) Bilateral clubfoot. (B) Casting for clubfoot in typical overcorrected position showing petalling of cast.

bilateral (both feet) or unilateral (one foot). The cause is unclear, although a hereditary factor is observed occasionally. A hypothesis that has received some acceptance proposes an arrested embryonic growth of the foot during the first trimester of pregnancy.

Clinical Presentation

Talipes equinovarus is detected easily in a newborn but must be differentiated from a persisting "position of comfort" assumed in utero. The positional deformity may be corrected easily by the use of passive exercise, but the true clubfoot deformity is fixed. The positional deformity should be explained to the parents at once to prevent anxiety.

Treatment

Nonsurgical Treatment. If treatment is started during the neonatal period, correction usually may be accomplished by manipulation and bandaging or by application of a cast. The cast often is applied while the newborn is still in the neonatal nursery. While the cast is applied, the foot is first moved gently into as nearly normal a position as possible. Force should not be used. If the family caregiver can be present to help hold the newborn while the cast is applied, the caregiver will have the opportunity to understand what is being done. The very young newborn gets satisfaction from sucking, so a pacifier helps prevent squirming while the cast is applied.

The cast is applied over the foot and ankle (and usually to midthigh) to hold the knee in right-angle flexion (Fig. 21-22B). Casts are changed frequently to provide gradual, atraumatic correction—every few days for the first several weeks, then every week or two. Treatment is continued usually for a matter of months until radiograph and clinical observation confirm complete correction.

Any cast applied to a child's body should have some type of waterproof material protecting the skin from the cast's sharp plaster edges. One method is to apply strips of adhesive vertically around the edges of the cast in a manner called "petaling" (Fig. 21-22B). To petal a cast, strips of adhesive are cut 2 inches or 3 inches long and 1 inch wide. One end is notched, and the other end is cut pointed to aid in smooth application. Family caregivers must be taught cast care.

After correction with a cast, a Denis Browne splint with shoes attached may be used to maintain the correction for another 6 months or longer (Fig. 21-23). After overcorrection has been attained, the child should wear a special clubfoot shoe, which is a laced shoe whose turning out makes it appear that the shoe is being worn on the wrong foot. The Denis Browne splint still may be worn at night, and the caregivers should carry out passive exercises of the foot. The older infant may resist wearing the splint, so family

● **Figure 21.23** A Denis Browne splint with shoes attached is used to correct clubfoot.

caregivers must be taught the importance of gentle, but firm, insistence that the splint be worn.

Surgical Treatment. Children who do not respond to nonsurgical measures, especially older children, need surgical correction. This approach involves several procedures, depending on the age of the child and the degree of the deformity. It may involve lengthening the Achilles tendon and operating on the bony structure for the child older than 10 years. Prolonged observation after correction by either means should be carried out, at least until adolescence; any recurrence is treated promptly.

Congenital Hip Dysplasia

Congenital hip dysplasia results from defective development of the acetabulum with or without dislocation. The malformed acetabulum permits dislocation, with the head of the femur becoming displaced upward and backward. The condition is difficult to recognize during early infancy. When there is a family history of the defect, increased observation of the young newborn is indicated. The condition is often bilateral and about seven times more common in girls than in boys.

Clinical Presentation

Early recognition and treatment before an infant starts to stand or walk are extremely important for successful correction. The first examination should be part of the newborn examination. Experienced examiners may detect an audible click when examining the newborn using the Barlow's sign and Ortolani's maneuver (see Chapter 13, Nursing Procedure 13-2). These tests, used together on one hip at a time, show a tendency for dislocation of the hip in adduction and abduction and should be conducted only by an experienced practitioner. The tests are effective only for the 1st month, after this time the clicks disappear. Signs that are useful after this include:

- Asymmetry of the gluteal skin folds (higher on the affected side) (Fig. 21-24A).

● *Figure 21.24* Congenital hip dislocation. (**A**) Asymmetry of the gluteal folds of the thighs. (**B**) Limited abduction of the affected hip. (**C**) Apparent shortening of the femur.

- Limited abduction of the affected hip (Fig. 21-24*B*). This is tested by placing the infant in a dorsal recumbent position with the knees flexed, then abducting both knees passively until they reach the examination table without resistance. If dislocation is present, the affected side cannot be abducted more than 45 degrees.
- Apparent shortening of the femur (Fig. 21-24*C*).

After the child has started walking, later signs include lordosis, swayback, protruding abdomen, shortened extremity, duck-waddle gait, and a positive Trendelenburg sign. To elicit this sign, the child stands on the affected leg and raises the normal leg. The pelvis tilts down, rather than up toward the unaffected side. X-ray studies usually are made to confirm the diagnosis in the older newborn. Uncorrected dislocation causes limping, easy fatigue, hip and low back discomfort, and postural deformities.

Treatment

Correction may be started in the newborn period by placing two or three diapers on the infant to hold the legs abducted, in a frog-like position. Cloth diapers work best for this purpose. Another treatment option, when the dislocation is discovered during the first few months, consists of manipulation of the femur into position and the application of a brace. The most common type of brace used is the Pavlik harness (Fig. 21-25). The primary care provider assesses the infant weekly while the infant is in the harness and adjusts the harness to align the femur gradually. Sometimes no additional treatment is needed.

If treatment is delayed until after the child has started to walk or if earlier treatment is ineffective, open reduction followed by application of a spica cast usually is needed. A spica or "hip spica cast," as it is

often called, covers the lower part of the body, from the waist down and either one or both legs, usually leaving the feet open. The cast maintains the legs in a frog-like position, with the hips abducted. There may be a bar placed between the legs to help support the cast. After the cast is removed, a metal or plastic brace is applied to keep the legs in wide abduction.

● Nursing Process in Caring for the Infant in an Orthopedic Device or Cast

ASSESSMENT

Although the actual hospitalization of the infant is relatively short (if no other abnormalities

● *Figure 21.25* Proper positioning of an infant in a Pavlik harness. The harness is composed of shoulder straps, stirrups, and a chest strap. It is placed on both legs, even if only one hip is dislocated.

require hospitalization), the nurse must teach the family about cast care or care of the infant in an orthopedic device such as a Pavlik harness. Determine the family caregiver's ability to understand and cooperate in the infant's care. Emotional support of the family is important.

The observation of the infant varies depending on the orthopedic device or cast used. Immediately after the application of a cast, observe for signs that the cast is drying evenly. Check the toes for circulation and movement. Check the skin at the edges of the cast for signs of pressure or irritation. If an open reduction has been performed, observe the child for signs of shock and bleeding in the immediate postoperative period.

SELECTED NURSING DIAGNOSES

- Acute Pain related to discomfort of orthopedic device or cast
- Risk for Impaired Skin Integrity related to pressure of the cast on the skin surface
- Risk for Delayed Growth and Development related to restricted mobility secondary to orthopedic device or cast
- Deficient Knowledge of family caregivers related to home care of the infant in the orthopedic device or cast

OUTCOME IDENTIFICATION AND PLANNING

Goals include relieving pain and discomfort, maintaining skin integrity, promoting growth and development, and increasing family knowledge about the infant's home care. Goals for the family focus on the desire for correction of the defect with minimal disruption to the infant's growth and development and care of the infant at home.

IMPLEMENTATION

Providing Comfort Measures. The infant may be irritable and fussy because of the restricted movement caused by the device or cast. Useful methods of soothing the infant include nonnutritive sucking, stroking, cuddling, and talking. If irritability seems excessive, check the infant for signs of irritation from the device or cast. The infant in a cast may be held after the cast is completely dry. Do not remove the harness unless specific permission for bathing is granted by the provider. Teach the family caregivers how to reapply the harness correctly. The infant in a Pavlik harness is not as difficult to handle as the infant in a cast.

Promoting Skin Integrity. For the first 24 to 48 hours after application of a cast, place the infant on

CULTURAL SNAPSHOT

Cradleboards are devices used as baby carriers and to provide security for newborns in some cultures. Using a cradleboard can sometimes aggravate hip dysplasia. The nurse can encourage the caregivers to use thick diapers, sometimes more than one, to help in keeping the hips in a slightly abducted position when the child is carried on a cradleboard. Cloth diapers work better than disposable diapers for this purpose.

a firm mattress and support position changes with firm pillows. When handling the cast, use the palms of the hands to avoid excessive pressure on the cast. Carefully inspect the skin around the cast edges for signs of irritation, redness, or edema. Petal the edges of the cast around the waist and toes and protect the cast with plastic covering around the perineal area. Take great care to protect the diaper area from becoming soiled and moist. If the covering becomes soiled, remove it, wash and dry thoroughly, then reapply or replace it. With the Pavlik harness, monitor the skin under the straps frequently and massage it gently to promote circulation. To relieve pressure under the shoulder straps, place extra padding in the area.

Avoid using powders and lotions because caking of the powder or lotion can cause areas of irritation. Daily sponge baths are important and must include close attention to the skin under the straps of the device or around the edge of the cast.

Observe the infant in a cast carefully for any restriction of breathing caused by tightness over the abdomen and lower chest area. Vomiting after a feeding may be an indication that the cast is too tight over the stomach. In either case, the cast may have to be removed and reapplied.

Prevent the older infant or child from pushing any small particles of food or toys down into the cast. Diapering can be a challenge for the infant in a cast. Disposable diapers are usually the most effective way to provide good protection of the cast and prevent leakage.

Providing Sensory Stimulation Because the infant will be in the device or cast for an extended period when much growth and development occur, provide him or her with stimulation of a tactile nature. Provide mobiles, musical toys, and stuffed toys. Do not permit the infant to cry for long periods. Keep feeding times relaxed. Hold the infant if possible and encourage interaction. Provide a pacifier if the infant desires it. Encourage activities that use the infant's free hands. The older infant may enjoy looking at picture books and interacting with siblings. Diversionary activities should include transporting the infant to other areas in the home or in the car. Strollers and car seats may be adapted to allow safe transportation.

Here's an idea. For older infants or toddlers in a hip spica cast, a wagon may provide a convenient and fun way to explore the environment, encourage stimulation, and promote independence.

Providing Family Teaching. Determine the family caregiver's knowledge and design a thorough teaching plan because the infant will be cared for at home for most of the time. Use complete explanations, written guidelines, demonstrations, and return demonstrations. Provide the family with a resource person who may be called when a question arises and encourage them to feel free to call that person. Make definite plans for return visits to have the device or cast checked. The caregiver needs to understand the importance of keeping these appointments. Provide a public or home health nurse referral when appropriate (see Nursing Care Plan 21-1: The Infant With an Orthopedic Cast).

EVALUATION: GOALS AND EXPECTED OUTCOMES

- **Goal:** The infant will show signs of being comfortable.
  Expected Outcomes: The infant is alert and content with no long periods of fussiness. The infant interacts with caregivers with cooing, smiling, and eye contact.
- **Goal:** The infant's skin will remain intact.
  Expected Outcomes: The infant's skin around the edges of the cast shows no signs of redness or irritation. The diaper area is clean, dry and intact, and protected from soiling.
- **Goal:** The infant will attain appropriate developmental milestones.
  Expected Outcomes: The infant responds positively to audio, visual, and diversionary activities. The infant shows age-appropriate development.
- **Goal:** The family caregivers will learn home care of the infant.
  Expected Outcomes: The family demonstrates care of the infant in the orthopedic device or cast, asks pertinent questions, and identifies a resource person to call.

Test Yourself
- How is congenital clubfoot treated?
- What three signs are seen in the infant with a congenital hip dysplasia?
- List five nursing interventions used to promote skin integrity for an infant in a cast.

Genitourinary Tract Defects

Most congenital anomalies of the genitourinary tract are not life threatening but may present social problems with lifelong implications for the child and family. Thus, early recognition and supportive, understanding care are essential.

Hypospadias and Epispadias

Hypospadias is a congenital condition in which the urethra terminates on the ventral (underside) surface of the penis, instead of at the tip. A cordlike anomaly (a **chordee**) extends from the scrotum to the penis, pulling the penis downward in an arc. Urination is not affected, but the boy cannot void while standing in the normal male fashion. Surgical repair is desirable between the ages of 6 and 18 months, before body image and castration anxiety become problems. Microscopic surgery makes early repair possible. Surgical repair is often accomplished in one stage and is often done as outpatient surgery. These newborns should not be circumcised because the foreskin is used in the repair. Severe hypospadias may require additional surgical procedures.

In epispadias, the opening is on the dorsal (top) surface of the penis. This condition often occurs with exstrophy of the bladder. Surgical repair is indicated.

Exstrophy of the Bladder

This urinary tract malformation occurs in 1 in 30,000 live births in the United States and is usually accompanied by other anomalies, such as epispadias, cleft scrotum, cryptorchidism (undescended testes), a shortened penis, and cleft clitoris. It also is associated with malformed pelvic musculature, resulting in a prolapsed rectum and inguinal hernias. Children with this defect have a widely split symphysis pubis and posterolaterally rotated hip sockets, causing a waddling gait.

In this condition, the anterior surface of the urinary bladder lies open on the lower abdomen (Fig. 21-26). The exposed mucosa is red and sensitive to touch and allows direct passage of urine to the outside. This condition makes the area vulnerable to infection and trauma.

NURSING CARE PLAN 21-1

The Infant With an Orthopedic Cast

Six-month-old Melissa Davis has right congenital hip dysplasia. After a trial with a Pavlik harness, she has been placed in a hip spica cast. The cast has just been applied. This is a new experience for her and her caregiver.

NURSING DIAGNOSIS
Acute Pain related to discomfort of hip spica cast

GOAL: The infant will show signs of being comfortable.

OUTCOME CRITERIA
• The infant is alert and contended.
• The infant has no long periods of fussiness.
• The infant interacts with caregivers by cooing, smiling, and eye contact.

NURSING INTERVENTIONS	*RATIONALE*
Check edges of cast for smoothness; petal edges of cast.	Rough edges can cause irritation and discomfort.
Soothe by stroking, cuddling, and talking to infant.	These comfort measures help the infant feel safe, secure, and loved and provide distraction from discomfort and restriction of cast.
Provide infant with a pacifier.	Nonnutritive sucking is a means of self-comfort.

NURSING DIAGNOSIS
Risk for Impaired Skin Integrity related to pressure of the cast on the skin surface

GOAL: The infant's skin will remain intact.

OUTCOME CRITERIA
• The infant's skin around the cast shows no signs of redness or irritation.
• The infant's skin in the diaper area is clean, dry, and intact with no signs of perineal redness of irritation.

NURSING INTERVENTIONS	*RATIONALE*
Place infant on firm mattress for 24 to 48 hours until cast is dry.	The cast is still pliable until dry. Undue pressure on any point must be avoided.
Use palms when handling damp cast.	Using palms instead of fingers prevents excessive pressure in any one area.
Petal all edges of cast.	Petalling provides a smooth edge along cast to avoid irritation.
Inspect skin around the cast edges for redness and irritation during each shift.	Early signs of irritation indicate areas that may need added protection.
Protect perineal area of cast with waterproof covering.	Urine and feces can easily cause irritation, skin breakdown, or a softened and malodorous cast.
Remove, wash, and thoroughly dry perineal covering if wet or soiled.	A clean, dry perineal cast protective covering decreases the problem of breakdown.

NURSING DIAGNOSIS
Risk for Delayed Growth and Development related to restricted mobility secondary to hip spica cast

GOAL: The infant will attain appropriate developmental milestones.

OUTCOME CRITERIA
• The infant responds positively to audio, visual, and diversional activities.
• The infant smiles, coos, and squeals in response to family caregivers.
• The infant shows age appropriate development.

(nursing care plan continues on page 542)

NURSING CARE PLAN 21-1 continued

The Infant With an Orthopedic Cast

NURSING INTERVENTIONS	RATIONALE
Provide mobiles, musical toys, stuffed toys, and toys infant can manipulate.	Visual, tactile, and auditory stimulation are important for infant development.
Encourage caregiver to interact with infant during feeding.	Interacting (babbling, cooing) with others in her or his environment encourages development.
Plan activities that include changes of environment such as moving to the playroom in the hospital or to a different room in the home.	Environmental variety provides increased visual, auditory, and tactile stimulation.

NURSING DIAGNOSIS
Deficient Knowledge of family caregivers related to the home care of the infant in a cast

GOAL: The family caregivers will learn home care of the infant.

OUTCOME CRITERIA
* The family caregivers demonstrate care of the infant in the hip spica cast.
* The family caregivers ask pertinent questions.
* The family caregiver identifies a resource person to call.

NURSING INTERVENTIONS	RATIONALE
Determine the family caregivers' knowledge level and design a teaching plan.	An effective teaching plan is tailored to begin with the knowledge base of the family.
Choose teaching methods most suited to family caregivers' recognized needs and learning style.	The family's ability to read, understand, and follow directions and their cognitive abilities affect the results.
Before discharge, schedule follow-up appointment for return visit to have the cast checked.	Scheduling the follow-up appointment emphasizes to family caregivers the importance of close follow-up.

Surgical closure of the bladder is preferred within the first 48 hours of life. Final surgical correction is completed before the child goes to school. If bladder repair is not done early in the child's life, the family caregivers must be taught how to care for this condition and how to deal with their feelings toward this less-than-perfect child. Their emotional reaction may be further complicated if the malformation is so severe that the sex of the child may be determined only by a chromosome test (see the following section on ambiguous genitalia).

A

B

● **Figure 21.26** Exstrophy of the bladder. (**A**) Prior to surgery, note the bright-red color of the bladder. (**B**) Following surgical repair.

Nursing care of the newborn with exstrophy of the bladder should be directed toward preventing infection, preventing skin irritation around the seeping mucosa, meeting the newborn's need for touch and cuddling, and educating and supporting the family during this crisis.

Ambiguous Genitalia

If a child's external sex organs did not follow a normal development in utero, at birth it may not be possible to determine by observation if the child is a male or female. The external sexual organs are either incompletely or abnormally formed. This condition is called ambiguous genitalia. Although rare, the birth of a newborn with ambiguous genitalia presents a highly charged emotional climate and has possible long-range social implications. Regardless of the cause, it is important to establish the genetic sex and the sex of rearing as early as possible, so that surgical correction of anomalies may occur before the child begins to function in a sex-related social role. Authorities believe that the newborn's anatomic structure, rather than the genetic sex, should determine the sex of rearing. It is possible to construct a functional vagina surgically and to administer hormones to offer an anatomically incomplete female a somewhat normal life. Currently it is impossible to offer comparable surgical reconstruction to males with an inadequate penis. Parents may feel guilt, anxiety, and confusion about their child's condition and need empathic understanding and support to help them cope with this emergency.

INBORN ERRORS OF METABOLISM

Disorders referred to as inborn errors of metabolism are hereditary disorders that affect metabolism. Inborn errors of metabolism include phenylketonuria, galactosemia, congenital hypothyroidism, maple syrup urine disease, and homocystinuria. Nursing care for the newborn involves prompt diagnosis and initiation of treatment. Family teaching might include dietary guidelines, information about the disorder, and genetic counseling. The family also needs support and information to prepare for the long-term care of a chronically ill child (see Chapter 32).

Phenylketonuria

Phenylketonuria (PKU) is a recessive hereditary defect of metabolism that, if untreated, causes severe mental retardation in most but not all affected children. It is uncommon, appearing in about 1 in 10,000 births. Children with this condition lack the enzyme that normally changes the essential amino acid phenylalanine into tyrosine.

As soon as the newborn with this defect begins to take milk (either breast or cow's milk), phenylalanine is absorbed in the normal manner. However, because the affected newborn cannot metabolize this amino acid, phenylalanine builds up in the blood serum to as much as 20 times the normal level. This build-up occurs so quickly that increased levels of phenylalanine appear in the blood after only 1 or 2 days of ingestion of milk. Phenylpyruvic acid appears in the urine of these newborns between the 2nd and the 6th week of life.

Most untreated children with this condition develop severe and progressive mental deficiency. The high levels of phenylalanine in the bloodstream and tissues cause permanent damage to brain tissues. The newborn appears normal at birth but begins to show signs of mental arrest within a few weeks. Therefore, this disorder must be diagnosed as early as possible, and the child must be placed immediately on a low-phenylalanine formula.

Clinical Presentation

Signs and Symptoms. Untreated newborns may experience frequent vomiting and have aggressive and hyperactive traits. Severe, progressive retardation is characteristic. Convulsions may occur, and eczema is common, particularly in the perineal area. There is a characteristic musty smell to the urine.

Laboratory and Diagnostic Test Results. Most states require newborns to undergo a blood test to detect the phenylalanine level. This screening procedure, the Guthrie inhibition assay test, uses blood from a simple heel prick. The test is most reliable after the newborn has ingested some form of protein. The accepted practice is to perform the test on the second or third day of life. If the newborn leaves the hospital before this time, the newborn is brought back to have the test performed. The test may be repeated in the third week of life if the first test was done before the newborn was 24 hours old. Health practitioners caring for newborns not born in a hospital are responsible for screening these newborns. When screening indicates an increased level of phenylalanine, additional testing is done to make a firm diagnosis.

Treatment and Nursing Care

Dietary treatment is required. A formula low in phenylalanine should be started as soon as the condition is detected; Lofenalac and Phenyl-free are low-phenylalanine formulas. Best results are obtained if the special formula is started before the newborn is 3 weeks of age. A low-phenylalanine diet is a very restricted one; foods to be omitted are breads, meat, fish, dairy products, nuts, and legumes. A nutritionist should supervise the diet carefully. The child remains on the diet at least into early adulthood, and it may even be recommended indefinitely. If a woman who has PKU decides to have a child and is not following a diet low in phenylalanine, she should return to following the dietary treatment for at least 3 months before becoming pregnant. The diet is continued through the pregnancy to help in preventing the child from being born with a mental impairment. Routine blood testing is done to maintain the serum phenylalanine level at 2 to 8 mg/dL.

Maintaining the newborn on the restricted diet is relatively simple compared with the problems that arise as the child grows and becomes more independent. As the child ventures into the world beyond home, more and more dietary temptations are available, and dietary compliance is difficult. The family and child need support and counseling throughout the child's developmental years. The length of time that the restrictions are necessary remains unclear. Although difficult, it seems best to follow the diet into adolescence.

Galactosemia

Galactosemia is a recessive hereditary metabolic disorder in which the enzyme necessary to convert galactose into glucose is missing. The newborns generally appear normal at birth but experience difficulties after ingesting milk (breast, cow's, or goat's) because one of the component monosaccharides of milk lactose is galactose.

Clinical Presentation

Early feeding difficulties with vomiting and diarrhea severe enough to produce dehydration and weight loss and jaundice are primary manifestations. Unless milk is withheld early, other difficulties include cataracts, liver and spleen damage, and mental retardation, with a high mortality rate early in life. A screening test (Beutler test) can be used to test for the disorder.

Treatment and Nursing Care

Galactose must be omitted from the diet, which in the young newborn means a substitution for milk. Nutramigen and Pregestimil are formulas that provide galactose-free nutrition for the newborn. The diet must continue to be free of lactose when the child moves on to table foods, but the diet allows more variety than does the phenylalanine-free diet.

Congenital Hypothyroidism

At one time referred to by the now unacceptable term "cretinism," congenital hypothyroidism is associated with either the congenital absence of a thyroid gland or the inability of the thyroid gland to secrete thyroid hormone. The incidence is about 1 in 5,000 births or about twice as common as PKU.

Clinical Presentation

Signs and Symptoms. The newborn appears normal at birth, but clinical signs and symptoms begin to be noticeable at about 6 weeks of life. The facial features are typical and include depressed nasal bridge, large tongue, and puffy eyes. The neck is short and thick (Fig. 21-27). The voice (cry) is hoarse, the skin is dry and cold, and the newborn has slow bone development. Two common features are chronic constipation and abdomen enlargement caused by poor muscle tone. The newborn is a poor feeder and often characterized as a "good" baby by the parent or caretaker because he or she cries very little and sleeps for long periods.

Laboratory and Diagnostic Test Results. Most states require a routine test for triiodothyronine (T_3) and thyroxine (T_4) levels to determine thyroid function in all newborns before discharge for early diagnosis of congenital hypothyroidism. This test is done as part of the heel-stick screening, which includes the Guthrie screening test for PKU.

Treatment and Nursing Care

The thyroid hormone must be replaced as soon as the diagnosis is made. Levothyroxine sodium, a synthetic thyroid replacement, is the drug most commonly used. Blood levels of T_3 and T_4 are monitored to prevent overdosage. Unless therapy is started in early infancy, mental retardation and slow growth occur. The later that therapy is started, the more severe the mental retardation. Therapy must be continued for life.

● **Figure 21.27** A newborn with congenital hypothyroidism; note the short, thick neck and enlarged abdomen.

Maple Syrup Urine Disease

Maple syrup urine disease (MSUD) is an inborn error of metabolism of the branched chain amino acids. It is autosomal recessive in inheritance. It is rapidly progressive and often fatal.

Clinical Presentation

The onset of MSUD occurs very early in infancy. In the 1st week of life, these newborns often have feeding problems and neurologic signs such as seizures, spasticity, and opisthotonos. The urine has a distinctive odor of maple syrup. Diagnosis is made through a blood test for the amino acids leucine, isoleucine, and valine. This is easily done at the same time the heel stick for PKU is performed.

Treatment and Nursing Care

Treatment of MSUD is dietary and must be initiated within 12 days of birth to be successful. The special formula is low in the branched chain amino acids. The special diet must be continued indefinitely.

CHROMOSOMAL ABNORMALITIES

Chromosomal abnormalities are often evident at birth and frequently cause physical and cognitive challenges for the child throughout life. There are various forms of chromosomal abnormalities, including nondisjunction, deletion, translocation, mosaicism, and isochromosome abnormalities.

The most common abnormalities are nondisjunction abnormalities, which occur when the chromosomal division is uneven. Normally during cell division of the cells of reproduction, the 46 chromosomes divide in half, with 23 chromosomes in each new cell. Nondisjunction abnormalities occur when a new cell has an extra chromosome (e.g., 24) or not enough chromosomes (e.g., 22). When this defective chromosome joins with a normal reproductive cell having 23 chromosomes, an abnormality occurs. Down syndrome, the most common chromosomal abnormality, most often is a result of chromosomal nondisjunction with an extra chromosome on chromosome 21. Two other common chromosomal abnormalities that may be seen include the Turner and Klinefelter syndromes, which are nondisjunction abnormalities occurring on the sex chromosomes.

Down Syndrome

Down syndrome is the most common chromosomal anomaly, occurring in about 1 in 700 to 800 births. Langdon Down first described the condition in 1866, but its cause was a mystery for many years. In 1932, it was suggested that a chromosomal anomaly might be the cause, but the anomaly was not demonstrated until 1959.

Down syndrome has been observed in nearly all countries and races. The old term "mongolism" is inappropriate and no longer used. Most people with Down syndrome have trisomy 21 (Fig. 21-28); a few have partial dislocation of chromosomes 15 and 21. A woman older than 35 years of age is at a greater risk of bearing a child with Down syndrome than is a younger woman, but children with Down syndrome are born to women of all ages. Older women and increasing numbers of younger women are choosing to undergo screening at 15 weeks' gestation for low maternal serum alpha-fetoprotein levels and high chorionic gonadotropin levels, which indicates the possibility of Down syndrome in the fetus. Amniocentesis and chorionic villus sampling are more accurate and will confirm the blood test results. These screening tests give women the option of aborting the fetus or continuing with the pregnancy and preparing themselves for the birth of a disabled child.

Clinical Presentation

All forms of the condition show a variety of abnormal characteristics. Mental status is usually within the moderate to severe range of retardation, with most children being moderately retarded. The most common anomalies include:

● **Figure 21.28** Karotype showing trisomy 21. Note three chromosomes in the 21 position.

- **Brachycephaly** (shortness of head)
- Retarded body growth
- Upward and outward slanted eyes (almond-shaped) with an epicanthic fold at the inner angle
- Short, flattened bridge of the nose
- Thick, fissured tongue
- Dry, cracked, fissured skin that may be mottled
- Dry and coarse hair
- Short hands with an incurved fifth finger
- A single horizontal palm crease (simian line)
- Wide space between the first and second toes
- Lax muscle tone (often referred to as "double jointed" by others)
- Heart and eye anomalies
- Greater susceptibility to leukemia than that of the general population

Not all these physical signs are present in all people with Down syndrome. Some may have only one or two characteristics; others may show nearly all the characteristics (Fig. 21-29).

Treatment and Nursing Care

The physical characteristics of the child with Down syndrome determine the medical and nursing management. Lax muscles, congenital heart defects, and dry skin contribute to a large variety of problems. The child's relaxed muscle tone may contribute to respiratory complications as a result of decreased respiratory expansion. The relaxed skeletal muscles contribute to late motor development. Gastric motility is also decreased, leading to problems with constipation. Congenital heart defects

and vision or hearing problems add to the complexities of the child's care.

In infancy, the child's large tongue and poor muscle tone may contribute to difficulty breast-feeding or ingesting formula and can cause great problems when the time comes to introduce solid foods. The family caregivers need support during these trying times. As the child gets older, concern about excessive weight gain becomes a primary consideration.

The family caregivers of the child with Down syndrome need strong support and guidance from the time the child is born. Early intervention programs have yielded some encouraging results, but depending on the level of cognitive impairment, the family may have to decide if they can care for the child at home or if other living arrangements need to be considered for the child. A cognitively impaired child who is undisciplined or improperly supervised may threaten the safety of others in the home and the neighborhood. Caring for the child may demand so much sacrifice from other family members that the family structure may be significantly affected. However, with consistent care, patience, and guidelines, families of children with Down syndrome often find joy and pleasure in the gentle and loving nature of the child.

Turner Syndrome

The newborn with Turner syndrome has one less X chromosome than normal. Characteristics of Turner syndrome include short stature, low set ears, a broad-based neck that appears webbed and short, a low-set

A   **B**

● **Figure 21.29** Typical features of a child with Down syndrome: (**A**) facial features; (**B**) horizontal palm crease (simian line).

hairline at the nap of the neck, broad chest, an increased angle of the arms, and edema of the hands and feet. These children frequently have congenital heart defects as well. Females are most often affected by Turner syndrome and, with the exception of pubic hair, do not develop secondary sex characteristics.

Children with Turner syndrome have normal intelligence but may have visual-spatial concerns, learning disabilities, problems with social interaction, and may lack physical coordination. Growth hormones are given to increase the height, as well as the hormonal levels, but females with Turner syndrome rarely can become pregnant.

Klinefelter Syndrome

The presence of an extra X chromosome causes Klinefelter syndrome. The syndrome is most commonly seen in males. Characteristics are not often evident until puberty, when the child does not develop secondary sex characteristics. The testes are usually small and do not produce mature sperm. Increased breast size and a risk of developing breast cancer are frequently seen.

Boys with Klinefelter syndrome often have normal intelligence but frequently have behavior problems, show signs of immaturity and insecurity, and have difficulty with memory and processing. Hormone replacements of testosterone may be started in the early teens to promote normal adult development.

KEY POINTS

- A failure of the maxillary and premaxillary processes to fuse during fetal development can cause a cleft lip on one or both sides of the lip or a cleft palate, in which the tissue in the roof of the mouth does not fuse properly.
- Early signs that a newborn may have an esophageal fistula include frothing and excessive drooling and periods of respiratory distress with choking and cyanosis.
- The greatest preoperative danger for the newborn with tracheoesophageal atresia is the possibility of aspiration and pneumonitis, as well as respiratory distress.
- Diaphragmatic hernias occur when abdominal organs are displaced into the left chest through an opening in the diaphragm. If the cardiac portion of the stomach slides into the area above the diaphragm, a hiatal hernia is caused. A rare occurrence, the omphalocele is seen when the abdominal contents protrude through the umbilical cord and form a sac lying on the abdomen. If the end of the umbilical cord does not close completely and a por-

tion of the intestine protrudes through the opening, an umbilical hernia is formed. Inguinal hernias occur mostly in males when a part of the intestine slips into the inguinal canal.
- Spina bifida is caused when the spinal vertebrae fail to close and an opening is left where the spinal cord or meninges may protrude. Spina bifida occulta is seen when soft tissue is not involved and only a dimple in the skin may be seen. Spina bifida with meningocele occurs when the spinal meninges protrude through and forms a sac, and spina bifida with myelomeningocele occurs when both the spinal cord and meninges protrude. The later condition is the most difficult to treat because of the concern of complete paralysis below the lesion.
- If an obstruction in the circulation of cerebral spinal fluid (CSF) occurs, the condition is called "noncommunicating hydrocephalus." With communicating hydrocephalus, there is defective absorption of CSF. The most obvious symptom of hydrocephalus is the rapid increase in head circumference. Ventriculoperitoneal shunting (VP shunt) drains CSF from the brain into the peritoneal cavity. With ventriculoatrial shunting, the CSF is drained into the heart.
- Ventricular septal defects allow the blood to pass from the left to the right ventricle; in the atrial septal defect the blood flows from the left to the right atria. With a patent ductus arteriosus, blood is shunted from the aorta into the pulmonary artery. When coarctation of the aorta occurs there is a narrowing of the aortic arch and an obstruction of blood flow.
- Tetralogy of Fallot is a group of heart defects including pulmonary stenosis, ventricular septal defect, overriding aorta, and right ventricular hypertrophy. The child with Tetralogy of Fallot has cyanosis and low oxygen saturation. The severe and usually fatal defect, transposition of the great arteries, causes cyanosis and occurs because the aorta arises from the right ventricle, instead of the left, and the pulmonary artery arises from the left ventricle, instead of the right.
- Clubfoot, talipes equinovarus, and congenital hip dysplasia are the most common skeletal deformities in the newborn. Signs and symptoms of congenital dislocation of the hip include asymmetry of the gluteal skin folds, limited abduction of the affected hip and shortening of the femur. To treat hip dislocation, the femur is manipulated and a brace applied. A hip spica cast may be used after an open reduction, if necessary.
- Phenylketonuria is detected by doing a blood test called the Guthrie inhibition assay test to detect phenylalanine levels. Dietary treatment using a formula and diet low in phenylalanine is started and continued as the child gets older.

▶ Congenital hypothyroidism is detected by performing tests for triiodothyronine (T_3) and thyroxine (T_4) levels to determine thyroid function.

▶ If phenylketonuria, congenital hypothyroidism, and galactosemia are not treated, the newborn often has severe mental retardation.

▶ Down syndrome is sometimes called trisomy 21 because of the three-chromosome pattern seen on the 21st pair of chromosomes. Signs and symptoms seen in children with Down syndrome include brachycephaly (shortness of head); slowed growth; slanted (almond shaped) eyes; short, flattened nose; thick tongue; dry, cracked, fissured skin; dry and coarse hair; short hands with an incurved fifth finger; single horizontal palm crease (simian line); wide space between the first and second toes; lax muscle tone; heart and eye anomalies; and a greater susceptibility to leukemia.

REFERENCES AND SELECTED READINGS

Books and Journals

Finesilver, C. (2002). Down syndrome. *RN, 65*(11), 43–49.

Fishman, M. A. (1999). Developmental defects. In *Oski's pediatrics: Principles and practice* (3rd ed.). Philadelphia: Lippincott Williams & Wilkins.

Goldberg, M. J. (2001). Early detection of developmental hip dysplasia. *Pediatrics in Review, 22*(4), 131–134.

Gorlin, R. J. (1999). Craniofacial defects. In *Oski's pediatrics: Principles and practice* (3rd ed.). Philadelphia: Lippincott Williams & Wilkins.

Holmes, L. B. (1999). Congenital malformations. In *Oski's pediatrics: Principles and practice* (3rd ed.). Philadelphia: Lippincott Williams & Wilkins.

Lewanda, A. F., & Jabs, E. W. (1999). Dysmorphology: Genetic syndromes and associations. In *Oski's pediatrics: Principles and practice* (3rd ed.). Philadelphia: Lippincott Williams & Wilkins.

McDaniel, N. L. (2001). Heart ventricular and atrial septal defects. *Pediatrics in Review, 22*(8), 265.

North American Nursing Diagnosis Association (NANDA). (2001). *NANDA nursing diagnoses: Definitions and classification 2001–2002.* Philadelphia: Author.

Oxley, J. (2001). Are arm splints required following cleft lip/palate repair? *Pediatric Nursing, 13*(1) 27–30.

Pillitteri, A. (2003). *Maternal and child health nursing* (4th ed.). Philadelphia: Lippincott Williams & Wilkins.

Purnell, L., & Paulanda, B. (2003). *Transcultural health care: A culturally competent approach* (2nd ed.). Philadelphia: FA Davis.

Robinson, D., & Drumm, L. (2001). Maple syrup disease: A standard of nursing care. *Pediatric Nursing, 27*(3), 255.

Sommerlad, B. C. (2002). The management of cleft lip and palate. *Current Pediatrics, 12*(1), 36–42.

Springhouse nurse's drug guide (3rd ed.). (2000). Springhouse, PA: Springhouse Corporation.

Sparks, S., & Taylor, C. (2001). *Nursing diagnosis reference manual* (5th ed.). Springhouse, PA: Springhouse Corporation.

Suddaby, E. C. (2001). Contemporary thinking for congenital heart disease. *Pediatric Nursing, 27*(3), 233.

Wedge, J. H., et al. (2001). Congenital clubfoot. *Current Pediatrics, 11*(5), 332–340.

Wong, D. L., & Hockenberry-Eaton, M. (2001). *Wong's essentials of pediatric nursing* (6th ed.). St. Louis: Mosby.

Wong, D. L., Perry, S., & Hockenberry, M. (2002). *Maternal child nursing care* (2nd ed.). St. Louis: Mosby.

Websites
Spina Bifida
http://www.sbaa.org

Cleft Lip and Cleft Palate
http://www.cleft.org

WORKBOOK

NCLEX-STYLE REVIEW QUESTIONS

1. The nurse is doing an admission examination on a newborn with a diagnosis of hydrocephalus. If the following data were collected, which might indicate a common symptom of this diagnosis?

   a. Sac protruding on the lower back

   b. Respiratory rate of 30 breaths a minute

   c. Gluteal folds higher on one side than the other

   d. Head circumference of 18 inches

2. When collecting data during an admission interview and examination on a newborn, the nurse finds the newborn has cyanosis, dyspnea, tachycardia, and feeding difficulties. These symptoms might indicate the newborn has which of the following conditions?

   a. Spina bifida

   b. Tetralogy of Fallot

   c. Congenital rubella

   c. Hip dysplasia

3. In caring for a newborn who has had a cleft lip/cleft palate repair, the *highest* priority for the nurse is to

   a. document the time period the restraints are on and off.

   b. observe the incision for redness or drainage.

   c. teach the caregivers about dental care and hygiene.

   d. provide sensory stimulation and age-appropriate toys.

4. In planning care for an infant who had a spica cast applied to treat a congenital hip dysplasia, which of the following nursing interventions would be included in this newborn's plan of care?

   a. Inspect skin for redness and irritation.

   b. Change bedding and clothing every 4 hours.

   c. Weigh every morning and evening using same scale.

   d. Monitor temperature and pulse every 2 hours.

5. The nurse is caring for a newborn who has a myelomeningocele and has not yet had surgery to repair the defect. Which of the following

measures will be used to prevent the site from becoming infected? (Select all that apply.)

   a. Give antibiotics as a prophylactic measure.

   b. Cover the sac with a saline soaked sterile dressing.

   c. Maintain the newborn in a supine position.

   d. Place a plastic protective covering over the dressing.

   e. Change the dressing every 8 hours.

STUDY ACTIVITIES

1. Using the table below, list the common types of congenital heart defects. Include the description of the defect (chambers and parts of the heart involved), the blood flow characteristics, symptoms, and treatment.

Detect	Description of Defect	Blood Flow Characteristics	Symptoms	Treatment

2. Make a list of the maternal risk factors that may cause congenital heart defects. For each of these risk factors, state what could be done to decrease the occurrence of these risks.

3. Develop a teaching project by creating a mobile or gathering a collection of appropriate toys and activities that could be used for sensory stimulation with a newborn who is in an orthopedic cast. Present your project to your classmates and explain why and how these items would be appropriate to use for developmental stimulation.

4. Go to the following Internet site: http://www.pediheart.org

   a. Click on "Parent's Place."

   b. Click on "Prepare for Surgery."

   c. Read the section "Preparing Your Child for Surgery."

   d. Read the section "Helpful Parent Tips."

5. List eight tips to share with parents whose child is having heart surgery.

6. List three books that parents could use with the child who is having heart surgery.

CRITICAL THINKING: What Would You Do?

1. Diane's baby was born with a bilateral cleft lip and cleft palate. When you bring the baby to her for feeding, she breaks down and sobs uncontrollably.

   a. Describe what your immediate response would be.

   b. What feelings and emotions do you think Diane is experiencing?

   c. Write out an example of a therapeutic response you could make?

2. Cody was born with hydrocephalus and has been admitted to the pediatric unit to have a ventriculoperitoneal (VP) shunt placed. You walk into Cody's room after the pediatrician has discussed the procedure with Cody's parents. They seem anxious and begin asking you questions. How will you answer the following questions?

   a. What is hydrocephalus and what caused Cody to have the disorder?

   b. Why does Cody need to have a shunt and how does it work?

   c. What long-term problems will Cody have because of the disorder?

3. *Dosage calculation:* The nurse is preparing the preoperative medication of Demerol (meperidine) for an infant who is having a surgical procedure to correct a congenital heart defect. The infant weighs 9.9 pounds (9 pounds, 14.4 ounces). The usual dosage range of this medication is 1 to 2.2 mg per kg. Answer the following:

   a. How many kilograms does the infant weigh?

   b. What is the low dose of Demerol (in milligrams) that this infant could be given?

   c. What is the high dose of Demerol (in milligrams) that this infant could be given?

Health Promotion for Normal Growth and Development

Principles of Growth and Development

22

Principles of Growth and Development
    Foundations of Growth and Development
    Factors Related to Growth and Development
Influences on Growth and Development
    Genetics
    Nutrition
    Environment

The Nurse's Role Related to Growth and Development
Theories of Child Development
    Sigmund Freud
    Erik Erikson
    Jean Piaget
    Lawrence Kohlberg
    Other Theorists

STUDENT OBJECTIVES

On completion of this chapter, the student should be able to

1. Define growth, development and maturation.
2. Explain the terms cephalocaudal and proximodistal.
3. Explain how height and weight are used to monitor growth and development.
4. Discuss how tools for measuring standards of growth and development are used.
5. List three influences on a child's growth and development.
6. Describe environmental factors that can influence growth and development.
7. Discuss the role of the nurse in understanding growth and development.
8. List and discuss the six stages of psychosexual development according to Freud.
9. Describe Erikson's theory of psychosocial development.
10. Name the eight stages of Erikson's psychosocial development.
11. List the developmental tasks in each of Erikson's stages.
12. Identify and describe the four stages of Piaget's theory of cognitive development.
13. Discuss the ideas included in Kohlberg's developmental theory.

KEY TERMS

archetypes
cephalocaudal
cognitive development
development
developmental task
ego
egocentric
growth
id
latchkey child
libido
maturation
proximodistal
sublimation
superego
temperament

PRINCIPLES OF GROWTH AND DEVELOPMENT

The process of growth and development continues from conception all the way to death. There are periods of time when growth is more rapid than others and times when development is slowed. Growth and development is affected and influenced by many factors. Some basic foundations of growth and development are important for the nurse to understand when working with infants, children, and adolescents.

Foundations of Growth and Development

"Growth and development" refers to the total growth of the child from birth toward maturity. **Growth** is the physical increase in the body's size and appearance caused by increasing numbers of new cells. **Development** is the progressive change in the child toward maturity or **maturation,** completed growth and development. As children develop, their capacity to learn and think increases. Growth of the child follows an orderly pattern starting with the head and moving downward. This pattern is referred to as **cephalocaudal.** The child is able to control the head and neck before being able to control the arms and legs. Growth also proceeds in a pattern referred to as **proximodistal,** in which growth starts in the center and progresses toward the periphery or outside (see Fig. 22-1). Following this pattern, the child can control movement of the arms before being able to control movement of the hands. Another example of proximodistal growth is the ability to hold something in the hand before being able to use the fingers to pick up an object. The process of growth moves from the simple to complex. **Developmental tasks** or milestones are basic achievements associated with each stage of development. These tasks must be mastered to move successfully to the next developmental stage. Developmental tasks must be completed successfully at each stage for a person to achieve maturity.

Factors Related to Growth and Development

Each child has a pattern of growth that is unique to that child. These patterns are related to height and weight. Monitoring these patterns and recognizing deviations can be helpful in discovering medical issues and concerns. As the child is monitored and growth and development plotted and compared with the child's previous measurements, deviations can be noted and investigated.

Height

As the child grows, the height, or distance from the head to the feet, increases in a predictable pattern. The

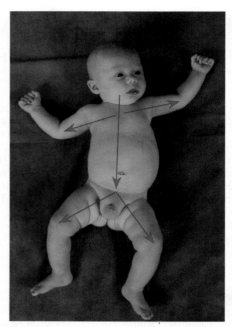

● **Figure 22.1** The pattern of growth starting with the head and moving downward is cephalocaudal. Proximodistal growth starts in the center and progresses outward.

changes in a child's height provide a concrete measurement of the child's growth. Although predictable, the increases in height are not uniform but often are seen in growth spurts or time periods when there is rapid growth and other periods of time when growth is slowed. The length of the infant and the increasing height of the child are measured routinely (see Chapter 28), and the patterns are monitored and plotted on a growth chart. The increase in height seen in children and adolescence is attributable to the skeletal growth that is taking place.

Weight

The weight gain of the child also progresses in a predictable pattern. Although for many different reasons there are variations in the weight of children the same age, the weight gain of each individual child is an important factor in the growth of the child. Patterns of weight increases are monitored and plotted on growth charts.

Standards of Growth

A growth chart with predictable patterns or growth curves is used to plot and monitor a child's growth through the years. These growth charts allow for comparison of children of the same age and sex. They also allow for comparison of the child's current measurements with the child's previous measurements. Standard growth charts are used to determine if the child's pattern is appropriate or if for some reason the child's growth is above or falls below a standardized normal range (see Appendix G). A

A PERSONAL GLIMPSE

Every time I had to take my baby to the pediatricians office for his well-baby checkup I would worry for days. The nurse would always weigh and measure him and look at the growth chart, then look at me with a curious look. Sometimes she would weigh him again and then just stare at me. I would ask what was wrong and she would say in an accusing voice, "Well, he is in the 95th percentile for height and in the 5th percentile for weight." She would start asking me questions like was I feeding him often enough, did he cry all the time, did he have a babysitter who took care of him while I worked or just why was he not gaining enough weight. I would get so upset because they acted like I was starving or neglecting my baby, and I knew I wasn't. Finally when he was 11 months old, it was discovered that he had a digestive problem and couldn't drink milk or eat wheat or oatmeal—his low weight didn't have anything to do with the way I was taking care of him. I started giving him soymilk, changed his diet and right away he started gaining weight. I was so relieved that now finally he was in a higher percentile on the growth chart. I will never forget how bad I felt when I was treated as if I was a neglectful mother, that was so hard. I am glad the disorder was discovered—by the time he was 21 he was 6 feet and 3 inches tall and weighed 190 pounds!

Diane

LEARNING OPPORTUNITY: What were the benefits in this situation of plotting this child's growth on a growth chart? What do you think this mother was feeling when she was in the pediatrician's office? What could the nurse have done to support this mother?

growth chart is used for comparison only and because a child does not fall into the "normal" range does not necessarily indicate that there is something of concern for that child.

Test Yourself

- Define growth, development, and maturation.

- What does cephalocaudal and proximodistal mean?

- Why is the child's height and weight plotted on a growth chart?

Standards of Development

Developmental screening is done by using standardized developmental tools such as the Denver Developmental Screening Test (DDST). Development in children occurs in a range of time, rather than at an exact time. Developmental screening offers information regarding any delays in what is considered a standard or normal pattern. Although one child might develop at a faster rate than another child, within a time range, both children will have mastered developmental tasks or milestones, thus following a normal and predictable pattern. It is important to recognize that developmental screening is used for the sake of comparison and does not automatically mean there is a concern if the child does not fit exactly into the standardized normal pattern.

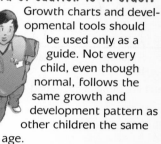

A word of caution is in order. Growth charts and developmental tools should be used only as a guide. Not every child, even though normal, follows the same growth and development pattern as other children the same age.

Body Proportions

From fetal life through adulthood body proportions vary and change. As the fetus develops and the child grows, the development of body systems and organs affects and changes the body proportions (see Fig. 22-2). In early fetal life the head is growing faster than the rest of the body and is thus proportionately larger. During infancy, the trunk portion of the body grows significantly. The legs grow rapidly during childhood, again changing the body proportions. As the child grows into an adolescent, the trunk portion grows and the body proportions are those of an adult.

INFLUENCES ON GROWTH AND DEVELOPMENT

There are many influences on the growth and development of a child. Prenatal factors that influence the fetus and child's growth and development include the mother's general health and nutrition, as well as her behaviors during pregnancy. These are covered in Chapters 5, 6, and 7. Genetic, nutritional, and environmental factors all affect the growth and development of the child.

Genetics

The science of genetics studies the ways in which normal and abnormal traits are transmitted from one generation to the next. The scientist Gregor Mendel did

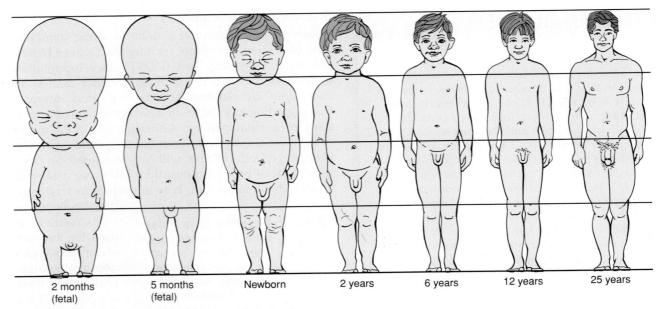

2 months (fetal)   5 months (fetal)   Newborn   2 years   6 years   12 years   25 years

● *Figure 22.2* From fetal life through adulthood the body proportions change.

experiments that proved each parent's individual characteristics could reappear unchanged in later generations. Human cells contain 46 chromosomes, consisting of 23 essentially identical pairs. At conception, the union of the sperm and egg forms a single cell. This cell is made up of one member of each pair contributed by the father and one member of each pair contributed by the mother. This combination determines the sex and inherited traits of the new organism.

The genetic makeup of each child helps determine characteristics such as the child's gender, race, eye color, height and weight. Growth and development of the child is influenced by these factors. For example, each child is genetically programmed to grow to be a certain height. With adequate nutrition and good health, most children will attain this height. Some diseases are genetically transmitted. If a child has a genetic predisposition to a certain disease, that child might not grow and develop as completely as a healthy child would. Physical and mental disorders can occur as a result of a child's genetic factors.

The child's heredity influences the physical as well as personality characteristics, including **temperament.** Temperament is the combination of all of an individual's characteristics, the way the person thinks, behaves and reacts to something that happens in his or her environment. Not all children react alike to situations. Depending on the child's temperament, one child might react to a situation with a quiet, shy response, whereas another child might react with acting out or aggressive behavior in the same situation. Children with differing temperaments might adapt in different time frames to new situations. One child might adapt quickly, whereas another child might adapt more slowly to the new situation. Characteristics that define a child's temperament include areas such as his or her activity level; the development of regular patterns, such as waking, eating, and elimination patterns, in their daily life; and how they approach and adapt to situations. Temperament also plays a part in a child's attention span and how easily they become distracted. All of these characteristics of temperament play a part in the child's development.

CULTURAL SNAPSHOT

Some cultural groups are more prone to certain diseases and disorders. Many of these are genetically passed from generation to generation. Being aware of these and sensitive to the concerns, fears, and feelings of people from various cultures helps the nurse remain supportive and objective.

Nutrition

The quality of a child's nutrition during the growing years has a major effect on the overall health and development of the child. It is important that the child have adequate amounts of food and nutrients for the body to grow. Nutrition is also a factor in the child's ability to resist infection and diseases. Motor skill development is influenced by inadequate, as well as excessive, food intake. Nutritional habits and patterns are established early in life, and these patterns are carried into adulthood, thus influencing the individual's growth, development, and health throughout life. Normal nutritional needs vary at each stage of development. In addition, at each stage of development variations in eating patterns, skills, and behaviors are seen. These aspects of nutrition are discussed in the chapters covering each of the stages of growth and development.

Environment

Many aspects of the child's environment affect growth and development. The family structures, including family size, sibling order, parent–child relationships, and cultural background all have an effect on the growth and development of the child. These topics are covered in Chapter 2.

The socioeconomic level of the family can affect the child, especially if there are not sufficient funds to provide adequate nutrition, childcare, and health care needs for the growing child. Play and entertainment are important environmental aspects in the development of a child. Other environmental factors that can affect growth and development include family homelessness and divorce; a latchkey situation, in which children come home from school to an empty house each day; and running away from home.

Good news. "Playing" is the job of every child! The use of movies, television, video games, computers and the Internet can have both positive and negative influences on the child. Children who have little or no supervision may not have the ability to recognize what is appropriate and healthy for their development.

Play and Entertainment

Throughout the stages of growth and development, the role and types of play differ. Through play children learn about themselves, the environment around them, and relationships with others. Various aspects of play, including the role, types, and functions of play, are discussed in each of the chapters covering the stages of growth and development.

The Homeless Family

A growing number of families are homeless in the United States. The causes of homelessness include job loss, loss of housing, drug addiction of adult caregivers, insufficient income, domestic turmoil, and separation or divorce. Single mothers with children make up an increasing number of these families. Many of these homeless single mothers and their families have multiple problems. Often there are higher rates of abuse, drug use, and mental health problems in homeless families. Many of these families lived with relatives for a time before being reduced to living in a car, an empty building, a welfare hotel, or perhaps a cardboard box. These families sometimes seek temporary housing in a shelter for the homeless. They often move from one living situation to another, living in a shelter for the time allowed and then moving elsewhere, only to return after a while to repeat the cycle.

Homelessness creates additional stresses for the family. Many homeless families have young children but have problems gaining entry into the health care system, even though these children are at high risk for developing acute and chronic conditions. Health care for these families commonly occurs as crisis intervention, instead of the more effective preventive intervention. Pregnant homeless women with their attendant problems receive little if any prenatal care, are poorly nourished, and bear low birth-weight infants. Most of the children of homeless families do not have adequate immunizations. Homeless children often have chronic illnesses at a higher rate than that of the general population. These chronic conditions may include anemia, heart disease, peripheral vascular disease, and neurologic disorders. Many homeless children have developmental delays, perform poorly when they attend school, and suffer from anxiety and depression in addition to having behavioral problems.

Many shelters available to the homeless are overcrowded, lack privacy (the bathroom facilities are used by many people), and have no personal bedding, or cribs for infants, and no facilities for cooking or refrigerating food. Because of limits to the length of stay, many families must move from one shelter to another. This adds to the problems these families face by contributing to a lack of consistency in the services and programs available to them.

Nurses can set the tone of the interaction between the homeless family and the health care facility. Establishing an environment in which the caregiver feels respected and comfortable is important. Focusing initially on the positive factors in the caregiver's relationship with the children alleviates some of the caregiver's guilt and fear of being criticized. Make every effort to offer down-to-earth suggestions and help the family in the most practical manner.

On the child's admission to the health care facility, the health care team performs a complete admission assessment. Ask the caregiver about the family's living arrangements; such information will help in the care and planning for the child. During this interview, the nurse may become aware of problems of other family members that need attention. When giving assistance and guidance, be careful to supplement, not take over, the family's functioning. For instance, tell the family how to go about getting a particular benefit and be certain they have complete and accurate information but do not take the steps for them. These families need to feel self-reliant and in control, and they need realistic solutions to their problems.

Outreach programs for the homeless have been established in many major cities. These programs conduct screening, treat acute illnesses, and help families contact local health care services when needed. Provide information to the family about any assistance that is available.

Divorce and the Child

Divorce has increased to the point where one in two marriages ends in divorce. About 50% of children experience the separation or divorce of their parents before they complete high school. Some children may experience more than one divorce because many of those who remarry divorce a second time. Divorce can be traumatic for children but may be better than the constant tension and turmoil that they have lived through in their home.

Children often feel responsible for the breakup and believe that it would not have occurred if they had just done the right thing or been good. On the other hand, children may blame one of the parents for deciding to end the marriage and causing the children grief and unhappiness. Children commonly feel unloved and, in a sense, feel that they too are being divorced. Counseling can help children to acknowledge and understand their anger and their need to blame one or the other parent. This process may take a considerable amount of time to resolve. Both parents should make every effort to eliminate the child's feeling of guilt and should avoid using the child as a spy or go-between with the estranged spouse. Parents must avoid trying to buy the affection of the children. This is especially true for the noncustodial parent, who must not shower the children with special gifts, trips, and privileges when the children are visiting.

Children should be encouraged to ask questions about the separation and divorce. A child who does not

ask questions may be afraid to ask for fear of retaliation by one of the parents. Children should be discouraged from thinking that they might be able to do something that would get the parents back together again. They must be helped to recognize the finality of the divorce. Plans for the children should be made (e.g., where and with whom the children will live, where they will go to school) and shared with the children as soon as possible. This can give the children a sense of security in their chaotic personal world. Each child's confidence and self-esteem must be strengthened through careful handling of the transition (Fig. 22-3).

When a child of a divorce is hospitalized, the nurse must be certain to have clear information about who is the custodial parent, as well as who may visit or otherwise contact the child. The custodial parent's instructions and wishes should be honored.

The nurse may encourage the child to express feelings of fear and guilt. The nurse also can help the child understand that other children have divorced parents. The school nurse may function as an advocate for a counseling program in the school setting that brings together children of divorces. During counseling, children can voice their fears and concerns and begin to work through them with the help of an objective counselor in a protected environment. One of the most important aspects of such groups is the reassurance the children get that they are not alone in this crisis.

When the custodial parent begins to date and plans to remarry, the child may again have strong emotions that must be worked through. If the remarriage brings together a blended family of children from the previous marriages of both adults, the children may need extra support in accepting the new stepparent and stepsiblings. Adults who seek preventive counseling when planning to form a stepfamily have greater success than do those who seek help only after problems are overwhelming.

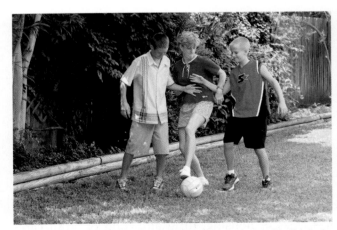

● **Figure 22.3** These children feel more secure and build their confidence as they enjoy time together with their newly divorced mother.

Children react in various ways to a parent's new marriage, depending in part on age. The new marriage may introduce additional problems of a new home, a new neighborhood, and a new school that can cause anxiety for any child. Although children should not be permitted to veto the parent's choice of a new partner, every effort should be made to help them adjust to this new family member and view the change in a non-threatening way.

The Latchkey Child

As a result of the increased number of families in which both parents work and the increase in single-parent families in which the parent must work, many children need after-school care and supervision; unfortunately, adequate or appropriate child care may not be readily available. A **latchkey child** is one who comes home to an empty house after school each day because the family caregivers are at work. The term was coined because this child often wears the house key around her or his neck. These children usually spend several hours alone before an adult comes home from work. The number of latchkey children may be as high as 10 million in the United States.

Latchkey children often have fears about being at home alone. When more than one child is involved and the older child is responsible for the younger one, conflicts can arise. The older child may have to assume responsibility that is beyond the normal expectations for the child's age. This can be a difficult situation for the caregivers and the children. The caregivers must carefully outline permissible activities and safety rules (Fig. 22-4). A plan should be in place to help the older child solve any arising problems that involve both children. The older child should not feel that the complete responsibility is on his or her shoulders, but rather that it is a shared responsibility with the caregiver. Some schools have after-school latchkey programs that pro-

vide safe activities for children. In addition, some communities have programs in which an adult telephones the child regularly every day after school, or there is a telephone hotline that the child can call (see Family Teaching Tips: Tips for Latchkey Children).

Despite concerns that latchkey children are more likely to become involved with smoking, stealing, or taking drugs, researchers have not found sufficient data to support this fear. Children who are given responsibility of this kind and who are recognized for their dependability usually live up to the expectations of the adults in their social environment.

Nurses must recognize the need for after-school services for these children and take an active role in the community to plan and support such services. Maintain a list of the facilities available to support families with latchkey children. The nurse can give caregivers guidance in planning children's after-school activities

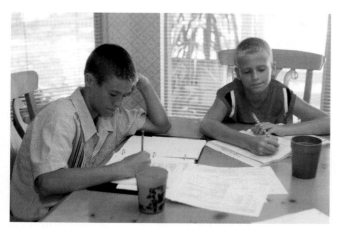

● *Figure 22.4* "Latchkey" children come home to an empty house after school. These boys have specific rules about activities to be done as they wait the arrival of their caregiver.

FAMILY TEACHING TIPS

Tips for Latchkey Children

- Teach the child to keep the key hidden and not show it to anyone.
- Plan with the child the routine to follow when arriving home; plan something special each day.
- Plan a telephone contact on the child's arrival home; either have the child call you or you call the child.
- Always let the child know if you are going to be delayed.
- Review safety rules with the child. Post them on the refrigerator as a reminder.
- Use a refrigerator chart to spell out daily responsibilities, and have the child check off tasks as they are completed.
- Let the child know how much you appreciate his or her responsible behavior.
- Have a trusted neighbor for backup if the child needs help; be sure the child knows the telephone number, and post it by the telephone.
- Post telephone emergency numbers that the child can use; practice when to use them.
- Teach the child to tell telephone callers that the caregiver is busy but never to say that the caregiver is not home.
- Teach the child not to open the door to anyone.
- Be specific about activities allowed and not allowed.
- Carefully survey your home for any hazards or dangerous temptations (e.g., guns, motorcycle, ATV, swimming pool). Eliminate them, if possible, or ensure that rules about them are clear.
- See if your community has a telephone friend program available for latchkey children.
- A pet can relieve loneliness, but give the child clear guidelines about care of the pet during your absence.

and offer support to the caregivers in their attempts to provide for their children.

The Runaway Child

In the United States, as many as 750,000 to 2 million adolescents run away from home each year. A child can be considered a runaway after being absent from home overnight or longer without permission from a family caregiver. Most children who run away from home are 10 to 17 years of age.

A child may run away from home in response to circumstances that he or she views as too difficult to tolerate. Physical or sexual abuse, alcohol or drug abuse, divorce, stepfamilies, pregnancy, school failure, and truancy may contribute to a child's desire to escape. However, some adolescents are not runaways but rather "throwaways" who have been forced to leave home and are not wanted by the adults in the home. Often the throwaways have been forced out of the home because their behavior is unacceptable to family caregivers or because of other family stresses, such as divorce, remarriage, and job loss.

Runaway or throwaway adolescents often turn to stealing, drug dealing, and prostitution to provide money for alcohol, drugs, food, and possibly shelter. Many of these adolescents live on the streets because they cannot pay for shelter; they avoid going to public shelters for fear of being found by police. They may become victims of pimps or drug dealers who use the adolescents for their own gain.

There are numerous programs to help runaways, especially in urban areas. The 24-hour-a-day National Runaway Switchboard (1-800-621-4000) is available to give runaways information and referral (website: http:// www.nrscrisisline.org). This service may help the runaway to find a safe place to stay and may provide counseling, shelter, health care, legal aid, message relay to the family, and transportation home if desired. Runaways are not forced to go home but may be encouraged to inform their family that they are all right. Other free hotline numbers are also available.

A sexually transmitted disease, pregnancy, acquired immunodeficiency syndrome (AIDS), or drug overdose are the usual reasons that runaways are seen at a health care facility. When caring for such a child, be nonjudgmental. Any indication of being disturbed or disgusted by the adolescent's lifestyle may end any chance of cooperation and cause the adolescent to refuse to give any additional information. Try to build a trusting relationship with the child. Remember that the runaway viewed his or her problems as so great that escaping was the only way to resolve them. Counseling is necessary to begin to resolve the problems.

Health teaching for the runaway must be suited to his or her lifestyle and must be at a level the child can understand. Without prying excessively, try to find out the runaway's living circumstances and adjust the teaching plans accordingly. Remember that the child's problems did not come about overnight, nor will they be resolved quickly. Caring for a runaway can be frustrating, challenging, and sometimes rewarding for the health care staff.

THE NURSE'S ROLE RELATED TO GROWTH AND DEVELOPMENT

The nurse must have an understanding of factors and influences, as well as normal or expected patterns related to the growth and development of the infant, child, and adolescent. Knowledge of growth and development will help the nurse working with the child in a well-child setting, during illness, or when a child is having surgery.

When interviewing the child and family caregiver, an understanding of growth and development will help the nurse ask appropriate questions in an effort to assess whether the child's development is within the normal range or if there are variations or abnormalities present. Knowledge of growth and development helps the nurse ask age-related questions, as well as answer the caregiver's questions regarding the child. In communicating with children, being aware of a child's language skills and development will enable the nurse to communicate at the child's level of understanding. Specific information about communicating with children at various stages of growth and development is discussed throughout this text.

Most nurses find this approach helpful. By using knowledge of growth and development the nurse is able to talk to the child at his or her level of development. Communicating with the child at his or her stage of development and level of understanding enables the nurse to quickly establish rapport and begin a trusting relationship with the child.

Much of the pediatric nurse's role is in teaching and working with family caregivers. Providing them with examples of normal growth and development and helping them anticipate safety and nutritional needs of their child is vital.

When working with a sick

This advice could be a lifesaver. An understanding of growth and development will help the nurse offer suggestions to the caregivers about what behaviors can be expected and what safety precautions need to be initiated for their child.

child or one with a disease or disorder, the nurse must be aware that the child's age and stage of growth and development can affect the way the child copes with the situation or responds to treatment. In developing a plan of care for any child, the nurse must use knowledge of growth and development to provide the best care for the child.

Test Yourself

- What are three commonly seen responses in children whose parents divorce?
- What are some concerns that might be expressed by caregivers of "latchkey" children?
- Why is it necessary for the nurse to understand growth and development?

THEORIES OF CHILD DEVELOPMENT

How a helpless infant grows and develops into a fully functioning independent adult has fascinated scientists for years. Four pioneering researchers whose theories in this area are widely accepted are Sigmund

Freud, Erik Erikson, Jean Piaget, and Lawrence Kohlberg (Table 22-1). Their theories present human development as a series of overlapping stages that occur in predictable patterns. These stages are only approximations of what is likely to happen in children at various ages, and each child's development may differ from these stages.

Sigmund Freud

Most modern psychologists base their understanding of children at least partly on the work of Sigmund Freud. His theories are concerned primarily with the **libido** (sexual drive or development). Although Freud did not study children, his work focused on childhood development as a cause of later conflict. Freud believed that a child who did not adequately resolve a particular stage of development would have a fixation (compulsion) that correlated with that stage. Freud described three levels of consciousness: the **id**, which controls physical need and instincts of the body; the **ego**, the conscious self, which controls the pleasure principle of the id by delaying the instincts until an appropriate time; and the **superego**, the conscience or parental value system. These consciousness levels interact to check behavior and balance each other. The psychosexual stages in Freud's theory are the oral, anal, phallic, latency, and genital stages of development.

TABLE 22.1	Comparative Summary of Theories of Freud, Erikson, Piaget, and Kohlberg			
Age (years)	Stage	Freud (Psychosexual Development)	Erikson (Psychosocial Development)	Piaget (Intellectual Development)	Kohlberg (Moral Development)
1	Infancy	Oral Stage	Trust vs. Mistrust	Sensorimotor Phase	Stage 0—Do what pleases me
2–3	Toddlerhood	Anal Stage	Autonomy vs. Shame		Preconventional Level Stage 1—Avoid punishment
4–6	Preschool (early childhood)	Phallic (infant genital) Oedipal Stage	Initiative vs. Guilt	Preoperational Phase	Preconventional Level Stage 2—Do what benefits me
7–12	School-age (middle childhood)	Latency Stage	Industry vs. Inferiority	Concrete Operational Phase	Conventional Level Stage 3 (Age 7–10)— Avoid disapproval Stage 4 (Age 10–12)— Do duty, obey laws
13–18	Adolescence	Genital Stage (puberty)	Identity vs. Role Confusion	Formal Operational Phase	Postconventional Level Stage 5 (Age 13)— Maintain respect of others Stage 6 (Age 15)— Implement personal principles

Note: In the table, the column headers are: Age (years), Stage, Freud (Psychosexual Development), Erikson (Psychosocial Development), Piaget (Intellectual Development), Kohlberg (Moral Development).

Oral Stage (Ages 0–2 Years)

The newborn first relates almost entirely to the mother (or someone taking a motherly role), and the first experiences with body satisfaction come through the mouth. This is true not only of sucking but also of making noises, crying, and breathing. It is through the mouth that the baby expresses needs, finds satisfaction and begins to make sense of the world.

Anal Stage (Ages 2–3 Years)

This stage is the child's first encounter with the serious need to learn self-control and take responsibility. Toilet training looms large in the minds of many people as an important phase in childhood. Because elimination is one of the child's first experiences of creativity, it represents the beginnings of the desire to mold and control the environment; this is the "mud pie period" in the child's life.

The child has pride in the product created. Cleanliness and this natural pride do not always go together, so it may be necessary to help direct this pride and interest into more acceptable behaviors. Playing with such materials as modeling clay, crayons, and dough helps put the child's natural interests to good use, a process called **sublimation.**

Phallic (Infant Genital) Stage (Ages 3–6 Years)

It is only natural that interest moves to the genital area as a source of pride and curiosity. To the child's mind, this area constitutes the difference between boys and girls, a difference that the child is beginning to be aware of socially. The superego begins to develop during this stage.

During this stage the child begins to understand what it means to be a boy or a girl. The child learns to identify with the parent of the same sex. (Fig. 22-5) At about this time, a boy begins to take pride in being a male and a girl in being a female. In many families, a new brother or sister also arrives, arousing the child's natural interest in human origins. The parents' reaction to the child's genital exploration may determine whether the child learns to feel satisfied with him or herself as a sexual being or is laden with feelings of guilt and dissatisfaction throughout life.

Freud hypothesized that this awareness of genital differences also leads to a time of conflict in the child's emotional relationships with parents. The conflict occurs between attachment to and imitation of the parent of the same sex and the appeal of the other parent. The boy who for years has depended on his mother for all his emotional and physical needs now is confronted by his desire to be a man (Oedipus complex). The girl, who has imitated her mother, now finds her father a real attraction (Electra complex). It is through contact with parents that the child learns to relate to the oppo-

● **Figure 22.5** The preschool child learns to identify with the parent of the same sex.

site sex. The child learns the interests, attitudes, concerns, and wishes of the opposite sex.

Latency Stage (Ages 6–10 Years)

The latency stage is the time of primary schooling, when the child is preparing for adult life but must await maturity to exercise initiative in adult living. It is the time when the child's sense of moral responsibility (the superego) is built, based on what has been taught through the parents' words and actions.

During this stage the child is involved with learning, developing cognitive skills, and actively participating in sports activities, with little thought given to sexual concerns. The child's main relationships are with peers of the same sex. Developing positive friendships at this stage helps the child learn about caring relationships.

When placed in an unfamiliar setting, children in this stage may become confused because they do not know what is expected of them. They need the sense of security that comes from approval and praise and usually respond favorably to a brief explanation of "how we do things here."

Genital Stage (Ages 11–13 Years)

Physical puberty is occurring at an increasingly early age, and social puberty occurs even earlier, largely because of the influence of sexual frankness on television and in movies and the print media. At puberty, all the child's earlier learning is concentrated on the powerful biological drive of finding and relating to a mate. In earlier societies, mating and forming a family occurred at a young age. Our society delays mating for many years after puberty, creating a time of confusion and turmoil during which biologic readiness must take second place to educational and economic goals. This is a sensitive period when privacy is important, and great uncertainty exists about relating to any members of the opposite crises. This development depends on a self-healing process within the person that helps counterbalance the stresses created by natural and accidental crises. The self-healing process is delayed by any major crisis, such as hospitalization, that interrupts normal development. Interruptions may cause regression to an earlier stage, such as the older child who begins to wet the bed when hospitalized.

Erik Erikson

Building on Freud's theories, Erikson described human psychosocial development as a series of tasks or crises. According to Erikson and Senn (1958), "children 'fall apart' repeatedly, and unlike Humpty Dumpty, grow together again," if they are given time and sympathy and are not interfered with.

Erikson formulated a series of eight developmental tasks or crises; the first five pertain to children and youth. To present a complete view of Erikson's theory, all eight tasks are presented. In each task, the person must master the central problem before moving on to the next one. Each task holds positive and negative counterparts, and each of the first five implies new developmental tasks for parents (Table 22-2).

Trust Versus Mistrust (Ages 0–1 Year)

The infant has no way to control the world other than crying for help and hoping for rescue. During the

This is critical to remember.
Trust has to be established and then reinforced at each stage of growth and development. The nurse helps the child build a trusting relationship by being consistent and responding appropriately to the child's needs at every age.

first year, the child learns whether the world can be trusted to give love and concern or only frustration, fear, and despair. The infant who is fed on demand learns to trust that cries, communicating a need, will be answered. The baby fed according to the nurse or caregiver's schedule does not understand the importance of routine but only that these cries may go unanswered.

Autonomy Versus Doubt and Shame (Ages 1–3 Years)

Even the smallest child wants to feel in control and needs to learn to perform tasks independently, even when this takes a long time or makes a mess. The toddler gains reassurance from self-feeding, from crawling or walking alone where it is safe, and from being free to handle materials and learn about things in the environment (Fig. 22-6).

A toddler exploring the environment begins to explore and learn about his or her body too. If caregivers react appropriately to this normal behavior, the

TABLE 22.2	Child and Parent Developmental Tasks According to Erikson		
Developmental Level	Basic Task	Stage of Parental Development	Parental Task
Infant	Trust	Learning to recognize and interpret infant's cues	To interpret cues and respond positively to the infant's needs; hold, cuddle, and talk to infant
Toddler	Autonomy	Learning to accept child's need for self-mastery	To accept child's growing need for freedom while setting consistent, realistic limits; offer support and understanding when separation anxiety occurs
Preschooler	Initiative	Learning to allow child to explore surrounding environment	To allow independent development while modeling necessary standards; generously praise child's endeavors to build child's self-esteem
School-Age	Industry	Learning to accept rejection without deserting	To accept child's successes and defeats, assuring child of acceptance to be there when needed without intruding unnecessarily
Adolescent	Identity	Learning to build a new life, supporting the emergence of the adolescent as an individual	To be available when adolescent feels need: provide examples of positive moral values; keep communication channels open; adjust to changing family roles and relationships during and after the adolescent's struggle to establish an identify.

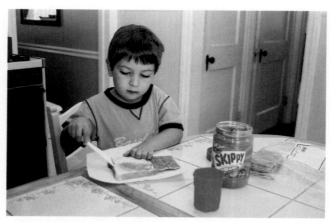

● *Figure 22.6* This toddler has a desire to do things independently, by himself.

● *Figure 22.7* The school-aged child enjoys activities that produce tangible results.

child will gain self-respect and pride. However, if caregivers shame the child for responding to this natural curiosity, the child may develop and sustain the belief that somehow the body is dirty, nasty, and bad.

Initiative Versus Guilt (Ages 3–6 Years)

During this period, the child engages in active, assertive play. Steadily improving physical coordination and expanding social skills encourage "showing off" to gain adult attention and, the child hopes, approval. The preschool child, still self-centered, plays alone, although in the company of other children; interaction comes later. These children want to know what the rules are and enjoy "being good" and the adult approval that action gains. During this time, the child develops a conscience and accepts punishment for doing wrong because it relieves feelings of guilt.

Children in this phase of development generally do not have a concept of time. The child needs a familiar frame of reference to understand when something is going to happen. For example, the parent or caregiver may say, "I will be back when your lunch comes" or "I will be back when the cartoons come on TV." Explaining that it is time for "Mommy and Daddy to go to work" might help an unhappy child realize that the parent or caregiver is not leaving because of any negative behavior of the child's.

Notice this difference. When working with children who have not fully developed a concept of time, explaining at the end of a shift that the nurse must go home to her own family may help the child understand and realize the nurse is not leaving because of any negative behavior of the child's.

Industry Versus Inferiority (Ages 6–12 Years)

Children begin to seek achievement in this phase. They learn to interact with others and sometimes to compete with them. They like activities they can follow through to completion and tangible results (Fig. 22-7).

Competition is healthy as long as the standards are not so high that the child feels there is no chance of winning. Praise, not criticism, helps the child to build self-esteem and avoid feelings of inferiority. It is important to emphasize that everyone is a unique person and deserves to be appreciated for his or her own special qualities.

Identity Versus Role Confusion (Ages 12–18 Years)

Adolescents are confronted by marked physical and emotional changes and the knowledge that soon they will be responsible for their own lives. The adolescent develops a sense of being an independent person with unique ideals and goals and may feel that parents, caregivers, and other adults refuse to grant that independence. Adolescents may break rules just to prove that they can. Stress, anxiety, and mood swings are typical of this phase. Relationships with peers are more important than ever.

Intimacy Versus Isolation (Early Adulthood)

This is the period during which the person tries to establish intimate personal relationships with friends and an intimate love relationship with one person. Difficulty in establishing intimacy results in feelings of isolation.

Generativity Versus Self-Absorption (Young and Middle Adulthood)

For many people, this phase means marriage and family, but for others it may mean fulfillment in some other way—a profession, a business career, or a religious vocation. The person who does not find this fulfillment becomes self-absorbed or stagnant and ceases to develop socially.

Ego Integrity Versus Despair (Old Age)

This final phase is the least understood of all, for it means finding satisfaction with oneself, one's achievements, and one's present condition without regret for the past or fear for the future.

Jean Piaget

Freud and Erikson studied psychosexual and psychosocial development; Piaget brought new insight into **cognitive development** or intellectual development—how a child learns and develops that quality called intelligence. He described intellectual development as a sequence of four principal stages, each made up of several substages (Piaget, 1967). All children move through these stages in the same order, but each moves at his or her own pace.

Sensorimotor Phase (Ages 0–2 Years)

The newborn behaves at a sensorimotor level linked entirely to desires for physical satisfaction. The newborn feels, hears, sees, tastes, and smells countless new things and moves in an apparently random way. Purposeful activities are controlled by reflexive responses to the environment. For example, while nursing, the newborn gazes intently at the mother's face, grasps her finger, smells the nipple, and tastes the milk, thus involving all senses.

As the infant grows, an understanding of cause and effect develops. When random arm motions strike the string of bells stretched across the crib, the newborn hears the sound made and eventually can manipulate the arms deliberately to make the bells ring.

In the same way, newborns cannot understand words or even the tone of voice; only through hearing conversation directed to them can they pick out sounds and begin to understand (Fig. 22-8). As the infant produces verbal noises, the responses of those nearby are encouraging and eventually help the infant learn to talk.

Preoperational Phase (Ages 2–7 Years)

The child in this phase of development is **egocentric**; that is he or she cannot look at something from another's point of view. The child's interpretation of the world is from a self-centered point of view and in terms of what is seen, heard, or otherwise experienced directly.

This child has no concept of quantity; if it looks like more, it is more. Four ounces of juice poured into two glasses looks like more than four ounces in one glass. A sense of time is not yet developed; thus the preschooler

● *Figure 22.8* The infant responds to mother's voice and her facial expressions.

or early school-age child cannot always tell if something happened a day ago, a week ago, or a year ago.

Concrete Operations (Ages 7–11 Years)

During this stage, children develop the ability to begin problem solving in a concrete, systematic way. They can classify and organize information about their environment. Unlike in the preoperational stage, children begin to understand that volume or weight may remain the same even though the appearance changes. These children can consider another's point of view and can deal simultaneously with more than one aspect of a situation.

Formal Operations (Ages 12–15 Years)

The adolescent is capable of dealing with ideas, abstract concepts described only in words or symbols. The person of this age begins to understand jokes based on double meanings and enjoys reading and discussing theories and philosophies. Adolescents can observe then draw logical conclusions from their observations.

Lawrence Kohlberg

Each of the theorists focuses on one element in the development of children. Kohlberg's theory is about the development of moral reasoning in children. Moral development closely follows cognitive development because reasoning and abstract thinking (the ability to conceptualize an idea without physical representation) are necessary to make moral judgments. Kohlberg's theory is divided into three levels with two or three stages in each level.

Preconventional Level (Premoral Level)

During the first 2 years (stage 0), there is no moral sensitivity. This is a time of egocentricity; decisions are made with regard only to what pleases the child or makes him or her feel good and what displeases or hurts the child. The child is not aware of how his or her behavior may affect others. The child simply reacts to pleasure with love and to hurtful experiences with anger.

In stage 1, punishment and obedience orientation (ages 2 to 3 years), the child determines right or wrong by the physical consequence of a particular act. The child simply obeys the person in power with no understanding of the underlying moral principle.

In stage 2, naive instrumental self-indulgence (ages 4 to 7 years), the child views a specific act as right if it satisfies his or her needs. Children follow the rules to benefit themselves. They think, "I'll do something for you if you'll do something for me" and, on the other hand, "If you do something bad to me, I'll do something bad to you." This is basically the attitude of "an eye for an eye."

Think about this. When working with children who are in the process of developing a sense of right and wrong, it is important for the nurse to understand that the child thinks if they get punished for doing something, then it is wrong; if they do not get punished, they think the behavior is right or acceptable.

Conventional Level

As concrete operational thought develops, children can engage in moral reasoning. School-age children become aware of the feelings of others. Living up to expectations is a primary concern, regardless of the consequences.

In stage 3, "good-boy" orientation (ages 7 to 10 years), being "nice" is very important. Children want to avoid a guilty conscience. Pleasing others is very important.

In stage 4, law and order orientation (ages 10 to 12 years), showing respect to others, obeying the rules, and maintaining social order are the desired behaviors. "Right" is defined as something that finds favor with family, teachers, and friends. "Wrong" is symbolized by broken relationships.

Postconventional Level (Principled Level)

By adolescence, the child usually achieves Piaget's formal operational stage. To achieve the postconventional level, the adolescent must have attained the formal operational stage. As a result, many persons do not reach this level.

In stage 5, social contract orientation (ages 13 to 18 years), personal standards, and personal rights are defined by culturally accepted values. A person's rights must not be violated for the welfare of the group. The end no longer justifies the means. Laws are for mutual good, cooperation, and development.

Stage 6, personal principles, is not attained very frequently. The person who reaches this level does what he or she thinks is right without regard for legal restrictions, the cost to self, or the views of others. Because of this person's deep respect for life, he or she would not do anything that would intentionally harm him or herself or another.

Test Yourself

- What are the five stages of growth and development according to Freud?
- What are the tasks that must be mastered at each of the five stages of child development according to Erikson?
- How are Piaget and Kohlberg's theories of development similar?

Other Theorists

Freud, Erikson, Piaget, and Kohlberg are only four of the many researchers who have studied the development of children and families. During the 1940s and 1950s, Arnold Gesell studied many infants and talked with their parents concerning children's behavior. From his studies emerged a series of developmental landmarks that are still considered valid and the observation that children progress through a series of "easy" and "difficult" phases as they develop. For example, he labeled one period the "terrible twos," the time when a toddler begins to assert new mobility and coordination to gain parental attention, even if the attention is unfavorable. Knowing that these cycles are normal makes it easier for parents to cope.

Carl Jung's contribution to the study of child growth and development focused on the inner sequence of events that shape the personality. He emphasized that human development follows predetermined patterns called **archetypes**. These archetypes replace the instinctive behavior present in other animals. Interaction of the archetypes with the outside environment is evident throughout human life. For example, a normal child learns to suck, crawl, walk, and talk without any instruction, but the details of how the child does these things come from observation and imitation of others.

Jung believed that the first 3 years of a child's life are spent coordinating experiences and learning to make a conscious personality, a distinct person who is separate from the rest of the environment. In the following years, the child learns to make sense of the environment by associating new discoveries to a general approach to the world. Dreams and nightmares help express personality developments that for some reason do not find a conscious outlet.

Jung points out that what happens to a child is not so critical to the child's development as the responses to these happenings. A hospital experience may permanently scar a child's personality if the child's natural feeling of terror is overlooked. Hospitalization may be accepted and even become a point of pride, however, if carried out in an atmosphere of assurance and support of the child's emotional concern and the need for love and acceptance.

The interaction between inner development and the environment is particularly clear in studies of young children who have been deprived in some way. John Bowlby's studies of children who were not held or loved and Bruno Bettelheim's studies of children given good physical care but little or no emotional satisfaction indicate how vital psychological interaction is.

In recent years, the theories of Erikson, Piaget, and Kohlberg have been criticized for being gender specific to males and culturally specific to Caucasians. In response, several theorists have conducted research on the growth and development of females and varying ethnic groups. Most notably, Carol Gilligan researched the moral development of males and females, and Patricia Green sought to construct a "truly universal theory of development through the empirical and theoretical understanding of cultural diversity" (Cocking & Greenfield, 1994).

KEY POINTS

- Growth is the physical increase in the body's size. Development is the progressive changes in the child toward maturity, which is completed growth and development.
- Growth following an orderly pattern from the head downward is called cephalocaudal. When growth is proximodistal, it starts in the center and progresses outward.
- Height and weight are monitored and plotted on growth charts to provide a comparison of measurements and patterns of a child's growth.
- Growth charts and developmental assessment tools are used to compare a child's growth to other children of the same age and sex. They are also used to compare the child's current measurements with their previous measurements.
- Genetics, nutrition, and environment are all influences on a child's growth and development.

- A lower socioeconomic level, decreased caregiver time and involvement, and media exposure are environmental factors that may influence growth and development. Homelessness, divorce, latchkey situations, and running away from home are also factors that influence a child's growth and development.
- The nurse who understands normal growth and development is better able to develop an appropriate plan of care for the child, including the areas of communication, safety, and family teaching.
- According to Freud, in the oral stage of development the newborn experiences body satisfaction through the mouth. During the anal stage, the child begins to learn self-control and taking responsibility. The child finds a source of pride and develops curiosity regarding the body in the phallic stage. Moral responsibility and preparing for adult life occurs in the latency stage, and in the genital stage, puberty and the drive to find and relate to a mate occurs.
- Erikson's theory of psychosocial development sets out sequential tasks that the child must successfully complete before going on to the next stage.
- The stages of psychosocial development according to Erikson are:
  - Trust vs. Mistrust—the infant learns that his or her needs will be met.
  - Autonomy vs. Doubt and Shame—the toddler learns to perform independent tasks.
  - Initiative vs. Guilt—the child develops a conscience and sense of right and wrong.
  - Industry vs. Inferiority—the child competes with others and enjoys accomplishing tasks.
  - Identity vs. Identity Confusion—the adolescent goes through physical and emotional changes as he or she develops as an independent person with goals and ideas.
  - Intimacy vs. Isolation—the young adult develops intimate relationships.
  - Generativity vs. Self-Absorption—the middle-aged adult finds fulfillment in life.
  - Ego Integrity vs. Despair—the older adult is satisfied with life and the achievements attained.
- Piaget's four stages of cognitive development include the sensorimotor phase, in which the infant uses the senses for physical satisfaction. The young child in the preoperational phase sees the world from an egocentric or self-centered point of view. During the concrete operations phase, the child learns to problem solve in a systematic way, and in the formal operations phase, the adolescent has his or her own ideas and can think in abstract ways.
- Kohlberg's theory relates to the development of moral reasoning in children. The child progresses from making decisions with no moral sensitivity to making decisions based on personal standards and values.

REFERENCES AND SELECTED READINGS

Books and Journals

Barry, P. (2001). *Mental health and mental illness* (7th ed.). Philadelphia: Lippincott Williams & Wilkins.

Berger, K. S. (2001). *The developing person through the life span.* New York: Worth Publishers.

Bowlby, J. (1969). *Attachment.* New York: Basic Books.

Brazelton, T. B., & Greenspan, S. (2001). *The irreducible needs of children: What every child must have to grow, learn, and flourish.* Cambridge, MA: Perseus Publishing.

Cocking, R. R., & Greenfield, P. M. (eds.). (1994). *Cross-cultural roots of minority child development.* Hillside, NJ: Lawrence Erlbaum Associates.

Dudek, S. G. (2000). *Nutrition essentials for nursing practice* (4th ed.). Philadelphia: Lippincott Williams & Wilkins.

Erikson, E. H., & Senn M. J. E. (1958). *Symposium on the healthy personality.* New York: Macy Foundation.

Erikson, E. H. (1963). *Childhood and society* (2nd ed.). New York: Norton.

Gilligan, C. (1982). *In a different voice.* Cambridge, MA: Howard University Press.

McEvoy, M. (2003). Culture and spirituality as an integrated concept in pediatric care. *American Journal of Maternal Child Nursing, 28*(1), 39–43.

National Institute of Child Health and Human Development. *Biobehavioral Development: From cells to selves.* Retrieved January 24, 2004, from http://www.nichd.nih.gov/publications/

Piaget, J. (1967). *The language and thought of the child.* Cleveland: World Publishing.

Pillitteri, A. (2003). *Maternal and child health nursing* (4th ed.). Philadelphia: Lippincott Williams & Wilkins.

Schuster, C., & Ashburn, S. (1992). *The process of human development* (3rd ed.). Philadelphia: JB Lippincott.

Shives, L., & Isaacs, A. (2001). *Basic concepts of psychiatric–mental health* (5th ed.). Philadelphia: Lippincott Williams & Wilkins.

Wadsworth, B. J. (1984). *Piaget's theory of cognitive and affective development.* New York: Longman.

Wong, D. L., Perry, S., & Hockenberry, M. (2002). *Maternal child nursing care* (2nd ed.). St. Louis: Mosby.

Web Addresses

www.nacd.org

www.piaget.org

www.keepkidshealthy.com/growthcharts

WORKBOOK

NCLEX-STYLE REVIEW QUESTIONS

1. The nurse observes that during feeding the newborn looks at the mother's face and holds her finger. According to Piaget, these observations indicate the child is in which phase of development?

   a. Sensorimotor

   b. Preoperational

   c. Concrete operations

   d. Formal operations

2. The nurse is caring for a toddler who has recently turned 2 years old. Of the following behaviors by the toddler, which would indicate the toddler is attempting to become autonomous? The toddler

   a. cries when the caregiver leaves.

   b. walks alone around the room.

   c. "shows off" to get attention.

   d. competes when playing games.

3. In working with a preschool age child, which of the following statements made by the child's caregiver would indicate an understanding of this child's stage of growth and development?

   a. "My child always wants her own way."

   b. "Why won't my child play with other children?"

   c. "I will tell my child I will be back after lunch."

   d. "She doesn't know when she has done something wrong."

4. In an interview, a 9-year-old child makes the following statement to the nurse, "I like to play basketball, especially when we win." This statement indicates this child is developing which basic task of child development?

   a. Trust

   b. Autonomy

   c. Initiative

   d. Industry

5. In discussing needs of adolescents with family caregivers, the nurse explains that to support the adolescent in developing her or his own identity, it would be most important for the adolescent caregiver to

   a. respond to physical needs.

   b. praise the child's actions.

   c. accept the child's defeats.

   d. maintain open communication.

6. Many researchers have theories relating to the stages of growth and development. Which of the following stages of accepted theories relate to the preschool-age child, from ages 4 to 6 years? Select all that apply.

   a. Oral stage

   b. Phallic stage

   c. Initiative vs. guilt

   d. Preoperational phase

   e. Formal operational phase

   f. Preconventional level stage 2

7. Using the growth charts in Appendix G, plot the measurements of a male child who is 18 months old, 33 inches tall and weighs 26 pounds. What percentile is this child for height? _75_ Weight? _50_

STUDY ACTIVITIES

1. Using the following table, compare the theories of Freud, Erikson, Piaget, and Kohlberg regarding children who are in the early elementary school years.

	Name of Theorist	Main Ideas and Similarities Between Theorists' Ideas
Latency stage		
Industry stage		
Concrete operational stage		
Conventional level		

2. Erikson identified trust as the development task for the first stage of life. Discuss why successful accomplishment of this task is essential to the person's future happiness and adjustment.

3. Go to the following Internet site: http://www.dbpeds.org. Go to "Pediatric Development and Behavior." Under "Hot Topics," click on "Developmental Screening Module." Read the section regarding developmental screening.

   a. What is the main objective for doing developmental screening?

   b. Who should be screened using developmental screening tools?

   c. What are the 5 major pitfalls of developmental screening?

4. Go to the following Internet site: www.missingkids.org. On the left hand side of screen, click on the section "Education and Resources." Scroll down. Click on "Know the Rules: After-School Safety Tips for Children Who Are Home Alone." Read the section "Maturity . . . not age . . . should be determining factor."

   a. List two questions that parents should ask themselves when considering leaving a child at home alone.

   b. List six factors that a parent should consider before allowing a child to stay home alone.

CRITICAL THINKING: What Would You Do?

1. The mother of a 4-month-old infant brings the baby to the health care clinic for her well-baby check. The baby is measured and weighed and the measurements plotted on a growth chart. The baby is in the 75th percentile for height and the 60th percentile for weight. When the provider examines the baby, the notion of doing a developmental screening on the child is discussed.

   a. What will you explain to this mother when she asks you the purpose of the growth chart?

   b. How often will the baby's measurements be plotted on the growth charts?

   c. What will you expect to see after the child has had several measurements plotted?

   d. What is the purpose of doing a developmental screening?

2. A group of family caregivers is participating in a class discussing influences on a child's growth and development. If you were the nurse doing this teaching session, how would you answer the following questions?

   a. What influence does genetics have on growth and development?

   b. What are the effects of nutrition on a child's growth?

   c. What are some environmental factors that influence a child's development?

Growth and Development of the Infant: 28 Days to 1 Year

23

STUDENT OBJECTIVES

On completion of this chapter, the student should be able to

1. State the ages at which the (a) anterior fontanel and (b) posterior fontanel normally close.
2. State the ages at which the infant's birth weight (a) doubles and (b) triples.
3. Discuss the eruption of deciduous teeth: (a) approximate age of the first tooth, (b) first teeth to erupt, (c) factors that may interfere with eruption, and (d) role of fluoride in dental health.
4. State the age at which the child becomes aware of himself or herself as a person.
5. State the age when the fear of strangers usually appears.
6. Discuss one useful purpose of the game "Peek-a-Boo."
7. Explain the reason a baby tends to push food out of the mouth with the tongue.
8. Discuss the rationale for introducing new foods one at a time.
9. Discuss weaning: (a) the usual age when the baby becomes interested in a cup and (b) criteria to determine the appropriate time.
10. State the cause of bottle mouth caries.
11. Discuss ways to prevent bottle mouth caries.
12. List three foods to offer the infant who does not drink enough milk from a cup.
13. List eleven communicable diseases against which children are immunized.
14. State at what age immunizations are usually started.
15. Identify caregiver teaching that the nurse should present during routine health maintenance visits.
16. Describe early dental care for the infant.
17. Discuss important safety issues for the infant.
18. Discuss the family caregivers' role in the infant's hospital care.

KEY TERMS

bottle mouth or nursing bottle
  caries
deciduous teeth
extrusion reflex
pedodontist
primary circular reactions
seborrhea
secondary circular reactions

The 1-month-old infant has a busy year ahead. During this year, the infant grows and develops skills more rapidly than he or she ever will again. In the brief span of a single year, this tiny, helpless bit of humanity becomes a person with strong emotions of love, fear, jealousy, and anger and gains the ability to rise from a supine to an upright position and move about purposefully.

In the first year, both weight and height increase rapidly. During the first 6 months, the infant's birth weight doubles and height increases about 6 inches. Growth slows slightly during the second 6 months but is still rapid. By 1 year of age, the infant has tripled his or her birth weight and has grown 10 inches to 12 inches.

Thinking in terms of the "average" child is misleading. To determine if an infant is reaching acceptable levels of development, birth weight and height must be the standard to which later measurements are compared. A baby weighing 6 lb at birth cannot be expected to weigh as much at 5 or 6 months of age as the baby who weighed 9 lb at birth, but each is expected to double his or her birth weight at about this time. A growth graph is helpful to the nurse, pediatrician, or caregiver for charting a child's progress (Fig. 23-1).

Erikson's psychosocial developmental task for the infant is to develop a sense of trust. The development of trust occurs when the infant has a need and that need is meet consistently. The infant feels secure when the basic needs are meet. This stage creates the foundation for the developmental tasks of the next stages to be meet. If the infant does not receive food, love, attention, and comfort, the infant learns to mistrust the environment and those who are responsible for caring for the child.

PHYSICAL DEVELOPMENT

Despite the many factors, such as genetic background, environment, health, gender, and race, that affect growth in the first year of life, the healthy infant progresses in a predictable pattern. By the end of the year, the dependent infant who at 1 month of age had no teeth and could not roll over, sit, or stand blossoms into an emerging toddler with teeth who can sit alone, stand, and begin to walk alone. The growth seen in the prenatal development of the fetus continues.

Head and Skull

Head Circumference

At birth, an infant's head circumference averages about 13.75 inches (35 cm) and is usually slightly larger than the chest circumference. The chest measures about the same as the abdomen at birth. At about 1 year of age, the head circumference has grown to about 18 inches (47 cm). The chest also grows rapidly, catching up to the head circumference at about 5 to 7 months of age. From then on, the chest can be expected to exceed the head in circumference.

Fontanels and Cranial Sutures

The posterior fontanel is usually closed by the second or third month of life. The anterior fontanel may

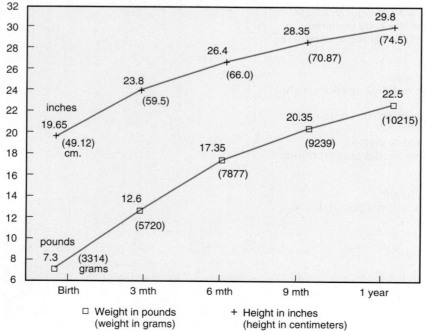

Height and Weight First Year
(50th percentile)

□ Weight in pounds
(weight in grams)

+ Height in inches
(height in centimeters)

● **Figure 23.1** Chart of infant growth representing an infant in the midrange birth-weight 7.3 lb (3314 g) and birth length 19.65 inches (49.12 cm). Infants of different races vary in average size. Asian infants tend to be smaller, African American infants larger.

increase slightly in size during the first few months of life. After the sixth month it begins to decrease in size, closing between the 12th and the 18th months. The sutures between the cranial bones do not ossify until later childhood.

Skeletal Growth and Maturation

During fetal life, the skeletal system is completely formed in cartilage at the end of 3 months' gestation. Bone ossification and growth occur during the remainder of fetal life and throughout childhood. The pattern of maturation is so regular that the "bone age" can be determined by radiologic examination. When the bone age matches the child's chronologic age, the skeletal structure is maturing at a normal rate. To avoid unnecessary exposure to radiation, radiologic examination is performed only if a problem is suspected.

Eruption of Deciduous Teeth

Calcification of the primary or **deciduous teeth** starts early in fetal life. Shortly before birth, calcification begins in the permanent teeth that are the first to erupt in later childhood. The first deciduous teeth, usually the lower central incisors, usually erupt between 6 and 8 months of age (Fig. 23-2).

Babies in good health who show normal development may differ in the timing of tooth eruption. Some

families show a tendency toward very early or very late eruption without having other signs of early or late development. Some infants may become restless or fussy from swollen, inflamed gums during teething. A cold teething ring may be helpful in soothing the baby's discomfort. Teething is a normal process of development and does not cause high fever or upper respiratory conditions.

Nutritional deficiency or prolonged illness in infancy may interfere with calcification of both the deciduous and the permanent teeth. The role of fluoride in strengthening calcification of teeth has been well documented. The American Dental Association recommends administration of fluoride to infants and children in areas where the fluoride content of drinking water is inadequate or absent.

Test Yourself

- When does an infant's birth weight double? Triple?

- When does the posterior fontanel close? Anterior fontanel?

- When do the first deciduous teeth erupt? Which teeth usually erupt first?

Circulatory System

In the first year of life, the circulatory system undergoes several changes. During fetal life, high levels of hemoglobin and red blood cells are necessary for adequate oxygenation. After birth, when oxygen is supplied through the respiratory system, hemoglobin decreases in volume, and red blood cells gradually decrease in number until the third month of life. Thereafter, the count gradually increases until adult levels are reached.

Obtaining an accurate blood pressure measurement in an infant is difficult. Electronic or ultrasonographic monitoring equipment is often used (see Chapter 28). The average blood pressure during the first year of life is 85/60 mm Hg. However, variability is expected among children of the same age and body build.

An accurate determination of the infant's heart beat requires an apical pulse count. A pediatric stethoscope with a small-diameter diaphragm is placed over the left side of the chest in a position where the heart beat can be clearly heard (Fig 23-3). A count is then taken for 1 full minute (see Chapter 28). During the first year of life, the average apical rate ranges from 70 (asleep) to 150 (awake) beats per minute and as high as 180 beats per minute while the infant is crying.

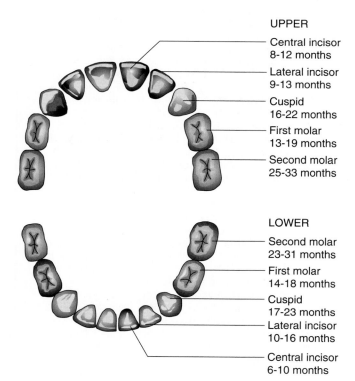

UPPER

Central incisor
8-12 months

Lateral incisor
9-13 months

Cuspid
16-22 months

First molar
13-19 months

Second molar
25-33 months

LOWER

Second molar
23-31 months

First molar
14-18 months

Cuspid
17-23 months

Lateral incisor
10-16 months

Central incisor
6-10 months

● **Figure 23.2** Approximate ages for the eruption of deciduous teeth.

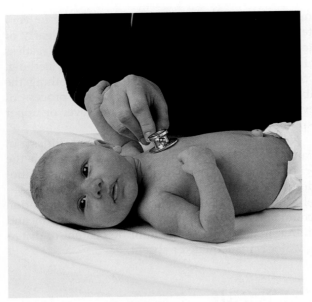

● *Figure 23.3* A pediatric stethoscope is used to clearly hear the heart beat of the infant.

Body Temperature and Respiratory Rate

Body temperature follows the average normal range after the initial adjustment to postnatal living. Respirations average 30 breaths per minute, with a wide range (20 to 50 breaths per minute) according to the infant's activity.

Neuromuscular Development

As the infant grows, nerve cells mature and fine muscles begin to coordinate in an orderly pattern of development. Naturally, the family caregivers are full of pride in the infant who learns to sit or stand before the neighbor's baby does, but accomplishing such milestones early means little. Each child follows a unique rhythm of progress within reasonable limits.

Average rates of growth and development are useful for purposes of making comparisons. Few landmarks call for special attention, and their absence may indicate the need for additional environmental stimulation. Do not emphasize routine developmental tables with family caregivers; a small time lag may be insignificant. A large time lag may require greater stimulation from the environment or a watchful attitude to discover how overall development is proceeding.

Figure 23-4 and Table 23-1 summarize the accepted norms in physical, psychosocial, motor, language, and cognitive growth and development in the first year of life.

PSYCHOSOCIAL DEVELOPMENT

The give-and-take of life is experienced by the infant who actively seeks food to fulfill feelings of hunger. The infant begins to develop a sense of trust when fed on demand. However, the infant eventually learns that not every need is met immediately on demand. Slowly the infant becomes aware that something or someone separate from oneself fulfills one's needs. Gradually, as a result of the loving care of family caregivers, the infant learns that the environment responds to desires expressed through one's own efforts and signals. The infant is now aware that the environment is separate from self.

Caregivers who expect too much too soon from the infant are not encouraging optimal development. Rather than teaching the rules of life before the infant has learned to trust the environment, the caregivers are actually teaching that nothing is gained by one's own activity and that the world does not respond to one's needs.

Conversely, caregivers who rush to anticipate every need give the infant no opportunity to test the environment. The opportunity to discover that through one's own actions the environment may be manipulated to suit one's own desires is withheld from the infant by these "smothering" caregivers. Family Teaching Tips: Infants From Birth to 1 Year suggests healthy child rearing patterns during infancy.

FAMILY TEACHING TIPS

Infants from Birth to 1 Year

First 6 weeks: Frequent holding of infant gives infant feeling of being loved and cared for. Rocking and soothing baby are important.

6 weeks to 3½ months: Continue to give infant feeling of being loved and cared for; respond to cries; provide visual stimulation with toys, pictures, mobiles, and auditory stimulation by talking and singing to baby; repeat sounds that infant makes to encourage vocal stimulation.

3½ to 5 months: Play regularly with baby; give child variety of things to look at; talk to baby; offer a variety of items to touch—soft, fuzzy, smooth, and rough—to provide tactile stimulation; continue to respond to infant's cries; move baby around home to provide additional visual and auditory stimulation; begin placing infant on floor to provide freedom of movement.

5 to 8 months: Continue to give infant feeling of being loved and cared for by holding, cuddling, and responding to needs; talk to infant; put infant on floor more often to roll and move about; fear of strangers is common at this age.

8 to 12 months: Accident-proof the house; give the infant maximum access to living area: supply infant with toys; stay close by to support infant in difficult situations; continue to talk to infant to provide language stimulation. The baby at this age loves surprise toys like jack-in-the-box and separation games like "Peek-a-Boo"; loves putting-in and taking-out activities. The child is developing independence, and temper tantrums may begin.

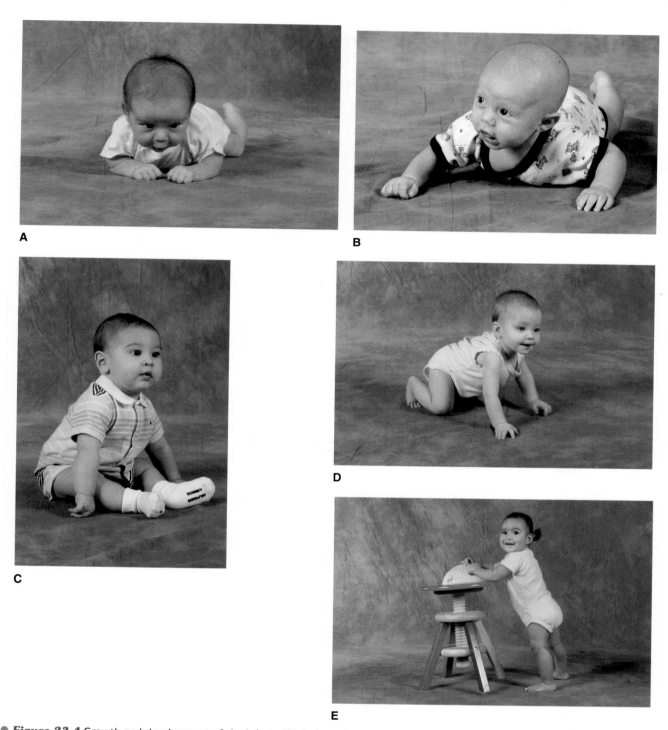

● *Figure 23.4* Growth and development of the infant. (**A**) At 4 weeks, this infant turns head when lying in a prone position. (**B**) At 12 weeks, this infant pushes up from a prone position. (**C**) At 21 weeks, the infant sits up but tilts forward for balance. (**D**) At 30 weeks, this infant is crawling around and on the go. (**E**) At 43 weeks, this infant is getting ready to walk.

No one is perfect, and every family caregiver misinterprets the infant's signals at times. The caregiver may be tired, preoccupied, or responding momentarily to his or her own needs. The caregiver may not be able to ease the infant's pain or soothe the restlessness, but this also is a learning experience for the baby.

As mentioned earlier, the infant's development depends on a mutual relationship with give and take between the infant and the environment in which the family caregivers play the most important role. Table 23-2 summarizes significant caregiver–infant interactions indicating positive behaviors.

TABLE 23.1	Growth and Development Chart: Birth to 1 Year					
Age	Physical	Personal-Social	Fine Motor	Gross Motor	Language	Cognition
Birth–4 wk	Weight gain of 5–7 oz (150–270 g) per wk Height gain of 1″ per mo first 6 mo Head circumference increase ½″ per mo Moro, Babinski, rooting, and tonic neck reflexes present	Some smiling Begins Erikson's stage of "trust vs. mistrust"	Grasp reflex very strong Hands flexed	Catches and holds objects in sight that cross visual field Can turn head from side to side when lying in a prone position (see Fig. 23-4A) When prone, body in a flexed position When prone, moves extremities in a crawling fashion	Cries when upset Makes enjoyment sounds during mealtimes	At 1 mo, sucking activity with associated pleasurable sensations
6 wk	Tears appear	Smiling in response to familiar stimuli	Hands open Less flexion noted	Tries to raise shoulders and arms when stimulated Holds head up when prone Less flexion of entire body when prone	Cooing predominant Smiles to familiar voices Babbling	**Primary circular reactions** Begins to repeat actions
10–12 wk	Posterior fontanel closes	Aware of new environment Less crying Smiles at significant others	No longer has grasp reflex Pulls on clothes, blanket, but does not reach for them	No longer has Moro reflex Symmetric body positioning Pumps arms, shoulders, and head from prone position (see Fig. 23-4B)	Makes noises when spoken to	Beginning of coordinated responses to different kinds of stimuli
16 wk	Moro, rooting, and tonic neck reflexes disappear; drooling begins	Responds to stimulus Sees bottle, squeals, laughs Aware of new environment and shows interest	Grasps objects with two hands Grasps objects in crib voluntarily and brings them to mouth Eye–hand coordination beginning	Plays with hands Brings objects to mouth Balances head and body for short periods in sitting position	Laughs aloud Sounds "n," "k," "g," and "b"	Likes social situations Defiant, bored if unattended
20 wk	May show signs of teething	Smiles at self in mirror Cries when limits are set or when objects are taken away	Holds one object while looking for another one Grasps objects wanted	Able to sit up (see Fig. 23-4C) Can roll over Can bear weight on legs when held in a standing position Able to control head movements	Cooing noises Squeals with delight	Visually looks for an object that has fallen

TABLE 23.1 (continued)	Growth and Development Chart: Birth to 1 Year					
Age	**Physical**	**Personal-Social**	**Fine Motor**	**Gross Motor**	**Language**	**Cognition**
24 wk	Birth weight doubles; weight gain slows to 3–5 oz (90–150 g) per wk Height slows to ½" per mo Teething begins with lower central incisors	Likes to be picked up Knows family from strangers Plays "Peek-a-Boo" Knows likes and dislikes Fear of strangers	Holds a bottle fairly well Tries to retrieve a dropped article	Tonic neck reflex disappears Sits alone in high chair, back erect Rolls over and back to abdomen	Makes sounds "guh," "bah" Sounds "p," "m," "b," and "t" are pronounced Bubbling sounds	**Secondary circular Reactions** Repeats actions that affect an object Beginning of object permanence
28 wk	Lower lateral incisors are followed in the next month by upper central incisors	Imitates simple acts Responds to "no" Shows preferences and dislikes for food	Holds cup Transfers objects from one hand to the other	Reaches without visual guidance Can lift head up when in a supine position	Babbling decreases Duplicates "ma-ma" and "pa-pa" sounds	
32 wk	Teething continues	Dislikes diaper and clothing change Afraid of strangers Fear of separating from mother	Adjusts body position to be able to reach for an object May stand up while holding on	Crawls around (see Fig. 23-4D) Pulls toy toward self	Combines syllables but has trouble attributing meaning to them	
40 wk-1 yr	Birth weight tripled; has six teeth; Babinski reflex disappears Anterior fontanel closes between now and 18 mo	Does things to attract attention Tries to follow when being read to Imitates parents Looks for objects not in sight	Holds tools with one hand and works on it with another Puts toy in box after demonstration Starts blocks Holds crayon to scribble on paper	Stands alone; begins to walk alone (see Fig. 23-4E) Can change self from prone to sitting to standing position	Words emerge Says "da-da" and "ma-ma" with meaning	Coordination of secondary schemes; masters barrier to reach goal, symbolic meanings

During the first few weeks of life, actions such as kicking and sucking are simple reflex activities. In the next sequential stage, reflexes are coordinated and elaborated. For example, in early infancy hand movements are random (Fig. 23-5A). The infant finds that repetition of chance movements brings interesting changes, and in the latter part of the first year these acts become clearly intentional (see Fig. 23-5B). The infant expects that certain results follow certain actions.

The smiling face looking down is soon connected by the infant with the pleasure of being picked up, fed, or bathed. Anyone who smiles and talks softly to the infant may make that small face light up and cause squirming of anticipation. In only a few weeks, however, the infant learns that one particular person is the main source of comfort and pleasure.

An infant cannot apply abstract reasoning but understands only through the five senses. As the infant matures enough to recognize the mother or primary

TABLE 23.2	Criteria of Positive Caregiver–Infant Interactions	
Area of Interaction	**Positive Caregiver Response**	
Feeding	Offers infant adequate amounts and proper types of food and prepares food appropriately	
	Holds infant in comfortable, secure position during feeding	
	Burps infant during or after feeding	
	Offers food at a comfortable pace for infant	
Stimulation	Provides appropriate nonaggressive verbal stimulation to infant	
	Provides a variety of tactile experiences and touches infant in caring ways other than during feeding times or when moving infant away from danger	
	Provides appropriate toys and interacts with infant in a way satisfying to infant	
Rest and sleep	Provides a quiet, relaxed environment and a regular, scheduled sleep time for infant	
	Makes certain infant is adequately fed, warm and dry before putting down to sleep	
Understanding of infant	Has realistic expectations of infant and recognizes infant's developing skills and behavior	
	Has realistic view of own parenting skills	
	View of infant's health condition similar to the view of medical or nursing diagnosis	
Problem-solving initiative	Motivated to manage infant's problems; diligently seeks information about infant; follows through on plans involving infant	
Interaction with other children	Demonstrates positive interaction with other children in home without aggression or hostility	
Caregiver's recreation	Seeks positive outlets for own recreation and relaxation	
Parenting role	Expresses satisfaction with parenting role; expresses positive attitudes	

caregiver, the infant becomes fearful when this person disappears. To the infant, out of sight means out of existence, and the infant cannot tolerate this. For the infant, self-assurance is necessary to confirm that objects and people do not cease to exist when out of sight. This is a learning experience on which the infant's entire attitude toward life depends.

Think about this. The ancient game of "Peek-a-Boo" is a universal example of this learning technique. It is also one of the joys of infancy as the child affirms the ability to control the disappearance and reappearance of self. In the same manner by which the infant affirms self-existence, the existence of others is confirmed, even when they are temporarily out of sight.

NUTRITION

During the first year of life, the infant's rapid growth creates a need for nutrients greater than at any other time of life. The Academy of Pediatrics Committee on Nutrition has endorsed breast-feeding as the best method of feeding infants.

Most of the infant's requirements for the first 4 to 6 months of life are supplied by either breast milk or commercial infant formulas. Nutrients that may need to be supplemented are vitamins C and D, iron, and fluoride. Breast-fed infants need supplements of iron, as well as vitamin D, which can be supplied as vitamin drops. Most commercial infant formulas are enriched with vitamins C and D. Some infant formulas are fortified with iron. Infants who are fed home-prepared formulas (based on evaporated milk) need supplemental vitamin

A

B

● *Figure 23.5* (**A**) In the early stages of infancy, hand movements are random. (**B**) Later in infancy, hand movements are coordinated and intentional.

C and iron; however, evaporated milk has adequate amounts of vitamin D, which is unaffected by heating in the preparation of formula. Vitamin C can be supplied in orange juice or juices fortified with vitamin C.

Fluoride is needed in small amounts (0.25 mg/day) for strengthening calcification of the teeth and preventing tooth decay. A supplement is recommended for breast-fed and commercial formula-fed babies and for those whose home-prepared formulas are made with water that is deficient in fluoride. Vitamin preparations are available combined with fluoride.

Addition of Solid Foods

The time or order requirement for starting foods is not exact. However, at about 4 to 6 months of age, the infant's iron supply becomes low and supplements of iron-rich foods are needed. Guidelines for introducing new foods into an infant's diet are provided in Table 23-3.

Infant Feeding

The infant knows only one way to take food: namely, to thrust the tongue forward as if to suck. This is called the **extrusion** (protrusion) **reflex** (Fig. 23-6) and has the effect of pushing solid food out of the infant's mouth. The process of transferring food from the front of the mouth to the throat for swallowing is a complicated skill that must be learned. The eager, hungry baby is puzzled over this new turn of events and is apt to become frustrated and annoyed, protesting loudly and clearly. Taking the edge off the very hungry infant's appetite by giving part of the formula is best before proceeding with this new experience. If the family caregivers understand that pushing food out with the tongue does not mean rejection, their patience will be rewarded.

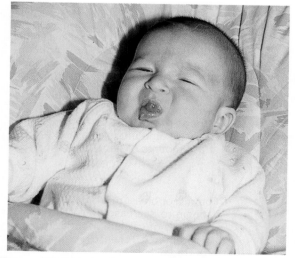

● **Figure 23.6** A baby thrusts the tongue forward using the extrusion reflex. This causes food to be pushed out of the mouth.

The baby's clothing (and the caregiver's as well) needs protection when the baby is held for a feeding. A small spoon fits the infant's mouth better than a large one and makes it easier to put food further back on the tongue—but not far enough to make the baby gag. If the food is pushed out, the caregiver must catch it and offer it again. The baby soon learns to manipulate the tongue and comes to enjoy this novel way of eating. To avoid the danger of aspiration, the caregiver must quiet an upset or crying baby before proceeding with feeding.

Foods are started in small amounts, 1 or 2 tsp daily. Babies like their food smooth, thin, lukewarm, and bland. The choice of mealtime does not matter. It works best, at first, to offer one new food at a time, allowing 4 or 5 days before introducing another so that the baby becomes accustomed to it. This method also helps determine which food is responsible if the baby has a reaction to a new food.

When teeth start erupting, anytime between 4 and 7 months of age, the infant appreciates a piece of zwieback or hard toast to practice chewing. At about 9 or 10 months of age, after a few teeth have erupted, chopped foods can be substituted for pureed foods. Breast milk or formula gradually is replaced with whole milk as the infant learns to drink from a cup. This change takes some time because the infant continues to derive comfort from sucking at the breast or bottle. Infants need fat and should not be given reduced-fat milk (skim, 1%, or 2%).

Preparation of Foods

Various pureed baby foods, chopped junior foods, and prepared milk formulas are available on the market. These products save caregivers much preparation time, but many families cannot afford them. No matter which type of food is used, family caregivers should read food labels carefully to avoid foods that have undesirable additives, especially sugar and salt.

The nurse can point out that vegetables and fruits can be cooked and strained or pureed in a blender and are as acceptable to the baby as commercially prepared baby foods. Baby foods prepared at home should be made from freshly prepared foods, not canned, to avoid commercial additives. Labels of frozen foods used should be checked for added sugar, salt, or other unnecessary ingredients. Excess blended food can be stored in the freezer in ice cube trays for future use. Cereals may be cooked and formulas may be prepared at home as well. Instead of purchasing junior foods, the caregiver can substitute well-cooked, unseasoned table foods that have been mashed or ground.

Preparation and storage of baby food at home require careful sanitary practices. All equipment used in the preparation of the infant's food must be carefully cleaned with hot, soapy water and rinsed thoroughly.

TABLE 23.3	Suggested Feeding Schedule for the First Year of Life		
Age	**Food Item**	**Amount***	**Rationale**
Birth–6 mo	Human milk or iron-fortified formula	Daily totals 0–1 mo 18–24 oz 1–2 mo 22–28 oz 2–3 mo 25–32 oz 3–4 mo 28–32 oz 4–5 mo 27–39 oz 5–6 mo 27–45 oz	Infants' well-developed sucking and rooting reflexes allow them to take in milk and formula. Infants do not accept semisolid food because their tongues protrude when a spoon is put in their mouths. They cannot transfer food to the back of the mouth. Human milk needs supplementation.
	Water	Not routinely recommended	Small amounts may be offered under special circumstances (e.g., hot weather, elevated bilirubin level, or diarrhea).
4–6 mo	*Iron-fortified infant cereal;[†] begin with rice cereal (delay adding barley, oats, and wheat until 6th mo)	4–8 tbsp after mixing	At this age, there is a decrease of the extrusion reflex, the infant can depress the tongue and transfer semi-solid food from a spoon to the back of the pharynx to swallow it.
	*Unsweetened fruit juices;[†‡] plain, vitamin C–fortified	2–4 oz	Cereal adds a source of iron and B vitamins; fruit juices introduce a source of vitamin C.
	Dilute juices with equal parts of water		Delay orange, pineapple, grapefruit, or tomato juice until 6th mo.
	Human milk or iron-fortified formula	Daily totals 4–5 mo 27–39 oz 5–6 mo 27–45 oz	Do not offer water as a substitute for formula or breast milk, but rather as a source of additional fluids.
	Water	As desired	
7–8 mo	*Fruits, plain strained; avoid fruit desserts	1–2 tbsp	Teething is beginning; thus, there is an increased ability to bite and chew.
	*Yogurt[†]		
	*Vegetables,[†] plain strained; avoid combination meat and vegetable dinners	5–7 tbsp	Vegetables introduce new flavors and textures.
	*Meats,[†] plain strained; avoid combination or high-protein, dinners	1–2 tbsp	Meat provides additional iron, protein, and B vitamins.
	*Crackers, toast, zwieback[†]	1 small serving	
	Iron-fortified infant cereal or enriched cream of wheat	4–6 tbsp	
	Fruit juices[‡]	4 oz	
	Human milk or iron-fortified formula	24–32 oz	Iron-fortified formula or iron supplementation with human milk is still needed because the infant is not consuming significant amounts of meat.
	Water	As desired	May introduce a cup to the infant.
9–10 mo	*Finger foods[†]—well-cooked, mashed, soft, bite-sized pieces of meat and vegetables	In small servings	Rhythmic biting movements begin; enhance this development with foods that require chewing.
	Iron-fortified infant cereal or enriched cream of wheat	4–6 tbsp	Decrease amounts of mashed foods as amounts of finger foods increase.
	Fruit juices[‡]	4 oz	
	Fruits	6–8 tbsp	
	Vegetables	6–8 tbsp	
	Meat, fish, poultry, yogurt, cottage cheese	4–6 tbsp	Formula or breast milk consumption may begin to decrease; thus, add other sources of calcium, riboflavin, and protein (e.g., cheese, yogurt, and cottage cheese).
	Human milk or iron-fortified formula	24–32 oz	
	Water	As desired	

TABLE 23.3 (continued)	Suggested Feeding Schedule for the First Year of Life		
Age	**Food Item**	**Amount***	**Rationale**
11–12 mo	Soft table foods† as follows: Cereal; iron-fortified infant cereal; may introduce dry, unsweetened cereal as a finger food	4–6 tbsp	Motor skills are developing; enhance this development with more finger foods.
	Breads; crackers, toast, zwieback	1 or 2 small servings	Rotary chewing motion develops; thus, child can handle whole foods that require more chewing.
	Fruit juice‡	4 oz	
	Fruit: soft, canned fruits or ripe banana, cut up, peeled raw fruit as the infant approaches 12 mo	½ cup	Infant is relying less on breast milk or formula for nutrients; a proper variety of solid foods (fruits, vegetables, starches, protein sources, and dairy products) will continue to meet the young child's needs.
	Vegetables: soft cooked, cut into bite-sized pieces	½ cup	
	Meats and other protein sources: strips of tender, lean meat, cheese strips, peanut butter	2 oz or ½ cup chopped	Delay peanut butter until 12th month.
	Mashed potatoes, noodles		
	Human milk or iron-fortified infant formula	24–30 oz	
	Water	As desired	

*Amounts listed are daily totals and goals to be achieved gradually. Intake varies depending on the infant's appetite.
†New food items for age group.
(Adapted from Twin Cities District Dietetic Association. *Manual of clinical nutrition*, with permission from its publisher, Chronimed Publishing, 13911 Ridgedale Dr, Minneapolis, MN 55343,1994:54–56.)
‡The Committee on Nutrition of the American Academy of Pediatrics recommends that fruit juices be introduced when infant can drink from a cup.

Some families prefer to spend more money for convenience and economize elsewhere, but no one should be made to feel that a baby's health or well-being depends on commercially prepared foods.

The healthy baby's appetite is the best index of the proper amount of food. Healthy babies enjoy eating and accept most foods, but they do not like strongly flavored or bitter foods. If the baby shows a definite dislike for any particular food, forcing it may develop into a battle of wills. A dislike for a certain food is not always permanent, and the rejected food may be offered again later. The important point is to avoid making an issue of likes or dislikes. The caregiver also should avoid introducing any personal attitudes about food preferences.

Self-feeding

The infant has an overpowering urge to investigate and to learn. At around 7 or 8 months of age, the baby may grab the spoon from the caregiver, examine it, and mouth it. The baby also sticks fingers in the food to feel the texture and to bring it to the mouth for tasting (Fig. 23-7). This is an essential, although messy, part of the learning experience.

After preliminary testing, the infant's next task is to try self-feeding. The baby soon finds that the motions involved in getting a spoon right side up into the mouth are too complex, so fingers become favored over the spoon. However, the infant returns to the

● *Figure 23.7* Eating by yourself is a messy business but so much fun!

spoon again until he or she eventually succeeds in getting some food from spoon to mouth at least part of the time. The nurse can help family caregivers understand that all this is not deliberate messiness to be forbidden but rather a necessary part of the infant's learning.

Weaning the Infant

Weaning, either from the breast or bottle, must be attempted gradually without fuss or strain. The infant is still testing the environment. The abrupt removal of a main source of satisfaction—sucking—before basic distrust of the environment has been conquered may prove detrimental to normal development. The speed with which weaning is accomplished must be suited to each infant's readiness to give up this form of pleasure for a more mature way of life.

At the age of 5 or 6 months, the infant who has watched others drink from a cup usually is ready to try a sip when it is offered. The infant seldom is ready at this point, however, to give up the pleasures of sucking altogether. Forcing the child to give up sucking creates resistance and suspicion. Letting the infant set the pace is best.

An infant who takes food from a dish and milk from a cup during the day may still be reluctant to give up a bedtime bottle. However, the infant must never be permitted to take a bottle of formula, milk, or juice to bed. **Pedodontists** (dentists who specialize in the care and treatment of children's teeth) discourage the bedtime bottle because the sugar from formula or sweetened juice coats the infant's teeth for long periods and causes erosion of the enamel on the deciduous teeth, resulting in a condition known as **bottle mouth** or **nursing bottle caries**. This condition can also occur in infants who sleep with their mother and nurse intermittently throughout the night. In addition to the caries, liquid from milk, formula, or juice can pool in the mouth and flow into the eustachian tube, causing otitis media (ear infection) if the infant falls asleep with the bottle.

Good judgment is in order. A bottle of plain water or a pacifier can be used if the infant needs the comfort of sucking at bedtime.

A few babies resist drinking from a cup. Milk needs (calcium, vitamin D) may be met by offering yogurt, custard, cottage cheese, and other milk products until the infant becomes accustomed to the cup. The caregiver should be cautioned not to use honey or corn syrup to sweeten milk because of the danger of botulism, which the infant's system is not strong enough to combat.

During the second half of the first year, the infant's milk consumption alone is not likely to be sufficient to meet caloric, protein, mineral, and vitamin needs.

Test Yourself

- What nutrients may need to be supplemented for the infant?
- Why is fluoride given to an infant?
- Why is one new food at a time introduced?
- What might occur if the infant is given a bottle of formula at bedtime?

Women, Infants, and Children Food Program

Women, Infants, and Children (WIC) is a special supplemental food program for pregnant, breast-feeding, or postpartum women and infants and children as old as 5 years of age. This federal program provides nutritious supplemental foods, nutrition information, and health care referrals. It is available free of charge to persons who are eligible based on financial and nutritional needs and who live in a WIC service area. The family's food stamp benefits or school children's breakfast and lunch program benefits are unaffected. The foods prescribed by the program include iron-fortified infant formula and cereal, milk, dry beans, peanut butter, cheese, juice, and eggs. These foods may be purchased with vouchers or distributed through clinics. To encourage the use of WIC services, many health care facilities give WIC information to eligible mothers during prenatal visits or at the time of delivery.

HEALTH PROMOTION AND MAINTENANCE

Routine checkups, immunizations, family teaching, and education about accident prevention are important aspects of health promotion and maintenance. Immunizations and frequent well-baby visits help ensure good health. Family teaching and accident prevention help caregivers provide the best care for their rapidly growing child.

Routine Checkups

During the first year of life, at least six visits to the health care facility are recommended. These are essentially considered well-baby visits and usually occur at 2 weeks, 2 months, 4 months, 6 months, 9 months, and 12 months. During these visits, the nurse collects data regarding the infant's growth and development, nutrition, and sleep, the caregiver–infant relationship, and any potential problems. The infant's weight, height, and head circumference are documented, and the infant receives immunizations to guard against disease. Family teaching, particularly for first-time caregivers, is an integral part of health promotion and maintenance.

Immunizations

Every infant is entitled to the best possible protection against disease. Obviously, infants cannot take proper precautions, so family caregivers and health professionals must be responsible for them. This care extends beyond the daily needs for food, sleep, cleanliness, love, and security to a concern for the infant's future health and well-being. Protection is available against a number of serious or disabling diseases, such as diphtheria, tetanus, pertussis, hepatitis A and B, polio, measles, mumps, German measles (rubella), varicella (chickenpox), and Haemophilus influenzae meningitis and pneumococcal disease, making it unnecessary to take chances with a child's health because of inadequate immunization.

Immunization Schedule

The American Academy of Pediatrics, through its committee on the control of infectious diseases and the Advisory Committee on Immmunization Practices for the Centers for Disease Control (CDC), has recommended a schedule of immunizations for healthy children living in normal conditions (Table 23-4). Additional recommendations are made for children who live in certain regions and areas or who have certain risk factors. Immunizations should be given within the prescribed timetable unless the child's physical condition makes this impossible. An immunization need not be postponed if the child has a cold but should be postponed if the child has an acute febrile condition or a condition causing immunosuppression or if he or she is receiving corticosteroids, radiation, or antimetabolites.

Side effects vary with the type of immunization but usually are minor in nature. The most common side effect is a low-grade fever within the first 24 to 48 hours and possibly a local reaction, such as tenderness, redness, and swelling at the injection site. The child may be fussy and eat less than usual. These reactions are treated symptomatically with acetaminophen for

---

TABLE 23.4 Recommended Childhood Immunization Schedule

Age ▶ Vaccine ▼	Birth	1 mo	2 mos	4 mos	6 mos	12 mos	15 mos	18 mos	24 mos	4–6 yrs	11–12 yrs	13–18 yrs
Hepatitis B	Hep B #1		Hep B #2			Hep B #3				Hep B series		
Diphtheria, Tetanus, Pertussis			DTaP	DTaP	DTaP			DTaP		DTaP	Td	
Haemophilus influenzae Type b			Hib	Hib	Hib	Hib						
Inactivated Polio			IPV	IPV		IPV				IPV		
Measles, Mumps, Rubella						MMR #1				MMR #2	MMR #2	
Varicella						Varicella				Varicella		
Pneumococcal			PCV	PCV	PCV	PCV				PCV	PPV	
Hepatitis A										Hepatitis A series		
Influenza						Influenza (yearly)						

Range of recommended ages · Catch-up vaccination · Preadolescent assessment

Vaccines below this line are for selected populations

This schedule indicates the recommended ages for routine administration of currently licensed childhood vaccines, as of December 1, 2003, for children through age 18 years. Any dose not given at the recommended age should be given at any subsequent visit when indicated and feasible. Indicates age groups that warrant special effort to administer those vaccines not previously given. Additional vaccines may be licensed and recommended during the year. Licensed combination vaccines may be used whenever any components of the combination are indicated and the vaccine's other components are not contraindicated. Providers should consult the manufacturer's package inserts for detailed recommendations.

Approved by the Advisory Committee on Immunization Practices (www.cdc.gov/nip/acip), the American Academy of Pediatrics (www.aap.org), and the American Academy of Family Physicians (www.aafp.org).

This advice could save the day. Preparing caregivers by giving information regarding common side effects following immunizations may be helpful in decreasing the caregivers' anxiety and concerns. A written information sheet gives the caregiver something to refer to at home if the child has a side effect.

the fever and cool compresses to the injection site. The child is encouraged to drink fluids, and holding and cuddling is comforting to the child. The parents are encouraged to call the provider if they are concerned, if there are any other reactions, or if these symptoms don't go away within about 48 hours.

Many children do not get their initial immunizations in infancy and may not get them until they reach school age, when immunizations are required for school entrance. Health care personnel should make every effort to encourage parents to have their children immunized in infancy to avoid the danger of possible epidemic outbreaks. For instance, measles outbreaks resulting in the deaths of children have been increasing at an alarming rate because of inadequate immunization. Serious illnesses, permanent disability, and deaths from inadequate immunizations are senseless and tragic. Answer any questions the caregiver may have about immunizations. Remember, however, that the caregiver has a right to refuse immunization if he or she has been fully informed about immunizations and any possible reactions. Maintain a nonjudgmental viewpoint throughout the discussion.

Test Yourself

- Discuss the reasons immunizations are given.
- What are the diseases that children can be immunized against?

Family Teaching

Because mothers are discharged so early after giving birth, every opportunity to perform teaching and promote healthy baby care should be used. Well-baby visits provide an opportunity to ask the caregiver about concerns and to provide teaching. During well visits, offer guidance to help caregivers prepare for the many changes that occur with each developmental level. Discuss normal growth and development milestones but emphasize that these milestones vary from infant to infant. The infant's overall progress is the most important concern, not when he or she accomplishes a given task as compared with another infant or a developmental table. Discuss any infant sleep and activity concerns that the caregiver has. Encourage the caregiver to seek information about any other problems, worries, or anxieties he or she has. Provide ample time and opportunity for the caregivers to ask questions and gain information. A perceptive nurse not only asks if the caregiver has concerns but also suggests possible topics that may need to be reinforced. Some of those topics are discussed here.

Bathing the Infant

A daily bath is unnecessary but is desirable and soothing in very hot weather. Placing the baby into a small tub for a bath, rather than giving a sponge bath, may have a soothing and comforting effect as long as the baby is healthy and has no open skin areas. The small tub or large basin bath is described in the Family Teaching Tips: Small Tub Bath.

The bathing procedure is essentially the same for the older infant. When old enough to sit and move about freely, the infant may enjoy the regular bathtub, but often this is frightening to him or her. Splashing about in a small tub may be more fun, especially with a floating toy. An infant in a tub should always be held securely (Fig. 23-8). If possible, time should be scheduled so that bathing is a leisurely process, a time for the caregiver and baby to enjoy. The procedure for sponge baths is discussed in Chapter 15. As noted in Chapter 16, regular shampooing is important to prevent seborrheic dermatitis (cradle cap), which is caused by a collection of **seborrhea**, yellow crusty patches of lesions on the scalp.

Scented or talcum powder should not be used after the bath; powder tends to cake in creases, causing irritation, and may cause respiratory problems when inhaled by the infant. Scented powders and lotions cause allergic reactions in some babies. In any case, a clean baby has a sweet smell without the use of additional fragrances. Excessively dry skin may benefit from the application of lanolin or A and D Ointment, but oils are believed to

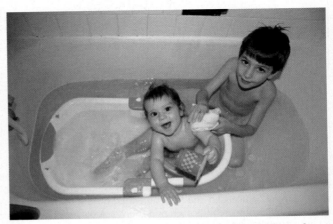

● *Figure 23.8* Bath time can be an enjoyable experience for the infant.

FAMILY TEACHING TIPS

Small Tub Bath

Make sure room is warm and draft-free. Wash hands, put on protective covering, and assemble the following equipment:
- Large basin or small tub
- Mild soap
- Nonsterile protective gloves
- Clean cotton balls
- Soft washcloth
- Large soft towel or small cotton blanket
- Clean diaper and clothes for infant

Fill tub with several inches of warm water (95°–100°F [35°–37°C]). This is comfortably warm to the elbow. Place basin or tub in crib or other protected surface.

Never turn from the baby during bathing. *Always* keep at least one hand holding the infant.

PROCEDURE

Wash the infant's head and face at the beginning of the bath, following the procedure for a sponge bath (see Chap. 8). A mild shampoo may be used for the infant over 1 month old, but soap is adequate.

After drying the head, undress the infant and examine for skin rashes or excoriations. Wearing protective gloves, remove diaper and wipe any feces from diaper area.

Place infant in tub and soap the body while supporting infant's head and shoulders on your arm. If infant's skin is dry, soap may be eliminated or a prescribed soap substitute used.

If the baby is enjoying the experience, make it a leisurely one by engaging the infant in talk, paddling in the water, and playing for a few extra minutes. When finished, lift infant from tub, place on dry towel and pat dry with careful attention to folds and creases (underarms, neck, perineal area).

After the bath, gently separate the female infant's labia and cleanse with moistened cotton balls and clean water, wiping from *front to back* to avoid bacterial contamination from the anal region. Circumcised male infants need only be inspected for cleanliness. Uncircumcised males may have the foreskin gently retracted to remove smegma and accumulated debris. The foreskin is gently replaced. Do not force foreskin if not easily retracted, but document and report this occurrence.

block pores and cause infection. Various medicated ointments are available for excoriated skin areas.

After the bath, the baby's fingernails need to be inspected and cut, if long. Otherwise, the baby may scratch his or her face during random arm movements. The nails should be cut straight across with great care. While cutting, hold the arm securely and the hand firmly.

Caring for the Diaper Area

To prevent diaper rash, soiled diapers should be changed frequently. Check every 2 to 4 hours while the infant is awake to see if the diaper is soiled. Waking the baby to change the diaper is not necessary. Cleanse the diaper area with water and a mild soap if needed (see Family Teaching Tips: Preventing and Treating Diaper Rash in Chapter 40). Commercial diaper wipes also may be used, but they are an added expense (Fig. 23-9).

Diapers are available in various sizes and shapes. The choice of cloth versus disposable diapers is controversial: disposable diapers have an environmental impact, but cloth diapers are inconvenient and associated with a higher risk of infection. Whatever the type, size, and folding method used, there should be no bunched material between the thighs. Two popular cloth diaper styles are the oblong strip pinned at the sides or the square diaper folded kite-fashion. The latter has the advantage of being useful for different ages and sizes. When folding a cloth diaper for a boy, the excess material is folded in the front; for a girl, it is folded to the back. Safety pins must always be closed when they are used to fasten the diaper. When removed, they must be closed and placed out of the infant's reach.

For the older infant, the diaper must be fastened snugly at the hips and legs to prevent feces from running out the open spaces. Cleaning a soiled crib and a

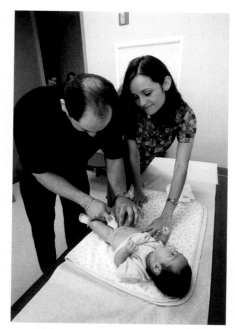

● *Figure 23-9* While Dad is changing his child's diaper, the nurse takes this opportunity to provide teaching on care of the diaper area.

smeared baby once or twice serves as an effective reminder!

Dressing the Infant

Dressing an infant can sometimes create a dilemma, especially for the first-time caregiver. Sometimes merely getting clothes on the baby is difficult. For instance, babies tend to spread their hands when the caregiver is trying to put on a top with long sleeves. The easiest way to put an infant's arm into a sleeve is to work the sleeve so that the armhole and the opening are held together, then to reach through the armhole and pull the arm through the opening. Clothing should not bind but should allow freedom of movement and be appropriate for the weather.

One rule of thumb is to dress the infant with the same amount of clothing that the adult finds comfortable. Overdressing in hot weather can cause overheating and prickly heat (miliaria rubra; see Chapter 40). In very hot weather, a diaper may be sufficient. When the infant begins to crawl, long pants help protect the knees from becoming chafed from the rug or flooring. When dressing the infant to go outdoors in cold weather, a head covering is important because infants lose a large amount of heat through their heads. In hot, sunny weather, the infant should not spend much time in the direct sun because the infant's skin is tender and burns easily.

Choosing shoes for the infant can be a problem for the new caregiver. Infants do not need hard-soled shoes; in fact, health care providers often recommend that infants be allowed to go barefoot and wear shoes only to protect them from harsh surfaces. Shoes with stiff soles actually hamper the development of the infant's foot. Sneakers made with a smooth lining with no rough surfaces to irritate the infant's foot are a good choice. They should be durable and flexible and have ample room in the toe. Properly made moccasins also are a good choice. High-topped shoes are unnecessary. Socks should provide plenty of toe room. Shoes should be replaced frequently as the infant's feet grow.

Promoting Sleep

Most infants sleep 10 to 12 hours at night and take 2 to 3 naps during the day. Each child develops his or her own sleeping patterns, and these vary from child to child. Caregivers often have concerns about their child's sleep needs and patterns. Infants should not have pillows placed in bed with them because of the possibility of suffocation. Sleep habits and patterns vary, but a consistent bedtime routine is usually helpful in establishing healthy sleeping patterns and in preventing sleep problems. Placing the child in the crib while awake and letting the child fall asleep in the crib creates good sleeping habits. In addition, this will often prevent the child from

CULTURAL SNAPSHOT

In some cultures it is a common and accepted practice for some or all of the children in the family to sleep in the bed with the parents.

waking up when he or she is moved from the position or place he or she has fallen asleep. Using the crib for sleeping only, not for play activities, helps the child associate the bed with sleep, rather than play. Sleep disturbances may be learned behaviors. Any concern expressed by the caregiver needs to be explored in depth. With the older child, bedtime rituals, consistent limits, and use of a reward system may decrease bedtime and sleep concerns and problems.

Dental Care

When teething begins in the second half of the first year, the caregiver can start practicing good dental hygiene with the infant. Initially the caregiver can rub the gums and newly erupting teeth with a clean, damp cloth while holding the infant in the lap. This time can be made pleasant by talking or singing to the infant. Brushing the teeth with a small, soft brush usually is not started until several teeth have erupted. Gentle cleansing with plain water is adequate. Toothpaste is not recommended at this stage because the infant will swallow too much of it.

Accident Prevention

Discussing safety issues with caregivers is important. Provide information about car safety and child-proofing and preventing aspiration, falls, burns, poisoning, and bathing accidents. Remind caregivers that the infant is developing rapidly and safety precautions should stay one step ahead of the infant's developmental abilities. Older children in the family should be taught to be watchful for possible dangers to the infant, and caregivers must be alert to potential dangers that may be introduced by the sibling, such as unsafe toys, rough play, or jealous harmful behavior (see Family Teaching Tips: Infant Safety).

Test Yourself

- List the areas of family teaching that are important for the caregivers of infants.
- What are the areas of concern for the safety of an infant?

FAMILY TEACHING TIPS

Infant Safety

Be one step ahead of child's development and pre-pared for the next stage.

ASPIRATION/SUFFOCATION

* Always hold bottle when feeding, **never** prop bottle.
* Crib and playpen bars should be spaced no more than 2-3/8 inches apart.
* Check toys for loose or sharp parts or small buttons.
* Keep small articles (such as buttons, marbles, safety pins, lint, balloons) off the floor and out of infant's reach.
* Store products such as baby powder out of child's reach.
* Keep plastic bags out of child's reach.
* Do not use pillows in a crib.
* Avoid giving child foods such as hot dogs, grapes, nuts, candy, and popcorn.
* Remove bibs at nap and bed times.
* Do not tie pacifier on a string around the child's neck.

FALLS

* Never leave child unattended on a high surface, such as a high chair, bed, couch, or countertop.
* Place gates at the tops and bottoms of stairways.
* Raise crib rails and be sure they are securely locked.

MOTOR VEHICLE

* Place infant in an approved infant car carrier in the back seat when in a car. Follow the manufacturer's instructions regarding the age and size of the infant regarding placement of the carrier (rear or front facing)
* Never leave child unattended in a car.

DROWNING

* Never leave child alone in the bathtub, or near any water, including toilets, buckets, or swimming pools.
* Fence and use locked gates around swimming pools.

BURNS/INJURIES

* Cover unused plugs with plastic covers.
* Keep electrical cords out of sight.
* Remove tablecloths or dresser scarves that child might grasp and pull.
* Pad sharp corners of low furniture or remove them from child's living area.
* Turn household hot water to a safe temperature—120°F (48.8°C).

POISONING

* Check toys for nontoxic material.
* Move all toxic substances (cleaning fluids, deter-gents, insecticides) out of reach and keep them in locked areas.
* Remove any houseplants that may be poisonous.
* Protect child from inhaling lead paint dust (from remodeling) or chewing on surfaces painted with lead paint.
* Place medicines in locked cupboards; remind family and friends (especially those with grown children or no children) to do the same.

THE INFANT IN THE HEALTH CARE FACILITY

Hospitalization, however brief, hampers the infant's normal pattern of living. Disruption occurs even if a family caregiver stays with the infant during hospital-ization. All or most of the sick infant's energies may be needed to cope with the illness. If given sufficient affection and loving care and if promptly restored to the family, however, the infant is not likely to suffer any serious psychological problems. Long-term hospi-talization, though, may present serious problems, even with the best of care.

Illness itself is frustrating; it causes pain and dis-comfort and limits normal activity, none of which the infant can understand. If the hospital atmosphere is emotionally unresponsive and offers little if any cud-dling or rocking, the infant may fail to respond to treat-ment, despite cleanliness and proper hygiene. Touch-ing, rocking, and cuddling a child are essential ele-ments of nursing care (Fig. 23-10).

Hospitalization may have other adverse effects. The small infant matures largely as a result of physical development. If hindered from reaching out and responding to the environment, the infant becomes apathetic and ceases to learn. This situation is particu-larly apparent when restraints are necessary to keep the child from undoing surgical procedures or dress-ings or to prevent injury. The child in restraints needs an extra measure of love and attention and the use of every possible method to provide comfort. Spending time, playing music in the room, or encouraging some-one to stay with the infant might help to make the infant more comfortable.

A PERSONAL GLIMPSE

By the time my second son Noah was 6 months old, my husband and I were relaxed and confident parents. Perhaps too much so! Noah had just begun crawling. "We need to dig out the gates," I said to my husband, Richard. He agreed. However, we didn't do it right away, being busy with two kids and work.

Shortly afterward, Richard was working in our upstairs office. Noah was playing underfoot. I opened the door to the office and walked in to put something away. On my way out, I carelessly left the door open. I went downstairs to the kitchen and began coloring with my older son Jacob. A few minutes later Noah crawled past my husband and out into the hallway. Richard was reading e-mail and didn't notice.

Then I heard something heavy and hard tumbling down the stairs and knocking into the walls, followed by my husband's screaming. I ran to the foyer and found Noah wailing face down on the hardwood floors. I fell to the ground, scooped him up, rocked him, and began crying. Will he be OK? Did he break anything? How could I be so careless? Why didn't we put the gates up? Why am I such a bad parent? I should have known better.

In the end Noah was fine. His cheek was bruised, and his arm was sore. My husband and I were shaken, but we were OK too. The gates went up that afternoon!

Darlene

LEARNING OPPORTUNITY: What would you say to these parents to support and reassure them? What recommendations would you make to caregivers regarding safety in the home?

● **Figure 23.10** Holding and cuddling can ease the discomfort and fear of the hospital experience.

and looking directly at the infant, thus helping to provide comfort during a time of stress. After the procedure, the infant may benefit from rocking, cuddling, singing, stroking, and other comfort measures that the family caregivers may provide. If the family caregivers are unavailable or can spend only limited time with the infant, the nursing staff must meet these emotional needs.

Parent–Nurse Relationship

The nurse's relationship with family caregivers is extremely important. The hospitalized infant needs continued stimulation, empathetic care, and loving attention from family caregivers. Encourage caregivers to feed, hold, diaper, and participate in their infant's care as much as they can. Through conscientious use of the nursing process, collect data regarding the needs of the caregivers and the infant and plan care with these needs in mind. Identify and acknowledge the caregivers' apprehensions and develop plans to resolve or eliminate them. Make arrangements for rooming-in for the family caregiver, if possible. Family caregivers often are sensitive to changes in their infant that may help to identify discomfort, pain, or fear. Caregivers may sometimes assist during treatments and other procedures by stroking, talking to,

KEY POINTS

▶ The posterior fontanel closes by the 2nd or 3rd month and the anterior fontanel closes between the 12th and 18th months.

▶ An infant's birth weight doubles by age 6 months and triples by 1 year.

▶ The first tooth usually erupts between 6 and 8 months. Family history, nutritional status, and prolonged illness affect the eruption of teeth. Fluoride is recommended to strengthen calcification of teeth.

▶ Between the ages of 6 and 7 months, most children develop a fear of strangers.

▶ The game "Peek-a-Boo" is useful in affirming self-existence to the infant and that even when temporarily out of sight, others still exist.

▶ Infants have a tendancy to push solid food out of their mouths with their tongue thrust forward because of the extrusion reflex.

⬧ New foods are introduced one at a time determine the food responsible if the infant has a reaction.

⬧ An infant can be gradually weaned to a cup as her/his desire for sucking decreases, usually around the age of 1 year.

⬧ Bottle mouth caries can occur when an infant is given a bottle at bedtime; the sugar from the formula causes erosion of the tooth enamel.

⬧ To prevent bottle mouth caries, a bottle of plain water or a pacifier for sucking can be given at bedtime.

⬧ If an infant resists drinking milk from a cup, calcium and vitamin D needs can be meet by giving foods such as yogurt, custard, and cottage cheese.

⬧ Children are immunized against hepatitis B virus, diphtheria, tetanus, pertussis, *Haemophilus influenzae* type b, polio, measles, mumps, rubella, varicella (chickenpox), and pneumococcal disease. In addition, they may be immunized against the hepatitis A virus.

⬧ Immunizations are begun shortly after birth.

⬧ During routine health maintainance visits caregivers are given teaching regarding normal growth and development milestones, sleep patterns, bathing, diapering, dressing, dental care, and safety.

⬧ Infants' gums and teeth should be cleaned with a clean, damp cloth and plain water.

⬧ Accident prevention for the infant includes closely watching the infant and monitoring the environment for safety hazards.

⬧ When an infant is hospitalized, the family caregiver can give the child stimulation and care and attention by feeding, holding, and diapering the infant.

REFERENCES AND SELECTED READINGS

Books and Journals

Berger, K. S. (2001). *The developing person through the life span.* New York: Worth Publishers.

Brazelton, T. B., & Greenspan, S. (2001). *The irreducible needs of children: What every child must have to grow, learn, and flourish.* Cambridge, MA: Perseus Publishing.

Dudek, S. G. (2000). *Nutrition essentials for nursing practice* (4th ed.). Philadelphia: Lippincott Williams & Wilkins.

Halsey, N. A., & Asturias, E. J. (1999). Immunization. In *Oski's pediatrics: Principles and practice* (3rd ed.). Philadelphia: Lippincott Williams & Wilkins.

Hockenberry, M. J., Wilson, D., Winkelstein, M. L., & Kline, N. E. (2003). *Wong's nursing care of infants and children* (7th ed.). St. Louis: Mosby.

Mera, K., & Hackley, B. (2003). Childhood vaccines: How safe are they. *American Journal of Nursing, 103*(2), 79.

Niederhauser, V., Baruffi, G., & Heck, R. (2001). Parental decision-making for the varicella vaccine. *Journal of Pediatric Health Care, 15*(5), 236.

Pillitteri, A. (2003). *Maternal and child health nursing* (4th ed.). Philadelphia: Lippincott Williams & Wilkins.

Spock, B., et al. (1998). *Dr. Spock's baby and child care.* New York: Pocket Books.

Wong, D. L., & Hess, C. (2000). *Wong and Whaley's clinical manual of pediatric nursing* (5th ed.). St. Louis: Mosby.

Wong, D. L., Perry, S., & Hockenberry, M. (2002). *Maternal child nursing care* (2nd ed.). St. Louis: Mosby.

Web Addresses
www.cdc.gov
www.kidshealth.org/parent/growth
www.drspock.com

Child Passenger Safety
www.nhtsa.dot.gov

WORKBOOK

NCLEX-STYLE REVIEW QUESTIONS

1. The nurse would expect an infant who weighs 7 pounds 2 ounces at birth to weigh approximately how many pounds at 6 months of age?

   a. 10 pounds

   b. 14 pounds

   c. 17 pounds

   d. 21 pounds

2. In caring for a 4-month-old infant, which of the following actions by the infant would the nurse note as appropriate for a 4-month-old infant? The infant

   a. grasps objects with two hands.

   b. holds a bottle well.

   c. tries to pick up a dropped object.

   d. transfers an object from one hand to the other.

3. When assisting with a physical exam on an infant, the nurse would expect to find the posterior fontanel closed by what age?

   a. 3 months

   b. 5 months

   c. 8 months

   d. 10 months

4. In teaching a group of parents of infants, the nurse would teach the caregiver that between 6 and 8 months of age, which of the following teeth usually erupt?

   a. First molars

   b. Upper lateral incisors

   c. Lower central incisors

   d. Cuspid

5. To obtain an accurate heart rate in an infant, which of the following would be the *most* important for the nurse to do?

   a. Take an apical pulse.

   b. Count the pulse rate for 30 seconds.

   c. Use a regular stethoscope.

   d. Check when infant is quiet.

6. An infant had the following intake in the 12 hours after receiving immunizations. Calculate the 12-hour intake for this infant.

   Pedialyte, 4 oz

   Rice cereal, 4 tbsp.

   Dilute apple juice, 3 oz

   Applesauce, ½ cup

   Iron-fortified formula, 8 oz

   Yogurt, 1/4 cup

   Crackers, 4 small

   Iron-fortified formula, 5 oz

   Strained vegetables, 1 jar

   Iron-fortified formula, 7 oz.

   12-hour intake ___810 cc___

STUDY ACTIVITIES

1. List and compare the fine motor and gross motor skills in each of the following ages:

	4 weeks old	24 weeks old	32 weeks old
Fine motor skills			
Gross motor skills			

2. Answer the following regarding immunizations:

   a. By the time the infant is 1 year old, immunizations will have been given to prevent which diseases?

   b. How many doses of the hepatitis B vaccine are recommended?

   c. What are the two most common side effects of immunizations? How are these treated?

3. List five safety tips important in the infant stage of growth and development.

4. Go to the following Internet site: http://www.cdc.gov

   At "Centers for Disease Control," click on "Health Topics A–Z." Click on "Immunization." Click on "Vaccines." Go to: "Are your child's shots up to date?" (children's schedule). Go to "Childhood Immunization Schedule," and click on the current immunization schedule and answer the following questions:

a. What is the date of this immunization schedule?

b. Compare the information on this site to Table 23-4. What is the same? What are the differences?

c. Why do you think these changes in the immunization schedule have been made?

CRITICAL THINKING: What Would You Do?

1. Tony Ricardo brings 6-month-old Essie for a routine checkup. You are responsible for formulating a plan for the visit.

   a. What characteristics would you observe for during the physical examination?

   b. What immunizations will the child need at this visit (assuming he is up to date)?

c. What nutritional factors and guidelines will you observe for and teach?

d. What other age-appropriate teaching will you do with Essie's father?

2. As you review nutrition with Mr. Ricardo, he states that Essie loves her bedtime bottle.

   a. What will you teach Mr. Ricardo regarding this practice?

   b. What suggestions will you make to help prevent the problems that often result from bedtime bottles?

3. At Nicole's 6-month checkup, her mother tells you that Nicole doesn't like the baby food and she just spits it out.

   a. What will you tell Nicole's mother to help her understand what is happening?

   b. What other information about feeding infants will you provide for this mother?

Growth and Development of the Toddler: 1 to 3 Years

Physical Development
Psychosocial Development
Behavioral Characteristics
Play
Discipline
Sharing With a New Baby
Nutrition

Health Promotion and Maintenance
Routine Checkups
Family Teaching
Accident Prevention
The Toddler in the Health Care Facility
Special Considerations

STUDENT OBJECTIVES

On completion of this chapter, the student should be able to

1. Identify characteristics of the age group known as the toddler.
2. State reasons parenting a toddler is often frustrating.
3. Describe physical growth that occurs during toddlerhood.
4. Define the following terms as they relate to the psychosocial development of the toddler: (a) negativism, (b) ritualism, (c) dawdling, and (d) temper tantrums.
5. List three reasons eating problems often appear in this age group.
6. Describe the progression of the toddler's self-feeding skills.
7. Describe the relationship between sweet foods and plaque formation on the teeth.
8. State the age when a child should be taught tooth brushing and explain why this is an appropriate age.
9. Discuss the purpose of the toddler's first dental visit and the ideal age for it.
10. State the physiologic development required for complete bowel and bladder control and the typical age when this development occurs.
11. Identify suggestions to aid in toilet training.
12. State why accident prevention is a primary concern when caring for a toddler.
13. State the four leading causes of accidental death of toddlers.
14. List preventive measures for each of the leading causes of accidental death of toddlers.
15. List eight types of medications most commonly involved in childhood poisonings.
16. List information that should be gathered in a social assessment when a toddler is admitted to the hospital.

KEY TERMS

autonomy
dawdling
discipline
negativism
parallel play
punishment
ritualism
temper tantrum

oon after a child's first birthday, important and sometimes dramatic changes take place. Physical growth slows considerably; mobility and communication skills improve rapidly; and a determined, often stubborn little person begins to create a new set of challenges for the caregivers. "No" and "want" are favorite words. Temper tantrums appear.

During this transition from infancy to early childhood, the child learns many new physical and social skills. With additional teeth and better motor skills, the toddler's self-feeding abilities improve and include the addition of a new assortment of foods. Left unsupervised, the toddler also may taste many nonfood items that may be harmful, even fatal.

This transition is a time of unpredictability: one moment, the toddler insists on "me do it;" the next moment, the child reverts to dependence on the mother or other caregiver. While seeking to assert independence and achieve autonomy, the toddler develops a fear of separation. The toddler's curiosity about the world increases, as does his or her ability to explore. Family caregivers soon discover that this exploration can wreak havoc on orderly routine and a well-kept house and that the toddler requires close supervision to prevent injury to self or objects in the environment (Fig. 24-1). The toddler justly earns the title of "explorer."

Toddlerhood can be a difficult time for family caregivers. Just as parents are beginning to feel confident in their ability to care for and understand their infant, the toddler changes into a walking, talking person whose attitudes and behaviors disrupt the entire family.

Accident-proofing, safety measures, and firm but gentle discipline are the primary tasks for caregivers of toddlers. Learning to discipline with patience and understanding is difficult but eventually rewarding. At the end of the toddlerhood stage, the child's behavior generally becomes more acceptable and predictable.

Erikson's psychosocial developmental task for this age group is **autonomy** (independence) while overcoming doubt and shame. In contrast to the infant's task of building trust, the toddler seeks independence, wavers between dependence and freedom, and gains self-awareness. This behavior is so common that the stage is commonly referred to as the "terrible twos," but it is just as often referred to as the "terrific twos" because of the toddler's exciting language development, the exuberance with which he or she greets the world, and a new-found sense of accomplishment. Both aspects of being 2 years old are essential to the child's development, and caregivers must learn how to manage the fast-paced switching between anxiety and enthusiasm.

PHYSICAL DEVELOPMENT

Toddlerhood is a time of slowed growth and rapid development. Each year the toddler gains 5 to 10 lb (2.26 to 4.53 kg) and about 3 inches (7.62 cm). Continued eruption of teeth, particularly the molars, helps the toddler learn to chew food. The toddler learns to stand alone and to walk (Fig. 24-2) between the ages of

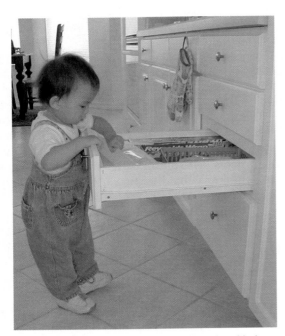

● *Figure 24.1* This curious toddler explores in a kitchen drawer while mom supervises closely.

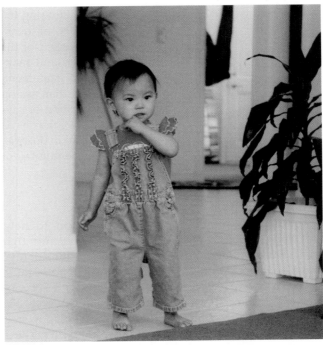

● *Figure 24.2* The toddler is proud of her ability to stand and walk.

1 and 2 years. During this time, most children say their first words and continue to improve and refine their language skills. By the end of this period, the toddler may have learned partial or total toilet training.

The rate of development varies with each child, depending on the individual personality and the opportunities available to test, explore, and learn. Significant landmarks in the toddler's growth and development are summarized in Table 24-1.

PSYCHOSOCIAL DEVELOPMENT

The toddler develops a growing awareness of self as a being, separate from other people or objects. Intoxicated with newly discovered powers and lacking experience, the child tends to test personal independence to the limit.

Behavioral Characteristics

Negativism, ritualism, dawdling, and temper tantrums are characteristic behaviors seen in toddlers.

Negativisim

This age has been called an age of **negativism**. Certainly the toddler's response to nearly everything is a firm "no," but this is more an assertion of individuality than of an intention to disobey. Limiting the number of questions asked of the toddler and making a statement, rather than asking a question or giving a choice, is helpful in decreasing the number of negative responses from the child.

Here's a helpful hint. Limiting the number of questions asked and offering a choice to the toddler will help decrease the number of "no" responses. For example the question, "Are you ready for your bath?" might be replaced by saying, "It is bathtime. Do you want to take your duck or your toy boat to the tub with you?"

Ritualism

Ritualism, employed by the young child to help develop security, involves following routines that make rituals of even simple tasks. At bedtime, all toys must be in accustomed places, and the caregiver must follow a habitual practice. This passion for a set routine is not found in every child to the same degree, but it does provide a comfortable base from which to step out into new and potentially dangerous paths. These practices often become more evident when a sitter is in the home, especially at bedtime. This gives the child some measure of security when the primary caregiver is absent.

Dawdling

Dawdling, wasting time or being idle, serves much the same purpose. The young child must decide between following the wishes and routines of the caregiver and asserting independence by following personal desires. Because he or she is incapable of making such a choice, the toddler compromises and tries both. If the task to be done is an important one, the caregiver with a firm and friendly manner should help the child to follow along the way he or she should go; otherwise, dawdling can be ignored within reasonable limits.

Temper Tantrums

Temper tantrums, an aggressive display of temper where the child reacts with rebellion to the wishes of the caregiver, spring from the many frustrations that are natural results of a child's urge to be independent. Add to this a child's reluctance to leave the scene for necessary rest, and frequently the frustrations become too great. Even the best of caregivers may lose patience and show a temporary lack of understanding. The child reacts with enthusiastic rebellion, but this, too, is a phase that must be lived through while the child works toward becoming an individual.

Reasoning, scolding, or punishing during a tantrum is useless. A trusted person who remains calm and patient needs to be nearby until the child gains self-control. After the tantrum is over, help the child relax by diverting attention with a toy or

Remaining calm is a must. It is not easy to handle a small child who drops to the floor screaming and kicking in rage in the middle of the supermarket or the sidewalk, nor are comments from onlookers at all helpful. The best a caregiver can do is pick up the out-of-control child as calmly as possible and carry him or her to a quiet, neutral place to regain self-control. The caregiver must ensure the child's safety by remaining near but ignoring the child's behavior.

CULTURAL SNAPSHOT

A common cultural belief is that children are to respect their elders, be quiet and humble, and often to be "seen and not heard." This may create a problem for the toddler who is attempting to express his or her independence and having a "temper tantrum."

TABLE 24.1	Growth and Development: The Toddler				
Age (months)	Personal–Social	Fine Motor	Gross Motor	Language	Cognition
12–15	Begins Erikson's stage of "autonomy versus shame and doubt" Seeks novel ways to pursue new experiences Imitations of people are more advanced	Builds with blocks; finger paints Able to reach out with hands and bring food to mouth Holds a spoon Drinks from a cup	Movements become more voluntary Postural control improves; able to stand and may take few independent steps	First words are not generally classified as true language. They are generally associated with the concrete and are usually activity-oriented.	Begins to accommodate to the environment, and the adaptive process evolves
18	Extremely curious Becomes a communicative social being Parallel play Fleeting contacts with other children "Make-believe" play begins	Better control of spoon; good control when drinking from cup Turns page of a book Places objects in holes or slots	Walks alone; gait may still be a bit unsteady Begins to walk sideways and backward	Begins to use language in a symbolic form to represent images or ideas that reflect the thinking process Uses some meaningful words such as "hi," "bye-bye," and "all gone" Comprehension is significantly greater	Demonstrates foresight and can discover solutions to problems without excessive trial-and-error procedures Can imitate without the presence of a model (deferred imitation)
24	Language facilitates autonomy Sense of power from saying "no" and "mine" Increased independence from mother	Turns pages of a book singly Adept at building a tower of six or seven cubes When drawing, attempts to enclose a space	Runs well with little falling Throws and kicks a ball Walks up and down stairs one step at a time	Begins to use words to explain past events or to discuss objects not observably present Rapidly expands vocabulary to about 300 words; uses plurals	Enters preconceptual phase of cognitive development State of continuous investigations Primary focus is egocentric
36	Basic concepts of sexuality are established Separates from mother more easily Attends to toilet needs	Copies a circle and a straight line Grasps spoon between thumb and index finger Holds cup by handle	Balances on one foot; jumps in place; pedals tricycles	Quest for information furthered by questions like "why," "when," "where," and "how" Has acquired the language that will be used in the course of simple conversation during adult years	Preconceptual phase continues; can think of only one idea at a time; cannot think of all parts in terms of the whole

some other interesting distraction. However, do not yield the point or give in to the child's whim. That would tell the child that to get whatever he or she wants, a person need only throw oneself on the floor and scream. The child would have to learn painfully later in life that people cannot be controlled in this manner.

These tantrums can be accompanied by head banging and breath holding. Breath holding can be frightening to the caregiver, but the child will shortly lose consciousness and begin breathing. Head banging can cause injury to the child, so the caregiver needs to provide protection.

The caregiver should try to be calm when dealing with a toddler having a tantrum. The child is out of control and needs help to regain control; the adult must maintain self-control to reassure the child and provide security.

Play

The toddler's play moves from the solitary play of the infant to **parallel play,** in which the toddler plays alongside other children but not with them (Fig. 24-3). Much of the playtime is filled with imitation of the people the child sees as role models: adults around him or her, siblings, and other children. Toys that involve the toddler's new gross motor skills, such as push-pull toys, rocking horses, large blocks, and balls, are popular. Fine motor skills are developed by use of thick crayons, play dough, finger paints, wooden puzzles with large pieces, toys that fit pieces into shaped holes, and cloth books. Toddlers enjoy talking on a play telephone and like pots, pans, and toys such as brooms, dishes, and lawn mowers that help them imitate the adults in their environment and promote socialization. The toddler cannot share toys until the later stage of toddlerhood, and adults should not make an issue of sharing at this early stage.

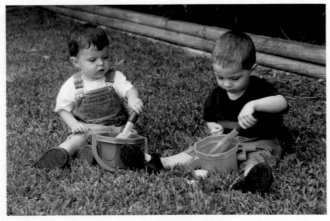

● *Figure 24.3* Toddlers engaged in parallel play.

Toys should be carefully checked for loose pieces and sharp edges to ensure the toddler's safety. Toddlers still put things into their mouths; therefore, small pieces that may come loose, such as small beads and buttons, must be avoided.

For an adult, staying quietly on the sidelines and observing the toddler play can be a fascinating revelation of what is going on in the child's world. However, the adult must intervene if necessary to avoid injury.

> ### Test Yourself
> - What does autonomy mean? How does the toddler develop autonomy?
> - What type of play is typically seen in the toddler?
> - List examples of parallel play?

Discipline

The word "discipline" has come to mean punishment to many people, but the concepts are not the same. To **discipline** means to train or instruct to produce a particular behavior pattern, especially moral or mental improvement, and self-control. **Punishment** means penalizing someone for wrongdoing. Although all small children need discipline, the need for punishment occurs much less frequently.

The toddler learns self-control gradually. The development from an egotistic being, whose world exists only to give self-satisfaction, into a person who understands and respects the rights of others is a long, involved process. The child cannot do this alone but must be taught.

Two-year-old children begin to show some signs of accepting responsibility for their own actions, but they lack inner controls because of their egocentricity. The toddler still wants the forbidden thing but may repeat "no, no, no" while reaching for a desired treasure, recognizing that the act is not approved. Although the child understands the act is not approved, the desire is too strong to resist. Even at this age, children want and need limits. When no limits are set, the child develops a feeling of insecurity and fear. With proper guidance, the child gradually absorbs the restraints and develops self-control or conscience.

Consistency and timing are important in the approach that the caregiver uses when disciplining the child. The toddler needs a lot of help during this time. People caring for the child should agree on the methods of discipline and should all operate by the same rules, so that the child knows what is expected. This need for consistency can cause disagreement for family caregivers who have experienced different types of child rearing themselves. The caregivers may be confused by this child who had been a sweet, loving baby and now has turned into a belligerent little being who throws tantrums at will.

This period can be challenging to adults. The child needs to learn that the adults are in control and will help the child to gain self-control while learning to be independent. When the toddler hits or bites another child, calmly remove the offender from the situation. Negative messages such as "You are a bad boy for hitting Jamal" or "Bad girl! You don't bite people" are not helpful. Instead, use messages that do not label the child as bad but label the act as unacceptable, such as "Biting hurts—be gentle."

Notice the difference. Praise children for good behavior with attention and verbal comments and, when possible, ignore negative behavior.

Another useful method for a child who is not cooperating or who is out of control is to send the child to a "time out" chair. This should be a place where the child can be alone but observed without other distractions. The duration of the isolation should be limited—1 minute per year of age is usually adequate. Warn the child in advance of this possibility, but only one warning per event is necessary.

"Extinction" is another discipline technique effective with this age group. If the child has certain undesirable behaviors that occur frequently, ignore the behavior. Do not react to the child as long as the behavior is not harmful to the child or others. Be consistent, and never react in any way to that particular behavior. Act as though you do not hear the child. However, when the child responds acceptably in a situation in which the undesirable behavior was the usual response, be sure to compliment the child. Suppose, for example that the child screams or makes a scene when you won't buy cookies in the grocery store. If, after you have practiced extinction, the child talks in a normal voice on another visit to the grocery store, compliment the child's "grown-up" behavior.

Spanking or other physical punishment usually does not work well because the child is merely taught that hitting or other physical violence is acceptable, and the child who is spanked frequently becomes immune to it.

Sharing With a New Baby

The first child has the caregivers' undivided attention until a new baby arrives, often when the first child is a toddler. Preparing a child just emerging from babyhood for this arrival is difficult. Although the toddler can feel the mother's abdomen and understand that this is where the new baby lives, this alone does not give adequate preparation for the baby's arrival. This real baby represents a rival for the mother's affection.

As in many stressful situations, the toddler frequently regresses to more infantile behavior. The toddler who no longer takes milk from a bottle may need or want a bottle when the new baby is being fed. Toilet training, which may have been moving along well, may regress with the toddler having episodes of soiling and wetting.

The new infant creates considerable change in the home, whether he or she is the first child or the fifth. In homes where the previous baby is displaced by the newcomer, however, some special preparation is necessary. Moving the older child to a larger bed some time before the new baby appears lets the toddler take pride in being "grown up" now.

Preparation of the toddler for a new brother or sister is helpful but should not be intense until just before the expected birth. Many hospitals have sibling classes for new siblings-to-be that are scheduled shortly before the anticipated delivery. These classes, geared to the young child, give the child some tasks to do for the new baby and discuss both negative and positive aspects of having a new baby in the home. Many books are available to help prepare the young child for the birth and that explore sibling rivalry.

Probably the greatest help in preparing the child of any age to accept the new baby is to help the child feel that this is "our baby" not just "mommy's baby" (Fig. 24-4). Helping to care for the baby, according to the child's ability, contributes to a feeling of continuing importance and self-worth.

The displaced toddler almost certainly will feel some jealousy. With careful planning, however, the mother can reserve some time for cuddling and playing with the toddler just as before. Perhaps the toddler may profit from a little extra parental attention for a time. The toddler needs to feel that parental love is just

● *Figure 24.4* The toddler is meeting her new baby brother.

as great as ever and that there is plenty of room in the parents' lives for both children.

The child should not be made to grow up too soon. The toddler should not be shamed or reproved for reverting to babyish behavior but should receive understanding and a bit more love and attention. Perhaps the father or other family member can occasionally take over the care of the new baby while the mother devotes herself to the toddler. The mother also may plan special times with the toddler when the new infant is sleeping and the mother has no interruptions. This approach helps the toddler feel special.

NUTRITION

Eating problems commonly appear between the ages of 1 and 3 years. These problems occur for a number of reasons, such as

- The child's growth rate has slowed; therefore, he or she may want and need less food than before. Family caregivers need to know that this is normal.
- The child's strong drive for independence and autonomy compels an assertion of will to prove his or her individuality both to self and others.
- A child's appetite varies according to the kind of foods offered. "Food jags," the desire for only one kind of food for a while, are common.

To minimize these eating problems and ensure that the child gets a balanced diet with all the proteins, carbohydrates, minerals, and vitamins essential for health and well-being, meals should be planned with an understanding of the toddler's developing feeding skills. Family Teaching Tips: Feeding Toddlers offers guidance for toddler mealtimes. Messiness is to be expected and prepared for when learning begins; it gradually diminishes as the child gains skill in self-feeding. At 15 months, the toddler can sit through meals, prefers finger feeding, and wants to self-feed. He or she tries to use a spoon but has difficulty with scooping and spilling. The 15-month-old grasps the cup with the thumb and forefinger but tilts the cup instead of the head. By 18 months, the toddler's appetite decreases. The 18-month-old has improved control of the spoon, puts spilled food back on the spoon, holds the cup with both hands, spills less often, and may throw the cup when finished if no one is there to take it. At 24 months, the toddler's appetite is fair to moderate. The toddler at this age has clearly defined likes and dislikes and food jags. The 24-month-old grasps the spoon between the thumb and forefinger, can put food on the spoon with one hand, continues to spill, and accepts no help ("Me do!"). By 30 months, refusals and preferences are less evident. Some tod-

dlers at this age hold the spoon like an adult, with the palm turned inward. The cup, too, may be handled in an adult manner. The 30-month-old tilts the head back to get the very last drop. A sample daily food plan is provided in Table 24-2.

HEALTH PROMOTION AND MAINTENANCE

Two important aspects of health promotion and maintenance for the toddler are routine checkups and accident prevention. Routine checkups help protect the

FAMILY TEACHING TIPS

Feeding Toddlers

- Serve small portions, and provide a second serving when the first has been eaten. One or 2 teaspoonfuls is an adequate serving for the toddler. Too much food on the dish may overwhelm the child.
- There is no *one* food essential to health. Allow substitution for a disliked food. Food jags where toddlers prefer one food for days on end are common and not harmful. If the child refuses a particular food such as milk, use appropriate substitutes such as pudding, cheese, yogurt, and cottage cheese. Avoid a battle of wills at mealtime.
- Toddlers like simply prepared foods served warm or cool, *not* hot or cold.
- Provide a social atmosphere at mealtimes; allow the toddler to eat with others in the family. Toddlers learn by imitating the acceptance or rejection of foods by other family members.
- Toddlers prefer foods that they can pick up with their fingers; however, they should be allowed to use a spoon or fork when they want to try.
- Try to plan regular mealtimes with small nutritious snacks between meals. Do not attach too much importance to food by urging the child to choose what to eat.
- Dawdling at mealtime is common with this age group and can be ignored unless it stretches to unreasonable lengths or becomes a play for power. Mealtime for the toddler should not exceed 20 minutes. Calmly remove food without comment.
- Do not make desserts a reward for good eating habits. It gives unfair value to the dessert and makes vegetables or other foods seem less desirable.
- Offer regularly planned nutritious snacks such as milk, crackers and peanut butter, cheese cubes, and pieces of fruit. Plan snacks midway between meals and at bedtime.
- Remember that the total amount eaten each day is more important than the amount eaten at a specific meal.

TABLE 24.2	Suggested Daily Food Guidelines for the Toddler	
Food Items	Daily Amounts*	Comments/Rationale
Cooked eggs	3–5/wk	Good source of protein. Moderate use is recommended because of high cholesterol content in egg yolk.
Breads, cereal, rice, pasta: whole-grain or enriched	6 or more servings (e.g., ½ slice bread, ¼ cup cereal, ¼ cup rice, 2 crackers, ¼ cup noodles)	Provide thiamine, niacin, and, if enriched, riboflavin and iron. Encourage child to identify and appreciate a wide variety of foods.
Fruit juices; fruit—canned or small pieces	2–4 child-sized servings (e.g., ½ cup juice, ¼–½ cup fruit pieces)	Use those rich in vitamins A and C; also source of iron and calcium. Self-feeding enhances the child's sense of independence.
Vegetables	3–5 child-sized servings (e.g., ¼–⅓ cup)	Include at least one dark-green or yellow vegetable every other day for vitamin A.
Meat, fish, poultry, cottage cheese, peanut butter, dried peas and beans	2–3 child-sized servings (e.g., 1 oz meat, ¼ cup cottage cheese, 1–2 tbsp peanut butter)	Source of complete protein, iron, thiamine, riboflavin, niacin, and vitamin B_{12} Nuts and seeds should not be offered until after age 3 when risk of choking is minimal.
Milk, yogurt, cheese	4–6 child-sized servings (e.g., 4–6 oz milk, ½ cup yogurt, 1 oz cheese)	Cheese, cottage cheese, and yogurt are good calcium and riboflavin sources. Also sources of calcium, phosphorus, complete protein, riboflavin, and niacin and vitamin D if milk is fortified
Fats and sweets	In moderation	May interfere with consumption of nutrient-rich foods. Chocolate should be delayed until the child is 1 year old.
Salt and other seasonings	In moderation	Children's taste buds are more sensitive than those of adults. Salt is a learned taste, and high intakes are related to hypertension.

*Amounts are daily totals and goals to be achieved gradually.
Adapted from Dudek, SG. (2000) *Nutrition essentials for nursing practice* (4th ed). Philadelphia: Lippincott Williams & Wilkins.

toddler's health and ensure continuing growth and development. The nurse can encourage good health through family teaching, support of positive parenting behaviors, and reinforcement of the toddler's achievements. Toddlers need a stimulating environment and the opportunity to explore it. This environment, however, must be safe to help prevent accidents and infection. Give caregivers information regarding accident prevention and home safety.

Routine Checkups

The child is seen at 15 months for immunization boosters and at least annually thereafter. Routine physical checkups include assessment of growth and development, oral hygiene, toilet training, daily health care, the caregiver–toddler relationship, and parenting

skills. Interviews with caregivers, observations of the toddler, observations of the caregiver–toddler interaction, and communication with the toddler are all effective means to elicit this information. Remember that caregiver interpretations may not be completely accurate. Communicate with the toddler on his or her level and offer only realistic options.

Current immunizations should be administered (see Table 23-4 in Chapter 23). Table 24-3 details nursing measures that may be implemented to ensure optimal health practices.

Family Teaching

The toddler is learning rapidly about the world in which she or he lives. As part of that process, the toddler learns about everyday care needed for healthy

TABLE 24.3	Guidelines for Health Promotion in the Toddler	
Developmental Characteristics of Toddler (2–3 Yr)	Possible Deviations From Health	Nursing Measures to Ensure Optimal Health Practices
Self-feeding (foods and objects more accessible for mouthing, handling, and eating)	Inadequate nutritional intake Accidental poisoning Gastrointestinal disturbances: Instability of gastrointestinal tract Infection from parasites (pinworm)	Diet teaching Childproofing the home Careful handwashing (before meals, after toileting) Avoidance of rich foods Observe for perianal itching (Scotch tape test, administer anthelmintic)
Toilet training	Constipation (if training procedures are too rigid) Urinary tract infection (especially prevalent in girls due to anatomic structure and poor toilet habits)	Teaching toileting procedures Urinalysis when indicated (e.g., burning) Teaching hygiene (at the onset of training, instruct girls to wipe from front to back, and wash hands to prevent cross-infection)
Increased socialization	Increased prevalence of upper respiratory infections (immune levels still at immature levels)	Hygienic practices (e.g., use of tissue or handkerchief, not drinking from same glass) Immunizations for passive immunity against communicable disease
Primary dentition	Caries with resultant infection or loss of primary as well as beginning permanent teeth	Oral hygiene, regular tooth brushing, dental examination at 2½–3 years Proper nutrition to ensure dentition
Sleep disturbances	Lack of sleep may cause irritability, lethargy, decreased resistance to infection	Teaching regarding recommended amounts of sleep (12–14 h in first year, decreasing to 10–12 h by age 3); need for rituals to enhance transition process to bedtime; possibility of need for nap; setting bedtime limits

growth and development. The toddler's urge for independence and the caregiver's response to that urge play an important part in everyday life with the toddler. Some of these activities are included in the following discussion.

Bathing

Toddlers generally love to take a tub bath. Setting a regular time each day for the bath helps give the toddler a sense of security about what to expect. Although the toddler can sit well in the tub, he or she should never be left alone. An adult must supervise the bath continuously to prevent an accident. The toddler enjoys having tub toys to play with. Avoid using bubble bath, especially for little girls, because it can create an environment that encourages the growth of organisms that cause bladder infections. A bath often is relaxing and may help the toddler quiet down before bedtime.

Dressing

By their second birthday, toddlers take an active interest in helping to put on their clothes. They often begin around 18 months by removing their socks and shoes

whenever they choose. This behavior can be frustrating to the caregiver but if accepted as another small step in development, the caretaker may feel less frustration. Between the ages of 2 and 3 years, the toddler can begin by putting on underpants, shirts, or socks (Fig. 24-5).

● **Figure 24.5** Getting dressed by himself is a fun morning activity for this 3-year-old boy.

Often the clothing ends up backwards, but the important thing is that the toddler accomplished the task. Encourage the caregiver to take a relaxed attitude as the toddler learns to dress him or herself. If clothes must be put on correctly, the caregiver should try to do it without criticizing the toddler's job. The caregiver should warmly acknowledge the toddler's accomplishment of putting on a piece of clothing that he or she may have struggled with for some time. Roomy clothing with easy buttons; large, smooth-running zippers; or Velcro is easier for the toddler to handle.

As in late infancy, shoes need to be worn primarily to protect the toddler's feet from harsh surfaces. Sneakers are still a good choice. Avoid hard-soled shoes. High-topped shoes are unnecessary.

Dental Care

Dental caries (cavities) are a major health problem in children and young adults. Sound teeth depend in part on sound nutrition. The development of dental caries is linked to the effect the diet has on the oral environment.

Bacteria that act in the presence of sugar and form a film, or dental plaque, on the teeth cause tooth decay. People who eat sweet foods frequently accumulate plaque easily and are prone to dental caries. Sugars eaten at mealtime appear to be neutralized by the presence of other foods and, therefore, are not as damaging as between-meal sweets and bedtime bottles. Foods consisting of hard or sticky sugars, such as lollipops and caramels that remain in the mouth for longer periods, tend to cause more dental caries than those eaten quickly. Sugarless gum or candies are not as harmful.

When the child is about 2 years of age, he or she should be taught to brush the teeth or at least to rinse the mouth after each meal or snack. Because this is the period when the toddler likes to imitate others, the child is best taught by example. Plain water should be used until the child has learned how to spit out toothpaste. An adult should also brush the toddler's teeth until the child becomes experienced. One good method is to stand behind the child in front of a mirror and brush the child's teeth. In addition to cleaning adequately, this also helps the child learn how it feels to have the teeth thoroughly brushed. The use of fluoride toothpaste strengthens tooth enamel and helps to prevent tooth decay, particularly in communities with unfluoridated water. An adult should supervise the use of fluoride toothpaste; the child should use only a small pea-sized amount. The physician may recommend supplemental fluoride, but families on limited incomes may find this difficult to afford. A fluoride supplement is a medication and should be treated and stored as such. Fluoride also can be applied during regular visits to the dentist, but the greatest benefit to the tooth enamel occurs before the eruption of the teeth.

The first visit to the dentist should occur at about 2 years of age just so the child gets acquainted with the dentist, staff, and office. A second visit might be a good time for a preliminary examination, and subsequent visits twice a year for checkups are recommended.

Pay attention to the little details. It is important for the nurse to teach the caregivers the importance of proper care of the child's baby teeth.

If there are older siblings, the toddler can go along on a visit with them to help overcome the fears of a strange setting. Some clinics are recommending earlier visits to check the child and give dietary guidance. Children of low-income families often have poor dental hygiene and care, both because of the cost of care and parental lack of knowledge about proper care and nutrition. Some caregivers may believe it is unnecessary to take proper care of baby teeth because "they fall out anyway." The care and condition of the baby teeth affect the normal growth of permanent teeth, which are forming in the jaw under the baby teeth.

Toilet Training

Learning bowel and bladder control is an important part of the socialization process. In Western culture, a great sense of shame and disgust has been associated with body waste products. To function successfully in this culture, one must learn to dispose of body waste products in a place considered proper by society.

The toddler has been operating on the pleasure principle by simply emptying the bowel and bladder when the urge is present without thinking of anything but personal comfort. During toilet training, the child, who is just learning about control of the personal environment, finds that some of that control must be given up to please those most important people, the caregivers. The toddler now must learn to conform not only to please those special loved ones; to preserve self-integrity, the toddler must persuade himself or herself that this acceptance of the dictates of society is voluntary. These new routines make little sense to the child.

Timing. Timing is an important aspect of toilet training. To be able to cooperate in toilet training, the child's anal and uretheral sphincter muscles must have developed to the stage where the child can control them. Control of the anal sphincter usually develops first. The child also must be able to postpone the urge to defecate or urinate until reaching the toilet or potty and must be able to signal the need before the event. In addition, before toilet training can occur, the child must have a desire to please the caregiver by holding feces and urine, rather than satisfying his/her

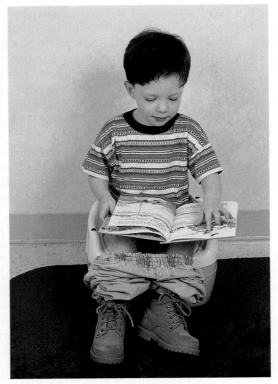

● **Figure 24.6** Toddlers will sit on the potty chair to please a caregiver.

own immediate need for gratification. This level of maturation seldom takes place before the age of 18 to 24 months.

At the start of toilet training, the child has no understanding of the uses of the potty chair, but to please the caregiver the child will sit there for a short time (Fig. 24-6). If the child's bowel movements occur at about the same time every day, one day a bowel movement will occur while the child is sitting on the potty. Although there is no sense of special achievement as yet, the child does like the praise and approval. Eventually the child will connect this approval with the bowel movement in the potty, and the child will be happy that the caregiver is pleased.

Give this a try. Offering small rewards, such as stickers, nutritious treats, or toys can be an encouragment to the child who is in the process of toilet training.

Generally the first indication of readiness for bladder training is when the child makes a connection between the puddle on the floor and something he or she did. In the next stage, the child runs to the caregiver and indicates a need to urinate, but only after it has happened. Sometimes the child who is ready for toilet training will pull on a wet or soiled diaper or even bring a clean diaper to the caregiver to indicate

they need a diaper change. Not much benefit is gained from a serious program of training until the child is sufficiently mature to control the urethral sphincter and reach the desired place. When the child stays dry for about 2 hours at a time during the day, sufficient maturity may be indicated.

Suggestions for Toilet Training. Suggestions for toilet training include

- A potty chair in which a child can comfortably sit with the feet on the floor is preferable. Most small children are afraid of a flush toilet.
- The child should be left on the potty chair for only a short time. The caregiver should be readily available but should not hover anxiously over the child. If a bowel movement or urination occurs, approval is in order; if not, no comment is necessary.
- Have the child wash her/his hands after sitting on the toilet or potty chair to instill good hygiene practices.
- Dressing the child in clothes that are easily removed and in training pants or "pull-up" type diapers and pants increases the child's success with training.
- Children love to copy and imitate others, and often, observing a parent or an older sibling gives the toddler a positive role model for toilet training.
- During the beginning stages of training, the child is likely to have a bowel movement or wet diaper soon after leaving the potty. This is not willful defiance and need not be mentioned.
- The potty chair should be emptied unobtrusively after the child has resumed playing. The child has cooperated and produced the product desired. If it is immediately thrown away, the child may be confused and not so eager to please the next time. However, some children enjoy the fun of flushing the toilet and watching as the materials disappear.
- Be careful not to flush the toilet while the child is sitting on it, this can be frightening to the child.
- The ability to feel shame and self-doubt appears at this age. Therefore, the child should not be teased about reluctance or inability to conform. This teasing can shake the child's confidence and cause feelings of doubt in self-worth.
- The caregiver should not expect perfection, even after control has been achieved. Lapses inevitably occur, perhaps because the child is completely absorbed in play or because of a temporary episode of loose stools. Occasionally a child feels aggression, frustration, or anger and may use this method to "get even." As long as the lapses are occasional, they should be ignored. If the lapses are frequent and persistent, however, the cause should be sought.

Each child follows an individual pattern of development, so no caregiver should feel embarrassed or ashamed because a child is still having accidents.

No one should expect the child to accomplish self-training, and family caregivers should be alert to the signs of readiness. Patience and understanding by the caregivers are essential. Complete control, especially at night, may not be achieved until the 4th or 5th year of age. Each child should be taught a term or phrase to use for toileting that is recognizable to others, clearly understood, and socially acceptable. This is especially true for children who are cared for outside the home.

Here's a tip for you. To help the child remember to use the toilet or potty chair, set a timer to sound at appropriate intervals. When the timer sounds, the child will be reminded to go to the bathroom.

Test Yourself

- List the areas of family teaching that are important for the caregivers of toddlers.

- What must develop in order for the toddler to be physically ready for toilet training? By what age are most children toilet trained?

Sleep

The toddler's sleep needs change gradually between the ages of 1 and 3 years. A total daily need for 12 to 14 hours of sleep is to be expected in the first year of toddlerhood, decreasing to 10 to 12 hours by 3 years. The toddler soon gives up a morning nap, but most continue to need an afternoon nap until sometime near the third birthday.

Rituals are a common part of bedtime procedures. A bedtime ritual provides structure and a feeling of security because the toddler knows what to expect and what is expected of him or her. The separation anxiety common in the toddler may contribute to some of the toddler's reluctance to go to bed. Family caregivers must be careful that the toddler does not use this to manipulate them and delay bedtime. Gentle, firm consistency by caregivers is ultimately reassuring to the toddler. Regular schedules with set bedtimes are important.

Check out this tip. Bedtime routines such as reading a story or having a quiet time are helpful in providing a calming end to a busy day for the toddler.

A PERSONAL GLIMPSE

My husband and I decided it was time to potty train our near 3-year-old son, William. We started by "introducing" him to the potty. In the morning, my husband would casually ask William if he'd like to sit on the potty. "No," he'd assert. Before a bath, I'd ask William if he would like to sit on the Elmo chair and get a treat. "No," he'd say again, "gimme back my diaper." Taking this as a sign that he wasn't ready, we decided to delay potty training. Then one day William followed our 5-year-old son, Jack, into the bathroom. From the other room I heard Jack say, "See, Will, this is how I use the potty." William, ever eager to please his brother, pulled up a step stool and mimicked Jack. Nothing happened, but William was starting to show interest. I praised them and gave them both a small treat. I suggested to Jack that he ask William to sit on the little potty while he sat on the big potty to "pee," which would be easier for William. "Got it," Jack said with two thumbs up. We resumed potty training. Jack took the lead in our family effort. A week later, Jack and William came bounding out of the bathroom together. "We did it," Jack exclaimed. "We did it," William repeated. "I go pee-pee like Jack!" Upon further inspection, I found that William had in fact successfully used the little potty. "High-five," Jack begged. "High-five," William dutifully repeated. "High-five all around," I giggled. We still have a long way to go, but we are making progress—all four of us together!

Melanie (and Joe)

LEARNING OPPORTUNITY: What behavioral characteristics commonly seen in the toddler did this child show? What would you suggest these parents do to praise and support both of their children in the toilet training process?

Accident Prevention

Toddlers are explorers who require constant supervision in a controlled environment to encourage autonomy and prevent injury. When supervision is inadequate or the environment is unsafe, tragedy often results; accidents are the leading cause of death for children between the ages of 1 and 4 years. Accidents involving motor vehicles, drowning, burns, poisoning, and falls are the most common causes of death. The number of motor vehicle deaths in this age group is more than three times greater than the numbers of deaths caused by burns or drowning. Family teaching can help minimize the risk for accident and injury.

● *Figure 24.7* Car seats are used for safety when toddlers ride in a vehicle.

Motor Vehicle Accidents

Many childhood deaths or injuries resulting from motor vehicle accidents can be prevented by proper use of restraints. Federally approved child safety seats are designed to give the child maximum protection if used correctly (Fig. 24-7). Adults must be responsible for teaching the child that seat belts are required for safe car travel and that he or she must be securely fastened in the car seat before the car starts. Adults in the car with a child should set the example by also using seat belts. Many toddlers are killed or injured by moving vehicles while playing in their own driveways or garages. Caregivers need to be aware that these tragedies can occur and must take proper precautions at all times. See Family Teaching Tips: Preventing Motor Vehicle Accidents.

Drowning

Although drowning of young children is often associated with bathtubs, the increased number of home swimming pools has added significantly to the number of accidental drownings. Often these pools are fenced on three sides to keep out nonresidents but are bordered on one side by the family home, making the pool accessible to infants and toddlers. Even small plastic wading pools hold enough water to drown an unsupervised toddler. Any family living near a body of water, no matter how small, must not leave a mobile infant or toddler unattended even for a moment. Even a small amount of water, such as that in a bucket, may be enough to drown a small child.

FAMILY TEACHING TIPS

Preventing Motor Vehicle Accidents

- Never start the car until the child is securely in the car seat.
- If the child manages to get out of the car seat or unfasten it, pull over to the curb or side of the road as soon as possible, turn off the car, and tell the child that the car will not go until he or she is safely in the seat. Children love to go in the car, and they will comply if they learn that they cannot go unless in the car seat.
- Never permit a child to stand in a car that is in motion.
- Teach the toddler to stop at a curb and wait for an adult escort to cross the street. An older child should be taught to look both ways for traffic. Start this as a game with toddlers, and continually reinforce it.
- Teach the child to cross only at corners.
- Begin in toddlerhood to teach awareness of traffic signals and their meanings. As soon as the child recognizes color, he or she can tell you when it is all right to cross.
- Never let a child run into the street after a ball.
- Teach a child never to walk between parked cars to cross.
- As a driver, always be on the alert for children running into the street when in a residential area.

Burns

Burn accidents occur most often as scalds from immersions and spills and from exposure to uninsulated electrical wires or live extension cord plugs. Children also are burned while playing with matches or while left unattended in a home where a fire breaks out. Whether the fire results from a child's mischief, an adult's carelessness, or some unforeseeable event, the injuries, even if not fatal, can have long-term or permanent effects. Often burns can be prevented by following simple safety practices (see Family Teaching Tips: Preventing Burns).

Ingestion of Toxic Substances

The curious toddler wants to touch and taste everything. Left unsupervised, the toddler may sample household cleaners, prescription or over-the-counter drugs, kerosene, gasoline, peeling lead-based paint chips, or dust particles. Poisoning is still the most common medical emergency in children, with the highest incidence between the ages of 1 and 4 years.

Caregivers need continual reminders about the possibility of childhood poisoning. Even with precautionary labeling and "child-resistant" packaging of medication and household cleaners, children display

FAMILY TEACHING TIPS

Preventing Burns

- Do not let electrical cords dangle over a counter or table. Repair frayed cords. Newer small appliances have shorter cords to prevent dangling.
- Cover electrical wall outlets with safety caps.
- Turn handles of pans on the stove toward the back of the stove. If possible, place pans on back burners out of the toddler's reach.
- Place cups of hot liquid out of reach. Do not use overhanging tablecloths that toddlers can pull.
- Use caution when serving foods heated in the microwave; they can be hotter than is apparent.
- Supervise small children at all times in the bathtub so they cannot turn on the hot water tap.
- Turn thermostat on home water heater down so that the water temperature is no higher than 120°F.
- Place matches in metal containers and out of reach of small children. Keep lighters out of reach of children.
- Never leave small children unattended by an adult or responsible teenager.

FAMILY TEACHING TIPS

Preventing Poisoning

- Keep medicines in their original containers in a locked cupboard. Do not rely on a high shelf being out of a child's reach.
- Never refer to medicines as candy.
- Discard unused medicines by a method that eliminates any possibility of access by children, other persons, or animals (e.g., flush them down the toilet).
- Replace safety caps properly, but do not depend on them to be childproof. Children can sometimes open them more easily than adults can.
- Keep a bottle of syrup of ipecac in a locked cupboard to induce vomiting if recommended by the poison control center.
- Keep the telephone number of the nearest poison control center posted near the telephone.
- Keep a chart with emergency treatment for poisoning in a handy permanent spot.
- Store household cleaning and laundry products out of children's reach.
- Never put kerosene or other household fluids in soda bottles or other drink containers.

amazing ingenuity in opening bottles and packages that catch their curiosity. Mr. Yuk labels are available from the nearest poison control center. The child can be taught that products are harmful if they have the Mr. Yuk label on them. However, labeling is not sufficient: all items that are in any way toxic to the child must be placed under lock and key or totally out of the child's reach.

Always exercise caution. The importance of careful, continuous supervision of toddlers and other young children cannot be overemphasized.

Preventive measures that should be observed by all caregivers of small children are listed in Family Teaching Tips: Preventing Poisoning.

The following medications are most commonly involved in cases of childhood poisoning:

- Acetaminophen
- Salicylates (aspirin)
- Laxatives
- Sedatives
- Tranquilizers
- Analgesics
- Antihistamines
- Cold medicines
- Birth control pills

Test Yourself

- What are the major causes of accidents in the toddler?
- List measures caregivers of toddlers should be taught to prevent accidents.

THE TODDLER IN THE HEALTH CARE FACILITY

Although hospitalization is difficult and frightening for a child of any age, the developmental stage of the toddler intensifies these problems. When planning care, the nurse must keep in mind the toddler's developmental tasks and needs. The toddler, engaged in trying to establish self-control and autonomy, finds that strangers seem to have total power; this eliminates any control on the toddler's part. Add these fears to the inability to communicate well, discomfort from pain, separation from family, the presence of unfamiliar people and surroundings, physical restraint, and uncomfortable or frightening procedures, and the toddler's reaction can be clearly understood.

As part of the child's admission procedure, a social assessment survey should be completed by interviewing the family caregiver who has accompanied the child to the facility. Usually part of the standard pediatric nursing assessment form, the social assessment covers eating habits and food preferences, toileting habits and terms used for toileting, family members and the names the child calls them, the name the child is called by family members, pets and their names, favorite toys, sleeping or napping patterns and rituals, and other significant information that helps the staff better plan care for the toddler (see Fig. 28-2 in Chapter 28). This information should become an indispensable part of the nursing care plan. Using this information, the nurse should develop a nursing care plan that provides opportunities for independence for the toddler whenever possible.

Separation anxiety is high during the toddler age. As discussed in detail in Chapter 29, the stages of protest and despair are common. Acknowledge these stages and communicate to the child that it is acceptable to feel angry and anxious at being separated from the primary family caregiver, the person foremost in the child's life. Never interpret the toddler's angry protest as a personal attack. Many facilities encourage family involvement in the child's care to minimize separation anxiety. The mother is often the family member who stays with the child, but in many families other members who are close to the child may take turns staying. Having a family caregiver with the toddler can be extremely helpful. Do not, however, neglect caring for the toddler who has a loved one present. In many families, it is impossible for the family caregiver to stay with the child for any of a number of reasons. These children need extra attention and care. All children should be assigned a constant caregiver while in the facility, but this is especially important for the toddler who is alone (Fig. 24-8).

The nurse assigned to the toddler will become a surrogate parent while caring for the child. Maintaining as much as possible the pattern, schedule, and rituals that the toddler is used to helps to provide some measure of security to the child. This is a time when the toddler needs the security of a beloved thumb or other "lovey," a favorite stuffed animal or blanket. The nurse needs to recognize that the toddler uses this to provide self-comfort (Fig. 24-9). The lovey may be well worn and dirty, but the toddler finds great reassurance in having it to snuggle or cuddle. Do not ridicule the child for its unkempt appearance, and make every effort to allow the toddler to have it whenever desired.

When the family caregiver must leave the toddler, it may be helpful for the adult to give the child some personal item to keep until the adult returns. The caregiver can tell the child he or she will return "when the cartoons come on TV" or "when your lunch comes." These are concrete times that the toddler will probably understand.

● *Figure 24.8* The nurse may become a surrogate parent for the hospitalized toddler.

Special Considerations

The busy toddler just learning to use the toilet, self-feed, and be disciplined presents a unique challenge to the staff nurse. The nurse must maintain control on the pediatric unit, promote safety, and help establish the toddler's sense of security while allowing the toddler's development to continue.

The toddler learning sphincter control is still dependent on familiar surroundings and the family caregiver's support. For this reason, some pediatric personnel automatically put toddlers back in diapers when they are admitted. This practice should be discouraged. Under the right circumstances and especially

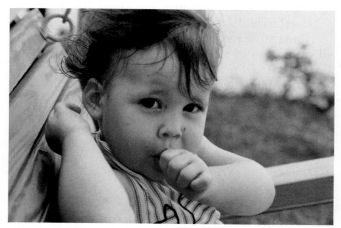

● *Figure 24.9* The toddler finds security and comfort in her "beloved" thumb.

with the caregiver's help, many of these children can maintain control. They at least should be given a chance to try. Potty chairs can be provided for the child when appropriate. The nursing staff must know the method and times of accomplishing toilet training used at home and must try to comply with them as closely as possible in the hospital.

Some limits are needed for the toddler, but be careful when setting them. Toddlers, like children of any age, need to feel that someone is in control and need limits set with love and understanding. A child who has been overindulged for a long time may need firm, calm statements of limits delivered in a no-nonsense but kind manner. Explaining what is going to be done, what is expected of the toddler, and what the toddler can expect from the nurse may be helpful. Sometimes the nurse may give some tactful guidance to the family caregiver to help set limits for the toddler. This is an area where experience helps the nurse to solve difficult problems. Discipline on the pediatric unit is discussed in Chapter 29.

A toddler's eating habits may loom large in the nurse's mind as a potential problem. In the hospital or clinic as at home, food can assume an importance out of proportion to its value and create unnecessary problems. Some helpful hints to minimize potential problems are

- View mealtime as a social event.
- Encourage self-feeding.
- Do not push the child to eat.
- Allow others to eat with the child.
- Offer familiar foods.
- Provide fluids in small but frequent amounts.

Eating concerns for the pediatric patient are fully discussed in Chapter 29.

Safety is a concern with all hospitalized children, but safety promotion for a toddler may be particularly challenging. The curious toddler needs to be watched with extra care but should not be unnecessarily prohibited from exploring and moving about freely. Safety in the hospital setting is discussed in detail in Chapter 29.

KEY POINTS

- The toddler tries to assert his or her independence, is curious about the world around him/her, and at times fears separation from caregivers.
- Because of the toddler's new-found independence, parenting can be frustrating and a challenge, especially related to creating a safe environment and disciplining the child.

- The toddler's physical growth slows while motor, social, and language development rapidly increase.
- Using negativism, the toddler often responds "no" to almost everything. To develop security, the toddler likes to follow specific sets of routines; this is referred to as "ritualism." Dawdling occurs when toddlers follow their own desires, rather than the caregiver's wishes and routines. Temper tantrums are an aggressive display of temper in which the child reacts with rebellion to the wishes of the caregiver.
- Eating problems occur in the toddler because of a slower growth rate, a drive for independence, "food jags," and variations in appetite.
- The toddler progresses from finger feeding and tilting the cup to being able to hold a spoon and handle a cup in an adult manner.
- Bacteria forms dental plaque on teeth because of the presence of sugar in foods. By the age of 2 years, a child often imitates others and can be taught to brush teeth by following the example of adults.
- The toddler should visit the dentist at about the age of 2 years to be introduced to the process of a dental checkup.
- Toilet training can be started when the child's sphincter muscles have developed enough so the child can control them; this usually occurs at age 18 to 24 months.
- Perfection should not be expected in toilet training. To aid in training, the child is put on a potty chair and left for only a short time. If the child has a bowel movement or urinates after leaving the potty, this is ignored. The child should not be teased, and the potty chair should not be emptied until the child has gone back to playing or other activities.
- The leading causes of death in toddlers are accidents involving motor vehicles, drowning, burns, poisons and falls. Supervision and prevention of accidents is especially important because of the exploring nature of the toddler.
- Toddlers should always be secured in a car seat when in a motor vehicle. Supervision is important when toddlers are near motor vehicles, streets, bathtubs, and swimming pools. Toxic substances should be stored out of reach and in child-proofed containers.
- The most common medications involved in child poisonings are acetaminophen, aspirin, laxatives, sedatives, tranquilizers, analgesics, antihistamines, cold medicines, and birth control pills.
- When a toddler is hospitalized, it is important to know their specific habits, terms used, patterns, and rituals.

REFERENCES AND SELECTED READINGS

Books and Journals

Banks, M. (2001). Fluoridated water: Nature's cavity fighter. *Community Health Forum, 2*(6), 12–15.

Berger, K. S. (2001) *The developing person through the life span.* New York: Worth Publishers.

Brazelton, T. B., & Greenspan, S. (2001). *The irreducible needs of children: What every child must have to grow, learn, and flourish.* Cambridge, MA: Perseus Publishing.

Bufalini, M. (2001). Dental health life cycle. *Community Health Forum, 2*(6), 36–38.

Dudek, S. G. (2000). *Nutrition essentials for nursing practice* (4th ed). Philadelphia: Lippincott Williams & Wilkins.

Gaylord, N. (2001). Parenting classes: From birth to 3 years. *Journal of Pediatric Health Care, 15*(4), 179.

Hockenberry, M. J., Wilson, D., Winkelstein, M. L., & Kline, N. E. (2003). *Wong's nursing care of infants and children* (7th ed.). St. Louis: Mosby.

Monsen, R. (2001). Giving children control and toilet training. *Journal of Pediatric Nursing, 16*(5), 375.

Pillitteri, A. (2003). *Maternal and child health nursing* (4th ed). Philadelphia: Lippincott Williams & Wilkins.

Spock, B. et al. (1998). *Dr. Spock's baby and child care.* New York: Pocket Books.

Starr, N. (2001). Kids and car safety: Beyond car seats and seat belts. *Journal of Pediatric Health Care, 15*(5), 257.

Wong, D. L., Perry, S., & Hockenberry, M. (2002). *Maternal child nursing care* (2nd ed.). St. Louis: Mosby.

Web Addresses

www.babycenter.com/toddler

Poison Control

www.aapcc.org

Accident Prevention

www.childrens.com

WORKBOOK

NCLEX-STYLE REVIEW QUESTIONS

1. The nurse is weighing a toddler who is 3 years old. If this child has had a typical pattern of growth and weighed 18 pounds at the age of 1 year, the nurse would expect this toddler to weigh approximately how many pounds?

   a. 22 pounds

   b. 30 pounds

   c. 36 pounds

   d. 42 pounds

2. The nurse is observing a group of 2-year-old children. Which of the following actions by the toddlers would indicate a gross motor skill seen in children this age?

   a. Turns pages of a book

   b. Uses words to explain an object

   c. Drinks from a cup

   d. Runs with little falling

3. The toddler-age child engages in "parallel play." The nurse observes the following behaviors in a room where children are playing with dolls and stuffed animals. Which of the following is an example of parallel play? Two children are

   a. sharing stuffed animals with each other.

   b. sitting next each other, each playing with her or his own doll.

   c. taking turns playing with the same stuffed animal.

   d. feeding the first doll, then feeding the second doll.

4. In preparing snacks for a 15-month-old toddler, which of the following would be the *best* choice for this age child?

   a. Small cup of yogurt

   b. Five or six green grapes

   c. Handful of dry cereal

   d. Three or four cookies

5. During the toddler years, the child attempts to become autonomous or independent. If the following statements were made by caregivers of 3-year-old children, which observation reflects that the child is developing autonomy?

   a. "When my child falls down, he always wants me to pick him up."

   b. "My child has temper tantrums when we go to the store."

   c. "Every night my child follows the same routine at bedtime."

   d. "My child uses the potty chair and is dry all day long."

6. The nurse is working with a group of caregivers of toddlers. The nurse explains that accident prevention and safety are very important when working with children. Which of the following statements is true regarding accidents and safety for the toddler?
   Check all that apply.

   a. Child car restraints are required for children.

   b. Accidents are the leading cause of death in children up to age 4 years.

   c. At least 5 to 6 inches of water is necessary for drowning to occur.

   d. Touching and tasting substances in the environment is a concern.

   e. Poisonous items should be kept in a locked area.

   f. Child-resistant packaging keeps children from opening any bottle.

STUDY ACTIVITIES

1. List and compare the fine motor and gross motor skills in each of the following ages:

	15 Months	24 Months	36 Months
Fine motor skills			
Gross motor skills			

2. Discuss the development of language seen in toddlerhood. Compare the language development of the 15-month-old child to the language development of the 36-month-old child.

3. List the four leading causes of accidents in toddlers. For each of these causes state three prevention tips that you could share with family caregivers of toddlers.

4. Go to the following Internet site: http://www.lee-bee.com
   At "Lee-Bee Motivational Charts," click on "Need help potty training your child?" Click on "When to start potty training" on left side of screen.

   a. What are the 15 common signs of toilet training readiness?

   b. After reading this section, what could you share with the caregivers of a toddler regarding potty training?

   c. What else is available on this site for caregivers of a toddler?

CRITICAL THINKING: What Would You Do?

1. You are in the supermarket with your 2-year-old niece, Lauren. She is having a loud, screaming temper tantrum because you won't buy some expensive cookies she wants. As you are trying to talk with her, she is yelling, "No, I want them."

   a. What are the reasons toddlers have temper tantrums?

   b. What is the best way to respond to a toddler who is having a temper tantrum? Why?

   c. What would you say to Lauren in this situation?

   d. What actions would you take during the temper tantrum? After the temper tantrum?

2. Marti complains to you that 2-year-old Tasha is very difficult to put to bed at night. Marti often just gives up and lets Tasha fall asleep in front of the television.

   a. What are some of the factors that might be affecting Tasha at bedtime?

   b. What would you explain to Marti regarding bedtime rituals and routines for toddlers?

   c. What would you suggest Marti do with Tasha at her bedtime?

3. Jed is a 26-month-old child whose family caregivers work outside the home. He goes to a day care center 3 days a week and is kept by his grandmother the other 2 days. Jed's mother asks you for advice in toilet training Jed.

   a. What questions would you ask Jed's mother regarding his physical readiness for toilet training?

   b. What suggestions will you offer regarding bowel training? Bladder training?

   c. How might the variety of caregivers Jed has affect his toilet training?

   d. What could Jed's mother do to provide consistency in toilet training for her child?

Growth and Development of the Preschool Child: 3 to 6 Years

25

Physical Development
Growth Rate
Dentition
Visual Development
Skeletal Growth
Psychosocial Development
Language Development
Development of Imagination
Sexual Development
Social Development

Nutrition
Health Promotion and Maintenance
Routine Checkups
Family Teaching
Accident Prevention
Infection Prevention
The Preschooler in the Health Care
Facility

STUDENT OBJECTIVES

On completion of this chapter, the student should be able to

1. State the major developmental task of the preschooler according to Erikson.
2. Describe the growth rate of the preschooler.
3. State the age at which 20/20 vision usually is attained.
4. Discuss the progression of language development in the preschooler.
5. List four factors that may delay language development.
6. Discuss the role of magical thinking and imagination in the preschooler.
7. Discuss the nurse's role in helping parents understand their preschooler's sexual curiosity.
8. Discuss masturbation in the preschool-age population.
9. List six types of play in which preschoolers engage; define each type.
10. Discuss aggression in the preschooler: (a) verbal aggression, (b) physical aggression, (c) parents' tasks, and (d) parents' example.
11. State the role of discipline for the preschooler: (a) caregiver behavior, (b) effect on child, and (c) effect on caregiver.
12. Discuss the special needs of the disadvantaged preschooler.
13. Discuss the value of Head Start programs.
14. State preschool nutritional needs, including (a) daily minimum needs, (b) appetite variations, (c) suggested snacks, and (d) television commercials and other influences.
15. State the recommended health maintenance schedule for the preschooler.
16. List guidelines for accident prevention in the preschool-age population.
17. List nine health teachings for the preschooler concerning prevention of infection.
18. Identify the preschool social characteristic that increases the risk of infection.

KEY TERMS

associative play
cooperative play
dramatic play
magical thinking
noncommunicative language
onlooker play
parallel play
solitary independent play
unoccupied behavior

Preschoolers are fascinating creatures. As their social circles enlarge to include peers and adults outside the family, preschoolers' language, play patterns, and appearance change markedly. Their curiosity about the world around them grows, as does their ability to explore that world in greater detail and see new meanings in what they find (Fig. 25-1). Preschoolers can be said to soak up information "like a sponge." "Why?" and "how?" are favorite words. This curiosity also means that accidents are still a serious concern.

At 3 years of age, the child still has the chubby, baby-face look of a toddler; by age 5, a leaner, taller, better-coordinated social being has emerged. The child works and plays tirelessly, "making things" and telling everyone about them. In children this age, exploring and learning go on continuously. They sometimes have problems separating fantasy from reality. According to Erikson, the developmental task of the preschool age is initiative versus guilt. Preschoolers often try to find ways to do things to help, but they may feel guilty if scolded when they fail because of inexperience or lack of skill.

PHYSICAL DEVELOPMENT

The physical development seen in the preschool child includes a slowed growth rate, changes in dentition and visual development, as well as skeletal growth changes, especially in the feet and legs.

Growth Rate

The preschool period is one of slow growth. The child gains about 3 to 5 lb each year (1.4 to 2.3 kg) and grows about 2.5 inches (6.3 cm). Because the increase in height is proportionately greater than the increase in weight, the 5-year-old child appears much thinner and less babyish than the 3-year-old child. Boys tend to be leaner than girls are during this time. Gross and fine motor skills continue to develop rapidly (Fig. 25-2). Balance improves and confidence emerges to try new activities. By age 5, the child generally can throw and catch a ball well, climb effectively, and ride a bicycle. Important milestones for growth and development are summarized in Table 25-1.

Dentition

By 6 years of age, the child's skull is 90% of its adult size. The deciduous teeth have completely emerged by the beginning of the preschool period. Toward the end

● **Figure 25.1** Preschoolers engage in meaningful play and are fascinated by what they find. They enjoy dressing up like the people they are playing.

of the preschool stage, these teeth begin to be replaced by permanent teeth. This is an event that most children anticipate as an indication that they are "growing up." Pictures of smiling 5- and 6-year-olds typically show missing front teeth (Fig. 25-3).

The age at which teeth erupt varies with individual children and with various ethnic and economic groups. Permanent teeth of African-American children erupt at least 6 months earlier than those of American children of European ancestry. The central incisors are usually the first to go, just as they were the first to erupt in infancy.

Visual Development

Although the preschooler's senses of taste and smell are acute, visual development is still immature at age 3. Eye-hand coordination is good, but judgment of distances generally is faulty, leading to many bumps and

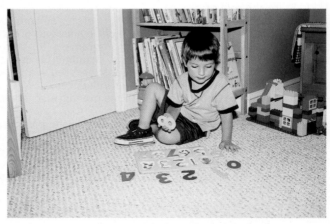

● **Figure 25.2** This 3-year-old child is developing fine motor skills, has good hand-eye coordination, and shows preference for using his right hand in putting a puzzle together.

TABLE 25.1	Growth and Development: The Preschooler				
Age (yr)	Personal–Social	Fine Motor	Gross Motor	Language	Cognition
3	Begins Erikson's stage of "initiative vs. guilt." Conscience develops. Shy with strangers and inept with peers. Sufficiently independent to be interested in group experiences with age mates (e.g., nursery school)	Able to button clothes Copies ○ and + Uses pencils, crayons, paints Shows preference for right or left hand (see Fig. 25-2)	Tends to watch motor activities before attempting them Can jump several feet Uses hands in broad movements Rides tricycle Negotiates stairs well	Vocabulary up to 1,000 words Articulates vowels accurately Talks a lot Sings and recites Asks many questions	Continues in pre-operational state (2–7 years) characterized by: 1. *Centration*, or the inability to attend to more than one aspect of a situation 2. *Egocentricity*, or the inability to consider the perception of others 3. The static and irreversible quality of thought that makes the child unable to perceive the processes of change
4	Boisterous and inflammatory Aggressive physically and verbally but developing behaviors to become socially acceptable Becomes socially acceptable Accepts punishment for wrongdoing because it relieves guilt	Can use scissors; copies a square Adds three parts to stick figures	Has some hesitation but tends to try feats beyond ability Greater powers of balance and accuracy Hops on one foot; can control movements of hands	Vocabulary of about 1,500 words Constant questions Sentences of four or five words Uses profanity Reports fantasies as truth	Reality and fantasy are not always clear to the preschooler. Believes that words make things real— "magical thinking"
5	Initiates contacts with strangers and relates interesting little tales Interested in telling and comparing stories about self Peer relations are important ("best friends" abound) Responds to social values by assuming sex roles with rigidity	Ties shoelaces Copies a diamond and a triangle Prints a few letters or numbers May print first name Cuts food	Will not attempt feats beyond ability Throws and catches ball well Jumps rope Walks backward with heel to toe Skips and hops Adept on bicycle and climbing equipment	Vocabulary of 3,000 words Speech is intelligible Asks meanings of words Enjoys telling stories	Thinks feelings and thoughts can happen Intrusions into the body cause fear and anxiety (fear of mutilation and castration)

falls. During the preschool years, the child's vision should be checked to screen for amblyopia. Usually by age 6 the child has achieved 20/20 vision, but mature depth perception may not occur in some children until 8 to 10 years of age.

Skeletal Growth

Between the third and sixth birthdays, the greatest amount of skeletal growth occurs in the feet and legs. This contributes to the change from the wide-gaited, pot-bellied look of the toddler into the slim, taller

● *Figure 25.3* The smiling 6-year-old is often seen without front teeth.

figure of the 6-year-old child. In addition, the carpals and tarsals mature in the hands and feet, which contributes to better hand and foot control.

Test Yourself

- When do children start to loose their deciduous teeth?

- Give examples of fine motor skill development.

- Give examples of gross motor skill development.

PSYCHOSOCIAL DEVELOPMENT

The preschool age is characteristic of rapid language development. Imagination, sexual and social development, and a variety of types of play also characterize the preschool child's psychosocial development.

Language Development

Between the ages of 3 and 5 years, language development is generally rapid. Most 3-year-old children can construct simple sentences, but their speech has many hesitations and repetitions as they search for the right word or try to make the right sound. Stuttering can develop during this period but usually disappears within 3 to 6 months. By the end of the 5th year, preschoolers use long, rather complex sentences; their vocabulary will have increased by more than 1,500 words since the age of 2.

Preschoolers' use of language changes during this period. Three-year-old children often talk to themselves or to their toys or pets without any apparent purpose other than the pleasure of using words. Piaget called this "egocentric" or **noncommunicative language**. By 4 years of age, children increase their use of communicative language, using words to transmit information other than their own needs and feelings.

Here's a helpful hint. By using a calm, matter-of-fact response when a preschooler uses "naughty" or swear words, some of the power of using that type of language will be diffused. The child learns that this is not language to use in the company of others.

Four- and 5-year-olds delight in using "naughty" words or swearing. Bathroom words become favorites, and taunts such as "you're a big doo-doo" bring heady excitement to them. Caregivers may become concerned by this turn of events, but the child simply may be trying words out to test their impact.

Development of preschoolers' verbal abilities is summarized in Table 25-2.

One or more of the following may cause delays or other difficulties in language development:

- Hearing impairment or other physical problem
- Lack of stimulation
- Overprotection
- Lack of parental interest or rejection by parents

Good language skills are developed as the child is engaged regularly in conversation with caregivers and others. The conversation should be on a level that the child can understand. Reading to the child is an excellent method of contributing to language development. Talking with the child about the pictures in storybooks can enhance this. Praise, approval, and encouragement are all part of supporting attempts at communication.

Family and cultural patterns also influence language development. Some children come from bilingual families and are trying to learn the rules of both languages. Others may come from geographic or social communities that have dialects different from the general population.

Development of Imagination

Preschoolers have learned to think about something without actually seeing it—to visualize or imagine. This normal development, sometimes called **magical thinking**, makes it difficult for them to separate fantasy from reality. Preschoolers believe that words or thoughts can make things real, and this belief can have either positive or negative results. For example, in a moment of anger, a child may wish that a parent or a

TABLE 25.2	Verbal Mastery by Preschoolers	
Age (yr)	Characteristics of Language Usage	Vocabulary Size, Pattern, Comprehension, Rhythm
3–4	Loves to talk; talks a lot; makes up words; sings or recites own version of song; likes new words; asks many questions and wants answers. Not always logical in sentences and concepts. Uses four- or five-word phrases. Aggressive with words rather than actions.	Vocabulary of 900–1500 words; at 3 understands up to 3,600 words, up to 5,600 words by 4. By 4 years, speech understandable even with mispronunciations. May have hesitations, repetitions, and revisions while trying to imitate adult speech. Stuttering may occur but disappears within 3–6 months; may continue up to 2 years without being permanent.
4–5	Understands out-of-context words. Speech highly emotional. Difficulty finding right word; tells function rather than name of item. Changes subject rapidly. Boasts, brags, quarrels; loves "naughty" words. Relates fanciful tales.	Vocabulary of 3,000 words; understands up to 9,600 words by 5 years. Speech completely understandable.

sibling would die; if that person later is hurt, the child feels responsible and suffers guilt. The child needs reassurance that this is not so.

Imagination makes preschoolers good audiences for storytelling, simple plays, and television, as long as the characters and events are not too frightening or sad. When preschoolers see a television character die, they believe it is real and often cry. The child's television viewing should be supervised to avoid programs with negative impact or overstimulation.

During this stage, children often have imaginary playmates who are very real to them. This occurs particularly with only children for whom imaginary playmates fill times of loneliness. The imaginary friend often has the characteristics that the child might wish for. Sometimes the child blames the imaginary friend for breaking a toy or engaging in another act for which the child does not want to take responsibility. Caregivers need assurance that this is normal behavior.

The preschooler's active imagination often leads to a fear of the dark or nightmares. Consequently, problems with sleep are common (see the Sleep Needs section later in this chapter).

Sexual Development

The preschool period is the stage that Freud termed the "oedipal" or "phallic" (genital) period. During these years, children become acutely aware of their sexuality, including sexual roles and organs. They generally develop a strong emotional attachment to the parent of the opposite sex. Children's curiosity about their own genitalia and those of peers and adults may make parents uncomfortable and evoke responses that indicate to the child that sex is dirty and something to be ashamed and guilty about.

Despite today's abundance of sexually oriented literature, many families find it difficult to deal with the young child's questions and actions. Nurses can help caregivers understand that the child's sexual

A PERSONAL GLIMPSE

We had just returned from a weekend visit to my parent's house. My 2-year-old was sleeping quietly. I was in the laundry room doing the laundry from our weekend trip and my 5-year-old (Kayla) was playing in the family room (or so I thought). Suddenly I heard a loud crashing sound that came from the kitchen. I asked, "What was that?" "Nothing Mom." I asked again, "What WAS that?" and headed toward the kitchen. When I got to the kitchen I discovered what the sound had been—the entire sugar canister was empty—the canister on its side, rolling on the floor with the contents all over the cabinet and kitchen floor. Clearly, SOMETHING had happened. I called to Kayla to come to the kitchen. This time I said, "Kayla, tell me how this happened." She told me, "I was playing Legos and Sandy (her imaginary friend) was making cookies just like at Gramma's house and Sandy was getting the sugar and then it was all over the floor." As I looked at the mess she continued, "Like last time Sandy got the toothpaste all over the wall, only this time it was in the kitchen." As upset as I was at having to clean the mess, I thought it was creative of Kayla to use her "imaginary friend" as the mess maker.

Ann

LEARNING OPPORTUNITY: What would you tell this mother regarding preschoolers and imaginary friends? What would you suggest this mother should say to respond to her child in this situation?

curiosity is a normal, natural part of total curiosity about oneself and the surrounding world. The informed, understanding parent can help children develop positive attitudes toward sexuality and toward themselves as sexual human beings.

In addition to responsible teaching of sexual information, the caregiver also should teach the child about "good touch" and "bad touch." The child needs to understand that no one should touch the child's body in a way that is unpleasant.

Masturbation

Exploration of the genitalia is as natural for the preschooler as thumb sucking is for the infant. It is one way the child learns to perceive the body as a possible source of pleasure and is the beginning of the acceptance of sex as natural and pleasurable.

Caregivers can be reassured that this is not uncommon behavior, and a calm, matter-of-fact response to the child found masturbating is the most effective approach. The child should be helped to understand that masturbation is not an activity that is appropriate in public. If the child seems to be masturbating excessively, counseling may be needed, especially if the child's life has been unsettled in other aspects.

Social Development

Preschoolers are outgoing, imaginative, social beings. They play vigorously and, in the process, learn about the world in which they live. As they gain control over their environment, preschoolers try to manipulate it, and this may lead to conflict with caregivers. Preschool children are delightful to watch as they go about the business of growing and learning.

Play

Play activities are one way that children learn. Normally by 3 years of age, children begin imitative play, pretending to be the mommy, the daddy, a policeman, a cowboy, an astronaut, or some well-known person or television character (Fig. 25-4). Caregivers can gain good insight into the way their child interprets family behavior by watching the child play. Listening to a preschooler scold a doll or stuffed animal for "bothering me while I'm busy talking on the phone" lets the adults hear how they sound to the child.

Watch out! Preschoolers love to imitate adults. Dressing up like Mommy or Daddy is a favorite play activity. Listening to a preschooler gives adults an idea of how they sound to the preschooler!

● **Figure 25.4** Imaginative play is common; this preschooler pretends to be a "cowboy."

Preschoolers engage in various types of play: dramatic, cooperative, associative, parallel, solitary independent, onlooker, and unoccupied behavior. **Dramatic play** allows a child to act out troubling situations and to control the solution to the problem. This is important to remember when teaching children who are going to be hospitalized. Using dolls and puppets to explain procedures makes the experience less threatening.

Drawing is another form of play through which children learn to express themselves. During the preschool years as fine motor skills improve, children's drawings become much more complex and controlled and can be revealing about the child's self-concept and perception of the environment.

In **cooperative play**, children play in an organized group with each other as in team sports. **Associative play** occurs when children play together and are engaged in a similar activity but without organization, rules, or a leader, and each child does what she or he wishes. In **parallel play**, children play alongside each other but independently. Although common among toddlers, parallel play exists in all age groups—for example, in a preschool classroom where each student is working on an individual project or craft. **Solitary independent play** means playing apart from others without making an effort to be part of the group or group activity. Watching television is one form of **onlooker play** in which there is observation without participation. In **unoccupied behavior**, the child may be daydreaming or fingering clothing or a toy without apparent purpose.

Children need all types of play to aid in their total development. Too much of one kind may signal a problem; for example, a youngster who spends most of the time unoccupied may be troubled, depressed, or not stimulated. Cooperative play helps to develop social interaction skills and often physical health.

Too much onlooker play, particularly television viewing, means that children are missing the benefits of other kinds of play and may be forming strong, highly inaccurate impressions of people and their behaviors. The amount of time that preschoolers spend watching television should be limited, and interactive play should be encouraged.

Test Yourself

- What is magical thinking? Why do preschoolers have imaginary friends?

- Who do preschool children imitate when they are playing?

- List the types of play seen in the preschool-age child.

Aggression

Temper tantrums are an early form of aggression. The preschooler with newly developed language skills uses words aggressively in name calling and threats. Four-year-old children use physical aggression as well; they push, hit, and kick in an effort to manipulate the environment. The family caregivers' task during these years is to help the child understand that the anger and frustration that result in aggressive behavior are normal but need to be handled differently because aggressive behavior is not socially acceptable.

Children who come from unhappy home situations are likely to be more aggressive than children from a comfortable family situation. Their caregivers have served as role models, and their aggressive behavior toward each other has said to the child, "this is acceptable."

Discipline

Family caregivers need to remember that preschoolers are developing initiative and a sense of guilt. They want to be good and follow instructions, and they feel bad when they do not, even if they are not physically punished. Discipline during this time should strive to teach the child a sense of responsibility and inner control. All the child's caregivers must understand and agree to the limits and disci-

● *Figure 25.5* Although he may not like it, quiet solitude helps the preschooler develop inner control.

pline measures for the child. If one caregiver says "no" and another one says "yes," the child soon learns to play one against the other, leading to confusion about limits. Spanking and other forms of physical punishment remove the responsibility from the child. Taking away a privilege from a child who has misbehaved until he or she can demonstrate that there has been an improvement in behavior is much more effective. Because the child's concept of time is not clear, the period should be comparatively brief (Fig. 25-5). Table 25-3 presents some examples of the effects of caregivers' positive and negative responses.

Nursery School or Day Care Experience

Group experiences with peers and adults outside the immediate family are important to a child's development. However, the transition to new experiences, new people, and new surroundings can be threatening to some preschoolers. Children vary in their willingness or ability to handle new situations; being introduced gradually according to individual readiness produces the most satisfactory adjustment. Some children spend only a few hours each week in a nursery school or other day care program; others must spend a great deal more time away from home and family because the adult family members work outside the home. The family should understand that this probably means that the child will demand more of their attention during the hours when they are together. As the child grows older and the attachment to peers becomes

TABLE 25.3	Effects of Positive and Negative Caregiver Behavior		
Behavior		**Effect on Child**	**Effect on Adult**
Attending only to desired behaviors Calm reasoning with expression of dislike of behavior Physical restraint with adult present Isolation of child for a period of time equal to 1 min per year of age Withholding of desired treats, outings, presents		Development of inner control	Feelings of adequacy as a parent
Yelling, screaming, and implying guilt and punishment Telling child that he or she is bad Physical punishment		Development of fears and compulsive behaviors	Feelings of guilt and inadequacy
Giving treats, presents, or food for lack of undesired behavior Physical punishment Threatening punishment from God or other authority figure		Development of control based on external forces	Feelings of being manipulated by child

stronger, family caregivers sense a decrease in the need for adult attention and a greater sense of independence in the child.

The Disadvantaged Child

Discussions of normal growth and development assume that children come from a secure, well-adjusted home in which there is ample opportunity for social, cultural, and intellectual enrichment. Many children, however, are deprived of such a background for many reasons. This population is the one most likely to have health problems and to need health services.

Children who have not been able to achieve a sense of security and trust, for whatever reason, need special understanding, warm acceptance, and intelligent guidance to grow into self-accepting people. Society is gradually awakening to the needs of these children and is trying to provide enriched nursery school and kindergarten experiences for those whose home life cannot do this for them.

Recognition that environmental enrichment is often unavailable in families with limited social, cultural, and economic resources led to the establishment of Head Start programs. Head Start programs are funded by federal and local money and are free to the children enrolled. Children in such programs have an opportunity to broaden their horizons through varied experiences and to increase their understanding of the world in which they live. Family caregiver participation is a central component of the Head Start concept and often has a positive effect on other children in the household. In some programs, teachers go into the home to help the caregiver teach the young child motor, cognitive, self-help, and language skills. Counseling and referral services are also provided through Head Start programs. Children who have had a background of Head Start enrichment are better prepared to enter kindergarten or first grade and compete successfully with their peers.

NUTRITION

The preschool period is not a time of rapid growth, so children do not need large quantities of food. Nevertheless, protein needs continue to remain high to provide for muscle growth. The preschooler's appetite is erratic; at one sitting the preschooler may devour everything on the plate, and at the next meal he or she may be satisfied with just a few bites. Portions are smaller than adult-sized portions, so the child may need to have meals supplemented with nutritious snacks (Box 25-1). Note that certain snacks are recommended only for the older child to avoid any danger of choking. The preschooler generally best accepts frequent, small meals with snacks in between.

BOX 25.1	Suggested Snacks for the Preschooler

Raw vegetables: carrots,* cucumbers, celery,*green beans, green pepper, mushrooms, turnips, broccoli, cauliflower, tomatoes
Fresh fruits: apples, oranges, pears, peaches, grapes,* cherries,* melons
Unsalted whole-grain crackers
Whole-grain bread: cut to finger-sized sticks; plain, toasted, or with peanut butter
Small sandwiches: cut into quarters
Natural cheese: cut into cubes
Cooked meat: cut into small chunks or sliced thinly
*Nuts**
*Sunflower seeds**
Cookies: made with lightly sweetened whole grains
*Plain popcorn**
Yogurt: plain or with fresh fruit added

* Children younger than 2 years of age may choke on nuts, seeds, popcorn, celery strings, or carrot sticks. Avoid these until preschool years and then always cut into small, bite-sized pieces.

Among the preschooler's favorites are soft foods, grain and dairy products, raw vegetables, and sweets. Television commercials for sugar-coated cereals, snacks, and fast foods of questionable nutritional value exert a powerful influence on the preschooler and can make supermarket shopping an emotional struggle between the caregiver and child. Caregivers should read labels carefully before making a purchase.

Preschoolers need guidance in choosing foods and are strongly influenced by the example of family members and peers. Food should never be used as a reward or bribe; otherwise, the child will continue to use food as a means to manipulate the environment and the behavior of others.

To meet the minimum daily requirements, the preschooler should have two or three glasses of milk each day and several small portions from each food group. Preschoolers have definite food preferences. They generally do not like highly spiced foods, often will eat raw vegetables but not cooked ones, and prefer plain foods, rather than casseroles. New foods may be accepted but should be introduced one at a time to avoid overwhelming the child.

The preschooler shows growing independence and skill in eating. The 3-year-old child tries to mimic adult behavior at the table but often reverts to eating with the fingers, spilling liquids, and squirming (Fig. 25-6). The 4-year-old is more skilled with the use of utensils, although an occasional misjudgment of

● **Figure 25.6** The preschooler may attempt to use a fork or spoon or revert to using fingers when eating.

abilities results in a mess. The 5-year-old uses utensils well, often can cut his or her own food, and can be taught to practice sophisticated table manners. Rituals such as using the same plate, cereal bowl, cup, or placemat may become important to the child's mealtime happiness.

HEALTH PROMOTION AND MAINTENANCE

Routine checkups, family teaching, as well as accident and infection prevention are all important aspects of health promotion and maintenance for the preschool child.

Routine Checkups

Preschoolers with up-to-date immunizations need boosters of diphtheria–tetanus–pertussis, polio vaccine, and measles–mumps–rubella (MMR) vaccine between 4 and 6 years of age. These are required as preschool boosters for entrance into kindergarten.

An annual health examination is recommended to monitor the child's growth and development and to screen for potential health problems. Recommended screening procedures include urinalysis, hematocrit, lead level, tuberculin skin testing, and Denver Developmental Screening Test. The preschool child needs to be told in advance about the upcoming examination. Use simple explanations and provide an opportunity for the child to ask questions and voice anxieties. A number of books available through public libraries are excellent for this purpose. Children who attend nursery school or a day care program are sometimes required to have an annual examination, but children who stay at home may not have this advantage. Particular attention should be paid to the child's vision and hearing so that any problems can be treated before he or she enters school at age 5 or 6. A semiannual dental examination is also recommended.

Family Teaching

The nurse can use routine checkups and any other opportunities to teach caregivers about common aspects of everyday life with a preschooler. Preschoolers are busy learning and showing initiative as they are involved in their day-to-day lives. Preschoolers are usually a pleasure to be around because they are so eager to learn anything new and are full of questions.

Bathing

Although preschoolers view themselves as "grown-up," they still need continual supervision while bathing. The caregiver should run the bath water. The hot water heater should be turned to no higher than 120°F (49°C) to avoid the danger of burns. Children should be taught to leave the faucets alone. Preschoolers can generally wash themselves with supervision. Ears, necks, and faces are spots that often need extra attention. Hands and fingernails often get soaked clean in the tub, but fingernails do need to be checked by the caregiver.

Preschoolers cannot wash their own hair, so this can be a time of tension between the child and caregiver. Shampooing in the tub with a nonirritating children's shampoo may work best. The child can lean the head back, look at the ceiling, and hold a washcloth on the forehead to keep water and soap from getting into the eyes. Shampoo protectors (clear plastic brims with no crowns) can be purchased if desired.

Bath time can be rather lengthy if the preschooler gets involved in playing with bath toys. This is something the caregiver can negotiate if limits need to be set. Some children this age are interested in taking a shower and may do so with adult supervision.

When washing their hands before meals or before or after going to the bathroom, preschoolers often wash only the fronts while totally ignoring the backs. If not supervised, the child may use only cold water and no soap. Again, the caregiver should turn the water on to a warm temperature to avoid burns.

Dental Care

The preschool child needs to be supervised in tooth brushing. Although the preschooler can brush well, the caregiver should check the cleanliness of the child's teeth. The caregiver should be responsible for flossing because the preschooler does not have the necessary motor skills. To help prevent tooth decay, the preschooler should be encouraged to eat healthy snacks such as fruits, raw vegetables, and natural cheeses, rather than candy, cakes, or sugar-filled gum. The use of fluoridated water or fluoride supplements should be continued.

Dressing

The preschooler may have definite ideas about what he or she wants to wear. Giving the child the opportunity to choose what to wear each day is an excellent way to begin fostering a sense of control and to help the child learn to make decisions. Preschoolers do not have very good taste in what matches, so some interesting outfits may result! Nevertheless, the child should be permitted to make these choices, and the caregivers (as well as older siblings and other adults) should accept the choices without negative comments. When it does matter—for the adults–how the child is dressed, the best plan is to give the child limited choices that will suit the occasion.

Toileting

By the preschool years, almost all children have succeeded in toilet training, although an occasional accident may occur. When the child does have an accident, treating it in a matter-of-fact way and providing the child with clean, dry clothing is best. The preschooler needs continual reminders to wash the hands before and after toileting. Little girls should be taught to wipe from front to back. Preschoolers may still need to be checked for careful wiping, especially after a bowel movement.

Bed-wetting is not uncommon for young preschoolers and is not a concern unless it continues past the age of 5 to 7 (see Chapter 38 for further discussion).

Sleep Needs

Preschoolers are often ready to give up their nap. This may depend partially on it if they go to a preschool program that has a rest time. Often preschoolers will just curl up and fall asleep on a chair, a couch, or the floor. Bedtime can still be a challenge, but leading up to it with a period of quiet activities or stories encourages the child to wind down for the day.

Creativity can be useful. One mother solved the problem of her child's fear of going to sleep in an interesting fashion. The child was afraid of a monster in the closet or under the bed. The mother acknowledged the child's fears and purchased a spray can of room air freshener. At bedtime, she ceremoniously sprayed around the room, in the closet, and under the bed. She assured the child that it was a special spray to kill monsters, just like bug spray kills bugs. The child was reassured and slept without fear.

Dreams and nightmares are common during the preschool period. Caregivers need to explain that "it was only a dream" and offer love and understanding until the fear has subsided. Fear of the dark is another common problem during these years. Children may be afraid to go to sleep in a dark bedroom. These are very real fears to the child. A small night light may be reassuring to the child.

Accident Prevention

Adults caring for preschoolers need to be just as attentive as they are with toddlers because a child's curiosity at this stage still exceeds his or her judgment. Burns, poisoning, and falls are common accidents. Preschoolers are often victims of motor vehicle accidents either because they dart into the street or driveway or fail to wear proper restraints. All states have laws that define safety seat and restraint requirements for children. Adults must teach and reinforce these rules. One primary responsibility of adults is always to wear seat belts themselves and to make certain that the child always is in a safety seat or has a seat belt on when in a motor vehicle. A child can be calmly taught that the vehicle "won't go" unless the child is properly restrained.

By the age of 5, many preschoolers move from riding a tricycle to riding a bicycle. If the preschooler is not already wearing a bicycle helmet, it is important to educate caregivers that safety helmets are a necessary safety precaution. Lightweight, child-sized safety helmets that fit properly can be purchased, and the child should be taught that the helmet must be worn when riding a bike (Fig. 25-7). Adults who wear helmets provide the best incentive to children. Safety rules for bicycle riding should be reinforced. The preschool child should be limited to protected areas for riding and should have adult supervision.

The preschool age is an excellent time to begin teaching safety rules. The rules for crossing the street and playing in an area near traffic are of vital importance. Adults who care for preschool children should be careful to serve as good role models. These safety rules should extend into all aspects of the child's life. See Family Teaching Tips: Preschooler Safety Teaching.

Test Yourself

- What are the major causes of accidents in the preschool child?

- List measures preschoolers should be taught to prevent accidents.

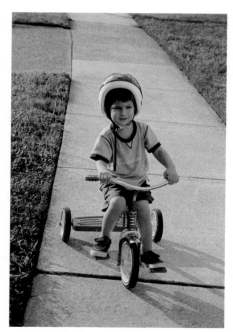

● **Figure 25.7** This preschooler has learned to always wear a proper safety helmet.

FAMILY TEACHING TIPS

Preschoolers Safety Teaching

- Look both ways before crossing the street.
- Cross the street only with an adult.
- Watch for cars coming out of driveways.
- Never play behind a car or truck.
- Watch for cars or trucks backing up.
- Wear a safety helmet when bike riding.
- Learn your name, address, and phone number.
- Stay away from strange dogs.
- Stay away from any dog while it's eating.
- Take only medicine that your caregiver gives you.
- Don't play with matches or lighters.
- Stay away from fires.
- Don't run near a swimming pool.
- Only swim when with an adult.
- Don't go anywhere with someone you don't know.
- Don't let anyone touch you in a way you don't like.

Infection Prevention

Preschoolers who enjoy sound nutrition and adequate rest, exercise, and shelter usually are not seriously affected by simple childhood infections. Children who live in less than adequate economic circumstances, however, can be severely threatened by even a simple illness, such as diarrhea or chickenpox. Immunizations are available for many childhood communicable diseases, but some caregivers do not have their children immunized until it is required for entrance to school. As a result, some children suffer unnecessary illnesses.

Preschoolers are just learning to share, and that can mean sharing infections with the entire family— and playmates as well. Teaching them basic precautions can help prevent the spread of infections. See Family Teaching Tips: Teaching to Prevent Infections.

FAMILY TEACHING TIPS

Teaching to Prevent Infections

- Cover your mouth when coughing or sneezing.
- Throw away tissues used for nose blowing.
- Wipe carefully after bowel movements (girls wipe front to back).
- Wash hands after going to bathroom or blowing your nose.
- Wash hands before eating.
- Do not share food that you've partly eaten.
- If food or an eating utensil falls on the floor, wash it right away.
- Do not drink from another person's cup.
- Do not share a toothbrush with someone else.

THE PRESCHOOLER IN THE HEALTH CARE FACILITY

The preschooler may view hospitalization as an exciting new adventure or as a frightening, dangerous experience, depending on the preparation by caregivers and health professionals. As mentioned, play is an effective way to let children act out their anxieties and to learn what to expect from the hospital situation. Preschoolers are frightened about intrusive procedures; therefore, it is preferable to take the temperature with an oral or tympanic thermometer, rather than with a rectal one.

Some nurses find this approach helpful. Children are less anxious about procedures if they are allowed to handle equipment beforehand and perhaps "use" it on a doll or another toy.

The hospitalized preschooler may revert to bed-wetting but should not be scolded for it. The nurse should assure the family that this is normal. Explanations of where the bathrooms are and how to use the call light or bell to get help can help avoid problems with bed-wetting. If a child is afraid of the dark, a night light can be provided.

Hospital routines should follow home routines as closely as possible. The child should be allowed to participate in the care, even though this may take longer. All procedures should be carefully explained to the child in words appropriate for the child's age; repeat the information as necessary.

● *Figure 25.8* This hospitalized child can enjoy age-appropriate activities, even when on bed rest.

If the child is ambulatory and not on infection-control precautions, the playroom can offer diversionary activities. If not, play materials can be provided for use in bed (Fig. 25-8)

KEY POINTS

▶ According to Erikson, the major developmental task for the preschool-age group is initiative versus guilt.

▶ During the preschool years, psychosocial growth is substantial but physical growth slows.

▶ By the age of 6, children usually have achieved 20/20 vision.

▶ Language develops rapidly during the preschool period, progressing from the ability to use simple sentences at age 3 to telling sometimes long and involved stories by age 5.

▶ Language development may be delayed because of hearing impairment or physical problems, lack of stimulation, overprotection, or lack of parental support.

▶ Magical thinking and imagination contribute to fears and anxieties of the preschooler because these make it difficult for the child to separate fantasy from reality. Caregivers must acknowledge these concerns, be patient with explanations, and offer reassurance to the child.

▶ A preschooler's sexual curiosity and exploration of her or his genitalia is normal. A calm, understanding caregiver can help the child develop positive attitudes about herself/himself as a sexual being.

▶ Dramatic play allows for acting out troubling situations, cooperative play is seen when children play in organized groups, and associative play occurs when there is no organization or rules, but children are engaged in a similar activity. When children play apart from others, it is solitary independent play; watching TV is a form of onlooker play; and in unoccupied play the child is often daydreaming without specific purpose.

▶ The preschooler may show verbal aggression by name calling and physical aggression by pushing, hitting, or kicking. The caregiver serves as a role model and disciplines by setting limits and helping the child to develop inner control and take responsibility for his/her actions.

▶ The disadvantaged child who has not been able to develop a sense of trust needs understanding, acceptance, and guidance to develop appropriately. Programs such as Head Start give children opportunities to promote development.

▶ Even though the preschool child has a decreased and erratic appetite, adequate protein, nutritious snacks, and avoidance of foods that lack nutritional value are important.

♦ Preschoolers should have annual routine checkups to monitor growth, receive immunizations, and for screening.

♦ Seat belt use, wearing bicycle safety helmets, and practicing street safety will help in prevention of accidents in the preschooler. Stranger, fire, and swimming safety should also be taught.

♦ The preschooler learns to share with family and playmates and in the process often shares infections. To prevent infection, the child istaught to cover his or her mouth when coughing or sneezing, proper disposal of tissues, correct wiping after bowel movements, good hand washing, and not to share cups, utensils, food, or toothbrushes.

REFERENCES AND SELECTED READINGS

Books and Journals
Berger, K. S. (2001). *The developing person through the life span.* New York: Worth Publishers.

Brazelton, T. B. (2001). *Touchpoints three to six: Your child's emotional and behavioral development.* Cambridge, MA: Perseus Publishing.

Brazelton, T. B., & Greenspan, S. (2001). *The irreducible needs of children: What every child must have to grow, learn, and flourish.* Cambridge, MA: Perseus Publishing.

Dudek, S. G. (2000). *Nutrition essentials for nursing practice* (4th ed.). Philadelphia: Lippincott Williams & Wilkins.

Dworkin, P. (2000). *Pediatrics* (4th ed.). Philadelphia: Lippincott Williams & Wilkins.

Hockenberry, M. J., Wilson, D., Winkelstein, M. L., & Kline, N. E. (2003). *Wong's nursing care of infants and children* (7th ed.). St. Louis: Mosby.

Pillitteri, A. (2003). *Maternal and child health nursing* (4th ed.). Philadelphia: Lippincott Williams & Wilkins.

Spock, B., et al. (1998). *Dr. Spock's baby and child care.* New York: Pocket Books.

Wong, D. L., Perry, S., & Hockenberry, M. (2002). *Maternal child nursing care* (2nd ed.). St. Louis: Mosby.

Web Addresses
Head Start Programs
http://www2.acf.dhhs.gov/programs/hsb
www.ecewebguide.com
www.earlychildhood.com

WORKBOOK

NCLEX-STYLE REVIEW QUESTIONS

1. The nurse is assisting with a well-child visit for a 5 ½-year-old child. This child's records show that at the age of 3 years, this child weighed 32 pounds, was 35.5 inches tall, had 20 teeth, and slept 11 hours a day. If this child is following a normal pattern of growth and development, which of the following would the nurse expect to find in this visit? The child

   a. weighs 54 pounds.

   b. measures 40 inches in height.

   c. has two permanent teeth.

   d. sleeps 2 hours for a morning nap.

2. In working with a group of preschool children, which of the following activities would this age child *most* likely be doing?

   a. Pretending to be television characters.

   b. Playing a game with large balls and blocks.

   c. Participating in a group activity.

   d. Collecting stamps or coins.

3. The nurse is talking with a group of caregivers of preschool-age children. Which of the following statements made by a caregiver would require further data collection?

   a. "My child calls her sister bad names when she doesn't get her way."

   b. "She told me her imaginary friend broke my favorite picture frame."

   c. "My son always wants to eat cookies for lunch and for snacks."

   d. "Even when his friends are over to play, he wants to play by himself."

4. A caregiver of a preschool-age child says to the nurse, "My 4-year-old touches her genitals sometimes when she is resting." Which of the following statements would be appropriate for the nurse to respond?

   a. "Masturbation is embarrassing to the parents; scolding the child will stop the behavior."

   b. "When children are angry or upset, they often masturbate."

   c. "When this age child masturbates, it can be unhealthy and dangerous."

   d. "Masturbation is a normal behavior, so providing another activity for the child would be appropriate."

5. In teaching caregivers of preschool children, the nurse would reinforce that which of the following would be *most* important for this age group? The preschool child should

   a. brush and floss teeth after snacks and meals.

   b. cover mouth when coughing or sneezing.

   c. be screened for amblyopia.

   d. wear a seat belt when riding in a vehicle.

6. In working with the preschool-age child and this child's family, teaching regarding prevention of infection is important. Which of the following are true regarding prevention of infection? Select all that apply:

   a. Girls should be taught to wipe from front to back after a bowel movement.

   b. Sharing foods or utensils with family members is acceptable.

   c. It is important to wash hands after coughing, sneezing, or blowing your nose.

   d. Each person should have her/his own toothbrush and use only that one.

   e. When washing hands, cold water works as well as warm water.

STUDY ACTIVITIES

1. List and compare the fine motor skills, gross motor skills, and language development in each of the following ages:

	3 Years	4 Years	5 Years
Fine motor skills			
Gross motor skills			
Language development			

2. Describe the guidelines you would give a family to help children develop good eating habits and encourage the trying of new foods. Write a 1-day menu, including snacks, for a preschooler.

3. You are working with the staff in a day care facility to help them develop activities for their preschool program. Using your knowledge of preschool growth and development, make a list of behaviors you would teach the staff to look for in the preschooler. What activities would you suggest to encourage normal preschool growth and development?

4. Go to the following Internet site: http://www.childrens.com/patients_families/healthinfo/

   In the search box, where it says "Choose," drop down to "Dental & Oral Health." Click on the "Go" circle. On the right side of the screen, click on "Preschool and School-aged Problems." On the right side of the screen, click on "Tooth Decay."

   a. Who is at risk for tooth decay?

   b. Look at the section "Smart Snacking." List three things you would suggest a caregiver to consider when choosing a snack for a preschool child.

   c. Read the section "Preventing Tooth Decay." What five things suggested can be done to prevent tooth decay in the preschooler?

CRITICAL THINKING: What Would You Do?

1. Clara has noticed her 5-year-old son Ted masturbating. She is upset and comes to you for help.

   a. What reactions and concerns might Clara express regarding masturbation in her preschool child?

   b. What will you tell Clara to help her understand preschoolers and masturbation?

   c. What actions would you suggest for Clara to do when she notices Ted is masturbating?

2. Jenny reports that her 3½-year-old daughter, Krista, wakes up screaming in the middle of the night. This is causing the family to lose sleep.

   a. What concerns do you think Jenny might have regarding this situation?

   b. What characteristics of a preschooler might be causing Krista to wake up at night screaming?

   c. What would you suggest Jenny do and say to Krista when this happens?

3. A group of caregivers of 4-year-olds are discussing their children and the behaviors they are noticing. One of the caregivers states, "My child is so frustrating." Several of the other caregivers nod their heads in agreement.

   a. What characteristics of preschoolers might lead to these caregivers' feelings of frustration?

   b. What explanations would you offer these caregivers as to the reasons they are seeing these behaviors in their children?

   c. How would you suggest these caregivers respond when they feel frustrated by these preschoolers?

Growth and Development of the School-Age Child: 6 to 10 Years

Physical Development
  Growth
  Dentition
  Skeletal Growth
Psychosocial Development
  The Child From Ages 6 to 7 Years
  The Child From Ages 7 to 10 Years
Nutrition

Health Promotion and
  Maintenance
    Routine Checkups
    Family Teaching
    Health Education
    Accident Prevention
The School-Age Child in the Health
  Care Facility

STUDENT OBJECTIVES

On completion of this chapter, the student should be able to

1. Discuss the physical growth patterns during the school-age years.
2. Describe dentition in this age group.
3. State the major developmental task of the school-age group according to Erikson.
4. State factors that may deter successful completion of the developmental task of industry versus inferiority.
5. Discuss the importance of "gangs" to the 7- to 8-year-old child.
6. Identify nutritional influences on the school-age child, including (a) family attitudes, (b) mealtime atmosphere, (c) snacks, and (d) school's role.
7. List three factors that contribute to obesity in the school-age child.
8. State two appropriate ways to help an obese child control weight.
9. Describe practices that contribute to good dental hygiene for this age group.
10. State the usual amount of sleep the school-age child needs.
11. Discuss the need for sex education in the school-age group: (a) family's role, (b) school's role, and (c) others' role.
12. Identify common inhalant products that children may use as deliriants.
13. Discuss principles that a family caregiver can use to teach children about substance abuse.
14. Describe safety education appropriate for the school-age group.
15. State several factors that may influence the school-age child's hospital experience.
16. Briefly describe the progression in the 6- to 10-year-old child's concept of biology: (a) birth, (b) death, (c) human body, (d) health, and (e) illness.

KEY TERMS

classification
conservation
decentration
deliriants
epiphyses
hierarchical arrangement
inhalants
reversibility
scoliosis

The first day of school marks a major milestone in a child's development, opening a new world of learning and growth. Between the ages of 6 and 10 years, dramatic changes occur in the child's thinking process, social skills, activities, attitudes, and use of language. The squirmy, boisterous 6-year-old child with a limited attention span bears little resemblance to the more reserved 10-year-old child who can become absorbed in a solitary craft activity for several hours.

Moving from the small circle of family into the school and community, children begin to see differences in their own lives and the lives of others. They constantly compare their families with other children's families and observe the way other children are disciplined, the foods they eat, the way they dress, and their homes. Every aspect of lifestyle is subject to comparison.

Most children reach school age with the necessary skills, abilities, and independence to function successfully in this new environment. They can feed and dress themselves, use the primary language of their culture to communicate their needs and feelings, and separate from their caregivers for extended periods. They show increasing interest in group activities and in making things. Children of this age work at many activities that involve motor, cognitive, and social skills. Success in these activities provides the child with self-confidence and a feeling of competence. Erikson's developmental task for this age group is industry versus inferiority. Children who are unsuccessful in completing activities during this stage, whether from physical, social, or cognitive disadvantages, develop a feeling of inferiority.

The health of the school-age child is no longer the exclusive concern of the family but of the community as well. Before admittance, most schools require that children have a physical examination and that immunizations meet state requirements. Generally this is a healthy period in the child's life, although minor respiratory disorders and other communicable diseases can spread quickly within a classroom. Few major diseases have their onset during this period. Accidents still pose a serious hazard; therefore, safety measures are an important part of learning.

PHYSICAL DEVELOPMENT

The physical development of the school-age child includes changes in weight and height, as well as changes in dentition and the eruption of permanent teeth. The school-age child's skeletal growth and changes are evident during this time period.

Growth

Between the ages of 6 and 10 years, growth is slow and steady. Average annual weight gain is about 5 to 6 lb (2 to 3 kg). By age 7, the child weighs about seven times

as much as at birth. Annual height increase is about 2.5 inches (6 cm). This period ends in the preadolescent growth spurt in girls at about age 10 and in boys at about age 12.

Dentition

At about age 6, the child starts to lose the deciduous ("baby") teeth, usually beginning with the lower incisors. At about the same time, the first permanent teeth, the 6-year molars, appear directly behind the deciduous molars (Fig. 26-1). These 6-year molars are of the utmost importance: they are the key or pivot teeth that help to shape the jaw and affect the alignment of the permanent teeth. If these molars are allowed to decay so severely that they must be removed, the child will have dental problems later. (More information on care of the teeth is given later in this chapter.)

Skeletal Growth

The 6-year-old's silhouette is characterized by a flatter, but still protruding abdomen and lordosis (sway-back). By the time the child has reached the age of 10 years, the spine is straighter, the abdomen flatter, and the body generally more slender and long-legged (Fig. 26-2).

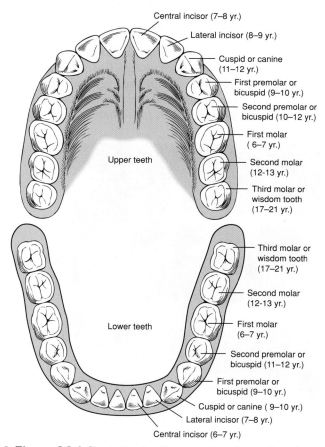

Central incisor (7–8 yr.)
Lateral incisor (8–9 yr.)
Cuspid or canine (11–12 yr.)
First premolar or bicuspid (9–10 yr.)
Second premolar or bicuspid (10–12 yr.)
First molar (6–7 yr.)
Second molar (12-13 yr.)
Third molar or wisdom tooth (17–21 yr.)

Upper teeth

Third molar or wisdom tooth (17–21 yr.)
Second molar (12-13 yr.)
First molar (6–7 yr.)
Second premolar or bicuspid (11–12 yr.)
First premolar or bicuspid (9–10 yr.)
Cuspid or canine (9–10 yr.)
Lateral incisor (7–8 yr.)
Central incisor (6–7 yr.)

Lower teeth

● **Figure 26.1** Chart showing the sequence of eruption of permanent teeth.

● *Figure 26.2* (*Left*) Profile of a 6-year-old showing protuberant abdomen. (*Right*) Profile of a 10-year-old showing flat abdomen and four curves of adult-like spine.

Bone growth occurs mostly in the long bones and is gradual during the school years. Cartilage is being replaced by bone at the **epiphyses** (growth centers at the end of long bones and at the wrists). Skeletal maturation is more rapid in girls than in boys and in African-American children than in whites. Growth and development of the school-age child is summarized in Table 26-1 (see also Fig. 26-3).

Test Yourself

- Why is the health of a child's first permanent molars important?
- What are the growth centers at the end of the long bones and wrist called?

PSYCHOSOCIAL DEVELOPMENT

A sense of duty and accomplishment occupies the years from 6 to 10. During this stage the child is interested in engaging in meaningful projects and seeing them through to completion. The child applies the energies earlier put into play toward accomplishing tasks and often spends numerous sessions on one project. With these attempts come the refinement of motor, cognitive, and social skills and development of a positive sense of self. Some school-age children, however, may not be ready for this stage because of environmental deprivation, a dysfunctional family, insecure attachment to parents, immaturity, or other reasons. Entering school at a disadvantage, these children may not be ready to be productive. Excessive or unrealistic goals set by a teacher or caregiver who is insensitive to this child's needs will defeat such a

A

B

● *Figure 26.3* (**A**) This 6-year-old enjoys cutting shapes with safety scissors. (**B**) This 6-year-old shows off his ability to hop on one foot. Photo by B. Proud.

TABLE 26.1	Developmental Milestones for the School-Age Child					
Age (yr)	Physical	Motor	Personal-Social	Language	Perceptual	Cognitive
6	Average height 45 inches (116 cm) Average weight 46 lb (21 kg) Loses first tooth (upper incisors) Six-year molars erupt Food "jags" Appetite increased	Tie shoes Can use scissors (see Fig. 26-3A) Runs, jumps, climbs, skips Can ride bicycle Can't sit for long periods Cuts, pastes, prints, draws with some detail	Increased need to socialize with same sex Egocentric— believes everyone thinks as they do Still in pre- operational stage until age 7	Uses every form of sentence structure Vocabulary of 2,500 words Sentence length about 5 words	Knows right from left May reverse letters Can discriminate vertical horizontal, and oblique Perceives pictures in parts or whole but not both	Recognizes simple words Conservation of number Defines objects by use Can group according to an attribute to form subclasses
7	Weight is seven times birth weight Gains 4.4–6.6 lb/yr (2–3 kg) Grows 2–2.5 inches/yr (5–6 cm)	More cautious Swims Printing smaller than 6-year- old's Activity level lower than 6-year-old's	More cooperative Same-sex play group and friends Less egocentric	Can name day, month, season Produces all language sounds	b, p, d, q confusion resolved Can copy a diamond	Begins to use simple logic Can group in ascending order Grasps basic idea of addition and subtraction Conservation of substance Can tell time
8	Average height 49.5 inches (127 cm) Average weight 55 lb (25 kg)	Movements more graceful Writes in cursive Can throw and hit a baseball Has symmetric balance and can hop (see Fig. 26-3B)	Adheres to simple rules Hero worship begins Same-sex peer group	Gives precise definitions Articulation near adult level	Can catch a ball Visual acuity 20/20 Perceives pictures in parts and whole	Increasing memory span Interest in causal relation Conservation of length Can put thoughts in a chronologic sequence
9-10	Average height 51.5–53.5 inches (132–137 cm) Average weight 59.5–77 lb (27–35 kg)	Good coordination Can achieve the strength and speed needed for most sports	Enjoys team competition Moves from group to best friend Hero worship intensifies	Can use language to convey thoughts and look at other's point of view	Eye–hand coordination almost perfect	Classifies objects Understands explanations Conservation of area and weight Describes characteristics of objects Can group in descending order

child and possibly lead to the child's feeling inferior, rather than self-confident.

When environmental support is adequate, several personality development tasks should be completed during these years. These tasks include developing coping mechanisms, a sense of right and wrong, a feeling of self-esteem, and an ability to care for oneself.

During the school-age years, the child's cognitive skills develop; at about the age of 7 years, the child enters the concrete operational stage identified by Piaget. The skills of **conservation** (the ability to recognize that a change in shape does not necessarily mean a change in amount or mass) are significant in this stage. This begins with the conservation of numbers, when the child understands that the number of cookies does not change even though they may be rearranged, along with the conservation of mass, when the child can see that an amount of cookie dough is the same whether in ball form or flattened for baking. This is followed by conservation of weight, in which the child recognizes that a pound is a pound, regardless of whether plastic or bricks are weighed. Conservation of volume (for instance, a half-cup of water is the same amount regardless of the shape of the container) does not come until late in the concrete operational stage, at about 11 or 12 years of age.

Each child is a product of personal heredity, environment, cognitive ability, and physical health. Every child needs love and acceptance, with understanding, support, and concern when mistakes are made. Children thrive on praise and recognition and will work to earn them (see Family Teaching Tips: Guiding Your School-Age Child).

This is important. The school-age child needs consistent rules, positive attention, and clear expectations in order to develop self-confidence.

The Child From Ages 6 to 7 Years

Children in the age group of 6 to 7 years are still characterized by magical thinking—believing in the tooth fairy, Santa Claus, the Easter Bunny, and others. Keen imaginations contribute to fears, especially at night, about remote, fanciful, or imaginary events. Trouble distinguishing fantasy from reality can contribute to lying to escape punishment or to boost self-confidence.

Children who have attended a day care center, preschool, kindergarten, or Head Start program usually make the transition into first grade with pleasure, excitement, and little anxiety. Those without that experience may find it helpful to visit the school to experience separation from home and caregivers and to try getting along with other children on a trial basis. Most 6-year-old children can sit still for short periods of time and understand about taking turns. Those who have not matured sufficiently for this experience will find school unpleasant and may not do well.

Group activities are important to most 6-year-old children, even if the groups include only two or three children. They delight in learning and show an intense interest in every experience. Judgment about acceptable and unacceptable behavior is not well developed and possibly results in name calling and the use of vulgar words.

FAMILY TEACHING TIPS

Guiding Your School-Age Child

- Give your child consistent love and attention. Try to see the situation through your child's eyes. Do your best to avoid a hostile or angry reaction toward your child.
- Know where your child is at all times and who his or her friends are. Never leave your child home alone.
- Encourage your child to become involved in school and community activities. Become involved with your child's activities whenever possible. Encourage fair play and good sportsmanship.
- Show your children good examples by your behavior toward others.
- Never hit your children. Physical punishment shows them that it is all right to hit others and that they can solve problems in that way.
- Use positive nonphysical methods of discipline such as
  - "Time out"—1 minute per year is an appropriate amount of time.
  - "Grounding"—don't permit them to play with friends or take part in a special activity.
  - Take away a special privilege.
- Set these limits for brief periods only. Consistency is extremely important in setting these restrictions.
- Be consistent. Make a reasonable rule, let your child know the rule, and then stick with it. You can involve your children in helping to set rules.
- Treat your child with love and respect. Always try to find the "positives" and praise the child for those behaviors. Don't treat your child in a manner that you would not use with an adult friend.
- Let the child know what you expect of him or her. Children who have responsibilities (age-appropriate) learn self-discipline and self-control.
- When you have a problem with your child, try to sit down and solve it together. Help him or her figure out ways to solve problems nonviolently.

Between the ages of 6 and 8 years, children begin to enjoy participating in real-life activities, such as helping with gardening, housework, and other chores. They love making things, such as drawings, paintings, and craft projects (Fig. 26-4).

The Child From Ages 7 to 10 Years

Between the seventh and eighth birthdays, children begin to shake off their acceptance of parental standards as the ultimate authority and become more impressed by the behavior of their peers. Interest in group play increases, and acceptance by the group or gang is

● *Figure 26.4* A 6-year-old works with her grandfather on a woodworking project.

● *Figure 26.5* This 8-year-old girl enjoys being part of a sports team.

tremendously important. These groups quickly become all-boy or all-girl groups and are often project oriented, such as Scout troops or athletic teams. Private clubs with homemade clubhouses, secret codes, and languages are popular. Individual friendships also are formed, and "best friends" are intensely loyal, if only for short periods. Table games, arts and crafts requiring skill and dexterity, computer games, school science projects, and science fairs are popular, as are more active pursuits. This period includes the beginning of many neighborhood team sports, including Little League, softball, football, and soccer (Fig. 26-5). Both boys and girls are actively involved in many of these sports.

Even though parents are no longer considered the ultimate authority, their standards have become part of the child's personality and conscience. Although the child may cheat, lie, or steal on occasion, he or she suffers considerable guilt if he or she learns that these are unacceptable behaviors.

Important changes occur in a child's thinking processes at about age 7 years, when there is move-

ment from preoperational, egocentric thinking to concrete, operational, decentered thought. For the first time, children can see the world from someone else's point of view. **Decentration** means being able to see several aspects of a problem at the same time and to understand the relation of various parts to the whole situation. Cause-and-effect relations become clear; consequently, magical thinking begins to disappear.

During the seventh or eighth year, children have an increased understanding of the conservation of continuous quantity. Understanding conservation depends on **reversibility**, the ability to think in either direction. Seven-year-old children can add and subtract, count forward and backward, and see how it is possible to put something back the way it was. A 7- or 8-year-old can understand that illness is probably only temporary, whereas a 6-year-old may think it is permanent.

Another important change in thinking during this period is **classification**, the ability to group objects into a **hierarchical arrangement** (grouping by some common system). Children in this age group love to collect sports cards, insects, rocks, stamps, coins, or anything else that strikes their fancy. These collections may be only a short-term interest, but some can develop into lifetime hobbies.

This tip will be fun and useful.

The school-age child loves to collect and count objects. Checking the child's pockets after school can be quite an adventure!

CULTURAL SNAPSHOT

In some cultures children are pressured to achieve high scores in school, as well as on college entrance exams, to bring value and pride to the family and culture. These children sometimes are pushed to study rather than to play and have normal relationships with their peers.

Test Yourself

- How is the developmental task of industry attained in the school-age child?

- What sex are most of the school-age child's friends and play groups?

NUTRITION

As coordination improves, the child becomes increasingly active and requires more food to supply necessary energy. The nutritional needs of the school-age child should be met by choosing foods from all the food groups with the appropriate number of servings from each group in the child's daily diet (Table 26-2). Increased appetite and a tendency to go on food "jags" are typical of the 6-year-old child. This stage soon passes and is unimportant if the child generally gets the necessary nutrients. As the child's tastes develop, once-disliked foods may become favorites unless earlier battles have been waged over the food. Children are more likely to learn to eat most foods if everyone else accepts them in a matter-of-fact way.

Children learn by the examples that caregivers and others set for them. They will accept more readily the importance of manners, calm voices, appropriate table conversation, and courtesy if they see them carried out consistently at home. To keep mealtime a positive and pleasant time, mealtime should never be used for nagging, finding fault, correcting manners, or discussing a poor report card. Hygiene should be taught in a cheerful but firm manner, even if the child must leave

Offering choices can make a difference. Allowing the child to express food dislikes and permitting refusal of a disliked food item is usually the best way to handle the school-age child.

TABLE 26.2	Daily Nutritional Needs of the 6- to 10-year-old	
Food Group	**Number of Servings Daily**	**Examples of Serving Sizes**
Bread, cereal, rice and pasta group (especially whole grains)	9	1 slice bread ½ hamburger bun or English muffin a small roll, biscuit, muffin 3 or 4 small or 2 large crackers ½ cup cooked cereal, rice, pasta 1 oz ready-to-eat cereal
Vegetable group	4	½ cup cooked vegetables ½ cup chopped raw vegetables 1 cup leafy raw vegetables such as lettuce or spinach
Fruit group	3	1 apple, banana, orange ½ grapefruit a melon wedge ¾ cup juice ½ cup berries ½ cup cooked or canned fruit ¼ cup dried fruit
Milk, yogurt, cheese—milk group	2 or 3	1 cup milk 8 oz yogurt 1½ oz natural cheese 2 oz processed cheese
Meat, poultry, fish, dry beans, eggs, and nuts group	2 for a total of 6 oz	Total 6 oz a day—lean meat, poultry, fish Count as 1 oz 1 egg ½ cup cooked beans 2 tablespoons peanut butter
Fats and sweets	Use sparingly, after recommended foods have been eaten	

Adapted from the U.S. Department of Agriculture. (2000). *Home and garden bulletin*. No. 232, 5th ed.

the table more than once to wash his or her hands adequately.

Most children prefer simple, plain foods and are good judges of their own needs if they are not coaxed, nagged, bribed, rewarded, or influenced by television commercials. Disease or strong emotions may cause loss of appetite. Forcing the child to eat is not helpful and can have harmful effects.

Caregivers must carefully supervise children's snacking habits to be sure that snacks are nutritious and not too frequent. Children should avoid junk food; continual nibbling can cause lack of interest at mealtime. They should be encouraged to eat a good breakfast to provide the energy and nutrients needed to perform well in school. Children need a clearly planned schedule that allows time for a good breakfast and tooth brushing before leaving for school.

Obesity can be a concern during this age. Some children may have a genetic tendency to obesity; environment and a sedentary lifestyle also play a part. In many families, children are urged to "clean your plate" or are encouraged to belong to the "clean plate club." In addition, many families now eat fast foods several times a week, which reinforces the problem because fast foods tend to have high fat and calorie content and contribute to obesity. Other children, especially in the later elementary grades, can be unkind to overweight children by teasing them, not choosing them in games, or avoiding them as friends. The child who becomes sensitive to being overweight is often miserable.

Encouraging physical activity and limiting dietary fat intake to 35% of total calories will help control the child's weight. Popular fad diets must be avoided because they do not supply adequate nutrients for the growing child. Caregivers must avoid nagging and creating feelings of inferiority or guilt because the child may simply rebel. The child who is pressured too much to lose weight may become a food sneak, setting up patterns that will be harmful later in life. In addition, anorexia nervosa (see Chapter 41) has become a problem for some girls in the older school-age group.

Health teaching at school should reinforce the importance of a proper diet. Family and cultural food patterns are strong, however, and tend to persist despite nutrition education. Some families are making a positive effort to reduce fat and cholesterol when preparing meals. Most schools have subsidized lunch programs for eligible children, and some have breakfast programs. These provide well-balanced meals, but often children eat only part of what they are offered. Some families post the school lunch menu on the refrigerator or kitchen bulletin board so that children can decide whether to eat the school's lunch or pack their own on any particular day. This way the child can avoid lunches he or she dislikes or simply refuses to eat. School-age children are old enough to be at least partially responsible for preparing their own lunch.

Test Yourself

- List the factors that may contribute to obesity in the school-age child.
- What can be suggested as ways to control a school-age child's weight?

HEALTH PROMOTION AND MAINTENANCE

The school years are generally healthy years for most children. However, routine health care and health education, including health habits, safety, sex education, and substance abuse, are very important aspects of well-planned health promotion and maintenance programs for school-age children.

Routine Checkups

The school-age child should have a physical examination by a physician or other health care provider every year. Additional visits are commonly made throughout the year for minor illness. The school-age child should visit the dentist at least twice a year for a cleaning and application of fluoride (Fig. 26-6).

Most states have immunization requirements that must be met when the child enters school. A booster of tetanus-diphtheria vaccine is recommended every

● *Figure 26.6* This school-age child visits the dentist twice a year.

A   B

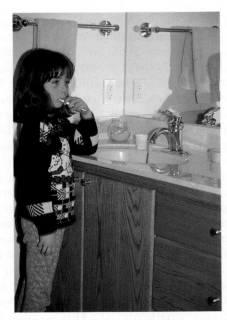

● *Figure 26.7* Scoliosis checkup. (**A**) Viewing from the back, the examiner checks the symmetry of the girl's shoulders. She will also look for a prominent shoulder blade, an unequal distance between the girl's arms and waist, a higher or more prominent hip, and curvature of the spinal column. (**B**) With the child bending over and touching her toes, the examiner checks for a curvature of the spinal column. She will also look for a rib hump.

10 years throughout life. In addition, physical and dental examinations may be required at specific intervals during the elementary school years. During a physical examination at about the age of 10 to 11 years, the child is initially examined for signs of **scoliosis** (lateral curvature of the spine). The child is monitored on an ongoing basis and re-examined during adolescence (Fig. 26-7; refer to Chapter 39). Vision and hearing screening should be performed before entrance to school and on a periodic basis (annual or biannual) thereafter. The school nurse often conducts these examinations.

Elementary school children generally are healthy, with only minor illnesses that are usually respiratory or gastrointestinal in nature. The leading cause of death in this age group continues to be accidents.

Family Teaching

The school-age child generally incorporates healthy habits into his or her daily routine, but reinforcement by caregivers is still needed. Education for the care of the teeth with particular attention to the 6-year molars is important. Proper dental hygiene includes a routine inspection and conscientious brushing after meals. A well-balanced diet with plenty of calcium and phosphorus and minimal sugar is important to healthy teeth. Foods containing sugar should be eaten only at mealtimes and should be followed immediately by proper brushing (Fig. 26-8).

Exercise and sufficient rest also are important during this period. Caregivers need to help school-age children to balance their rest needs and their extracurricular activities. Extracurricular activities help the child remain fit, bond with peers, and establish positive, lifelong attitudes toward exercise. The school-age child needs 10 to 12 hours of sleep per night. The 6-year-old needs 12 hours of sleep and should be provided with a quiet time after school to recharge after a busy day in the classroom. The nurse should take an opportunity to highlight these important aspects of daily health care to both the caregivers and child.

● *Figure 26.8* The school-age child needs encouragement to brush after meals and at bedtime as part of a good dental hygiene program.

Health Education

Health teaching in the home and at school is essential. Caregivers have a responsibility to teach the child about basic hygiene, sexual functioning, substance abuse, and accident prevention. Schools must include these topics in the curriculum because many families are not informed well enough to cover them adequately. Some schools offer health classes taught by a health educator at each grade level. In other schools, health and sex education are integrated into the curriculum and taught by each classroom teacher. Nurses should become active in their community to ensure that these kinds of programs are available to children.

Sex Education

Children learn about femininity and masculinity from the time they are born. Behaviors, attitudes, and actions of the men and women in the child's life, especially their actions toward the child and toward each other, form impressions in the child that last a lifetime. The proper time and place for formal sex education have been very controversial. Part of the problem seems to be that many people automatically think that sex education means just adult sexuality and reproduction. However, sex education includes helping children develop positive attitudes toward their own bodies, their own sex, and their own sexual role to achieve optimum satisfaction in being a boy or a girl.

In some schools, sex education is limited to one class, usually in the fifth grade, in which children are shown films about menstruation and their developing bodies. Often these are taught in separate classes for boys and girls. Some health educators strongly recommend that sex education should be started in kindergarten and developed gradually over the successive grades. Learning about reproduction of plants and animals, about birth and nurturing in other animals, and about the roles of the male and the female in family units can lead to the natural introduction of human reproduction, male and female roles, families, and nurturing. If all children grew up in secure, loving, ideal families, much of this could be learned at home. However, many children do not have this type of home, so they need healthy, positive information to help them develop healthy attitudes about their own sexuality. Feelings of self-worth woven into these lessons help children feel good about themselves and who they are.

Caregivers who feel uncomfortable discussing sex with their children may find it helpful to use books or pamphlets available for various age groups. Generally a female caregiver finds it easier to discuss sex with a girl, and a male caregiver feels more comfortable with a boy. This can pose special problems for the single caregiver with a child of the opposite sex. Again, printed materials may be helpful. Nurses may be called on to help a caregiver provide information and must be comfortable with their own sexuality to handle these discussions well.

At a young age, children are exposed to a large amount of sexually provocative information through the media. Children who do not get accurate information at home or at school will learn what they want to know from their peers; this information is often inaccurate, which makes sex education even more urgent. In addition, the United States Centers for Disease Control currently recommends that elementary school children be taught about acquired immunodeficiency syndrome (AIDS) and how it is spread. Many school districts are working hard to integrate this information into the health curriculum at all grade levels in a sensitive, age-appropriate manner.

Substance Abuse

In addition to nutrition, health practices, safety, and sex education, school-age children also need substance abuse education. Programs that teach children to "just say no" are one way that children can learn that they are in control of the choices they make regarding substance abuse. Children as young as elementary school age may try cigarette smoking, chewing tobacco, alcohol, and other substances. Teaching children the unhealthy aspects of tobacco and alcohol use and drug abuse should be started in elementary school as a good foundation for more advanced information in adolescence.

A PERSONAL GLIMPSE

When we had the program on drugs at school, I learned some things. Like when you take drugs, you can get sick or even die. In one part of the lesson, we watched a video where a kid took drugs and almost died and during the other part the school nurse showed us samples of drugs. Even though I leaned about drugs from the program, I think that all children should be taught this subject by their parent or guardian.

Stephen, age 10

LEARNING OPPORTUNITY: What do you think is the most effective way to teach school-age children about the dangers of substance abuse? List some ways you can help to reduce substance abuse among school-age children.

BOX 26.1	Common Products Inhaled as Deliriants

Model glue
Rubber cement
Cleaning fluids
Kerosene vapors
Gasoline vapors
Butane lighter fluid
Paint sprays
Paint thinner
Varnish
Shellac
Hair spray
Nail polish remover
Liquid typing correction fluid
Propellant in whipped-cream spray cans
Aerosol paint cans
Upholstery-fabric-protection spray cans
Solvents

Test Yourself

- How is a child screened for scoliosis? At what age is a child usually initially examined for signs of scoliosis?

- List substances that school-age children might abuse.

Accident Prevention

As stated, accidents continue to be a leading cause of death during this period. Even though school-age children do not require constant supervision, they must be taught certain safety rules and practice them until they are routine (Fig. 26-9). They should understand the

Children may experiment with **inhalants** (substances whose volatile vapors can be abused) because they are readily available and may seem no more threatening than an innocent prank. Inhalants classified as **deliriants** contain chemicals that give off fumes that can produce symptoms of confusion, disorientation, excitement, and hallucinations. Many inhalants are commonly found in the home (Box 26-1). The fumes are mind altering when inhaled. The child initially may experience a temporary high, giddiness, nausea, coughing, nosebleed, fatigue, lack of coordination, or loss of appetite. Overdose can cause loss of consciousness and possible death from suffocation by replacing oxygen in the lungs or depressing the central nervous system, thereby causing respiratory arrest. Permanent damage to the lungs, the nervous system, or the liver can result. Children who experiment with inhalants may proceed to abuse other drugs in an attempt to get similar effects. Addiction occurs in younger children more rapidly than in adults.

Family caregivers must work to develop a strong, loving relationship with the children in the family, teach the children the family's values and the difference between right and wrong, set and enforce rules for acceptable behavior of family members, learn facts about drugs and alcohol, and actively listen to the children in the family (see Family Teaching Tips: Guidelines to Prevent Substance Abuse). An excellent reference for family caregivers is *Growing Up Drug Free: A Parent's Guide to Prevention*, which is published by the United States Department of Education and can be ordered free by calling the Department of Education's toll-free number, (800) 624-0100, or via the Internet at http://www.ed.gov/offices/OESE/SDFS/.

FAMILY TEACHING TIPS

Guidelines to Prevent Substance Abuse

- Openly communicate values by talking about the importance of honesty, responsibility, and self-reliance. Encourage decision-making. Help children see how each decision builds on previous decisions.
- Provide a good role model for the child to copy. Children tend to copy parent's habits of smoking and drinking alcohol and attitudes about drug use, whether they are over-the-counter, prescription, or illicit drugs.
- Avoid conflicts between what you say and what you do. For example, don't ask the child to lie that you are not home when you are or encourage the child to lie about age when trying to get a lower admission price at amusement centers.
- Talk about values during family times. Give the child "what if" examples, and discuss the best responses when faced with a difficult situation. For example, "What would you do if you found money that someone dropped?"
- Set strong rules about using alcohol and other drugs. Make specific rules with specific punishments. Discuss these rules and the reasons for them.
- Be consistent in applying the rules that you set.
- Be reasonable; don't make wild threats. Respond calmly and carry out the expected punishment.
- Get the facts about alcohol and other drugs, and provide children with current, correct information. This helps you in discussions with children and also helps you to recognize symptoms if a child has been using them.

(From U.S. Department of Education. (1998). Washington, DC: Author.)

● *Figure 26.9* Helmets are an important aspect of bike safety. Parents can be role models for their children by also wearing bike helmets.

communicate better with health care providers, understand cause and effect, and tolerate longer separations from their family.

Nurses who care for school-age children should understand how concepts about birth, death, the body, health, and illness change between the ages of 6 and 10 years (Table 26-3). All procedures must be explained to children and their families; showing the equipment and materials to be used (or pictures of them) and outlining realistic expectations of procedures and treatments are helpful. Children's questions, including those about pain, should be answered truthfully. Children of this age have anxieties about looking different from other children. An opportunity to verbalize these anxieties will help a child deal with them. School-age children need privacy more than younger children do and may not want to have physical contact with adults; this wish should be respected. Boys may be uncomfortable having a female nurse bathe them, and girls may feel uncomfortable with a male nurse. These attitudes should be recognized and handled in a way that ensures as much privacy as possible.

function of traffic lights. Family members should obey traffic lights as a matter of course because example is the best teacher for any child. Every child should know her or his full name, the caregivers' names, and his or her own home address and telephone number. Children should be taught the appropriate way to call for emergency help in their community (911 in a community that has such a system). Many communities have safe-home programs that designate homes where children can go if they have a problem on the way home from school. These homes are clearly marked in a way that children are taught to recognize. In many communities, local police officers or firefighters are interested in coming into the classroom to help teach safety. Children benefit from meeting police officers and understanding that the officer's duty is to help children, not to punish them. Safety rules should be stressed at home and at school. Family Teaching Tips: Safety Topics for Elementary School-Age Children summarizes important safety considerations for school-age children.

THE SCHOOL-AGE CHILD IN THE HEALTH CARE FACILITY

Increased understanding of their bodies, continuing curiosity about how things work, and development of concrete thinking all contribute to helping school-age children understand and accept a health care experience better than younger children do. They can

FAMILY TEACHING TIPS

Safety Topics for Elementary School-Age Children

- Traffic signals and safe pedestrian practices
- Safety belt use for car passengers
- Bicycle safety
  a. Wear a helmet.
  b. Use hand signals.
  c. Ride with traffic.
  d. Be sure others see you.
- Skateboard and skating safety
  a. Wear a helmet.
  b. Wear elbow and knee pads.
  c. Skate only in safe skating areas.
- Swimming safety
  a. Learn to swim.
  b. Never swim alone.
  c. Always know the water depth.
  d. Don't dive head first.
  e. No running or horseplay at a pool.
- Danger of projectile toys
- Danger of all-terrain vehicles
- Use of life jacket when boating
- Stranger safety
  a. Who is a stranger?
  b. Never accept a ride from someone you don't know.
  c. If offered a ride, check the vehicle license number and try to remember it.
  d. Never accept food or gifts from someone you don't know.
- Good touch and bad touch.

TABLE 26.3	Children's Concept of Biology		
Concept	6 to 8 Years	8 to 10 Years	Implications for Nursing
Birth	Gradually see babies as the result of three factors: social and sexual intercourse and biogenetic fusion Tend to see baby as emerging from female only; many still see baby as manufactured by outside force—created whole Boys less knowledgeable about baby formation than girls	Begin to put three components together; recognize that sperm and egg come together but may not be sure why Fewer discrepancies in knowledge based on sex differences	Cultural and educational factors play a part in development of where babies come from. Nurse should assess children's ideas about birth and if they can understand where babies come from and how before teaching. Explanations about roles of both parents can begin, but the idea of sperm and egg union may not be understood until 8 or 9 years of age.
Death	May be viewed as reversible Animism (attribution of life) may be seen in some children; death is viewed as result of outside force Experiences with death facilitate concept development.	Considered irreversible Ideas about what happens after death unclear; related to concreteness of thinking and socio-religious upbringing	Change from vague view of death as reversible and caused by external forces to awareness of irreversibility and bodily causes Fears about death more common at 8; adults should be alert to this. Explanations about death, the fact that their thoughts will not cause a death, and they will not die (if illness is not fatal) are needed.
Human body	Know body holds everything inside Use outside world to explain Aware of major organs Interested in visible functions of body	Can understand physiology; use general principles to explain body functions; interested in invisible functions of body	Cultural factors may play a part in ability and willingness to discuss bodily functions. Educational programs can be very effective because of natural interest Assess knowledge of body by using diagrams before teaching.
Health	See health as doing desired activities List concrete practices as components of health Many do not see sickness as related to health; may not consider cause and effect	See health as doing desired activities Understand cause and effect Believe it is possible to be part healthy and part not at the same time; can reverse from health to sickness and back to health	Need assistance in seeing cause and effect Capitalize on positiveness of concept; health lets you do what you really want to do. Young children who are sick may feel they will never get well again.
Illness	Sick children may see illness as punishment; evidence suggests that healthy children do not see illness as punishment. Highly anxious children more likely to view illness as disruptive. Sickness is a diffuse state; rely on others to tell them when they are ill	Same as 6–8 years of age; can identify illness states, report bodily discomfort, recognize that illness is caused by specific factors	Social factors play a part in illness concept. Recognize that some see illness as punishment. Encourage self-care and self-help behavior, especially in older children.

● *Figure 26.10* School-age children still like to listen to stories, in either the hospital or the home setting.

Family caregivers may feel guilty about the child's need for hospitalization and, as a result, may overindulge the child. The child may regress in response to this, but this regression should not be encouraged. Sometimes the family needs as much reassurance as the child does.

Discipline and rules have a place on a pediatric unit. Families and children must be informed about the rules as part of the admission routine. Opportunities for interaction with peers, learning situations, and doing crafts and projects can help make the child's experience more tolerable (Fig. 26-10).

KEY POINTS

▶ Physical growth is slow and steady during the school-age years. The child begins to lose deciduous teeth and the first permanent teeth appear at about 6 years of age.

▶ According to Erikson, the developmental task of school-age children is industry versus inferiority. The child engages in many activities using motor, cognitive, and social skills. Success in these activities is necessary for the child to develop a sense of competency.

▶ Even though family is still a major influence, the school-age child has a need to be accepted by groups of peers, often spends time in activities with children of the same sex, and enjoys team sports and completing projects.

▶ By allowing expression of food likes and dislikes and by setting good examples, caregivers can help the school-age child develop good nutrition habits to be followed at home and school for meals as well as snacks.

▶ Obesity in the school-age child can be related to genetic, environmental, or sedentary lifestyle factors. Appropriate physical activity, limiting fat intake, and positive caregiver support can be helpful in decreasing obesity.

▶ A well-balanced diet with adequate calcium and phosphorus, brushing after meals, and eating foods containing sugar only at mealtimes contribute to good dental health.

▶ The school-aged child needs 10 to 12 hours of sleep each night.

▶ Sex education regarding sexuality, reproduction, and positive attitudes regarding sexuality are important roles that families and schools often share.

▶ Substance abuse is an ever-increasing concern during this age, especially the use of products that can be inhaled and used as deliriants. Family caregivers must make every effort to be alert to children's use of inhalants, deliriants, alcohol, or tobacco and to talk with the school-age child about the abuse of substances.

▶ Safety issues for the school-age child include teaching regarding traffic safety, especially in bicycle riding and skateboarding, seat belt use, and stranger safety.

▶ Children's interest in science creates a fascination with their bodies and how they work. The hospitalized child needs explanations and privacy.

▶ The changes in a school-aged child's understanding of birth, death, the human body, health, and illness influence the child's view of his or her own health care. The nurse needs to understand these concepts to plan nursing care for the school-age child.

REFERENCES AND SELECTED READINGS

Berger, K. S. (2001). *The developing person through the life span* (5th ed.). New York: Worth Publishers.

Brazelton, T. B., & Greenspan, S. (2001). *The irreducible needs of children: What every child must have to grow, learn, and flourish*. Cambridge, MA: Perseus Publishing.

Brown, R. L., et al. (2002). All-terrain vehicle and bicycle crashes in children: Epidemiology and comparison of injury severity. *Journal of Pediatric Surgery, 37*(3), 375–380.

Counseling about bicycle safety. (2001). *Pediatrics in Review, 22*(9), 321–322.

Craven, R. F., & Hirnle, C. J. (1999). *Fundamentals of nursing* (3rd ed.). Philadelphia: Lippincott Williams & Wilkins.

Dudek, S. G. (2000). *Nutrition essentials for nursing practice* (4th ed.). Philadelphia: Lippincott Williams & Wilkins.

McClowry, S. G. (2002). The temperament profiles of school-age children. *Journal of Pediatric Nursing, 17* (1), 3–10.

Pillitteri, A. (2003). *Maternal and child health nursing* (4th ed.). Philadelphia: Lippincott Williams & Wilkins.

Sanford, C. C. (2001). Delivering health care to children on their turf: An elementary school school-based wellness center. *Journal of Pediatric Health Care, 15*(3), 132.

Schmidt, C. K. (2001). Development of children's body knowledge, using knowledge of the lungs as an exemplar. *Issues in Comprehensive Pediatric Nursing, 24*(3), 177–191.

Spock, B., et al. (1998). *Dr. Spock's baby and child care.* New York: Pocket Books.

Wong, D. L. (1998). *Whaley and Wong's nursing care of infants and children* (6th ed.). St. Louis: Mosby.

Wong, D. L., Perry, S., & Hockenberry, M. (2002). *Maternal child nursing care* (2nd ed.). St. Louis: Mosby.

Web Addresses
Substance abuse
www.toughlove.org

Family support groups
http://home.earthlink.net/famanon/index.html
www.keepkidshealthy.com/schoolage

WORKBOOK

NCLEX-STYLE REVIEW QUESTIONS

1. The nurse is assisting with a well-child visit for a 7-year-old. This child's records show that at birth this child weighed 7 pounds 8 ounces. At the age of 6 years, this child was 45 inches tall. If this child is following a normal pattern of growth and development, which of the following would the nurse expect to find in this visit? The child

   a. weighs 54 pounds.

   b. measures 50 inches in height.

   c. has four molars in the lower jaw.

   d. has an apical pulse of 60 beats a minute.

2. In working with a group of school-age children, which of the following activities would this age child most likely be doing?

   a. Pretending to be television characters

   b. Playing a game with large balls

   c. Participating in a group activity

   d. Telling stories about themselves

3. During the school-age years, according to Erikson, the child is in the stage of growth and development known as industry versus inferiority. If the caregivers of a group of children made the following statements, which statement reflects that the child is developing industry?

   a. "When my child falls down, he tries so hard to just get up and not cry."

   b. "My child was so excited when she finished her science project all by herself."

   c. "Every night my child follows the same routine at bedtime."

   d. "My child loves to make up stories about tall, big buildings."

4. In teaching caregivers of school-age children, the nurse would reinforce that which of the following would be most important for this age group? The school-age child should be

   a. encouraged to brush teeth.

   b. taught basic sex education.

   c. screened for scoliosis.

   d. required to wear a bicycle helmet.

5. The nurse is teaching a group of caregivers of school-age children about the importance of setting a consistent bedtime for the school-age child. Which of the following statements made by a caregiver indicates an understanding of the sleep patterns and needs of the school-age child?

   a. "My child sleeps between 11 and 12 hours a night."

   b. "She stays up late when she takes a nap after school."

   c. "My son doesn't even know when he is tired."

   d. "My teenage child doesn't sleep as much as my 9-year-old does."

6. In working with the school-age child and this child's family, teaching is an important role of the nurse. Which of the following are important to teach the school-age child and family? Select all that apply:

   a. Food "jags" are common at this age.

   b. Eating foods that are disliked is important

   c. Obesity can be a concern at this age

   d. Scoliosis screening should be done

   e. Foods containing sugar can be eaten as snacks

   f. Sex education is best taught in the home

STUDY ACTIVITIES

1. List and compare the motor skills, social skills, and cognitive development in each of the following ages:

	6 Years	7 Years	8 Years	9–10 Years
Motor skills				
Social skills				
Cognitive development				

2. Make a safety poster or teaching aid to use in an elementary school classroom. Perhaps you can make this a class project and donate the posters to your pediatric unit or nearby school.

3. Survey your home and make a list of all the products available that a child could use as an inhalant for a deliriant effect.

4. Go to the following Internet site: http://arizonachildcare.org/childproof/bicyclesfty.html Read the section "General Tips of Bicycle Safety."

   a. List seven things that you would check when following this bike safety checklist.

   b. Describe how a bicycle helmet works.

   c. After reading this site, how would you answer the parent of a school-age child who asks, "Does my child really need a bicycle helmet?"

CRITICAL THINKING: What Would You Do?

1. Delsey, the mother of 6-year-old Jasmine, is upset because Jasmine is a picky eater and often does not want to eat what Delsey has prepared.

   a. What eating patterns are seen in most school-age children?

   b. What information would you share with Delsey about the normal nutrition requirements for Jasmine?

   c. What suggestions would you give Delsey regarding what she might offer Jasmine at meal and snack times?

   d. How could Delsey involve Jasmine in developing good nutritional patterns?

2. Steve, the primary family caregiver of 8-year-old Rebekah, feels that he should offer her sex education and asks for your advice.

   a. What topics need to be included in sex education for the school-age child?

   b. How would you suggest Steve go about giving his daughter the sex education she needs?

   c. What resources would you offer to Steve to help him in teaching his daughter?

   d. Why is it important for the family to be part of the sex education training of a child?

3. You have been asked to teach a school-age program regarding substance abuse, including alcohol and tobacco use.

   a. What areas would you include in your teaching plan?

   b. What would be the most effective teaching methods for you to use to present this material to school-age children?

   c. What questions and concerns would you anticipate from these children?

Growth and Development of the Adolescent: 11 to 18 Years

27

STUDENT OBJECTIVES

On completion of this chapter, the student should be able to

1. State the age of (a) the preadolescent and (b) the adolescent.
2. Describe the psychosocial development of the preadolescent.
3. Name the physical changes that make the child appear uncoordinated in early adolescence.
4. List the secondary sexual characteristics that appear (a) in adolescent boys and (b) in adolescent girls.
5. State (a) the major cognitive task of the adolescent according to Piaget and (b) the psychosocial task according to Erikson.
6. Explain some problems that adolescents face when making career choices today.
7. Explain the role of intimacy in the preparation for long-term relationships.
8. Discuss the adolescent's need to conform to peers.
9. Discuss the influence of peer pressure on psychosocial development.
10. Discuss adolescent body image and associated problems.
11. Name the nutrients commonly deficient in the diets of adolescents.
12. Discuss the aspects of sexual maturity that affect the need for health education in the adolescent.
13. Discuss the issues that the adolescent faces in making decisions related to sexual responsibility and substance use.
14. State factors that may influence the adolescent's hospital experience.

KEY TERMS

early adolescence
heterosexual
homosexual
malocclusion
menarche
nocturnal emissions
orthodontia
puberty

"**A**dolescence" comes from the Latin word meaning "to come to maturity," a fitting description of this stage of life. The adolescent is maturing physically and emotionally, growing from childhood toward adulthood, and seeking to understand what it means to be grown up.

Early adolescence (preadolescence, pubescence) begins at about age 10 in girls and about age 12 in boys with a dramatic growth spurt that signals the advent of **puberty** (reproductive maturity). During this stage, the child's body begins to take on adult-like contours, the primary sex organs enlarge, secondary sexual characteristics appear, and hormonal activity increases. This early period ends with the onset of menstruation in the female and the production of sperm in the male. The bone growth that began during intrauterine life continues through adolescence and is usually completed by the end of this period.

Adolescents are fascinated and sometimes fearful and confused by the changes occurring in their bodies and their thinking processes. They begin to look grown up, but they do not have the judgment or independence to participate in society as an adult. These young people are strongly influenced by their peer group and often resent parental authority. Roller-coaster emotions characterize this age group, as does intense interest in romantic relationships (Fig. 27-1).

The adolescent years can be a time of turmoil and uncertainty that creates conflict between family caregivers and children. If these conflicts are resolved, normal development can continue. Unresolved conflicts

● *Figure 27.1* Intense interest in the opposite sex characterizes adolescence.

● *Figure 27.2* The development of self-identity in adolescence involves developing interests and talents and becoming emotionally independent.

can foster delays in development and prevent the young person from maturing into a fully functioning adult.

Body image is critical to adolescents. Health problems that threaten body image, such as acne, obesity, dental or vision problems, and trauma, can seriously interfere with development.

During this period, teens are engaged in a struggle to master the developmental tasks that lead to successful completion of this stage and the development of their own personal identity. Erikson describes this stage as "identity versus role confusion." Adolescents confront marked physical and emotional changes and the knowledge that soon they will be responsible for their own lives. They develop a sense of being independent people with unique ideals and goals (Fig. 27-2). If parents, caregivers, and other adults refuse to grant that independence, adolescents may break rules just to prove that they can. Stress, anxiety, and mood swings are typical of this phase and add to the feelings of role confusion.

PREADOLESCENT DEVELOPMENT

During the period between 10 and 12 years of age, the rate of growth varies greatly in boys and girls. This variability in growth and maturation can be a concern to the child who develops rapidly or the one who develops more slowly than his or her peers. Children of this age do not want to be different from their friends. The developmental characteristics of the preadolescent child in late school age stage overlap with those of early adolescence; nevertheless there are unique characteristics to set this stage apart (Table 27-1).

Physical Development

Preadolescence begins in the female between the ages of 9 and 11 years and is marked by a growth spurt that

TABLE 27.1	Growth and Development of the Preadolescent: 10 to 13 Years				
Physical	**Motor**	**Personal-Social**	**Language**	**Perceptual**	**Cognitive**
Average height 56¾ inches–59 inches (144–150 cm) Average weight 77-88 lb (35-40 kg) Pubescence may begin Girls may surpass boys in height Remaining permanent teeth erupt	Refines gross and fine motor skills May have difficulty with some fine motor coordination due to growth of large muscles before that of small muscle growth; hands and feet are first structures to increase in size; thus, actions may appear uncoordinated during early preadolescence Can do crafts Uses tools increasingly well	Attends school primarily for peer association Peer relationships of greatest importance Intolerant of violation of group norms Can follow rules of group and adapt to another point of view Can use stored knowledge to make independent judgments	Fluent in spoken language Vocabulary 50,000 words for reading; oral vocabulary of 7,200 words Uses slang words and terms, vulgarities, jeers, jokes, and sayings	Can catch or intercept ball thrown from a distance Possible growth spurts may cause myopia	Begins abstract thinking Conservation of volume Understands relations among time, speed, and distance Ability to sympathize, love, and reason are all evolving Right and wrong become logically clear

lasts for about 18 months. Girls grow about 3 inches each year until **menarche** (the beginning of menstruation), after which growth slows considerably. Early in adolescence, girls begin to develop a figure, the pelvis broadens, and axillary and pubic hair begins to appear along with many changes in hormone levels. The variation between girls is great and often is a cause for much concern by the "early bloomer" or the "late bloomer." Young girls who begin to develop physically as early as 9 years of age are often embarrassed by these physical changes. In girls, the onset of menarche marks the end of the preadolescent period.

Boys enter preadolescence a little later, usually between 11 and 13 years of age, and grow generally at a slower, steadier rate than do girls. During this time, the scrotum and testes begin to enlarge, the skin of the scrotum begins to change in coloring and texture, and sparse hair begins to show at the base of the penis. Boys who start their growth spurt later often are concerned about being shorter than their peers. In boys, the appearance of **nocturnal emissions** ("wet dreams") is often used as the indication that the preadolescent period has ended.

Preparation for Adolescence

Preadolescents need information about their changing bodies and feelings. Sex education that includes infor-

mation about the hormonal changes that are occurring or will be occurring is necessary to help them through this developmental stage.

Girls need information that will help them handle their early menstrual periods with minimal apprehension. Most girls have irregular periods for the first year or so; they need to know that this is not a cause for worry. They have many questions about protection during the menstrual period and the advisability of using sanitary pads or tampons. They may fear that "everybody will know" when they have their first period and must be allowed to express this fear and be reassured.

Boys also need information about their bodies. Erections and nocturnal emissions are topics they need to discuss, as well as the development of other male secondary sex characteristics.

Both boys and girls need information about changes in the opposite sex, including discussions that address their questions. This kind of information helps them increase their understanding of human sexuality. School programs may provide a good foundation for sex education, but each preadolescent needs an adult to turn to with particular questions. Even a well-planned program does not address all the needs of the preadolescent. The best school program begins early and builds from year to year as the child's needs progress (see Chapter 26).

Preadolescence is an appropriate time for discussions that will help the young teen resist pressures to become sexually active too early. Family caregivers may turn to a nurse acquaintance for guidance in preparing their child. Perhaps the most important aspect of discussions about sexuality is that honest, straightforward answers must be given in an atmosphere of caring concern. Children whose need for information is not met through family, school, or community programs will get their information—often inaccurate—from peers, movies, television, or other media.

ADOLESCENT DEVELOPMENT

Adolescence spans the ages of about 13 to 18 years. Some males do not complete adolescence until they are 20 years old. The rate of development during adolescence varies greatly from one teen to another. It is a time of many physical, emotional, and social changes. During this period, the adolescent is engaged in a struggle to master the developmental tasks that lead to successful completion of this stage of development (Table 27-2). Completion of the developmental tasks of earlier developmental stages is a prerequisite for the completion of these tasks.

Physical Development

Rapid growth occurs during adolescence. Girls begin growing more rapidly during the preadolescent period and achieve 98% of their adult height by the age of 16. Boys start their growth spurt, period of rapid growth, around 13 years of age and may continue to grow until 20 years of age. The skeletal system's rapid growth, which outpaces muscular system growth, causes the long and lanky appearance of many teens and contributes to the clumsiness often seen during this age.

During the first menstrual cycles, ovulation does not usually occur because increased estrogen levels are needed to produce an ovum mature enough to be released. However, at 13 to 15 years of age, the cycle becomes ovulatory, and pregnancy is possible. The girl's breasts take on an adult appearance by age 16, and pubic hair is curly and abundant.

By the age of 16 years, the penis, testes, and scrotum are adult in size and shape, and mature spermatozoa are produced. Male pubic hair also is adult in appearance and amount. After age 13, muscle strength and coordination develop rapidly. The larynx and vocal cords enlarge, and the voice deepens. The "change of voice" makes the teenage male's voice vary unexpectedly, which occasionally causes embarrassment for the teen.

Psychosocial Development

Adolescence is a time of transition from childhood to adulthood. Between the ages of 10 and 18 years, adolescents move from Freud's latency stage to the genital stage, from Erikson's industry versus inferiority to identity versus role confusion, and from Piaget's concrete operational thinking to formal operational thought. They develop a sense of moral judgment and a system of values and beliefs that will affect their entire lives. The foundation provided by family, religious groups, school, and community experiences is still a strong influence, but the peer group exerts tremendous power. Trends and fads among adolescents dictate clothing choices, hairstyles, music, and other recreational choices (Fig. 27-3). The adolescent whose family caregivers make it difficult to conform are adding another stress to an already emotion-laden period. Peer pressure to experiment with potentially dangerous practices, such as drugs, alcohol, and reckless driving, also can be strong; adolescents may need careful guidance and understanding support to help resist this peer influence.

Personality Development

Erikson considered the central task of adolescence to be the establishment of identity. Adolescents spend a lot of time asking themselves, "Who am I as a person? What will I do with my life? Marry? Have children? Will I go to college? If so, where? If not, why not? What kind of career should I choose?"

Adolescents are confronted with a greater variety of choices than ever before. Sex role stereotypes have been shattered in most careers and professions. More women are becoming lawyers, physicians, plumbers, and carpenters; more men are entering nursing or choosing to become house-husbands while their wives earn the primary family income. Transportation has made greater geographic mobility possible, so that many youngsters can spend summers or a full school year in a foreign country, plan to attend college thousands of miles from home, and begin a career in an even more remote location. Making decisions and choices is never simple. With such a tremendous variety of options, it is understandable that adolescents often are preoccupied with their own concerns.

When identity has been established, generally between the ages of 16 and 18 years, adolescents seek intimate relationships, usually with members of the opposite sex. Intimacy, which is mutual sharing of one's deepest feelings with another person, is impossible unless both persons have established a sense of trust and a sense of identity. Intimate relationships are a preparation for long-term relationships, and people

TABLE 27.2	Developmental Tasks of Adolescence	
Basic Task	**Associated Tasks**
Appreciate own uniqueness*	Identify interests, skills, and talents Identify differences from peers Accept strengths and limitations Challenge own skill levels
Develop independent internal identity*	Value self as a person Separate physical self from psychological self Differentiate personal worth from cultural stereotypes Separate internal value from societal feedback
Determine own value system*	Identify options Establish priorities Commit self to decisions made Translate values into behaviors Resist peer and cultural pressures to conform to their value system Find comfortable balance between own and peer/cultural standards, behaviors, and needs
Develop self-evaluation skills*	Develop basis for self-evaluation and monitoring Evaluate quality of products Assess approach to tasks and responsibilities Develop sensitivity to intrapersonal relationships Evaluate dynamics of interpersonal relationships
Assume increasing responsibility for own behavior*	Quality of work, chores Emotional tone Money management Time management Decision making Personal habits Social behaviors
Find meaning in life	Accept and integrate meaning of death Develop philosophy of life Begin to identify life or career goals
Acquire skills essential for adult living	Acquire skills essential to independent living Develop social and emotional abilities and temperament Refine sociocultural amenities Identify and experiment with alternatives for facing life Acquire employment skills Seek growth-inducing activities
Seek affiliations outside of family	Seek companionship with compatible peers Affiliate with organizations that support uniqueness Actively seek models or mentors Identify potential emotional support systems Differentiate between acquaintances and friends Identify ways to express sexuality
Adapt to adult body functioning	Adapt to somatic (body) changes Refine balance and coordination Develop physical strength Consider sexuality and reproduction issues

* Tasks deemed crucial to continued maturation

who fail to achieve intimacy may develop feelings of isolation and experience chronic difficulty in communicating with others.

Most intimate relationships during adolescence are **heterosexual**, or between members of the opposite sex.

Sometimes, however, young people form intimate attachments with members of the same sex, or **homosexual** relationships. Because our culture is predominately heterosexual and is still struggling with trying to understand homosexual relationships, these relationships can

● **Figure 27.3** For many teens, hanging out with friends is an important way to share common interests and gain a sense of belonging.

cause great anxiety for family caregivers and children. Although some parts of American society are beginning to accept homosexual relationships as no more than another lifestyle, prejudice still exists. So great a stigma has been attached to homosexuality that many adolescents fear they are homosexual if they are uncomfortable about heterosexual intimacy. However, this discomfort is normal as adolescents move from same-sex peer group activities to dating peers of the opposite sex.

Body Image

Body image is closely related to self-esteem. Seeing one's body as attractive and functional contributes to a positive sense of self-esteem. During adolescence, the desire not to be different can extend to feelings about one's body and can cause adolescents to feel that their bodies are inadequate even though they are actually healthy and attractive.

American culture tends to equate a slender figure with feminine beauty and acceptability and a lean, tall, muscular figure with masculine virility and strength. Adolescents, particularly males, who feel that they are underdeveloped suffer great anxiety. Adolescent girls have even undergone plastic surgery to augment their breasts to relieve this anxiety. Girls in this age group often feel that they are too fat and try strange, nutritionally unsound diets to reduce their weight. Some literally starve themselves. Even after their bodies have become emaciated, they truly believe that they are still fat and, therefore, unattractive. This condition is called *anorexia nervosa* and is discussed further in Chapter 41.

Adolescents need to establish a positive body image by the end of their developmental stage. Because bone growth is completed during adoles-

cence, a person's height will remain basically the same throughout adult life even though weight can fluctuate greatly. Tall girls who long to be petite and boys who would like to be 6 feet tall may need guidance and support to bring their expectations in line with reality and learn to have positive feelings about their bodies and accept them the way they are.

Test Yourself

- What are the secondary sex characteristics that develope in the (a) adolescent boy and the (b) adolescent girl?

- Why is body image so important for the adolescent?

NUTRITION

Nutritional requirements are greatly increased during periods of rapid growth in adolescence. Adolescent boys need more calories than do girls throughout the growth period. Appetites increase, and most teens eat frequently. Families with teenage boys often jokingly say that they cannot keep the refrigerator filled. Nutritional needs are related to growth and sexual maturity, rather than age.

Even though adolescents understand something about nutrition, they may not relate this understanding to their dietary habits. Their accelerated growth rate and increased physical activities for some mean that they need more food to meet their energy requirements. Because adolescents are seeking to establish their independence, their food choices are sometimes not wise and tend to be influenced by peer preference, rather than parental advice. Teens frequently skip meals, especially breakfast, snack on foods that provide empty calories, and eat a lot of fast foods. The era of fast food meals has given adolescents easy access to high-calorie, nutritionally unbalanced meals. Too many fast-food meals and nutritionally empty snacks can result in nutritional deficiencies (Fig. 27-4).

When good nutritional habits have been established in early childhood, adolescent nutrition is likely to be better balanced than when nutritional teaching has been insufficient. Being part of a family that practices sound nutrition helps ensure that occasional lapses into sweets, fast foods, and other peer group food preferences will not create serious deficiencies. Nutrients that are often deficient in the teen's diet include calcium; iron; zinc; vitamins A, D, and B_6; and folic acid. Calcium needs increase during skeletal growth. Girls need additional iron because of losses during menstruation. Boys also need additional iron during this growth period (Table 27-3).

● *Figure 27.4* Teens are always hungry, but often choose convenient junk foods, which lack nutritional value.

In their quest for identity and independence, some adolescents experiment with food fads and diets. Adolescent girls, worried about being fat, fall prey to a variety of fad diets. Athletes also may follow fad diets that may include supplements in the belief that these diets enhance bodybuilding. These diets often include increased amounts of protein and amino acids that cause diuresis and calcium loss. Carbohydrate loading, which some practice during the week before an athletic event, increases the muscle glycogen level to two to three times normal and may hinder heart function. A meal that is low in fat and high in complex carbohydrates eaten 3 to 4 hours before an event is much more appropriate for the teen athlete.

Adolescents need a balanced diet consisting of three servings from the milk/dairy group, two or three servings (6 to 7 oz total) from the meat group, three or four servings from the fruit group, four or five servings from the vegetable group, and 9 to 11 servings from the grain group (Fig. 27-5). Adolescents often resist pressure from family members to eat balanced meals; all family caregivers can do is to provide nutritious meals and snacks and regular mealtimes. A good example may be the best teacher at this point. A refrigerator stocked with ready-to-eat nutritious snacks can be a good weapon against snacking on empty calories.

Families with low incomes may have difficulty providing the kinds of foods that meet the requirements for a growing teen. These families need help to learn how to make low-cost, nutritious food selections and plan adequate meals and snacks. The nurse can be instrumental in helping them plan appropriate food purchases. For instance, the nurse might recommend fruit and vegetable stores or farm stands that accept food stamps.

Ethnic and Cultural Influences

Culture also influences adolescent food choices and habits. For example, many Mexican-Americans are accustomed to having their big meal at noon. When school lunches do not provide such a heavy meal, the Mexican-American adolescent may supplement the lunch with sweets or fast foods. In the Asian community, milk is not a popular drink; this can result in a calcium deficiency. Many Asians are lactose intolerant;

TABLE 27.3	Food Sources of Nutrients Commonly Deficient in Preadolescent and Adolescent Diets
Common Nutrient Deficiencies	**Food Sources**
Vitamin A	Liver, whole milk, butter, cheese; sources of carotene such as yellow vegetables, green leafy vegetables, tomatoes, yellow fruits
Vitamin D	Fortified milk, egg yolk, butter
Vitamin B_6 (pyridoxine)	Chicken, fish, peanuts, bananas, pork, egg yolk, whole-grain cereals
Folate (folic acid)	Green leafy vegetables, enriched cereals, liver, dried peas and beans, whole grains
Calcium	Milk, hard cheese, yogurt, ice cream, small fish eaten with bones (e.g., sardines), dark-green vegetables, tofu, soybeans, calcium-enriched orange juice
Iron	Lean meats, liver, legumes, dried fruits, green leafy vegetables, whole-grain and fortified cereals
Zinc	Oysters, herring, meat, liver, fish, milk, whole grains, nuts, legumes

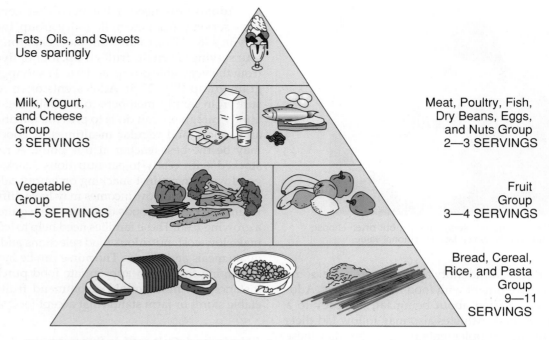

Fats, Oils, and Sweets
Use sparingly

Milk, Yogurt,
and Cheese
Group
3 SERVINGS

Meat, Poultry, Fish,
Dry Beans, Eggs,
and Nuts Group
2—3 SERVINGS

Vegetable
Group
4—5 SERVINGS

Fruit
Group
3—4 SERVINGS

Bread, Cereal,
Rice, and Pasta
Group
9—11
SERVINGS

Smaller number of servings for Teen Girls—Larger number of servings for Teen Boys

What Counts as 1 Serving? ▶ The amount you eat may be more than one serving.
For example, a dinner portion of spaghetti would count as 2 or 3 servings.

Bread, Cereal, Rice & Pasta Group	**Vegetable Group**	**Fruit Group**	**Milk, Yogurt & Cheese Group**	**Meat, Poultry, Fish, Dry Beans, Eggs & Nuts Group**	**Fats & Sweets**
1 slice of bread	½ cup of chopped raw or cooked vegetables	1 piece of fruit or melon wedge	1 cup of milk or yogurt	2½ to 3 ounces of cooked lean meat, poultry, or fish	LIMIT CALORIES FROM THESE especially if you need to lose weight
½ cup of cooked rice or pasta	1 cup of leafy raw vegetables	¾ cup of juice	1½ ounces of natural cheese	Count ½ cup of cooked beans, or 1 egg, or 2 table-spoons of peanut butter as 1 ounce of lean meat	
½ cup of cooked cereal		½ cup of canned fruit	2 ounces of processed cheese		
1 ounce of ready-to-eat cereal		¼ cup of dried fruit			

● **Figure 27.5** Food guide pyramid adapted for adolescent girls and boys. (From United States Department of Agriculture.)

therefore, other products high in calcium, such as tofu (soybean curd), soybeans, and greens should be recommended to increase calcium intake.

Certain religions recommend a vegetarian diet; other persons follow a vegetarian diet for ecologic or philosophic reasons. If planned with care, vegetarian diets can provide needed nutrients. The most common types of vegetarian diets are the following:

- Semivegetarian includes dairy products, eggs, and fish; excludes red meat and possibly poultry.
- Lacto-ovovegetarian includes eggs and dairy products but excludes meat, poultry, and fish.
- Lactovegetarian includes dairy products and excludes meat, fish, poultry, and eggs.
- Vegan excludes all food of animal origin, including dairy products, eggs, fish, meat, and poultry.

Vegan diets may not provide adequate nutrients without careful planning. All vegetarians should include whole-grain products, legumes, nuts, seeds, and fortified soy substitutes if low-fat dairy products are unacceptable.

CULTURAL SNAPSHOT

Be alert to cultural dietary influences on the adolescent; take these into consideration when helping the adolescent and the family devise an adequate food plan.

HEALTH PROMOTION AND MAINTENANCE

Adolescents have much the same need for regular health checkups, protection against infection, and prevention of accidents as do younger children. They also have special needs that can best be met by health professionals with in-depth knowledge and understanding of adolescent concerns. The number of adolescent clinics and health centers has increased along with innovative health services, such as school-based clinics, crisis hotlines, homes for runaways, and rehabilitation centers for adolescents who have been involved with alcohol or other drugs or with prostitution. Staff members in these programs provide teens with services needed for healthy growth.

Routine Checkups

A routine physical examination is recommended at least twice during the teen years, although annual physical examinations are encouraged. At this time, a complete history of developmental milestones, school problems, behavioral problems, family relationships, and immunizations should be completed. Immunization for measles, mumps, and rubella (MMR) is given if the second dose of the MMR vaccine was not administered between 4 and 6 years of age. A urine pregnancy screening is advisable before the rubella vaccine is administered to a girl of childbearing age because administration of the vaccine during pregnancy can cause serious risks to the developing fetus. A booster of tetanus toxoid and diphtheria (Td) is given around 14 to 16 years of age (about 10 years after the last booster). If the teen has not been immunized with hepatitis B vaccine series, immunization also is recommended at this time. Any other immunizations that are incomplete should be updated. Tuberculin testing is included in at least one visit and, depending on the community, may be recommended at both visits if there is an interval of several years between visits.

Height, weight, and blood pressure are measured and recorded. Vision and hearing screening are done if they have not been part of a regular school screening program. Adolescents to the age of 16 years need to be screened for scoliosis. Thyroid enlargement should be checked through age 14. Sexually active girls must have a pelvic examination, screening for sexually transmitted diseases (STDs), and a Papanicolaou smear (Fig. 27-6). Urinalysis is performed on all female adolescents, and a urine culture is performed if the girl has any symptoms of a urinary tract infection, such as urgency or burning and pain on urination. A routine physical is an excellent time for the nurse to counsel the adolescent about sexual activity, STDs, and human immunodeficiency virus (HIV) infection.

Body piercing and tattoos are becoming more common in the adolescent population. Piercings are seen in ears, eyebrows, noses, lips, chins, breasts, navels—in almost every part of the body. Tattoos of all designs are seen in the adolescent. The adolescent with piercing and tattoos needs to be aware of the

A PERSONAL GLIMPSE

Every year around our birthdays, my little brother and I always go to our pediatrician's office. After being called by the nurse, we both go down to a tiny room with bright walls, baby pictures, and the kind of mobiles hung over a crib, the same kind of decorations that cover the entire office. I suppose the room itself is comforting, but then I have to strip down to my underwear right in front of my 6-year-old brother. To make matters worse, I have to put on a skimpy little gown that hardly covers my underwear and wait in a room with huge windows and blinds that don't close, overlooking the next building's parking lot. It's so embarrassing, having to climb up onto the examining table with a gown falling down underneath me. Why can't the gowns be longer? It isn't just 6-year-olds who have to wear them!

Jessica, age 12

LEARNING OPPORTUNITY: What do nurses and health care providers need to take into consideration regarding the privacy needs of adolescents? What specific things would you do in this situation to acknowledge and respect the needs of this adolescent girl?

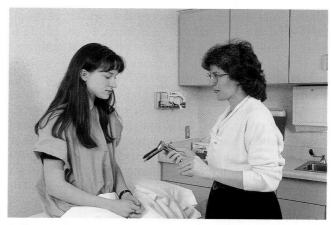

● *Figure 27.6* The adolescent is usually nervous about her first pelvic examination and Pap smear. Careful explanation by the nurse regarding these procedures may ease some of these fears.

signs and symptoms of infection (redness, swelling, warmness, drainage, discomfort) and that these must be reported immediately if they occur. Sharing needles for piercing or tattooing needs to be discussed, and the adolescent needs to be taught that sharing needles carries the same risks as sharing needles with IV drug users.

A little sensitivity is in order. Adolescents who are given privacy and respect feel safer to share their feelings and concerns with adults.

Adolescents must be given privacy, individualized attention, confidentiality, and the right to participate in decisions about their health care. They may feel uncomfortable and out of place in a pediatrician's waiting room, where most of the patients are 3 feet tall, or in a waiting room filled with adults. Some clinics and providers specialize in adolescent health care, but many adolescents do not have these facilities available to them.

Continuity of care helps build the adolescent's confidence in the service and the caregivers. Professionals dealing with teens should recognize that the physical symptoms offered as the reason for seeking care are often not the most significant problem about which the adolescent is concerned. An attitude of nonjudgmental acceptance on the part of health care personnel can often encourage the adolescent to ask questions and share feelings and concerns about a troubling matter. Adolescents may be accompanied to the health care facility by a family caregiver, but they need to have an opportunity to be interviewed alone. Questions must be asked in a way that is concrete and specific so that the adolescent will give direct answers. The interviewer must be alert to verbal and nonverbal clues.

Dental Checkups

Adolescents need continued regular dental checkups every 6 months. Dental **malocclusion** (improper alignment of the teeth) is a common condition that affects the way the teeth and jaws function. Correction of the malocclusion with dental braces improves chewing ability and appearance. The treatment of the malocclusion with dental braces is called **orthodontia**. Braces have become very common among adolescents because about half of them have malocclusions that can be corrected. Orthodontic treatment is usually started in early adolescence or late school age. The use of braces has become very widespread, and braces are readily accepted among teens, although many teens still feel awkward and self-conscious during their orthodontic treatment. Tongue piercing among adolescents has increased, and during dental checkups is a good time to discuss concerns of possible infections and teeth damage that can occur when an adolescent has a pierced tongue.

Family Teaching

The adolescent years are difficult for the maturing young person and often are just as difficult for the family caregiver. Caregivers must allow the independent teen to flourish while continuing to safeguard him or her from risky and immature behavior. Caregivers and adolescents struggle with issues related to sexuality, substance abuse, accidents, discipline, poor nutrition, and volatile emotions.

Learning about adolescent physical and psychosocial developments can help caregivers struggling to understand their teen. Caregivers will find information on sexuality and substance abuse enlightening and useful. Attending workshops or consulting counselors, teachers, religious leaders, or health care workers may enhance the caregiver's communication skills. Good communication between adolescents and their caregivers is essential to fostering healthy relationships between them. Caregivers may need both guidance in preparing their teen for adulthood and emotional support to feel successful in this difficult period. Take every opportunity to provide the family caregiver with information and support.

Health Education and Counseling

Before adolescents can take an active role in their own health care, they need information and guidance on the need for health care and how to meet that need most effectively. Education and counseling about sexuality, STDs, contraception, substance abuse, and mental health are a vital part of adolescent health care. Some of this teaching should and sometimes does come from family caregivers.

You can make the difference. Family caregivers' lack of information or discomfort in discussing certain topics with adolescents sometimes means that the job will have to be done by health professionals.

Sexuality

A good foundation in sex education can help the adolescent take pride in having reached sexual maturity; otherwise, puberty can be a frightening, shameful experience. Girls who have not been taught about menstruation until it occurs are understandably alarmed. Those who have been taught to regard it as "the curse," rather than an entrance into womanhood, will not have positive feelings about this part of their sexuality.

Boys who are unprepared for **nocturnal emissions** may feel guilty, believing that they have caused these "wet dreams" by sexual fantasies or masturbation. They need to understand that this is a normal occurrence and simply the body's method of getting rid of surplus semen.

Assuming that adolescents are adequately prepared for the events of puberty, sex education during adolescence can deal with the important issues of responsible sexuality, contraception, and venereal disease. More adolescents today are sexually active than ever, resulting in an alarmingly rapid increase in teenage pregnancies and STDs. The incidence of HIV infection is particularly increasing among adolescents.

Girls need to learn the importance of regular pelvic examinations and Pap smears and the technique for the monthly self-care procedure of breast self-examination (see Family Teaching Tips: Breast Self-Exam) (Fig. 27-7). Boys need to learn that testicular cancer is one of the most common cancers in young men between the ages of 15 and 34 years and must be taught how and when to perform testicular self-examination (see Family Teaching Tips: Testicular Self-Examination) (Fig. 27-8).

Adolescents' growing awareness of their sexuality, sexually provocative material in the media, and lack of acceptable means to gratify sexual desires make masturbation a common practice during adolescence. Unlike young children's genital exploration, adolescent masturbation can produce orgasm in the female and ejaculation in the male. Generally, it is a private and solitary activity, but occasionally it occurs with other members of the peer group. Health professionals recognize masturbation as a positive way to release sexual tension and increase one's knowledge of body sensations. The nurse can reassure adolescents that masturbation is common in both males and females and is a normal outlet for sexual urges.

Sexual Responsibility

Not all adolescents are sexually active, but the number of those who are increases with each year of age. Although abstinence is the only completely successful protection, all adolescents need to have information concerning safe sex practices to be prepared for the occasion when they wish to be sexually intimate with someone. Adolescents do not have a good record of using contraceptives to prevent pregnancy. Many teens give excuses such as "sex shouldn't be planned," because if it is planned, it is wrong or they feel guilty. They need to feel that it "just happened" in the heat of the moment, not because they really wanted or planned it. Many adolescents are beginning to realize that much more than pregnancy may be at risk, but their attitude of "it won't happen to me," which is typical of their developmental age, continues to contribute to their increasing sexual activity.

FAMILY TEACHING TIPS
Breast Self-Exam

The best time to do the breast self-exam is about a week after your period ends. The breast is not as tender or swollen at this point in the menstrual cycle.

1. Lie down with a pillow under your right shoulder. Place your right arm behind your head (see Fig. 27-7A).
2. Use the sensitive finger pads (where your fingerprints are, not the tips) of the middle three fingers on your left hand to feel for lumps in the right breast (see Fig. 27-7B). Use overlapping dime-sized circular motions of the finger pads to feel the breast tissue. Powder, oil, or lotion can be applied to the breast to make it easier for the fingers to glide over the surface and feel changes.
3. Use three different levels of pressure to feel the breast tissue. First, light pressure to just move the skin without jostling the tissue beneath, then medium pressure pressing midway into the tissue, and finally firm pressure to probe more deeply down to the chest and ribs or to the point just short of discomfort. Use each pressure level to feel the breast tissue before moving on to the next spot.
4. Move your fingers around the breast in an up and down pattern (called the vertical pattern), starting at an imaginary line drawn straight down your side from the underarm and moving across the breast to the middle of the chest bone (sternum or breastbone). Check the entire breast using each of the pressures described above. Completely feel all of the breast and chest area up under your armpit, up to the collarbone and all the way over to your shoulder to cover breast tissue that extends toward the shoulder (see Fig. 27-7C).
5. Repeat the exam on your left breast using the finger pads of your right hand, with a pillow under your left shoulder (see Fig. 27-7D).
6. While standing in front of a mirror with your hands pressing firmly down on your hips (this position shows more clearly any breast changes), look at your breasts for any change in size, shape, contour, dimpling of the skin, changes in the nipple, redness, or spontaneous nipple discharge (see Fig. 27-7, E and F).
7. Examine each underarm while sitting or standing, with your arm only slightly raised (raising your arm straight tightens the tissue and makes it difficult to examine). The upright position makes it easier to check the upper and outer parts of the breasts (toward your armpits). You may want to do this part of the exam while showering. It's easy to slide soapy hands over your skin, and to feel anything unusual (see Fig. 27-7G).

Breast self examination as revised and presented by the American Cancer Society. Retrieved from www.cancer.org, January 2004.

● *Figure 27.7* (**A**) Lie down with pillow under right shoulder. Place right arm behind head.
(**B**) Use the sensitive finger pads (where your fingerprints are, not the tips) of the middle three
fingers on left hand to feel right breast. (**C**) Move fingers around the breast in an up and down
vertical pattern, starting at an imaginary line drawn straight down the side from the underarm
and moving across the breast to the middle of the chest bone. (**D**) Repeat examine on left
breast using the finger pads of right hand. (**E**) While standing in front of a mirror, press hands
firmly down on hips and look for breast changes. (**F**) Look for changes in the nipple, redness or
spontaneous nipple discharge. (**G**) Examine each underarm while sitting or standing, with your
arm slightly raised. This may be done while showering.

FAMILY TEACHING TIPS

Testicular Self-Examination

1. Perform the examination once a month after a warm bath or shower. The scrotum is relaxed from the warmth. Select a day that is easy to remember such as the first or last day of the month.
2. Stand in front of a mirror, if possible, and look for any swelling on the skin of the scrotum.
3. Examine each testicle, one at a time, using both hands.
4. Place the index and middle fingers under the testicle and the thumbs on top. Roll each testicle gently between the thumbs and fingers. One testicle is normally larger than the other (see Fig. 27-8A).
5. The epididymis is the soft, tubelike structure located at the back of the testicle that collects and carries sperm. This must not be mistaken for an abnormal lump (see Fig. 27-8B).
6. Most lumps are found on the sides of the testicle, although they may also appear on the front. Report any lump to your health care provider at once.
7. Testicular cancer is highly curable when treated promptly.

Epididymis

Testicle

● **Figure 27.8** (**A**) Examine each testicle with index and middle fingers under testicle and thumbs on top; (**B**) cross section of scrotum showing position of the epididymis and the testicle.

Some adults continue to resist providing contraceptive information to adolescents in school, believing that such information encourages teens to become sexually active. However, as HIV infection becomes a greater threat to every sexually active person, this argument becomes harder to defend. Adolescents need contraceptive information to prevent pregnancy, but more importantly they need straightforward information about using condoms to protect them against HIV and other infections. Both male and female adolescents need this information, and girls must be advised to carry their own condoms if they believe that there is any possibility of having sexual intercourse.

When condoms are used consistently and correctly they are highly effective in preventing pregnancy and sexually transmitted diseases. Condoms used with spermicidal foam have an even greater effective rate. The safest condom is one made of latex with a prelubricated tip or reservoir and pretreated with nonoxynol-9 spermicide. Family Teaching Tips: Safe Condom Use and Figure 27-9 provide guidelines for use.

Other STDs that sexually active adolescents need to know about are syphilis, gonorrhea, genital herpes, genital warts, and chlamydial and trichomonal infections. Prevention of STDs is the primary aim of education for adolescents. If prevention proves ineffective,

however, the most important factor is referral for treatment. Many adolescents are reluctant to seek treatment, fearing that their family caregivers will discover their activity. Crisis hotlines are valuable resources to assure adolescents that treatment is vital for them and their partners and that confidentiality is ensured.

Health care personnel who work with adolescents seeking treatment for an STD must be nonjudgmental, supportive, and understanding. The adolescents need treatment and information about preventing spread of the STD to others, as well as how to prevent contracting another STD. See Chapter 40 for a thorough discussion of STDs and related nursing care.

Many adolescents are not sexually active, but most spend time dating or socializing with peers. In recent years the use of Rohypnol, also known as the "date rape drug," has become a concern for the adolescent. Rohypnol is not sold legally in the United States but is brought in from countries where it is sold legally. The drug, especially in combination with alcohol, causes memory loss, blackouts, and an inability to resist sexual attacks. Often the drug is secretly slipped into a person's drink. The drug has no taste or odor, but within a few minutes after ingesting the drug, the person feels dizzy, disoriented, and nauseated, then rapidly passes out. After several hours, the person awakens and has

FAMILY TEACHING TIPS

Safe Condom Use

1. Use a new condom each time.
2. The safest type of condom is prelubricated latex with a tip or reservoir pretreated with nonoxynol-9 spermicide.
3. If the condom is not pretreated, you may lubricate it with water or water-based lubricant such as K-Y Jelly *and* a spermicidal jelly or foam containing nonoxynol-9.
4. Do not use oil-based products such as mineral oil, cold cream, or petroleum jelly for lubrication; they may weaken the latex.
5. Put the condom on as soon as the penis is erect. Retract the foreskin if not circumcised, and unroll the condom over the entire length of the penis.
6. Leave a ½ inch space at the end. Press out the tip of the condom to remove air bubbles.
7. The outside of the condom may be lubricated as much as desired with a water-soluble lubricant.
8. If the condom starts to slip during intercourse, hold it on. Do not let it slip off. Condoms come in sizes; so if there is a problem with slipping, look for a smaller size.
9. After ejaculation, hold the rim of the condom at the base of the penis and withdraw before losing the erection.
10. Remove the condom and tie a knot in the open end. Dispose of it so that no one can come in contact with semen.
11. Heat can damage condoms. Store them in a cool, dry place.
12. Immediately after intercourse, both partners should wash off any semen or vaginal secretions with soap and water.

no memories of what happened while under the influence of the drug. The adolescent needs to be encouraged to stay aware and alert to avoid becoming a victim of date rape. He or she should be taught to avoid using alcohol and never to leave any drink unattended.

Substance Abuse

As adolescents search for identity and independence, they are susceptible to many pressures from society and their peers. Adolescents may experiment with substances that may be habit forming or addictive and ultimately will harm them. This may be done "just for kicks," to "go along with the crowd" (peer group), or to rebel against the authority of family caregivers or other adults. Some substances abused by adolescents also are abused by many adults; so to some adolescents, using these substances may appear sophisticated.

Alcohol and certain other drugs provide an escape, however brief, from pressures the adolescent may feel. Alcohol is the mind-altering substance most commonly abused by adolescents. Other substances that adolescents may abuse are tobacco (including smokeless tobacco), marijuana, cocaine or "crack," heroin, "Ecstacy," other street drugs, and prescription drugs. (See Chapter 41 for further discussion of substance abuse.) Adolescents can often obtain tobacco products, despite federal legislation to enforce strict age limitations on their sale.

Programs developed to educate students about substance abuse meet with varying success. Health care personnel must stress to adolescents that use of alcohol or mind-altering chemicals is often accompanied by irresponsible sexual behavior that could further complicate their lives. Chapter 41 discusses these problems in more detail.

● *Figure 27.9* Putting on a condom: (**A**) Press the air out ½ inch at the tip of the condom; (**B**) holding the tip of the condom, carefully roll it down the shaft of the erect penis; (**C**) be certain that the condom covers the full length of the penis, with the rim of the condom at the base of the penis.

A   B   C

Mental Health

The turmoil that adolescents experience while searching for self-esteem and self-confidence can cause stress that may lead to depression, suicide, and conduct disorders. Academic and social pressures add to that stress. The family also may be under stress due to unemployment or economic difficulties, separation, divorce, or death of a caregiver. Health care personnel must be sensitive to signs that the adolescent is having problems. Adolescents need the opportunity to ventilate their fears, concerns, and frustrations. The rapport between family caregivers and teens may not be such that the adolescent can express these feelings to the family. Many schools have mental health personnel on staff who can provide counseling when needed. Adolescents need counseling to work through troublesome situations and to avoid chronic mental health problems. Mental health assessment is an important part of the adolescent's total health assessment. With the increased use of computers and Internet sites, Internet safety is an important aspect of adolescent mental health. Parents need to be aware of their adolescent's computer activities and the sites they access, especially communication sites such as chat rooms. Discussions with adolescents regarding safety concerns on Internet sites help to increase their awareness and decrease potential dangers. See Family Teaching Tips: Internet Safety.

FAMILY TEACHING TIPS

Internet Safety

Signs that might indicate on-line risks in a child or adolescent:
- Spends large amounts of time on-line, especially at night
- Has pornography on computer
- Receives phone calls from adults you don't know
- Makes calls, especially long distance, to numbers you don't recognize
- Receives mail, gifts, packages from someone you don't know
- Turns computer monitor off or changes screen when you enter room
- Becomes withdrawn from family

To minimize on-line concerns:
- Communicate and talk with child; openly discuss concerns and dangers.
- Spend time with child on-line.
- Use blocking software and devices.
- Use caller ID to determine who is calling your child.
- Maintain access to child's on-line account and monitor activity.

Adapted from FBI publication, *A parent's guide to Internet safety, http://www.fbi.gov/publications/pguide/pguidee.htm*

Test Yourself

- What nutrients are often missing in the adolescent diet?

- List the topics of health education that should be discussed with the adolescent.

Accident Prevention

In every part of society, increasing numbers of adolescents are dying as a result of violence; this includes motor vehicle accidents, homicide, suicide, and other causes. Homicide ranks as the leading cause of death for 15- to 19-year-old minority youth, regardless of gender (Joffe, 1999). Statistics regarding adolescents are difficult to interpret, but death among adolescents is often related to risky behaviors (Fig. 27-10). These behaviors include the unintentional (motor vehicles, fires) as well as the intentional (violence, suicide) injuries, alcohol and other drug use, sexual behaviors, tobacco use, and dietary behaviors. Alcohol and other drugs are often involved in fatal accidents. Death is not the only negative outcome of violence: many adolescents are injured and hospitalized or treated in emergency departments, and many suffer psychological injury from being victims of violence.

Violence is also on the rise in schools—not just inner-city schools. Weapons are detected on students in schools all over the country. Guns and knives are the weapons most often found. The problem has become so serious that some schools have installed metal detectors to protect students.

Youth Ages 10 – 24

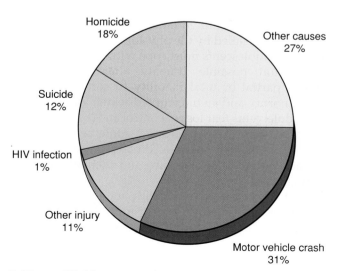

● *Figure 27.10* Leading causes of death for adolescents, many of which result from risk behaviors.

Adolescents also are victims of violence in their own homes in greater numbers than any other age group of children. Date rape and other violence in a dating relationship have become common.

Students have formed groups such as Students Against Drunk Driving to promote safety in driving (website: http://www.saddonline.com). Many schools provide support groups that help students to work through their grief after schoolmates have met with violent death.

Much work needs to be done to understand the reason for this increasing violence. One factor in adolescents is that they often act recklessly without benefit of mature judgment. Adolescents have relatively easy access to guns and often use them as a means to solve problems. Efforts to control and regulate gun sales are nationally discussed topics. Acts of terror and violence in our world increase the confusion and anxiety that adolescents have regarding conflicts and conflict resolution.

Nurses who have any contact with adolescents must make every effort to help them work through their problems in nonviolent ways. The nurse can become involved at the school or community level by becoming an advocate for adolescents and an educator to promote safe driving, as well as helmet wear and safety practices when using a motorcycle, all-terrain vehicle, bicycle, skateboard, or in-line skates. Nurses also can work with support groups that offer counseling to adolescents involved in date violence. As a community member and a health care worker, the nurse can provide a positive role model for adolescents.

THE ADOLESCENT IN THE HEALTH CARE FACILITY

When adolescents are hospitalized, it is usually because of a major health problem such as an injury from violence or from a motor vehicle accident, substance abuse, attempted suicide, or a chronic health problem intensified by the physiologic changes of adolescence. Adolescents must cope with the stress of hospitalization, possible dramatic alterations in body image, partial or total inability to conform to peer group norms, and an interrupted search for identity.

Adolescents fear loss of control and loss of privacy. Provide opportunities for the adolescent to make choices whenever possible. Protect the adolescent's privacy by providing screening and adequate covering during procedures.

Adolescents may react with anger and refuse to cooperate when their privacy or feelings of control are threatened. Be aware of this possible reaction and avoid labeling such an adolescent as a difficult patient.

The admission interview for an adolescent may be more successful if the family caregiver and the

This is critical to remember. In working with adolescents, as with all patients, clear, honest explanations about treatments and procedures are essential.

adolescent are interviewed separately. This provides the opportunity to gain information that the adolescent may not want to reveal in the presence of the family caregiver. Thoroughly explore the adolescent's developmental level, listen carefully with empathy to his or her concerns, encourage maximum participation in self-care, and provide sufficient information to make this participation possible.

During the admission interview, advise the adolescent of the unit's rules. Adolescents need to know what limits are set for their behavior while they are in the hospital. To share feelings and gain information, many find it helpful to discuss their health problem with a peer who has had the same or a related problem.

Adolescents need access to a telephone to contact peers and keep up social contacts. Recreation areas are important. In settings specifically designed for adolescents, recreation rooms can provide an area where teens can gather to do school work, play games and cards, and socialize. In many hospitals with adolescent units, video games as well as television are provided in each patient room. Access to a computer and electronic mail might also help the teen stay connected to peers. Supervision is important to decrease misuse of computer privileges. Teens are encouraged to wear their own clothes. They can be encouraged to shampoo and style their hair, and girls can wear their usual makeup.

The adolescent's health problem may require a lengthy hospitalization and intense rehabilitation efforts. Adequate preparation and guidance can help make that difficult experience easier and less damaging to normal growth and development.

Test Yourself

- What are the most frequent causes of accidents in adolescents?

- Give examples of how hospitalized adolescents can be given choices and control.

KEY POINTS

- The preadolescent period is between ages 10 and 12 years, and the ages from 13 to 18 years are known as adolescence.

- During the preadolescent years, children go through many physical and emotional changes on their way to adulthood. Offering preadolescents information about their changing bodies and feelings is important.
- The rapid growth of the skeletal system outpaces the growth of the muscular system, contributing to the clumsiness sometimes noted in the adolescent.
- Secondary sexual characteristics seen in the adolescent boy include penis, testes, and scrotum reaching adult size and shape, as well as pubic hair, increased strength, and a deepening of the voice. Adolescent girls develop breasts and pubic hair and begin ovulation and menstruation.
- According to Piaget the adolescent moves from concrete operational thinking to formal operational thought. Erikson's stage of development in the adolescent is referred to as identity versus role confusion. The adolescent's task is to establish his or her own identity and to find a place in society.
- Changing sex role stereotypes, geographic mobility, and abundant career opportunities and options add to the adolescent's difficulties in making a career choice.
- Intimacy or mutual sharing of deep feelings with another person occurs when people have developed trust and their own sense of identity. Intimate relationships in adolescents help in preparation for long-term relationships.
- In trying to develop their own sense of self and identity adolescents begin the process of separating from family caregivers. The peers exert influence, and the adolescent feels a need to conform and to "fit" with peers. This peer pressure may be extremely influential in affecting the adolescent's attitudes and behaviors. A strong support system is important to help the adolescent through this stressful stage of development.
- Body image and self-esteem are closely related, and the adolescent struggles with wanting to be attractive and accepted. This drive can create anxiety in the adolescent, which can lead to unhealthy behavior, practices, and conditions.
- Adolescent diets are often deficient in calcium; iron; zinc; vitamins A, D, and B_6; and folic acid.
- Health education in the adolescent needs to include information regarding sexuality, sexual responsibility, STDs and contraception, as well as teaching about substance abuse and mental health issues and concerns. Adolescents are faced with peer pressure, personal values and beliefs, and societal influences in making decisions related to sexual responsibility and substance use.
- In the health care facility, the adolescent fears loss of control and loss of privacy. The nurse caring for the hospitalized adolescent must be sensitive to the adolescent's needs, provide supportive care, and encourage as much participation by the adolescent as possible. Health problems that threaten the adolescent's body image may threaten the satisfactory completion of developmental tasks.

REFERENCES AND SELECTED READINGS

Books and Journals

Berger, K. S. (2001). *The developing person through the life span* (5th ed.). New York: Worth Publishers.

Brazelton, T. B., & Greenspan, S. (2001). *The irreducible needs of children: What every child must have to grow, learn, and flourish.* Cambridge, MA: Perseus Publishing.

Deering, C. G., & Jennings, C. D. (2002). Communicating with children and adolescents. *American Journal of Nursing, 102*(3), 34–42.

Dudek, S. G. (2000). *Nutrition essentials for nursing practice* (4th ed.). Philadelphia: Lippincott Williams & Wilkins.

Dworkin, P. (2000). *Pediatrics* (4th ed.). Philadelphia: Lippincott Williams & Wilkins.

Fehrenbach, M. J. (2002). *Tongue piercing.* Retrieved July 2, 2004, from http://www.dhed.net/patient.html#tongue

Hockenberry, M. J., Wilson, D., Winkelstein, M. L., & Kline, N. E. (2003). *Wong's nursing care of infants and children* (7th ed.). St. Louis: Mosby.

Joffe, A. (1999). Introduction to adolescent medicine. In *Oski's pediatrics: Principles and practice* (3rd ed.). Philadelphia: Lippincott Williams & Wilkins.

Nagai, A., & Siktberg, L. (2001). Osteoporosis prevention in female adolescents: Calcium intake and exercise participation. *Pediatric Nursing, 27*(2), 132.

Nicoll, L. (2001). *Nurse's guide to the Iinternet* (3rd ed.). Philadelphia: Lippincott Williams & Wilkins.

Norris, A. E., & Beaton, M. M. (2002). Who knows more about condoms? A comparison between nursing students, education students and at-risk adolescents. *American Journal of Maternal/Child Nursing, 27*(2), 103.

Pillitteri, A. (2003). *Maternal and child health nursing* (4th ed.). Philadelphia: Lippincott Williams & Wilkins.

Spock, B., et al. (1998). *Dr. Spock's baby and child care.* New York: Pocket Books.

Wong, D. L., Perry, S., & Hockenberry, M. (2002). *Maternal child nursing care* (2nd ed.). St. Louis: Mosby.

Web Addresses
Testicular Exam/Cancer
http://www.cancerlinkusa.com

Breast Self-Exam
www.cancer.org

Drug-Resistance Activities
www.health.org/features/kidsarea

WORKBOOK

NCLEX-STYLE REVIEW QUESTIONS

1. The nurse is assisting with a physical exam on a 12-year-old girl. Her record indicates that at age 9 she was 51 inches tall and weighed 72 pounds. Which of the following would the nurse *most likely* find if the child were following a normal pattern of growth and development? The adolescent

   a. weighs 94 pounds.

   b. measures 53 inches in height.

   c. has a small amount of pubic hair.

   d. has well-developed breasts.

2. The nurse is working with a group of caregivers of adolescents who are discussing normal adolescent growth and development. Which of the following statements made by a caregiver would indicate a need for follow-up?

   a. "He wants to be a nurse after he finishes college."

   b. "She has her own money to spend now because she has a job."

   c. "My son has been spending at least half an hour to 1 hour in front of the mirror the last 3 months getting ready for school."

   d. "My daughter is so slim and trim, she has lost 10 pounds in the last 6 weeks."

3. The nurse is teaching a group of adolescent girls about good nutrition habits and eating foods that will help to increase the deficient nutrients in the adolescent diet. Which of the following statements made by the girls in the group is correct?

   a. "Eating lots of broccoli will help increase the iron in my diet."

   b. "If I drink three glasses of milk each day, I will get plenty of vitamin C."

   c. "Even though I don't like eggs, if I eat four eggs a week I will get enough calcium."

   d. "I am sure I get enough vitamin A since I eat bread at every meal."

4. In working with adolescent children, the nurse would know that if the adolescents were following normal development patterns, this age child would be *most* likely be involved in which of the following activities?

   a. Working to establish a career

   b. Playing a board game with siblings

   c. Participating in a activities with peers

   d. Volunteering in community projects

5. The nurse is discussing teenage substance abuse with a group of caregivers of adolescent children. If the caregivers make the following statements, which statement is the *most* accurate regarding substance abuse in teens?

   a. "Every teenager experiments with substances."

   b. "The most common drugs used by teenagers is alcohol."

   c. "It won't really hurt teenagers if they try tobacco."

   d. "Even teenagers need a release from the pressures they face."

6. The nurse is teaching a group of adolescent girls how to perform a breast self-exam. Which of the following actions should the nurse teach regarding the breast self-exam?

   Select all that apply.

   a. Perform the breast exam each month.

   b. Do the breast exam just before your period starts.

   c. Use the tips of the fingers to exam the breast.

   d. Use the same pattern to feel every part of the breast.

   e. Stand in front of a mirror to look for changes in breasts

   f. Examine the breasts while in the bathtub.

STUDY ACTIVITIES

1. List and compare the 15-year-old female and the 15-year-old male in regard to physical development, psychosocial development, personality development, and their feelings about body image.

Area of Development	15-Year-Old Female	15-Year-Old Male
Physical development		
Psychosocial development		
Personality development		
Body image		

2. Mattie is the mother of 13-year-old Chantal. Chantal has decided she will not eat meat or poultry because animals had to be killed to obtain it. Mattie is concerned about Chantal's nutrition. Develop a teaching plan, including a menu for a day for Mattie. Be sure your plan provides nutrients often deficient in adolescents and that supports Chantal in her choice to not eat meat and poultry.

3. You are working with a group of adolescents in a school-based clinic and plan to have a discussion about substance abuse and sexually transmitted diseases. Make a list of questions that you think the adolescents might want to ask but are uncomfortable asking. Discuss with your peers the answers you could give to each of these questions.

4. Go to the following Internet site:

   http://www.kidshealth.org/teen

   Click on "Your Body" on the left side of the screen. Under the section "Skin Stuff," click on "Is Body Piercing Safe." Read this section and answer the following.

   a. List 10 risks related to body piercing.

   b. Why is it a concern to pierce the tongue? Eyebrow? Nose?

   c. What makes piercing the ears less of a concern?

   d. What specifically can make piercing more safe?

CRITICAL THINKING: What Would You Do?

1. You have the opportunity to talk with a group of 16-year-old girls. The topics you have decided to focus on during this talk are breast self-examination and Pap smears.

   a. What are the reasons adolescent girls should do a breast self-exam and have routine Pap smears?

   b. What steps will you teach these girls to follow when doing a breast self-exam?

   c. What areas of concern would you anticipate these girls would have regarding breast self-exams and Pap smears?

   d. What would your responses to these concerns be?

2. Jamal is an adolescent athlete. He has told you he is planning to use a carbohydrate-loading diet before a big track meet.

   a. What reasons do you think Jamal will give you for wanting to follow this diet before his track meet?

   b. What concerns would you share with Jamal about his plan?

   c. What alternate suggestions and guidance could you offer to Jamal that would be more appropriate for him to follow?

3. Fifteen-year-old Caitlin is in a group discussing condom use. She scornfully tells you that girls don't need to know anything about condoms.

   a. How would you respond to Caitlin?

   b. What are your ideas regarding what you think should and should not be part of health education in high school settings?

   c. What are your rationales for your ideas for question b?

Foundations of Pediatric Health Care

Assessment of the Child
(Data Collection)

STUDENT OBJECTIVES

On completion of this chapter, the student should be able to

1. Describe the process for collecting subjective data from caregivers and children.
2. Define chief complaint.
3. Explain the purpose of doing a review of systems when gathering data.
4. State how the caregiver may be involved in collecting objective data about the child.
5. Compare observations indicating health or illness in children.
6. Discuss the reasons that height and weight are assessed on an ongoing basis.
7. Discuss the appropriate use of developmental tables.
8. List the types of patients on whom a rectal temperature should not be taken.
9. Identify the five types of respiratory retractions and the location of each.
10. State the purpose of pulse oximetry.
11. Name three methods of obtaining blood pressure.
12. Explain the reason a physical exam is performed.
13. Discuss the process of assisting with or performing a physical examination.
14. Identify the purpose of using the Glasgow coma scale for neurologic assessment.

KEY TERMS

nutrition history
personal history
pinna
point of maximum impulse (PMI)
school history
social history
symmetry

W hether the setting is a hospital or other health care facility, it is important to gather information regarding the child's history and current status. Although data collection is continuous throughout a child's care, most data are collected during the interview, the physical examination, and from the results of diagnostic tests and studies.

COLLECTING SUBJECTIVE DATA

Information spoken by the child or family is called *subjective data*. Interviewing the family caregiver and child allows the nurse to collect information that can be used to develop a plan of care for the child. Communicating with the child and family caregiver requires knowledge of growth and development and an understanding of communication techniques. See Appendix J for further information regarding communicating with children of all ages and family caregivers.

Think about this. The interview process is goal directed, unlike a social conversation. The focus is on the child and caregiver and their needs.

Conducting the Client Interview

Most subjective data are collected through interviewing the family caregiver and the child. The interview helps establish relationships between the nurse, the child, and the family. Listening and using appropriate communication techniques help promote a good interview. Listening and using appropriate communication techniques help promote a good interview (see Appendix J). Using focused questions and allowing time for answering will help the child and family feel comfortable.

A little sensitivity is in order. A private, quiet setting decreases distractions during the interview.

The nurse should be introduced to the child and caregiver and the purpose of the interview stated. A calm, reassuring manner is important to establish trust and comfort. Past experiences with health care may influence the interview. The caregiver and the nurse should be comfortably seated, and the child should be included in the interview process (Fig. 28-1). The child may sit on the caregiver's lap or, if a crib is available, the child can be placed in the crib with the side rails up. This will help to ensure the safety of the infant or child during the interview.

● *Figure 28.1* The child sits on the caregiver's lap during the interview process.

Interviewing Family Caregivers

The family caregiver provides most of the information needed in caring for the child, especially the infant or toddler. Rather than simply asking the caregiver to fill out a form, the nurse may ask the questions and write down the answers; this process gives the opportunity to observe the reactions of the child and the caregiver as they interact with each other and answer the questions. In addition, this eases the problem of the caregiver who cannot read or write. The nurse must be non-judgmental, being careful not to indicate disapproval by verbal or nonverbal responses. While gathering information about the child's physical condition, the nurse also must allow the caregiver to express concerns and anxieties. If a certain topic seems uncomfortable for the caregiver to discuss in front of the child, that topic should be discussed later when the child cannot hear what is being said.

Here's a helpful hint. Age-appropriate toys and activities to keep young children occupied will allow the caregiver to focus on the questions asked.

Interviewing the Child

It is important that the preschool child and the older child be included in the interview. Use age-appropriate

CULTURAL SNAPSHOT

Being aware of the primary language spoken and using an interpreter when needed will help in gaining accurate information. Various cultural patterns, such as avoiding eye contact, should be noted and respected.

questions when talking with the child. Showing interest in the child and what she or he says helps both the child and caregiver to feel comfortable. By being honest when answering the child's questions, the nurse establishes trust with the child.

Check out this tip. Using a doll or stuffed animal that the child is familiar with can help involve the child in the interview process.

Using stories or books written at a child's level helps with understanding what the child is thinking or feeling. The child's comments should be listened to attentively, and the child should be made to feel important in the interview.

Interviewing the Adolescent

Adolescents can provide information about themselves; interviewing them in private often encourages them to share information that they might not contribute in front of their caregivers. This is especially true when asking questions of a sensitive nature, such as information regarding drug use or the adolescent's sexual practices.

Test Yourself

- Define subjective data. How does the nurse collect subjective data?

- Why is it important to interview the family caregiver when caring for children?

- In what ways does interviewing the adolescent differ from interviewing the child?

Obtaining a Client History

When a child is brought to any health care setting, it is important to gather information regarding the child's current condition, as well as medical history. This information is used to develop a plan of care for the child. In obtaining information from the child and caregiver, the nurse is developing a relationship, as well as noting what the child and family know and understand about the child's health. Observations of the caregiver–child relationship can also provide important information.

Biographical Data

To begin obtaining a client history, the nurse collects and records identifying information about the child, including the child's name, address, and phone number, as well as information regarding the caregiver. This information is part of the legal record and should be treated as confidential. A questionnaire often is used to gather information, such as the child's nickname, feeding habits, food likes and dislikes, allergies, sleeping schedule, and toilet-training status. Any special words the child uses or understands to indicate needs or desires, such as words used for urinating and bowel movements, would be included on the questionnaire. Figure 28-2 provides an example of an assessment form that may be used to collect information.

Chief Complaint

The reason for the child's visit to the health care setting is called the *chief complaint*. In a well-child setting, this reason might be a routine check or immunizations, whereas an illness or other condition might be the reason in another setting. The caregiver's primary concern is his or her reason for seeking health care for the child. To best care for the child, it is important to get the most complete explanation of what brought the child to the health care setting. Repeating the caregiver's statement regarding the child's chief complaint will help to clarify that the nurse has correctly heard what the caregiver has said.

History of Present Health Concern

To help the nurse discover the child's needs, the nurse elicits information about the current situation, including the child's symptoms, when they began, how long the symptoms have been present, a description of the symptoms, their intensity and frequency, and treatments to this time. The nurse should ask the questions in a way that encourages the caregiver to be specific. This is also the time for the nurse to ask the caregiver about any other concerns regarding the child.

Health History

Information regarding the mother's pregnancy and prenatal history are included in obtaining a health history for the child. Any occurrences during the delivery can contribute to the child's health concerns. The child's mother is usually the best source of this information. Other areas the nurse asks questions about include common childhood, serious, or chronic illnesses; immunizations and health maintenance; feeding and nutrition; as well as hospitalizations and injuries.

Family Health History

Some diseases and conditions are seen in families and are important in prevention, as well as detection, for the child. The caregiver can usually provide information regarding family health history. The nurse uses this information to do preventative teaching with the child and family. Certain risk factors in families contribute to the development of health care concerns; risk

PEDIATRIC NURSING ASSESSMENT FORM

1. Name _____ Date/Time of Admission _____ Via _____

2. Birth Date _____ Information obtained from:_____ Relationship to child _____

3. Child's legal guardian: _____ Child's Nickname: _____

VITAL SIGNS	Temp	Apical Pulse	Radial Pulse	Respirations	BP	Height	Weight	Head Circum

CURRENT CHIEF COMPLAINT/DIAGNOSIS:
Symptoms and Duration

Child's/Caregivers' Understanding of Condition:

PREVIOUS ILLNESS/INJURIES/DIAGNOSIS:
Illness, Symptoms, and Duration

Injuries or Surgery:

Anesthesia Complications?

Allergies and Reactions:	Immunizations	Dates:	Exposure to Infectious Disease Date
	DTaP (DT)		(chicken pox, measles, etc.)
	Polio		
	Hepatitis B		
	Hib (type)		
	MMR (measles, mumps, rubella)		
	TB skin test Result		

Medications: Name:	Dose	Frequency	Time of Last Dose

Child's reaction to previous hospitalizations: _____

Special fears of child about hospitalization? _____

Family History: (Check all that apply—indicate relationship to child)

____ Cancer _____	____ Seizures _____	____ TB _____
____ Heart disease _____	____ Asthma _____	____ Anesthesia complications_____
____ Allergy _____	____ Smoking _____	____ Other (specify) _____
____ Diabetes _____	____ Hypertension _____	_____

● *Figure 28.2* A sample pediatric nursing assessment form.

Living Facilities (check)

_____ House   _____ Apartment   _____ Trailer   _____ Steps to travel?_____

Who does child live with? _____

Names, ages, of siblings in home_____

Names, ages of other children in home _____

Other persons in home _____

Special interests, toys, games, hobbies: _____

_____

Security object:_____ Was it brought to hospital? _____

Bowel/Bladder Habits:

Toilet Training(if applicable)

Started	_____ Yes	_____ No	
Completed	_____ Yes	_____ No	

Diapers:

Day	_____ Yes	_____ No
Night	_____ Yes	_____ No

Potty Chair:	_____ Yes	_____ No
Toilet:	_____ Yes	_____ No
Bedwetter:	_____ Yes	_____ No

Terms Used for:

Bowel Movement _____   Urination _____

Frequency of BM _____ Color _____ Consistency _____

Does child have problems with diarrhea or constipation?_____

_____

Does child have urinary frequency, burning, discomfort: _____ Yes _____ No

If yes, please explain:_____

_____

_____

Patterns of:

Sleep/rest:

Bedtime_____ Wakeup _____

Nap ____ Yes ____ No — When? _____

Activity:

Does infant roll over? _____

Does child stand/walk? _____

Does child climb? _____

Does child dress self? _____

Does child go up and down stairs? _____

Does child talk in formed sentences? _____

Eating Habits:

Does child: Feed self ____ Yes ____ No

Does child need help to eat? _____

Food and beverage:

Likes:_____

_____

Dislikes: _____

_____

Usual appetite? _____

Appetite now? _____

Last time child had food or beverage: _____

Items brought to hospital:

Glasses	_____ Yes	_____ No
Contacts	_____ Yes	_____ No
Hearing Aid	_____ Yes	_____ No
Dentures	_____ Yes	_____ No
Braces	_____ Yes	_____ No
Retainer	_____ Yes	_____ No
Special bottle	_____ Yes	_____ No
Own pacifier	_____ Yes	_____ No

Does child smoke or drink alcoholic beverages? _____ Yes _____ No

If yes, please give details _____

_____

Does child use street drugs? _____ Yes _____ No

If yes, please give details_____

_____

Other behavior habits of the child (Please check)

Thumbsucking _____ ; Nailbiting _____ ; Headbanging _____

Rituals (Explain) _____

_____

Disposition (Describe)_____

_____

Skin Assessment:

_____ Jaundice _____ Cyanosis _____ Pallor _____ Redness

_____ Cool _____ Warm _____ Clammy _____ Dry

_____ Normal appearance

Describe: (Location and character)

Rash _____

Abrasions _____

Lacerations _____

Contusions _____

Respiratory Assessment:

____ Clear ____ Stridor ____ Rales (___moist, ___ dry) ____ Wheezing

____ Rhonchi ____ Retractions (type) _____

____ Coughing, Sneezing ____ Nasal Discharge (describe) _____

Child/Caregiver oriented to unit? _____ Yes _____ No; understanding verbalized by child _____ , caregiver _____

Reviewed safety measures with child _____ , caregiver _____ ; understanding verbalized by child _____ , caregiver _____

Additional information nursing staff should know:

● **Figure 28.2** Continued

factors addressed early in a child's life can often be monitored or changed to decrease the child's risk of getting these diseases or conditions.

Test Yourself

- Why is it important to collect biographical data when developing a plan of care for a child?
- Explain what is meant by the "chief complaint."
- What are the reasons it is important for the nurse to ask about a child's present, past, and family health history?

Review of Systems for Current Health Problem

Pay attention to the details. Using a head-to-toe approach is an organized way to gather subjective data.

While the nurse is collecting subjective data, the caregiver or child is asked questions about each body system. Information is gathered that helps to focus the physical exam, as well as to get an overall picture of the child's current status. The body system involved in the chief complaint is reviewed in detail. As other body systems are discussed, it is important to reassure the caregiver that the chief complaint has not been forgotten or ignored. In doing a review of the body systems, the nurse needs to include the areas listed in Table 28-1.

Allergies, Medications, and Substance Abuse

Allergic reactions to any foods, medications, or any other known allergies should be discussed to prevent the child being given any medications or substances that might cause an allergic reaction. Medications the child is taking or has taken, whether prescribed by a care provider or over the counter, are recorded. This information will help avoid the possibility of over-medicating or causing drug interactions. It is important, especially in the adolescent, to assess the use of substances such as tobacco, alcohol, or illegal drugs (substance abuse is discussed in Chapters 27 and 44).

This could save a life. Always discuss a child's allergies with the caregiver. Document this information in the child's record.

Lifestyle

School history includes information regarding the child's current grade level and academic performance, as well as behavior seen at school. The child's interactions with teachers and peers often give insight into areas of concern that might affect the child's health.

Social history offers information about the environment that the child lives in, including the home setting, parent's occupations, siblings, family pets, religious affiliations, and economic factors. The persons who live in the home and those who care for the child are important data, especially in cases of separation or divorce.

Personal history relates to data collected about such things as the child's hygiene and sleeping and elimination patterns. Activities, exercise, special interests, and the child's favorite toys or objects are

TABLE 28.1	Review of Systems
Areas to Be Reviewed	
General	Weight gain or loss, fatigue, colds, illnesses, behavior changes, edema
Skin	Itching, dryness, rash, color change
Head and neck	Headache, dizziness, injury, stiff neck, swollen neck glands
Eyes	Drainage, trouble focusing or seeing, rubbing, redness
Ears	Pulling, pain, drainage, difficulty hearing
Nose, mouth, throat	Nosebleeds, drainage, trouble breathing, toothache, sore throat, trouble swallowing
Chest and lungs—respiratory	Coughing, wheezing, shortness of breath, sputum, breast development, pain
Heart—cardiovascular	Cyanosis, fatigue, anemia, heart murmurs
Abdomen—gastrointestinal	Nausea, vomiting, pain
Genitalia and rectum	Pain or burning when voiding, blood in urine or stool, constipation, diarrhea
Back and extremities Musculoskeletal	Extremities—pain, difficult movement, swollen joints, broken bones, muscle sprains
Neurologic	Seizures, loss of consciousness

included. Questions about relationships and how the child emotionally handles certain situations can help in understanding the child. Any behaviors such as thumb sucking, nail biting, or temper tantrums are discussed.

Nutrition history of the child offers information regarding eating habits and preferences, as well as nutrition concerns that might indicate illness.

Developmental Level

Gathering information about the child's developmental level is done by asking questions directly related to growth and development milestones. These milestones are discussed in detail in the growth and development chapters (see Chapters 23–27) of this text. Knowing normal development patterns will help the nurse determine if there are concerns that should be further assessed regarding the child's development.

COLLECTING OBJECTIVE DATA

The collection of objective data includes the nurse doing a baseline measurement of the child's height, weight, blood pressure, temperature, pulse, and respiration. Data are also collected by examination of the body systems. Often the exam for a child is not done in a head-to-toe manner as in adults but rather in an order that takes the child's age and developmental needs into consideration. Aspects of the exam that might be more traumatic or uncomfortable for the child are done last.

This advice could save the day. Examining the nose and mouth may be uncomfortable and traumatic for the child; save these for last.

The procedure of the physical exam may be familiar from previous health care visits. If comfortable with helping, the caregiver may be involved in helping with the data collection. For example, the caregiver might help take a young child's temperature and obtain a urine specimen. Arrangements should be made so that the caregiver also may be present, if possible, for tests or examinations that need to be performed. Included in this initial exam is an inspection of the child's body. All observations are recorded. The nurse carefully documents any finding that is not within normal limits and describes in detail any unusual findings.

The nurse conducts or assists in conducting a complete physical exam with special attention to any symptoms that the caregiver has identified. The nurse's primary role in the complete assessment may be to support the child. All the information gathered is used to plan the child's care.

Test Yourself

- What approach should the nurse use to do a review of systems in a child?
- Explain why this approach is used.
- What is included when collecting information about the child's lifestyle?
- Define objective data. How does the nurse collect objective data?

General Status

The nurse uses knowledge of normal growth and development to note if the child appears to fit the characteristics of the stated age. Interactions the child has with caregivers and siblings provide the nurse information about these relationships. The child's overall general appearance, facial expressions, speech, and behavior are noted as the nurse begins collecting information about the child.

Observing General Appearance

Observing physical appearance and condition can give clues to the child's overall health. The infant or child's face and body should be symmetrical (i.e., well balanced). Observe for nutritional status, hygiene, mental alertness, and body posture and movements. Examine the skin for color, lesions, bruises, scars, and birthmarks. Observe hair texture, thickness, and distribution.

Noting Psychological Status and Behavior

Carefully observing the child's behavior and recording those observations provide vital clues to a child's condition. Observation of behavior should include factors that influenced the behavior and how often the behavior is repeated. Physical behavior, as well as emotional and intellectual responses, should be noted. Also consider the child's age and developmental level, the abnormal environment of the health care facility, and if the child has been hospitalized previously or otherwise separated from family caregivers. It is important to note if the behavior is consistent or unpredictable and any apparent reasons for changed behavior.

Observation of the infant's behavior is critical because infants cannot articulate information regarding their health status. Characteristic behaviors of the healthy infant compared with behaviors that may indicate signs of illness are shown in Table 28-2. The nurse must be cautious when using the type of information shown in such a table because occasional evidence of one or more of the behaviors may not be significant.

Any instance of behavior indicating illness needs to be documented and further evaluated in light of the behavior frequency, as well as the child's usual behavior. If the caregiver has indicated in the interview or on further questioning that this behavior is not out of the ordinary for the child, it may not be indicative of a problem.

TABLE 28.2	Comparison of Observations of an Infant's Physical and Emotional Behavior	
Observation	**Healthy Activity**	**Behavior Indicating Illness***
Activity	Constantly active; some infants are more intense and curious than others.	Lies quietly; little or no interest in surroundings; may stay in the same position
State of muscular tension	Muscular state is tense; grasp is tight; head is raised when prone; kicks are vigorous. When supine, there is a space between the mattress and the infant's back.	Lies relaxed with arms and legs straight and lax; makes no attempt to turn or raise head if placed in prone position; does not move about in crib
Constancy of reaction	Shows a constancy in reaction; does not regress in development; peppy and vigorous; interested in food; responds to caregiver's presence or voice	Not as peppy as usual; responds to discomfort and pain in apathetic manner; turns away from food that had once interested; turns head and cries instead of usual response
Behavior indicating pain	Appreciates being picked up Activity is not restlessness. Shows activity in every part of body	Cries or protests when handled; seems to want to be left alone. May cry when picked up, but settles down after being held for a time, indicating something hurts when moved Turns head fretfully from side to side; pulls ear or rubs head; turns and rolls constantly; seemingly to try to get away from pain
Cry	Strong, vigorous cry	Weak, feeble cry or whimper High-pitched cry; shrill cry may indicate increased intracranial pressure
Skin color	Healthy tint to skin; nail beds, oral mucosa, conjunctivae, and tongue are reddish-pink	Light-skinned babies may show unusual pallor or blueness around the eyes and nose. All babies may have dark or cyanotic nail beds; pale oral mucosa, conjuctivae, and tongue.
Appetite or feeding pattern	Exhibits an eagerness and impatience to satisfy hunger	May show indifference toward formula; sucks half-heartedly; vomits feeding; habitually regurgitates. May exhibit discomfort after feeding
Bizarre behavior		Any behavior that differs from expected for level of development; unusually good, or passive when in strange surroundings; responds with rejection to every overture, friendly or otherwise; extremely clinging, never satisfied with amount of attention received

*Any *one* manifestation in itself may not be significant. The important thing is whether this behavior is consistent with this particular child or is a change from previous behavior. The significance depends greatly on the constancy of the behavior.

A

B

● *Figure 28.3* (**A**) The nurse keeps a hand close to the infant while weighing. (**B**) The older child can be measured for weight and height on a standing scale.

Measuring Height and Weight

The child's height and weight are helpful indicators of growth and development. Height and weight should be measured and recorded each time the child has a routine physical examination, as well as at other health care visits. These measurements must be charted and compared with norms for the child's age (see Appendix G). Plotting the child's growth on a growth chart gives a good indication of the child's health status. This process gives a picture of how the child is progressing and often indicates wellness. Although the charts are indicators, the size of other family members,

the child's illnesses, general nutritional status, and developmental milestones also must be considered.

In a hospital setting, the infant or child should be weighed at the same time each day on the same scales while wearing the same amount of clothing. The infant is weighed nude, lying on an infant scale, or when the infant is big enough to sit, the child can be weighed while sitting. The nurse must keep a hand within 1 inch of the child at all times to be ready to protect the child from injury (Fig. 28-3A). The scale is covered with a fresh paper towel or clean sheet of paper as a means of infection control (Nursing Procedure 28-1). A child

Nursing Procedure 28.1
Weighing the Infant or Child

EQUIPMENT

Scale appropriate for child's age and ability to sit or stand
Disposable paper covering for scale
Paper and pen to record weight
Cleaning solution and equipment, according to facility policy

PROCEDURE

1. Explain procedure to child and family caregiver.
2. Wash hands.
3. Place paper on scale.
4. Balance scale to a reading of "0."

5. Weigh the hospitalized child at the same time, using same scale, same amount of clothing each time child is weighed.
6. Weigh infant with no clothing, older child in underwear or lightweight gown; child should not wear shoes.
7. **Always** hold one hand within 1 inch of the child for safety.
8. Pick up the child or have older child step off scale.
9. Remove and discard paper scale cover.
10. Read the weight on the scale.
11. Record the weight on paper to be transferred to permanent document.
12. Clean the scale according to the facility's policy.
13. Report weight as appropriate.

who can stand alone steadily is weighed on platform-type scales. The child should be weighed without shoes. Bed scales may be used if the child cannot get out of bed. Weights are recorded in grams and kilograms or pounds and ounces.

The child who can stand usually is measured for height at the same time. The standing scales have a useful, adjustable measuring device (Fig. 28-3B). To measure the height of a child who is not able to stand alone steadily, usually under the age of about 2, place the child flat, with the knees held flat, on an examining table. Measure the child's height by straightening the child's body and measuring from the top of the head to the bottom of the foot. Sometimes examining tables have a measuring device mounted along the side of the table. If not, the measurement can be done by making marks on the paper table covering and then measuring between the marks. Height is recorded in centimeters or inches according to the practice of the health care facility; the nurse must know which measuring system is used.

Measuring Head Circumference

The head circumference is measured routinely in children to the age of 2 or 3 years or in any child with a neurologic concern. A paper or plastic tape measure is placed around the largest part of the head just above the eyebrows and around the most prominent part of the back of the head (Fig. 28-4). This measurement is recorded and plotted on a growth chart kept to monitor the growth of the child's head. During childhood the chest exceeds the head circumference by 2–3 inches.

Figure 28.4 Measuring the head circumference.

Vital Signs

Vital signs, including temperature, pulse, respirations, and blood pressure, are taken at each visit and compared with the normal values for children of the same age, as well as to that child's previous recordings. In a hospital setting, the vital signs are closely monitored and recorded; any changes are reported. Keeping in mind the child's developmental needs will increase the nurse's ability to take accurate vital sign measurements. It will usually be less traumatic for the infant if the nurse counts the respirations before the child is disturbed, then takes the pulse and the temperature.

Temperature

The method of measuring a child's temperature commonly is set by the policy of the health care setting. The temperature can be measured by the oral, rectal, axillary, or tympanic method. Temperatures are recorded in Celsius or Fahrenheit, according to the policy of the health care facility. A normal oral temperature range is 36.4°C to 37.4°C (97.6°F to 99.3°F). A rectal temperature

A PERSONAL GLIMPSE

I am 11 years old, and I have already been in the hospital for four surgeries. I think I could be a nurse. One time a student nurse and her teacher came to do my vital signs. The teacher left, and the student named Joan told me I was her first patient ever. She tried three of those electronic thermometers to take my temperature, but she said they were all broken. Then she tried to take my blood pressure with the blood pressure machine and she said it was broken. Then she used another blood pressure cuff, and this time she put it on backwards. I knew it was wrong, but I just let her pump it up and up until it exploded off my arm. I laughed, but she almost cried. I showed her how to do it right, and she seemed pretty glad that she finally got it to work. I was kind of happy when she left because I didn't know if I could teach her everything. A little while later she came back with her teacher and the teacher said, "Joan is going to give you your shot." "Uh Oh!" I thought, "here comes trouble." I just held my breath and hoped she won't do that wrong too. It wasn't too bad. Later, before she went home she brought me a pear. I am pretty sure she was relieved the day was over and I was too.

Abigail, age 11

LEARNING OPPORTUNITY: What could this student nurse have done to be better prepared to take care of this patient? What feelings do you think this child might have had when the nurse came in with the medication?

A   B

● *Figure 28.5* (**A**) Many facilities use a tympanic thermometer sensor to take the child's temperature. (**B**) Taking an axillary temperature on a newborn. (© B. Proud.)

is usually 0.5° to 1.0° higher than the oral measurement. An axillary temperature usually measures 0.5° to 1.0° lower than the oral measurement. The temperature measurement taken by the tympanic method is in the same range as the oral method. Any deviation from the normal range of temperature should be reported. Temperatures vary according to the method by which they are taken, so it is important to record the method of temperature measurement, as well as the measured temperature.

Mercury thermometers have been replaced by mercury-free glass thermometers, electronic, tympanic membrane, and digital devices, which accurately measure temperatures. Electronic thermometers have oral and rectal probes. The nurse should be careful to select the correct probe when using the thermometer.

Warning! Some caregivers might still have a mercury thermometer at home. Advise them to replace the glass mercury thermometer with a nonmercury thermometer, which can easily be purchased at many pharmacies or super stores.

Oral Temperatures. In pediatrics, oral temperatures usually are taken only on children older than 4 to 6 years of age who are conscious and cooperative. Oral thermometers should be placed in the side of the child's mouth. The child should not be left unattended while any temperature is being taken.

Tympanic Temperatures. Tympanic thermometers are now used in many health care settings to measure temperature (Fig. 28-5*A*). The tympanic thermometer records the temperature rapidly (registering in about 2 seconds), is noninvasive, and causes little disturbance to the child. A tympanic measurement often can be obtained without awakening a sleeping infant or child. Tympanic thermometers are used according to the manufacturer's directions and the facility's policy. A disposable speculum is used for each child.

Rectal Temperatures. Rectal temperatures may be taken in children but usually only if another method cannot be used. They are not desirable in the newborn because of the danger of irritation to the rectal mucosa or in children who have had rectal surgery or who have diarrhea. When a rectal temperature is taken, the end of the thermometer should be lubricated with a water-soluble lubricant. The child is placed in a prone position, the buttocks are gently separated with one hand, and the thermometer is inserted gently about ¼ to ½ inch into the rectum. If the nurse feels any resistance, he or she should remove the thermometer immediately, take the temperature by some other method, and notify the physician about the resistance. The nurse must keep one hand on the child's buttocks and the other on the thermometer during the entire time the rectal thermometer is in place. An electronic thermometer is removed as soon as it signals a recorded temperature.

Axillary Temperatures. Axillary temperatures are taken on newborns and on infants and children with diarrhea or when a rectal temperature is contraindicated. When taking an axillary temperature on an infant or child, the nurse must be certain to place the thermometer tip well into the armpit and bring the child's arm down close to the body (Fig. 28-5B). The nurse must check to see that there is skin-to-skin contact with no clothing in the way. The thermometer is left in place until the electronic thermometer signals.

Pulse

Counting an apical rate is the preferred method to determine the pulse in an infant or young child. The nurse should try to accomplish this while the child is quiet.

The apical pulse should be counted before the child is disturbed for other procedures. A child can be held on the caregiver's lap for security for the full minute that the pulse is counted.

Some nurses find this tip helpful. When checking an apical pulse, approach the child in a soothing, calm, quiet manner.

The stethoscope is placed between the child's left nipple and sternum. A radial pulse may be taken on an older child. This pulse may be counted for 30 seconds and multiplied by two. A pulse that is unusual in quality, rate, or rhythm should be counted for a full minute. Any rate that deviates from the normal rate should be reported. Pulse rates vary with age: from 100 to 180 beats per minute for a neonate (birth to 30 days old) to 50 to 95 beats per minute for the 14- to 18-year-old adolescent (Table 28-3).

Cardiac monitors are used to detect changes in cardiac function. Many of these monitors have a visual display of the cardiac actions. Electrodes must be placed properly to obtain accurate readings of the cardiac system. The skin is cleansed with alcohol to remove oil, dirt, lotions, and powder. Alarms are set to maximum and minimum settings above and below the

● **Figure 28.6** It is important for the nurse to frequently check the cardiopulmonary monitor, settings, and electrode sites. (© B. Proud.)

child's resting heart rate. The electrode sites must be checked every 2 hours to detect any skin redness or irritation and to determine that the electrodes are secure. The child's cardiac status must be checked immediately when the alarm sounds (Fig. 28-6). Sometimes the monitor used will monitor both cardiac and respiratory function. Apnea monitors, which monitor respiratory function, are discussed later in this chapter.

Respirations

Respirations of an infant or young child also must be counted during a quiet time. The child can be observed while lying or sitting quietly. Infants are abdominal breathers; therefore, the movement of the infant's abdomen is observed to count respirations. The older child's chest can be observed much as an adult's would be. The infant's respirations must be counted for a full minute because of normal irregularity. The chest of the infant or young child must be observed for retractions that indicate respiratory distress. Retractions are noted as substernal (below the sternum), subcostal (below the ribs), intercostal (between the ribs), suprasternal (above the sternum), or supraclavicular (above the clavicle) (Fig. 28-7).

Pulse Oximetry. Pulse oximetry measures the oxygen saturation of arterial hemoglobin. The probe of the oximetry unit can be taped to the toe or finger or clipped on the earlobe (Fig. 28-8). The pulse oximetry is taken and recorded with the other vital signs. In certain situations the probe is left in place to continually monitor the oxygen saturation. The site is changed at least every 4 hours to prevent skin irritation. In an infant, the foot may be used. The site should be checked every 2 hours to ensure that the probe is secure and tissue perfusion is adequate. Alarms can be set to sound when oxygen saturation registers lower than a predetermined limit. At the beginning of each shift and after transport of the patient, the nurse must

TABLE 28.3	Normal Pulse Ranges in Children	
Age	Normal Range	Average
0–24 hr	70–170 bpm	120 bpm
1–7 d	100–180 bpm	140 bpm
1 mo	110–188 bpm	160 bpm
1 mo–1 y	80–180 bpm	120–130 bpm
2 y	80–140 bpm	110 bpm
4 y	80–120 bpm	100 bpm
6 y	70–115 bpm	100 bpm
10 y	70–110 bpm	90 bpm
12–14 y	60–110 bpm	85–90 bpm
14–18 y	50–95 bpm	70–75 bpm

bpm = beats per minute

● *Figure 28.7* Sites of respiratory retraction.

● *Figure 28.9* Apnea monitor being used in a hospital setting. (© B. Proud.)

check that alarms are accurately set and have not been inadvertently changed. This is true for all types of monitors.

Apnea Monitor. An apnea monitor detects the infant's respiratory movement. Electrodes or a belt are placed on the infant's chest where the greatest amount of respiratory movement is detected; the electrodes are attached to the monitor by a cable. An alarm is set to sound when the infant does not breathe for a predetermined number of seconds.

Warning. Respond immediately when the alarm on the apnea monitor sounds. The child must be observed to determine what caused the alarm to sound.

These monitors can be used in a hospital setting and often are used in the home for an infant who is at risk for apnea or who has a tracheostomy (Fig. 28-9). Family caregivers are taught to stimulate the infant when the monitor sounds and to perform cardiopulmonary resuscitation if the infant does not begin breathing.

Blood Pressure

For children 3 years of age and older, blood-pressure monitoring is part of routine and ongoing data collection. Children of any age who come to a health care facility should have a baseline blood pressure taken. It is important for the nurse to offer the child an explanation of the procedure in terms the young child can understand. First taking a blood pressure on a stuffed animal or doll will further show the child the procedure is not one to be feared.

Try this approach. Referring to the blood pressure cuff as "giving your arm a hug" will help in the explanation of taking the blood pressure.

Obtaining a blood pressure measurement in an infant or small child is difficult, but equipment of the proper size helps ease the problem. The most common sites used to obtain a blood pressure reading in children are the upper arm, lower arm or forearm, thigh and calf or ankle (Fig. 28-10). When the upper arm is used, the cuff should be wide enough to cover about two thirds of the upper arm and long enough to encircle the extremity without overlapping. If other sites are used, the size of the cuff is determined by the size of the extremity; a smaller cuff is used on the forearm, whereas a larger cuff is used on the thigh or calf.

The blood pressure is taken by the auscultation, palpation, or Doppler or electronic method (Nursing

● *Figure 28.8* The pulse oximetry sensor measuring the oxygen saturation in the older child.

● *Figure 28.10* Sites in the child where blood pressure may be measured.

Procedure 28-2). The Doppler method is used with increasing frequency to monitor pediatric blood pressure, but the cuff still must be the correct size. Electronic blood pressure recording devices are used frequently in health care settings and provide accurate measurement. Normal blood pressure values gradually increase from infancy through adolescence (Table 28-4).

Test Yourself

- How is comparing behaviors seen in a healthy child to behaviors that might indicate illness helpful in caring for the child?

- Why should height and weight be routinely measured and monitored in children?

- What is the purpose in doing pulse oximetry when obtaining vital signs?

- Describe the methods used to obtain a blood pressure in a child.

TABLE 28.4	Normal Blood-Pressure Ranges (mm Hg)	
Age	Systolic	Diastolic
Newborn—12 hr (<1,000 g)	39–59	16–36
Newborn—12 hr (3,000 g)	50–70	24–45
Newborn—96 hr (3,000 g)	60–90	20–60
Infant	74–100	50–70
Toddler	80–112	50–80
Preschooler	82–110	50–78
School-age	84–120	54–80
Adolescent	94–140	62–88

Providing a Physical Examination

Data are also collected by examining the body systems of the child. The nurse does the physical exam or assists the health care provider in doing the physical exam.

Head and Neck

The head's general shape and movement should be observed. **Symmetry** or a balance is noted in the features of the face and in the head. Observe the child's ability to control the head and the range of motion. To see full range of motion, ask the older child to move her or his head in all directions. In the infant the nurse gently moves the head to observe for any stiffness in the neck. The nurse feels the skull to determine if the fontanels are open or closed and to check for any swelling or depression.

Eyes. Observe the eyes for symmetry and location in relationship to the nose. Note any redness, evidence of rubbing, or drainage. Ask the older child to follow a light to observe her or his ability to focus. An infant will also follow a light with his or her eyes. Observe pupils for equality, roundness, and reaction to light. Neurologic considerations will be discussed later in this chapter. Routine vision screening is done in school or clinic settings. Screening helps identify vision concerns in children; with early detection, appropriate visual aids can be provided.

Ears. The alignment of the ears is noted by drawing an imaginary line from the outside corner of the eye to the prominent part of the child's skull; the top of the ear, known as the **pinna**, should cross this line (Fig. 28-11). Ears that are set low often indicate mental retardation (see Chapter 34). Note the child's ability to hear during normal conversation. A child who speaks loudly, responds inappropriately, or does not speak clearly may have hearing difficulties that should be explored. Note any drainage or swelling.

Nose, Mouth, and Throat. The nose is in the middle of the face. If an imaginary line were drawn down

Nursing Procedure 28.2
Methods for Measuring Pediatric Blood Pressure

EQUIPMENT

Stethoscope, pediatric preferred
Blood pressure cuff, appropriate size for child
    Wide enough to cover 2/3 of child's upper arm
    Long enough to encircle child's arm
Doppler or electronic monitor
Paper and pen to record blood pressure

PROCEDURE

1. Explain procedure to child and family caregiver.
2. Wash hands.
3. Allow child to handle equipment when appropriate.
4. Use terminology appropriate to child's age.
5. Encourage preschool or school-age child to use equipment to "take" blood pressure on a doll or stuffed animal.
6. Record blood pressure on paper to be transferred to permanent document.
7. Report blood pressure as appropriate.

AUSCULTATION

1. Place the correct size of cuff on the infant's or child's bare arm.

2. Locate the artery by palpating the antecubital fossa.
3. Inflate the cuff until radial pulse disappears or about 30 mm Hg above expected systolic reading.
4. Place stethoscope lightly over the artery and slowly release air until pulse is heard.
5. Record readings as in adults.

PALPATION

1. Follow steps 1 and 2 above.
2. Keep the palpating finger over the artery and inflate the cuff as above.
3. The point at which the pulse is felt is recorded as the systolic pressure.

DOPPLER OR ELECTRONIC MONITOR

1. Obtain the monitor, dual air hose, and proper cuff size.
2. If monitor is not on a mobile stand, be certain that it is placed on a firm surface.
3. Plug in monitor (unless battery-operated) and attach dual hose if necessary.
4. Attach appropriate-size blood pressure cuff and wrap around child's limb.
5. Turn on power switch. Record the reading.

---

the middle, both sides of the nose should be symmetrical. Flaring of the nostrils might indicate respiratory distress and should be reported immediately. Observe for swelling, drainage, or bleeding. To observe the

mouth and throat, have the older child hold her or his mouth wide open and move the tongue from side to side. With the infant or toddler, use a tongue blade to see the mouth and throat. Gently place the tongue blade on the side of the tongue to hold it down. Observe the mucous membranes for color, moisture, and any patchy areas that might indicate infection. Observe the number and condition of the child's teeth. The lips should be moist and pink. Note any difficulty in swallowing.

Chest and Lungs

Chest measurements are done on infants and children to determine normal growth rate. Take the measurement at the nipple level with a tape measure. Observe the chest for size, shape, movement of the chest with breathing, and any retractions (see respirations in this chapter). In the older school-age child or adolescent, note evidence of breast development. Evaluate respiratory rate, rhythm, and depth. Report any noisy or grunting respirations. Using a stethoscope, the nurse listens to breath sounds in each lobe of the lung, anterior and posterior, while the child inhales and exhales. Describe, document, and report absent or diminished breath sounds, as well as unusual sounds such as crackling or wheezing. If the child is coughing or bringing up sputum, record the frequency, color, and consistency of sputum.

≤10 degrees

● **Figure 28.11** Normal alignment of the ear in the child.

Heart

In some infants and children, a pulsation can be seen in the chest that indicates the heart beat. This point is called the **point of maximum impulse** (PMI). This point is where the heart beat can be heard the best with a stethoscope. The nurse listens for the rhythm of the heart sounds and counts the rate for 1 full minute. Abnormal or unusual heart sounds or irregular rhythms might indicate the child has a heart murmur, heart condition, or other abnormality that should be reported. The heart is responsible for circulating blood to the body. To determine the heart function's effectiveness, the nurse assesses the pulses in various parts of the body (Fig. 28-12). Other indicators of good cardiac function are included in this textbook's discussions of specific disorders.

Abdomen

The abdomen may protrude slightly in infants and small children. To describe the abdomen, divide the area into four sections and label sections with the terms left upper quadrant (LUQ), left lower quadrant (LLQ), right upper quadrant (RUQ), and right lower quadrant (RLQ). Using a stethoscope, the nurse listens for bowel sounds or evidence of peristalsis in each section of the abdomen and records what is heard. The umbilicus is observed for cleanliness and any abnormalities. Infants and young children sometimes have protrusions in the umbilicus or inguinal canal that are called hernias. Hernias are discussed in Chapter 21. Report a tense or firm abdomen or unusual tenderness.

Genitalia and Rectum

When inspecting the genitalia and rectum, it is important to respect the child's privacy and take into account the child's age and the stage of growth and development.

Sensitivity is essential. Keeping the child covered as much as possible when examining the genitalia and rectum is important in respecting the child's privacy.

While wearing gloves, the nurse inspects the genitalia and rectum. Observe the area for any sores or lesions, swelling, or discharge. In male children the testes descend at varying times during childhood; if the testes cannot be palpated, this information should be reported. The nurse needs to be aware that unusual findings, such as bruises in soft tissue, bruises with a clear outline of an object, or unexplained injuries, might indicate child abuse and should be further investigated (see Chapter 41).

Back and Extremities

The back should be observed for symmetry and for the curvature of the spine. In infants the spine is rounded and flexible. As the child grows and develops motor skills, the spine further develops. Screening is done in school-age children to detect abnormal curvatures of the spine such as scoliosis (see Chapter 39). Note gait and posture when the child enters or is walking in the room. The extremities should be warm, have good color, and be symmetrical. By observing the child's movements during the exam, the nurse notes range of motion, movement of the joints, and muscle strength. In infants, examine the hips and report any dislocation or asymmetry of gluteal skin folds. These could indicate a congenital hip dislocation (see Chapter 21).

Neurologic

Assessing the neurologic status of the infant and child is the most complex aspect of the physical exam. All the body systems function in relationship to the nervous system. The practitioner in the health care

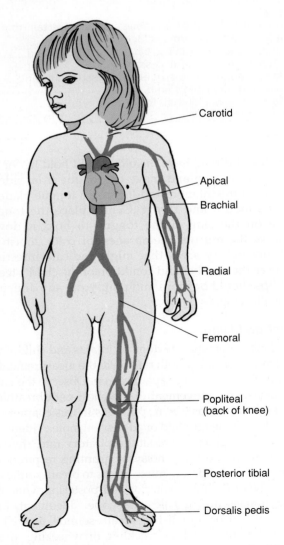

Carotid

Apical

Brachial

Radial

Femoral

Popliteal
(back of knee)

Posterior tibial

Dorsalis pedis

● *Figure 28.12* Sites in the child where pulses can be felt.

GLASGOW COMA SCALES			MODIFIED COMA SCALE FOR INFANTS		
ACTIVITY	BEST RESPONSE		ACTIVITY	BEST RESPONSE	
Eye Opening	Spontaneous	4	Eye Opening	Spontaneous	4
	To speech	3		To speech	3
	To pain	2		To pain	2
	None	1		None	1
Verbal	Oriented	5	Verbal	Coos, babbles	5
	Confused	4		Irritable	4
	Inappropriate words	3		Cries to pain	3
	Nonspecific sounds	2		Moans to pain	2
	None	1		None	1
Motor	Follows commands	6	Motor	Normal spontaneous movements	6
	Localizes pain	5		Withdraws to touch	5
	Withdraws to pain	4		Withdraws to pain	4
	Abnormal flexion	3		Abnormal flexion	3
	Extend	2		Abnormal extension	2
	None	1		None	1

PUPIL SIZE:

6mm ● 5mm ● 4mm ●
3mm ● 2mm ● 1mm ●

REACTION: **N**−normal, **S**−sluggish, **F**−fixed

DATE	TIME	PUPIL SIZE		PUPIL REACTION		EXTREMITY MOVEMENT/ RESPONSE				GLASGOW COMA SCALE			VITAL SIGNS		
		R	L	R	L	RA	LA	RL	LL	VERBAL RESP.	MOTOR RESP.	EYE OPENING	BP	PULSE	RESP.

GUIDE TO NEUROLOGIC EVALUATION

Pupils

Pupils should be examined in dim light

1. Compare each pupil with the size chart and record pupil size.
2. Use a bright flashlight to check the reaction of each pupil. Hold the flashlight to the outer aspect of the eye. While watching the pupil, turn the flashlight on and bring it directly over the pupil. Record the reaction. Repeat for the other eye. Report if either pupil is fixed or dilated.

Extremities

1. Observe the child for quality and strength of muscle tone in each upper extremity. Have child squeeze nurse's hand. Have child raise arms. Ask child to turn palms up, then palms down. Infant is observed for movement and position of arms when stroked or lightly pinched.
2. The child should be able to move each leg on command, and push against nurse's hands with each foot. Infant is observed for movement of legs and feet when stroked or lightly pinched.
3. Score the extremities using the motor scale appropriate for age (below).

Glasgow Coma Scale

Assess each response according to age

Eye opening

4 Opens eyes spontaneously when approached
3 Opens eyes to spoken or shouted speech
2 Opens eyes only to painful stimuli (nail bed pressure)
1 Does not open eyes in response to pain

Verbal

5 Oriented to time, place, person; infant responds by cooing and babbling, recognizes parent
4 Talks, not oriented to time, place, person; infant irritable, doesn't recognize parent
3 Words senseless, unintelligible; infant cries in response to pain
2 Responds with moaning and groaning, no intelligible words; infant moans to pain
1 No response

Motor

6 Responds to commands; infant smiles, responds
5 Tries to remove painful stimuli with hands; infant withdraws from touch
4 Attempts to withdraw from painful stimuli; infant withdraws from pain source
3 Flexes arms at elbows and wrists in response to pain (decorticate rigidity)
2 Extends arms at elbows in response to pain (cerebrate rigidity)
1 No motor response to pain

Check infant's fontanelle for bulging and record results

● *Figure 28.13* Neurologic flow sheet and neurologic evaluation guide.

setting assesses the neurologic status of the child by doing a complete neurologic exam. This exam includes detailed examination of the reflex responses, as well as the functioning of each of the cranial nerves. The practitioner will perform a neurologic exam on children after a head injury or seizure or on children who have metabolic conditions, such as diabetes mellitus, drug ingestion, severe hemorrhage, or dehydration, that might affect neurologic status. A neurologic assessment is done to determine the level of the child's neurologic functioning. The nurse often is responsible for using neurologic assessment tools to monitor a child's neurologic status after the initial neurologic exam. The nurse uses a neurologic assessment tool such as the Glasgow coma scale. The use of a standard scale for monitoring permits the comparison of results from one time to another and from one examiner to another. Using this tool, the nurse monitors various aspects of the child's neurologic functioning (Fig. 28-13). If a child is hospitalized with a neurologic concern, the neurologic status is monitored closely, and a neurologic assessment tool is used every 1 or 2 hours to observe for significant changes.

Assisting With Common Diagnostic Tests

Diagnostic tests and studies often are done to further evaluate the subjective and objective data collected. These diagnostic tests help the practitioner to determine more clearly the nature of the child's concern. The needs of the infant or child during these studies vary greatly from child to child. The role of the nurse in assisting with common diagnostic tests is discussed in Chapter 30.

Test Yourself

- Explain the term symmetry and the importance of observing for symmetry when doing a physical exam on a child.

- What does the term *point of maximum impulse* (PMI) mean and how does it relate to the physical exam in children?

- What is included when doing a neurologic exam on a child?

KEY POINTS

- Interviewing the caregiver and the child is important to collect subjective data regarding the child.

- The chief complaint is the reason the child was brought to the health care setting and should be fully explored with the child and caregiver.

- When doing a review of systems, the nurse asks questions about each of the body systems using a head-to-toe approach to gather data to get an overall picture of the child's current status.

- The caregiver may be involved in collecting objective data by being a support to the child, as well as assisting with tasks such as obtaining a temperature or urine specimen.

- Indicators that might indicate possible illness in children include the child being quieter or less active than usual, crying or acting uncomfortable, refusing to eat, exhibiting behaviors that are different from expected for the child's level of development, and having changes in skin coloration.

- Height and weight are assessed on an ongoing basis because they are good indicators of the child's growth and development, as well as the child's health status.

- Developmental tables are used to establish a standard to compare an individual child's growth progress.

- A rectal temperature should not be taken on newborns, on children who have had rectal surgery or who have diarrhea, or if any resistance is noted when inserting the thermometer.

- Respiratory retractions are substernal (below the sternum), subcostal (below the ribs), intercostal (between the ribs), suprasternal (above the sternum), or supraclavicular (above the clavicle).

- Pulse oximetry is done to measure the oxygen saturation of arterial hemoglobin.

- Blood pressure can be obtained by auscultation, palpation and Doppler or electronic methods.

- To collect objective data, a physical exam is done on a child using the knowledge of normal growth and development as a basis for the exam. Unlike the head-to-toe exam in the adult, the exam in the child proceeds from the less traumatic areas to be examined to the areas that are more traumatic or uncomfortable to the child.

- The Glasgow coma scale is used as a tool for neurologic assessment and to consistently monitor the child's neurologic functioning.

REFERENCES AND SELECTED READINGS

Books and Journals

Barone, M. A., & Rowe P. C. (1999). Pediatric procedures. In *Oski's pediatrics: Principles and practice* (3rd ed.). Philadelphia: Lippincott Williams & Wilkins.

Craven, R. F., & Hirnle, C. J. (1999). *Fundamentals of nursing* (3rd ed.). Philadelphia: Lippincott Williams & Wilkins.

Gaynor, S. (2000). Pandora's box: Educational materials resources assessment. *Journal of Child and Family Nursing, 3*(2), 163–164.

Heery, K. (2000). Straight talk about the patient interview. Nursing. Retrieved from http://www.findarticles.com.

Hockenberry, M. J., Wilson, D., Winkelstein, M. L., & Kline, N. E. (2003). *Wong's nursing care of infants and children* (7th ed.). St. Louis: Mosby.

Houlder, L. C. (2000). Evidence-based practice: The accuracy and reliability of tympanic thermometry compared to rectal and axillary sites in young children. *Pediatric Nursing, 26*(3), 31–34.

Karch, A. M. (2003). *2004 Lippincott's nursing drug guide.* Philadelphia: Lippincott Williams & Wilkins.

Knies, R. C. (2001). Temperature measurement in acute care: The who, what, where, when, how, why and wherefore. Retrieved July 2, 2004, from www.allnurses.com.

Multon, A. H., Blactop, J., & Hall, C. M. (2001). Temperature taking in children. *Journal of Child Health Care, 5*(1), 5–10.

Pillitteri, A. (2003). *Maternal and child health nursing* (4th ed.). Philadelphia: Lippincott Williams & Wilkins.

Wetzel, G. V. (1999). Red flags in common pediatric symptoms. *The American Journal of Maternal/Child Nursing, 24*(1), 37.

Wong, D. L., Perry, S., & Hockenberry, M. (2002). *Maternal child nursing care* (2nd ed.). St. Louis: Mosby.

Web Addresses
http://health.discovery.com

Pediatric Assessment
www.solutions-etc.com/PAO
www.nurseone.com

WORKBOOK

NCLEX-STYLE REVIEW QUESTIONS

1. The nurse is doing an admission interview with a toddler and the child's caregiver. Which of the following statements that the nurse makes to the caregiver indicates the nurse has an understanding of this child's growth and development needs?

   a. "You can sit in one chair and your child can sit in the other chair."

   b. "It would be best if you let the child play in the playroom while we are talking."

   c. "If you would like to hold your child on your lap, that would be fine."

   d. "I can find someone to take your child for a walk for a while."

2. When interviewing an adolescent, which of the following is the *most* important for the nurse to keep in mind. The adolescent

   a. will be able to give accurate details regarding her or his history.

   b. may feel more comfortable discussing some issues in private.

   c. may have a better understanding if books and pamphlets are provided.

   d. will be more cooperative if age-appropriate questions are asked.

3. In taking vital signs on a 6-month-old infant, the nurse obtains the following vital sign measurements. Which set of vital signs would the nurse be *most* concerned about?

   a. Pulse 90 bpm, temperature 36.9°C, blood pressure 80/50 mm Hg

   b. Pulse 114 bpm, temperature 37.6°C, blood pressure 88/60 mm Hg

   c. Pulse 148 bpm, temperature 38.0°C, blood pressure 92/62 mm Hg

   d. Pulse 162 bpm, temperature 38.5°C , blood pressure 96/56 mm Hg

4. When doing a physical exam on an infant, an understanding of this child's developmental needs are recognized when the exam is done by examining the

   a. heart before the abdomen.

   b. chest before the nose.

   c. extremities before the eyes.

   d. neurologic status before the back.

5. The nurse is measuring an 18-month-old child's height and weight. Which of the following actions should the nurse implement? The nurse should: Select all that apply.

   a. plot the measurements on a growth chart.

   b. wear a gown and mask during the procedure

   c. keep a hand within 1 inch of the child.

   d. encourage the parent to gently hold the child's legs.

   e. have the child wear the same amount of clothing each time the procedure is done.

   f. cover the scale with a clean sheet of paper before placing the child on the scale.

6. The nurse is performing an assessment on a child who has a respiratory condition. Identify the area where the nurse will observe this child for substernal respiratory retractions by marking an X on the spot where substernal retractions are noted.

7.

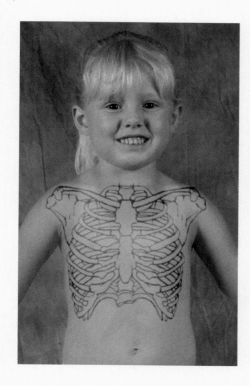

STUDY ACTIVITIES

1. Explain the step-by-step procedure you would follow to take vital signs on a 3-month-old infant. List the order in which you would take the vital signs and explain why you would do them in that order.
2. For each of the following body parts or systems, write a question that would be appropriate to ask a patient or caregiver when doing a review of systems as part of an interview.

Body Part or System	Question to Be Asked
General	
Skin	
Head and neck	
Eyes	
Ears	
Nose, mouth, throat	
Chest and lungs—respiratory	
Heart—cardiovascular	
Abdomen—gastrointestinal	
Genitalia and rectum	
Back and extremities	
Musculoskeletal	
Neurologic	

3. List four methods of taking a temperature and describe each method. Give an example of a reason that each method might be used to take a child's temperature.
4. Go to the following Internet site: http://www.meddean.luc.edu/lumen/DeptWebs/emschild/stndrd-teaching.htm
Download "Initial Pediatric Assessment Teaching Tool." Scroll down to section III "General Approach to the Stable Pediatric Patient."

   a. List five suggestions for the nurse to use in approaching the pediatric patient. Scroll down to section V "Initial Inspection."

   b. List five observations that the nurse would make when first approaching the child.

CRITICAL THINKING: What Would You Do?

1. You are conducting an interview with the caregiver of a preschool-age child.

   a. What would you discuss with the caregiver?

   b. What would you say and do with the caregiver to get the important information you need to care for the child?

   c. What would you say to the preschool-age child during the interview with the caregiver?

2. As the nurse in a pediatric outpatient setting, you are responsible for obtaining the child's height and weight at each visit.

   a. What would you explain to the caregiver when you are asked why the height and weight of a child are measured at each health care visit?

   b. What information would you record and document on the child's growth record?

   c. What is the purpose and significance of plotting height and weight on a pediatric growth chart?

3. You are assisting in doing a physical exam on a toddler.

   a. What is the process of doing a physical exam on a child?

   b. How does the exam on a child differ from that of an adult?

   c. What are the most important considerations to keep in mind when doing a physical exam on a child?

Care of The Hospitalized Child

STUDENT OBJECTIVES

On completion of this chapter, the student should be able to

1. List nine possible influences on the family's response to a child's illness.
2. Explain the family caregivers' role in preparing a child for hospitalization.
3. Describe the benefits of rooming-in.
4. Identify four ways that pathogens are transmitted and give an example of each.
5. State the role that handwashing plays in infection control.
6. Describe how the nurse can help ease the feelings of isolation a child may have when segregated because of transmission-based precautions.
7. Identify and differentiate the three stages of response to separation seen in the child.
8. Describe how a preadmission visit helps to prepare the child for hospitalization.
9. State the role of the caregiver in the child's admission process.
10. Discuss the need for written discharge instructions for the caregiver.
11. State how family members should react to the child just discharged from the hospital during this period of adjustment.
12. Describe how health professionals can help the adjustment of the child scheduled for surgery.
13. Discuss variations in preoperative preparation for children, including skin, gastrointestinal, urinary, and medication preparation.
14. Identify behavioral characteristics that may indicate an infant or a young child is having pain.
15. Discuss the purpose of a hospital play program.
16. State how stress affects the frequency of accidents and how this relates to a child's hospitalization.

KEY TERMS

anuria
child-life program
patient-controlled analgesia
play therapy
rooming-in
therapeutic play

ospitalization may cause anxiety and stress at any age. Fear of the unknown is always threatening. The child who faces hospitalization is no exception. Children are often too young to understand what is happening or are afraid to ask questions. Short hospital stays occur more frequently than extended hospitalization, but even during a short stay the child is often apprehensive. In addition, the child may pick up on the fears of family caregivers, and these negative emotions may hinder the child's progress.

The child's family suffers stress for a number of reasons. The cause of the illness, its treatment, guilt about the illness, past experiences of illness and hospitalization, disruption in family life, the threat to the child's long-term health, cultural or religious influences, coping methods within the family, and financial impact of the hospitalization all may affect how the family responds to the child's illness. Although some of these are concerns of the family and not specifically the child, they nevertheless influence how the child feels.

This is important to keep in mind. Children are tuned in to the feelings and emotions of their caregivers. By supporting the caregiver, the child is also being supported.

The child's developmental level also plays an important role in determining how he or she handles the stress of illness and hospitalization. The nurse who understands the child's developmental needs may significantly improve the child's hospital stay and overall recovery (Fig. 29-1). Many hospitals have a **child-life program** to make hospitalization less threatening for children and their parents. These programs are usually under the direction of a child-life specialist whose background is in psychology and early childhood development. This person works with nurses, physicians, and other health team members to help them meet the developmental, emotional, and intellectual needs of hospitalized children. The child-life specialist also works with students interested in child health care to help further their education. Sometimes, however, the best way to ease the stress of hospitalization is to ensure that the child has been well prepared for the hospital experience.

THE PEDIATRIC HOSPITAL SETTING

Early Childhood Education About Hospitals

Hospitals are part of the child's community, just as police and fire departments are. When the child is capable of understanding the basic functions of community resources and the people who staff them, it is time for an explanation. Some hospitals have regular open house programs for healthy children. Children may attend with parents or caregivers or in an organized community or school group. A room is set aside where children can handle equipment, try out call bells, try on masks and gowns, have their blood pressure taken to feel the squeeze of the blood pressure cuff, and see a hospital pediatric bed and compare it with their bed at home. Hospital staff members explain simple procedures and answer children's questions (Fig. 29-2). A tour of the pediatric department, including the playroom, may be offered. Some hospitals have puppet shows or show slides or videos about admission and care. Child-life specialists, nurses, and volunteers help with these orientation programs.

Families are encouraged to help children at an early age develop a positive attitude about hospitals. The family should avoid negative attitudes about hospitals. Young children need to know that the hospital is more than a place where "mommies go to get babies"; it is also important to avoid fostering the view of the hospital as a place where people go to die. This is a particular concern if the child knows someone who died in the hospital. A careful explanation of the person's illness and simple, honest answers to questions about the death are necessary.

● **Figure 29.1** Holding and rocking the younger child helps alleviate the anxiety of hospitalization, especially when caregivers are not able to be with the child.

● **Figure 29.2** A nurse helps children learn what to expect from hospitalization during a prehospital program. (© B. Proud.)

● **Figure 29.3** Rooming-in helps alleviate separation anxiety for both the child and the caregiver.

The Pediatric Unit Atmosphere

An effort by pediatric units and hospitals to create friendly, warm surroundings for children has produced many attractive, colorful pediatric settings. Walls are colorful, often decorated with murals, wallpaper, photos, and paintings specifically designed for children. Curtains and drapes in appealing colors and designs are often coordinated with wall coverings.

Good News. In pediatric units, furniture is attractive, appropriate in size, and designed with safety in mind. A variety of colors helps decrease the child's anxiety.

The staff members of the pediatric unit often wear colored smocks, colorful sweatshirts, or printed scrub suits. Research has shown that children react with greatest anxiety toward the traditional white uniform. Children often are encouraged to wear their own clothing during the day. Colorful printed pajamas are provided for children who need to wear hospital clothing.

Treatments are performed in a treatment room, not in the child's room. Using a separate room to perform procedures promotes the concept that the child's bed is a "safe" place. All treatments, with no exceptions, should be performed in the treatment room to reassure the child.

A playroom or play area is a vital part of all pediatric units. The playroom should be a place that is safe from any kind of procedures. Some hospitals provide a person trained in therapeutic play to coordinate and direct the play activities.

Most pediatric settings provide **rooming-in** facilities, where the caregiver can stay in the room with the child, and encourage parents or family caregivers to visit as frequently as possible (Fig. 29-3). This approach helps minimize the separation anxiety of the young child in particular. Caregivers are involved in much of the young child's care.

Here's a helpful tip. Caregivers can be supportive and helpful in the pediatric unit. They provide comfort and reassurance to the child.

Many pediatric units use primary nursing assignments so that the same nurse is with a child as much as possible. This approach gives the nurse the opportunity to establish a trusting relationship with the child.

Planning meals that include the child's favorite foods, within the limitations of any special dietary restrictions, may perk up a poor appetite. In addition when space permits, several children may eat together at a small table. Younger children can be seated in high chairs or other suitable seats and should always be supervised by an adult. Meals should be served out of bed, if possible, and in a pleasant atmosphere. Some pediatric units use the playroom to serve meals to ambulatory children.

Test Yourself

- What are some of the reasons the child and family of a hospitalized child might suffer from stress?

- What are some advantages of children having an opportunity to tour or visit a hospital setting before they are hospitalized?

- Describe some differences that might be seen between a pediatric unit and an adult hospital unit.

A PERSONAL GLIMPSE

Hi my name is Jenni. I am 15 years old and would like to tell you about my experience in the hospital.

I am an asthmatic. I have been since my early childhood because of allergies to many things. Whenever I get a cold, it sometimes aggravates my asthma. I recently had an episode where I needed to be hospitalized because of an asthma attack.

I don't like hospitals. I could not wait until I was released. The IV hurt and needed to be put back in. The nurse had dry, scaly hands. It looked like she worked on a farm and then came to work at the hospital. The food was not too great either, not like Pizza Hut or McDonald's.

The person who made the whole ordeal tolerable was the respiratory therapist. I needed regular nebulizer treatments, and it was a dream when he came into the room. Yes, he was good looking, but what made the difference was his personality and sense of humor. It makes a big difference when it seems as if the staff person wants to be there and really cares, rather than being cared for by someone who is there just because it's a job and can't wait until the shift ends.

Jenni, age 15 years

LEARNING OPPORTUNITY: What do you think are three important behaviors by the nurse or health care professional that indicate to a patient that he or she is cared about as a person?

Pediatric Intensive Care Units

A child's admission to a pediatric intensive care unit (PICU) may be overwhelming for both the child and the family, especially if the admission is unexpected. Highly technical equipment, bright lights, and the crisis atmosphere may be frightening. Visiting may be restricted. The many stressors present increase the effects on the child and the family. PICU nurses should take great care to prepare the family for how the child will look when they first visit. The family should be given a schedule of visiting hours so that they may plan permitted visits. Visiting hours should be flexible enough to accommodate the child's best interests. The family should be encouraged to bring in a special doll or child's toy to provide comfort and security. The child's developmental level must be assessed so that the nursing staff can provide appropriate explanations and reassurances before and during procedures. Positive reinforcements, such as stickers and small badges, may provide symbols of courage. The nurse also needs to interpret technical information for family members. The nurse should promote the relationship between the family caregiver and the child as much as possible. The caregiver should be encouraged to touch and talk to the child. If possible the caregiver may hold and rock the child; if not, he or she can comfort the child by caressing and stroking.

Infection Control in the Pediatric Setting

Infection control is important in the pediatric setting. The ill child may be especially vulnerable to pathogenic (disease-carrying) microorganisms. Precautions must be taken to protect the children, families, and personnel. Microorganisms are spread by contact (direct, indirect, or droplet), vehicle (food, water, blood, or contaminated products), airborne (dust particles in the air), or vector (mosquitoes, vermin) means of transmission. Each type of microorganism is transmitted in a specific way, so precautions are tailored to prevent the spread of specific microorganisms.

The United States Centers for Disease Control and Prevention and the Hospital Infection Control Practices Advisory Committee publish guidelines for isolation practices in hospitals. The guidelines include two levels of precautions: standard precautions and transmission-based precautions. Health care facilities follow these guidelines (see Appendix A).

Standard Precautions

Standard precautions blend the primary characteristics of universal precautions and body substance isolation. Standard precautions apply to blood; all body fluids, secretions, and excretions, except sweat; nonintact skin; and mucous membranes. Standard precautions are geared toward reducing the risk of transmission of microorganisms from recognized or unrecognized sources of infection in hospitals. Standard precautions are used in the care of all patients.

Transmission-Based Precautions

Transmission-based precautions pertain to patients documented or suspected to have highly transmissible or other pathogens that require additional precautions beyond those covered under standard precautions. Transmission-based precautions include three types: airborne precautions, droplet precautions, and contact precautions. They may need to be combined to cover certain diseases. The infection control guidelines are presented in Standard and Transmission-

This is critical to remember.
Handwashing is the cornerstone of all infection control. The nurse must wash his or her hands conscientiously between seeing each patient, even when gloves are worn for a procedure.

Based Precautions in Appendix A. See Nursing Care Plan 29-1: Care for the Child Placed on Transmission-Based Precautions.

NURSING CARE PLAN 29.1

Care for the Child Placed on Transmission-Based Precautions

TS is a 5-year-old girl who has a highly infectious illness resulting from an airborne microorganism. The child is placed on Airborne Transmission-Based Precautions.

NURSING DIAGNOSIS
Risk for Loneliness related to transmission-based precautions

GOAL: The child will have adequate social contact.

EXPECTED OUTCOMES
• The child interacts with nursing staff and family.
• The child visits with friends and family via telephone.

NURSING INTERVENTIONS	RATIONALE
Identify ways in which the child can communicate with staff, family, and friends.	Frequent contact with family and staff helps to decrease the child's feeling of isolation.
Facilitate the use of telephone for the child to talk with friends.	Use of the telephone helps child feel connected with her friends.
Suggest family caregivers ask the child's preschool friends to send notes and drawings.	Notes, photos, and drawings are concrete signs to the child that her friends are thinking of her. It helps her stay in touch with her preschool.

NURSING DIAGNOSIS
Deficient Diversional Activity related to monotony of restrictions

GOAL: The child will be engaged in age-appropriate activities.

EXPECTED OUTCOMES
• The child participates in age-appropriate activities.
• The child approaches planned activities with enthusiasm.

NURSING INTERVENTIONS	RATIONALE
Gather a collection of age-appropriate books, puzzles, and games. Consult with play therapist if available.	A variety of appropriate activities provide diversion and entertainment without boredom.
Encourage family caregivers to engage the child in activities she enjoys. Audiotapes can be made for (or by) playmates.	Family caregivers can use visiting time to help alleviate the monotony of isolation. Audiotapes make friends seem closer.
Plan nursing care to include time for reading or playing a game with the child.	Activities with a variety of persons (besides family caregivers) are welcome to the child.
Encourage physical exercise within the restrictions of the child's condition.	Physical activity helps to improve circulation and feelings of well-being.

NURSING DIAGNOSIS
Powerlessness related to separation resulting from required precautions

GOAL: The child will have control over some aspects of the situation.

EXPECTED OUTCOMES
• The child will make choices about some of her daily routine.
• The child's family caregivers and the staff keep their promises about planned activities.

NURSING INTERVENTIONS	RATIONALE
Include the child in planning for daily activities such as bath routine, food choices, timing of meals and snacks, and other flexible activities.	The child will feel some control over her life if she is included in ways where she can have a choice.
Maintain the schedule after making the plan.	Keeping the schedule reinforces for the child that she really does have some control.
Plan a special activity with the child each day and keep your promise.	When the child can depend on the word of those in control, she is reassured about her own value.

The child who is segregated because of transmission-based precautions is subject to social isolation. Feelings of loneliness and depression are common. Every effort must be made to help reduce these feelings. The child must not think that being in a room alone is a punishment. The nurse can arrange to spend extra time in the room when performing treatments and procedures. While in the room, the nurse might read a story, play a game, or just talk with the child, rather than going quickly in and out of the room.

Family caregivers should be encouraged to spend time with the child. The nurse might help them with gowning and other necessary precaution procedures so that they become more comfortable in the situation. Caregivers may need to have the precaution measures reviewed, including handwashing, gowning, and masking as necessary. The nurse may encourage the family to bring the child's favorite dolls, stuffed animals, or toys. Most of these items can be sterilized after use. For the older child, electronic toys may help provide stimulation to ease the loneliness. The child should be encouraged to make phone calls to friends or family members to keep up social contacts. For the school-age child, family caregivers might be encouraged to contact the child's teacher so that classmates can send cards and other school items to keep the child involved. If the child's room has a window, move the bed so the child can see outside.

If masks or gloves are part of the necessary precautions, the child may experience even greater feelings of isolation. Before putting on the mask, the nurse should allow the child to see his or her face; that process will help the child easily identify the nurse. Gloves prevent the child from experiencing skin-to-skin contact; the nurse should talk to the child to draw out any of the youngster's feelings about this. Explaining at the child's level of understanding why gloves are necessary may help the child accept them. Gowns on the staff are generally not upsetting to the child, but the child may be bothered by the fact that caregivers must wear gowns. If this is the case, a careful explanation should help the child accept this. No matter what precautions are necessary, the nurse should always be alert to the child's loneliness and sadness and should be prepared to meet these needs.

Importance of Caregiver Participation

Research has shown that separating young children from their family caregivers, especially during times of stress, may have damaging effects. Young children have no concept of time, so separation from their primary caregivers is especially difficult for them to understand.

Three characteristic stages of response to the separation have been identified: protest, despair, and denial. During the first stage (protest), the young child cries, often refuses to be comforted by others, and constantly seeks the primary caregiver at every sight and sound. When the caregiver does not appear, the child enters the second stage—despair—and becomes apathetic and listless. Health care personnel often interpret this as a sign that the child is accepting the situation, but this is not the case; the child has given up.

In the third stage—denial—the child begins taking interest in the surroundings and appears to accept the situation. However, the damage is revealed when the caregivers do visit: the child often turns away from them, showing distrust and rejection. It may take a long time before the child accepts them again, and even then remnants of the damage linger. The child may always have a memory of being abandoned at the hospital. Regardless of how mistaken they may be, childhood impressions have a deep effect.

Rooming-in helps remove the hospitalized child's hurt and depression. Although separation from primary caregivers is thought to cause the greatest upset in children younger than 5 years of age, children of all ages should be considered when setting up a rooming-in system.

One advantage of rooming-in is the measure of security the child feels as a result of the caregiver's care and attention. The primary caregiver may participate in bathing, dressing, and feeding, preparing the child for bed, and providing recreational activities. If treatments are to be continued at home, rooming-in creates an excellent opportunity for the caregiver to observe and practice before leaving the hospital.

Nursing judgment is in order.
Rooming-in should not be used to relieve staff shortage. The role of the caregiver is to help the child feel safe and secure.

Rules should be clearly understood before admission, and facilities for caregivers should be clearly explained. The hospital may provide a foldout bed or reclining chair in the child's room. Provision for meals should be explained to the caregiver.

The nursing staff should be careful to avoid creating a situation in which they appear to be expecting the primary caregivers to perform as health care technicians. The primary caregiver's basic role is to provide security and stability for the child.

Many pediatric units also have recognized the importance of allowing siblings to visit the ill child. This policy benefits both the ill child and the sibling. The sibling at home may be imagining a much more serious illness than is actually the case. Visiting policies usually require that a family adult accompany and be responsible for the child and that the visiting period is not too long. There also should be a policy requiring that the visiting sibling does not have a cold or other contagious illness and has up-to-date immunizations.

The nursing staff also should be aware of the caregiver's needs. The caregiver needs to be encouraged to take a break, leave for a meal, or to occasionally go home, if possible, for a shower and rest. The child may be given a possession of the caregiver's to help reassure him or her that the caregiver will return. Having a way to contact the family quickly gives the family freedom with the reassurance they can be easily contacted. This is particularly useful during periods when the caregivers must wait for procedures, surgery, or other activities.

This advice could be a lifesaver.

Some hospitals have established a program in which family caregivers receive pagers so that they can leave the immediate area of the child's room or waiting area but can be quickly paged to return if needed. Having caregivers' mobile phone numbers easily accessible is also helpful in contacting them.

| BOX 29.1 | Guidelines to Orient Child to Pediatric Unit |

1. Introduce the primary nurse.
2. Orient to the child's room:
   a. Demonstrate bed, bed controls, side rails.
   b. Demonstrate call light.
   c. Demonstrate television; include cost, if any.
   d. Show bathroom facilities.
   e. Explain telephone and rules that apply.
3. Introduce to roommate(s); include families.
4. Give directions to or show "special" rooms:
   a. Playroom—rules that apply, hours available, toys or equipment that may be taken to child's room.
   b. Treatment room—explain purpose.
   c. Unit kitchen—rules that apply.
   d. Other special rooms.
5. Explain pediatric rules; give written rules if available:
   a. Visiting hours, who may visit.
   b. Mealtimes, rules about bringing in food.
   c. Bedtimes, naptimes, or quiet time.
   d. Rooming-in arrangements.
6. Explain daily routines:
   a. Vital signs routine.
   b. Bath routine.
   c. Other routines.
7. Provide guidelines for involvement of family caregiver.

Test Yourself

- Why is infection control especially important in the pediatric setting?

- Explain the difference between standard precautions and transmission-based precautions.

- Why is caregiver participation important in the pediatric hospital setting?

ADMISSION AND DISCHARGE PLANNING

Although admission may be a frightening experience, the child feels in much better control of the situation if the person taking the child to the hospital has explained where they are going and why and has answered questions truthfully. When the caregiver and the child arrive on the nursing unit, they should be greeted in a warm, friendly manner and taken to the child's room or to a room set aside specifically for the admission procedure. The caregiver and the child need to be oriented to the child's room, the nursing unit, and regulations (Box 29-1).

Planned Admissions

Preadmission preparation may make the experience less threatening and the adjustment to admission as smooth as possible. Children who are candidates for hospital admission may attend open house programs or other special programs that are more detailed and specifically related to their upcoming experience. It is important for family caregivers and siblings to attend the preadmission tour with the future patient to reduce anxiety in all family members.

During the preadmission visit, children may be given surgical masks, caps, shoe covers, and the opportunity to "operate" on a doll or other stuffed toy specifically designed for teaching purposes (Fig. 29-4). Many hospitals have developed special coloring books to help prepare children for tonsillectomy or other specific surgical procedures. These books are given to children during the preadmission visit or sent to children at home before admission. Questions may be answered and anxieties explored during the visit. Children and their families often are hesitant to ask questions or

● *Figure 29.4* The child who is going to have surgery may act out the procedure on a doll, thereby reducing some of her fear. (© B. Proud.)

express feelings; the staff must be sensitive to this problem and discuss common questions and feelings. Children are told that some things will hurt but that doctors and nurses will do everything they can to make the hurt go away. Honesty must be a keynote to any program of this kind. The preadmission orientation staff also must be sensitive to cultural and language differences and make adjustments whenever appropriate.

Emergency Admissions

Emergencies leave little time for explanation. The emergency itself is frightening to the child and the family, and the need for treatment is urgent. Even though a caregiver tries to act calm and composed, the child often may sense the anxiety. If the hospital is still a great unknown, it will only add to the child's fear and panic. If the child has even a basic understanding about hospitals and what happens there, the emergency may seem a little less frightening.

In an emergency, physical needs assume priority over emotional needs. When possible, the presence of a family caregiver who can conceal his or her own fear often is comforting to the child; however, the child may be angry that the caregiver does not prevent invasive procedures from being performed. Sometimes, however, it is impossible for the caregiver to stay with the child. A staff member may use this time to collect information about the child from the family member. This helps the family member to feel involved in the child's care.

Emergency department nurses must be sensitive to the needs of the child and the family. Recognizing the child's cognitive level and how it affects the child's reactions is important. In addition, the staff must

explain procedures and conduct themselves in a caring, calm manner to reassure both the child and the family.

The Admission Interview

An admission interview is conducted as soon as possible after the child has been admitted. See Chapter 28 for specific information related to the client interview and history. During the interview, an identification bracelet is placed on the child's wrist. If the child has allergies, an allergy bracelet must be placed on the wrist as well. The child must be prepared for even this simple procedure with an explanation of why it is necessary.

The nurse who receives the child on the pediatric unit should be friendly and casual, remembering that even a well-informed child may be shy and suspicious of excessive friendliness.

Through careful questioning, the interviewer tries to determine what the family's previous experience has been with hospitals and health care providers. It is also important to ascertain how much the caregiver and the child understand about the child's condition and their expectations of this hospitalization, what support systems are available when the child returns home, and any disturbing or threatening concerns on the part of the caregiver or the child. These findings, in addition to the client history and physical exam (see Chapter 28), form the basis for the patient's total plan of care while hospitalized.

The child who reacts with fear to well-meaning advances and who clings to the caregiver is telling the nurse to go more slowly with the acquaintance process. Children who know that the caregiver may stay with them are more quickly put at ease.

The Admission Physical Examination

After the child has been oriented to the new surroundings by perhaps clinging to the family caregiver's hand or carrying a favorite toy or blanket, the caregiver may undress the child for the physical examination. This procedure may be familiar from previous health care visits. If comfortable with helping, the caregiver may stay with the child while the physical exam is being completed. See Chapter 28 for specific information related to the physical exam.

Discharge Planning

Planning for the child's discharge and care at home begins early in the hospital experience. Nurses and other health team members must assess the levels of understanding of the child and family and their abilities to learn about the child's condition and the care necessary after the child goes home. Giving medications, using special equipment, and enforcing necessary restrictions must be discussed with the person who will be the primary caregiver and with one other person, if possible. It is necessary to provide specific, written instructions for reference at home; the anxiety and strangeness of hospitalization often limit the amount of information retained from teaching sessions. The nurse must be certain the caregiver can understand the written materials too. If the treatment necessary at home appears too complex for the caregiver to manage, it may be helpful to arrange for a visiting nurse to assist for a period after the child is sent home.

Shortly before the child is discharged from the hospital, a conference may be arranged to review information and procedures with which the family caregivers must become familiar. This conference may or may not include the child, depending on his or her age and cognitive level. Questions and concerns must be dealt with honestly, and a resource such as a telephone number the caregiver can call should be offered for questions that arise after discharge.

The return home may be a difficult period of adjustment for the entire family. The preschool child may be aloof at first, followed by a period of clinging, demanding behavior. Other behaviors, such as regression, temper tantrums, excessive attachment to a toy or blanket, night waking, and nightmares, may demonstrate fear of another separation. The older child may demonstrate anger or jealousy of siblings. The family may be advised to encourage positive behavior and avoid making the child the center of attention because of the illness. Discipline should be firm, loving, and consistent. The child may express feelings verbally or in play activities. The family may be reassured that this is not unusual.

THE CHILD UNDERGOING SURGERY

Surgery frightens most adults, even though they understand why it is necessary and how it helps correct their health problem. Young children do not have this understanding and may become frightened of even a minor surgical procedure. If they are properly prepared, older children and adolescents are capable of understanding the need for surgery and what it will accomplish.

Many health care facilities have outpatient surgery facilities that are used for minor procedures and permit the patient to return home the day of the operation. These facilities reduce or eliminate the separation of parents and children, one of the most stressful factors in surgery for infants and young children. Whether admitted for less than 1 day or for several weeks, the child who has surgery needs sympathetic and thorough preoperative and postoperative care. When the child is too young to benefit from preoperative teaching, explanations should be directed to family caregivers to help relieve their anxiety and to prepare them to participate in the child's care after surgery.

Preoperative Care

Specific physical and psychological preparation of the child and the family varies according to the type of surgery planned. General aspects of care include patient teaching, skin preparation, preparation of the gastrointestinal and urinary systems, and preoperative medication.

Patient Teaching

The child admitted for planned surgery probably has had some preadmission preparation by the physician and family caregivers. Many families, however, have an unclear understanding of the surgery and what it involves, or they may be too anxious to be helpful.

Balance is the order of the day. If possible, preoperative teaching should be conducted in short sessions, rather than trying to discuss everything at once.

The health professionals involved in the child's care must determine how much the child knows and is capable of learning, help correct any misunderstandings, explain the preparation for surgery and what the surgery will "fix," as well as how the child will feel after surgery. This preparation must be based on the child's age, developmental level, previous experiences, and caregiver support. All explanations should be clear and honest and expressed in terms the child and the family caregivers can understand. Questions should be encouraged to ensure that the child and the family caregivers correctly understand all the information.

Therapeutic play, discussed later in this chapter, is useful in preparing the child for surgery. Using drawings to identify the area of the body to be operated on helps the child have a better understanding of what is going to happen.

Children need to be prepared for standard preoperative tests and procedures, such as radiographs and blood and urine tests. Nurses may explain the reason for withholding food and fluids before surgery so children do not feel they are being neglected or punished when others receive meal trays.

Surgery and surgical procedures are feared in some cultures. Anxiety over anesthesia and being "put to sleep" causes such concern in some cultures that surgery is refused. Careful explanations of procedures and the benefits to the patient are important. Using an interpreter when language barriers exist is helpful.

Children sometimes interpret surgery as punishment and should be reassured that they did not cause the condition. They also fear mutilation or death and must be able to explore those feelings, while recognizing them as acceptable fears. Children deserve careful explanation that the physician is going to repair only the affected body part.

It is important to emphasize that the child will not feel anything during surgery because of the special sleep that anesthesia causes. Describing the postanesthesia care unit (PACU or wake-up room) and any tubes, bandages, or appliances that will be in place after surgery lets the child know what to expect. If possible, the child should be able to see and handle the anesthesia mask (if this is the method to be used) and equipment that will be part of the postoperative experience.

Role playing, adjusted to the child's age and understanding, is helpful. This approach may include a trip on a stretcher and pretending to go to surgery. If the child requests, the nurse or play leader can pretend to be the patient.

The older child or adolescent may have a greater interest in the surgery itself, what is wrong and why, how the repair is done, and the expected postoperative results. Models of a child's internal organs or individual organs, such as a heart, are useful for demonstration, or the patient may be involved in making the drawing (Fig. 29-5).

A child needs to understand that several people will be involved in preoperative, surgical, and postoperative care. If possible, staff members from the anesthesia department and the operating room, recovery room, or the ICU should visit the child before surgery. Explaining what the people will be wearing (caps, masks, and gloves) and what equipment will be used (including bright lights) helps make the operating room experience less frightening. A preoperative tour of the ICU or PACU is also helpful.

Most patients experience postoperative pain, and children should be prepared for this experience. They also need to know when they may expect to be allowed to have fluids and food after surgery.

Children should be taught to practice coughing and deep-breathing exercises. Deep-breathing practice may be done with games that encourage blowing. Teaching children to splint the operative site with a pillow helps reassure them that the sutures will not break and allow the wound to open (Fig. 29-6).

Children should be told where their family will be during and after surgery, and every effort should be made to minimize separation. Family caregivers should be encouraged to be present when the child leaves for the operating room.

Skin Preparation

Depending on the type of surgery, skin preparation may include a tub bath or shower and certainly includes special cleaning and inspection of the operative site. Shaving needed as part of the preparation usually is performed in the operating room. If fingers or toes are involved, the nails are carefully trimmed.

● *Figure 29.5* Before surgery, these children work with a child-life specialist using a model of the body organs.

● *Figure 29.6* The preoperative teaching this adolescent received helps him splint his abdomen after surgery.

The operative site may be painted with a special antiseptic solution as an extra precaution against infection, depending on the physician's orders and the procedures of the hospital.

Gastrointestinal and Urinary System Preparation

The surgeon may order a cleansing enema the night before surgery (see Chapter 30). An enema is an intrusive procedure and must be explained to the child before it is given. If old enough, the child should understand the reason for the enema.

Some nurses find this approach helpful. The child who is NPO might have a better understanding of why they are NPO if they are told that food and drink are being withheld to prevent an upset stomach.

Children usually receive nothing by mouth (NPO) 4 to 12 hours before surgery because food or fluids in the stomach may cause vomiting and aspiration, particularly during general anesthesia.

The NPO period varies according to the child's age; infants become dehydrated more rapidly than older children and thus require a shorter NPO period before surgery. Pediatric NPO orders should be accompanied by an intravenous (IV) fluid initiation order. Loose teeth are also a potential hazard and should be counted and recorded according to hospital policy.

In some instances, urinary catheterization may be performed before surgery, but usually it is done while the child is in the operating room. The catheter is often removed immediately after surgery but can be left in place for several hours or days. Children who are not catheterized before surgery should be encouraged to void before the administration of preoperative medication.

Preoperative Medication

Depending on the physician's order, preoperative medications usually are given in two stages: a sedative is administered about 1.5 to 2 hours before surgery, and an analgesic-atropine mixture may be administered immediately before the patient leaves for the operating room. When the sedative has been given, the lights should be dimmed and noise minimized to help the child relax and rest. Family caregivers and the child should be aware that atropine could cause a blotchy rash and a flushed face.

Preoperative medication should be brought to the child's room when it is time for administration. At that time, the child is told that it is time for medication and that another nurse has come along to help the child hold still. Medication should be administered carefully and quickly because delays only increase the child's anxiety.

If hospital regulations permit, family caregivers should accompany the child to the operating room and wait until the child is anesthetized. If this is impossible, the nurse who has been caring for the child can go along to the operating room and introduce the child to personnel there.

Postoperative Care

During the immediate postoperative period, the child is cared for in the PACU or the surgical ICU. Meanwhile the room in the pediatric unit should be prepared with appropriate equipment for the child's return. Depending on the type of surgery performed, it may be necessary to have suctioning, resuscitation, or other equipment at the bedside.

When the child has been returned to the room, nursing care focuses on careful observation for any signs or symptoms of complications: shock, hemorrhage, or respiratory distress. Vital signs are monitored according to postoperative orders and recorded. The child is kept warm with blankets as needed. Dressings, IV apparatus, urinary catheters, and any other appliances are noted and observed. An IV flow sheet is begun that documents the type of fluid, the amount of fluid to be absorbed, the rate of flow, any additive medications, the site, and the site's appearance and condition. The IV flow sheet may be separate or incorporated into a general flow sheet for the pediatric patient. The first voiding is an important milestone in the child's postoperative progress because it indicates the adequacy of blood flow and indicates possible urinary retention.

This is critical to remember. A child's intake and output after surgery should be measured, recorded, and reported.

Any irritation or burning also should be noted, and the physician should be notified if **anuria** (absence of urine) persists longer than 6 hours.

Postoperative orders may provide for ice chips or clear liquids to prevent dehydration; these may be administered with a spoon or in a small medicine cup. Frequent repositioning is necessary to prevent skin breakdown, orthostatic pneumonia, and decreased circulation. Coughing, deep breathing, and position changes are performed at least every 2 hours (Fig. 29-7).

Pain Management

Pain is a concern of postoperative patients in any age group. Most adult patients can verbally express the pain they feel, so they request relief. However, infants and young children cannot adequately express themselves

● *Figure 29.7* The nurse is encouraging this child to deep breathe following surgery by using a pinwheel device.

increased pulse rate and blood pressure, sweating palms, dilated pupils, flushed or moist skin, and loss of appetite, also may indicate pain.

Various tools have been devised to help children express the amount of pain they feel and allow nurses to measure the effectiveness of pain management efforts. These tools include the faces scale, the numeric scale, and the color scale. The first two scales are useful primarily with children 7 years of age and older (Fig. 29-8). To use the color scale, the young child is given crayons ranging from yellow to red or black. Yellow represents no pain, and the darkest color (or red) represents the most pain. The child selects the color that represents the amount of pain felt.

Pain medication may be administered orally, by routine intramuscular or IV routes, or by **patient-controlled analgesia**, a programmed IV infusion of narcotic analgesia that the child may control within set limits. A low-level dose of analgesia may be administered, with the child able to administer a bolus as needed. Patient-controlled analgesia may be used for children 7 years of age or older who have no cognitive impairment and undergo a careful evaluation. Intramuscular injections are avoided if possible because injections can be traumatic and painful for the child. Vital signs must be monitored, and the child's level of consciousness must be documented frequently following the standards of the facility.

Comfort measures should be used along with the administration of analgesics. The child is encouraged to become involved in activities that may provide distraction (Fig. 29-9). Such activities must be appropriate for the child's age, level of development, and interests. No child should be allowed to suffer pain unnecessarily. Appropriate nonpharmacologic comfort measures may include position changes, massage, distraction, play, soothing touch, talk, coddling, and affection.

and need help to tell where or how great the pain is. Longstanding beliefs that children do not have the same amount of pain that adults have or that they tolerate pain better than adults have contributed to undermedicating infants and children in pain. Research has shown that infants and children do experience pain (Gallo, 2003)

Nursing judgment is in order. Some children may try to hide pain because they fear an injection or because they are afraid that admitting to pain will increase the time they have to stay in the hospital.

The nurse must be alert to indications of pain, especially in young patients. Careful assessment is necessary—for example, noting changes in behavior such as rigidity, thrashing, facial expressions, loud crying or screaming, flexion of knees (indicating abdominal pain), restlessness, and irritability. Physiologic changes, such as

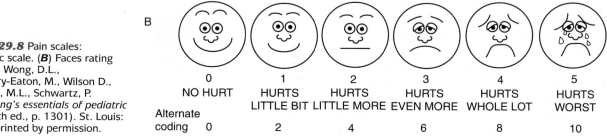

● *Figure 29.8* Pain scales: (*A*) Numeric scale. (*B*) Faces rating scale. From Wong, D.L., Hockenberry-Eaton, M., Wilson D., Winkelstein, M.L., Schwartz, P. (2001). *Wong's essentials of pediatric nursing*, (6th ed., p. 1301). St. Louis: Mosby. Reprinted by permission.

● *Figure 29-9* Distraction supplements pain control while a child is using PCA.

Surgical Dressings

Postoperative care includes close observation of any dressings for signs of drainage or hemorrhage and reinforcing or changing dressings as ordered. Wet dressings can increase the possibility of contamination; clean, dry dressings increase the child's comfort. If there is no physician's order to change the dressing, the nurse is expected to reinforce the moist original dressing by covering it with a dry dressing and taping the second dressing in place. If bloody drainage is present, the nurse should draw around the outline of the drainage with a marker and record the time and date. In this way the amount of additional drainage can be assessed when the dressings are inspected later.

Supplies needed for changing dressings vary according to the wound site and the physician's orders that specify the sterile or antiseptic technique to be used. Detailed procedures for these techniques and the supplies to be used can be found in the facility's procedures manual.

As with all procedures, the nurse must explain to the child what will be done and why before beginning the dressing change. Some dressing changes are painful; if so, the child should be told that it will hurt and should be praised for behavior that shows courage and cooperation.

Patient Teaching

Postoperative patient teaching is as important as preoperative teaching. Some explanations and instructions given earlier must be repeated during postoperative care because the child's earlier anxiety may have prevented thorough understanding. Now that tubes, restraints, and dressings are part of the child's reality, they need to be discussed again: why they are important and how they affect the child's activities.

Family caregivers want to know how they can help care for the child and what limitations are placed on the child's activity. If caregivers know what to expect and how to aid in their child's recovery, they will be cooperative during the postoperative period.

As the child recuperates, the caregivers and child should be encouraged to share their feelings about the surgery, any changes in body image, and their expectations for recovery and rehabilitation.

When the sutures are removed, the nurse should reassure the child that the opening has healed and the child's insides will not "fall out," which is a common fear.

Before the child is discharged from the hospital, teaching focuses on home care, use of any special equipment or appliances, medications, diet, restrictions on activities, and therapeutic exercise (Fig. 29-10). Caregivers should demonstrate the procedures or repeat information so the nurse can determine if learning has occurred. The nursing process is used to assess the needs of the child and the family to plan appropriate postoperative care and teaching.

> ## Test Yourself
> - Why is preoperative teaching important for the child and family caregivers?
> - What preparation procedures might the child have before surgery?
> - What factors are important in pain management for the child after surgery?
> - What might be included in postoperative teaching for the child and family?

● *Figure 29.10* The nurse uses charts with pictures to perform patient teaching before the child goes home.

THE HOSPITAL PLAY PROGRAM

Play is the business of children and a principal way in which they learn, grow, develop, and act out feelings and problems. Playing is a normal activity; the more it can be part of hospital care, the more normal and more comfortable this environment becomes.

Play helps children come to terms with the hurts, anxieties, and separation that accompany hospitalization. In the hospital playroom, children may express frustrations, hostilities, and aggressions through play without the fear of being scolded by the nursing staff. Children who keep these negative emotions bottled up suffer much greater damage than do those who are allowed to express them where they may be handled constructively. Children must feel secure enough in the situation to express negative emotions without fear of disapproval.

Children, however, must not be allowed to harm themselves or others. Although it is important to express acceptable or unacceptable feelings, unlimited permissiveness is as harmful as excessive strictness. Children rely on adults to guide them and set limits for behavior because this means the adults care about them. When behavior correction is necessary, it is important to make it clear that the child's action, not the child, is being disapproved.

The Hospital Play Environment

An organized and well-planned play area is of considerable importance in the overall care of the hospitalized child. The play area should be large enough to accommodate cribs, wheelchairs, IV poles, and children in casts. It should provide a variety of play materials suitable for the ages and needs of all children. The child chooses the toy and the kind of play needed or desired; thus the selection and kind of play may usually be left unstructured (Fig. 29-11). However, all children should participate, and the play leaders should ignore no one.

If possible, adolescents should have a separate recreation room or area. Ideally, this is an area where adolescents may gather to talk, play pool or table tennis, drink soft drinks (if permitted), and eat snacks. Tables and chairs should be provided to encourage interaction among the adolescents. Television with a videocassette tape player, computer games, and shuffleboard are also desirable (Fig. 29-12). These activities should be in an area away from young children. Rules may be clearly spelled out and posted. If adolescents must share the same recreation area with younger children, the area should be referred to as the "activity center," rather than the "playroom."

Although a well-equipped playroom is of major importance in any pediatric department, some children cannot be brought to the playroom, or some play programs may be cut because of cost-containment efforts. In these situations, nurses must be creative in providing play opportunities for children. Children may act out their fantasies and emotions in their own cribs or beds if materials are brought to them and someone (a nurse, student, or volunteer) is available to give them needed support and attention.

● **Figure 29.11** Children occupied in a hospital playroom. It is important to provide age-appropriate activities for younger and older children.

● *Figure 29.12* This adolescent enjoys playing on the computer in the adolescent room on the pediatric unit.

Children in isolation may be given play material, provided infection control precautions are strictly followed.

Therapeutic Play

The nurse should understand the difference between play therapy and therapeutic play. **Play therapy** is a technique of psychoanalysis that psychiatrists or psychiatric nurse clinicians use to uncover a disturbed child's underlying thoughts, feelings, and motivations to help understand them better. The therapist might have the child act out experiences using dolls as the participants in the experience.

Therapeutic play is a play technique that may be used to help the child have a better understanding of what will be happening to him or her in a specific situation. For instance, the child who will be having an IV started before surgery might be given the materials and encouraged to "start" an IV on a stuffed animal or doll. By observing the child, the nurse can often note concerns, fears, and anxieties the child might express. Therapeutic play is a play technique that play therapists, nurses, child-life specialists, or trained volunteers may use to help the child express feelings, fears, and concerns (Fig. 29-13).

The play leader should be alert to the needs of the child who is afraid to act independently as a result of strict home discipline. Even normally sociable children may carry their fears of the hospital environment into the playroom. It could be some time before timid, fearful, or nonassertive children feel free enough to take advantage of the play opportunities. Too much enthusiasm on the part of the play leader in trying to get the child to participate may defeat the purpose and make the child withdraw. The leader must decide carefully whether to initiate an activity for a child or let the child advance at a self-set pace.

Often other children provide the best incentive by doing something interesting, so that the timid child forgets his or her apprehensions and tries it, or another child says, "Come and help me with this," and soon the other child becomes involved. A fearful child trusts a peer before trusting an adult, who represents authority. Naturally this fact does not mean that the adult ignores the child's presence. The leader shows the child around the playroom, indicating that the children are free to play with whatever they wish and that the leader is there to answer questions and to help when a child wishes help.

When group play is initiated, the leader may invite but not insist that the timid child participate. The leader must give the child time to adjust and gain confidence.

Play Material

Play material should be chosen with safety in mind; there should be no sharp edges and no small parts that can be swallowed or aspirated. Toys and equipment should be inspected regularly for broken parts or sharp edges.

One important playroom function is that it gives the child opportunities to dramatize hospital experiences. One section of the playroom containing hospital equipment, miniature or real, gives the child an opportunity to act out feelings about the hospital environment and treatments. Stethoscopes, simulated thermometers, stretchers, wheelchairs, examining tables, instruments,

Exercise caution. Constant supervision of children while they are playing is necessary for safety.

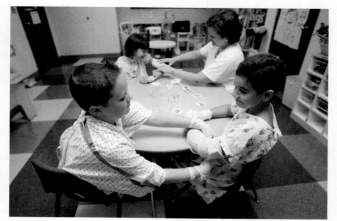

● *Figure 29.13* This group of children is involved in therapeutic play with the supervision of the child-life specialist.

bandages, and other medical and hospital equipment are useful for this purpose.

Dolls or puppets dressed to represent the people with whom the child comes in contact daily—a boy, girl, infant, adult family members, nurses, physicians, therapists, and other personnel—should be available. Hospital scrub suits, scrub caps, isolation-type gowns, masks, or other types of uniforms may be provided for children to use in acting out their hospital experiences. These simulated hospitals also serve an educational purpose: they may help a child who is to have surgery, tests, or special treatments to understand the procedures and why they are done.

Other useful materials include clay, paints, markers, crayons, stamps, stickers, sand art, cut-out books, construction paper, puzzles, building sets, and board games. Tricycles, small sliding boards, and seesaws may be fun for children who can be more physically active. Books for all age groups are also important.

Sometimes only a little imagination is needed to initiate an interesting playtime. Table 29-1 suggests activities for various age levels, most of which may be played in the child's room. These are especially useful for the child who cannot go to the playroom.

Puppets play an important part in the children's department. The use of hand puppets does much to orient or reassure a hospitalized child. The doctor or nurse puppet on the play leader's hand answers questions (and discusses feelings) that the puppet on the child's hand has asked. A child often finds it easier to express feelings, fears, and questions through a puppet than to verbalize them directly. A ready sense of magic can let the child make believe that the puppet is really expressing things that he or she hesitates to ask.

SAFETY

Safety is an essential aspect of pediatric nursing care. Accidents occur more often when people are in stressful situations; infants, children, and their caregivers experience additional stress when a child is hospitalized. They are removed from a familiar home environment, faced with anxieties and fear, and must adjust to

TABLE 29.1	Games and Activities Using Materials Available on a Nursing Unit
Age	**Activity**
Infant	Make a mobile from roller gauze and tongue blades to hang over a crib.
	Ask the pharmacy or central supply for different size boxes to use for put-in, take-out toys. (Do not use round vials from pharmacy; if accidentally aspirated, these can completely occlude the airway.)
	Blow up a glove as a balloon; draw a smiling face on it with a marker. Hang it out of infant's reach.
	Play "patty cake," "So Big," "Peek-a-boo."
Toddler	Ask central supply for boxes to use as blocks for stacking.
	Tie roller gauze to a glove box for a pull toy.
	Sing or recite familiar nursery rhymes such as "Peter, Peter, Pumpkin Eater."
Preschool	Play "Simon Says" or "Mother, May I?"
	Draw a picture of a dog; ask child to close eyes; add an additional feature to the dog; ask child to guess the added part, repeat until a full picture is drawn.
	Make a puppet from a lunch bag or draw a face on your hand with a marker.
	Cut out a picture from a newspaper or a magazine (or draw a picture); cut it into large puzzle pieces.
	Pour breakfast cereal into a basin; furnish boxes to pour and spoons to dig.
	Furnish chart paper and a magic marker for coloring.
	Make modeling clay from 1 cup salt, ½ cup flour, ½ cup water from diet kitchen.
	Play "Ring-Around-the-Rosey" or "London Bridge."
School-age	Play "I Spy" or charades.
	Make a deck of cards to play "Go Fish" or "Old Maid"; invent cards such as Nicholas Nurse, Doctor Dolittle, Irene Intern, Polly Patient.
	Play "Hangman."
	Furnish scale or table paper and a magic marker for a hug drawing or sign.
	Hide an object in the child's room and have the child look for it (have the child name places for you to look if the child cannot be out of bed).
Adolescent	Color squares on a chart form to make a checker board.
	Have adolescent make a deck of cards to use for "Hearts" or "Rummy."
	Compete to see how many words the adolescent can make from the letters in his or her name.
	Compete to guess whether the next person to enter the room will be a man or woman, next car to go by window will be red or black, and so forth.
	Compete to see who can name the characters in current television shows or movies.

BOX 29.2	Safety Precautions for Pediatric Units

- Cover electrical outlets.
- Keep floor dry and free of clutter.
- Use tape or Velcro closures when possible.
- Always close safety pins when not in use.
- Inspect toys (child's or hospital's) for loose or small parts, sharp edges, dangerous cords, or other hazards.
- Do not permit friction toys where oxygen is in use.
- Do not leave child unattended in high chair.
- Keep crib sides up all the way except when caring for child.
- If the crib side is down, keep hand firmly on infant at all times.
- Use crib with top if child stands or climbs.
- Always check temperature of bath water to prevent burns.
- Never leave infant or child unattended in bath water.
- Keep beds of ambulatory children locked in low position.
- Turn off motor of electric bed if young children might have access to controls.
- Always use safety belts or straps for children in infant seats, feeding chairs, strollers, wheelchairs, or stretchers.
- Use restraints only when necessary.
- When restraints are used, remove and check for skin integrity, circulation, and correct application at least every hour or two.
- Never tie a restraint to the crib side; tie to bed frame only.
- Keep medications securely locked in designated area; children should never be permitted in this area.
- Set limits and enforce them consistently; do not let children get out of control.
- Place needles and syringes in sharps containers; make sure children have no access to these containers.
- Always pick up any equipment after a procedure.
- Never leave scissors or other sharp instruments within child's reach.
- Do not allow sleepy family caregivers to hold a sleeping child as they may fall asleep and drop the child.

opening is in their bodies, the oxygen tent, or elsewhere in the pediatric unit. Careful observation to eliminate dangers may prevent the toddler from having access to small objects. Toddlers are also often climbers and must be protected from climbing and falling. Toddlers and preschoolers must be watched to protect them from danger. Nurses also must encourage family members to keep the crib sides up when not directly caring for the infant in the crib. One unguarded moment may mean that the infant falls out of a crib. Box 29-2 presents a summary of pediatric safety precautions.

Test Yourself

- Why is play an important part of the hospitalization of children?
- Explain the difference between play therapy and therapeutic play.
- What is the most important factor to keep in mind when choosing play materials as well as other activities on the pediatric unit?

KEY POINTS

▶ The cause of the illness, its treatment, guilt about the illness, past experiences of illness and hospitalization, disruption in family life, the threat to the child's long-term health, cultural or religious influences, coping methods within the family, and financial impact of the hospitalization all may affect how the family responds to the child's illness.

▶ The family caregivers' role in preparing a child for hospitalization includes helping the child develop a positive attitude about hospitals, hospitalization, and illness and giving children simple, honest answers to their questions.

▶ Rooming-in facilities allow and encourage the caregiver to stay in the room with the child. This helps minimize the child's concerns with separation from the caregiver, increases the child's feelings of security, and helps to decrease the stress of hospitalization.

▶ Microorganisms are spread by contact (direct, indirect, or droplet), vehicle (food, water, blood, or contaminated products), airborne (dust particles in the air), or vector (mosquitoes, vermin) means.

▶ Handwashing is the cornerstone of all infection control. The nurse must wash his or her hands conscientiously between seeing each patient, even when gloves are worn for a procedure.

▶ The nurse can help ease the feelings of isolation in a child who is placed on transmission-based precautions by spending extra time in the room

an unfamiliar schedule. Consciously assessing every situation for accident potential, the pediatric nurse must have safety in mind at all times.

The environment should meet all the safety standards appropriate for other areas of the facility, including good lighting, dry floors with no obstacles that may cause falls, electrical equipment checked for hazards, safe bath and shower facilities, and beds in low position for ambulatory patients.

The child's age and developmental level must be considered. Toddlers are explorers whose developmental task is to develop autonomy. Toddlers love to put small objects into equally small openings, whether the when performing treatments and procedures, reading a story, playing a game, or talking with the child.

- The three stages of response to separation seen in the child include protest, in which the child cries, refuses to be comforted, and constantly seeks the primary caregiver. When the caregiver does not appear, the child enters the second stage—despair—and becomes apathetic and listless. The third stage is denial, in which the child begins taking interest in the surroundings and appears to accept the situation.

- Preadmission education helps prepare the child for hospitalization and helps make the experience less threatening. During the preadmission visit the child may be given surgical masks, caps, shoe covers, coloring books, and even the opportunity to "operate" on a doll or other stuffed toy specifically designed for teaching purposes.

- The family caregiver is a vital participant in the care of an ill child. The caregiver participates in the admission interview and should be included in the planning of nursing care.

- Discharge planning includes teaching the child and the family about the care needed after discharge from the hospital. Discharge teaching should include verbal and written instructions to reference once the child is at home. The nurse must be certain that instructions are fully understood.

- After discharge the family should encourage positive behavior and avoid making the child the center of attention because of the illness. Discipline should be firm, loving, and consistent.

- Health professionals can help the adjustment of the child scheduled for surgery by determining how much the child knows and is capable of learning, helping correct any misunderstandings, explaining the preparation for surgery, and explaining how the child will feel after surgery. This preparation must be based on the child's age, developmental level, previous experiences, and caregiver support.

- Preoperative preparation for the child may include skin preparation, such as a tub bath or shower, shaving the surgical site, administering enemas, keeping the child NPO, urinary catheterization, and administering preoperative medications.

- Pain in children may be indicated by behaviors such as rigidity, thrashing, facial expressions, loud crying or screaming, flexion of knees (indicating abdominal pain), restlessness, and irritability. Physiologic changes, such as increased pulse rate and blood pressure, sweating palms, dilated pupils, flushed or moist skin, and loss of appetite, also may indicate pain.

- Play is the principal way in which children learn, grow, develop, and act out feelings and problems.

In hospital play programs, children may express frustrations, hostilities, and aggressions through play without the fear of being scolded.

- Infants, children, and their caregivers experience stress when a child is hospitalized, which may increase the frequency of accidents. Safety is an essential aspect of pediatric care. Children must be protected from hazards. Understanding the growth and development levels of each age group helps the nurse be alert to possible dangers for each child.

REFERENCES AND SELECTED READINGS

Books and Journals

Gallo, A. M. (2003). The fifth vital sign: Implementation of the neonatal infant pain scale. *Journal of Obstetrics, Gynecologic and Neonatal Nursing, 32*(2), 199–206.

Helgadottir, H. L. (2000). Pain management practices in children after surgery. *Journal of Pediatric Nursing, 15*(5), 334–340.

Hockenberry, M. J., Wilson, D., Winkelstein, M. L., & Kline, N. E. (2003). *Wong's nursing care of infants and children* (7th ed.). St. Louis: Mosby.

Karch, A. M. (2003). *2004 Lippincott's nursing drug guide*. Philadelphia: Lippincott Williams & Wilkins.

Kristensson-Hallstrom, I. (2000). Parental participation in pediatric surgical care. *AORN Journal, 71*(5), 1021–1029.

Merkel, S., et al. (2002). Pain assessment infants and young children: The FLACC scale. *AJN, 102*(10), 55.

Miles, M. S. (2003). Support for parents during a child's hospitalization. *American Journal of Nursing, 103*(2), 62–64.

Nettina, S. (2001). *The Lippincott manual of nursing practice* (7th ed.). Philadelphia: Lippincott Williams & Wilkins.

O'Connor-Von, S. (2000). Preparing children for surgery—an integrative research review. *AORN Journal, 71*(2), 334–343.

Pasero, C. (2002). Pain assessment in infants and young children: Premature infant pain profile. *American Journal of Nursing, 102*(9), 105.

Pillitteri, A. (2003). *Maternal and child health nursing* (4th ed.). Philadelphia: Lippincott Williams & Wilkins.

Salantera, L. S. (2000). Nursing students' knowledge of and views about children in pain. *Nurse Education Today, 20*(7), 539–547.

Siwula, C. M. (2003). Managing pediatric emergencies: No small matter. *Nursing 2003, 33*(2), 48–51.

Wong, D. L. (1998). *Whaley and Wong's nursing care of infants and children* (6th ed.). St. Louis: Mosby.

Wong, D. L., Perry, S., & Hockenberry, M. (2002). *Maternal child nursing care* (2nd ed.). St. Louis: Mosby.

Web Addresses

www.vh.org/VCH

www.faculty.fairfield.edu/fleitas (click on "Band-Aides and Blackboards: When Chronic Illness Goes to School")

http://health.discovery.com

WORKBOOK

NCLEX-STYLE REVIEW QUESTIONS

1. When caring for a child in a pediatric setting, which of the following actions by the nurse indicates an understanding of standard precautions. The nurse

   a. carries used syringes immediately to the sharps container in the medication room.

   b. wears one pair of gloves while doing all care for a patient.

   c. leaves an isolation gown hanging inside the patient's room to reuse for the next treatment or procedure.

   d. cleans reusable equipment before using it for another patient.

2. When discussing postoperative pain management with a caregiver of a school-age child, which of the following statements by the caregiver indicates a need for further teaching?

   a. "My child can push the PCA pump button without any help."

   b. "After the last surgery they gave my child pain medicine shots in the leg."

   c. "Talking or singing seems to decrease the amount of pain medication my child needs."

   d. "I am relieved to know my child will have less pain than adults do."

3. A 5-year-old child placed on transmission-based precautions has a nursing diagnosis of "Risk for loneliness" as part of the child's care plan. Which of the following would best help the child cope with the loneliness?

   a. Talking to the child about how he or she feels being alone

   b. Answering the call light over the intercom immediately

   c. Encouraging the child to talk to friends on the telephone

   d. Providing age-appropriate activities that can be played alone

4. The hospitalized child away from her or his home and normal environment goes through stages of separation. Which of the following behaviors might indicate the child is in the "denial" stage of separation? The child

   a. cries loudly even when being held by the nurse.

   b. searches for the caregiver to arrive.

   c. ignores caregivers when they visit.

   d. quietly lies in the crib when no one is in room.

5. After the discharge of a preschool-age child from the hospital, which of the following behaviors by the child might indicate he or she is afraid of another separation? The child

   a. plays with siblings for long periods of time.

   b. carries a favorite blanket around the house.

   c. requests to go visit the nurses at the hospital.

   d. wakes up very early in the morning.

6. The nurse is following standard precautions when caring for a child on the pediatric unit when the nurse does which of the following? Select all that apply.

   a. Washes hands when gloves are removed.

   b. Wears gloves when touching contaminated articles.

   c. Cleans reusable equipment with hot water before using on another patient.

   d. Removes needle from syringe immediately after medication administration.

   e. Wears protective eye covering when secretions are likely to splash.

   f. Removes disposable gown promptly if soiling has occurred.

STUDY ACTIVITIES

1. Design an ideal teen activity room. List all furniture and equipment you would have, and state the use(s) for each.
2. Discuss how rooming-in can be helpful in discharge planning.
3. Plan an orientation visit for a group of preschoolers from a nursery school. Check and use what is available in the pediatric unit where you have your clinical experience.
4. Go to the following Internet site: www.findarticles.com
   Go to the space next to "for" and type in "Hospitalization." Scroll down to "Hospitalization—

Admittance" to a hospital as a patient. Read down to the section "Books and Videos for Children."

a. Make a list of books you would recommend to caregivers of children who are planning a hospital admission.

b. Make a list of videos available to show to children who are preparing for a hospital admission.

CRITICAL THINKING: What Would You Do?

1. Your neighbor's daughter, 3-year-old Angela, is going to be admitted to the pediatric unit for tests and possible surgery.

a. What will you say to Angela to help prepare her for the tests that will be done?

b. What activities will you suggest Angela's mother might do to prepare her daughter for this event?

c. What will you tell Angela when she asks you what surgery is?

2. Edgar, the 4-year-old son of migrant workers, is hurt in a farming accident. You are working in the emergency department when he is brought in for treatment. His grandmother, who speaks little English, is with him.

a. What will you include in Edgar's plan of care that will help both the child and his grandmother?

b. What can you do to further communication between you, Edgar, and his grandmother?

3. On a playground, you hear a child's caregiver say, "If you don't stop that, you're going to hurt yourself and end up in the hospital!"

a. What are your feelings about this statement?

b. What would you say if you had the opportunity to respond to this caregiver after this statement was made?

c. What statement do you think would have been more appropriate for the caregiver to say in this situation?

Procedures and Treatments

STUDENT OBJECTIVES

On completion of this chapter, the student should be able to

1. Discuss the importance of preparing a child for a procedure or treatment.
2. List the responsibilities of the nurse when preparing a child for a procedure or treatment.
3. Describe the responsibilities of the nurse after a procedure or treatment.
4. List safety measures to consider when using restraints.
5. Describe methods of holding a child.
6. List four methods of reducing an elevated body temperature.
7. Explain the reason for monitoring accurate intake and output when caring for children.
8. State how a nasogastric tube is measured to determine how far it is inserted.
9. Explain the reason that stomach contents are aspirated before a gastric tube feeding is done.
10. Discuss what is done with contents aspirated from the stomach.
11. Describe the reasons that gavage feedings or gastrostomy tubes might be used in children.
12. List the methods used to administer oxygen to children.
13. Discuss the use of hot or cold therapy in relationship to circulation.
14. Describe three ostomies that are created that relate to elimination.
15. Describe four methods of collecting a urine specimen.
16. Discuss the role of the nurse in assisting with procedures related to diagnostic tests and studies.

KEY TERMS

clove hitch restraint
colostomy
elbow restraint
gastrostomy tube
gavage feedings
ileostomy
jacket restraint
mummy restraint
papoose board
tracheostomy
urostomy

NURSE'S ROLE IN PREPARATION AND FOLLOW-UP

The role of the nurse in performing or assisting with procedures and treatments includes following guidelines set by the health care institution. These guidelines include the preparation before the procedure, as well as the follow-up needed when the procedure is completed. The nurse is responsible for following facility policies and ensuring patient safety before, during, and after all procedures and treatments.

Preparation for Procedures

The emotional support and information the nurse offers often help to decrease anxiety for the child and family. Following the facility's policies regarding legal and safety factors is part of the nurse's responsibility, especially when working with children.

Psychological or Emotional Support

Many procedures in highly technological health care facilities may be frightening and painful to children. The nurse can be an important source of comfort to children who must undergo these procedures, even though it is

Here's an important tip. When the caregiver's anxiety and concerns decrease, the child in turn often will have less anxiety.

difficult to assist with or perform procedures that cause discomfort or pain. It is also important for the nurse to explain the procedure and purpose of the procedure or treatment to the caregiver.

The child who is old enough to understand the purpose of the procedure and the expected benefit must have the procedure explained; he or she should be encouraged to ask questions and should be given complete answers (Fig. 30-1). Infants can be soothed and comforted before and after the procedure.

The nurse caring for toddlers has a greater opportunity to explain procedures than does the nurse caring for infants, but at best the nurse will be only imperfectly understood. Even when toddlers grasp the words, they aren't likely to understand the meaning. The reality is the pain that occurs.

Sometimes children's interest can be diverted so that they may forget their fear. They must be allowed to cry if necessary, and they should always be listened to and have their questions answered. It takes maturity and experience on the nurse's part to know exactly which questions are stalling techniques and which call for firmness and action. Children need someone to take charge in a kind, firm manner that tells them the

● *Figure 30.1* The nurse explains the procedure to the older child in a calm, reassuring manner and allows him to ask questions. This open communication helps minimize the child's stress related to the procedure.

decision is not in their hands. They are too young to take this responsibility for themselves.

Nurses have conflicting feelings about the merit of giving some reward after a treatment. Careful thought is necessary. This has nothing to do with the child's behavior. If a reward is given, it is not a reward for being brave or good or big; it is simply a part of the entire treatment. The unpleasant part is mitigated by the pleasant.

Good news. Children given a lollipop or a small toy after an uncomfortable procedure tend to remember the experience as not totally bad.

An older person's reward is contemplating the improved health that the procedure may provide, but the child does not have sufficient reasoning ability to understand future benefits.

Test Yourself

- What are two important responsibilities of the nurse who is performing or assisting with procedures and treatments?
- Why is emotional support from the nurse important for the child and family?

Legal and Safety Factors

When the nurse is preparing to perform or assist with any procedures or treatments, he or she follows certain steps no matter what the health care setting is. Most procedures require a written order before they are done. Orders should be clarified when needed. The child must always be identified before any treatment or procedure. The nurse identifies the child by checking the child's ID band and verifies that information by having the child or caregiver state the child's name. If consent is needed, the form is completed, signed, and witnessed. As stated earlier, the procedure is discussed with the child and family caregiver, and questions are answered. Washing hands before and after any procedure helps prevent or control the spread of microorganisms. The nurse gathers the needed supplies and equipment and reviews the steps for beginning the procedure. Safety for the child (see Chapter 29) is a priority. Standard precautions are followed for all procedures (see Appendix A).

Follow-up for Procedures

When the procedure is completed, the child is left in a safe position with side rails raised and bed lowered. For the older child, the call light is put within her or his reach. Comforting and reassuring the child is important, particularly if the procedure has been uncomfortable or traumatic. The caregiver might have concerns or questions that need to be discussed. Equipment and supplies are removed and disposed of properly. Contaminated linens are handled according to facility policy. If a specimen is to be taken to another department, the specimen is labeled with the patient's name, identifying information, and the type of specimen in the container. The appropriate facility policies are followed. Often paperwork must go with the specimen, and certain precautions are taken to prevent any exposure from the specimen. Documentation includes the procedure, the child's response, and the description and characteristics of any specimen obtained. If specimens were sent to another department in the facility, this information is also recorded.

Test Yourself

- Explain why written orders are required before doing a procedure.

- How does the nurse identify the child before a procedure is done?

- What are the important factors for the nurse to remember for a child after a procedure?

PERFORMING PROCEDURES RELATED TO POSITION

Safety is the nurse's most important responsibility when performing procedures related to positioning a

child. The child's safety and comfort must be a priority when using restraints or transporting children. Safety is also an important factor when holding or positioning children for sleep.

Restraints

Restraints often are needed to protect a child from injury during a procedure or an examination or to ensure the infant's or child's safety and comfort. Restraints should never be used as a form of punishment. The procedure for the health care setting must be followed when using restraints. Many settings require a written order and have a set procedure of releasing the restraint at least every 2 hours and documenting this. When possible, restraining by hand is the best method. However, mechanical restraints must be used to secure a child during IV infusions, to protect a surgical site from injury, such as cleft lip and cleft palate, or when restraint by hand is impractical.

Be careful. Safety is ALWAYS a priority when performing any procedure on children. The importance of observing a child closely cannot be overemphasized.

Various types of restraints may be used. Whatever the type of restraint, however, caution is essential (Fig. 30-2). Close and conscientious observation is a necessary part of nursing care. The nurse also must be alert to family concerns when the child is in restraints. Explanations about the need for restraints will help the family understand and be cooperative. The caregiver may wish to restrain the child physically to prevent the use of restraints, and this action is often possible. Each situation must be judged individually.

Mummy Restraints and Papoose Boards

Mummy restraints are used for an infant or small child during a procedure. This device is a snug wrap that is effective when performing a scalp venipuncture, inserting a nasogastric tube, or performing other procedures that involve only the head or neck. **Papoose boards** are used with toddlers or preschoolers.

Clove Hitch Restraints

Clove hitch restraints are used to secure an arm or leg, most often when a child is receiving an IV infusion. The restraint is made of soft cloth formed in a figure eight. Padding under the restraint is desirable if the child puts any pull on it. The site should be checked and loosened at least every 2 hours. Commercial restraints also are available for this purpose. This restraint should be secured to the lower part of the crib

● *Figure 30.2* (**A**) Clove hitch restraint. (**B**) Jacket restraint. (**C**) Elbow restraint. (**D**) Commercial elbow restraint. (**E**) Mummy restraint. (**F**) Papoose board.

or bed, not to the side rail, to avoid possibly causing injury when the side rail is raised or lowered.

Elbow Restraints

Elbow restraints often are made of muslin in two layers. Pockets wide enough to hold tongue depressors are placed vertically in the width of the fabric. The top flap folds over to close the pockets. The restraint is wrapped around the child's arm and tied securely to prevent the child from bending the elbow. Care must be taken that the elbow restraints fit the child properly. They should not be too high under the axillae. They may be pinned

to the child's shirt to keep them from slipping. Commercially made elbow restraints may also be used.

Jacket Restraints

Jacket restraints are used to secure the child from climbing out of bed or a chair or to keep the child in a horizontal position. The restraint must be the correct size for the child. A child in a jacket restraint should be checked frequently to prevent him or her from slipping and choking on the neck of the jacket. Ties must be secure to the bed frame, not the sides, so that the jacket is not pulled when the sides are moved up and down.

A   **B**   **C**

● *Figure 30.3* Positions to hold an infant or child: (**A**) horizontal position, (**B**) upright position, (**C**) football hold.

Test Yourself

- What are the different types of restraints used in children?
- When are each of the different types of restraints used?

Transporting

When moving infants and small children in a health care setting, the safety of the child is the biggest concern. It is best to carry the infant or place him or her in a crib or bassinet.

Have some fun with this. When transporting a child, a wagon ride is functional, as well as enjoyable for the child.

Often in pediatric settings wagons are used to transport children.

The toddler may be transported in a crib with high side rails or a high-topped crib. Strollers or wheelchairs are used when the child is able to sit. Older children are placed on stretchers or may be moved in their beds. Seat belts or safety straps should be used when the child is being transported. Often a hospitalized child who is in traction, which cannot be removed, can go to the playroom or other areas in the hospital in this manner.

Holding

When a child is held, it is most important to be sure the child is safe and feels secure. The three most common methods of holding a child are the horizontal position,

upright position, or the football hold (Fig. 30-3). When holding an infant, always support the head and back. During and after feedings, the infant to be burped is sometimes held in a sitting position on the lap. The infant is held leaning forward against the nurse's hand while the nurse's thumb and finger support the infant's head. This leaves the other hand free to gently pat the infant's back (Fig. 30-4).

Sleeping

Infants should be positioned on their backs or supported on their sides for sleeping. The nurse working

● *Figure 30.4* The nurse holds the infant in a sitting position to burp the baby.

with family caregivers teaches and reinforces this information. These positions seem to have decreased the incidence of crib death or sudden infant death syndrome (see Chapter 20) in infants.

PERFORMING PROCEDURES RELATED TO ELEVATED BODY TEMPERATURE

Significant alterations in body temperature can have severe consequences for children. "Normal" body temperature varies from 97.6°F (36.4°C) orally to 100.3°F (37.9°C) rectally. The body temperature generally should be maintained below 101°F (38.3°C) orally or 102°F (38.9°C) rectally, although the health care facility or practitioner may set lower limits. Methods used to reduce fever include maintaining hydration by encouraging fluids and administering acetaminophen. Because of their ineffectiveness in reducing fever and the discomfort they cause, tepid sponge baths are no longer recommended for reducing fever. Because many children have a fever but do not need hospitalization, family caregivers need instructions on fever reduction (see Family Teaching Tips: Reducing Fever).

Control of Environmental Factors

Excess coverings should be removed from the child with fever to permit additional cooling through evaporation. Changing to lightweight clothes, removing clothes, lowering the room temperature, or applying cool compresses to the forehead may help to lower the temperature. If a child begins to shiver, whatever is being used to lower the temperature should be stopped. Shivering indicates the child is chilling, which will cause the body temperature to increase.

FAMILY TEACHING TIPS

Reducing Fever

- Do not overdress or heavily cover child. Diaper, light sheet, or light pajamas are sufficient.
- Encourage child to drink fluids.
- Keep room environment cool.
- Use acetaminophen or other antipyretics according to the care provider's directions. Do not give aspirin.
- Wait for 30 minutes and take temperature again.
- Call care provider at once if child's temperature is 105°F (40.6°C) or higher.
- Call care provider if child has history of febrile seizures.

Cooling Devices

A cooling device may be used to lower an elevated temperature. A hypothermia pad or blanket lowers or maintains the body temperature. The child's temperature is monitored closely and checked frequently with a regular thermometer. The blanket is always covered before being placed next to the child's skin so moisture can be absorbed from the skin. The baseline temperature and additional temperature measurements are documented, as well as information regarding the child's response to the treatment.

PERFORMING PROCEDURES RELATED TO FEEDING AND NUTRITION

Monitoring the intake of fluids and nutrients is important in both maintaining and promoting appropriate growth in children. The nurse is responsible for accurately documenting both a child's intake and output. If a child is unable to consume adequate amounts of fluid or foods, gavage or gastrostomy feedings are given to meet the child's nutrient needs and promote normal growth.

Intake and Output

Accurately measuring and recording intake and output are especially important in working with the ill or hospitalized child to monitor and maintain the child's fluid balance. In a well-child setting, the caregiver can provide information about the child's usual patterns of intake and output. With the ill or hospitalized child, more exact measurements of fluid intake and output are required. In many settings these measurements are recorded as often as every hour, and a running total is kept to closely monitor the child.

Oral fluids, feeding tube intake, IV fluids, and foods that become liquid at room temperature are all measured and recorded (Fig. 30-5). Urine, vomitus, diarrhea, gastric suctioning, and any other liquid drainage are measured and considered output. The color and characteristics of the output are described and recorded.

To measure the output of an infant wearing a diaper, the wet diaper is weighed, and the weight of the dry diaper is subtracted before the amount is recorded.

Gavage Feeding

Sometimes infants or children who have had surgery or have a chronic or serious condition are unable to take adequate food and fluid by mouth and must receive nourishment by means of gavage feedings. **Gavage feedings** provide nourishment directly through a tube passed into the stomach. This procedure is particularly appropriate in infants but also may

● **Figure 30.5** The nurse offers the child room temperature liquids that will be recorded as intake.

● **Figure 30.6** Measurement of tubing for nasogastric tube insertion.

be used in the older child. If gavage feedings are not well tolerated, the nurse should report it and await alternate orders from the provider.

Whether the tube is inserted nasally (nasogastric) or orally (orogastric), the measurement is the same: from the tip of the child's nose to the earlobe and down to the tip of the sternum (Fig. 30-6). This length may be marked on the tube with tape or a marking pen. The end of the tube to be inserted should be lubricated with sterile water or water-soluble lubricating jelly, never an oily substance because of the danger of oil aspiration into the lungs.

To prepare the child for gavage feeding, elevate the head and place a rolled-up diaper behind the neck. Turn the head and align the body to the right.

After the tube is inserted, it is important to verify its position to ensure that the tube is in the stomach (Fig. 30-7A). The most accurate method of confirming placement of the tube is to check the pH of the fluids aspirated. The pH of gastric contents is acidic, rather than alkaline, which would be noted if the fluid were respiratory in nature. If stomach contents are aspirated, these should be measured and replaced and, in a very small infant, subtracted from the amount ordered for that particular feeding. Positioning of the tube can also be verified by inserting 1 to 5 mL of air (using an Asepto syringe) and listening with a stethoscope. If the tube is properly placed, gurgling or growling sounds will be heard as air enters the stomach.

A

B

● **Figure 30.7 (A)** Nasogastric tube placement. **(B)** Adhesive tape used to secure nasogastric tube.

● *Figure 30.8* The nasogastric tube can be secured by gently placing the tubing behind the child's ear and taping the tubing to the child's cheek.

The nurse may hold the tube in place if it is going to be removed immediately after the feeding. If the tube is left in position for further use, it should be secured to the child's nose using adhesive tape (Fig. 30-7*B*). The tube may be further secured and more comfortable for the child if the excess tubing is gently placed behind the ear and secured to the child's cheek (Fig. 30-8). The correct position must be verified before each feeding.

The feeding syringe is inserted into the tube, and the feeding, which has been warmed to room temperature, is allowed to flow by gravity. The entire feeding should take 15 to 20 minutes, after which the infant must be burped and the child positioned on the right side for at least 1 hour to prevent regurgitation and aspiration.

The nurse should record the following items on the patient's chart:

- The type and amount of contents aspirated by the nurse.
- The amount of feeding given.
- The child's tolerance for the procedure.
- The positioning of the child after completion.

The feeding tube and any leftover feeding should be discarded at the completion of the procedure.

Gastrostomy Feeding

Children who must receive tube feedings over a long period may have a **gastrostomy tube** surgically inserted through the abdominal wall into the stomach (Fig. 30-9). This procedure is performed under general anesthesia. It also is used in children who have obstructions or surgical repairs in the mouth, pharynx, esophagus, or cardiac sphincter of the stomach or who are respirator dependent.

The surgeon inserts a catheter, usually a Foley or mushroom, that is left unclamped and connected to gravity drainage for 24 hours. Meticulous care of the wound site is necessary to prevent infection and irritation. Until healing is complete, the area must be covered with a sterile dressing. Ointment, Stomadhesive, or other skin preparations may be ordered for application to the site. The child may need to be restrained to prevent pulling on the catheter, which may cause leakage of caustic gastric juices.

Procedures for positioning and feeding the child with a gastrostomy tube are similar to those for gavage feedings. The residual stomach contents are aspirated, measured, and replaced at the beginning of the procedure. The child's head and shoulders are elevated during the feeding. After each feeding, the child is placed on the right side or in Fowler's position.

When regular oral feedings are resumed, the tube is surgically removed, and the opening usually closes spontaneously.

For long-term gastrostomy feedings, a gastrostomy button may be inserted. Some advantages of buttons are that they are more desirable cosmetically, are simple to care for, and cause less skin irritation.

Test Yourself

- When might a cooling device be used?
- Why is it important to monitor and document a child's intake?
- When are gavage or gastrostomy feedings used?
- What is the difference between a gavage tube and a gastrostomy tube?

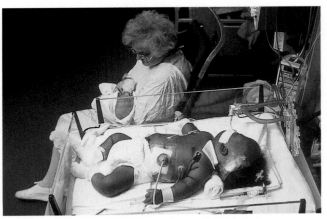

● *Figure 30.9* A gastrostomy tube is placed when long-term feedings will be needed.

PERFORMING PROCEDURES RELATED TO RESPIRATION

Oxygen administration, nasal and oral suctionings, and caring for the child with a tracheostomy are procedures the nurse might be called on to perform for the child with a respiratory condition. The nurse is responsible for monitoring and maintaining adequate oxygenation.

Oxygen Administration

Oxygen is administered to treat symptoms of respiratory distress or when the oxygen saturation level in the blood is below normal (see Chapter 28 for measurement of O_2 saturation). Depending on the child's age and oxygen needs, many different methods are used to deliver oxygen. The infant is often given oxygen while in an isolette or incubator. Infants, as well as older children, might have oxygen administered by nasal cannula or prongs, mask, or via an oxygen hood (Table 30-1). Oxygen tents may also be used to deliver oxygen. The oxygen concentration is more difficult to maintain in the tent because it is opened many times throughout the day. The tent is frightening to children, so they must be reassured frequently (Fig. 30-10).

Don't forget. An advantage of using an oxygen tent for the toddler and school-age child is that no device has to be put over the child's nose or face.

● **Figure 30.10** The child in the oxygen tent must be reassured often.

Whatever equipment is used to administer oxygen, the procedure and equipment must be explained to the child and the caregiver. Letting the child hold and feel the equipment and flow of oxygen through the device helps decrease the child's fear and anxiety about the procedure. The device warms and humidifies oxygen to prevent the recipient's nasal passages from becoming dry. The nurse closely monitors children receiving oxygen therapy; when oxygen is to be discontinued, it is done so gradually. Equipment is checked frequently to ensure proper functioning, cleanliness, and correct oxygen content. Exposure to high concentrations of oxygen can be dangerous to small infants and children with other respiratory diseases. Many times children are cared for in a home setting while receiving

TABLE 30.1	**Methods of Oxygen Administration**	
Method	Age or Reason to Use	Nursing Concerns When Using
Isolette/incubator	Newborn or infant	
Nasal prongs/cannula	Many sizes available	Not humidified; causes dryness
	Nasal prongs fit into child's nose	Keep nasal prongs clean and clear of secretions
	Toddlers may pull out of nose, other method better	Monitor nostrils for irritation
Mask	Various sizes available	Not used in comatose children
	Covers mouth and nose, not eyes	
	Humidified, decreases dryness	
Hood	Fits over head and neck of child	May be frightening for child
	Clear so child can be seen	
Oxygen tent/croupette	Equipment does not come in contact with face	Difficult to see child in tent
	Allows for movement inside tent	Difficult for child to see out
		Child feels isolated
		Change clothing and linen often
		Keep siderails up
Tracheostomy	Used in emergencies or when long-term oxygen is needed	Must be kept clean with airway patent
		Suction when needed

FAMILY TEACHING TIPS

Oxygen Safety

- Keep equipment clean. Dirty equipment can be a source of bacteria.
- Use signs noting that oxygen is in use.
- Give good mouth care. Use swabs and mouthwash.
- Offer fluids frequently.
- Keep nose clean.
- Don't use electric or battery-powered toys.
- Don't allow smoking, matches, or lighters nearby.
- Don't keep flammable solutions in room.
- Don't use wool or synthetic blankets.

oxygen. The nurse teaches the family caregiver regarding oxygen administration, equipment, and safety measures (see Family Teaching Tips: Oxygen Safety).

Nasal/Oral Suctioning

Excess secretions in the nose or mouth can obstruct the infant or child's airway and decrease respiratory function. Coughing often clears the airway, but when the infant or child is unable to remove secretions, the nurse must remove secretions by suctioning. A bulb syringe is used to remove secretions from the nose and mouth (Fig. 30-11). Sterile normal saline drops may be used to loosen dried nasal secretions. Nasotracheal suctioning with a sterile suction catheter may be needed if secretions cannot be removed by other methods.

● *Figure 30.11* A bulb syringe is used to remove secretions from the nose and mouth.

Tracheostomy

A **tracheostomy** is a surgical procedure in which an opening is made into the trachea so that a child with a respiratory obstruction can breathe. A tracheostomy is performed in emergency situations or in conditions in which infants or children have a blocked airway. Children with a tracheostomy are cared for initially in a hospital setting; children with a long-term condition often are cared for at home. The tracheostomy tube is suctioned to remove mucus and secretions and to keep the airway patent. The plastic or metal tracheostomy tube must be cleaned often to decrease the possibility of infection. Care of the skin around the site will prevent breakdown. A tracheostomy collar or mist tent provides moisture and humidity. The tracheostomy prevents the child from being able to cry or speak, so the nurse must closely monitor and find alternative methods of communicating with the child.

PERFORMING PROCEDURES RELATED TO CIRCULATION

After a provider has written an order for heat or cold therapy, the nurse is responsible for applying the treatment, closely monitoring the effects of the treatment, and documenting those observations.

Heat Therapy

The local application of heat increases circulation by vasodilatation and promotes muscle relaxation, thereby relieving pain and congestion. It also speeds the formation and drainage of superficial abscesses.

Artificial heat should never be applied to the child's skin without a specific order. Tissue damage can occur, particularly in fair-skinned people or those who have experienced sensory loss or impaired circulation. Children should be closely monitored, and none should receive heat treatments longer than 20 minutes at a time, unless specifically ordered by the provider.

Warning. If towels are used to provide moist heat, they should not be warmed in the microwave because the microwave may unevenly heat the towels, which in turn may burn the child.

Moist heat produces faster results than does dry heat and is usually applied in the form of a warm compress or soak.

Dry heat may be applied by means of an electric heating pad, a K-pad (a unit that circulates warm water through plastic-enclosed tubing), or a hot water bottle. Many children have been burned because of the improper use of hot water bottles; therefore, these devices are not recommended. Electric heating pads and K-pads should be covered with a pillowcase, towel, or stockinette. Documentation includes the application type, start time, therapy duration, and the skin's condition before and after the application.

Cold Therapy

As with heat, a provider must order the use of cold applications. In addition to reducing body temperature (see the section on Cooling Devices), the local application of cold also may help prevent swelling, control hemorrhage, and provide an anesthetic effect. Intervals of about 20 minutes are recommended for both dry cold (ice bag and commercial instant-cold preparation) and moist cold (compress, soak, and bath) treatments. Dry cold applications should be covered lightly to protect the child's skin from direct contact. Because cold decreases circulation, prolonged chilling may result in frostbite and gangrene.

The child's skin must be inspected before and after the cold application to detect skin redness or irritation. Documentation includes the application type, start time, therapy duration, and the skin's condition before and after the application.

Detailed instructions for the therapeutic application of cold and heat may be obtained in the procedures manual of each facility and from manufacturers of commercial devices.

Test Yourself

- What are some methods used for the administration of oxygen to children?

- What is a tracheostomy and when would one be used?

- For what reasons might heat therapy be used?

- For what reasons might cold therapy be used?

PERFORMING PROCEDURES RELATED TO ELIMINATION

The nurse in the pediatric setting might be responsible for performing procedures related to elimination. The nurse might administer an enema to a child as a treatment or as a preoperative procedure. When a child has a colostomy, ileostomy, or urostomy, the nurse cares for

the ostomy site and documents the output from the ostomy.

Enema

The pediatric nurse may administer an enema to an infant or child as treatment for some disorders or before a diagnostic or surgical procedure. The procedure can be uncomfortable and threatening, so it is important for the nurse to discuss the procedure with the child before giving the enema. The type and amount of fluid, as well as the distance the tube is inserted, vary according to age. The tube is well lubricated with a water-soluble jelly before insertion. Because the infant or younger child cannot retain the solution, the nurse holds the buttock for a short time to prevent the fluid from being expelled. A diaper or bedpan is used and the child's back and head are supported by a pillow. With an explanation before the procedure, the older child can usually hold the solution. A bedpan or bathroom should be available before the enema is started.

Ostomies

Infants and children may have an ostomy created for various disorders and conditions. A **colostomy** is made by bringing a part of the colon through the abdominal wall to create an outlet for fecal material elimination. Colostomies can be temporary or permanent. A new colostomy may be left to open air or a bag, pouch, or appliance used to collect the stool. An **ileostomy** is a similar opening in the small intestine. The drainage from the ileostomy contains digestive enzymes, so the stoma must be fitted with a collection device to prevent skin irritation and breakdown. It is important to teach the child or caregiver how to care for the stoma and skin with any ostomy. Preventing skin breakdown is a priority. A **urostomy** may be created to help in the elimination of urine. Ostomy bags should be checked for leakage, emptied frequently, and changed when needed. A variety of collection bags and devices are available to be used with ostomies. The products used and the procedure for changing the bags or appliances should be reviewed and institution procedures followed. The output from any ostomy is recorded accurately.

PERFORMING PROCEDURES FOR SPECIMEN COLLECTION

The nurse is often responsible for collecting or assisting in the collection of specimens. Standard precautions (see Appendix E) are followed in collecting and transporting specimens, no matter what the source of the specimen.

Nose and Throat Specimen

Specimens from the nose and throat are used to help diagnose infection. To collect a specimen, the nose or the back of the throat and tonsils are swabbed with a special collection swab. The swab is placed directly into a culture tube and taken to the lab for analysis. If epiglottitis (Chapter 35) is suspected, a throat culture should not be done because of possible trauma and airway occlusion. To diagnose respiratory syncytial virus (RSV) (Chapter 35), a nasal washing may be done. A small amount of saline is instilled into the nose; then the fluid is aspirated and placed into a sterile specimen container.

Urine Specimens

Urine is collected for a variety of reasons, including urinalysis, urine cultures, specific gravity, and dipsticking urine for glucose, protein, and pH.

This advice could save the day! When requesting a specimen, the nurse uses the word the child knows to identify urination, such as "pee-pee" or "potty," so the child will understand.

Several methods can be used to obtain specimens. To monitor the intake and output, all urine is collected and measured, whether voided into a diaper, urinal, bedpan, or toilet collection device (see intake and output). If urine specimens are needed for diagnostic purposes, other methods of collection may be used. Cotton balls can be placed in the diaper of an infant; the urine squeezed from the cotton ball can be collected and used for many urine tests. Because toddlers and young children cannot usually void on command, they should be offered fluids 15 to 20 minutes before the urine specimen is needed. Offering privacy to the older child and adolescent is important when obtaining a urine specimen.

In preparation for collecting a urine specimen, the infant or child is positioned so that the genitalia are exposed and the area can be cleansed. On the male patient, the tip of the penis is wiped with a soapy cotton ball, followed by a rinse with a cotton ball saturated with sterile water or wiped with a commercial cleaning pad (Fig. 30-12A). In the female patient, the labia majora are cleansed front to back using one cotton pad for each wipe. The labia minora are then exposed and cleansed in the same fashion (Fig. 30-12B). The area is rinsed with a cotton ball saturated with sterile water. The male or female genitalia are permitted to air-dry before collection methods are followed (see below).

After the collection, the specimen may be sent to the laboratory in the plastic collection container or in a specimen container preferred by the laboratory. Appropriate documentation includes the time of specimen collection, the amount and color of the urine, the test to be performed, and the condition of the perineal area.

Collection Bag

To collect a urine specimen from infants and toddlers who are not potty trained, a pediatric urine collection bag is used (Fig. 30-13). For the collection bag to stay in place, the skin must be clean, dry, and free of lotions, oils, and powder. The device is a small, plastic bag with a self-adhesive material to apply it to the child's skin. The paper backing is removed from the urine collection container, and the adhesive surface is applied over the penis in the male and the vulva in the female.

● **Figure 30.12** (**A**) The nurse cleans the penis of the child, being sure to pull back on the foreskin. (**B**) The nurse cleans the perineal area of the female from front to back.

● **Figure 30.13** The skin must be clean and dry in order for the urine collection bag to adhere to the child's skin.

The child's diaper is replaced. Usually within a short period of time, the child will void and the specimen can be obtained. The collection device should be removed as soon as the child voids.

Clean Catch

If a urine specimen is needed for a culture, the older child may be able to cooperate in the collection of a midstream specimen. Instruct the child as to the procedure so she or he understands what to do. The genital area is cleaned (as above), the child urinates a small amount, stops the flow, then continues to void into a specimen container.

Catheterization

Occasionally children must be catheterized to obtain a specimen, particularly if a sterile specimen is required. If the catheter is only needed to get a specimen, often a small sterile feeding tube is used. If an indwelling or Foley catheter is needed after catheterization, the catheter is left in place, the balloon inflated, and a collection bag attached.

24-Hour Urine Collection

Timed urine collections are sometimes done for a period of as long as 24 hours. The caregiver can often assist the nurse and should be instructed in the procedure. The urine is kept on ice in a special bag or container during the collection time period. At the end of the timed collection, the entire specimen is sent to the lab.

Stool Specimens

Stool specimens are tested for various reasons, including the presence of occult blood, ova and parasites, bacteria, glucose, or excess fat. The nurse puts on gloves, uses a tongue blade to collect these specimens from a diaper or bedpan, and places the specimens in clean specimen containers. Stool specimens must not be contaminated with urine, and they must be labeled and delivered to the laboratory promptly. Documentation includes the time of specimen collection; stool color, amount, consistency, and odor; the test to be performed; and the skin condition.

ASSISTING WITH PROCEDURES RELATED TO COLLECTION OF BLOOD AND SPINAL FLUID

One role of the pediatric nurse is to assist with procedures performed on children. The nurse might assist with the collection of blood samples or in holding and supporting a child during a lumbar puncture.

Blood Collection

Blood tests are part of almost every hospitalization experience and many times must be done in other settings to help with diagnosis. Although laboratory personnel or a physician usually obtains the specimens, the nurse must be familiar with the general procedure to explain it to the child. The nurse may be

A PERSONAL GLIMPSE

I have been sick so many times that I don't know which one to write about. When I had hepatitis, I was very sick for a very long time. I missed a lot of school. I had to get blood tests, urine tests, and medications all the time, and I slept a lot because I felt tired all the time. Every time I had to get a blood test I would cry because I didn't want to go. After a very long time, I got well enough to go back to school, but I couldn't play any gym games or activities because I couldn't get hit in my belly.

Justin, age 9 years

LEARNING OPPORTUNITY: What approach would be appropriate for the nurse to take with this patient if he were to become ill again and need medical care? What would you say to him before any treatment or procedure was done?

● *Figure 30.14* (**A**) Position of infant for jugular venipuncture. (**B**) Position of infant for femoral venipuncture.

asked to help hold or restrain the child during the procedure. Blood specimens are obtained either by pricking the heel, great toe, earlobe, or finger or by venipuncture. In infants, the jugular or scalp veins are most commonly used; sometimes the femoral vein is used (Fig. 30-14). In older children, the veins in the arm are used.

Lumbar Puncture

When analysis of cerebrospinal fluid is necessary, a lumbar puncture is performed. During this procedure, the nurse must restrain the child in the position shown in Figure 30-15 until the procedure is com-

pleted. The nurse grasps the child's hands with the hand that has passed under the child's lower extremities and holds the child snugly against his or her chest. This position enlarges the intervertebral spaces for easier access with the aspiration needle. Children undergoing this procedure may be too young to understand the nurse's explanation. The nurse should tell the child, however, that it is important to hold still and the child will have help to do this. The lumbar puncture is performed with strict asepsis. A sterile dressing is applied when the procedure is complete. The child must remain quiet for 1 hour after the procedure. Vital signs, level of consciousness, and motor activity should be monitored frequently for several hours after the procedure.

ASSISTING WITH PROCEDURES RELATED TO DIAGNOSTIC TESTS AND STUDIES

A variety of health care personnel in the radiology, nuclear imaging, and other departments of the health care setting perform many diagnostic tests and procedures. These diagnostic studies include x-rays, arteriograms, computed tomography (CT) scans, intravenous pyelograms, bone or brain scans, electrocardiograms (EKGs), electroencephalograms (EEGs), magnetic resonance imaging (MRI) scans, and cardiac catheterizations. The nurse's role often is to teach and prepare the child and the caregiver for the procedures to be done. After orders have been written, the nurse requests and schedules the tests or studies to be done. The required paperwork is completed and consents are signed. If the child must receive nothing by mouth (be NPO) before the study, the nurse ensures that the NPO status is maintained. Any allergies are clarified and documented on

● *Figure 30.15* Position of child for lumbar puncture. (© B. Proud.)

the consent and requisition forms. During the procedure, the nurse might be called on to support and comfort or restrain the child. After the procedure, the nurse performs and documents the care needed.

Test Yourself

- How do a colostomy, an ileostomy, and a urostomy differ?

- How are nose and throat specimens obtained?

- Describe various methods for obtaining urine specimens in children.

- What are the reasons a stool specimen might be obtained?

KEY POINTS

- Preparation of the child for procedures and treatments gives the child and family support and information and helps to decrease their anxiety.

- The responsibilities of the nurse when preparing a child for a procedure or treatment include supporting and teaching the child and family, as well as following guidelines and policies of the health care setting.

- After any procedure or treatment, the nurse has the responsibility of ensuring the child is in a safe position, comforting and reassuring the child, answering questions, and following documentation and procedure policies of the health care setting.

- When restraints are necessary, care and caution, including regular, careful observation, must be taken to protect the child from injury. Restraints should never be used as a form of punishment, and explanations about the need for restraints must be given to the family caregivers.

- The three most common methods of holding a child are the horizontal position, upright position, or the football hold. When holding an infant, the head and back should always be supported.

- Four methods of reducing an elevated body temperature include not overdressing or heavily covering child, encouraging the child to drink fluids, keeping the room environment cool, and using acetaminophen or other antipyretics, according to the provider's instructions.

- Accurately measuring and recording intake and output are especially important in working with the ill or hospitalized child to monitor and maintain the child's fluid balance.

- A nasogastric tube is measured from the tip of the child's nose to the earlobe and down to the tip of the sternum to determine how far it should be inserted. It is important to verify the position of a gastric tube before it is used for feeding to ensure that the tube is in the stomach. If stomach contents are aspirated when checking placement, these should be measured and replaced.

- If a child cannot take adequate food and fluid by mouth, gavage feedings may be used. If feedings are needed for a long period of time, a gastrostomy tube may be inserted.

- The infant often receives oxygen while in an isolette or incubator. Other methods of oxygen administration include nasal cannula or prongs, mask, or an oxygen hood. Oxygen tents may also be used to deliver oxygen to children.

- The local application of heat increases circulation by vasodilatation and promotes muscle relaxation, thereby relieving pain and congestion. It also speeds the formation and drainage of superficial abscesses. The local application of cold may help prevent swelling, control hemorrhage, and provide an anesthetic effect.

- A colostomy is created as an outlet for fecal material elimination. An ileostomy is a similar opening in the small intestine, and the drainage contains digestive enzymes. A urostomy may be created to help in the elimination of urine.

- To collect a urine specimen from an infant, cotton balls are placed in the diaper, and urine squeezed from the cotton ball can be used. Other ways to collect a urine specimen include using a pediatric urine collection bag or collecting a midstream specimen.

- The nurse's role in assisting with procedures and diagnostic tests and studies is often one of supporting the child, as well as the caregiver. The nurse's role includes teaching and preparing the child and the caregiver for the procedure, completing required paperwork, getting consents signed, maintaining NPO status, clarifying allergies, and documenting what has been done.

REFERENCES AND SELECTED READINGS

Books and Journals

Barone, M. A., & Rowe, P. C.. (1999). Pediatric procedures. In *Oski's pediatrics: Principles and practice* (3rd ed.). Philadelphia: Lippincott Williams & Wilkins.

Champi, C., & Gaffney-Yocum, P. (2001). Managing febrile seizures in children. *Dimensions of Critical Care Nursing, 20*(5).

Chandler, T. (2000). Oxygen saturation monitoring. *Pediatric Nursing, 12*(8), 37–42.

Hockenberry, M. J., Wilson, D., Winkelstein, M. L., & Kline, N. E. (2003). *Wong's nursing care of infants and children* (7th ed.). St. Louis: Mosby.

Karch, A. M. (2003). *2004 Lippincott's nursing drug guide.* Philadelphia: Lippincott Williams & Wilkins.

Pillitteri, A. (2003). *Maternal and child health nursing* (4th ed.). Philadelphia: Lippincott Williams & Wilkins.

Springhouse (2001). Handbook of nursing procedures. Springhouse, PA: Springhouse Corp.

Wilson, L. (2000). Nurse-assisted PEG in pediatric patients. *Gastroenterology Nursing, 23*(3), 121.

Wong, D. L., & Hess, C. (2000). *Wong and Whaley's clinical manual of pediatric nursing* (5th ed.). St. Louis: Mosby.

Wong, D. L., Perry, S., & Hockenberry, M. (2002). *Maternal child nursing care* (2nd ed.). St. Louis: Mosby.

Woodring, B. C. (2001). Humane treatment of children. *Journal of Child and Family Nursing, 4*(3), 232–236.

Web Addresses
www.wwnurse.com
www.nursetonurse.com
http://nursing.about.com/library/blhowto.htm

WORKBOOK

NCLEX-STYLE REVIEW QUESTIONS

1. When the nurse is performing or assisting the care provider in doing a treatment, which of the following actions by the nurse would be the *highest* priority? The nurse

   a. explains the procedure to the child.

   b. gathers the needed supplies.

   c. identifies the child before beginning the procedure.

   d. documents the procedure immediately after completion.

2. The nurse is inserting a nasogastric tube on a toddler. Which of the following restraints would be the *most* appropriate for the nurse to use with this child during this procedure?

   a. Mummy restraint

   b. Clove hitch restraint

   c. Elbow restraint

   d. Jacket restraint

3. After giving instructions to the child's caregiver regarding methods used to reduce an elevated temperature, the caregiver makes the following statements. Which statement would require follow-up by the nurse?

   a. "The last time my child had shots I gave her Tylenol."

   b. "When my older child had a fever, I always gave him a cold bath."

   c. "I never have had trouble getting my child to drink juice."

   d. "My child does not like lots of blankets over her."

4. When caring for a 3½-year-old child who is receiving oxygen in an oxygen tent, which of the following toys or activities would be best to offer this child?

   a. A radio playing soothing music

   b. Age-appropriate books

   c. A favorite blanket belonging to the child

   d. Board games the child can play alone

5. The practical nurse is participating in the development of a plan of care for a child who has a new ileostomy. Of the following nursing diagnoses, which would be the *highest* priority for this child?

   a. Risk for altered development

   b. Ineffective family coping

   c. Bowel incontinence

   d. Risk for impaired skin integrity

6. The nurse needs to calculate the intake and output during the 7 a.m. to 7 p.m. shift. The child is being given supplemental gavage feedings in addition to the child's oral intake. The child had a bowl of cereal with 2 ounces of milk and a 3-ounce glass of orange juice for breakfast. At 10:00 a.m. the child voided 75 cc of urine. The child refused lunch and was given a gavage feeding of 120 cc of supplemental feeding. Early in the afternoon the child had an emesis of 50 cc. Throughout the afternoon the child sucked on 4 ounces of ice chips. At 3:00 p.m. the child had 25 cc of apple juice and several crackers. At 4 p.m. the child voided 45 cc of urine and had a small formed stool. The child again refused to eat any supper and was given a 120-cc gavage feeding. Calculate the child's 12-hour intake and output.

STUDY ACTIVITIES

1. Using the table below, list the types of restraints, describe each restraint, and explain the purpose of using this type of restraint in the pediatric patient.

Type of Restraint	Description	Purpose

2. Develop a teaching plan to be used in teaching a group of caregivers about caring for a child who has a fever. Include in your plan when and how to take a temperature, what to do to reduce the fever, and when it would be important for the caregiver to call the health care provider.

3. Make a list of games and activities that a child who is in an oxygen tent could play or do. Develop

a game or activity that would be appropriate to use with a child who is in an oxygen tent.

4. Go to the following Internet site: www.vh.org/Providers/Simulations/ VirtualPedsPatients/PedsVPHome.html

   Go to "The Virtual Pediatric Patient."

   Scroll down to and click on "Case 7—A Child With a Fever."

   Read the sections discussing the patient and the problem.

   Read the section "Approach to the Child with Fever."

   a. List six "common" causes of fever in children.

   b. At what body temperature is it considered that a child has an elevation?

CRITICAL THINKING: What Would You Do?

1. Three-year-old Denise has an elevated temperature of 104.4°F (40.2°C).

   a. What specific steps would you follow in caring for this child?

   b. What explanations would you give this child and caregiver about what you are doing?

   c. What would be your highest priority for this child?

   d. What complication would you be most concerned about for this child?

2. The caregiver of a 2-year-old child seems upset when you enter the patient's room. The child has a feeding tube in place, as well as an intravenous line. The caregiver says, "My child does not like to have her hands tied down. Why don't you just untie her?"

   a. What explanation would you give to the caregiver?

   b. What could you do to help reassure this caregiver?

   c. What could you do to support this child?

3. You are the nurse on the pediatric unit teaching a group of your peers about caring for children who are in oxygen tents.

   a. What will you teach regarding the reasons the child might be in an oxygen tent versus receiving oxygen by a different method?

   b. What factors must be considered when providing activities for a child who must be in an oxygen tent?

   c. Why must these factors be considered?

Medication Administration and Intravenous Therapy

Medication Administration
Computing Dosages
Oral Medication
Intramuscular Medication
Other Routes of Medication
  Administration

Intravenous Therapy
Fundamentals of Fluid Balance
Intravenous Fluid Administration
Intravenous Medication
Intravenous Sites
Infusion Control

STUDENT OBJECTIVES

On completion of this chapter, the student should be able to

1. Identify the six "rights" of medication administration.
2. Convert pounds to kilograms of body weight to use in pediatric dosage calculation.
3. Calculate low and high dosages of medications using body weight.
4. Identify seven routes of medication administration.
5. Identify the muscle preferred for intramuscular injections in the infant.
6. Differentiate between intracellular fluid and extracellular fluid.
7. Explain the reason it is important to maintain fluid balance in children.
8. Identify the reasons IV fluids might be administered to children.
9. State the reason a control chamber or buretrol is used in pediatric intravenous infusions.
10. Discuss what needs to be observed for and monitored when a child has an IV.

KEY TERMS

acid-base balance
acidosis
alkalosis
azotemia
body surface area method
electrolytes
extracellular fluid
extravasation
homeostasis
induration
intermittent infusion device
interstitial fluid
intracellular fluid
intravascular fluid
total parenteral nutrition
West nomogram

MEDICATION ADMINISTRATION

Caring for children who are ill challenges every nurse to function at the highest level of professional competence. Giving medications is one of the most important nursing responsibilities.

This is critical to remember.

Medication administration calls for accuracy, precision, and considerable psychological skill.

Basic to administering medications to a person of any age are the following six "rights" of medication administration:

- The right medication. Check the drug label to confirm that it is the correct drug. Do not use a drug that is not clearly labeled. Check the expiration date of the drug.
- The right patient. Check the identification bracelet each time that a medication is given to confirm identification of the patient. In settings where such bracelets are not worn, always verify the child's name with the caregiver.
- The right dose. Always double-check the dose by calculating the dosage according to the child's weight. Question the order if it is unclear. Have another qualified person double-check any time that a divided dosage is to be given or for insulin, digoxin, and other agents governed by the facility's policy. Use drug references or check with a physician or pharmacist for the appropriateness of the dose. Orders must be questioned before the drug is given.
- The right route. Give the drug only by the route ordered. Question the order if it is unclear or confusing. If a child is vomiting or a drug needs to be given by an alternate route, always get an order from the provider before administration.
- The right time. Administering a drug at the correct time helps to maintain the desired blood level of the drug. When giving a PRN medication, always check the last time it was given and clarify how much has been given during the past 24 hours.
- The right documentation. Recording the administration of the medication, especially PRN medications, is critical to avoiding potential errors in medication administration.

Administering medications to children is much more complex than these guidelines indicate. Accurate administration of medications to children is especially critical because of the variable responses to drugs that children have as a result of immature body systems. The nurse must understand the factors that influence or alter how the child absorbs, metabolizes, and excretes the medication, and any allergies the child has. The nurse is responsible for the administration of medications. It is also important to teach the patient and the family caregivers about the effects and possible side effects of medications given.

A word of caution is in order.

The nurse is legally liable for errors of medication.

Ten rules to guide the nurse in administering medications are presented in Box 31-1. The nurse should evaluate each child from a developmental point of view to administer medications successfully. Understanding, planning, and implementing nursing care that considers the child's developmental level and coping mechanisms contribute to administering medications with minimal trauma to the child (Table 31-1).

Medication errors can occur because nurses are human and not perfect. To admit an error is often difficult, especially if there has been carelessness concerning the rules. A person may be strongly tempted to adopt a "wait and see" attitude, which is the gravest error of all. Nurses must accept responsibility for their own actions. Serious consequences for the child may be avoided if a mistake is disclosed promptly.

BOX 31.1	Rules of Medication Administration in Children

- Never give a child a choice of whether or not to receive medicine. The medication is ordered and is necessary for recovery, therefore there is no choice to be made.
- Do give choices that allow the child some control over the situation, such as the kind of juice or the number of bandages.
- Never lie. Do not tell a child that an injection will not hurt.
- Keep explanations simple and brief. Use words that the child will understand.
- Assure the child that it is all right to be afraid and that it is okay to cry.
- Do not talk in front of the child as though he or she were not there. Include the child in the conversation when talking to family caregivers.
- Be positive in approaching the child. Be firm and assertive when explaining to the child what will happen.
- Keep the time between explanation and execution to a minimum. The younger the child, the shorter the time should be.
- Preparations such as setting up an injection, solutions, or instrument trays should be done out of the child's sight.
- Obtain cooperation from family caregivers. They may be able to calm a frightened child, persuade the child to take the medication, and achieve cooperation for care.

TABLE 31.1	Developmental Considerations in Medication Administration	
Age	Behaviors	Nursing Actions
Birth–3 mo	Reaches randomly toward mouth and has a strong reflex to grasp objects	The infant's hands must be held to prevent spilling of medications.
	Poor head control	The infant's head must be supported while medications are given.
	Tongue movement may force medication out of mouth	A syringe or dropper should be placed along the side of the mouth.
	Sucks as a reflex with stimulation	Use this natural sucking desire by placing oral medications into a nipple and administering in that manner.
	Stops sucking when full	Administer medications before feeding when infant is hungry. Be aware that some medications' absorption is affected by food.
	Responds to tactile stimulations	The likelihood that the medication is taken will increase if the infant is held in a feeding position.
3–12 mo	Begins to develop fine muscle control and advances from sitting to crawling	Medication must be kept out of reach to avoid accidental ingestion.
	Tongue may protrude when swallowing	Administer medication with a syringe.
	Responds to tactile stimuli	Physical comfort (holding) given after a medication is helpful.
12–30 mo	Advances from independent walking to running without falling	Allow the toddler to choose position for taking medication.
	Advances from messy self-feeding to proficient feeding with minimal spilling	Allow the toddler to take medicine from a cup or spoon.
	Has voluntary tongue control; begins to drink from a cup	Disguise medication in a small amount of corn syrup to decrease incidence of spitting out medication.
	Develops second molars	Chewable tablets may be an alternative.
	Exhibits independence and self-assertiveness	Allow as much freedom as possible. Use games to gain confidence. Use a consistent, firm approach. Give immediate praise for cooperation.
	Responds to sense of time and simple direction	Give direction to "Drink this now" and "Open your mouth."
	Responds to and participates in routines of daily living	Involve the family caregivers and include the toddler in medicine routines.
	Expresses feelings easily	Allow for expression through play.
30 mo–6 y	Knows full name	Ask the child his or her name before giving medicine.
	Is easily influenced by others when responding to new foods or tastes	Approach the child in a calm, positive manner when giving medications.
	Has a good sense of time and a tolerance of frustration	Use correct immediate rewards for the young child and delayed gratification for the older child.
	Enjoys making decisions	Give choices when possible.
	Has many fantasies; has fear of mutilation	Give simple explanations. Stress that the medication is not being given because the child is bad.
	Is more coordinated	Child can hold cup and may be able to master pill-taking.
	Begins to lose teeth	Chewable tablets may be inappropriate because of loose teeth.
6–12 y	Strives for independence	Give acceptable choices. Respect the need for regression during hospitalization.
	Has concern for bodily mutilation	Give reassurance that medication, especially injectables, will not cause harm. Reinforce that medications should be taken only when given by nurse or family caregiver.
	Can tell time	Include the child in daily schedule of medication. Make the child a poster of medications and time due so he or she can be involved in care.
	Is concerned with body image and privacy	Provide private area for administration of medication, especially injections.
	Peer support and interaction are important	Allow child to share experiences with others.
12+ years	Strives for independence	Write a contract with the adolescent, spelling out expectations for self-medication.
	Can understand abstract theories	Explain why medications are given and how they work.

TABLE 31.1 (continued)	Developmental Considerations in Medication Administration	
Age	Behaviors	Nursing Actions
12+ years	Decisions are influenced by peers	Encourage teens to talk with their peers in a support group. Work with teens to plan medication schedule around their activities. Differentiate pill-taking from drug-taking.
	Questions authority figures	Be honest and provide medication information in writing.
	Is concerned with sex and sexuality	Explain relationships among illness, medications, and sexuality. For example, emphasize, "This medication will not react with your birth-control pills."

Computing Dosages

Commercial unit-dose packaging sometimes does not include dosages for children, so the nurse must calculate the correct dosage. Two methods of computing dosages are used to determine accurate pediatric medication dosages. Nurses use these methods to clarify that dosages ordered are appropriate and accurate. The first method uses the child's weight to determine dosage. To use this method, the child's weight in kilograms must be calculated if the weight has been recorded in pounds. The second method uses the child's body surface area.

Test Yourself

- What are the six "rights" of medication administration?

- Why are the six "rights" especially important when administering medication to children?

- Why is it necessary for the nurse to always calculate and have another nurse double-check medication dosages for children?

Body Weight Method

The first method of computing dosages uses the child's weight. Often drug companies provide a dosage range of milligrams of a medication to number of kilograms the child weighs. To calculate an accurate dose for a child, the nurse uses the dosage range provided by the drug manufacturer. The child's weight in kilograms is used to calculate a safe dose range for that child.

Converting Pounds to Kilograms

To use the body weight method of dosage calculation, a child's weight recorded in pounds has to be converted into kilograms. To do this, set up a proportion using the number of pounds in a kilogram in one fraction and the known weight in pounds and the unknown weight in kilograms in the other fraction. For a child weighing 42 pounds, the conversion is set up as follows:

$$\frac{2.2 \text{ lbs}}{1 \text{ kg}} = \frac{42 \text{ lbs}}{X \text{ kg}}$$

The fractions are then cross-multiplied:

$$2.2 \text{ lb} \times X \text{ kg} = 1 \text{ kg} \times 42 \text{ lb}$$

The problem is solved for X. Divide each side by 2.2 and cancel the units that are in both the numerator and the denominator.

$$\frac{2.2 \text{ lb} \times X \text{ kg}}{2.2 \text{ lb}} = \frac{1 \text{ kg} \times 42 \text{ lb}}{2.2 \text{ lb}}$$

$$X = \frac{42}{2.2}$$

$$x = 19 \text{ kg}$$

(Adapted from *Springhouse Nurse's Drug Guide* [2000].)

The child who weighs 42 pounds weighs 19 kilograms.

Calculating Dosage Using Body Weight Method

After converting the child's weight into kilograms, a safe dose range for that child is calculated. For example, if a dosage range of 10 to 30 mg/kg of body weight is a safe dosage range and a child weighs 20 kg, calculate the low safe dose using the following:

$$\frac{10 \text{ mg}}{1 \text{ kg}} = \frac{X \text{ mg}}{20 \text{ kg}}$$

Cross multiply the fractions:

$$10 \text{ mg} \times 20 \text{ kg} = 1 \text{ kg} \times X \text{ mg}$$

Solve for X by dividing each side of the equation by 1 (canceling the units that are in both the numerator and the denominator):

$$\frac{10 \text{ mg} \times 20 \text{ kg}}{1 \text{ kg}} = \frac{1 \text{ kg} \times X \text{ mg}}{1 \text{ kg}}$$

$$200 \times 1 = 1X$$
$$200 = X$$

The low safe dose range of this medication for the child who weighs 20 kilograms is 200 milligrams.

To calculate the high safe dose for this child, use the following:

$$\frac{30 \text{ mg}}{1 \text{ kg}} = \frac{X \text{ mg}}{20 \text{ kg}}$$

Cross multiply the fractions:

$$30 \text{ mg} \times 20 \text{ kg} = 1 \text{ kg} \times X \text{ mg}$$

Solve for X by dividing each side of the equation by 1 (canceling the units that are in both the numerator and the denominator):

$$30 \text{ mg} \times 20 \text{ kg} = \frac{1 \text{ kg} \times X \text{ mg}}{1 \text{ kg}}$$

$$600 \times 1 = 1X$$
$$600 = X$$

The high safe dose range of this medication for the child who weighs 20 kilograms is 600 milligrams.

The safe dose range for this medication for the child who weighs 20 kg is 200 mg to 600 mg. (Adapted from *Springhouse Nurse's Drug Guide* [2000].)

Body Surface Area Method

The second formula used to calculate dosages is the **body surface area (BSA) method**. The **West nomogram,** commonly used to calculate BSA, is a graph with several scales arranged so that when two values are known, the third can be plotted by drawing a line with a straight edge (Fig. 31-1). The child's weight is marked on the right scale, the height on the left scale. Use a straight edge to draw a line between the two marks. The point where the lines cross the column labeled SA (surface area) is the BSA expressed in square meters (m²). The average adult BSA is 1.7 m²; thus, the formula to calculate the appropriate dosage for a child is

$$\text{Estimated child's dose} = \frac{\text{child's BSA (m}^2)}{1.7 \text{ (adult BSA)}}$$

● **Figure 31.1** West homogram for estimating body surface area of infants and young children. To determine the body surface area, draw a straight line between the point representing the child's height on the left scale to the child's weight on the right scale. The point at which this line intersects the middle scale is the child's body surface area in square meters.

For example, a child is 37 inches (95 cm) tall and weighs 34 lb (15.5 kg). The usual adult dose of the medication is 500 mg. Place and hold one end of a straight edge on the first column at 37 inches and move it so that it lines up with 34 lb in the far right column. On the SA column, the straight edge falls across 0.64 (m)². You are ready to do the calculation.

$$\frac{0.64}{1.7} = 0.38$$

You now know that the child's BSA is 0.38 that of the average adult. You are ready to calculate the child's dose by multiplying 0.38 times 500 mg.

$$0.38 \times 500 = 190$$

The child's dose is 190 mg.

After computing any dosage, the nurse should always have the computation checked by another staff person qualified to give medication or someone in the department who is delegated for this purpose. Errors are easy to make and easy to overlook. A second person should do the computation separately; then both results should be compared.

Oral Medication

Small babies who are hungry are not too particular about the taste of food. Almost anything liquid may be sucked through a nipple, including liquid medicines, unless they are bitter. Medications that are available in syrup or fruit-flavored suspensions are easily administered this way. Another method of administering oral medications is to drop them slowly into the child's mouth with a plastic medicine dropper or oral syringe. When using a syringe, place it on the side of the tongue and slowly drip the medication into the child's mouth (Fig. 31-2).

Elixirs contain alcohol and are apt to cause choking unless they are diluted. Syrups and suspensions are thick and may need dilution to ensure that the child gets the full dose. Always check with the pharmacist before diluting any medication.

When a child is old enough to swallow a pill, make sure that the pill is actually swallowed. When asked to open their mouths, children usually cooperate so well and open so wide that their tonsils can be inspected. While the mouth is open, the nurse can look under the tongue to be sure the medication is not hidden.

Check out this tip. When available, chewable tablets work well for the pre-school child.

It usually is best to give medicine in solution form to a small child. Tablets, if used, must be dissolved in water. Do not use orange juice for a solvent unless specifically ordered to do so; the child may always associate the taste of orange juice with the unpleasant medicine. If the medicine is bitter, corn syrup may disguise the taste. The child may develop a dislike for corn syrup, but that is not as important as a lifelong dislike of orange juice. Medications should not be given in food because if the child does not consume the entire amount of food, the dosage of medication will not be accurate. In addition, if given with food, the child may eventually associate the bad taste of the medication with food and may refuse to eat that food.

There is little excuse for restraining a small child and forcing a medication down the child's throat. The child can always have the last word and bring it up again. The danger of aspiration is real. Of even greater importance are the antagonism and helplessness that build up in the child subjected to such a procedure. A child's sense of dignity must be respected as much as that of an adult. Refer to Table 31-1 to review the developmental characteristics to be considered at each age. Family teaching tips for administering oral medications at home are provided in the accompanying Family Teaching Tips: Giving Oral Medications.

Intramuscular Medication

Children have the same fear of needles as do adults. Inexperienced nurses are reluctant to hurt children and often cause the pain they are trying to prevent by inserting the needle slowly. A swift, sure thrust with insertion is the best way to minimize pain, but the nurse must stay calm and sure and be prepared for the child's squirming. It is best to have a second nurse help hold the child if he or she is younger than school age or if this is his or her first injection.

Something to always remember. Whenever possible give injections and do treatments in the treatment room. Keep the bed and playroom "safe" places for the child.

The nurse may have a ready Band-Aid to cover the injection site. This technique prevents young children from worrying that they might "leak out" of the hole, and the bandage serves as a badge of courage or bravery for the older child.

Table 31-2 describes intramuscular injection sites, how to locate them, the suggested needle size, and the amount of medication to inject.

Other Routes of Medication Administration

With few variations, the principles of administering medications by other routes are much the same as those for adults. Eye, ear, and nose drops should be warmed to room temperature before being administered. The infant or young child may need to be

● *Figure 31.2* A syringe may be used to administer an oral medication by placing the syringe at the side of the tongue.

FAMILY TEACHING TIPS

Giving Oral Medications

Before giving the medication know
• The name of the medication
• What the drug is and what it is used for
• How the medication will help your child
• How often and for how long your child will need to take it
• If it should be taken with meals or on an empty stomach
• What the correct dose is and how it is given
• How soon the medication will start working
• What the possible side effects are and when the care provider should be called
• What to do if a dose is missed, spit up, or vomited
• If there are any concerns about your child taking this medication and other medications

When giving the medication
• Read the entire label and instructions each time it is given
• Check the medicine's expiration date
• Give the right dose at the right time interval
• Use a dosing instrument that will administer an exact dose such as the following:
  • Plastic medication cup
  • Hypodermic syringe without the needle
  • Oral syringe or dropper
  • Cylindrical dosing spoon
• Measure the medication carefully and read at eye level
• **ALWAYS** remove the cap on the syringe before giving the medication
• Throw the cap away or place it out of the reach of children
• Squirt it in the back of the child's mouth or along the side of the cheek (a little at a time)
• Blowing gently on your child's face after giving the medication will cause him to swallow, if the he is reluctant
• Make the medication more palatable by mixing it with a small amount of liquid or soft food (such as applesauce or yogurt); use only a small amount of food and make sure your child eats the entire portion. (*Always* check with your child's pharmacist before doing so, however, because the effectiveness of some drugs may be compromised.)
• *Never* tell your child the medication is candy to get the child to take it

After the medication is given
• **If the child is wheezing, has trouble breathing, or has severe pain after taking a medication, seek emergency help by calling 911 or going to the emergency department** immediately
• Watch closely for side effects or allergic reactions
• **ALWAYS** use child-resistant caps and store all medications in a safe place
• Refrigerate the medication if required to do so
• Don't give medication prescribed for one child to another child
• Keep a chart and mark it each time your child takes the medication

A PERSONAL GLIMPSE

When I was 5 years old I went to the doctor's office. I had to get shots my Mom said were for school. I don't know what they were for. I felt scared before I went. My Mom told me ideas to think about when I got the shots so I wouldn't think about it hurting. She told me to think about my puppy dog and flowers and sailing ships. The nurse told me it would hurt a little. It hurt when the nurse stuck a needle in my leg. It didn't hurt as much as I thought it would. The nurse was nice and told me I was a brave girl. I am glad I thought about my dog Cheeto. I was happy to go to kindergarten.

Adriel, age 6

LEARNING OPPORTUNITY: Why is it important to prepare children for medication administration? What would you include when teaching a child before giving IM injections?

restrained for safe administration. This restraint may be accomplished with a mummy restraint or the assistance of a second person. The nurse must realize that these are invasive procedures and that the young child may be resistant. Approaching the child with patience, explanations, and praise for cooperation helps gain the child's cooperation. Documentation must be completed after the administration of any medication.

Eye Drops or Ointment

The child is placed in a supine position. To instill the drops, the lower lid is pulled down to form a pocket, and the solution is dropped into the pocket (Fig. 31-3). The eye is held shut briefly, if possible, to help distribute the medication to the conjunctiva. Ointment is applied from the inner to the outer canthus with care not to touch the eye with the tip of the dropper or tube.

● *Figure 31.3* Administering eye drops (© B. Proud.)

TABLE 31.2	Intramuscular Injection Sites			
Muscle Site		**Needle Size**	**Maximum Amount**	**Procedures**
Vastus lateralis	Greater trochanter — Site of injection (vastus lateralis) — Knee joint	Infant: 25 gauge, ⅝ inch or 23 gauge, 1 inch Older: 22 gauge, 1 inch to 1.5 inches	1 mL 2 mL	This main thigh muscle is used almost exclusively in infants for intramuscular injections but is used frequently in children for all ages. Locate the trochanter (hip joint) and knee as landmarks. Divide the area between landmarks into thirds. Inject into the middle third section, using the lateral aspect. Inject at a 90-degree angle. The accompanying figure shows the vastus lateralis muscle.
Ventrogluteal	Iliac crest — Anterior superior iliac spine — Site of injection — Palm over greater trochanter	Assess child's muscle mass. 22–25 gauge, ⅝ inch to 1 inch Infant: Toddler: School-age and older:	½–¾ mL 1 mL 1½–2 mL	With thumb facing the front of child, place forefinger on the anterior superior iliac spine with middle finger on the iliac crest and the palm centered over the greater trochanter. Inject at a 90-degree angle below the iliac crest within the triangle defined. No important nerves are in this area. The accompanying figure shows how to locate the ventrogluteal intramuscular injection site.
Deltoid	Acromion process — Deltoid muscle	Not recommended for infants Older: 22–25 gauge, 0.5 inch to 1 inch	Small muscle limits amount to ½–1 mL	Expose entire arm. Locate the acromion process at the top of the arm. Give the injection in the densest part of the muscle below the acromion process and above the armpit. Not recommended for repeated injections. Can be used for one-time immunizations. Angle needle slightly toward the shoulder. The accompanying figure shows the location of the deltoid intramuscular injection site (marked by an X).

(table continues on page 732)

TABLE 31.2 (continued)	Intramuscular Injection Sites			
Muscle Site		**Needle Size**	**Maximum Amount**	**Procedures**

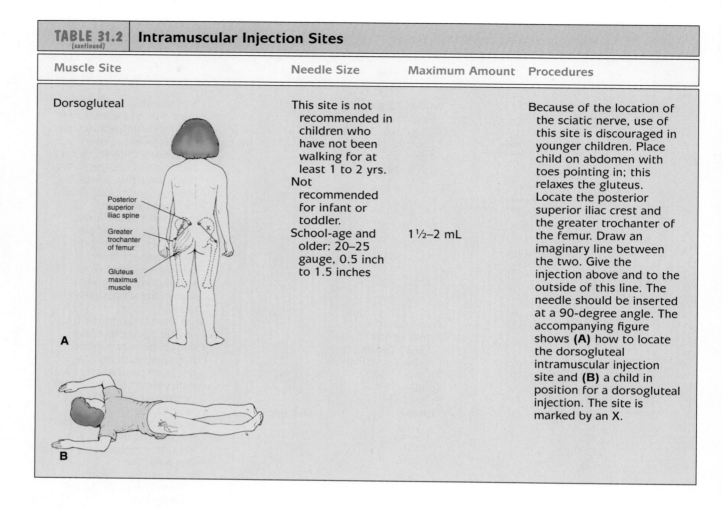

| Dorsogluteal | This site is not recommended in children who have not been walking for at least 1 to 2 yrs. Not recommended for infant or toddler. School-age and older: 20–25 gauge, 0.5 inch to 1.5 inches | 1½–2 mL | Because of the location of the sciatic nerve, use of this site is discouraged in younger children. Place child on abdomen with toes pointing in; this relaxes the gluteus. Locate the posterior superior iliac crest and the greater trochanter of the femur. Draw an imaginary line between the two. Give the injection above and to the outside of this line. The needle should be inserted at a 90-degree angle. The accompanying figure shows (A) how to locate the dorsogluteal intramuscular injection site and (B) a child in position for a dorsogluteal injection. The site is marked by an X. |

Labels on figure: Posterior superior iliac spine; Greater trochanter of femur; Gluteus maximus muscle; A; B

Nose Drops

Before nose drops are instilled, the nostrils should be wiped free of mucus. For instillation, an infant may be held in the nurse's arms with the head tilted over the arm. For a toddler or older child, the head may be placed over a pillow while the child is lying flat. The infant or child should maintain the position for at least 1 minute to ensure distribution of the medication.

Ear Drops

The infant or young child is placed in a side-lying position with the affected ear up. In an infant or toddler, the pinna (the outer part of the ear) is pulled down and back to straighten the ear canal. In a child older than 3 years of age, the pinna is pulled up and back, as with adults, to straighten the canal (Fig. 31-4). After instilling the drops, gently massage the area in front of the ear. The child should be kept in a position with the affected ear up for 5 to 10 minutes. A cotton pledget may be loosely inserted into the ear to prevent leakage of medication, but care should be taken to avoid blocking drainage from the ear.

Test Yourself

- What are some methods of administering oral medications to children?
- What sites are used in children to administer intramuscular injections?
- What is the procedure for administering eye drops to children?
- What are the important factors to remember when administering ear drops to children of different ages?

Rectal Medications

For the administration of rectal medications, the child is placed in a side-lying position, and the nurse must wear gloves or a finger cot. The suppository is lubricated, then inserted into the rectum, followed by a finger, up to the first knuckle joint. The little finger should

* To provide nutritional support
* To administer chemotherapy or anticancer drugs
* To administer pain medication

Candidates for IV therapy include children who have poor gastrointestinal absorption caused by diarrhea, vomiting, and dehydration; those who need a high serum concentration of a drug; those who have resistant infections that require IV medications; those with emergency problems; and those who need continuous pain relief.

Fundamentals of Fluid Balance

Maintenance of fluid balance in the body tissues is essential to health. Uncorrected, severe imbalance causes death, as in patients with serious dehydration resulting from severe diarrhea, vomiting, or loss of fluids in extensive burns. The fundamental concepts of fluid and electrolyte balance in body tissue are reviewed briefly to help the student understand the importance of adequate fluid therapy for the sick child.

Water

A continuous supply of water is necessary for life. At birth, water accounts for about 77% of body weight. Between ages 1 and 2 years, this proportion decreases to the adult level of about 60%.

In health, the body's water requirement is met through the normal intake of fluids and foods. Intake is regulated by the person's thirst and hunger. Normal body losses of fluid occur through the lungs (breathing) and the skin (sweating) and in the urine and feces. In the normal state of health, intake and output amounts balance each other, and the body is said to be in a state of **homeostasis** (a uniform state). Homeostasis signifies biologically the dynamic equilibrium of the healthy organism. This balance is achieved by appropriate shifts in fluid and electrolytes across the cellular membrane and by elimination of the end products of metabolism and excess electrolytes.

Body water, which contains electrolytes, is situated within the cells, in the spaces between the cells, and in the plasma and blood. Imbalance (failure to maintain homeostasis) may be the result of some pathologic process in the body. Some of the disorders associated with imbalance are pyloric stenosis, high fever, persistent or severe diarrhea and vomiting, and extensive burns. Retention of fluid may occur through impaired kidney action or altered metabolism.

Intracellular Fluid
Intracellular fluid is contained within the body cells. Nearly half the volume of body water in the infant is intracellular. Intracellular fluid accounts for about 40% of body weight in both infants and adults. Each cell must be supplied with oxygen and nutrients to keep

● *Figure 31.4* Positioning for administering ear drops. (**A**) In the child over 3-yrs-old, the pinna is pulled up and back. (© B. Proud) (**B**) In the child under 3-yrs-old, the pinna is pulled down and back. (Photo by Rick Brady.)

be used for insertion in infants. After the insertion of the suppository, the buttocks must be held tightly together for 1 or 2 minutes until the child's urge to expel the suppository passes.

INTRAVENOUS THERAPY

Fluids and medications are often administered intravenously (IV) to infants and children. Planning nursing care for the child receiving IV therapy requires knowledge of the physiology of fluids and electrolytes as well as the child's developmental level and an understanding of the emotional aspects of IV therapy for children. Intravenous therapy is commonly administered in the pediatric patient for the following reasons:

* To maintain fluid and electrolyte balance
* To administer antibiotic therapy

the body healthy. In addition, the body's water and salt levels must be kept constant within narrow parameters.

A semipermeable membrane that retains protein and other large constituents within the cell surrounds cells. Water, certain salts and minerals, nutrients, and oxygen enter the cell through this membrane. Waste products and useful substances produced within the cell are excreted or secreted into the surrounding spaces.

Extracellular Fluid

Extracellular fluid is situated outside the cells. It may be **interstitial fluid** (situated within the spaces or gaps of body tissue) or **intravascular fluid** (situated within the blood vessels or blood plasma). Blood plasma contains protein within the walls of the blood vessels and water and mineral salts that flow freely from the vascular system into the surrounding tissues.

Interstitial fluid (also called intercellular or tissue fluid) has a composition similar to plasma except that it contains almost no protein. This reservoir of fluid outside the body cells decreases or increases easily in response to disease. An increase in interstitial fluid results in edema. Dehydration depletes this fluid before the intracellular and plasma supplies are affected.

In the infant, about 25% to 35% of body weight is attributable to interstitial fluid. In the adult, interstitial fluid accounts for only about 15% of body weight (Fig. 31-5). Infants and children can become dehydrated in a short amount of time.

Fluid Distribution in Body

● *Figure 31.5* Graph indicating distribution on fluid in body compartments. Comparison between the infant and adult fluid distribution in body compartments shows that the adult total is about 60% of body weight, whereas the infant total is more than 70% of body weight.

In part, this dehydration occurs because of a greater fluid exchange caused by the rapid metabolic activity associated with infants' growth and because of the relatively larger ratio of skin surface area to body fluid volume, which is two or three times that of adults.

> **Remember this.** Infants and children become dehydrated much more quickly than do adults.

Because of these factors, the infant who is taking in no fluid loses an amount of body fluid equal to the extracellular volume in about 5 days, or twice as rapidly as does an adult. The infant's relatively larger volume of extracellular fluid may be designed to compensate partially for this greater loss.

Test Yourself

- What are five different reasons children might be given intravenous fluids?
- What are some disorders that might cause an imbalance of water in children?
- What is the difference between intracellular and extracellular fluid?

Electrolytes

Electrolytes are chemical compounds (minerals) that break down into ions when placed in water. An ion is an atom having a positive or a negative electrical charge. Important electrolytes in body fluids are sodium (Na^+), potassium (K^+), magnesium (Mg^{++}), calcium (Ca^{++}), chloride (Cl), phosphate (PO_4), and bicarbonate (HCO_3). Electrolytes have the important function of maintaining acid-base balance. Each water compartment of the body has its own normal electrolyte composition.

Acid-Base Balance

Acid-base balance is a state of equilibrium between the acidity and the alkalinity of body fluids. The acidity of a solution is determined by the concentration of hydrogen (H^+) ions. Acidity is expressed by the symbol pH. Neutral fluids have a pH of 7.0, acid fluids lower than 7.0, and alkaline fluids higher than 7.0. Normally, body fluids are slightly alkaline. Internal body fluids have a pH of 7.35 to 7.45. Body excretions, however, are products of metabolism and become acid; the normal pH of urine, for example, is 5.5 to 6.5.

Defects in the acid-base balance result either in **acidosis** (excessive acidity of body fluids) or **alkalosis** (excessive alkalinity of body fluids). Acidosis may occur in conditions such as diabetes, kidney failure, and diarrhea. Hypochloremic alkalosis may occur in pyloric stenosis because of the decrease in chloride concentration and increase in carbon dioxide.

In normal health, the fluid and electrolyte balance is maintained through the intake of a well-balanced diet. The kidneys play an important part in regulating concentrations of electrolytes in the various fluid compartments. In illness, the balance may be disturbed because of excessive losses of certain electrolytes. Replacement of these minerals is necessary to restore health and maintain life. When the infant or child can take sufficient fluids orally, that is the preferred route; often though it is necessary to administer fluids IV.

Intravenous Fluid Administration

Intravenous fluids are administered to provide water, electrolytes, and nutrients that the child needs. Total parenteral nutrition (TPN), chemotherapy, and blood products also are administered IV. **Total parenteral nutrition (TPN)** is the administration of dextrose, lipids, amino acids, electrolytes, vitamins, minerals, and trace elements into the circulatory system to meet the nutritional needs of a child whose needs cannot be met through the gastrointestinal tract.

These solutions are administered through a central intravenous access line. Medications may also be given through a central venous line. A central venous line passes directly into the subclavian vein through the jugular or subclavian vein. The line is inserted by surgical technique and is sutured into place. Caring for a child with a central venous line calls for skilled nursing care because of the danger of complications, such as contamination, thrombosis, dislodgement of the catheter, and **extravasation** (fluid escaping into surrounding tissue). The infant or child must be closely monitored for hyperglycemia, dehydration, or **azotemia** (nitrogen-containing compounds in the blood).

Vascular access ports (VAPs), including brands such as Port-A-Cath and Infus-A-Port, are small plastic devices that are implanted under the skin and are used for medication administration or for long-term fluid administration. Special needles are used to access these ports. The advantages of VAPs are that blood samples can be removed through the port, they are not visible, and do not need a dressing over them.

Peripheral vein TPN may occasionally be used on a short-term basis. Extra care must be taken to avoid infiltration because tissue sloughing may be severe.

For long-term administration of TPN or medications, a venous access device such as a Hickman, Broviac, or Groshong catheter may be inserted into the jugular or subclavian vein in a surgical procedure under anesthesia. These catheters may exit through a tunnel in the subcutaneous tissue on the right chest. Children can be discharged from the hospital on TPN therapy after family caregivers have been instructed in the care of the device, thus reducing hospital time and expense.

Dressing changes are routinely performed on the external site of a central venous device. The institution's policies must always be clarified and followed; often the practical nurse assists with this dressing change. This is a sterile procedure so sterile gloves and forceps are used. After the dressing change, the procedure is documented, as is skin condition, including any redness, swelling, drainage, or irritation.

Intravenous Medication

Intravenous medications often are administered to pediatric patients. Some drugs must be administered IV to be effective; in some patients the quick response gained from IV administration is important. Delivering medications IV is actually less traumatic than administering multiple intramuscular injections. Extra caution is necessary to observe for irritation of small pediatric veins from irritating medications. The nurse must double-check the medication label before hanging the IV fluid bottle to ensure that the medication is correct for the correct patient, that it is being administered at the correct time, and that it is not outdated.

Intravenous Sites

Site selection in the pediatric patient varies with the child's age. The best choice of sites is the one that least restricts the child's movements. Sites used include the hand, the wrist, forearm, the foot, and the ankle. The antecubital fossa, which restricts movement, is sometimes used only if other sites aren't available. The scalp vein may be used if no other site can be accessed. This site has an abundant supply of superficial veins in infants and toddlers. When a scalp vein is used, the child's hair is shaved over a small area; family caregivers can be reassured that the child's hair will grow back quickly. An inverted medicine cup or a paper cup with the bottom cut out is often taped over the site to protect it. The needle is stabilized with U-shaped taping, and a loop of the tubing is taped so that if the child pulls on the tubing, the loop will absorb the pull and the site will remain intact (Fig. 31-6*A* and *B*). The older infant's hands may need to be restrained.

If a site in the hand, foot, or arm is used, the limb should be stabilized on an armboard before insertion is attempted (Fig. 31-6*C* and *D*). These sites restrict the child's movement much more than the scalp site.

● **Figure 31.6** (**A**) Scalp vein IV site. (**B**) Paper cup taped over IV site for protection. (**C**) Armboard restraint used when IV site is in the hand. (**D**) Infant's leg taped to a sandbag to secure IV site in the leg.

The use of a plastic cannula or winged, small-vein needle has reduced the need for surgical cutdowns. In a surgical cutdown, a small incision is made, usually in the foot or hand, to provide access to a vein. A physician performs the cutdown procedure under sterile conditions.

Older children may be permitted some choice of site, if possible. The child should be involved in all aspects of the procedure within age-appropriate capabilities. The preschool child often can cooperate if given adequate explanation. Play therapy in preparation for IV therapy may be helpful. Honesty is essential with children of any age. The older school-age child and adolescent may have many questions that should be answered at his level of understanding. Family caregivers also need explanations and should be included in the preparation for the procedure. By their presence and reassurance, family caregivers may provide the emotional support the child needs and may help the child remain calm throughout the procedure.

In preparation for starting an IV line, the nurse must collect all the equipment that may be needed, including the IV tubing, any necessary extension tubing, the container of solution, the equipment to stabilize the site, a tourniquet, cleansing supplies used by the institution such as povidone-iodine or alcohol swabs, sterile gauze, adhesive tape, cling roll gauze, an IV pole, an infusion pump or controller, and a plastic cannula or winged small-vein needle usually between 21-gauge and 25-gauge (depending on the child's size).

Only nurses skilled in the procedure should start an IV infusion in children. An unskilled nurse should not attempt the procedure unless under the direct supervision of a person skilled in pediatric IV administration. It is sometimes difficult to gain access to children's small veins, and they may easily be "blown." Venipuncture requires practice and expertise. The staff nurse may serve as the child's advocate when the physician or IV nurse comes to start an infusion. The staff nurse who has cared for the child has the child's confidence and knows the child's preferences.

Infusion Control

A variety of IV infusion pumps are suitable for pediatric use. The rate of infusion for infants and children must be carefully monitored. To avoid overloading the circulation and inducing cardiac failure, the IV drip rate must be slow for the small child. Various adapting devices are available that decrease the size of the drop to a "mini" or "micro" drop of 1/50 mL or 1/60 mL, thus delivering 50 or 60 minidrops or microdrops per milliliter, rather than the 15 drops per milliliter of a regular set. Many IV sets also contain a control chamber (or buretrol) that holds 100 to 150 mL of fluid and is designed to deliver controlled volumes of fluid, avoiding the accidental entrance of too great a fluid volume into the child's system (Fig. 31-7).

Regardless of the control systems and safeguards, the child and the IV infusion should be monitored as frequently as every hour. The IV site must be checked to see that it is intact and observed for redness, pain, **induration** (hardness), flow rate, moisture at the site, and swelling. Documentation is sometimes done on an IV flow sheet that lists the flow rate, the amount in the bottle, the amount in the burette, the amount infused, and the condition of the site. It is important to accurately document IV fluid intake on any child undergoing IV therapy.

For the administration of an IV medication, a heparin lock or **intermittent infusion device** may be used (Fig. 31-8). This method allows the child more freedom and frees him or her from IV tubing between medication administrations. The veins on the back of the hand are often used for heparin lock insertion. Medication is administered through the lock; when the administration is completed, the needle and tubing are

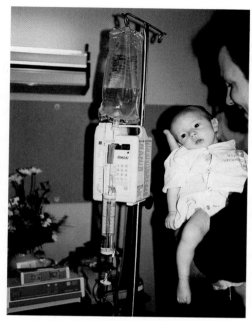

● *Figure 31.7* An infant with an infusion pump and an infusion chamber. The infusion chamber has a "mini" dropper to reduce the size of the drops.

removed and the heparin lock is flushed (Fig 31-9). A self-healing rubber stopper closes the heparin lock so that it does not leak between administrations. This method also may be used for a child who must have frequent blood samples drawn. The heparin lock is

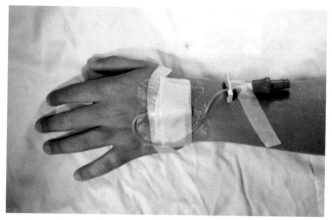

● *Figure 31.9* The heparin lock allows for more freedom of movement between uses.

flushed every 4 to 8 hours with saline or heparin, according to the facility's procedure.

Test Yourself

- What sites might be used for intravenous therapy in children?
- Why is it important to use an infusion control devices for IV therapy in children?

KEY POINTS

▶ The six "rights" of medication administration are basic to administering medications to anyone, but administering medications to children is much more complex because of their immature body systems and varying sizes. The six "rights" include the right medication, patient, dose, route, time, and documentation.

▶ When administering medications to children, the nurse should always calculate the child's weight in kilograms if the medication is ordered as a dose per kilogram. The nurse calculates the low and high dose of medications by using the child's body weight and always has another person check his or her computations of drug dosage before administering medications to children.

▶ The seven routes of medication administration are oral; intramuscular; eye, ear, and nose drops; rectal; and intravenous.

▶ The muscle preferred for intramuscular injections in the infant is the vastus lateralis.

▶ Intracellular fluid is contained within the body cells and makes up 40% of body weight in children and adults. Extracellular fluid is situated outside

● *Figure 31.8* Secondary administration through a volume control set into a heparin lock.

Administration spike

Air filter

Medicine port

Drip chamber

the cells and is either interstitial fluid (situated within the spaces or gaps of body tissue) or intravascular fluid (situated within the blood vessels or blood plasma).

◗ Maintaining fluid balance in the body tissues is essential to health. Severe imbalance can occur rapidly in children because they dehydrate much faster than do adults. Serious dehydration can result from diarrhea, vomiting, or loss of fluids in extensive burns.

◗ Intravenous (IV) fluids might be administered to children to provide water, electrolytes, and nutrients the child needs. Total parenteral nutrition (TPN), chemotherapy, and blood products also are administered IV. IV fluid administration requires careful observation of the child's appearance, vital signs, intake and output, and the fluid's flow rate. The flow rate is regulated by the use of a control chamber or buretrol. Intravenous infusion sites must be monitored to avoid infiltration and tissue damage.

REFERENCES AND SELECTED READINGS

Books and Journals

Hockenberry, M. J., Wilson, D., Winkelstein, M. L., & Kline, N. E. (2003). *Wong's nursing care of infants and children* (7th ed.). St. Louis: Mosby.

Johnson, C., & Horton, S. (2001). Owning up to errors: Put an end to the blame game. *Nursing, 31(6)*, 54.

Karch, A. M. (2003). *2004 Lippincott's nursing drug guide.* Philadelphia: Lippincott Williams & Wilkins.

Pillitteri, A. (2003). *Maternal and child health nursing* (4th ed.). Philadelphia: Lippincott Williams & Wilkins.

Roach, S., & Scherer, J. (2000). *Introductory clinical pharmacology* (6th ed). Philadelphia: Lippincott Williams & Wilkins.

Springhouse nurse's drug guide (3rd ed.). (2000). Springhouse, PA: Springhouse Corporation.

Steward, D. (2001). Taking the 'ouch' out of injection for children: Using distraction to decrease pain. *The American Journal of Maternal/Child Nursing, 26(2)*, 72–78.

Teplitsky, B. (2001). Avoiding the hazards of look-alike drug names. *Nursing, 31(9)*, 56.

VanHulle, V. C. (2001). Nurses' analgesic practices with hospitalized children. *Journal of Child and Family Nursing, 4(2)*, 79.

Wong, D. L., & Hess, C. (2000). *Wong and Whaley's clinical manual of pediatric nursing* (5th ed.). St. Louis: Mosby.

Wong, D. L., Perry, S., & Hockenberry, M.J. (2002). *Maternal child nursing care* (2nd ed.). St. Louis: Mosby.

WEB ADDRESSES

Drug Calculations
www.geocites.com/HotSprings/8517/Quiz/quiz.htm
    Nursing Library, Doing Two-Step Dosage Calculations, www.findarticles.com

WORKBOOK

NCLEX-STYLE REVIEW QUESTIONS

1. The pediatric nurse is administering medications to a 4-year-old child. Which of the following statements by the nurse indicates an understanding of the child's developmental level?

   a. "Your Mom will help me hold your hands."

   b. "Would you like orange or apple juice to drink after you take your medicine?"

   c. "You can make a poster of the schedule for all your medications."

   d. "This booklet tells all about how this medicine works."

2. The nurse is doing a dosage calculation for an infant who weighs 16 pounds. How many kilograms does the child weigh?

   a. 0.72 kg

   b. 1.7 kg

   c. 7.3 kg

   d. 9.0 kg

3. The dosage range of Demerol for a school-age child is 1.1 mg/kg to 1.8 mg/kg. Of the following, which dosage would be appropriate to give a school-age child who weighs 76 pounds?

   a. 24.4 mg

   b. 30.0 mg

   c. 60 mg

   d. 110 mg

4. When administering an IM injection to a 4-month-old infant, the *best* injection site to use would be the

   a. vastus lateralis.

   b. ventrogluteal.

   c. deltoid.

   d. dorsogluteal.

5. Infusion pumps and volume control devices are used when children are given IV fluids. The *most* important reason these devices are used is to

   a. regulate the rate of the infusion.

   b. decrease the size of the drops delivered.

   c. reduce the chance of infiltration.

   d. administer medications.

6. The nurse is administering an IM (intramuscular) injection using the vastus lateralis muscle. Mark an X on the location of the vastus lateralis muscle in this child's right leg.

Vastus lateralis muscle

STUDY ACTIVITIES

1. Catlin weighs 28.5 lb (13 kg) and measures 35.5 inches (90 cm). Find her BSA using the West nomogram. Calculate the dose of a medication for her if the adult dosage is 750 mg.

2. Describe how you would approach each of the following children when giving oral medications and intramuscular medications.

	Oral Medications	Intramuscular Medications
6-month-old Kristi		
18-month-old Jared		
3-year-old Sarah		
4½-year-old Miguel		
8-year-old Danika		
16-year-old Jon		

3. Identify each of the intramuscular injection sites, state how to locate each of the sites, and name the landmarks used.

4. Go to the following Internet site:

   www.findarticles.com

   Go to the space next to "for" and type in "Medication Errors DOSING ERROR."

   Scroll down to "Medication Errors DOSING ERROR."

   a. What does the author say should always be written before a decimal for doses that are less than 1?

   Scroll down to "RESPONDING TO ERRORS."

   b. List four disciplinary actions that can occur after a medication error.

CRITICAL THINKING: What Would You Do?

You have been asked to lead a discussion with a group of your peers about medicating children.

   a. What is the importance of following the six "rights" of medication administration?

   b. What do you think are the most important responsibilities of the nurse when medicating children?

   c. How does medicating children differ from medicating adults?

   d. What steps would you take if you discovered that you had made a medication error?

   e. What are your legal responsibilities related to medication errors?

The Child With a Chronic Health Problem

STUDENT OBJECTIVES

On completion of this chapter, the student should be able to

1. Identify 10 conditions that cause chronic illness.
2. Identify 10 concerns common to many families of a child with a chronic illness.
3. Describe economic pressures that can overwhelm families of chronically ill children.
4. Discuss the importance of respite care.
5. Identify positive and negative responses that well siblings may manifest in response to an ill sibling.
6. Identify several ways the nurse may encourage self-care by the child.
7. Describe how the nurse can help the family adjust to the child's condition.
8. Discuss general guidelines for preparing the family for home care of the child.

KEY TERMS

chronic illness
denial
gradual acceptance
overprotection
rejection
respite care
stigma

Chronic illness is a leading health problem in the United States. The numbers of chronically ill children are growing as more infants and children survive prematurity, difficult births, congenital anomalies, accidents, and illnesses that once were fatal. Most children experience only brief, acute episodes of illness; however, a significant number are affected by chronic health problems. Diseases that cause chronic illness in children include congenital heart disease, cystic fibrosis, juvenile arthritis, asthma, hemophilia, muscular dystrophy, leukemia and other malignancies, spina bifida, and immunodeficiency syndromes. When a family member has a chronic illness, the entire family is affected in many ways. Chronic illness may affect the child's physical, psychosocial, and cognitive development. Because nurses are usually involved from the early stages of diagnosis and the child and family have ongoing and long-term needs, the nurse can play a vital role in helping the family adjust to the condition.

COMMON PROBLEMS IN CHRONIC ILLNESS

Chronic illness is a condition of long duration or one that progresses slowly, shows little change, and often interferes with daily functioning. Specific chronic health problems of children are discussed in chapters throughout this text. Each requires individualized management based on the disease process and the abilities of the patient and family to understand and comply with the treatment regimen. All chronic health problems, however, create some common difficulties for patients and families; these are the focus of this chapter. Some of these concerns are

- Financial concerns, such as payment for treatment, living expenses at a distant health care facility, caregiver's job loss because of time not at work
- Administration of treatments and medications at home
- Disruption of family life, such as vacations, family goals, careers
- Educational opportunities for the child
- Social isolation because of the child's condition
- Family adjustments because of the disease's changing course
- Reaction of well siblings
- Stress among caregivers
- Guilt about and acceptance of the chronic condition
- Care of the child when family caregivers can no longer provide care

EFFECTS OF CHRONIC ILLNESS ON THE FAMILY

The diagnosis of a chronic health problem causes a crisis in the family, whether it happens during the first few hours or days of the child's life or much later. How families cope with chronic illness varies greatly from one family to another, but they all face many of the same problems.

Parents and Chronic Illness

When family caregivers learn of the child's diagnosis, their first reactions may be shock, disbelief, and denial. These reactions may last for a varied amount of time, from days to months. The initial response may be one of mourning for the "perfect" child they lost combined with guilt, blame, and rationalization. The caregivers may seek advice from other professionals and actually may go "shopping" for another physician, hoping to find the diagnosis is incorrect or not as serious as they have been told. They may refuse to accept the diagnosis or talk about it, or they may delay seeking or agreeing to treatment. Gradually, however, they adjust to the diagnosis. They may enter a period of chronic sorrow when they adapt to the child's state of chronic illness but do not necessarily accept it. They often waver between the stages, and they experience emotional highs and lows as they care for the child and meet the challenges of daily life. Families who have a strong support system usually are better able to meet these challenges.

Economic pressures can become overwhelming to the families of chronically ill children. If the family does not have adequate health insurance, the costs of treatment may be enormous. Away-from-home living costs may become a problem if the child must go to a distant hospital for further diagnosis or treatment. To keep health insurance benefits, a family caregiver may feel tied to a job, which creates additional stress. The time required to take the child to medical appointments can be excessive and may cause an additional threat to job security because of the time lost from the job.

Families must make many adjustments to care for the chronically ill child. The family caregivers may have to learn to perform treatments and give medications. Family life is often disrupted. Vacations may be nonexistent, and the family may be limited in how they can spend their leisure time. Families may have difficulty finding baby-sitters and have little opportunity for a break from the routine. Some families become isolated from customary social activities because of the responsibilities of caring for their child. **Respite care** (care of the ill child so that the caregivers can have a period of rest and refreshment) is often desperately needed but is not readily available in many communities. Families in which both parents work may have to forgo a second income so that one adult can stay home with the child.

As the child grows, concerns about education may become foremost among the caregivers' worries. These concerns include the availability of appropriate education, early learning opportunities, physical accessibility of the facilities, acceptance of the child by school personnel and classmates, inclusive versus segregated classes, availability and quality of homebound teaching, and general flexibility of the school's teachers and administrators. Few schools are prepared to accommodate treatments at school that would otherwise require the child to leave during the school day. Family caregivers often must become the child's advocate to preserve as much normalcy as possible in the child's educational experience.

As the child's condition changes, the family must make additional changes. All these stresses may strain a marriage, and couples may have little time left for each other when caring for a chronically ill child. Sometimes partners in relationships blame each other for the child's problems, which further strains the relationship. Single-parent families have significant needs to which health care personnel must be especially sensitive.

The Child and Chronic Illness

The child with a chronic illness may face many problems that interfere with normal growth and development. For example, the child who must be immobilized during school age while in the stage of industry versus inferiority cannot complete the tasks of industry, such as helping with household chores or working on special projects with siblings or peers. These problems vary with the diagnosis and condition. The child's attitude toward the condition is a critical element in its long-term management and the family's adjustment.

The child's response to the chronic condition is influenced by the response of family caregivers. Several typical responses have been identified: overprotection, rejection, denial, and gradual acceptance. Caregivers responding with **overprotection** try to protect the child at all costs: they hover, which prevents the child from learning new skills; they fail to use discipline; and they use any means to prevent the child from experiencing any frustration. Caregivers in **rejection** distance themselves emotionally from the child: although they provide physical care, they tend to scold and correct the child continuously. Caregivers in **denial** behave as though the condition does not exist, and they encourage the child to overcompensate for

A PERSONAL GLIMPSE

I am 16 years old and I was diagnosed with cystic fibrosis at birth. Every morning I wake up and have many things that I have to accomplish; taking a breathing treatment, having percussion done, and taking many pills. I guess it isn't so bad if you are used to doing it every day, but it is a bit annoying having the same routine all the time. I have been doing all of this for 16 years. I sometimes feel that I am very different from other people. My friends don't feel it is weird having me as a friend, but they know that I have this disease and they are afraid of what can happen to me. My friends don't treat me any different. I think that is the most important thing. It is good that I have friends who can care so much that they don't let it bother them.

I don't like it when I have to cough all the time; everyone stares at me. When I am in school, at lunch I have to take pills before I eat. Everyone is always asking me why I am taking the pills. Even when I go to a friend's house, I have to take my medication and get my percussions done. My friends usually help out with the percussions.

A lot of times I feel very lonely because I am the only one in my family that has this disease. No one knows what I am feeling, and that sometimes makes me very lonely and afraid. I have a twin brother who really cares for me a lot. When anyone asks about my illness, he is usually the person to explain it to them. He has always been there for me when I needed him. When I have to go in the hospital, he gets my work for me. We are very close. I am glad to have a brother like him.

I am very lucky to have a family that cares for me and loves me like they do. They are always helping me when I need percussions done and they are very supportive. I don't know what I would do without their help. They all took care of me when I couldn't. They still do now. I owe them a lot of credit. I love them very much and always will.

Gretchen, age 16

LEARNING OPPORTUNITY: Do you think this adolescent has accepted her disease? What are the things she shared that you think show that she has or has not accepted her condition? What are your thoughts about her family and friends?

any disabilities. Caregivers who respond with **gradual acceptance** take a common-sense approach to the child's condition; they help the child to set realistic goals for self-care and independence and encourage the child to achieve social and physical skills within his or her capability (Fig. 32-1).

Children often perceive any illness as punishment for a bad thought or action. The child's perception of

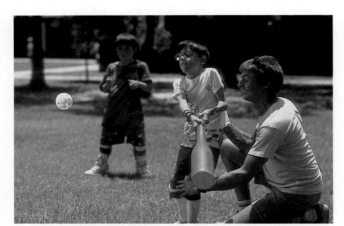

● *Figure 32.1* This father and brother encourage a child with a disability to participate in outdoor activities.

chronic illness is subject to this magical thinking as well, depending on the child's developmental stage at the time of diagnosis. This perception also is influenced by the attitudes of parents and peers and by whether or not the dysfunctional body part is visible. Problems such as asthma, allergies, and epilepsy are difficult for children to understand because "what's wrong" is inside, not outside.

The child's family, peers, and school personnel comprise the support system that can affect the child's adaptation. Sometimes the efforts necessary to meet the child's physical needs are so great that finding time and energy to meet the child's emotional needs can be difficult for members of the support team. The older child with a chronic illness also has developing sexual needs that should not be ignored but must be acknowledged and provided for.

Additional stresses continue to occur as the disease progresses. For instance, Hodgkin's disease can be successfully treated for a time with chemotherapy and radiation therapy, but this requires adding the side effects of treatment (steroid-induced acne, edema, and alopecia) to the disease manifestations of night sweats, chronic fatigue, pruritus, and gastrointestinal bleeding. The child with Duchenne muscular dystrophy gradually weakens, so that in adolescence he or she is wheelchair-bound, when peers are actively involved in sports and exploring sexual relationships. These stresses can add up to more than one young person can cope with for long.

Discrimination continues to be present in the life of the chronically ill child and the family. Discrimination can occur in relationships among children, and social exclusion of the chronically ill child is common. Physical barriers may present problems that families must struggle to help their child overcome. Sometimes hurtful discrimination is as simple as being stared at in public places.

Siblings and Chronic Illness

Some degree of sibling rivalry can be found in most families with healthy children, so it is not surprising that a child with a chronic health problem can seriously disrupt the lives of brothers and sisters. Much of the family caregivers' time, attention, and money are directed toward management of the ill child's problem. This can cause anger, resentment, and jealousy in the well siblings. The caregivers' failure to set limits for the ill child's behavior while maintaining discipline for the healthy siblings can cause further resentment. Some family caregivers unknowingly create feelings of guilt in the healthy children by overemphasizing the ill child's needs.

Siblings may feel **stigma** (embarrassment or shame) because of a brother or sister with a chronic illness, especially if the ill child has a physical disfigurement or apparent cognitive deficit. Siblings may choose not to tell others about the ill child or may be selective in whom they tell, choosing to tell only persons they can trust.

An older sibling is more likely to tell others than a younger one, perhaps because the older child tends to understand more about the illness and its effect.

Both positive and negative influences can be found in the behaviors of well siblings. Some siblings react with anger, hostility, jealousy, increased competition for attention, social withdrawal, and poor school performance. On the other hand, many siblings demonstrate positive behaviors such as caring and concern for the ill sibling, cooperating with family caregivers in helping care for the ill child, protecting the ill child from negative reaction of others, and including the ill child in activities with peers.

How well siblings react to a chronically ill sibling may ultimately depend on how the family copes with stress and how its members feel about one another. See Family Teaching Tips: Helping Siblings Cope With a

---

FAMILY TEACHING TIPS

Helping Siblings Cope With a Chronic Illness

- Find time for special activities with the healthy children.

- Explain the ill child's condition as simply as possible.

- Involve the healthy siblings in the care of the ill child according to his or her developmental ability.

- Set behavioral limits for all children in the family.

Chronic Illness for additional information. This delicate balance is challenging and takes great effort and caring for a family to sustain, but the results are well worth it.

Test Yourself

- What problems might the child with a chronic illness face?

- What effect does chronic illness have on the parents of the chronically ill child?

- What effect does chronic illness have on the siblings of the chronically ill child?

● Nursing Process in Caring for a Child With a Chronic Illness

ASSESSMENT

The assessment of the family and the child with a disability or chronic illness is an ongoing process by the health care team. The information and data collected are reviewed and updated with each visit the child makes to the health care facility. Include the child in the admission and ongoing interview processes if he or she is old enough and able to participate.

Something to think about! The child may have had many visits and treatments in the past that have left negative memories, so approach the child in a low-key, kind, gentle manner to gain cooperation.

Unless the child is newly diagnosed, the family caregivers may have a good understanding of the condition. Observe for evidence of the family's knowledge and understanding so that plans can be made to supplement it as needed.

During any interview with the child or family caregivers, determine how the family is coping with the child's condition and observe for the family's strengths, weaknesses, and acceptance of the diagnosis. Identify the needs that change with the child's condition and include them in planning care. Also consider needs that change with the child's growth and development.

Adjust the physical exam to correspond with the child's illness and current condition. Throughout the physical exam, make every effort to gain the child's cooperation and explain what is being done in terms that the child can understand. Praise the child for cooperation throughout the process to gain the child's (and the family caregivers') goodwill.

SELECTED NURSING DIAGNOSES

- Delayed Growth and Development related to impaired ability to achieve developmental tasks or family caregivers' reactions to the child's condition
- Self-Care Deficit related to limitations of illness or disability
- Anxiety related to procedures, tests, or hospitalization
- Risk for Social Isolation of the child or family related to the child's condition
- Anticipatory Grieving of family caregiver related to possible losses secondary to condition
- Interrupted Family Processes related to adjustment requirements for the child with chronic illness or disability
- Health-Seeking Behaviors by caregivers related to home care of the child

OUTCOME IDENTIFICATION AND PLANNING

Major goals for the chronically ill child are to accomplish growth and development milestones, perform self-care tasks, decrease anxiety, and experience more social interaction. Goals for the caregiver or family are to increase their social interaction; decrease their feelings of grief, anger, and guilt; increase their adjustment to living with a chronically ill child; and teach them about caring for the chronically ill or disabled child.

IMPLEMENTATION

Encouraging Optimal Growth and Development

The family caregivers may become overprotective and prevent the ill child from exhibiting growth and development appropriate for his or her age and disability. Help the caregivers recognize the child's potential and set realistic growth and development goals. Consistent care by the same staff helps to provide a sense of routine in which the child can be encouraged to have some control and perform age-appropriate tasks within the limitations of the disability. Set age-appropriate limits and enforce appropriate discipline.

Accomplish this gradually by displaying a kind and caring attitude. Give the child choices within the limits of treatments and other aspects of required care. Encourage the child to wear regular clothes, rather than stay in pajamas, to reduce feelings of being an invalid. Encourage the child to learn about the condition. Introducing the child to other children with the same or a similar condition can help dispel feelings that he or she is the only person with such a condition. An older child or adolescent benefits from social interaction with peers with and without disabilities (Fig. 32-2). Encourage family caregivers to help the adolescent join in age-appropriate activities. The adolescent also may need some help dressing or using makeup to improve his or her appearance and minimize any physical disability.

Promoting Self-care

To encourage the child to assist in self-care, devise aids to ease tasks. When appropriate, integrate play and toys into the care to help encourage cooperation. Do not expect the child to perform tasks beyond his or her capabilities. Make certain that the child is well rested before attempting any energy-taxing tasks. Remember these tasks are often hard work for the child. Praise and reward the child genuinely and generously for tasks attempted, even if they are not totally completed.

Try this! Use a chart or other visual aid with listed tasks as a tool to help the child reach a desired goal. Stickers can record the child's progress. School-age children often respond well to contracts: for instance, a special privilege or other incentive is awarded when a set number of stickers are earned.

Reducing Anxiety About Procedures and Treatments

Periodically the child may need to undergo procedures, tests, and treatments. The child may also be hospitalized frequently. Many of the procedures may be painful or at least uncomfortable. Explain the tests, treatments, and procedures to the child ahead of time and encourage the child to ask questions. Acknowledge to the child that a particular procedure is painful and help him or her to plan ways to cope with the pain. Advise family caregivers that they should also help the child to prepare for hospitalization ahead of time whenever possible.

Preventing Social Isolation

The chronically ill child may feel isolated from peers. When the child is hospitalized, consider arranging for contact with peers by phone, in writing, or through visits. Many pediatric units have special programs that help children deal with chronic conditions and the hospitalizations that occur with these conditions (Fig. 32-3). Encourage regular school attendance as soon as the child is physically able. If the child is a member of an inclusive classroom, suggest that the caregiver make arrangements with the school for rest periods as needed. Ask the child about interests; these may give some clues about suitable

Listen carefully! The child's discussions about social activities can help you gain insight into his or her feelings about socialization.

● **Figure 32.2** The adolescent with disabilities benefits from social interaction.

● **Figure 32.3** Ronald McDonald, a familiar face to many children, visits a hospitalized child who has a long-term illness.

after-school activities that will increase the child's interactions with peers. Make suggestions and confer with family caregivers to ensure that proposed plans are carried out.

A child who requires constant or frequent attention often can be exhausting for the family caregivers. The family with no close extended family and few close friends may find getting away for rest and relaxation, even for an evening, almost impossible. Help the family caregivers find resources for respite care. Any caregiver, no matter how devoted, needs to have a break from everyday cares and concerns. Refer the family to social services where they can get help. Sometimes a caregiver may feel that another person cannot care for the child adequately. Encourage this caregiver to express fears and anxieties about leaving the child. This helps the caregiver to work through some of these anxieties and feel more confident about getting away for a period of rest.

Aiding Caregivers' Acceptance of the Condition

When anyone suffers a serious loss, a grief reaction occurs. This is true of family caregivers when they first learn that their child has a chronic or disabling illness. Encourage family caregivers to express these feelings and help them to understand that this reaction is common and acceptable.

Denial is usually the first reaction that family caregivers have to the diagnosis. This is a time when they say, "How could this be?" or "Why my child?" Let them express their emotions, and respond in a nonjudgmental way. Staying with them and offering quiet, accepting support may be helpful. Statements such as "It will seem better in time" are inappropriate. Acknowledge the caregivers' feelings as acceptable and reasonable.

During the next stage, called guilt, listen to the caregivers express their feelings of guilt and remorse. Again, acknowledging their feelings is useful. Accept expressions of anger by family caregivers without viewing them as a personal attack. Using active listening techniques that reflect the caregivers' feelings, such as "You sound very angry," is a helpful method of handling these emotions.

Grief reactions also may occur when the family caregivers are informed that their child is deteriorating or has had a setback. Although caregivers usually cycle through these reactions much more quickly by this time, the same methods are useful.

Helping the Family Adjust to the Child's Condition

The family's adjustment to the condition is assessed during initial and ongoing interviews. Adjustment may depend on how recently the child has been diagnosed. After determining the family's needs, provide an opportunity for the family members to express their feelings and anxieties. Help them explore any feelings of guilt or blame about the child's condition. Encourage them to express doubts they may have about their ability to cope with the child's future. Help the caregivers look realistically at their resources, and give them suggestions about ways to cope. Serve as a role model when caring for the child, expressing a positive attitude toward the child and the illness or disability.

Question the family to determine the resources and support systems available to them. Remind them that these support systems may include immediate family members, extended family, friends, community services, and health care providers.

Encourage the caregivers to discuss the needs of the well siblings and their adjustment to the ill child's condition. Help the family meet the needs of the well siblings, and help the siblings feel comfortable with the ill child's problems and needs. Assist the family in setting reasonable expectations for all their children.

Planning for Home Care

Home care planning begins when the child is admitted to the health care facility and continues until discharge. Focus plans for care at home on the continuing care, medications, and treatments the child will need. During a health care visit or hospitalization, include family caregivers when caring for the child so that they become comfortable with the care. Children are often sent home with sophisticated equipment and treatments; therefore, demonstrate the use of the equipment and treatments and give the family caregivers a chance to perform the treatments under guidance and supervision. A discussion of the home's facilities may be appropriate to help the family accommodate any special needs the child may have. Give the caregivers a list of community services and organizations that they can turn to for help and support, including appropriate disease- or disability-specific organizations.

Teach the caregivers about growth and development guidelines so that they have a realistic concept of what to expect as the child develops. Throughout the child's stay, encourage caregivers to express their concerns to help solve whatever problems the family anticipates having while caring for the child at home. Give the family the name and telephone number of a contact person they can call for support.

You can make a difference!

Families face many hurdles while caring for a chronically ill child, but they are more likely to feel that they can competently face the future with the reassurance that help is just a telephone call away.

Caring for a chronically ill child can be an overwhelming task that requires cooperation by all involved with the child and the family. Family caregivers deserve all the help they can get (see Nursing Care Plan 32-1).

EVALUATION: GOALS AND EXPECTED OUTCOMES

- **Goal:** The child will achieve highest level of growth and development within constraints of illness, and the family caregivers will acknowledge appropriate growth and development expectations.
  Expected Outcome: The child attains growth and development milestones within her or his capabilities; the family caregivers acknowledge the child's capabilities, encourage the child, and set realistic goals for the child.
- **Goal:** The child will become involved in self-care activities.
  Expected Outcome: The child participates in self-care as appropriate for age and capabilities.
- **Goal:** The child's anxiety will be decreased.
  Expected Outcome: The child's anxiety is minimized as evidenced by cooperation with care and treatments.
- **Goal:** The child and the family will actively socialize with others.
  Expected Outcome: The child and family use opportunities to socialize with others; the family seeks and finds adequate respite care for the child.
- **Goal:** The family will deal with their feelings of anger, grief, guilt, and loss.
  Expected Outcome: The family caregivers express their feelings of guilt, fears, and anxieties, and they receive support while working toward accepting the child's condition.
- **Goal:** The family caregivers will adjust to the requirements of caring for the child with chronic illness or disability.
  Expected Outcome: The family caregivers express ways they can cope with their child's

condition and list the resources and support systems available to them.
- **Goal:** The family caregivers will actively participate in the child's home care.
  Expected Outcome: The family caregivers ask pertinent questions, contact support groups and community agencies for help, and demonstrate their ability to perform care and treatments.

Test Yourself

- How might a chronic illness affect a child's growth and development?
- What can the nurse do to help decrease the social isolation of the chronically ill child?
- Why is it important for the nurse to try to determine how the family and child are coping with a chronic illness?

KEY POINTS

▶ Diseases that cause chronic illness in children include congenital heart disease, cystic fibrosis, juvenile arthritis, asthma, hemophilia, muscular dystrophy, leukemia and other malignancies, spina bifida, and immunodeficiency syndromes.

▶ Concerns common to many families of a child with a chronic illness include financial, administration of treatments and medications at home, disruption of family life, educational opportunities for the child, social isolation, family adjustments, reaction of siblings, stress among caregivers, guilt about and acceptance of the chronic condition, and care of the child when family caregivers can no longer provide care.

▶ Economic pressures, such as adequate health insurance; away-from-home living costs; the stress of having to keep a job, especially when the child needs the caregiver's time and attention; and the threat to job security because of time away from the job, can become overwhelming to the families of chronically ill children.

▶ Respite care is important so that family caregivers can have time away from the ill child and a break in the routine. Time away will help keep the caregivers from becoming isolated and enable them to participate in normal social activities.

▶ Negative responses that well siblings may manifest in response to an ill sibling include anger, hostility, jealousy, increased competition for attention, social

(text continues on page 751)

NURSING CARE PLAN 32.1

The Chronically Ill Child and Family

CASE SCENARIO
Billy is a 10-year-old who has Duchenne muscular dystrophy. His condition has worsened and he has recently begun to use a walker. He has gradually begun to need more assistance in his activities of daily living. He has a sister who is 8 years old and a 5-year-old brother. Both parents live at home.

NURSING DIAGNOSIS
Delayed Growth and Development related to impaired ability to achieve developmental tasks or family caregivers' reactions to the child's condition

GOAL: The child will achieve the highest levels of growth and development within constraints of illness and the family caregivers will acknowledge appropriate growth and development expectations.

EXPECTED OUTCOME
- The child attains growth and development milestones within his capabilities.
- The family encourages the child to reach his potential.
- The family sets realistic developmental goals for the child.

NURSING INTERVENTIONS	*RATIONALE*
Encourage the child to participate in growth and development activities to the best of his abilities.	Milestones of growth and development are attained when activities are offered to help child develop those skills.
Discuss with the child's family the effects of overprotectiveness on his development.	Many families react to a child's long-term illness by shielding the child from challenges that the child could cope with if allowed to do so.
Help the child's family recognize his potential and help them to set realistic goals; encourage them to set age-appropriate limits for activities with appropriate discipline for violations.	Family caregivers may not know what to expect in terms of their child's development and may tend to overprotect the child, which prevents him from reaching his potential; it is important to allow him to reach for his potential without overprotection.

NURSING DIAGNOSIS
Self-Care Deficit related to limitations of illness or disability

GOAL: The child will become involved in self-care activities.

EXPECTED OUTCOME
- The child participates in self-care as appropriate for his age and capabilities.
- The child demonstrates evidence of using creative problem-solving techniques.
- The child demonstrates a positive outlook about his achievements.

NURSING INTERVENTIONS	*RATIONALE*
Generously praise any self-care the child performs; carefully avoid expecting him to do tasks beyond his capabilities.	Positive reinforcement gives the child self-confidence and pride in his accomplishments.
When the child finds a task difficult to accomplish, assist him by devising aids to help him with the task, rather than doing it for him.	Difficult accomplishments reinforce the importance of self-care and independence; demonstrating creative problem-solving techniques provides skills that the child can use in the future.
Encourage the child to carry out self-care appropriate for his age and stage of mobility; allow him to make as many choices as possible.	The child will have a better feeling of control and self-worth; he will be encouraged to try new things and not let his illness unnecessarily stop him.

NURSING DIAGNOSIS
Risk for Social Isolation of the child or family related to the child's condition

GOAL: The child and the family will actively socialize with others.

(nursing care plan continues on page 750)

NURSING CARE PLAN 32.1 continued

The Chronically Ill Child and Family

EXPECTED OUTCOME
- The child participates in activities with his peers.
- The child's family finds adequate respite care for Billy.
- The child's family gets away for a break with minimal anxieties.

NURSING INTERVENTIONS	RATIONALE
Encourage the family to establish and maintain the child's contacts with his peers. Advise the family that it may take advance planning and creative solutions for him to participate in activities such as team sports.	The child needs to feel that he is part of the world in which his schoolmates and friends are involved; he needs activities to look forward to.
Help family caregivers find resources for respite care by making referrals to social services or other resources as necessary.	Family caregivers who periodically get away from the responsibilities of caring for the child will be re-energized and return with a refreshed spirit.
Encourage the family caregivers to express anxieties about leaving the child with someone else.	Talking with the family about such fears helps them to work through anxieties, dismiss unrealistic fears, and make specific plans for legitimate ones. This helps the family to have a more restful time when away.

NURSING DIAGNOSIS
Interrupted Family Processes related to adjustment requirements for the child with chronic illness or disability

GOAL: The family caregivers will deal with their feelings of anger, grief, guilt, and loss.

EXPECTED OUTCOME
- The family members express fears and anxieties about the child's weakening condition.
- The family verbalizes a positive attitude to the child about his adaptations to his growing weakness.
- The child's family expresses feelings of guilt about his illness and deals with them positively.

NURSING INTERVENTIONS	RATIONALE
Provide opportunities for family members to express feelings, including fears about his or her weakening condition.	The family may need encouragement to talk about some of their fears and anxieties.
Maintain a positive but realistic attitude about the child's growing disabilities both when providing care and when discussing the impact of the child's illness on the family.	The nurse serves as a role model for the family; modeling a positive attitude will help family caregivers take the same approach.
Explore with the child's family their feelings of guilt.	The family needs to resolve their feelings of guilt.
Provide the family with resources and support systems. Encourage them to talk with their younger children about their feelings concerning the child's illness.	The family needs to use community resources and support systems to help them with the long-term needs of the entire family.

NURSING DIAGNOSIS
Health-Seeking Behaviors by caregivers related to home care of the child

GOAL: The family caregivers will actively participate in the child's home care.

EXPECTED OUTCOME
- The family members ask appropriate questions about the child's care.
- The family members demonstrate the ability to perform the child's care and treatment.
- The family members make contact with support groups and community services.

NURSING CARE PLAN 32.1 continued

The Chronically Ill Child and Family

NURSING INTERVENTIONS	RATIONALE
Explain and demonstrate any equipment used in the child's care; demonstrate treatments or therapy that the family will need to do at home; provide opportunities for practice under the guidance of a nurse or therapist.	Watching someone who knows how to perform a technique well and performing that technique yourself are very different matters. Practice and opportunities for questions are essential.
Provide the family with a list of community services and organizations where they can turn for help and support; include the name and telephone number of a contact person at the health care facility whom the family can call with questions or concerns.	Knowing whom to contact and how to reach that person gives the family reassurance that help is close by and increases their self-confidence about being able to handle their child's care.

withdrawal, and poor school performance. Positive responses many siblings demonstrate include caring and concern for the ill sibling, cooperating with family caregivers in helping care for the ill child, protecting the ill child from negative reaction of others, and including the ill child in activities with peers.

 • The nurse may encourage self-care by the child by devising aids to ease tasks, integrating play and toys into the care, praising the child for tasks attempted, being sure the child is well rested before attempting tasks, and by using charts, visual aids, and stickers as ways to reward the child.

 • The nurse can help the family adjust to the child's condition by encouraging the family caregivers to express their feelings of anger, guilt, fear, and remorse by responding in a nonjudgmental way. The family should be encouraged to express doubts they may have about their ability to cope with the child's future and to look realistically at their resources. The nurse can give suggestions about ways to cope, be a role model when caring for the child, and have a positive attitude.

 • Preparing the family for home care of the child may include having the family caregivers observe the nurse when caring for the child so that they become comfortable performing continuing care, using equipment, giving medications, and doing treatments when the child goes home.

REFERENCES AND SELECTED READINGS

Books and Journals

Balling, K., & McCubbin, M. (2001). Hospitalized children with chronic illness: Parental caregiving needs and valuing parental expertise. *Journal of Pediatric Nursing, 16*(2), 111.

Berger, K. S. (2001). *The developing person through the life span* (5th ed.). New York: Worth Publishers.

Brazelton, T. B., & Greenspan, S. (2001). *The irreducible needs of children: What every child must have to grow, learn, and flourish.* Cambridge, MA: Perseus Publishing.

Godshall, M. A. (2003). Caring for families of chronically ill kids. *RN, 66*(2), 30–35.

Hockenberry, M. J., Wilson, D., Winkelstein, M. L., & Kline, N. E. (2003). *Wong's nursing care of infants and children* (7th ed.). St. Louis: Mosby.

Hutton, N. (1999). Special needs of children with chronic illnesses. In *Oski's pediatrics: Principles and practice* (3rd ed.). Philadelphia: Lippincott Williams & Wilkins.

Karch, A. M. (2003). *2004 Lippincott's nursing drug guide.* Philadelphia: Lippincott Williams & Wilkins.

Keefe, S. (2002). Caring for children with disabilities. *Nursing Spectrum, 3*(5), 26–27.

Perry, D. F., & Ireys, H. T. (2001). Maternal perceptions of pediatric providers for children with chronic illnesses. *American Journal of Maternal/Child Nursing, 5*(1), 15–20.

Pillitteri, A. (2003). *Maternal and child health nursing* (4th ed.). Philadelphia: Lippincott Williams & Wilkins.

Sein, E. P. (2001). Chronic illness: The child and the family. *Current Paediatrics, 11*(1), 46–50.

Smucker, J. M. R. (2001). Managed care and children with special health care needs. *Journal of Pediatric Health Care, 15*(1), 3.

Wong, D. L., Perry, S., & Hockenberry, M. (2002). *Maternal child nursing care* (2nd ed.). St. Louis: Mosby.

Web Addresses

www.wish.org
www.fathersnetwork.org
www.coachart.org
www.kcdream.org

WORKBOOK

NCLEX-STYLE REVIEW QUESTIONS

1. In planning care for a child with a chronic illness, which of the following goals would *most likely* be part of this child's plan of care? The child will

   a. achieve the highest levels of growth and development.

   b. participate in age-appropriate activities.

   c. eat at least 75% of each meal.

   d. share feelings about changes in body image.

2. The nurse is working with the caregivers of a child who has a chronic illness. Of the following statements made by the child's caregivers, which statement is an example of the common response called overprotection?

   a. "My child was born with this and it will always be part of our lives."

   b. "She should be punished when she breaks things because she knows better."

   c. "I know I should let her try new activities, but she just gets frustrated."

   d. "My child just isn't what I expected when I decided to become a parent."

3. The nurse is working with the caregivers of a child who has a chronic illness. Of the following statements made by the child's caregivers, which statement is an example of the common response called acceptance?

   a. "My child was born with this and it will always be part of our lives."

   b. "She should be punished when she breaks things because she knows better."

   c. "I know I should let her try new activities, but she just gets frustrated."

   d. "My child just isn't what I expected when I decided to become a parent."

4. In working with families of children who have chronic illnesses, an important nursing intervention would be which of the following? The nurse would encourage the family members to

   a. refrain from talking about the condition.

   b. openly express their feelings.

   c. prevent the child from overhearing conversations.

   d. tell stories about themselves.

5. In working with siblings of children who have chronic illnesses, it is important for the nurse to recognize that in many cases the siblings

   a. may feel embarrassed about their brother's or sister's condition.

   b. are the primary caregiver for the sick child.

   c. excel in school in an effort to decrease the family stress.

   d. get jobs at a young age to help support the family.

6. When working with the family caregivers of a child with a chronic health concern, the nurse may note the family experiences a grief reaction before coming to an acceptance of the child's condition. Which of the following behaviors by the nurse would be helpful in working with these family caregivers? Select all that apply. The nurse

   a. encourages family to express their feelings.

   b. responds in a nonjudgmental way.

   c. states, "It won't be so hard as time goes on."

   d. reminds family that anger is inappropriate,

   e. stays quietly with family.

STUDY ACTIVITIES

1. Lena and Josh are the young parents of Nina, a 12-month-old girl with meningomyelocele (spina bifida). Nina must be catheterized at least four times a day and also has mobility problems. Explore some of the economic and other stresses that this young couple faces.

2. Using your local telephone book, make a list of agencies to which you could refer families for assistance and support in the care of a chronically ill child.

3. Eight-year-old Jason, a patient in your pediatric unit, is undergoing chemotherapy. He seems very lonely and sad, although his family visits him regularly. You decide he may need contact with children his own age. Describe plans that you will make to provide contact with peers.

4. Go to the following Internet site:

www.faculty.fairfield.edu/fleitas/contents.html

See "Bandaides and Blackboards."

Click on "Kids."

Click on the star next to the section "To tell or not to tell."

Read this section.

a. List five reasons kids choose *not* to tell others that they have a chronic health condition.

b. List five reasons kids choose *to tell* others that they have a chronic health condition.

CRITICAL THINKING: What Would You Do?

1. You are caring for 5-year-old Abby, who has cystic fibrosis. Her mother, Mattie, has been overprotective and has always done everything for her.

a. What will you do to involve Abby in caring for herself?

b. What will you say or do to help and encourage Mattie to encourage Abby to do more of her own care?

c. What are the reasons you think Mattie is overprotective of her child?

2. Nine-year-old Tyson is angry. He tells you that he hates his 6-year-old brother, Josh, who has Down syndrome.

a. What would you say to Tyson to begin a discussion with him about his feelings?

b. What are some of the factors you think might be causing Tyson to be angry?

c. What would you say or suggest if you had the opportunity to talk to Tyson and Josh's family caregiver?

3. Cassie is a 16-year-old girl with cerebral palsy. She wants to go to the school prom, but her family caregivers are very resistant to the idea. Cassie pleads with you to talk to them.

a. How will you approach this problem?

b. What are your responses to Cassie and to her caregivers?

The Dying Child

STUDENT OBJECTIVES

On completion of this chapter, the student should be able to

1. Describe the role of anticipatory grief in the grieving process.
2. Identify reasons why nurses may have difficulty working effectively with dying children.
3. Identify how a nurse can personally prepare to care for a dying child.
4. List the factors that affect the child's understanding of death.
5. Describe how a child's understanding of death changes at each developmental level.
6. State the importance of encouraging families to complete unfinished business.
7. Describe why a family may suffer excessive grief and guilt when a child dies suddenly.
8. Describe possible reactions in a child when a sibling dies.
9. Identify settings for caring for the dying child and the advantages and disadvantages of each.

KEY TERMS

anticipatory grief
hospice
thanatologist
unfinished business

The most difficult death to accept is the death of a child. We can accept that elderly patients have lived a full life and that life must end, but the life of a child still holds the hopes, dreams, and promises of the future. When a child's life ends early, whether abruptly, such as the result of an accident, or after a prolonged illness, we ask ourselves, "Why? What's the justice of this?"

Caring for a family facing the death of their child calls on all the nurse's personal and professional skills. It means offering sensitive, gentle, physical care and comfort measures for the child and continuing emotional support for the child, the family caregivers, and the siblings. This kind of caring demands an understanding of the nurse's own feelings about death and dying, knowledge of the grieving process that terminally ill patients and their families experience, and a willingness to become involved.

> ## You can make a difference.
>
> Caring for a dying child and his or her family is stressful but can also be extremely rewarding.

Like chronic illness, terminal illness creates a family crisis that can either destroy or strengthen the family as a unit and as individuals. Nurses and other health professionals who can offer knowledgeable, sensitive care to these families help to make the remainder of the child's life more meaningful and the family's mourning experience more healing. Helping a family struggle through this crisis and emerge stronger and closer can yield deep satisfaction.

Diagnosis of a fatal illness initiates the grieving process in the child and the family: denial and isolation, anger, bargaining, depression and acute grief, and finally, acceptance. Not every child or family will complete the process because each family, as well as each death, is personal and unique.

When death is expected, the family begins to mourn, a phenomenon called **anticipatory grief**. For some people, this shortens the period of acute grief and loss after the child's death. Unexpected death offers no chance for preparation, and grief may last longer and be more difficult to resolve.

Death is a tragic reality for thousands of children each year. Accidents are the leading cause of death in children between the ages of 1 and 14 years; cancer is the number one fatal disease in this age group (National Childhood Cancer Foundation, 2004). Nearly all these children leave behind at least one grieving family caregiver and perhaps brothers, sisters, and grandparents. Nurses who care for children and families must be prepared for encounters with the dying and the bereaved.

THE NURSE'S REACTION TO DEATH AND DYING

Health care workers often are uncomfortable with dying patients, so they avoid them and are afraid that the patients will ask questions they cannot or should not answer. These caregivers signal by their behavior that the patient should avoid the fact of his or her impending death and should keep up a show of bravery. In effect, they are asking the patient to meet their needs, instead of trying to meet the patient's needs.

Death reminds us of our own mortality, a thought with which many of us are uncomfortable. The thought that someone even younger than we are is about to die makes us feel more vulnerable.

> ## Something to think about.
> Every nurse needs to examine his or her own feelings about death and the reasons for these feelings.

How have you reacted to the death of a friend or a family member? When growing up, was talking and thinking about death avoided

A PERSONAL GLIMPSE

I am a student nurse. I am dying. I write this to you who are and will become nurses in the hope that by my sharing my feelings with you, you may someday be better able to help those who share my experience. . . . You slip in and out of my room, give me medications and check my blood pressure. Is it because I am a student nurse, myself, or just a human being, that I sense your fright? And your fears enhance mine. Why are you afraid? I am the one who is dying!

I know you feel insecure, don't know what to say, don't know what to do. But please believe me, if you care, you can't go wrong. Just admit that you care . . . Don't run away—wait—all I want to know is that there will be someone to hold my hand when I need it. . . . If only we could be honest, both admit our fears, touch one another. If you really care, would you lose so much of your valuable professionalism if you even cried with me? Just person to person? Then it might not be so hard to die in a hospital—with friends close by.

(American Journal of Nursing, 1970)

LEARNING OPPORTUNITY: Describe your feelings about the student nurse's story. How might this person's experience influence your approach to caring for the dying patient?

because of your family's attitudes? Admitting that death is a part of life and that patients should be helped to live each day to the fullest until death are steps toward understanding and being able to communicate with those who are dying. A workshop, conference, or seminar in which one's own feelings about life and death are explored is useful in preparing the nurse to care for the dying child and family (Box 33-1).

Learning to care for the dying patient requires talking with other professionals, sharing concerns, and comforting each other in stressful times. It calls for reading studies about death to discover how dying patients feel about their care, their illness, their families, and how they want to spend the rest of their lives. It also requires being a sensitive, empathic, nonjudgmental listener to patients and families who need to express their feelings, even if they may not be able to express them to each other. Caring for the dying is usually a team effort that may involve a nurse, a physician, a chaplain, a social worker, a psychiatrist, a hospice nurse, or a **thanatologist** (a person [sometimes a nurse] trained especially to work with the dying and their families), but the nurse often is the person who coordinates the care.

Test Yourself

- What does the term anticipatory grief mean?
- How is anticipatory grief helpful to the family who has lost a child by death?
- Why is it important for the nurse to examine his or her own feelings about death?

THE CHILD'S UNDERSTANDING OF DEATH

Stage of development, cognitive ability, and experiences all influence children's understanding of death. The death of a pet or a family member may be a child's first experience with death. How the family deals with the death has a great impact on the child's understanding of death, but children usually do not have a realistic comprehension of the finality of death until they near preadolescence. Although the dying child may be unable to understand death, the emotions of family caregivers and others alert the child that something is threatening his or her secure world. Dealing with the child's anxieties with openness and honesty restores the child's trust and comfort.

Developmental Stage

Infants and Toddlers

Infants and toddlers have little if any understanding of death. The toddler may fear separation from beloved caregivers but have no recognition of the fact that death is nearing and irreversible. A toddler may say, "Nana's gone bye-bye to be with God" or "Grampy went to heaven" and a few moments later ask to go visit the deceased person. This is an opportunity to explain to the child that Nana or Grampy is in a special place and cannot be visited, but the family has many memories of him or her that they will always treasure. The child should not be scolded for not understanding. Questions are best answered simply and honestly.

If the infant's or toddler's own death is approaching, family caregivers can be encouraged to stay with the child to provide comfort, love, and security. Maintaining

---

| **BOX 33.1** | **Questions to Cover in a Self-examination About Death** |

Some Considerations in the Resolution of Death and Dying

1. What was your first conscious memory of death? What were your feelings and reactions?
2. What is your most recent memory of death? How was it the same or different from your first memory?
3. What experience of death had the most effect on you? Why?

Get Comfortable and Imagine Now

You have just been told you have 6 months to live. What is your *first* reaction to that news?

3 months later—What relationships might require you to tie up loose ends? What unfinished business do you have to deal with? You and your significant other are trying to cope with the news. What changes occur in your relationship?

1 month remains—What do you need to have happen in the remaining time? What hopes, dreams, and plans can or need to be fulfilled?

1 week remains—You are very weak and barely have enough energy to talk. You don't even want to look at yourself. Nausea and vomiting are constant companions. Write a letter to the one person you feel would be the most affected by your dying.

24 hours remain—You are dying. Breathing is difficult; you feel very hot inside; overwhelming fatigue is ever-present. How would you like to spend this last day?

These questions can be used in a group with a hospice or other facilitator. They can be used to help heighten your awareness of yourself: who are you; how you have gotten to where you are today; what you are doing with your life and why; how you would change the way you live; your feelings about death in general, in relation to your friends and family, and in regard to your own death.

With permission from Ruth Anne Sieber, Hospice: The Bridge, Lewistown, PA.

routines as much as possible helps to give the toddler a greater sense of security.

Preschool Children

The egocentric thinking of preschool children contributes to the belief that they may have caused a person or pet to die by thinking angry thoughts. Magical thinking also plays an important part in the preschooler's beliefs about death. It is not unusual for a preschool child to insist on burying a dead pet or bird, then in a few hours or a day or two dig up the corpse to see if it is still there. This may be especially true if the child has been told that it will "go to heaven." Many preschoolers think of death as a kind of sleep; they do not understand that the dead person will not wake up. They may fear going to sleep after the death of a close family member because they fear that they may not wake up. Family caregivers must watch for this kind of reaction and encourage children to talk about their fears while reassuring them that they need not fear dying while sleeping. The child's feelings must be acknowledged as real, and the child must be helped to resolve them. The feelings must never be ridiculed.

A preschool child may view personal illness as punishment for thoughts or actions. Because preschoolers do not have an accurate concept of death, they fear separation from family caregivers. Caregivers can provide security and comfort by staying with the child as much as possible.

Test Yourself

- What does the toddler fear in relationship to death and dying?
- How does magical thinking in preschool children relate to their understanding of death?

School-age Children

The child who is 6 or 7 years old is still in the magical thinking stage and continues to think of death in the same way as the preschool child does. At about 8 or 9 years of age, children gain the concept that death is universal and irreversible. Around this age, death is personified—that is, it is given characteristics of a person and may be called the devil, God, a monster, or the bogeyman. Children of this age often believe they can protect themselves from death by running past a cemetery while holding their breath, keeping doors locked, staying out of dark rooms, staying away from funeral homes and dead people, or avoiding stepping on cracks in the sidewalk.

When faced with the prospect of their own death, school-age children usually are sad that they will be leaving their family and the people they love (Fig. 33-1).

● **Figure 33.1** School-age children are often sad when faced with their own death and leaving their family.

They may be apprehensive about how they will manage when they no longer have their parents around to help them. Often they view death as another new experience, like going to school, leaving for camp, or flying in an airplane for the first time. They may fear the loss of control that death represents to them and express this fear through vocal aggression. Family caregivers and nurses must recognize this as an expression of their fear and avoid scolding or disciplining them for this behavior. This is a time when the people close to the child can help him or her voice anxieties about the future and provide an outlet for these aggressive feelings. The presence of family members and maintenance of relatively normal routines help to give the child a sense of security. Family Teaching Tips: Talking to Children About Death provides help for caregivers in talking with their children about death.

Adolescents

Adolescents have an adult understanding of death but feel that they are immortal—that is, death will happen to others but not to them. This belief contributes to adolescents' sometimes dangerous, life-threatening behavior. This denial of the possibility of serious personal danger may contribute to an adolescent's delay in reporting symptoms or seeking help. Diagnosis of a life-threatening or terminal illness creates a crisis for the adolescent. To cope with the illness, the adolescent must draw on cognitive functioning, past experiences, family support, and problem-solving ability. The adolescent with a terminal illness may express helplessness, anger, fear of pain, hopelessness, and depression. Adolescents often try to live the fullest lives they can in the time they have.

FAMILY TEACHING TIPS

Talking to Children About Death

- Encourage children to talk about the topic of death
- Talk about the subject when the child wants to talk
- Share information at the child's level of understanding
- Listen to what the child is saying and to what they are asking
- Accept the child's feelings
- Be open, honest, and give simple, brief answers, especially when talking with the younger child
- Answer the question each time the child asks, sometimes children need to ask the same question more than once
- Say "I don't know" to questions you don't have answers for
- Use the words "death," "died," and "dying"
- Talk about death when less emotion is involved, such as dead flowers, trees, insects, birds
- Explain death in terms of the absence of things that occur in everyday life, such as when people die they don't breathe, eat, talk, think or feel

Adolescents may be upset by the results of treatments that make them feel weak and alter their appearance, such as alopecia, edema resulting from steroid therapy, and pallor. They may need assistance in presenting themselves as attractively as possible to their peers. Adolescents need opportunities to acknowledge their impending death and can be encouraged to express fears and anxieties and ask questions about death. Participating in their usual activities helps adolescents feel in control.

This is important to remember.
A child's understanding of death and dying is affected by the stage of growth and development the child is in, and the nurse must be aware of what the child may understand and think.

Test Yourself

- At what age does the child understand the concept that death is universal and irreversible?

- What belief do adolescents have regarding dying that allows them to sometimes participate in dangerous, life-threatening behaviors?

Experience With Death and Loss

Every death that touches the life of a child makes an impression that affects the way the child thinks about every other death, including his or her own. Attitudes of family members are powerful influences. Family caregivers must be able to discuss death with children when a grandparent or other family member dies, even though the discussion may be painful. Otherwise the child thinks that death is a forbidden topic; avoiding the subject leaves room for fantasy and distortion in the child's imagination.

Many books are available to help a child deal with loss and death. *A Balloon Story*, a simply produced 13-page coloring storybook by hospice nurse Ruth Anne Sieber, is an introduction to loss appropriate for the young child. This story of two children who go to a fair with their mothers is illustrated with large line drawings to color. The children each select and purchase a helium balloon of which they are quite proud. Unfortunately, Nathan's balloon slips from his hand and floats away forever. Nathan displays typical grief reactions of protest, anger, and finally acceptance (Fig. 33-2). Reading the story to a child provides the adult with the perfect opening to discuss loss. A small booklet for caregivers accompanies *A Balloon Story* and contains excellent guidelines for discussing death and loss with a child. *A Balloon*

● **Figure 33.2** Nathan cried and kept jumping and reaching after everyone else had given up. (Courtesy of Ruth Anne Sieber.)

Story can be obtained from Hospice: The Bridge, Lewistown Hospital, Lewistown, Pennsylvania 17044.

Another small booklet that is excellent to use with any age group is *Water Bugs and Dragonflies*. This story approaches life and death as stages of existence by illustrating that after a water bug turns into a dragonfly, he can no longer go back and tell the other curious water bugs what life is like in this beautiful new world to which he has gone. This story can serve as the foundation for further discussion about death (Fig. 33-3).

Available books on death vary in their approaches. A number of books focus on the death of an animal or pet. Many stories deal with death as a result of old age. Several books have an accident as the cause of death. Most of the books are fiction, but several nonfiction ones are available for older children (Box 33-2). There is no discussion of one's own death in these books, which is consistent with the Western philosophy of handling death as something that happens to others but not to oneself (Bowden, 1993).

Awareness of Impending Death

Children know when they are dying. They sense and fear what is going to happen, even if they cannot identify it by name. Their play activities, artwork, dreams, and symbolic language demonstrate this knowledge.

Family caregivers who insist that a child not learn the truth about his or her illness place health care professionals at a disadvantage because they are not free to help the child deal with fears and concerns. If caregivers permit openness and honesty in communication with a dying child, the health care staff can meet the child's needs more effectively, dispel misunderstandings, and see that the child and the family are able to resolve any problems or **unfinished business**. Completing unfinished business may mean spending more time with the child, helping siblings to understand the child's illness and impending death, and giving family members a chance to share their love with the child. Allowing openness does not mean that nurses and other personnel offer information not requested by the child but means simply that the child be given the information desired gently and directly in words the child can understand. The truth can be kind as well as cruel.

Adolescents usually are sensitive to what is happening to them and may need the nurse to be an advocate for them if they have wishes they want to fulfill before dying. An adolescent who senses the nurse's willingness and ability may discuss feelings that he or she is uncomfortable discussing with family members. The nurse can talk with the adolescent and work with the family to help them understand

Acceptance is not as hard as you think. When working with the child who is dying, as well as the child's family, honest, specific answers leave less room for misinterpretation and distortion.

A

In the s[t]ages of life we change

Nobody can live forever.

B

● *Figure 33.3* Drawings done by fourth-grade students after a presentation about death that included a reading of *Water Bugs and Butterflies*. (**A**) In the s[t]ages of life we change. At the center of the drawing is a pond with three lily pads. The stems at the end represent plants that waterbugs crawl up on before turning into dragonflies. (**B**) Nobody lives forever. (Courtesy of Ruth Anne Sieber.)

CULTURAL SNAPSHOT

Death and dying are not discussed openly in many cultures. In some cultures, the fact that a person is dying is discussed only in very private settings and often not with the dying individual. In front of the dying child for instance, the atmosphere might be jovial, with eating, joking, playing games, and singing.

| BOX 33.2 | Books About Death for Children | | | |

Author	Book	Publisher	Who Died	Age Appropriate
Blume, Judy	*Tiger Eyes*	Scarsdale, NY: Bradbury Press	Father	11–15
Bunting, E.	*The Happy Funeral*	New York: Harper and Row	Grandfather	3–7
Carrick, C.	*The Accident*	New York: Houghton Mifflin, Clarion Books	Dog	6–11
Claudy, A.F.	*Dusty Was My Friend*	Human Sciences Press	Friend	6–11
Edleman, Hope	*Motherless Daughters*	Dell Publishing Company	Mother	14 and up
Graeber, C.	*Mustard*	New York: MacMillian Publishing Co.	Cat	6–10
Hemery, Kathleen	*The Brightest Star*	Omaha, NE: Centering Corporation	Mother	4–8
Henkes, Kevin	*Sun & Spoon*	New York: Greenwillow Books	Grandmother	9–13
Hermes, P.	*You Shouldn't Have to Say Goodbye*	New York: Harcourt Brace Jovanovich	Mother	9–13
Hesse, K.	*Poppy's Chair*	New York: MacMillian Publishing Co.	Grandfather	6–11
Hickman, M.W.	*Last Week My Brother Anthony Died*	Abington Press	Brother	3–7
Holmes, Margaret Mudlaff, Sasha	*Molly's Mom Died*	Omaha, NE: Centering Corporation	Mother	5–9
Lorenzen, K.	*Lanky Longlegs*	New York: Atheneum. A Margaret K. McElderry Book	Brother	9–13
Lowden, Stephanie Golightly	*Emily's Sadhappy Season*	Omaha, NE: Centering Corporation	Father	4–8
Schotter, R.	*A Matter of Time*	New York: Collins Press	Mother	14 and up
Scrivani, Mark	*I Heard Your Mommy Died*	Omaha, NE: Centering Corporation	Mother	3–7
Scrivani, Mark	*I Heard Your Daddy Died*	Omaha, NE: Centering Corporation	Father	3–7
Scrivani, Mark	*When Death Walks In: For Teens Facing Grief*	Omaha, NE: Centering Corporation		13 and up
Shook-Hazen, B.	*Why Did Grandpa Die*	Racine, WI: Western Publishing Co.	Grandfather	3–7
Smith, D.B.	*A Taste of Blackberries*	Boston: Thomas Crowell Company	Friend	6–11
Thomas, J.R.	*Saying Goodbye to Grandma*	New York: Clarion Books	Grandmother	6–11
Tiffault, Benette	*A Quilt for Elizabeth*	Omaha, NE: Centering Corporation	Father	4–8
Vigna, Judith	*Saying Goodbye to Daddy*	Morton Grove, IL: Albert Whitman & Co.	Father	6–9

the adolescent's desires and needs. The nurse can call on hospice workers, social or psychiatric services, or a member of the clergy to help the family express and resolve their concerns and recognize the adolescent's needs.

THE FAMILY'S REACTION TO DYING AND DEATH

The death of a child sends feelings of shock, disbelief, and guilt through every family member. When a potentially fatal disease (such as acquired immunodeficiency syndrome, cystic fibrosis, or cancer) is diag-

nosed, anticipatory grief begins and continues until remission or death. When the disease rapidly advances, anticipatory grief may be short-lived as the child's death nears. In cases of accidental or sudden death, the family has no time to anticipate or begin grieving the loss of the child.

Grief for the death of a child is not limited in time but may continue for years. Sometimes professional counseling is necessary to help family members work through grief. The support of others who have experienced the same sort of loss can be helpful. Two national organizations founded to offer support are the Candlelighters Childhood Cancer Foundation (P.O. Box 498, Kensington, MD 20895-0498; 800-366-2223; http://www.candlelighters.org) and The Compassionate

Friends (P.O. Box 3696, Oak Brook, IL 60522-3696; 877-969-0010; http://www.compassionatefriends.org). These organizations have many local chapters.

Family Caregivers

Terminal illness and sudden or unexpected death represent two types of deaths for which family caregivers grieve.

Terminal Illness

The family caregivers of children in the final stages of a terminal illness may have had to cope with many hospital admissions between periods at home. During this time, the family may face decisions about the child's physical care, as well as learning to live with a dying child. As the child's condition deteriorates, the family can be encouraged to talk to their child about dying. This is a task they may find very difficult. Support from a religious counselor, hospice nurse, or social service or psychiatric worker can help them through this difficult task. Family caregivers can be encouraged to provide as much normalcy as possible in the child's schedule. School attendance and special trips can be encouraged within the child's capabilities and desires.

During this time, family caregivers may find themselves going through a grieving process of anger, depression, ambivalence, and bargaining over and over again. The caregivers may direct anger at the hospital staff, themselves (because of guilt), each other, or the child. Reassure the caregivers that this is a normal reaction but avoid taking sides.

If the child improves enough to go home again, parents may find that they tend to be overprotective of the child. As in chronic illness, this overprotective attitude reinforces the child's sick behavior and dependency and is usually accompanied by a lack of discipline. Failure to set limits accentuates the child's feelings of being different and creates problems with siblings. The child learns to manipulate family members, only to find that this kind of behavior does not bring positive results when attempted with peers or health care personnel.

When the child has to return to the hospital because of increasing symptoms, family caregivers may once again experience all stages of the grieving process. The family members dread the child's approaching death and fear that the child will be in great pain or may die when they are not present. Nurses can help relieve these fears by keeping the family informed about the child's condition, making the child as comfortable as possible, and reassuring the family members that they will be summoned if death appears to be near.

When death comes, it is perfectly appropriate to share the family's grief, crying with them then giving them privacy to express their sorrow. The nurse can stay with the family for a while, remaining quietly supportive with an attitude of a comforting listener. An appropriate comment may be, "I am so sorry" or "This is a very sad time." The nurse needs to keep the focus on the family's grief and what the nurse can do to support them.

A little sensitivity is in order. When a child dies it is not an appropriate time for the nurse to share personal experiences of loss.

The family may want to hold the child to say a final good-bye, and the nurse can encourage and assist them in this. Intravenous lines and other equipment can be removed to make holding the child easier. The family may be left alone during this time if they desire. The nurse must be sensitive to the family's needs and desires to provide them with comfort.

Sudden or Unexpected Death

During anticipatory grief, the family of a child with a terminal illness has an opportunity to complete any unfinished business. This can help them prepare for the child's death. However, when a child dies suddenly and unexpectedly, the family has not had the opportunity to go through anticipatory grief. Such a family may have excessive guilt and remorse for something they felt they left unsaid or undone. Even if a child has had a traumatic death with disfigurement, the family must be given the opportunity to be with, see, and hold the child to help with closure of the child's life. The nurse can prepare the family for seeing the child, explaining why parts of the body may be covered. Viewing the child, even if the body is severely mutilated, helps the family to have a realistic view of the child and aids in the grief process.

The family may face a number of decisions that must be made rather quickly, especially when the child's death is unexpected. Families of terminally ill children usually have made some plans for the child's death and may know exactly what they want done. However, when the child dies unexpectedly, decisions may be necessary concerning organ donation, funeral arrangements, and an autopsy. If the death has been the result of violence or is unexplained, law requires an autopsy, but there may be other reasons that an autopsy is desired. An autopsy might be helpful in finding causes and treatments for other children diagnosed with the same disease, especially if it is a diagnosis about which little research is available. Organ donation can be discussed with the family by the hospital's organ donor coordinator or other designated person. The family needs to be well informed and must be supported throughout these difficult decisions.

A PERSONAL GLIMPSE

As I sit here each morning after losing my little girl, I know I'll make it through another day. I know this because I told her every day how happy I was that she was my child. As she was developing into a young woman, I never forgot to say how gorgeous she looked. I also know in my heart I can sleep each night hereafter, because from the day I gave birth to her I told her to always come back to me. Don't get me wrong! I always worried endlessly, but I felt it was important for her not to know these fears. As parents we hope our kids will always do the right thing. I wanted my children, and still do Michael, to know that whatever they did or do I would stand behind them, beside them, and always in my heart near them. I spent every waking day with Nicole and Michael as they were growing. I enjoyed all their developmental years. I reveled in their games, ideas, and thoughts. I know now that I was growing vicariously through them. Not a day went by that I didn't want them with me. Maybe because of this I was not as good a wife as I should have been, but I can sleep at night knowing that I was and am a great mother to my children.

You are all saying how strong I am. This is not strength. This is the power of knowing I tried through it all to be supportive and share with them what little knowledge I had. I understood that these little bodies were given to me to mold and build into productive, loving, caring human beings and with that I held the future so that my grandchildren would be better people. Nicole would have definitely gone on to bigger and better things. I know her part in society would have made a difference. Her impact on the future would have changed things for the better. Cry? I really can't cry for I know my Nikki will never leave me. I'll always see her smile. I'll always remember her voice. I'll always remember all the little things she needed to cultivate to become the adult that she would have become.

Sunday night the skies were in such turmoil. I found deep solace in that for I knew that they were letting her in. She was probably fighting with others and found her way to the front of the line. I know in my heart that once she got there she began checking the situation carefully and assessing what needed to be done and the tasks that she wanted to take on to make a difference up there. How do I know this? The skies were rumbling, the lightning was crashing, and then a heavy downpour began. I knew the angels were crying—so happy and confused as to why someone with so much to give on Earth would be up in Heaven so early. This went on for a good 10 minutes. It was pouring like crazy and then in my Nikki's infinite wisdom she spoke to them, explained the stupidity of that night, and everyone settled down. I also found great comfort, for at this time the sun, which hadn't appeared all day, broke through the clouds and shined on me. I was sitting where she knows I always sit when I need quiet time and through an opening in these clouds she spoke directly to me and said "Ma, I'm here. It's okay. I tried to get home. I would have told you some of the things of how my night was. But, Ma, I screwed up and I'll be waiting here for all of you!" This, my friend, is what has given me comfort. To love has many different meanings, but I am by far a better person for having her in memories with me always. Thanks Nikki. I will always love you.

Marie (after losing her 16-yr-old daughter, Nicole, in a car accident)

LEARNING OPPORTUNITY: What are some of the experiences this mother shared that gave her strength in dealing with her daughter's death? What are your feelings about the death of a child or teenager?

The Child

The child who has a terminal illness also experiences anticipatory grief. Even young children are aware of the seriousness of their illness, this awareness often coming from the actions and emotions of the people around them. The child realizes that he is going to die and that there is no cure for him. Sadness and depression are common. The child may have fears about dying, as well as concerns for the family members who will be left behind. It is important for the child to have the opportunity to talk about her fears, anger, and concerns, as well as to be able to express her feelings about the joys and happiness in her life. When the child is ready to talk about these things, she should be encouraged to do so. The child needs support, honesty, and answers to questions regarding her illness, treatment, and prognosis. Children should be encouraged to express their feelings through crying, playing, acting out, or drawing. The child may have a fear that pain is a part of death and should be reassured that medications can be used to control pain and keep the child comfortable. Religious and spiritual beliefs can help the child deal with feelings regarding separation from family. Reassure the child that he will not be alone at the time of death.

The dying child may have a decreased level of consciousness, although hearing remains intact. Family members at the bedside and health care personnel may need to be reminded to avoid saying anything that would not be said if the child were fully conscious. Gentle touching and caressing may provide comfort to the child. Excellent nursing care is required. Medications for pain are given intravenously because they are poorly absorbed from muscle due to poor circulation. Mucous membranes are kept clean, and petroleum jelly (Vaseline) can be applied to the lips to prevent drying and cracking. The conjunctiva of the eyes can be moistened with normal saline eye drops, such as Artificial Tears, if drying occurs. The skin is kept clean and dry, and the child is turned and positioned regularly to provide comfort and to prevent skin breakdown. While caring for the child, the nurse should talk to the child and explain everything that is being done.

As death approaches, the internal body temperature increases; thus, dying patients seem to be unaware of cold even though their skin feels cool. Explain this to family members so they do not think the child needs additional covering. Just before death, the child who has remained conscious may become restless, followed by a time of peace and calm. The nurse and family members should be aware of these reactions and know that death is near.

Test Yourself

- Why is it important for the family of the dying child to refrain from being overprotective with the child?

- What feelings might the family of a child who dies suddenly and unexpectedly have?

- For what reason should caregivers and families never say anything in the presence of a comatose child that they would not say if the child were alert?

Siblings

The siblings of a child who is dying of a terminal illness have an opportunity to themselves go through a period of anticipatory grieving. If a sibling dies suddenly, the sibling begins the process of grief at the time of the death. Siblings may feel confused, lonely, and frightened about the sudden loss of their brother or sister. The unexpected change in the atmosphere of the household can be upsetting.

Just as in the case of chronic illness, siblings resent the attention given to the ill child and are angry about the disruption in the family. Reaction varies according to the sibling's developmental age and parental attitudes and actions. Younger children find it almost impossible to understand what is happening; it is difficult even for older children to grasp. Reaction to the illness and its accompanying stresses can cause classroom problems for school-age siblings; these may be incorrectly labeled as learning disabilities or behavioral disorders unless school personnel are aware of the family situation.

When the child dies, young siblings who are still prone to magical thinking may feel guilty, particularly if a strong degree of rivalry existed before the illness. These children need continued reassurance that they did not cause or help to cause their sibling's death.

The decision of whether or not a sibling should attend funeral services for the child may be difficult. Although there has been little research, the current thinking among many health professionals supports the presence of the sibling. The sibling may be encouraged to leave a token of love and good-bye with the child—a drawing, note, toy, or another special memento. Siblings can visit the dead child in privacy with few other mourners present. Dealing with the realities of the brother's or sister's death openly is likely to be more beneficial than avoiding the issue and allowing the sibling to use his or her imagination about death (Box 33-3).

| BOX 33.3 | **Guidelines for Helping Children Cope With Death** |

DO
- Know your own beliefs.
- Begin where the child is.
- Be there.
- Confront reality.
- Encourage expression of feelings.
- Be truthful.
- Include the child in family rituals.
- Encourage remembrance.
- Admit when you don't know the answer.
- Use touch to communicate.
- Start death education early, simply, using naturally occurring events.
- Recognize symptoms of grief, and deal with the grief.
- Accept differing reactions to death.

DON'T
- Praise stoicism (detached, unemotional behavior).
- Use euphemisms (mild expressions substituted for ones that might be offensive).
- Be nonchalant.
- Glamorize death.
- Tell fairy tales or half-truths.
- Close the door to questions.
- Be judgmental of feelings and behaviors.
- Protect the child from exposure to experiences with death.
- Encourage forgetting the deceased.
- Encourage the child to be like the deceased.

Courtesy of Alice Demi, President, Grief Education Institute, PO Box 623, Englewood, CO 80151.

SETTINGS FOR CARE OF THE DYING CHILD

The family's response to and acceptance of a child's death can be greatly influenced by where the child dies. In a hospital, the child may receive the most professional care and the most technologically advanced treatment, but having a child in the hospital can contribute to family separation, a feeling of loss of control, and a sense of isolation. An increasing number of families are choosing to keep the child at home to die.

Hospice Care

In medieval times, a **hospice** was a refuge for various travelers: not only those traveling through the countryside but the terminally ill who were leaving this life for another. Hospices often were operated by religious orders and became havens for the dying. The current hospice movement in health care began in England, when Dr. Cicely Saunders founded St. Christopher's Hospice in London in 1967. This institution has become the model for others in the United States and Canada, with an emphasis on sensitive, humane care for the dying. Hospice principles of care include relief of pain, attention to the needs of the total person, and absence of heroic life-saving measures.

The first hospice in the United States was the New Haven Hospice in Connecticut. Many communities now have hospice programs that may or may not be affiliated with a hospital. Some programs offer a hospice setting to which patients go in terminal stages of illness; others provide support and guidance for the patient and family while the patient remains in the hospital or is cared for at home. Most of these hospice programs are established primarily for adults, but some programs also accept children as patients.

Children's Hospice International, founded in 1983, is an organization dedicated to hospice support of children. Through an individualized plan of care, Children's Hospice addresses the physical, developmental, psychological, social, and spiritual needs of children and families in a comprehensive and consistent way. It serves as a resource and advocacy center, providing education for parents and professionals. The organization conducts seminars and conferences, publishes training manuals, and supports a clearinghouse of information available through a national hotline (1-800-24-CHILD). Its Internet Web page (http://www.chionline.org) provides information for adults and games, books, and an excellent list of websites for children.

Home Care

Caring for the dying patient, young or old, at home has become increasingly common in recent years. More families are choosing to keep their child at home during the terminal stage of illness. Factors that contribute to the decision to care for a child at home include

- Concerns about costs for hospitalization and non-medical expenses, such as the family's travel, housing, and food
- Stress from repeated family separations
- Loss of control over the care of the child and family life

Families feel that the more loving, caring environment of the home draws the family closer and helps to reduce the guilt that often is a part of bereavement. All family members can be involved to some extent in the child's care and in this way gain a feeling of usefulness. Family caregivers feel that they remain in control.

There are disadvantages, however. Costs that would have been covered by health insurance if the child were hospitalized may not be covered if the child is cared for at home. Caring for a dying child can be extremely difficult emotionally and physically. Not every family has someone who can carry out the procedures that may need to be performed regularly. In some instances, home nursing assistance is available, but this varies from community to community. Usually the home care nurse visits several days a week and may be on call the rest of the time. In some communities, hospice nurses may provide the teaching and support that families need.

Deciding whether or not to care for a dying child at home is an extremely difficult decision for a family. Family members need support and guidance from health care personnel when they are trying to make the decision, after the decision is made, and even after the child dies.

Hospital Care

Dying in a hospital has limitations and advantages. The child and the family may find support from others in the same situation. Family members may not have the physical or emotional strength to cope with total care of the child at home, but they can participate in care supported by the hospital staff (Fig. 33-4). Hospital care is much more expensive, but this may not be important to some families, especially those with health insurance. The hospital is still the culturally accepted place to die, and this is important to some persons. Patients and families who choose hospital care need to know that they have rights and can exert some control over what happens to them.

● *Figure 33.4* The nurse helps support the dying child in the hospital setting.

Test Yourself

- What are the principles of hospice care for the dying child?

- What factors contribute to the decision to care for a dying child at home?

- What might be helpful for the family of a dying child, if the child is hospitalized?

● Nursing Process for the Dying Child

ASSESSMENT

The assessment of the terminally ill child and family is an ongoing process developed over a period of time by the health care team. The health care team assessment covers the child's developmental level, the influence of cultural and spiritual concerns, the family's support system, present indications of grieving (e.g., anticipatory grief), interactions among family members, and unfinished business. To understand the child's view of death, consider the child's previous experiences, developmental level, and cognitive ability.

SELECTED NURSING DIAGNOSES

Nursing diagnoses for the dying child include those appropriate for the child's illness, as well as the following, which are specific to the dying process:

- Acute Pain related to illness and weakened condition
- Risk for Social Isolation related to terminal illness
- Anxiety related to condition and prognosis
- Compromised Family Coping related to approaching death
- Powerlessness of family caregivers related to inability to control child's condition

OUTCOME IDENTIFICATION AND PLANNING

The goals set and the planning done to meet those goals depend on the stage of the illness, the child's and the family's acceptance of the illness, and their attitudes and beliefs about death and dying. Major goals for the child include minimizing pain, diminishing feelings of abandonment by peers and friends, and relieving anxiety about the future. Goals for the family include helping cope with the impending death and identifying feelings of powerlessness.

IMPLEMENTATION

Relieving Pain and Discomfort
The child may be in pain for many reasons, such as chemotherapy; nausea, vomiting, and gastrointestinal cramping; pressure caused by positioning; or constipation. Until the child is comfortable and relatively pain free, all other nursing interventions are fruitless: pain becomes the child's primary focus until relief is provided. Nursing measures to relieve pain may include positioning, using pillows as needed; changing linens; providing conscientious skin and mouth care; protecting skin surfaces from rubbing together; offering back rubs and massages; and administering antiemetics, analgesics, and stool softeners as appropriate.

Providing Appropriate Social Interactions
Encourage the child's siblings and friends to maintain contact. Provide opportunities for peers to visit, write, or telephone, as the child is able. Read to the child and engage in other activities that he or she finds interesting and physically tolerable. When possible, encourage the child to make decisions to foster a feeling of control. Explain all procedures and how they will affect the child. Provide the child with privacy,

but do not neglect him or her. Provide ample periods of rest. Continue to talk to and tell the child what you are doing, even though the child may seem unresponsive.

Easing the Child's Anxiety

Ask family caregivers about the child's understanding of death and previous experiences with death. Observe how the child exhibits fear, and ask family caregivers for any additional information. Encourage the child to use a doll, a pillow, or another special "warm fuzzy" for comfort. Use words such as "dead" or "dying" if appropriate in conversation because this may give the child an opening to talk about death. Nighttime is especially frightening for children because they often think they will die at night. Provide company and comfort, and be alert for periods of wakefulness when the child may need someone to talk to. Be honest and straightforward, and avoid injecting your beliefs into the conversation. If appropriate, read a book about death to the child to initiate conversation (although ideally this would have been done much earlier in the child's care).

Helping the Family Cope

Family caregivers may need encouragement to discuss their feelings about the child. Emotions and fears must be acknowledged and caregivers reassured that their reactions are normal. The support of a member of the clergy may be helpful during this time. Help family members contact their own spiritual counselor, or offer to contact the hospital chaplain if the family desires. Encourage family caregivers to eat and rest properly so they will not become ill or exhausted themselves. Explain the child's condition to the family and answer any questions. The family can be reassured that everything is being done to keep the child as comfortable and pain free as possible. Interpret signs of approaching death for the family.

If appropriate, ask the family about the siblings: what they know, how much they understand, and if the family has discussed the approaching death. Offer to help the caregivers talk with siblings.

Helping the Family Feel Involved in the Child's Care

Respond to the family's need to feel some control over the situation by suggesting specific measures they can perform to provide comfort for the child, such as positioning, moistening lips, and reading or telling a favorite story. Encourage the caregivers to talk to the child even if the child does not respond. Discourage

whispered conversations in the room. Encourage and help the family to carry out cultural customs if they wish. Help the family complete any unfinished business on the agenda; this may include the need for the child to go home to die. Help family contact support persons such as hospice workers or social services. (See Nursing Care Plan 33-1.)

EVALUATION: GOALS AND EXPECTED OUTCOMES

- **Goal:** The child will have minimal pain.
  Expected Outcome: The child rests quietly and denies pain when asked.
- **Goal:** The child will have social interaction with others.
  Expected Outcome: Within physical capabilities the child engages in activities with peers, family, and others.
- **Goal:** The child will express feelings of anxiety and use available supports to cope with anxiety.
  Expected Outcome: The child keeps a "warm fuzzy" close by for comfort and talks about death to the nurse or family. When awake at night, the child is comforted by the presence of someone to talk to.
- **Goal:** The family members will develop ways to cope with the child's approaching death.
  Expected Outcome: The family members express their feelings; identify signs that indicate approaching death; use available support systems and people. The siblings visit and talk about their feelings regarding the approaching death of their sister or brother.
- **Goal:** The family members will be involved in the child's care to decrease feelings of powerlessness.
  Expected Outcome: The family members provide comfort measures for the child, talk to the child, and complete unfinished business with the child.

KEY POINTS

- Anticipatory grief shortens the period of acute grief and loss after the child's death.
- Nurses and other health care workers often are uncomfortable with dying patients because they are afraid that the patients will ask questions they cannot or should not answer. In addition death reminds us of our own mortality, a thought with

NURSING CARE PLAN 33.1

The Dying Child and Family

CASE SCENARIO
JR is a 7-year-old who has a terminal illness. She is not expected to live more than a few more weeks. She has a brother who is 10 and a sister who is 4. A family member is with her continuously.

NURSING DIAGNOSIS
Acute Pain related to illness and weakened condition

GOAL: The child will have minimal pain.

EXPECTED OUTCOME
- The child has uninterrupted periods of quiet rest.
- Using a pain scale, the child indicates that she experiences relief from pain.

NURSING INTERVENTIONS	*RATIONALE*
Pain relief must be the primary focus of all nursing care until the child is comfortable. Administer pain relief medication, but also include such nursing measures as positioning, providing back rubs and massages, changing linens, providing conscientious skin and mouth care, and protecting skin surfaces from rubbing together to increase child's comfort.	Pain is the child's primary focus; until pain is relieved, all other nursing interventions are fruitless. Each child's pain experience is unique, and it may vary from one time to another. Some measures may relieve pain in one situation but not another. Discover the measures that work most frequently for this child.

NURSING DIAGNOSIS
Risk for Social Isolation related to terminal illness

GOAL: The child will have social interaction with others.

EXPECTED OUTCOME
- The child engages in social interaction with her classmates and other peers.
- The family caregivers and others play games with or read to child within her physical limitations.
- The caregivers talk with child when giving care regardless of her apparent level of consciousness.

NURSING INTERVENTIONS	*RATIONALE*
Encourage child's siblings and peers (including school friends) to maintain contact; provide opportunities for such contact by arranging for convenient visiting hours, providing paper and pens for writing, and making a telephone available. Spend time with and talk to the child, even when you are not sure she is responsive.	The child needs to feel that she is not cut off from everyone and everything. This helps relieve boredom and also diverts the child's attention from her condition. Hearing is often the last sense to shut down; the child will feel reassured by your voice and presence.

NURSING DIAGNOSIS
Anxiety related to condition and prognosis

GOAL: The child will express feelings of anxiety and use available supports to cope with anxiety.

EXPECTED OUTCOME
- The child talks to her family or the nurse about death.
- The child has a "warm fuzzy" close by.
- The child freely expresses her fears about dying, especially fears about nighttime.

NURSING INTERVENTIONS	*RATIONALE*
Discuss with the family the child's understanding of death, and note how she exhibits fear. Use straightforward terminology when discussing death.	The child may or may not have discussed death with the family, and it is important for the nurse to respond to the child appropriately. The nurse is able at the same time to get a sense of how family members view the child's death and what sort of help they may need to discuss the topic with their child and each other.

(nursing care plan continues on page 768)

NURSING CARE PLAN 33.1 continued

The Dying Child and Family

NURSING INTERVENTIONS	RATIONALE
Encourage the child to keep a favorite object or "warm fuzzy" for comfort and reassurance. Provide company and comfort particularly at night. Keep a night light on to ease anxieties.	Many children think they will die at night; periods of wakefulness are common. If the child is left alone, fears may compound. A night light provides some sense of security.

NURSING DIAGNOSIS
Compromised Family Coping related to approaching death

GOAL: The family members will develop ways to cope with the child's approaching death.

EXPECTED OUTCOME
- The family caregivers express their feelings and anxieties.
- The family caregivers contact a spiritual advisor for support.
- The family caregivers identify signs in the child that indicate approaching death.

NURSING INTERVENTIONS	RATIONALE
Encourage family caregivers to discuss their feelings about the child and to acknowledge their fears and emotions; reassure them that their reactions are normal.	It may be very difficult for family members to talk about their child's death; they may feel they need to "keep up a brave front" for the child and siblings. However, it is important for them to acknowledge the death and begin to express some of their emotions.
Help the family contact their spiritual advisor or a hospital chaplain, if they desire.	The support of a spiritual counselor, particularly one known to the family, may be helpful.
Help the family recognize and acknowledge signs of the child's impending death. Help them talk with her siblings.	Acknowledging the impending signs of death helps the family caregivers to be realistic about the approaching death. They also may need support and guidance to know how to talk with the other children.
Make sure family caregivers are resting and eating adequately.	The family caregivers must avoid exhaustion; lack of sleep and inadequate nutrition will only make it harder for them to cope.

NURSING DIAGNOSIS
Powerlessness of family caregivers related to inability to control child's condition

GOAL: The family members will be involved in child's care to decrease feelings of powerlessness.

EXPECTED OUTCOME
- The family caregivers provide comfort measures for the child.
- The family caregivers talk with child and complete unfinished business with her.

NURSING INTERVENTIONS	RATIONALE
Suggest specific care measures that family members might perform to comfort the child; encourage the family to carry out cultural practices if they desire.	Caregivers need to feel they are doing something to help their child; performing meaningful cultural customs helps the family express feelings and provides a feeling of continuity.
Explain "unfinished business" to the family and encourage them to complete any unfinished business on their agenda.	Discussion of unfinished business provides another opportunity for family members to engage in meaningful activity with their child before the child's death.
Encourage family members to talk to the child even when she seems unresponsive.	The child may be able to hear voices even when unable to respond; family caregivers will feel better when they can still communicate love and support.

which many of us are uncomfortable. Nurses need to examine their own feelings about death and the reasons for these feelings.

♦ The nurse can personally prepare to care for dying children by exploring her/his own feelings about life and death. Attending a workshop, conference, or seminar in which one's own feelings about death are explored, talking with other professionals, sharing concerns, and comforting each other in stressful times and reading studies about death to discover how dying patients feel about their situation also can be helpful for the nurse in preparing to work with dying patients.

♦ Factors that affect the child's understanding of death include his/her stage of development, cognitive ability, experiences, and how the family deals with death. Most children do not understand the finality of death until they near preadolescence.

♦ Infants and toddlers have little understanding of death; the toddler may fear separation but has no recognition of the fact that death is nearing and irreversible. The preschool child may believe that death happens because of angry thoughts. Magical thinking about death and thinking of death as a kind of sleep are seen in children preschool age until about 8 or 9 years of age. Children after age 9 gain the concept that death is universal and irreversible. Adolescents have an adult understanding of death but feel that they are immortal—that is, death will happen to others but not to them.

♦ It is important for families to complete unfinished business by spending time with the dying child, helping siblings to understand the child's illness and impending death, and giving family members a chance to share their love with the child. Openness and honest answers given to the child in words the child can understand leave less room for misinterpretation and distortion.

♦ When a child dies suddenly, a family may suffer excessive grief and guilt for something they felt they left unsaid or undone.

♦ When a sibling dies, possible reactions seen in children depend on the stage of development of that sibling. Young siblings find death impossible to understand. School-age siblings may have classroom problems, behavioral disorders, and feelings of guilt about the death of their sibling. Dealing with the realities of the brother's or sister's death openly is likely to be more beneficial than avoiding the issue.

♦ Settings for caring for the dying child include the home, hospice, and hospital settings. The home provides a loving, caring environment and may decrease costs and family separations. Home settings may prevent some expenses from being covered and may be difficult emotionally and physically for the family. Hospice principles of care include relief of pain, attention to the needs of the total person, and absence of heroic life-saving measures. In the hospital setting the child and the family may find support from others in the same situation, support from the hospital staff, and technologically advanced treatment. Hospital care is much more expensive, but this may not be important to some families. The hospital is still the culturally accepted place to die, but having a child in the hospital can contribute to family separation, a feeling of loss of control, and a sense of isolation.

REFERENCES AND SELECTED READINGS

Books and Journals

Anonymous. (1970). *American Journal of Nursing, 70*(2), 335.

Berger, K. S. (2001). *The developing person through the life span* (5th ed.). New York: Worth Publishers.

Bowden, V. R. (1993). Children's literature: The death experience. *Pediatric Nursing, 19*(1), 17–21.

Brazelton, T. B., & Greenspan, S. (2001). *The irreducible needs of children: What every child must have to grow, learn, and flourish.* Cambridge, MA: Perseus Publishing.

Busch, T., & Kimble, C. S. (2001). Grieving children: Are we meeting the challenge? *Pediatric Nursing, 27*(4), 414.

Hockenberry, M. J., Wilson, D., Winkelstein, M. L., & Kline, N. E. (2003). *Wong's nursing care of infants and children* (7th ed.). St. Louis: Mosby.

Karch, A. M. (2003). *2004 Lippincott's nursing drug guide.* Philadelphia: Lippincott Williams & Wilkins.

Pillitteri, A. (2003). *Maternal and child health nursing* (4th ed.). Philadelphia: Lippincott Williams & Wilkins.

Ritchie, M. A. (2001). Psychosocial nursing care for adolescents with cancer. *Issues in Comprehensive Pediatric Nursing, 24*(3), 165–175.

Wong, D. L., Perry, S., & Hockenberry, M. (2002). *Maternal child nursing care* (2nd ed.). St. Louis: Mosby.

Web Addresses

http://www.candlelighters.org
http://compassionatefriends.org
http://www.chionline.org
http://www.hospicenet.org
http://www.nccf.org/childhoodcancer/facts.asp

WORKBOOK

NCLEX-STYLE REVIEW QUESTIONS

1. While the nurse is working with the family of a child who is terminally ill, the child's siblings make the following statements to the nurse. Which statement is an example of the stage of grief referred to as bargaining?

    a. "I just want him to come to my birthday party next month."

    b. "It makes me mad that they said my brother is going to die."

    c. "I think he will get well now that he has a new medicine."

    d. "When he dies at least he won't have any more pain."

2. When working with the family of a child who is terminally ill, the child's siblings make the following statements to the nurse. Which statement is an example of the stage of grief referred to as denial?

    a. "I just want him to come to my birthday party next month."

    b. "It makes me mad that they said my brother is going to die."

    c. "I think he will get well now that he has a new medicine."

    d. "When he dies at least he won't have any more pain."

3. The nurse is working with a group of 4- and 5-year-old children who are talking about death and dying. One child in the group recently experienced the death of the family pet. Which of the following statements would the nurse expect a 5-year-old child to say about the death of the pet?

    a. "I think he was sad to leave us."

    b. "He's only a little dead."

    c. "A monster came and took him during the night."

    d. "I will be real good so I won't die."

4. The nurse is discussing the subject of death and dying with a group of adolescents. Which of the following statements made by an adolescent would be expected considering her or his stage of growth and development?

    a. "I always hold my breath and run past the cemetery to protect myself."

    b. "It would be sad to die because my girlfriend would really miss me."

    c. "Others die in car wrecks, but even if I had a wreck, I wouldn't be killed."

    d. "It makes me nervous to go to sleep. I am afraid I won't wake up."

5. The nurse is with a family whose terminally ill child has just died. Which of the following statements made by the nurse would be the *most* therapeutic statement?

    a. "It will not hurt as much as time passes."

    b. "My sister died when I was a teenager. I know how you feel."

    c. "I will leave the call light here. Call me if you need me."

    d. "This is a really sad and difficult time."

6. The family of a child with a terminal illness might go through a process known as anticipatory grief. Which of the following might occur during this process? Choose all that apply. The family

    a. has an opportunity to complete unfinished business.

    b. can prepare for the eventual death of the child.

    c. will not have feelings of guilt or remorse.

    d. may begin the process of preparing for the funeral

    e. help the child's siblings deal with the coming death.

STUDY ACTIVITIES

1. List and compare thoughts and ideas a child of each of the following ages would most likely have regarding death and dying:

Toddler	Preschool	School-age	Adolescent

2. Research your community to find the procedure for organ donation. Make arrangements for a speaker from the organization to discuss organ donation with your class. If such a person is not available, research organ donation on the Internet and share your findings with your class.

3. Survey your community to see if there is a hospice available. Describe how it functions. Find out if it accepts children as patients and if there are any restrictions concerning children. Discuss your findings with your peers.

4. Go to the following Internet site:
   http://dying.about.com

   Click on "Grieving Child."

   Click on "How children deal with the death of a sibling."

   a. List some statements that well-meaning friends and relatives often say to children who are grieving.

   b. List four ideas of ways that adults can help a child who has lost a sibling.

   Click on "Talking to children about death." Read this section.

c. List the normal children's reactions to death for each stage of growth and development.

d. State suggestions of ways to help a child deal with the death of a sibling.

CRITICAL THINKING: What Would You Do?

1. The Andrews family has an 8-year-old daughter with a terminal illness.

   a. What factors do you think the family needs to consider when deciding if they will care for the child at home?

   b. What feelings do you think the family might be dealing with?

2. The Andrews decide they cannot care for the child at home.

   a. What are your feelings about this decision?

   b. What you would say to this family to support them in their decision.

The Child With a Major Illness

The Child With Sensory/Neurologic Disorders

STUDENT OBJECTIVES

On completion of this chapter, the student will be able to

1. Discuss ways the infant and child's eyes, ears, and nervous system differs from the adult's.
2. List five types of vision impairment.
3. Describe treatment for bacterial conjunctivitis.
4. Differentiate between a child who is hard of hearing and one who is deaf.
5. Describe the behavior of the child with acute otitis media.
6. List four complications of *Haemophilus influenzae* meningitis.
7. Describe the nursing care specific to a child at high risk for seizures.
8. Describe (a) simple partial motor seizures, (b) simple partial sensory seizures, and (c) complex partial (psychomotor) seizures.
9. Describe (a) tonic-clonic seizures, (b) absence seizures, (c) atonic or akinetic seizures, (d) myoclonic seizures, and (e) infantile spasms.
10. Describe cerebral palsy.
11. Discuss the causes of cerebral palsy: (a) prenatal, (b) perinatal, and (c) postnatal.
12. Differentiate between spastic and athetoid cerebral palsy.
13. Identify the health care professionals involved in the care of the child with cerebral palsy.
14. List the causes of mental retardation: (a) prenatal, (b) perinatal, and (c) postnatal.

KEY TERMS

absence
amblyopia
astigmatism
ataxia
aura
binocular vision
cataract
clonus
conjunctivitis
diplopia
dysarthria
esotropia
exotropia
external hordeolum
febrile seizures
goniotomy
hyperopia
lacrimation
myopia
myringotomy
nuchal rigidity
opisthotonos
orthoptics
partial
photophobia
purpuric rash
refraction
strabismus

Neurologic disorders can be caused by many different factors. Nerve cells do not regenerate, and complications from these disorders can be serious and permanent. If neurologic damage has occurred, the role of the nurse is often one of support and guidance to the child and family dealing with the neurologic disorder.

Children learn about the world they live in through their senses. Any disorder related to the eyes and ears can have significant impact on the normal growth and development of the child.

GROWTH AND DEVELOPMENT OF THE EYES, EARS, AND NERVOUS SYSTEM

The Nervous System

The nervous system is the communication network of the body. The central nervous system is made up of the brain and spinal cord. The peripheral nervous system is made up of the nerves throughout the body. A fluid known as cerebral spinal fluid (CSF) flows through the chambers of the brain and through the spinal cord, serving as a cushion and protective mechanism for nerve cells.

> **Maybe this will jog your memory on an exam.** Cerebral spinal fluid (CSF) continually forms, circulates and is reabsorbed. Many neurologic disorders relate to this aspect of the functioning of the nervous system.

Nerves go from the brain and spinal cord to all parts of the body. Information is quickly transmitted from the central nervous system. Stimuli of all types cause signals called nerve impulses to occur. These nerve impulses activate, coordinate, integrate, and control all of the body functions.

A part of the peripheral nervous system, the autonomic nervous system, regulates the involuntary functions of the body, such as the heart rate. At birth the nervous system is immature. As the child grows, the quality of the nerve impulses sent through the nervous system develops and matures. As these nerve impulses become more mature, the gross and fine motor skills seen in the child increase in complexity. The child becomes more coordinated and able to develop motor skills.

Sensory Organs

The eyes and ears are specialized organs of the nervous system. These organs transmit impulses to the central nervous system.

Eyes

The eye is a sense organ that detects light, the stimuli, from the environment. Parts of the eye respond to the light and produce and transmit a nerve impulse to the brain. That information and image is interpreted in the brain, and thus the person "sees" the object.

Newborns do not focus clearly but will stare at a human face directly in front of them. By 2 months of age, the infant can focus and follow an object with the eyes (Fig. 34-1). By 7 months of age, depth perception has matured enough so that the infant can transfer objects back and forth between his hands. Visual acuity of children gradually increases from birth, when the visual acuity is usually between 20/100 and 20/400 until about 7 years of age, when most children have 20/20 vision. (Traboulsi & Maumenee, 1999).

Ears

Ears function as the sense organ of hearing, as well as the organ responsible in part for equilibrium and balance. Sounds waves, vibrations, and fluid movements create nerve impulses that are ultimately distinguished in the brain as sounds.

The ear is made up of the external, middle, and inner ear. The eardrum or tympanic membrane is in the external ear. In the middle ear, the eustachian tube connects the throat with the middle ear. In infants and young children, this tube is straighter, shorter, and wider than in the older child and adult. Hearing in children is acute, and the infant will respond to sounds within the 1st month of life.

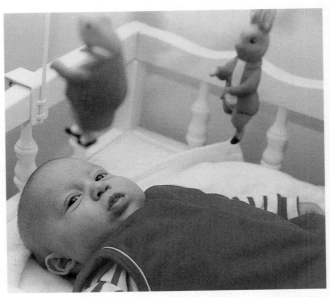

● **Figure 34.1** A two-month-old focusing on a simple mobile.

VISION IMPAIRMENT

Good vision is essential to a child's normal development. How well a child sees affects his or her learning process, social development, coordination, and safety. One in 1,000 children of school age has serious vision impairment. The sooner these impairments are corrected, the better a child's chances are for normal or near-normal development.

Children with vision impairments are classified as sighted with eye problems, partially sighted, or legally blind.

Types of Vision Impairment

Among sighted children with eye problems, errors of **refraction** (the way light rays bend as they pass through the lens to the retina) are the most common. About 10% of school age children have **myopia** (nearsightedness), which means that the child can see objects clearly at close range but not at a distance. When proper lenses are fitted, vision is corrected to normal. If uncorrected, this defect may cause a child to be labeled inattentive or retarded. Myopia tends to be seen in families and often progresses into adolescence then levels off.

Hyperopia (farsightedness) is a refractive condition in which the person can see objects better at a distance than close up. It is common in young children and often persists into the first grade or even later. The ocular specialist examining the child must decide whether or not corrective lenses are needed on an individual basis. Usually correction is not needed in a preschooler. Teachers and parents should be aware of the considerable eye fatigue that may result from efforts at accommodation for close work.

Astigmatism, which may occur with or without myopia or hyperopia, is caused by unequal curvatures in the cornea that bend the light rays in different directions; this produces a blurred image. Slight astigmatism often does not require correction; moderate degrees usually require glasses for reading and watching television and movies; severe astigmatism requires glasses at all times.

Children with partial sight have a visual acuity between 20/20 and 20/200 in the better eye after all necessary medical or surgical correction. These children also have a high incidence of refractive errors, particularly myopia. Eye injuries also cause loss of vision, as do conditions such as cataracts, which can be improved by treatment but result in diminished sight.

Good news. The incidence of maternal rubella causing blindness in infants has decreased since the immunization for MMR has been given.

Blindness is legally defined as a corrected vision of 20/200 or less or peripheral vision of less than 20° in the better eye. Many causes of blindness, such as retrolental fibroplasia (caused by excessive oxygen concentrations in newborns) and trachoma, a viral infection, have been reduced or eliminated. Maternal infections are still a common cause of blindness.

Between the ages of 5 and 7 years, children begin to form and retain visual images; they have memory with pictures. Children who become blind before 5 years of age are missing this crucial element in their development.

Blindness can seriously hamper the child's ability to form human attachments; learn coordination, balance, and locomotion; distinguish fantasy from reality; and interpret the surrounding world. How well the blind child learns to cope depends on the family's ability to communicate, teach, and foster a sense of independence in the child.

Clinical Manifestations and Diagnosis

Squinting and frowning while trying to read a blackboard or other material at a distance, tearing, red-rimmed eyes, holding work too close to the eyes while reading or writing, and rubbing the eyes are all signs of possible vision impairment. Although blindness is likely to be detected in early infancy, partial sightedness or correctable vision problems may go unrecognized until a child enters school, unless vision screening is part of routine health maintenance (Fig. 34-2).

A simple test kit for young children is available for home use by family caregivers or visiting nurses (Fig. 34-3). This kit is an adaptation of the Snellen E chart used for testing children who have not learned to read. The child covers one eye and then points the fingers in the same direction as the "fingers" on each E, beginning with the largest. Some examiners refer to these as "legs on a table."

● **Figure 34.2** Vision screening on a preschool child as part of a routine exam.

Lighthouse flash-card vision test. This test may be obtained from the New York Association for the Blind, 111 East 59th Street, New York, New York 10022.

● *Figure 34.3* Home testing kit. This allows the young child to take the test in more familiar surroundings. The test may be obtained at www.preventblindness org/children or by calling 1-800-331-2020.

The Snellen chart is a familiar test in which the letters on each line are smaller than those on the line above. If the child can read the 20-foot line standing 20 feet away from the chart, visual acuity is stated as 20/20. If the child can read only the line marked 100, acuity is stated as 20/100. The chart should be placed at eye level with good lighting and in a room free from distractions. One eye is tested at a time, with the other eye covered.

Picture charts for identification also are used but are not considered as accurate. An intelligent child can memorize the pictures and guess from the general shape without being able to see distinctly.

Treatment and Education

Significant medical and surgical advances have occurred in the treatment of cataracts, strabismus, and amblyopia.

Did you know? Normal visual acuity in the preschool age child is 20/30.

The earlier the child is treated, the better the child's chances of adequate vision for normal development and function. Errors of refraction are usually correctable. Corrective lenses for minor vision impairments should be prescribed early and checked regularly to be sure they still provide adequate correction.

Children who are partially sighted or totally blind benefit from association with normally sighted children. In most communities, education for these special children is provided within the regular school or in special classes that offer the child more specialized equipment and instruction.

Specialized equipment includes printed material with large print, pencils with large leads for darker lines, tape recordings, magnifying glasses, and keyboards. For children with a serious impairment whose participation in regular activities is sharply curtailed, talking books, raised maps, and Braille equipment are needed as well. These devices prevent isolation of the visually impaired child and minimize any differences from the other children.

Nursing Care for the Visually Impaired Child

Children with a visual impairment have the same needs as other children, and these should not be overlooked. The child who is blind needs emotional comfort and sensory stimulation, much of which must be communicated by touch, sound, and smell. It is important for the nurse to explain sounds and other sensations that are new to the child and to let him or her touch the equipment that will be used in procedures. A tactile tour of the room helps orient the child to the location of furniture and other facilities.

Nurses and other personnel must identify themselves when they enter the room and must tell the child when they leave. Explanations of what is going to happen reduce the child's fear and anxiety and the possibility of being startled by an unexpected touch. The child with a visual impairment should be involved with as many peers and their activities as possible. The child also should be encouraged to be as independent as possible. One step is to provide the child with finger foods and encourage self-feeding after orienting the child to the plate. A small bowl, instead of a plate, is

Be careful. Awareness of safety hazards is particularly important when caring for the blind or partially sighted child.

useful so that food can be scooped against the side to get it on the spoon. Eating can be a time-consuming and messy affair, but it is essential to the growth of independence in all children that they have the opportunity to learn to feed themselves.

EYE CONDITIONS

Cataracts, congenital infantile glaucoma, and strabismus are disease conditions that may need to be dealt with during childhood. Eye injuries can occur when children are exploring their environment or playing. In addition, eye infections may occur because exploring hands can easily carry infectious organisms to the eyes.

Cataracts

A **cataract** is a development of opacity in the crystalline lens that prevents light rays from entering the eye. Congenital cataracts may be hereditary, or they may be complications of maternal rubella infection during the 1st trimester of pregnancy. Cataracts also may develop later in infancy or childhood from eye injury or from metabolic disturbances such as galactosemia and diabetes.

Surgical extraction of the cataracts can be performed at an early age. With early removal, the prognosis for good vision is improved. The child is fitted with a contact lens. If only one eye is affected, the "good" eye is patched to prevent amblyopia (see discussion in the section on strabismus). As the child gets older, numerous lens changes are needed to modify the strength of the lens.

Glaucoma

Glaucoma may be of the congenital infantile type, occurring in children younger than 3 years; of the juvenile type, showing clinical manifestations after 3 years; or of the secondary type, resulting from injury or disease. Increased intraocular pressure caused by overproduction of aqueous fluid causes the eyeball to enlarge and the cornea to become large, thin, and sometimes cloudy. Untreated, the disease slowly progresses to blindness. Pain may be present.

Goniotomy (surgical opening into Schlemm's canal) provides drainage of the aqueous humor and is

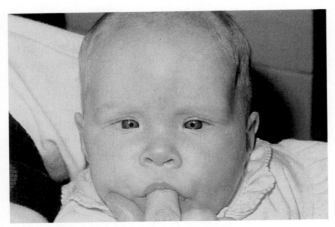

● *Figure 34.4* Strabismus in an infant.

often effective in relieving intraocular pressure. Goniotomy may need to be performed multiple times to control intraocular pressure. Surgery is performed as early as possible to prevent permanent damage.

Strabismus

Strabismus is the failure of the two eyes to direct their gaze at the same object simultaneously. This condition is commonly called "squint" or "crossed eyes" (Fig. 34-4).

Normally, **binocular (normal) vision** is maintained through the muscular coordination of eye movements, so that a single vision results. In strabismus, the visual axes are not parallel, and **diplopia** (double vision) results. In an effort to avoid seeing two images, the child's central nervous system suppresses vision in the deviant eye, causing **amblyopia** (dimness of vision from disuse of the eye), which is sometimes called "lazy eye."

A wide variation in the manifestation of strabismus exists; there are lateral, vertical, and mixed lateral and vertical types. There may be monocular strabismus, in which one eye deviates while the other eye is used; or alternating strabismus, in which deviation alternates from one eye to the other. The term **esotropia** is used when the eye deviates toward the other eye; **exotropia** denotes a turning away from the other eye (Fig. 34-5).

Treatment depends on the type of strabismus present. In monocular strabismus, occlusion of the better eye by patching to force the use of the deviating eye should be initiated at an early age. Patching is continued for weeks or months. The younger the child is, the more rapid the improvement. The patching may be for set periods of time or be continuous, depending on the child's age. For example, the older child usually needs continuous periods of patching, whereas the younger one may respond quickly to short periods of patching.

Some nurses find this approach helpful. For the child who must have one eye patched, the child is encouraged to use the unpatched eye. Activities such as doing puzzles, drawing, and sewing should be promoted.

Glasses can correct a refractive error if amblyopia is not present. **Orthoptics** (therapeutic ocular muscle exercises) to improve the quality of vision may be prescribed to supplement the use of glasses or surgery.

Early detection and treatment of strabismus are essential for a successful outcome. Surgery on the eye muscle to correct the defect is necessary for children who do not respond to glasses and exercises. Many children need surgery after amblyopia has been corrected. The surgical correction is believed to be necessary before the child reaches age 6 years or the visual damage may be permanent. However, some authorities believe that correction can be successful up to age 10 years.

Eye Injury and Foreign Objects in the Eye

Eye injuries are fairly common, particularly in older children. Ecchymosis of the eye (black eye) is of no great importance unless the eyeball is involved. A penetrating wound of the eyeball is potentially serious—BB shots in particular are dangerous—and requires the ophthalmologist's attention. With any history of an injury, a thorough examination of the entire eye is necessary.

Sympathetic ophthalmia may follow perforation wounds of the globe, even if the perforations are small. Sympathetic ophthalmia, an inflammatory reaction of the uninjured eye, often includes **photophobia** (intolerance to light), **lacrimation** (secretion of tears), pain, and some

A   B

● *Figure 34.5* Strabismus. (A) Esotropia. (B) Exotropia.

A word of caution is in order. Cotton-tipped applicators should not be used to remove small objects that have lodged inside the eyelid because of the danger of sudden movement and possible perforation of the eye.

dimness of vision. The retina may become detached, and atrophy of the eyeball may occur. Prompt and skillful treatment at the time of the injury is essential to avoiding involvement of the other eye.

Small foreign objects, such as specks of dust that have lodged inside the eyelid, may be removed by rolling the lid back and exposing the object. If the object cannot be easily removed with a small piece of moistened cotton or soft clean cloth or flushed out with saline solution, the child should be seen by a care provider.

Eye Infections

External hordeolum, known commonly as a stye, is a purulent infection of the follicle of an eyelash generally caused by *Staphylococcus aureus*. Localized swelling, tenderness, pain, and a reddened lid edge are present. The maximal tenderness is over the infected site. The lesion progresses to suppuration, with eventual discharge of the purulent material. Warm saline compresses applied for about 15 minutes three or four times daily give some relief and hasten resolution, but recurrence is common. The stye should never be squeezed. Antibiotic ointment may help prevent accompanying conjunctivitis and recurrence.

Conjunctivitis is an acute inflammation of the conjunctiva. In children, a virus, bacteria, allergy, or foreign body may be the cause. Most commonly, conjunctivitis is caused by bacteria. The purulent drainage, a common characteristic, can be cultured to determine the causative organism. Because of the danger of spreading infection, bacterial conjunctivitis is treated with ophthalmic antibacterial agents, such as erythromycin, bacitracin, sulfacetamide, and polymyxin. Because ointments blur vision, eye drops are used during the day and ointments are used at night. Before medication is applied, warm moist compresses can be used to remove the crusts that form on the eyes. The child who has bacterial conjunctivitis should be kept separate from other children until the condition has been treated. The use of separate washcloths and towels and disposable tissues is important in preventing spread of infection among family members.

Nursing Care for the Child Undergoing Eye Surgery

When a child undergoes eye surgery, sensory deprivation is possible. Anyone experiencing sensory depri-

vation finds it difficult to stay in touch with reality, and a child whose eyes are covered is particularly vulnerable. Nurses who have not experienced this deprivation do not always appreciate the implications of not being able to see. A child who wakens from surgery to total darkness may go into a state of panic. Observation of the child returning from surgery may reveal panic and anxiety evidenced by trembling and nervousness. The child needs a family caregiver or loved one to stay during the time when vision is restricted.

The child needs to be as well prepared for the event as possible. However, the small child has no experience to help in understanding what actually is going to happen. The darkness, pain, and total strangeness of the situation can be overwhelming. Using play can be helpful. For example, one preoperative preparation might be to play a game with a blindfold to help the child become accustomed to having his or her eyes covered (Fig. 34-6).

Restraints should not be used indiscriminately. However, most small children need some reminder to keep their hands away from the affected eye unless someone is beside them to prevent them from rubbing it or from removing eye dressings. Elbow restraints are useful, although they do not prevent rubbing the eye with the arm. Flannel strips applied to the wrists in clove-hitch fashion can be tied to the bed sides in such a manner as to allow freedom of arm movement but to prevent the child from causing damage to the operative site.

The nurse should speak to the child to alert him or her as the nurse approaches. The child needs tactile stimulation; therefore, after speaking, the nurse would do well to stroke or pat the child. If permitted, the nurse may hold the child for additional reassurance.

● **Figure 34.6** Pretending to be a pirate enables this toddler to find enjoyment in wearing an eye patch.

HEARING IMPAIRMENT

Hearing loss is one of the most common disabilities in the United States, with as many as 33 children a day born with a hearing impairment (Ansel, Landa, & Luethke, 1999). Depending on the degree of hearing loss and the age at detection, a child's development can be moderately to severely impaired. Development of speech, human relationships, and understanding of the environment all depend on the ability to hear. Infants at high risk for hearing loss should be screened when they are between 3 and 6 months of age.

Hearing loss ranges from mild (hard of hearing) to profound (deaf) (Table 34-1). A child who is hard of hearing has a loss of hearing acuity but can learn speech and language by imitating sounds. A deaf child has no hearing ability.

TABLE 34.1	Levels of Hearing Impairment
Decibel Level	**Hearing Level Present**
Slight (<30 dB)	Unable to hear whispered word or faint speech No speech impairment present May not be aware of hearing difficulty Achieves well in school and home by compensating by leaning forward, speaking loudly
Mild (30–50 dB)	Beginning speech impairment may be present Difficulty hearing if not facing speaker; some difficulty with normal conversation
Moderate (55–70 dB)	Speech impairment present; may require speech therapy Difficulty with normal conversation
Severe (70–90 dB)	Difficulty with any but nearby loud voice Hears vowels easier than consonants Requires speech therapy for clear speech May still hear loud sounds such as jets or a train
Profound (>90 dB)	Hears almost no sound

From Pillitteri, A. (2003). *Maternal and child health nursing* (4th ed.). Philadelphia: Lippincott Williams & Wilkins.

Types of Hearing Impairment

There are four types of hearing loss: conductive, sensorineural, mixed, and central.

Conductive Hearing Loss

In this type of impairment, middle ear structures fail to carry sound waves to the inner ear. Conductive hearing loss is most often the result of chronic serous otitis media or other infection and can make hearing levels fluctuate. Chronic middle ear infection can destroy part of the eardrum or the ossicles, which leads to conductive deafness. This type of deafness is seldom complete and responds well to treatment.

Sensorineural (Perceptive) Hearing Loss

This type of hearing loss may be caused by damage to the nerve endings in the cochlea or to the nerve pathways leading to the brain. It is generally severe and unresponsive to medical treatment. Diseases such as meningitis and encephalitis, hereditary or congenital factors, and toxic reactions to certain drugs (such as streptomycin) may cause sensorineural hearing loss. Maternal rubella is believed to be one of the common causes of sensorineural deafness in children.

Mixed Hearing Loss

Some children have both conductive and sensorineural hearing impairments. In these instances, the conduction level determines how well the child can hear.

Central Auditory Dysfunction

Although this child may have normal hearing, damage to or faulty development of the proper brain centers makes the child unable to use the auditory information received.

Clinical Manifestations

Mild to moderate hearing loss often remains undetected until the child moves outside the family circle into nursery school or kindergarten. The hearing loss may have been gradual, and the child may have become such a skilled lip reader that neither the child nor the family is aware of the partial deafness.

Don't be too quick to judge. Caregivers and teachers should be aware of the possibility of hearing loss in children who appear to be inattentive and noisy and who create disturbances in the classroom.

Certain reactions and mannerisms characterize a child with hearing loss. The child should be observed for an apparent inability to locate a sound and a turning of the head to one side when listening. The child who fails to comprehend when spoken to, who gives inappropriate answers to questions, who consistently turns up the volume on the television or radio, or who cannot whisper or talk softly may have hearing loss.

Diagnosis

Children who are profoundly deaf are more likely to be diagnosed before 1 year of age than are children with mild to moderate hearing losses. The child who is suspected of having a hearing loss should be referred for a complete audiologic assessment, including pure-tone audiometric, speech reception, and speech discrimination tests. Children with sensorineural impairment generally have a greater loss of hearing acuity, which may vary from slight to complete, in the high-pitched tones. Children with a conductive loss are more likely to have equal losses over a wide range of frequencies.

A child's hearing should be tested at all frequencies by a pure-tone audiometer in a soundproof room. Speech reception and speech discrimination tests measure the amount of hearing impairment for both speech and communication. Accurate measurements usually can be made in children as young as 3 years of age if the test is introduced as a game.

Infants and very young children must be tested in different ways. An infant with normal hearing should be able to locate a sound at 28 weeks, imitate sounds at 36 weeks, and associate sounds with people or objects at 1 year of age. A commonly used screening test for very young children uses noisemakers of varying intensity and pitch. The examiner stands beside or behind the child who has been given a toy. As the examiner produces sounds with a rattle, buzzer, bell, or other noisemaker, a hearing child is distracted and turns to the source of the new sound, whereas a deaf child does not react in a particular way.

Deafness, mental retardation, and autism are sometimes incorrectly diagnosed because the symptoms can be similar. Deaf children may fail to respond to sound or develop speech because they cannot hear. Mentally retarded or autistic children may show the same lack of response and development, even though they do not have a hearing loss.

Treatment and Education

When the type and degree of hearing loss have been established, the child or even infant may be fitted with a hearing aid. Hearing aids are helpful only in conductive deafness, not in sensorineural or central auditory dysfunction. These devices only amplify sound; they do not localize or clarify it. Many models are available including those that are worn in the ear or behind the

● **Figure 34.7** A young deaf girl learns to use the computer with the help of a speech therapist.

ear, incorporated in glasses, or worn on the body with a wire connection to the ear. FM receiver units also are available that can broadcast the speaker's voice from a greater distance and cut out the background noise. When the FM transmitter is turned off, this type of unit functions as an ordinary hearing aid.

It is believed that deaf children can best be taught to communicate by a combination of lip reading, sign language, and oral speech (Fig. 34-7). The family members are the child's first teachers; they must be aware of all phases of development—physical, emotional, social, intellectual, and language—and seek to aid this development.

A deaf child depends on sight to interpret the environment and to communicate. Thus it is important to be sure that the child's vision is normal and, if it is not, to correct that problem. The probability is twice as great that the child with a hearing loss also will have some vision impairment. Training in the use of all the other senses—sight, smell, taste, and touch—makes the deaf child better able to use any available hearing. Some researchers believe that most deaf children do have some hearing ability.

Preschool classes for deaf children exist in many large communities. These classes attempt to create an environment in which a deaf child can have the same experiences and activities that normal preschoolers have. Children are generally enrolled at age 2.5 years.

The John Tracy Clinic in Los Angeles, founded in 1943, is dedicated to young children (birth through age 5 years) born with severe hearing loss or those who have lost hearing through illness before acquiring speech and language. The clinic's purpose is "to find, encourage, guide, and train the parents of deaf and hard-of-hearing children, first in order to reach and help the children, and second to help the parents themselves." With early diagnosis and intervention, hearing-impaired children can develop language and communication skills in the critical preschool period that enable many of them to speech-read and to speak. All services to parents and children are free. Full audiologic testing, parent–child education, demonstration nursery school, parent education classes, and parent groups are offered. Many medical residents, nurses, and allied health care professionals come to observe the model programs at the clinic to see the benefits of early diagnosis.

The clinic also provides a correspondence course for parents. Three courses are available for deaf infants, deaf preschoolers, and deaf-blind children. These courses, which are provided in both English and Spanish and include written materials and videotapes, guide parents in encouraging their child to develop auditory awareness, speech-reading skills, and expressive language. Information about the clinic can be obtained by calling toll-free (800) 522-4582 or on the Internet at http://www.johntracyclinic.org.

Federal law requires free and appropriate education for all disabled children. Children with a hearing loss who cannot successfully function in regular classrooms are provided with supplementary services (speech therapist, speech interpreter, signer) in special classrooms or in a residential school.

Nursing Care for the Deaf Child

When the deaf child is in a health care facility, the child's primary caregiver should be present during the stay. Caregiver presence is encouraged to help the child communicate needs and feelings, not as a convenience to the nursing staff.

The deaf child's anxiety about unfamiliar situations and procedures can be greater than that of the child with normal hearing. When speaking to the deaf child, stand or sit face to face on the child's level. Be certain that a deaf child can see you before you touch him or her. Demonstrate each procedure before it is performed, showing the child the equipment or pictures of the equipment to be used. Follow demonstrations with explanations to be sure the child understands. Keep a night light in the child's room because sight is a critical sense to the deaf child.

A little sensitivity is in order. To understand the deaf child's helpless feeling, imagine being in a soundless, dark room. Be sure the child's room is well lighted.

Hearing aids are expensive, so learning how to take care of and maintain them is important. Put the aid in a safe place when the child is not wearing it. Check linens before putting them into the laundry so as not to discard a hearing aid along with the dirty linens.

Use family members as important resources to learn about the child's habits and communication patterns. In many communities signing classes are available for those working with hearing-impaired children and adults.

Test Yourself

- What are five types of vision impairment?
- What term is commonly used to describe strabismus?
- What are four types of hearing loss?
- What are four examples of nursing interventions used when working with deaf children.

OTITIS MEDIA

Otitis media is one of the most common infectious diseases of childhood. Two in three children have at least one episode of otitis media by the time they are 1 year old (Kline, 1999). The eustachian tube in an infant is shorter and wider than in the older child or adult (Fig. 34-8). The tube is also straighter, thereby allowing nasopharyngeal secretions to enter the middle ear more easily. *Haemophilus influenzae* is an important causative agent of otitis media in infants and children.

Clinical Manifestations

A restless infant who repeatedly shakes the head and rubs or pulls at one ear should be checked for an ear infection. These behaviors often indicate that the infant is having pain in the ears. Older children can express and describe the pain they are experiencing. In addition to pain, symptoms may include fever, irritability, and hearing impairment. Vomiting or diarrhea may occur.

Diagnosis

Examination of the ear with an otoscope is done in the infant by pulling the ear down and back to straighten the ear canal. In the older child, the ear is pulled up and back. The exam reveals a bright-red, bulging eardrum in otitis media. Spontaneous rupture of the eardrum may occur, in which case there will be purulent drainage, and the pain caused by the pressure build-up in the ear will be relieved. If present, purulent

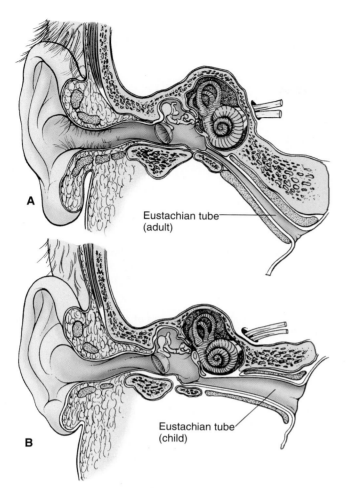

● *Figure 34.8* Comparison of the eustachian tube in the adult (*A*) and the infant (*B*).

drainage is cultured to determine the causative organism and appropriate antibiotic.

Treatment and Nursing Care

Antibiotics are used during the period of infection and for several days after to prevent mastoiditis or chronic infection. A 10-day course of amoxicillin is a common treatment. Most children respond well to antibiotics.

Some children have repeated episodes of otitis media. Children with chronic otitis media may be put on a prophylactic course of an oral penicillin or sulfonamide drug. **Myringotomy** (incision of the eardrum) may be performed to establish drainage and to insert tiny tubes into the tympanic membrane to facilitate drainage. In most cases, the tubes eventually fall out spontaneously. Attention to chronic otitis media is essential because permanent hearing loss can result from frequent occurrences.

Mastoiditis, infection of the mastoid sinus, is a possible complication of untreated acute otitis media. Mastoiditis was much more common before the advent of antibiotics. Currently it is seen only in children who have an untreated ruptured eardrum or inadequate treatment (through noncompliance of caregivers or improper care) of an acute episode.

Most infants and children with otitis media are cared for at home; therefore, a primary responsibility of the nurse is to teach the family caregivers about prevention and the care of the child (see Family Teaching Tips: Otitis Media).

FAMILY TEACHING TIPS

Otitis Media

The eustachian is a connection between the nasal passages and the middle ear. The eustachian tube is wider, shorter, and straighter in the infant, allowing organisms from respiratory infections to travel into the middle ear to cause infection (otitis media).

PREVENTION

• Hold infant in an upright position or with head slightly elevated while feeding to prevent formula from draining into the middle ear through the wide eustachian tube.
• Never prop a bottle.
• Do not give infant a bottle in bed. This allows fluid to pool in the middle ear, encouraging organisms to grow.
• Protect child from exposure to others with upper respiratory infections.
• Protect child from passive smoke; don't permit smoking in child's presence.
• Remove sources of allergies from the home.
• Observe for clues to ear infection: shaking head, rubbing or pulling at ears, fever, combined with restlessness or screaming and crying.
• Be alert to signs of hearing difficulty in toddlers and preschoolers. This may be the first sign of an ear infection.
• Teach toddler or preschooler gentle nose blowing.

CARE OF CHILD WITH OTITIS MEDIA

• Have child with upper respiratory infection who shows symptoms of ear discomfort checked by a health care professional.
• Complete the entire amount of antibiotic prescribed, even though the child seems better.
• Use heat (such as a heating pad on low setting) to provide comfort, but an adult must stay with the child.
• Soothe, rock, and comfort child to help relieve discomfort. The child is more comfortable sleeping on side of infected ear.
• Give pain medications (such as acetaminophen) as directed. Never give aspirin.
• Provide liquid or soft foods; chewing causes pain.
• Know that hearing loss may last up to 6 months after infection.
• Schedule follow-up with hearing test as advised.

INSERTION OF FOREIGN BODIES INTO THE EAR OR NOSE

Children, especially toddlers and preschool-age children, may insert small objects into their ears or noses.

This is important and can be dangerous! Children often put small objects such as peas or beans, crumpled paper, beads, and small toys into their ears or noses.

Irrigation of the ear may remove small objects, except paper, which becomes impacted as it absorbs moisture. The physician generally uses small forceps to remove objects not dislodged by irrigation.

The child may have placed a foreign body in the nose just inside the nares, but manipulation may push it in further. If the object remains in the nose for any length of time, infection may occur. When the object is discovered, a care provider should inspect with a speculum and remove the object.

TABLE 34.2	Staging of Reye Syndrome
Stage	**Symptoms Seen in Stage**
Stage I	Lethargic, vomiting, follows verbal commands, normal posture
Stage II	Combative or stuporous, inappropriate verbalizing, normal posture
Stage III	Comatose, decorticate posture and response to pain
Stage IV	Comatose, decerebrate posture and response to pain
Stage V	Comatose, flaccid, seizures, no papillary response, no response to pain

Adapted from the National Institutes of Health Staging System, Louis, P. T. (1999). Reye syndrome. In *Oski's pediatrics: Principles and practice* (3rd ed). Philadelphia: Lippincott Williams & Wilkins.

REYE SYNDROME

Reye syndrome (rhymes with "eye") is characterized by acute encephalopathy and fatty degeneration of the liver and other abdominal organs. It occurs in children of all ages but is seen more frequently in young school-age children than in any other age group. Reye syndrome usually occurs after a viral illness, particularly after an upper respiratory infection or varicella (chickenpox). Administration of aspirin during the viral illness has been implicated as a contributing factor. As a result, the American Academy of Pediatrics recommends that aspirin or aspirin compounds not be given to children with viral infections.

Clinical Manifestations

The symptoms appear within 3 to 5 days after the initial illness. The child is recuperating unremarkably when symptoms of severe vomiting, irritability, lethargy, and confusion occur. Immediate intervention is needed to prevent serious insult to the brain, including respiratory arrest (Table 34-2).

Diagnosis

The history of a viral illness is an immediate clue. Liver function tests, including aspartate aminotransferase (AST; serum glutamic oxaloacetic transaminase [SGOT]), alanine aminotransferase (ALT; serum glutamic pyruvic transaminase (SGPT]), lactic dehydrogenase (LDH), and serum ammonia levels, are elevated because of poor liver function. The child is hypoglycemic and has delayed prothrombin time.

Treatment and Nursing Care

The child with Reye syndrome often is cared for in the intensive care unit because the disease may rapidly progress. Medical management focuses on supportive measures—improving respiratory function, reducing cerebral edema, and controlling hypoglycemia. The specific treatment is determined by the staging of the symptoms (refer to Table 34-2). The nurse carefully observes the child for overall physical status and any change in neurologic status. This is essential in evaluating the progression of the illness. Accurate intake and output determinations are necessary to determine when fluids need to be adjusted to control cerebral edema and prevent dehydration. Osmotic diuretics (e.g., mannitol) may be administered to reduce cerebral edema. The nurse monitors the blood glucose level and bleeding time. Low blood glucose levels can lead to seizures quickly in young children, and a prolonged bleeding time can indicate coagulation problems as a result of liver dysfunction.

This hospitalization period is a traumatic time for family members, so the nurse must give them opportunities to deal with their feelings. In addition, the family must be kept well informed about the child's care. Having a child in intensive care is a frightening experience, and every effort must be made to reassure the family with sincerity and honesty.

Since the American Academy of Pediatrics made its recommendation to avoid giving aspirin to children, especially during viral illnesses, the number of cases of Reye syndrome has steadily decreased. The prognosis for children with Reye syndrome is greatly improved with early diagnosis and vigorous treatment. The nurse is responsible for teaching family caregivers to avoid the use of aspirin.

Don't! Don't give children aspirin, especially if they have a viral illness.

HAEMOPHILUS INFLUENZAE *MENINGITIS*

Purulent meningitis in infancy and childhood is caused by a variety of agents, including meningococci, the tubercle bacillus, and the *Haemophilus influenzae* type B bacillus. Of these, the most common form is *H. influenzae* meningitis. Transmission of the infection varies. For example, meningococcal and *H. influenzae* meningitis are spread by means of droplet infection from an infected person; all other forms are contracted by invasion of the meninges via the bloodstream from an infection elsewhere.

Peak occurrence of *H. influenzae* meningitis is between the ages of 6 and 12 months. It is rare during the first 2 months of life and is seldom seen after the 4th year. Purulent meningitis is an infectious disease. In addition to standard precautions, droplet transmission precautions should be observed for 24 hours after the start of effective antimicrobial therapy or until pathogens can no longer be cultured from nasopharyngeal secretions. Current immunizations include the Hib vaccine, given at 2 months and repeated at 4, 6, and 12 months, which offers protection against the bacterium. (See Chapter 23, Table 23-4.)

Clinical Manifestations

The onset may be either gradual or abrupt after an upper respiratory infection. Children with meningitis may have a characteristic high-pitched cry, fever, and irritability. Other symptoms include headache, **nuchal rigidity** (stiff neck) that may progress to **opisthotonos** (arching of the back), and delirium. Projectile vomiting may be present. Generalized convulsions are common in children. Coma may occur early, particularly in the older child. Meningococcal meningitis, which tends to occur as epidemics in older children, produces a **purpuric rash** (caused by bleeding under the skin) in addition to the other symptoms.

Diagnosis

Early diagnosis and treatment are essential for uncomplicated recovery. A lumbar puncture (spinal tap) is performed promptly whenever symptoms raise a suspicion of meningitis. For accurate results, the procedure is done before antibiotics are administered. The nurse assists by holding the child in the proper position (Fig. 34-9). The spinal fluid is under increased pressure, and laboratory examination of the fluid reveals increased protein and decreased glucose content. Early in the disease, the spinal fluid may be clear, but it rapidly becomes purulent. The causative organism usually can be determined from stained smears of the spinal fluid, enabling specific medication to be started early without waiting for growths of organisms on culture media.

Treatment

The child is initially isolated and treatment is started using intravenous (IV) administration of antibiotics. Third-generation cephalosporins, such as ceftriaxone

A

B

● *Figure 34.9* Two positions for a lumbar puncture. (**A**) Knee-chest position for young infant. The nurse can hold the infant securely. (**B**) Sitting position. Small infant is held in a sitting position, the knees flexed on the abdomen, and the nurse holds the elbow and knee in each hand, flexing the spine.

(Rocephin), are commonly used, often in combination with other antibiotics. Antibiotics chosen for treatment depend on sensitivity studies. Later in the disease, medications may be given orally. Treatment depends on the progress of the condition and continues as long as there is fever or signs of subdural effusion or otitis media. The administration of IV steroids early in the course has decreased the incidence of deafness as a complication. If seizures occur, anticonvulsants are often given.

Subdural effusion may complicate the condition in children during the course of the disease. Fluid accumulates in the subdural space between the dura and the brain. Needle aspiration through the open suture lines in the infant or bur holes in the skull of the older child are used to remove the fluid. Repeated aspirations may be required.

Complications of *H. influenzae* meningitis with long-term implications are hydrocephalus, nerve deafness, mental retardation, and paralysis. The risk of complications is lessened when appropriate medication is started early in the disease.

Test Yourself

- What is the physiologic reason otitis media occurs more often in young children than in older children and adults?

- What has greatly decreased the incidence of Reye syndrome?

- How can *H. influenzae* meningitis be prevented?

● Nursing Process for the Child With Meningitis

ASSESSMENT

The child with meningitis is obviously extremely sick, and the anxiety level of the family caregivers is understandably high. Be patient and sensitive to their feelings when doing an interview. Obtain a complete history with particular emphasis on the present illness, including any recent upper respiratory infection or middle ear infection. Information on other children in the family and their ages is also important.

The physical exam of the child includes obtaining temperature, pulse, and respirations; use a neurologic evaluation tool to monitor neurologic status, including the child's level of

consciousness (see the section on neurologic evaluation, Chapter 28). Examine the infant for a bulging fontanelle and measure the head circumference for a baseline. Perform this exam after the lumbar puncture is completed and IV fluids and antibiotics are initiated because those procedures take precedence over everything else.

SELECTED NURSING DIAGNOSES

- Decreased Intracranial Adaptive Capacity related to infection and seizure activity
- Risk for Aspiration related to decreased level of consciousness
- Risk for Injury related to seizure activity
- Risk for Deficient Fluid Volume related to vomiting, fever, and fluid restrictions
- Excess Fluid Volume related to syndrome of inappropriate antidiuretic hormone
- Deficient Knowledge of family caregivers related to airborne transmission exposure to others
- Compromised Family Coping related to the child's condition and prognosis

OUTCOME IDENTIFICATION AND PLANNING

The goals for the child with meningitis include monitoring for complications related to neurologic compromise, preventing aspiration, keeping the child safe from injury during a seizure, and monitoring fluid balance. The goals for the family include teaching ways of preventing the transmission of infection and promoting family coping. Plan the nursing care according to these goals. Include interventions such as eliminating the infection by administering antibiotics and observing for signs of increased intracranial pressure.

IMPLEMENTATION

Monitoring for Complications
Because of the child's neurologic status, the child is closely monitored for signs of increased intracranial pressure (IICP), including increased head size, headache, bulging fontanelle, decreased pulse, vomiting, seizures, high-pitched cry, increased blood pressure, change in eyes, level of consciousness or in pupil response, and irritability or other behavioral changes. Vital signs also require close monitoring. An increase in blood pressure, decrease in pulse, change in neurologic signs, or signs of respiratory distress must be reported at once. Measure the infant's head circumference at least every 4 hours to detect complications of subdural effusion or obstructive hydrocephalus. The child's room

should be quiet and darkened to decrease stimulation that may cause seizures. While in the room, speak softly, avoid sudden movements, move quietly, and raise and lower side rails carefully. The head of the bed can be elevated.

Preventing Aspiration

Position the child in a side-lying position with the neck supported for comfort and the head elevated. Remove pillows, blankets, and soft toys that might obstruct the airway. Watch for and remove excessive mucus as much as possible. Use suction sparingly.

Promoting Safety

Keep the child under close observation. Implement seizure precautions and observe the child for seizure activity. At least every 2 hours monitor vital signs, neurologic signs, and observe for change only in level of consciousness. Pad the crib sides, and keep sharp or hard items out of the crib.

Don't forget. During a seizure stay with the child, protect the child from injury, but *DO NOT* restrain him or her.

Loosen any tight clothing (see Nursing Process for the Child at Risk for Seizures later in this chapter).

Monitoring Fluid Balance

Fluid balance is an important aspect of this child's care. Strict intake and output measurements are critical. Methods of reducing fever may be used as needed. Administer IV fluids while observing and monitoring the IV infusion site and following safety precautions to maintain the site.

The infectious process may increase secretion of the antidiuretic hormone produced by the posterior pituitary gland. As a result, the child may not excrete urine adequately, and body fluid volume excess will occur, further emphasizing the need for strict measurement of intake and output. Also monitor daily weight and electrolyte levels. Signs for concern that must be reported immediately are decreased urinary output, hyponatremia, increased weight, nausea, and irritability. The child is placed on fluid restrictions if these signs occur.

Providing Family Teaching Regarding Spread of Infection

H. influenzae is a highly contagious organism that may spread to other people by means of droplet transmission. Droplet transmission precautions must be maintained for the first 24 hours after the antibiotic is administered. Staff members and family caregivers must follow proper precautions, including standard precautions. Meticulous handwashing also is key. Other children in the family may need to be examined to determine if they should receive prophylactic antibiotics.

Promoting Family Coping

Teach the caregivers isolation procedures and good handwashing technique and encourage them to stay with their child, if possible. Support family caregivers through every step of the process. Their anxiety about procedures, the child's seizures and condition, and the possible complications are all serious concerns. Family caregivers must be included and made to feel useful. If they are not too apprehensive, help them find small things they can do for their child. Keep them advised about the child's progress at all times.

EVALUATION: GOALS AND EXPECTED OUTCOMES

- **Goal:** The child will have a normal neurologic status.
  Expected Outcome: The child's vital signs are within normal limits and neurologic status is stable.
- **Goal:** The child's airway will remain patent and clear.
  Expected Outcome: The child's position is side-lying with neck supported and head elevated; airway remains patent with no aspiration of saliva or vomitus.
- **Goal:** The child will remain free from injury.
  Expected Outcome: The child is free from bruises, abrasions, concussions, or fractures during seizure activity.
- **Goal:** The child will maintain normal fluid balance.
  Expected Outcome: The child's intake and output are within normal limits; temperature is 98.6°F to 100° F (37°C to 37.8°C); there are no signs of dehydration.
- **Goal:** The child will maintain normal weight and have adequate urinary output.
  Expected Outcome: The child's weight and electrolyte levels are within normal limits; hourly urine output is 2 to 3 mL/kg.
- **Goal:** The family caregivers follow measures to prevent the transmission of *H. influenzae* bacteria to others.
  Expected Outcome: The family caregivers identify measures for preventing the spread of bacteria and discuss the need for isolation of the ill child.
- **Goal:** The family caregivers' anxiety will decrease.

Expected Outcome: The family caregivers verbalize understanding of the disease process and relate the child's progress throughout the crisis.

ACUTE OR NONRECURRENT SEIZURES

A seizure (convulsion) may be a symptom of a wide variety of disorders. In children between the age of 6 months and 3 years, **febrile seizures** are the most common. Febrile seizures usually occur in the form of a generalized seizure early in the course of a fever. Although commonly associated with high fever (102°F to 106°F [38.9°C to 41.1°C]), some children appear to have a low seizure threshold and convulse when a fever of 100°F to 102°F (37.8°C to 38.9°C) is present. These seizures are often one of the initial symptoms of an acute infection somewhere in the body.

Less common causes of convulsions are intracranial infections, such as meningitis, toxic reactions to certain drugs or minerals such as lead, metabolic disorders, and various brain disorders.

Clinical Manifestations

A seizure may occur suddenly without warning; however, restlessness and irritability may precede an episode. The body stiffens, and the child loses consciousness. In a few seconds, clonic movements occur. These movements are quick, jerking movements of the arms, legs, and facial muscles. Breathing is irregular, and the child cannot swallow saliva.

Diagnosis

Immediate treatment is based on the presenting symptoms. Further evaluation is made after the urgency of the seizure has passed.

Treatment

Emergency care to protect the child during the seizure is the primary concern. If the seizure activity continues, diazepam (Valium) may be administered IV to control the seizure. Acetaminophen is administered to reduce the temperature.

● Nursing Process for the Child at Risk for Seizures

ASSESSMENT

During the family caregiver interview, ask about any history of seizure activity. Have the care-givers describe any previous episodes, including the child's temperature, how the child behaved immediately before the seizure, movements during the seizure, and any other information they believe to be relevant. Ask about the presence of any fever during the present illness and any indications of seizure activity before this admission. Promptly institute seizure precautions. A child whose fever or other symptoms indicate that a seizure may be anticipated should be placed under constant observation.

During the physical exam, obtain a baseline temperature. Using a neurologic tool, observe the child's neurologic status, and make other observations appropriate for the present illness.

Selected Nursing Diagnoses
- Risk for Aspiration during seizure related to decreased level of consciousness
- Risk for Injury related to uncontrolled muscular activity during seizure
- Compromised Family Coping related to the child's seizure activity
- Deficient Knowledge of caregivers related to seizure prevention and precautions during seizures

OUTCOME IDENTIFICATION AND PLANNING

The immediate goals for the child during a seizure are preventing aspiration and preventing injury. Goals for the family include promoting coping and increasing knowledge about seizures. With safety in mind, develop the nursing plan of care according to these goals.

IMPLEMENTATION

Preventing Aspiration
When convulsions begin, position the child to one side to prevent aspiration of saliva or vomitus. Remove blankets, pillows, or other items that may block the child's airway. Oxygen and suction equipment must be readily available for emergency use.

Do you know the why of it? If a child has a seizure, do not put anything in the child's mouth.

Promoting Safety
Keep the child who has a history of seizures under close observation. Pad the crib sides, and keep sharp or hard items out of the crib. Do not, however, completely hide the view of the surroundings outside the crib because this could

make the child feel isolated. During the seizure, stay with the child to protect, but not restrain, him or her. Loosen any tight clothing. If the child is not in bed when the seizure starts, move him or her to a flat surface.

Document the seizure completely after the episode. Document the type of movements (rigidity, jerking, twitching), the body parts involved, the duration of the seizure, pulse and respirations, the child's color, and any deviant eye movements or other notable signs.

Promoting Family Coping

A convulsion or seizure is very frightening to family caregivers. With a calm, confident attitude, reassure caregivers that the child is in good hands. Explain that febrile seizures are not uncommon in small children. Reassure caregivers that the provider will evaluate the child to determine if the seizure has any cause other than nervous system irritation resulting from the high fever.

Providing Family Teaching

Teach family caregivers seizure precautions so that they can handle a seizure that occurs at home. Also instruct them on what observations to make during a seizure so that they can report these to the physician to help in evaluating the child. Explain methods to control fever, cautioning caregivers to avoid using aspirin for fever reduction. Refer to Family Teaching Tips: Reducing Fever, in Chapter 30, when teaching caregivers how to reduce fevers at home.

EVALUATION: GOALS AND EXPECTED OUTCOMES

- **Goal:** The child's airway will remain patent throughout the seizure.
  Expected Outcome: The child's airway is patent with no aspiration of saliva or vomitus.
- **Goal:** The child will remain free from injury during the seizure.
  Expected Outcome: The child is free from bruises, abrasions, concussions, or fractures after the seizure.
- **Goal:** The family caregivers' anxiety will be reduced.
  Expected Outcome: The family caregivers verbalize their concerns and relate an understanding of febrile seizures.
- **Goal:** The family caregivers will verbalize an understanding of seizure precautions.
  Expected Outcome: The family caregivers state methods to reduce fevers and handle seizures at home.

SEIZURE DISORDERS

Seizure disorders, also referred to as convulsive disorders, are common in children and may result from a variety of causes. A common form of seizures is the acute febrile seizure that occurs with fevers and acute infections. Epilepsy, on the other hand, is a recurrent and chronic seizure disorder. Epilepsy can be classified as primary (idiopathic), with no known cause, or secondary, resulting from infection, head trauma, hemorrhage, tumor, or other organic or degenerative factors. Primary epilepsy is the most common; its onset generally is between ages 4 and 8 years.

Clinical Manifestations

Seizures are the characteristic clinical manifestation of both types of epilepsy and may be either partial (focal) or generalized. **Partial** seizures are limited to a particular area of the brain; generalized seizures involve both hemispheres of the brain.

Partial Seizures

Manifestations of partial seizures vary depending on the area of the brain from which they arise. Loss of consciousness or awareness may not occur. Partial seizures are classified as simple partial motor, simple partial sensory, or complex partial (psychomotor).

Simple Partial Seizures
Simple partial motor seizures cause a localized motor activity such as shaking of an arm, leg, or other part of the body. These may be limited to one side of the body or may spread to other parts.

Simple partial sensory seizures may include sensory symptoms called an **aura** (a sensation that signals an impending attack) involving sight, sound, taste, smell, touch, or emotions (a feeling of fear, for example). The child may also have numbness, tingling, paresthesia, or pain.

Complex Partial Seizures
Complex partial seizures, also called psychomotor seizures, also begin in a small area of the brain and change or alter consciousness. They cause memory loss and staring. Nonpurposeful movements, such as hand rubbing, lip smacking, arm dropping, and swallowing, may occur. After the seizure the child may sleep or be confused for a few minutes. The child is often unaware of the seizure. These can be the most difficult seizures to control.

Generalized Seizures

Types of generalized seizures include tonic-clonic (formerly called grand mal), **absence** (formerly called petit mal), atonic or akinetic (formerly called "drop attacks"), myoclonic, and infantile spasms.

Tonic-Clonic Seizures

Tonic-clonic seizures consist of four stages: the prodromal period, which can be days or hours; the aura, which is a warning, immediately before the seizure; the tonic-clonic movements; and the postictal stage. Not all these stages occur with every seizure: the seizure may just begin with a sudden loss of consciousness. During the prodromal period the child might be drowsy, dizzy, or have a lack of coordination. If the seizure is preceded by an aura, it is identified as a generalized seizure secondary to a partial seizure. The aura may reflect in which part of the brain the seizure originates. Young children may have difficulty describing an aura but may cry out in response to it. In the tonic phase the child's muscles contract, the child may fall, and the child's extremities may stiffen. The contraction of respiratory muscles during the tonic phase may cause the child to become cyanotic and appear briefly to have respiratory arrest. The eyes roll upward and the child might utter a guttural cry. The initial rigidity of the tonic phase changes rapidly to generalized jerking muscle movements in the clonic phase. The child may bite the tongue or lose control of bladder and bowel functions. The jerking movements gradually diminish then disappear, and the child relaxes. The seizure can be brief, lasting less than 1 minute, or it can last 30 minutes or longer. The period after the tonic-clonic phase is called the postictal period. The child may sleep soundly for several hours during this stage or return rapidly to an alert state. Many have a period of confusion, and others experience a prolonged period of stupor.

Absence Seizures

Absence seizures rarely last longer than 20 seconds. The child loses awareness and stares straight ahead but does not fall. The child may have blinking or twitching of the mouth or an extremity along with the staring. Immediately after the seizure, the child is alert and continues conversation but does not know what was said or done during the episode. Absence seizures can recur frequently, sometimes as often as 50 to 100 a day. If seizures are not fully controlled, the caregiver needs to be especially aware of dangerous situations that might occur in the child's day such as crossing a street on the way to school. These seizures often decrease significantly or stop entirely at adolescence.

Atonic or Akinetic Seizures

These cause a sudden momentary loss of consciousness, muscle tone, and postural control and can cause the child to fall. They can result in serious facial, head, or shoulder injuries. They may recur frequently, particularly in the morning. After the seizure the child can stand and walk as normal.

Myoclonic Seizures

Myoclonic seizures are characterized by a sudden jerking of a muscle or group of muscles, often in the arms or legs without loss of consciousness. Myoclonus occurs during the early stages of falling asleep in people who do not have epilepsy.

Infantile Spasms

Infantile spasms occur between 3 and 12 months of age, almost always indicate a cerebral defect, and have a poor prognosis despite treatment. These seizures occur twice as often in boys as in girls and are preceded or followed by a cry. Muscle contractions are sudden, brief, symmetric, and accompanied by rolling eyes. Loss of consciousness does not always occur.

Status Epilepticus

Status epilepticus is the term used to describe a seizure that lasts longer than 30 minutes or a series of seizures in which the child does not return to his or her previous normal level of consciousness.

This advice could be a life-saver. Status epilepticus is an emergency situation and requires immediate treatment.

Immediate treatment will decrease the likelihood of permanent brain injury, respiratory failure, or even death.

Diagnosis

The types of seizures can be differentiated through the use of EEG (electroencephalography), video and ambulatory EEG, skull radiography, CT (computed tomography), MRI (magnetic resonance imaging), a brain scan, and physical and neurologic assessments. The child's seizure history is an important part of determining the diagnosis.

Treatment

The main goal of treatment, complete control of seizures, can be achieved for most people through the use of anticonvulsant drug therapy. A number of anticonvulsant drugs are available (see Table 34-3). The choice of drug is made based on its effectiveness in controlling seizures and side effects and on its degree of toxicity. Chewable or tablet forms of the medications are often used because suspensions separate and sometimes are not shaken well, causing the possibility of inaccurate dosage. The oldest and most popular drug is phenytoin (Dilantin). It can cause hypertrophy of the gums (gingival hyperplasia) after prolonged use.

A few children may be candidates for surgical intervention when the focal point of the seizures is in an area of the brain that is accessible surgically and is

TABLE 34.3 Antiepileptic-Anticonvulsive Therapeutic Agents

Drug	Indication	Side Effects	Nursing Implications
Carbamazepine (Tegretol)	Generalized tonic-clonic, simple partial, complex partial	Drowsiness, dry mouth, vomiting, double vision, leukopenia, GI upset, thrombocytopenia	There may be dizziness and drowsiness with initial doses. This should subside within 3–14 days.
Clonazepam (Klonopin)	Absence seizures, generalized tonic-clonic, myoclonic, simple partial, complex partial	Double vision, drowsiness, increased salivation, changes in behavior, bone marrow depression	Obtain periodic liver function tests and complete blood count. Monitor for drowsiness, lethargy.
Ethosuximide (Zarontin)	Absence seizures, myoclonic	Dry mouth, anorexia, dizziness, headache, nausea, vomiting, GI upset, lethargy, bone marrow depression	Use with caution in hepatic or renal disease.
Phenobarbital (Luminol)	Generalized tonic-clonic, myoclonic, simple partial, complex partial	Drowsiness, alteration in sleep patterns, irritability, respiratory and cardiac depression, restlessness, headache	Alcohol can enhance the effects of phenobarbital. Monitor blood levels of drug. Liver function studies are necessary with prolonged use.
Phenytoin (Dilantin)	Generalized tonic-clonic, simple partial, complex partial	Double vision, blurred vision, slurred speech, nystagmus, ataxia, gingival hyperplasia, hirsutism, cardiac arrhythmias, bone marrow depression	Alcohol, antacids, and folic acid decrease the effect of phenytoin. Instruct the child or caregiver to notify the dentist that he or she is taking phenytoin to monitor hyperplasia of the gums. Inform the child or caregiver that the drug may color the urine pink to red-brown.
Primidone (Mysoline)	Generalized tonic-clonic, simple partial, complex partial	Behavior changes, drowsiness, hyperactivity, ataxia, bone marrow depression	Adverse effects are the same as for phenobarbital. Sedation and dizziness may be severe during initial therapy; dosage may need to be adjusted by the physician.
Valproic acid (Depakene)	Absence, generalized tonic-clonic, myoclonic, simple partial, complex partial	Nausea, vomiting, or increased appetite, tremors, elevated liver enzymes, constipation, headaches, depression, lymphocytosis, leukopenia, increased prothrombin time	Physical dependency may result when used for prolonged period. Tablets and capsules should be taken whole. Elixir should be taken alone, not mixed with carbonated beverages. Increased toxicity may occur with administration of salicylates (aspirin).

General Nursing Considerations With Anticonvulsant Therapy
General nursing considerations with anticonvulsant therapy that apply to all or most of drugs given to children include:
1. Warn the patient and family that patients should avoid activities that require alertness and complex psychomotor coordination (e.g., climbing).
2. Medication can be given with meals to minimize gastric irritation.
3. The anticonvulsant medications should not be discontinued abruptly as this can precipitate status epilepticus.
4. Anticonvulsant medications generally have a cumulative effect, both therapeutically and adversely.
5. Alcohol ingestion increases the effects of anticonvulsant drugs, exaggerating central nervous system depression.
6. Many of the drugs can cause bone marrow depression (leukopenia, thrombocytopenia, neutropenia, megaloblastic anemia). Regular complete blood cell counts, including WBCs, RBCs, and platelets, are necessary to evaluate bone marrow production.
7. The child should receive periodic blood tests to monitor therapeutic levels as opposed to toxic levels.

not an area critical to functioning. If the cause of the seizures is a tumor or other lesion, surgical removal is sometimes possible.

Ketogenic diets (high in fat and low in carbohydrates and protein) cause the child to have high levels of ketones, which helps to reduce seizure activity. These diets are prescribed, but long-term maintenance is difficult because the diets are difficult to follow and are unappealing to the child.

Nursing Care

In the hospital or home setting, keeping the child safe during a seizure is the highest priority. The caregiver of a child who has a seizure disorder needs to be taught how to prevent injury if the child has a seizure (see Family Teaching Tips: Precautions Before and During Seizures). In the hospital setting, the side rails are padded; objects that could cause harm are kept away from the bed; oxygen and suction are kept at the bedside; and the side rails are in the raised position and the bed lowered when the child is sleeping or resting.

If the child begins having a seizure, the child is placed on her or his side with the head turned toward one side. The nurse stays calm and removes any objects from around the child, protects the child's head, and loosens tight clothing. During the seizure, the nurse notes

- Time the seizure started
- What the child was doing when the seizure began
- Any factor present just before the seizure (bright light, noise)
- Part of the body where seizure activity began
- Movement and parts of the body involved
- Any cyanosis
- Eye position and movement
- Incontinence of urine or stool
- Time seizure ended
- Child's activity after the seizure

When the seizure is over, the nurse should monitor the child, closely paying attention to his or her level of consciousness, motor functions, and behavior. The nurse documents the information noted during the seizure activity.

Be sure to ask. The child may be able to describe the aura or sensation that occurred just before a seizure.

If the child is able to describe the aura, this information is important to document.

Education and counseling of the child and the family caregivers are important parts of nursing care. They need complete, accurate information about the disorder and the results that can be realistically expected from treatment. Epilepsy does not lead inevitably to mental retardation, but continued and uncontrolled seizures do increase its possibility. Thus, early diagnosis and control of seizures are very important.

Although the outlook for a normal, well-adjusted life is favorable, the nurse should inform the child and family about restrictions that may be encountered. Children with epilepsy should be encouraged to participate in physical activities but should not participate in sports in which a fall could cause serious injury. In many states a person with uncontrolled epilepsy is legally forbidden to drive a motor vehicle; this could limit choice of vocation and lifestyle. Despite attempts to educate the general public about epilepsy, many people remain prejudiced about this disorder, and this can limit the epileptic person's social and vocational acceptance.

CEREBRAL PALSY

Cerebral palsy (CP) is a group of disorders arising from a malfunction of motor centers and neural pathways in the brain. It is one of the most complex of the common permanent disabling conditions and often can be accom-

---

FAMILY TEACHING TIPS

Precautions Before and During Seizures

BEFORE

- Have child swim with a companion.
- Have child use protective helmet and padding for bicycle riding, skate boarding.
- Supervise when using power equipment.
- Carry or wear medical ID bracelet.
- Discuss the child's condition with teachers and school nurse.
- Know factors that trigger seizure activity.

DURING

- Stay calm.
- Move furniture or objects that could cause injury.
- Turn child on side with head turned to one side.
- Remove glasses.
- Protect child's head.
- Don't restrain.
- Don't try to put anything between child's teeth.
- Keep people from crowding around child.
- After seizure, notify care provider for follow-up.
- If seizures continue without stopping, call for emergency help.

panied by seizures, mental retardation, sensory defects, and behavior disorders. Research in this area is directed at adapting biomedical technology to help people with cerebral palsy cope with the activities of daily living and achieve maximum function and independence.

Causes

Although the cause of CP cannot be identified in many cases, several causes are possible. It may be caused by damage to the parts of the brain that control movement; this damage generally occurs during the fetal or perinatal period, particularly in premature infants.

Common *prenatal* causes are

- Any process that interferes with the oxygen supply to the brain, such as separation of the placenta, compression of the cord, or bleeding
- Maternal infection (e.g., cytomegalovirus, toxoplasmosis, rubella)
- Nutritional deficiencies that may affect brain growth
- Kernicterus (brain damage caused by jaundice) resulting from Rh incompatibility
- Teratogenic factors such as drugs and radiation

Common *perinatal* causes are

- Anoxia immediately before, during, and after birth
- Intracranial bleeding
- Asphyxia or interference with respiratory function
- Maternal analgesia (e.g., morphine) that depresses the sensitive neonate's respiratory center
- Birth trauma
- Prematurity because immature blood vessels predispose the neonate to cerebral hemorrhage

About 10% to 20% of cases occur after birth. Common *postnatal* causes are

- Head trauma (e.g., due to a fall, motor vehicle accident)
- Infection (e.g., encephalitis, meningitis)
- Neoplasms
- Cerebrovascular accident

Prevention

Because brain damage in CP is irreversible, prevention is the most important aspect of care. Prevention of CP focuses on

- Prenatal care to improve nutrition, prevent infection, and decrease the incidence of prematurity
- Perinatal monitoring with appropriate interventions to decrease birth trauma
- Postnatal prevention of infection through breastfeeding, improved nutrition, and immunizations
- Protection from trauma of motor vehicle accidents, child abuse, and other childhood accidents

Clinical Manifestations and Types

Difficulty in controlling voluntary muscle movements is one manifestation of the central nervous system damage. Seizures, mental retardation, hearing and vision impairments, and behavior disorders often accompany the major problem. Delayed gross motor development, abnormal motor performance (e.g., poor sucking and feeding behaviors), abnormal postures, and persistence of primitive reflexes are other signs of CP. Diagnosis of CP seldom occurs before 2 months of age and may be delayed until the 2nd or 3rd year, when the toddler attempts to walk and caregivers notice an obvious lag in motor development. Diagnosis is based on observations of delayed growth and development through a process that rules out other diagnoses.

Several major types of CP occur; each has distinctive clinical manifestations.

Spastic Type

This is the most common type and is characterized by

- A hyperactive stretch reflex in associated muscle groups
- Increased activity of the deep tendon reflexes
- **Clonus** (rapid involuntary muscle contraction and relaxation)
- Contractures affecting the extensor muscles, especially the heel cord
- Scissoring caused by severe hip adduction. When scissoring is present, the child's legs are crossed and the toes are pointed down (Fig. 34-10). When standing, the child is on her or his toes. It is difficult for this child to walk on the heels or run.

Athetoid Type

Athetoid CP is marked by involuntary, uncoordinated motion with varying degrees of muscle tension. Children with this disorder are constantly in motion, and

● **Figure 34.10** The physical therapist works with a child who has cerebral palsy. Note the scissoring of the legs.

the whole body is in a state of slow, writing muscle contractions whenever voluntary movement is attempted. Facial grimacing, poor swallowing, and tongue movements causing drooling and **dysarthria** (poor speech articulation) also are present. These children are likely to have average or above-average intelligence, despite their abnormal appearance. Hearing loss is most common in this group.

Ataxic Type

Ataxia is essentially a lack of coordination caused by disturbances in the kinesthetic and balance senses. The least common type of CP, ataxic CP may not be diagnosed until the child starts to walk: the gait is awkward and wide-based.

Rigidity Type

This type is uncommon and is characterized by rigid postures and lack of active movement.

Mixed Type

Children with signs of more than one type of CP, termed mixed type, are usually severely disabled. The disorder may have been caused by postnatal injury.

Diagnosis

Children with CP may not be diagnosed with certainty until they have difficulties when attempting to walk. They may show signs of mental retardation, attention deficit disorder, or recurrent convulsions. Computed tomography, magnetic resonance imaging, and ultrasonography for infants before closure of skull sutures may be used to help determine the cause of CP.

Treatment and Special Aids

Treatment of CP focuses on helping the child to make the best use of residual abilities and achieve maximum satisfaction and enrichment in life. A team of health care professionals—physician, surgeon, physical therapist, occupational therapist, speech therapist, and perhaps a social worker—works with the family to set realistic goals. Dental care is important because enamel hypoplasia is common, and children whose seizure disorders are controlled with phenytoin (Dilantin) are likely to develop gingival hypertrophy. Medications such as baclofen, diazepam, and dantrolene may be used to help decrease spasticity.

Physical Therapy

Body control needed for purposeful physical activity is learned automatically by a normal child but must be consciously learned by a child who has problems with physical mobility (Fig. 34-11). Physical therapists attempt to teach activities of daily living that the child has been unable to accomplish. Methods must be

● *Figure 34.11* During a physical therapy session, this boy with CP works hard to take a step forward. His mom stays by his side to encourage him.

suited to the needs of each child, as well as to the general needs arising from the condition. These methods are based on principles of conditioning, relaxation, use of residual patterns, stimulation of contraction and relaxation of antagonistic muscles, and others. Various techniques are used. Because there are many variations in the disabilities caused by CP, each child must be considered individually and treated appropriately.

Orthopedic Management

Braces are used as supportive and control measures to facilitate muscle training, to reinforce weak or paralyzed muscles, or to counteract the pull of antagonistic muscles. Various types are available; each is designed for a specific purpose. Orthopedic surgery sometimes is used to improve function and to correct deformities, such as the release of contractures and the lengthening of tight heel cords.

Technological Aids for Daily Living

Biomedical engineering, particularly in the field of electronics, has perfected a number of devices to help make the disabled person more functional and less dependent on others. The devices range from simple items, such as wheelchairs and specially constructed toilet seats, to completely electronic cottages furnished with a computer (even including a voice synthesizer), a tape recorder, a calculator, and other equipment that facilitates independence and useful study or work. Many of these devices can be controlled by a mouth

● *Figure 34.12* Feeding techniques to promote jaw control.

stick, which is an extremely useful feature for people with poor hand coordination.

A child who has difficulty maintaining balance while sitting may need a high-backed chair with side pieces and a foot platform. Feeding may be a challenge, so caregivers may need help finding a method that works for feeding their child. Sometimes controlling and stabilizing the jaw will help with feeding (Fig. 34-12). Feeding aids include spoons with enlarged handles for easy grasping or with bent handles that allow the spoon to be brought easily to the mouth. Plates with high rims and suction devices to prevent slipping enable a child to eat with little assistance. Covered cups set in holders with a hole in the lid to admit a straw help a child who does not have hand control (Fig. 34-13). The severely disabled child may need a nasogastric or gastrostomy tube.

Manual skill can be aided by games that must be manipulated, such as pegboards and cards.

Computer programs have been designed to enable these children to communicate and improve their learning skills. Special keyboards, joysticks, and electronic devices help the child to have fun and gain a sense of achievement while learning. Computers also have expanded the opportunities for future employment for these children.

Good news. Keyboarding is an ego-boosting alternative for a child whose disability is too severe to permit legible writing.

Nursing Care

The child with CP may be seen in the health care setting at any age level. Interview and observe the child and the family to determine the child's needs, the level of development, and the stage of family acceptance, and to set realistic long-range goals. The child with a new diagnosis and the family may have more potential nursing diagnoses than the child and family who have been successfully dealing with CP for a long time.

To ease the change of environment, the nurse needs to communicate with the family to learn as much as possible about the child's activities at home. The child should be encouraged to maintain current self-care activities and set goals for attaining new ones. Positioning to prevent contractures, providing modified feeding utensils, and suggesting appropriate educational play activities are all important aspects of the child's care. If the child has been admitted for surgery, the child and family need appropriate preoperative and postoperative teaching, emotional support, and assistance in setting realistic expectations. The family may need help to explore educational opportunities for the child.

Like any chronic condition, CP can become a devastating drain on the family's emotional and financial resources. The child's future depends on many variables: family attitudes; economic and therapeutic resources; the child's intelligence; and the availability of competent, understanding health care professionals. Some children, when given the emotional and physical support they

A   **B**   **C**

● *Figure 34.13* Feeding aids and devices: (**A**) cups; (**B**) utensils; (**C**) dishes.

need, can achieve a satisfactory degree of independence. Some have been able to attend college and find fulfilling work. Vocational training is also available to an increasing number of these young people. Some people with CP will always need a significant amount of nursing care with the possibility of institutionalized care when their families can no longer care for them.

The outlook for these children and their families is improving, but a great deal of work remains to be done. Working as a community member, the health care professional can play a vital role in promoting educational opportunities, rehabilitation, and acceptance for disabled children.

Test Yourself

- What are seven types of seizures seen in children?
- What 10 factors should the nurse document after a seizure?
- What is the difference between the five types of cerebral palsy?

MENTAL RETARDATION

Mental retardation is defined in the *Diagnostic and Statistical Manual of Mental Disorders* (DSM-IV-TR) (American Psychiatric Association, 2000) using two criteria: significantly subaverage general intellectual functioning—an intelligence quotient (IQ) of 70 or lower—and concurrent deficits in adaptive functioning. Adaptive functioning refers to how well people can meet the standards of independence (activities of daily living) and social responsibility expected for their age and the cultural group to which they belong. Mental retardation often occurs in combination with other physical disorders.

Causes

Many factors can cause mental retardation. Prenatal causes include

- Inborn errors of metabolism, such as phenylketonuria, galactosemia, or congenital hypothyroidism. Damage often can be prevented by early detection and treatment.
- Prenatal infection, such as toxoplasmosis or cytomegalovirus. Microcephaly, hydrocephalus, cerebral palsy, and other brain damage can result from intrauterine infections.
- Teratogenic agents, such as drugs, radiation, and alcohol, can have devastating effects on the central nervous system of a developing fetus.
- Genetic factors—inborn variations of chromosomal patterns—result in a variety of deviations, the most common of which is Down syndrome.

Perinatal causes of mental retardation include birth trauma, anoxia from various causes, prematurity, and difficult birth. In some instances, prenatal factors may have influenced the perinatal complications.

Postnatal causes include

- Poisoning such as lead poisoning. Children who develop encephalopathy from chronic lead poisoning usually have significant brain damage.
- Infections and trauma, such as meningitis convulsive disorders, and hydrocephalus.
- Impoverished early environment, such as inadequate nutrition and a lack of sensory stimulation. Emotional rejection in early life may do irreparable damage to a child's ability to respond to the environment.

Clinical Manifestations of the Mentally Retarded Child

About 3% of all children born in the United States have some level of cognitive impairment. About 20% of these are so severely retarded that diagnosis is made at birth or during the 1st year. Most of the other children have retardation diagnosed when they begin school.

The most common classification of mental retardation is based on IQ. Although controversy exists about the validity of tests that measure intelligence, this system is still the most useful for grouping these children.

The child with an IQ of 70 to 50 is considered mildly mentally retarded. This child is a slow learner but can acquire basic skills. The child can learn to read, write, and do arithmetic to a fourth- or fifth-grade level but is slower than average in learning to walk, talk, and feed himself or herself. Retardation may not be obvious to casual acquaintances. With support and guidance, this child usually can develop social and vocational skills adequate for self-maintenance. About 80% of retarded children are classified in this category.

The moderately retarded child with an IQ of 55 to 35 has little, if any, ability to attain independence and academic skills and is referred to as trainable. Motor development and speech are noticeably delayed, but training in self-help activities is possible. This child may be able to learn repetitive skills in sheltered workshops. Some children may learn to travel alone, but few become capable of assuming complete self-maintenance. This category accounts for about 10% of retarded children.

The child considered severely retarded tests in the IQ range of 40 to 20. This child's development is markedly delayed during the 1st year of life. The child cannot learn academic skills but may be able to learn some self-care activities if sensorimotor stimulation is begun early. Eventually this child will probably learn to walk and develop some speech; however, a sheltered environment and careful supervision always will be required.

The profoundly retarded child has an IQ lower than 20. This child has minimal capacity for functioning and needs continuing care. Eventually the child may learn to walk and develop a primitive speech but will never be able to perform self-care activities. Only about 1% of retarded children are in this category.

Treatment and Education

Knowledge about teaching children with cognitive impairment has increased dramatically, and new teaching methods have been yielding encouraging results. Mildly and moderately retarded people are taught to perform tasks that enable them to achieve some degree of independence. More and better services are being provided for all cognitively impaired children and adults.

The child with cognitive impairment may not be identified until well into the preschool stage, because slow development often can be excused in one way or another. The family may be the best judge of the child's development, and health care personnel must listen carefully to any concerns or questions that caregivers express.

When family members are faced with the fact that their child is retarded, they need to go through a grieving process, as do family members of any other child with a serious disorder. They need to mourn the loss of the normal child that was expected and resolve to give this child the best opportunities to develop his or her potential.

A PERSONAL GLIMPSE

The mother of a developmentally delayed child knows her child has a problem before any doctor notices. Visually my son looked perfect. There were no outward signs of retardation. He was a beautiful baby but he was often ill—severe croup, pneumonia, bronchitis, grand mal seizures due to fever, hospital stays, EEGs, spinal taps, tests and more tests—but he always bounced back, much better than his parents recovered.

Slowly I started to notice that he was not the same as other kids his age. His vocabulary was Mom and DaDa where other 3 year olds were starting to put words together into little sentences. Everyone said he didn't talk because I spoiled him and got him everything he needed before he asked for it. I would try to believe people, including doctors, who would say, "Don't worry; you are just being an overprotective mother. Your son will be fine." You try to hide from the truth but slowly you realize you have to get others to see what you see. You have to get help for your child—someone has to listen to you.

Finally I forced my pediatrician to try some physical dexterity tests. My son failed these tests. I heard the doctor say the words that broke my heart: "I am sorry. I thought you were just another hysterical mother—but there is something wrong with your child. We must schedule him for more testing." Then I cried.

Patricia

LEARNING OPPORTUNITY: What are some feelings parents of children diagnosed with mental retardation might have? What are some ways that the nurse can support the mother and the child in the above situation?

Early diagnosis and intervention are important tools to use in the care of the cognitively impaired child. Tests done during infancy are difficult to administer and the results are inaccurate, but they may provide the family with some idea about the child's potential. The family must be aware that these are only predictions based on unreliable test data.

The child is usually kept at home in the family environment. The current philosophy of care for such a child is to approach teaching in an aggressive manner by encouraging learning in a supportive home environment where the child can relate closely to a few people whose role is to stimulate and encourage maximum development. The individual attention, security, and sense of belonging to a family are important factors in every child's growth and development.

● Nursing Process for the Child With Cognitive Impairment

ASSESSMENT

The child who has a cognitive impairment is seen in the health care setting for diagnosis, treatment, and follow-up, as well as the usual health maintenance visits. During these visits, health care personnel may be challenged to communicate with the child. A thorough interview with the child's caregiver can be helpful in learning about the child and family. Listen carefully to the caregiver, paying particular attention to any comments or concerns he or she has.

The interview and physical exam may be lengthy and detailed, depending partially on the circumstances of the child's primary need for health care. Aside from the data collection needed as dictated by the current health care needs, the nurse also needs information about the child's habits, routines, and personal terminology (such as nicknames and toileting terms). Be careful to communicate at the child's level of understanding, and do not talk down to the child during the interview. Treat the child with respect. This approach helps gain cooperation from both the family and the child. Arrange the initial interview and physical exam so that they can be conducted in an unhurried atmosphere that avoids placing undue stress on the child or the family.

SELECTED NURSING DIAGNOSES

- Bathing/Hygiene, Dressing/Grooming, Feeding, and Toileting Self-Care Deficit related to cognitive or neuromuscular impairment (or both)
- Impaired Verbal Communication related to impaired receptive or expressive skills
- Delayed Growth and Development related to physical and mental disability
- Risk for Injury related to physical or neurologic impairment (or both)
- Compromised Family Coping related to emotional stress or grief
- Risk for Social Isolation (family or child) related to fear of and embarrassment about the child's behavior or appearance

OUTCOME IDENTIFICATION AND PLANNING

The major goals for the cognitively impaired child depend entirely on the child's abilities as determined during data collection and the interview. Common goals include promoting self-care (within the child's ability), fostering communication with caregivers and nurses, promoting growth and development to reach the highest level of functioning (within the child's ability), and preventing injury. The goals for the family include promoting family coping and preventing social isolation.

IMPLEMENTATION

Promoting Self-care

Teaching the mentally retarded child can be time-consuming, frustrating, challenging, and rewarding. When the child is first seen in a health care setting, a teaching program that reflects his or her developmental level must be

Most nurses find this approach helpful. Patience is one of the most important aspects of teaching a cognitively impaired child.

designed. Be certain that all personnel who care for the child and any involved family members are aware of the program. Break each element of care to be taught into small segments and repeat those steps over and over.

Use praise generously, and give small material rewards as useful tools to aid in teaching. Challenge the child, but make the immediate small goals realistic and attainable. Brushing teeth, brushing or combing the hair, bathing, washing the hands and face, feeding oneself, dressing independently, and basic safety are all self-care areas in which the child needs instruction and positive reinforcement.

Teaching the cognitively impaired child requires the same principles used in teaching any child: work at a level appropriate to the stage of the child's maturation, not the chronological age. If the child has physical disabilities in addition to retardation, the rate of physical development is also affected. One factor that makes the child with cognitive impairment different from the average child is the lack of ability to reason abstractly. This prevents transfer of learning or application of abstract principles to varied situations. Learning takes place by habit formation and emphasizing the "three Rs": routine, repetition, and relaxation. Most cognitively impaired children increase in mental age, although slowly and to a limited level. Therefore, each child needs to be watched for evidence of readiness for a new skill.

Environmental stimulation is essential for development in all children, but the cognitively impaired child needs much more environmental enrichment than does the average child. Suggested activities for providing this enrichment are summarized in Table 34-4.

Whether at home or in a health care facility, the child with cognitive impairment needs to know which behaviors are acceptable and which are unacceptable. Discipline is as important to this child as to any other. The limited ability of these children to adapt to varying circumstances makes consistent discipline essential, with instructions given in simple, direct, concise language. Using a positive approach with many examples and demonstrations achieves better results than a constant stream of "don't touch" or "stop that."

Obedience is an important part of discipline, especially for the child with faulty reasoning

TABLE 34.4	Examples of Developmental Stimulation and Sensorimotor Teaching for Retarded Infants and Young Children
Developmental Sequence	**Possible Activities to Encourage Development**
Sitting	
1. Sit with support in caregiver's lap	Hold child in sitting position on lap, supporting under armpits. Do several times a day, gradually lessening the support.
2. Sit independently when propped	Place child in sitting position against firm surface with pillow behind the back and on either side. Leave the child alone several times a day.
3. Sit with increasingly less support	Allow child to sit on equipment that provides increasingly less support such as baby swing, feeder, walker, high chair.
4. Sit in chair without assistance	Place child in a chair with arms. Provide balance support at first, then gradually withdraw. Leave for 10 minutes at a time.
5. Sit without support	Place child on floor. Gradually withdraw assistance.
Self-Feeding	
1. Sucking	Encourage child to suck by putting food on pacifier, putting a drop on tongue, and so forth.
2. Drink from a cup	Put small amount of fluid in a baby cup. Raise cup to mouth by placing hands under child.
3. Grasp piece of food and place in mouth	Place bit of favorite food in child's hand. Guide hand and food to mouth. Gradually reduce support.
4. Transfer food from spoon to mouth	Move spoon to child's mouth with hand supporting baby's. Gradually withdraw support.
5. Scoop up food and transfer to mouth	Have child hold spoon by handle, scoop up food, and transfer to mouth. Do not allow child to use fingers. Progress from bowl to flat plate.
Stimulation of Touch	
1. Body sensation	Hold, cuddle, rock child.
2. Explore environment through touch	Brush skin with objects of various textures (feathers, silk, sandpaper). Place objects of different textures near child. Move hand to object.
3. Explore environment through mouth	Give child objects that can be chewed. Guide hand to mouth at first.
4. Explore tactile sensations	Expose child to hard, soft, warm, and cold objects.
5. Explore with water	Place hands or feet in water.

ability, but the objectives of discipline should be much broader than simply obedience. The child needs to know what to expect and finds security and support in routines and consistency. Use kindness, love, understanding, and physical comforting as a major part of discipline.

If discipline is needed, be certain it follows the misdeed immediately so that the cause-and-effect relationship is clear. Taking the child away from the group for a short time may help restore self-control. If the child is using misbehavior to get attention, praise and approval for good behavior may eliminate the need for wrongdoing.

Fostering Communication Skills

The child with cognitive impairment often has major problems with language skills. The child may have problems forming various speech sounds because of an enlarged tongue or other physical deviations, including hearing impairment. These problems can frustrate attempts at communication. In addition, the child may not be able to process the spoken word, which compounds communication problems. A speech therapist can evaluate the child and develop a program to help caregivers work with the child to improve both the child's understanding of what is said and the child's ability to use language.

Promoting Growth and Development
Self-care Deficit

The child with cognitive impairment often has physical disabilities that affect growth and development. All but the most profoundly impaired children go through the sequence of normal development with delays at each stage; their abilities level off as the children reach the limits of their capabilities. A cognitively impaired child proceeds according to mental age, rather than chronological age. Thus, an impaired 6-year-old child may be functioning on a mental level of 2 years, and the expected behavior must be essentially that of a 2-year-old child. Teach the family caregivers about the important landmarks of normal growth and development to help them understand the progressive nature of maturation and to improve planning for the child.

Preventing Injury

The child with cognitive impairment has faulty reasoning ability and a short attention span. As a result, the caregivers must be responsible for protecting the child. The health care facility and the home must be made safe. Teach elementary safety rules and reinforce them continuously.

Promoting Family Coping

Before effective treatment can begin, the family must accept the reality of the child's problem and must want to cope with the difficult task of helping the child develop to his or her full potential. Diagnosis made at birth or during the 1st year affords the greatest hope of early acceptance and beginning education and training.

The family's first reaction to learning that the child may have cognitive impairment is grief because this is not the perfect child of their dreams. A parent may feel shame, assuming that he or she cannot produce a perfect child. Some rejection of the child is almost inevitable, at least in the initial stages, but this must be worked through for the family to cope. Some parents compensate for their early hostile feelings by overprotection or overconcern, making the child unnecessarily helpless and perhaps taking out their anger and frustration on the normal siblings. The family begins to function effectively only when the caregivers accept the child as another family member to be helped, loved, and disciplined.

Preventing Social Isolation

Family members need to know that their feelings are normal. Talking with other families of impaired children can offer some of the best support and guidance as caregivers seek information to help them deal with the problem. One group that includes both families and health care professionals is the National Association of Retarded Citizens, a volunteer organization with chapters in many communities (website http://www.thearc.org). The National Down Syndrome Society is another excellent resource for the family of a child with Down syndrome (website http://www.ndss.org). Participating in the Special Olympics is a good way for children to begin to gain self-confidence.

EVALUATION: GOALS AND EXPECTED OUTCOMES

- **Goal:** The child will develop skills to meet self-care needs within her or his ability.
  Expected Outcome: The child practices basic hygiene habits, as well as dressing/grooming, feeding, and toileting skills within his or her abilities with support and supervision.
- **Goal:** The child's communication skills will improve.
  Expected Outcome: The child can communicate basic needs to staff and family.
- **Goal:** The child will attain the milestones of his or her stage of growth and development according to mental age; family caregivers ver-

balize an understanding of the child's level of development.

Expected Outcome: The child attains the highest level of functioning for his or her mental age; family caregivers identify the child's developmental level and set realistic goals.

- **Goal:** The child will be free from injury by caregivers and will learn basic safety rules.

  Expected Outcome: The child remains free from injury and cooperates with basic safety rules within his or her abilities.

- **Goal:** The family will effectively cope with the child's diagnosis.

  Expected Outcome: The family verbalizes feelings, mourns the loss of the "perfect child," and provides appropriate care to help the child reach optimum functioning.

- **Goal:** The family will interact with social groups and support networks.

  Expected Outcome: The family freely voices feelings and concerns about the child, makes contact with support systems, and establishes relationships with families of other cognitively impaired children.

HEAD INJURIES

Head injuries are a significant cause of serious injury or death in children of all ages. The primary cause of a head injury varies with the child's age. Toddlers and young children may receive a head injury from a fall or child abuse; school-age children and adolescents usually experience such an injury as a result of a bicycling, in-line skating, or motor vehicle accident.

Children, especially young children seem to receive many head injuries. Fortunately most of them are not serious, but they are often frightening to the caregiver. If a scalp laceration is involved, the caregiver can be quite alarmed by the amount of bleeding because of the large blood supply to the head and scalp. The caregiver can apply an ice pack and pressure until the bleeding is controlled. Applying ice cubes in a zip-closure sandwich bag wrapped in a washcloth works well at home. An open wound should be cleaned with soap and water and a sterile dressing applied. For an injury without a break in the skin, the caregiver can apply ice for an hour or so to decrease the amount of swelling.

The caregiver should observe the child for at least 6 hours for vomiting or a change in the child's level of consciousness. If the child falls asleep, he or she should be awakened every 1 to 2 hours to determine that the level of consciousness has not changed. No analgesics or sedatives should be administered during this period of observation. The child's pupils are checked for reaction to light every 4 hours for 48 hours. The caregiver should notify the health care provider immediately if the child vomits more than three times, has pupillary changes, has double or blurred vision, has a change in level of consciousness, acts strange or confused, has trouble walking, or has a headache that becomes more severe or wakes him or her from sleep; these instructions should be provided in written form to the caregiver.

TABLE 34.5	Summary of Basic Life Support Maneuvers in Infants and Children	
Maneuver	Infant (<1 y)	Child (1 to 8 y)
Airway	Head tilt-chin lift (unless trauma present) Jaw thrust	Head tilt-chin lift (unless trauma present) Jaw thrust
Breathing		
Initial	2 breaths at 1 to 1½ s/breath	2 breaths at 1 to 1½ s/breath
Subsequent	20 breaths/min	20 breaths/min
Circulation		
Pulse check	Brachial/femoral	Carotid
Compression area	Lower half of sternum	Lower half of sternum
Compression width	2 or 3 fingers	Heel of 1 hand
Compression depth	About ½–1 inch	About 1–1½ inch
Rate	At least 100/min	100/min
Compression-ventilation ratio	5:1 (pause for ventilation)	5:1 (pause for ventilation)
Foreign body airway obstruction	Back blows/chest thrusts	Heimlich maneuver

Adapted from American Heart Association. (2001). *Basic life support for healthcare providers*. Dallas, TX: Author.

A. Opening the airway with the head tit-chin lift maneuver. One hand is used to tilt the head, extending the neck. The index finger of the rescuer's other hand lifts the mandible outward by lifting or the chin. Head tilt should not be performed it cervical spine injury is suspected.

B. Opening the airway with the jaw-thrust maneuver. The airway is opened by lifting the angle of the mandible. The rescuer uses two or three fingers of each hand to lift the jaw while other fingers guide the jaw upward and outward.

C. Rescue breathing in an infant. The rescuer's mouth covers the infant's nose and mouth, creating a seal. One hand performs head tilt while the other hand lifts the infant's jaw. Avoid head tilt if the infant has sustained head or neck trauma.

D. Rescue breathing in a child. The rescuer's mouth covers the mouth of the child creating a mouth-to-mouth seal. One hand maintains the head tilt; the thumb and forefinger of the same hand are used to pinch the child's nose.

E. Locating and palpating the carotid artery pulse in the child.

F. Palpating the brachial artery pulse

G. Cardiac compressions. Top: Infant supine on palm of the rescuer's hand. Bottom: Performing CPR while carrying the infant or small child. Note that the head is kept level with the torso. (Compare with H).

H. Locating proper finger position for chest compression in infant. Note that the rescuer's other hand is used to maintain head position to facilitate ventilation.

I. Locating hand position for chest compression in child.

J. Lift fingers to avoid pressing on child's ribs. Note that the hand not performing chest compressions is used to maintain head position to facilitate ventilation.

● **Figure 34.14** Cardiopulmonary resuscitation. (Adapted from American Heart Association [2001] *Basic life support for healthcare providers.* Dallas, TX: Author.)

Family caregivers are wise to take the child to a health care facility to have the injury evaluated if they have any doubt about its seriousness. Complications of head injuries with or without skull fractures can include cerebral hemorrhage, cerebral edema, and increased intracranial pressure. These conditions require highly skilled intensive care, and victims are usually cared for in a pediatric neurologic or intensive care unit.

Shaken baby syndrome, a form of child abuse that can cause head injury without external signs of head trauma, is discussed in Chapter 41.

Test Yourself

• What is the most common way to classify mental retardation?

• What is usually seen in the growth and development of a child with cognitive impairment?

• After a head injury, what should be monitored closely for several hours?

DROWNING

Drowning is the second leading cause of accidental death in children. Toddlers and older adolescents have the highest actual rate of death from drowning. Drowning in children often occurs when the child has been left unattended in a body of water. Infants more commonly drown in a bathtub; toddlers and preschoolers drown in pools or small bodies of water. A pail of water may become something for the toddler to investigate, which could lead to accidental death. Many drowning deaths in this age group occur in home pools, including spas, hot tubs, and whirlpools. Drowning in older children often occurs because the child is playing or acting in an unsafe manner.

A responsible adult must continuously supervise all infants and young children when they are near any source of water. Older children and adolescents should not play alone around any body of water. Swimming in undesignated swimming areas, such as creeks, quarries, and rivers, is especially hazardous for older children and adolescents.

When a drowning victim of any age is discovered, cardiopulmonary resuscitation (CPR) should be started immediately and continued until the victim can be transported to a medical facility for additional care. Intensive care is carried out according to the patient's needs. All adults who care for children in any capacity must learn CPR and be ready to perform it immediately (see Table 34-5 and Fig. 34-14 on previous pages.).

KEY POINTS

▸ Vision impairment includes myopia (nearsightedness), hyperopia (farsightedness), astigmatism, partial sight, or blindness.

▸ Bacterial conjunctivitis is treated with ophthalmic antibacterial agents such as erythromycin, bacitracin, sulfacetamide, and polymyxin.

▸ A child who is hard of hearing has a loss of hearing but is able to learn speech and language. A child who is deaf has no hearing ability.

▸ The child with acute otitis media is usually restless, shakes the head, and rubs or pulls at the ear. The child may also have fever, irritability, and hearing impairment.

▸ The four complications of *Haemophilus influenzae* meningitis are hydrocephalus, nerve deafness, mental retardation, and paralysis.

▸ Nursing care for the child at high risk for seizures includes monitoring for complications, such as signs of increased intracranial pressure (IICP), as well as preventing aspiration, keeping the child safe, monitoring intake and output, and supporting the child's family.

▸ A simple partial motor seizure causes a localized motor activity, such as shaking of an arm, leg, or other body part. Simple partial sensory seizures may include sensory symptoms, called an aura, which signals an impending attack. Complex partial (psychomotor) seizures begin in a small area of the brain and can cause memory loss and staring.

▸ Tonic-clonic seizures consist of four stages. In the prodromal period the child may be drowsy or dizzy. An aura is a warning and occurs immediately before the seizure. During the tonic phase the muscles contract and the extremities stiffen. The initial rigidity of the tonic phase changes to generalized jerking muscle movements in the clonic phase. The jerking movements gradually diminish then disappear. Sleep usually occurs during the postictal stage.

▸ In absence seizures there is lose of awareness and eye blinking or twitching, but the child does not fall. After the seizure, the child is alert and continues conversation. Atonic or akinetic seizures cause a sudden momentary loss of consciousness, muscle tone, and postural control, and the child may fall. In myoclonic seizures, there is a sudden jerking of a muscle or group of muscles, often in the arms or legs. Infantile spasms usually indicate a cerebral defect and consist of muscle contractions and rolling of the eyes.

▸ Cerebral palsy is a group of disorders arising from a malfunction of motor centers and neural pathways in the brain, often accompanied by seizures, mental retardation, sensory defects, and behavior disorders.

▸ Prenatal causes of cerebral palsy include oxygen deprivation, maternal infection, nutritional deficiencies, Rh incompatibility, and teratogenic agents, such as drugs and radiation. Perinatal causes include anoxia, intracranial bleeding, asphyxia, maternal analgesia, trauma, and prematurity. Postnatal head trauma, infection, neoplasms, or cerebrovascular accident can also cause CP.

▸ Spastic type CP is characterized by a hyperactive stretch reflex in associated muscle groups, increased activity of the deep tendon reflexes, clonus, contractures of the extensor muscles especially the heel cord, and scissoring caused by hip adduction. Athetoid type CP is marked by involuntary, uncoordinated motion with muscle tension; the child is in constant motion.

▸ Health care professionals involved in the care of the child with cerebral palsy include a physical therapist, as well as individuals who specialize in orthopedic and technological aids to help in activities of daily living.

▸ Prenatal causes of mental retardation include inborn errors of metabolism; prenatal infection; teratogenic agents, such as drugs, radiation, and alcohol; and genetic factors. Birth trauma, anoxia, prematurity, and difficult birth are perinatal causes. Postnatal causes include poisoning such as lead poisoning, infections, trauma, inadequate nutrition, and a lack of sensory stimulation.

▸ Head injuries are a significant cause of serious injury or death in children of all ages. The primary cause of a head injury varies with the child's age. Toddlers and young children may receive a head injury from a fall or child abuse; school-age children and adolescents usually experience such an injury as a result of a bicycling, in-line skating, or motor vehicle accident.

▸ Drowning is the second leading cause of accidental death in children. Toddlers and older adolescents have the highest actual rate of death from drowning. Drowning in children often occurs when the child has been left unattended in a body of water.

REFERENCES AND SELECTED READINGS

Books and Journals

American Heart Association. (2001). *Basic life support for healthcare providers*. Dallas, TX: Author.

American Psychiatric Association. (2000). *Diagnostic and statistical manual of mental disorders*, 4th ed., text revision. Washington, DC: Author.

Ansel, B. M., Landa, R. M., & Luethke, L. E. (1999). Development and disorders of speech, language and hearing. In *Oski's pediatrics: Principles and practice* (3rd ed.). Philadelphia: Lippincott Williams & Wilkins.

Accardo, P. J., & Capute, A. J. (1999). Mental retardation. In *Oski's pediatrics: Principles and practice* (3rd ed.). Philadelphia: Lippincott Williams & Wilkins.

Hagerman, R. J. (1999). *Neurodevelopmental disorders: Diagnosis and treatment*. New York: Oxford University Press.

Hall-Long, B. A. Schell, K., & Corrigan, V. (2001). Youth safety education and injury prevention program. *Pediatric Nursing, 27*(2), 141.

Hockenberry, M. J., Wilson, D., Winkelstein, M. L., & Kline, N. E. (2003). *Wong's nursing care of infants and children* (7th ed.). St. Louis: Mosby.

Kamienski, M. C. (2003). Reye syndrome. *American Journal of Nursing, 103*(7), 54–57.

Karch, A. M. (2003). *2004 Lippincott's nursing drug guide*. Philadelphia: Lippincott Williams & Wilkins.

Kline, M. K. (1999). Otitis media. In *Oski's pediatrics: Principles and practices* (3rd ed.). Philadelphia: Lippincott Williams & Wilkins.

Naslund, J. (2001). Modes of sensory stimulation. *Physiotherapy, 87*(8), 13–23.

North American Nursing Diagnosis Association (NANDA). (2001). *NANDA nursing diagnoses: Definitions and classification 2001–2002*. Philadelphia: Author.

Parini, S. (2001). Eight faces of meningitis. *Nursing, 31*(8), 51.

Pillitteri, A. (2003). *Maternal and child health nursing* (4th ed.). Philadelphia: Lippincott Williams & Wilkins.

Smeltzer, S. C., & Bare, B. G. (2003). *Textbook of medical–surgical nursing* (10th ed.). Philadelphia: Lippincott Williams & Wilkins.

Sparks, S., & Taylor, C. (2001). *Nursing diagnosis reference manual* (5th ed.). Springhouse, PA: Springhouse Corporation.

Traboulsi, E. I., & Maumenee, I. H. (1999). Eye problems. In *Oski's pediatrics: Principles and practices* (3rd ed.). Philadelphia: Lippincott Williams & Wilkins.

Wong, D. L., Perry, S., & Hockenberry, M. (2002). *Maternal child nursing care* (2nd ed.). St. Louis: Mosby.

Web Addresses
Epilepsy
www.efa.org

Hearing Loss
www.johntracyclinic.org

Mental Retardation
www.aamr.org

Reye Syndrome
http://www.reyessyndrome.org

WORKBOOK

NCLEX-STYLE REVIEW QUESTIONS

1. If a child has a febrile seizure, the *highest* priority for the nurse is to

   a. document the child's behavior during the seizure.

   b. teach the caregivers about fever reduction methods.

   c. protect the child during the seizure activity.

   d. reassure the caregivers that seizures are common.

2. After discussing ways to lower a fever with the caregiver of an infant, the caregiver makes the following statements. Which statement requires further teaching?

   a. "I won't give my child baby aspirin when she has a fever."

   b. "I know I need to dress my baby lightly if she has a fever."

   c. "When my baby has a fever, I will sponge her in cool water for 20 minutes."

   d. "I need to recheck my baby's temperature until it is below 101."

3. The nurse admits a child with a diagnosis of meningitis. The child is being monitored for signs of increased intracranial pressure (IICP). Of the following signs and symptoms which would *most* likely be seen in the child with IICP?

   a. High-pitched cry, headache

   b. Itching, swelling around eyes

   c. Weight gain or loss

   d. Decreased head size, sunken fontanel

4. The nurse has admitted a 6-year-old child who has received a diagnosis of a seizure disorder and has frequent tonic-clonic seizures. Which of the following are characteristics of tonic-clonic seizures? Select all that apply. The seizure activity:

   a. might be preceded by a sight, sound, taste or smell.

   b. is usually limited to one side of the body.

   c. involves a phase in which the muscles are rigid.

   d. causes memory loss and staring.

   e. involves a phase in which there are jerking muscle movements.

   f. often is followed by a loss of control of bowel and bladder.

5. The nurse has admitted a 9-year-old child who is blind. Of the following nursing actions, which be would important for the nurse to implement? Select all that apply. The nurse should:

   a. identify self when entering the room.

   b. quietly walk out of the room when he or she leaves.

   c. involve the child in activities with younger children.

   d. encourage the child to be as independent as possible.

   e. provide the child with only finger foods.

   f. encourage self-feeding after orienting the child to the plate.

STUDY ACTIVITIES

1. Research your community for financial resources, supplies and equipment, and support groups available to children and families with the following disorders. Complete the following table and share the information with your peers.

Condition	Financial Resources	Supplies Equipment	Support Groups
Vision impairment Hearing impairment Cerebral palsy Mental retardation			

2. Create a poster or teaching aid to be used in teaching family caregivers of children who have seizure disorders. Include safety precautions, what to do when a child has a seizure and after the seizure, and medication considerations.

3. Go to the following Internet site: http://www.preventblindness.org. On the left side of the screen, click on "Children." Click on "Eye Tests."

Click on "The Pointing Game."

a. What are the steps to follow in administering this eye test to children?

Click on "Back."

Click on "Distance Vision Test."

b. Print a copy of the Distance Vision Chart.

c. Following the instructions given, administer the distance vision test to a preschooler.

d. What did you discover about this child's vision?

CRITICAL THINKING: What Would You Do?

1. Four-year-old Todd is blind. You are the nurse helping with his care. He is going to have surgery and will be hospitalized for 3 to 4 days.

   a. What will you do to orient him to the pediatric unit?

   b. What things will you teach him and do to prepare him for his hospital stay?

   c. What age-appropriate activities will you offer to him before and after surgery?

2. You are caring for 10-year-old Missy, who has a mild hearing impairment. She and her father have returned to the pediatric clinic for a follow-up visit.

   a. What information do you need to ask Missy's father that will help you in communicating with Missy?

   b. What will you do to adapt your nursing care to improve your communication with her?

3. You and your friend are working with a group of children with physical limitations. One of the children has cerebral palsy. Your friend asks you if cerebral palsy is inherited and if it can be prevented.

   a. What explanation will you give your friend regarding the causes of cerebral palsy?

   b. How will you answer the question regarding whether or not CP can be prevented?

   c. What will you tell your friend about the types of cerebral palsy that children might have?

4. Dosage calculation: An infant with a diagnosis of otitis media is being treated with amoxicillin. The child weighs 13.2 pounds. The usual dosage of this medication is 40 mg/kg per day in divided doses every 8 hours. Answer the following:

   a. How many kilograms does the child's weigh?

   b. How much amoxicillin will be given in a 24-hour time period?

   c. How many milligrams per dose will be given?

   d. How many doses will the child receive in a day?

5. Dosage calculation: A school-age child with a diagnosis of a seizure disorder is being treated with Dilantin. The child weighs 58 pounds. The child is being given a dose of 6 mg/kg a day in three divided doses. Answer the following:

   a. How many kilograms does the child's weigh?

   b. How many milligrams of Dilantin will the child receive in a 24-hour period of time?

   c. How many milligrams of Dilantin will the child receive in each dose?

   d. If the dose is increased by 20 mg a dose, how many milligrams will then be in each dose?

   e. How many milligrams will the child receive in a 24-hour period after the dose has been increased?

The Child With Respiratory Disorders

STUDENT OBJECTIVES

On completion of this chapter, the student should be able to

1. Discuss ways the infant and child's respiratory system differs from the adult's system.
2. Name the most common complication of acute nasopharyngitis.
3. State the most common complication of a tonsillectomy and list the signs requiring observation.
4. Describe the usual treatment for spasmodic laryngitis.
5. Discuss acute laryngotracheobronchitis, including the symptoms and treatment.
6. List factors that can trigger an asthma attack.
7. Describe the physiologic response that occurs in the respiratory tract during an asthma attack.

KEY TERMS

achylia
adenoids
circumoral
coryza
croup
dysphagia
emetic
hypochylia
metered-dose inhaler

STUDENT OBJECTIVES

8. Discuss the medications most commonly used in the treatment of pneumonia.
9. Identify the basic defect in cystic fibrosis.
10. State the major organs affected by cystic fibrosis.
11. Name the most common type of complication in cystic fibrosis.
12. List the diagnostic procedures used to diagnose cystic fibrosis.
13. Describe the dietary and pulmonary treatment of cystic fibrosis.
14. Discuss how tuberculosis is detected.

KEY TERMS

nebulizer
stridor
teratogenicity
tonsils
wheezing

Respiratory disorders in infants and children are common. They range from mild to serious, even life threatening. They can be acute or chronic in nature. Sometimes these problems require hospitalization, which interrupts development of the child–family relationship and the child's patterns of sleeping, eating, and stimulation. Although the illness might be acute, if recovery is rapid and the hospitalization brief, the child probably will experience few, if any, long-term effects. However, if the condition is chronic or so serious that it requires long-term care, both child and family may suffer serious consequences.

GROWTH AND DEVELOPMENT OF THE RESPIRATORY SYSTEM

The respiratory system is made up of the nose, pharynx, larynx, trachea, epiglottis, bronchi, bronchioles, and the lungs. These structures are involved in the exchange of oxygen and carbon dioxide and the distribution of the oxygen to the body cells. Tiny, thin-walled sacs called alveoli are responsible for distributing air into the bloodstream. It is also through the alveoli that carbon dioxide is removed from the bloodstream and exhaled through the respiratory system. The air that enters the body is cleansed, warmed, and humidified by the structures and organs found in the respiratory system.

This is critical to remember. The diameter of the infant and child's trachea is about the size of the child's little finger. This small diameter makes it extremely important to be aware that something can easily be lodged in this small passageway and the child's airway can become obstructed.

Respiratory problems occur more often and with greater severity in infants and children because of their immature body defenses and small, undeveloped anatomic structures.

The respiratory tract grows and changes until the child is about 12 years of age. During the first 5 years, the airway increases in length not in diameter.

The infant and young child have shorter necks, narrower airways, and the structures are closer together. This leads to the possibility of respiratory obstruction, especially if there is edema, swelling, or increased mucus in the airways. The ability to breath through the mouth when the nose is blocked is not automatic but develops as the child's neurologic development increases.

This is important. Because the infant is a nose breather, it is essential to keep the nasal passages clear to enable the infant to breath and to eat.

The tonsillar tissue is enlarged in the early school-age child, but the pharynx, which contains the tonsils, is still small, so the possibility of obstruction of the upper airway is more likely. In children older than 2 years, the right bronchus is shorter, wider, and more vertical than the left.

Think about this. If the child inhales a foreign body, it is more likely to be drawn into the right bronchus, rather than the left.

Infants use the diaphragm and abdominal muscles to breathe. Beginning at about age 2 to 3 years, the child starts using the thoracic muscles to breath. The change from using abdominal to using thoracic muscles for respiration is completed by the age of 7 years. Because accessory muscles are used for breathing, weakness of these muscles can cause respiratory failure (Fig. 35-1).

ACUTE NASOPHARYNGITIS (COMMON COLD)

The common cold is one of the most common infectious conditions of childhood. The young infant is as susceptible as the older child but generally is not exposed as frequently.

The illness is of viral origin such as rhinoviruses, Coxsackievirus, respiratory syncytial virus (RSV),

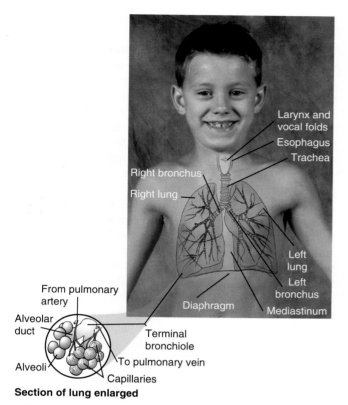

Larynx and
vocal folds
Esophagus
Trachea
Right bronchus
Right lung
Left
lung
Left
bronchus
Diaphragm
Mediastinum
From pulmonary
artery
Alveolar
duct
Terminal
bronchiole
To pulmonary vein
Alveoli
Capillaries

Section of lung enlarged

● *Figure 35.1* Anatomy of the child's respiratory tract.

influenza virus, parainfluenza virus, or adenovirus. Bacterial invasion of the tissues might cause complications such as ear, mastoid, and lung infections. The child appears to be more susceptible to complications than is an adult. The infant should be protected from people who have colds because complications in the infant can be serious.

Clinical Manifestations

The child older than the age of 3 months usually develops fever early in the course of the infection, often as high as 102°F to 104°F (38.9°C to 40°C). Younger infants usually are afebrile. The child sneezes and becomes irritable and restless. The congested nasal passages can interfere with nursing, increasing the infant's irritability. Because the older child can mouth breathe, nasal congestion is not as great a concern as in the infant. The child might have vomiting or diarrhea, which might be caused by mucous drainage into the digestive system.

Diagnosis

This nasopharyngeal condition might appear as the first symptom of many childhood contagious diseases, such as measles, and must be observed carefully. The common cold also needs to be differentiated from allergic rhinitis.

Treatment and Nursing Care

The child with an uncomplicated cold may not need any treatment in addition to rest, increased fluids and adequate nutrition, normal saline nose drops, suction with a bulb syringe, and a humidified environment. In the older child, acetaminophen or children's ibuprofen can be administered as an analgesic and antipyretic. Aspirin is best avoided. If the nares or upper lip become irritated, cold cream or petrolatum (Vaseline) can be used. The child needs to be comforted by holding, rocking, and soothing. If the symptoms persist for several days, the child must be seen by a physician to rule out complications such as otitis media.

ALLERGIC RHINITIS (HAY FEVER)

Allergic rhinitis in children is most often caused by sensitization to animal dander, house dust, pollens, and molds. Pollen allergy seldom appears before 4 or 5 years of age.

Clinical Manifestations

A watery nasal discharge, postnasal drip, sneezing, and allergic conjunctivitis are the usual symptoms of allergic rhinitis. Continued sniffing, itching of the nose and palate, and the "allergic salute," in which the child pushes his or her nose upward and backward to relieve itching and open the air passages in the nose, are common complaints. Because of congestion in the nose, there is back pressure to the blood circulation around the eyes, and dark circles are visible under the eyes (Fig. 35-2). Headaches are common in older children.

● *Figure 35.2* Back pressure to blood circulation around the eyes leads to dark areas under the eyes in the child with allergic rhinitis.

Treatment and Nursing Care

When possible, offending allergens are avoided or removed from the environment. Antihistamine-decongestant preparations, such as Dimetapp, Actifed, and others, can be helpful for some patients. Hyposensitization can be implemented, particularly if antihistamines are not helpful or are needed chronically. Parents should be taught the importance of avoiding allergens and administering antihistamines to decrease symptoms.

TONSILLITIS AND ADENOIDITIS

Tonsillitis is a common illness in childhood resulting from pharyngitis. A brief description of the location and functions of the tonsils and adenoids serves as an introduction to the discussion of their infection and medical and surgical treatments.

A ring of lymphoid tissue encircles the pharynx, forming a protective barrier against upper respiratory infection. This ring consists of groups of lymphoid tonsils, including the faucial, the commonly known **tonsils;** pharyngeal, known as the **adenoids;** and lingual tonsils. Lymphoid tissue normally enlarges progressively in childhood between the ages of 2 and 10 years and shrinks during preadolescence. If the tissue itself becomes a site of acute or chronic infection, it may become hypertrophied and can interfere with breathing, may cause partial deafness, or may become a source of infection in itself.

Clinical Manifestations and Diagnosis

The child with tonsillitis may have a fever of 101°F (38.4°C) or more, a sore throat, often with dysphagia (difficulty swallowing), hypertrophied tonsils, and erythema of the soft palate. Exudate may be visible on the tonsils. The symptoms vary somewhat with the causative organism. Throat cultures are performed to diagnose tonsillitis and the causative organism. Frequently the cause of tonsillitis is viral, although beta-hemolytic streptococcal infection also may be the cause.

Treatment and Nursing Care

Medical treatment of tonsillitis consists of analgesics for pain, antipyretics for fever, and an antibiotic in the case of streptococcal infection. A standard 10-day course of antibiotics is recommended. Stress the importance of completing the full prescription of antibiotic to ensure that the streptococcal infection is eliminated. A soft or liquid diet is easier to swallow, and the child should be encouraged to maintain good fluid intake. A cool-mist vaporizer may be used to ease respirations.

Tonsillectomies and adenoidectomies are controversial. One can be performed independent of the other, but they are often done together. No conclusive evidence has been found that a tonsillectomy in itself improves a child's health by reducing the number of respiratory infections, increasing the appetite, or improving general well-being. Currently, tonsillectomies generally are not performed unless other measures are ineffective or the tonsils are so hypertrophied that breathing and eating are difficult. Tonsillectomies are not performed while the tonsils are infected. The adenoids are more susceptible to chronic infection. An indication for adenoidectomy is hypertrophy of the tissue to the extent of impairing hearing or interfering with breathing. Performing only an adenoidectomy if the tonsil tissue appears to be healthy is an increasingly common practice. Tonsillectomy is postponed until after the age of 4 or 5 years, except in the rare instance when it appears urgently needed. Often when a child has reached the acceptable age, the apparent need for the tonsillectomy has disappeared.

● Nursing Process for the Child Having a Tonsillectomy

ASSESSMENT

Much of the preoperative preparation, including complete blood count, bleeding and clotting time, and urinalysis, is done on a preadmission outpatient basis. In many facilities, the child is admitted on the day of surgery or the procedure is done in a day surgery setting. Psychological preparation is often accomplished through preadmission orientation. Acting out the forthcoming experience, particularly in a group, with the use of puppets, dolls, and play-doctor or play-nurse material helps the child develop security. The amount and the timing of preparation before admission depend on the child's age. The child may become frightened about losing a body part. Telling the child that the troublesome tonsils are going to be "fixed" is a much better choice than saying that they are going to be "taken out." Include the child and the caregiver in the admission interview. Ask about any bleeding tendencies because postoperative bleeding is a concern. Carefully explain all procedures to the child and be sensitive to the child's apprehension. Take and record vital signs to establish a baseline for postoperative monitoring. The temperature is an important part of the data collection to determine that the child has no upper respiratory infection. Observe the child for loose teeth that could cause a problem during administration of anesthesia; document findings.

SELECTED NURSING DIAGNOSES

- Risk for Aspiration postoperatively related to impaired swallowing and bleeding at the operative site
- Acute Pain related to surgical procedure
- Deficient Fluid Volume related to inadequate oral intake secondary to painful swallowing
- Deficient Knowledge related to caregivers understanding of postdischarge home care and signs and symptoms of complications

OUTCOME IDENTIFICATION AND PLANNING

The major postoperative goals for the child include preventing aspiration; relieving pain, especially while swallowing; and improving fluid intake. The major goal for the family is to increase knowledge and understanding of post-discharge care and possible complications. Design the plan of care with these goals in mind.

IMPLEMENTATION

Preventing Aspiration Postoperatively

Immediately after a tonsillectomy, place the child in a partially prone position with head turned to one side until the child is completely awake. This position can be accomplished by turning the child partially over and by flexing the knee where the child is not resting to help maintain the position. Keeping the head slightly lower than the chest helps facilitate drainage of secretions. Avoid placing pillows under the chest and abdomen, which may hamper respiration. Encourage the child to expectorate all secretions, and place an ample supply of tissues and a waste container near him or her. Discourage the child from coughing. Check vital signs every 10 to 15 minutes until the child is fully awake, and then check every 30 minutes to 1 hour. Note the child's preoperative baseline vital signs to interpret the vital signs correctly. Hemorrhage is the most common complication of a tonsillectomy. Bleeding is most often a concern within the first 24 hours after surgery and the 5th to 7th postoperative day. During the 24 hours after surgery, observe, document, and report any unusual restlessness or anxiety, frequent swallowing, or rapid pulse that may indicate bleeding. Vomiting dark, old blood may be expected, but bright, red-flecked emesis or oozing indicates fresh bleeding.

Observe the pharynx with a flashlight each time vital signs are checked. Bleeding can occur when the clots dissolve between the 5th and 7th postoperative days if new tissue is not yet present. Because the child is cared for at home by this time, the family should be given information concerning signs and symptoms for which to watch.

Providing Comfort and Relieving Pain

Apply an ice collar postoperatively; however, remove the collar if the child is uncomfortable with it. Administer pain medication as ordered. Liquid acetaminophen with codeine is often prescribed. Rectal or intravenous analgesics may be used. Encourage the caregiver to remain at the bedside to provide soothing reassurance. Crying irritates the raw throat and increases the child's discomfort; thus, it should be avoided if possible. Teach the caregiver what may be expected in drainage and signs that should be reported immediately to the nursing staff.

Encouraging Fluid Intake

When the child is fully awake from surgery, give small amounts of clear fluids or ice chips. Synthetic juices, carbonated beverages that are "flat," and frozen juice popsicles are good choices.

Avoid irritating liquids such as orange juice and lemonade. Milk and ice cream products tend to cling to the surgical site and make swallowing more difficult; thus they are poor choices, despite the old tradition of offering ice cream after a tonsillectomy. Continue administration of intravenous fluid and record intake and output until adequate oral intake is established.

Here's a helpful hint. After a tonsillectomy, offer the child liquids that are not red in color to eliminate confusion with bloody discharge.

Providing Family Teaching

The child typically is discharged on the day of or the day after surgery if no complications are present. Instruct the caregiver to keep the child relatively quiet for a few days after discharge. Recommend giving soft foods and nonirritating liquids for the first few days. Teach family members that if at any time after the surgery they note any signs of hemorrhage (bright red bleeding, frequent swallowing, restlessness), they should notify the care provider. Provide written instructions and telephone numbers before discharge. Advise the caregivers that a mild earache may be expected about the 3rd day.

Evaluation: Goals and Expected Outcomes

- **Goal:** The child's airway will remain patent after surgery.
  Expected Outcomes: The child's airway is open and clear and the child expectorates saliva and drainage with no aspiration.
- **Goal:** The child will show signs of being comfortable.
  Expected Outcomes: The child rests quietly and does not cry; the pulse rate is regular and normal for age; and the child states that pain is lessened.
- **Goal:** The child's fluid intake will be adequate for age.
  Expected Outcomes: The child's skin turgor is good, mucous membranes are moist, and hourly urinary output is at least 20 to 30 mL. Parenteral fluids are maintained until the child's oral fluid intake is adequate.
- **Goal:** Family caregivers will verbalize an understanding of postdischarge care.
  Expected Outcomes: Family caregivers give appropriate responses when questioned about care at home, can state signs and symptoms of complications, and ask appropriate questions for clarification.

CROUP SYNDROMES

Croup is not a disease but a group of disorders typically involving a barking cough, hoarseness, and inspiratory **stridor** (shrill, harsh respiratory sound). The disorders are named for the respiratory structures involved. Acute laryngotracheobronchitis, for instance, affects the larynx, trachea, and major bronchi.

SPASMODIC LARYNGITIS

Spasmodic laryngitis occurs in children between ages 1 and 3 years. The cause is undetermined; it may be of infectious or allergic origin, but certain children seem to develop severe laryngospasm with little, if any, apparent cause.

Clinical Manifestations and Diagnosis

The attack may be preceded by <u>coryza</u> (runny nose) and hoarseness or by no apparent signs of respiratory irregularity during the evening. The child awakens after a few hours of sleep with a bark-like cough, increasing respiratory difficulty, and stridor. The child becomes anxious, restless, and markedly hoarse. A low-grade fever and mild upper respiratory infection may be present.

This condition is not serious but is frightening both to the child and the family. The episode subsides after a few hours; little evidence remains the next day when an anxious caregiver takes the child to the physician. Attacks frequently occur 2 or 3 nights in succession.

Treatment and Nursing Care

Humidified air is helpful in reducing laryngospasm. Taking the child into the bathroom and opening the hot water taps with the door closed is a quick method for providing moist air, if the water runs hot enough. The physician may prescribe an **emetic** (an agent that causes vomiting) in a dosage less than that needed to produce vomiting; this usually gives relief by helping to reduce spasms of the larynx. Humidifiers may be used in the child's bedroom to provide high humidity. Cool humidifiers are recommended, but vaporizers also may be used. If a vaporizer is used, caution must be taken to place it out of the child's reach to protect the child from being burned. Cool-mist humidifiers provide safe humidity. Humidifiers and vaporizers must be cleaned regularly to prevent the growth of undesirable organisms. Sometimes the spasm is relieved by exposure to cold air—when, for instance, the child is taken out into the night to go to the emergency department or to see the care provider.

Good news. Although frightening to the child and family, spasmodic laryngitis is not serious and can often be lessened quickly by taking the child into the bathroom, shutting the door and turning on the hot water tap. This fills the room with steam or humidified air and relieves the child's symptoms.

It is important to explain which symptoms can be treated at home (hoarseness, croupy cough, and inspiratory stridor) and which symptoms might indicate a more serious condition in which the child needs to be seen by the care provider (continuous stridor, use of accessory muscles, labored breathing, lower rib retractions, restlessness, pallor, and rapid respirations). The family must be aware that recurrence of these conditions may occur.

ACUTE LARYNGOTRACHEOBRONCHITIS

Laryngeal infections are common in small children, and they often involve tracheobronchial areas as well. Acute laryngotracheobronchitis (bacterial tracheitis or laryngotracheobronchitis) may progress rapidly and become a serious problem within a matter of hours. The toddler is the most frequently affected age group. This condition is usually of viral origin, but bacterial invasion, usually staphylococcal, follows the original infection. It generally occurs after an upper respiratory infection with fairly mild rhinitis and pharyngitis.

Clinical Manifestations and Diagnosis

The child develops hoarseness and a barking cough with a fever that may reach 104°F to 105°F (40°C to 40.6°C). As the disease progresses, marked laryngeal edema occurs, and the child's breathing becomes difficult; the pulse is rapid, and cyanosis may appear. Heart failure and acute respiratory embarrassment can result.

Treatment and Nursing Care

The major goal of treatment for acute laryngotracheobronchitis is to maintain an airway and adequate air exchange. Antimicrobial therapy is ordered. The child is placed in a supersaturated atmosphere, such as a croupette or some other kind of mist tent that also can include the administration of oxygen. To achieve bronchodilation, racemic or nebulized epinephrine may be administered, usually by a respiratory therapist. Nebulization is usually administered every 3 or 4 hours. Nebulization often produces relief. This rapid improvement results from vasoconstriction. However, the child requires careful observation for the reappearance of symptoms.

If necessary, intubation with a nasotracheal tube may be performed for a child with severe distress unrelieved by other measures. Tracheostomies, once performed frequently, are rarely performed today; intubation is preferred. Antibiotics are administered parenterally initially and continued after the temperature has normalized.

Close and careful observation of the child is important. Observation includes checking the pulse, respirations, and color, listening for hoarseness and stridor, and noting any restlessness that may indicate an impending respiratory crisis. Pulse oximetry is used to determine the degree of hypoxia.

EPIGLOTTITIS *Emergency Situation*

Epiglottitis is acute inflammation of the epiglottis (the cartilaginous flap that protects the opening of the larynx). Commonly caused by *Haemophilus influenzae* type B, epiglottitis most often affects children ages 2 to 7 years. The epiglottis becomes inflamed and swollen with edema. The edema decreases the ability of the epiglottis to move freely, which results in blockage of the airway and creates an emergency.

Clinical Manifestations and Diagnosis

The child may have been well or may have had a mild upper respiratory infection before the development of a sore throat, **dysphagia** (difficulty swallowing), and a high fever of 102.2°F to 104°F (39°C to 40°C). The dysphagia may cause drooling. A tongue blade should never be used to initiate a gag reflex because complete obstruction may occur. The child is very anxious and prefers to breathe by sitting up and leaning forward with the mouth open and the tongue out. This is called the "tripod" position (Fig. 35-3). Immediate emergency attention is necessary.

Treatment and Nursing Care

The child may need endotracheal intubation or a tracheostomy if the epiglottis is so swollen that intubation cannot be performed. Moist air is necessary to help reduce the inflammation of the epiglottis. Pulse oximetry is required to monitor oxygen requirements. Antibiotics are administered intravenously (IV). After 24 to 48 hours of antibiotic therapy, the child may be extubated. Antibiotic therapy usually is continued for 10 days. This condition is not common, and it is extremely frightening for the child and the family.

● *Figure 35.3* The "tripod" position of the child with epiglottitis.

ACUTE BRONCHIOLITIS/ RESPIRATORY SYNCYTIAL VIRUS INFECTION

Acute bronchiolitis (acute interstitial pneumonia) is most common during the first 6 months of life and is rarely seen after the age of 2 years. Most cases occur in infants who have been in contact with older children or adults with upper respiratory viral infections. It usually occurs in the winter and early spring.

Acute bronchiolitis is caused by a viral infection. The causative agent in more than 50% of cases has been shown to be RSV. Other viruses associated with the disease are parainfluenza virus, adenoviruses, and other viruses not always identified.

The bronchi and bronchioles become plugged with thick, viscid mucus, causing air to be trapped in the lungs. The child can breathe air in but has difficulty expelling it. This hinders the exchange of gases, and cyanosis appears.

Clinical Manifestations

The onset of dyspnea is abrupt, sometimes preceded by a cough or nasal discharge. There are a dry and persistent cough, extremely shallow respirations, air hunger, and often marked cyanosis. Suprasternal and subcostal retractions are present. The chest becomes barrel-shaped from the trapped air. Respirations are 60 to 80 breaths per minute.

Fever is not extreme, seldom higher than 101°F to 102°F (38.3°C to 38.9°C). Dehydration may become a serious factor if competent care is not given. The infant appears apprehensive, irritable, and restless.

Diagnosis

Diagnosis is made from clinical findings and can be confirmed by laboratory testing (ELISA, enzyme-linked immunosorbent assay) of the mucus obtained by direct nasal aspiration or nasopharyngeal washing.

Treatment and Nursing Care

The child is usually hospitalized and treated with high humidity by mist tent (see Chapter 30, Fig. 30-10), rest, and increased fluids. Oxygen may be administered in addition to the mist tent. Monitoring of oxygenation may be done by means of capillary blood gases or pulse oximetry. Antibiotics are not prescribed because the causative organism is a virus. Intravenous fluids often are administered to ensure an adequate intake and to permit the infant to rest. The hospitalized child is placed on contact transmission precautions to prevent the spread of infection.

Ribavirin (Virazole) is an antiviral drug that may be used to treat certain children with RSV. It is administered as an inhalant by hood, mask, or tent. The American Academy of Pediatrics states that the use of ribavirin must be limited to children at high risk for severe or complicated RSV, such as children with chronic lung disease, premature infants, transplant recipients, and children receiving chemotherapy. Ribavirin is classified as a category X drug, signifying a high risk for **teratogenicity** (causing damage to a fetus). Health care personnel and others may inhale the mist that escapes into the room, so care must be taken when the drug is administered.

Warning. Women who might be pregnant should stay out of the room where ribavirin is being administered.

For children who are at high risk for getting RSV and having serious complications, there are some new drugs available that may be given to prevent RSV. These are administered only in specific cases and are given intravenously or intramuscularly.

Test Yourself

- What is the most common complication after a tonsillectomy?
- What is a fast and effective way to reduce laryngospasm for the child with croup?
- What is a complication often seen in the infant with a respiratory infection?
- What is the causative agent in many cases of bronchiolitis?

ASTHMA

Asthma is a spasm of the bronchial tubes caused by hypersensitivity of the airways in the bronchial system and inflammation that leads to mucosal edema and mucus hypersecretion. Asthma is also sometimes referred to as reactive airway disease. This reversible obstructive airway disease affects millions of people in the United States, including 5% to 10% of all U.S. children.

Asthma attacks are often triggered by a hypersensitive response to allergens. In young children, asthma may be a response to certain foods. Asthma is often triggered by exercise, exposure to cold weather, and irritants such as wood-burning stoves, cigarette smoke, dust, pet dander, and foods such as chocolate, milk, eggs, nuts, and grains. Infections, such as bronchitis and upper respiratory infection, can provoke asthma attacks. In children with asthmatic tendencies, emotional stress or anxiety can trigger an attack. Some children with asthma may have no evidence of an immunologic cause for the symptoms.

Asthma can be either intermittent, with extended periods when the child has no symptoms and does not need medication, or chronic, with the need for frequent or continuous therapy. Chronic asthma affects the child's school performance and general activities and may contribute to poor self-confidence and dependency. Asthma is the most common single cause of school absence (Eggleston, 1999).

Spasms of the smooth muscles cause the lumina of the bronchi and bronchioles to narrow. Edema of the mucous membranes lining these bronchial branches and increased production of thick mucus within them combine with the spasm to cause respiratory obstruction (Fig. 35-4).

Clinical Manifestations

The onset of an attack might be very abrupt or it might progress over several days, as evidenced by a dry, hacking cough; **wheezing** (the sound of expired air being pushed through obstructed bronchioles); and difficulty breathing. Asthma attacks often occur at night and awaken the child from sleep. The child must sit up and is totally preoccupied with efforts to breathe. Attacks might last for only a short time or might continue for several days. Thick, tenacious mucus might be coughed up or vomited after a coughing episode. In some asthmatic patients, coughing is the major symptom, and wheezing occurs rarely if at all. Many children no longer have symptoms after puberty, but this is not predictable. Other allergies may develop in adulthood.

Diagnosis

The history and physical examination are of primary importance in diagnosing asthma. When observing the child's breathing, dyspnea and labored breathing may be noted, especially on expiration. When listening to the child's lung sounds (auscultation), the examiner hears wheezing, which is often generalized over all lung fields. Mucus production may be profuse. Pulmonary function tests are valuable diagnostic tools and indicate the amount of obstruction in the bronchial airways, especially in the smallest airways of the lungs. A definitive diagnosis of asthma is made when the obstruction in the airways is reversed with bronchodilators.

Treatment

Children and their families must be taught to recognize the symptoms that lead to an acute attack so that they can be treated as early as possible. These symptoms include respiratory retractions and wheezing and an increased amount of coughing at night, in the early morning, or with activity. Use of a peak flow meter is an objective way to measure airway obstruction, and children as young as 4 or 5 years of age can be taught to use one (Family Teaching Tips: How to Use a Peak Flow Meter; Fig. 35-5). A peak flow diary should be maintained and also can include symptoms, exacerbations, actions taken, and outcomes. Families must make every effort to eliminate any possible allergens from the home.

Did you know? Prevention is the most important aspect in the treatment of asthma.

The goals of asthma treatment include preventing symptoms, maintaining near normal lung function and activity levels, preventing recurring exacerbations and hospitalizations, and providing the best medication treatment with the fewest adverse effects. Depending on the frequency and severity of symptoms and exacerbations, a stepwise approach to the treatment of asthma is used to manage the disease. The steps are used to determine combinations of medications to be used (Table 35-1).

Medications used to treat asthma are divided into two categories: quick-relief medications for immediate treatment of symptoms and exacerbations and long-term

Cross section of normal bronchiole

Smooth muscle in spasm

Bronchiole

Alveoli

Thick mucous secretions

Cross section of bronchiole constricted during asthma attack

● **Figure 35.4** Bronchiole airflow obstruction in asthma.

FAMILY TEACHING TIPS

How to Use a Peak Flow Meter

INTRODUCTION

Your child cannot feel early changes in the airway. By the time the child feels tightness in the chest or starts to wheeze, he or she is already far into an asthma episode. The most reliable early sign of an asthma episode is a drop in the child's peak expiratory flow rate, or the ability to breathe out quickly, which can be measured by a peak flow meter. Almost every asthmatic child over the age of 4 years can and should learn to use a peak flow meter (Figs. *A* and *B*.)

(*A*) The Assess peak flow meter. (*B*) The Mini-Wright peak flow meter.

A   B

STEPS TO ACCURATE MEASUREMENTS

1. Remove gum or food from the mouth.
2. Move the pointer on the meter to zero.
3. Stand up and hold the meter horizontally with fingers away from the vent holes and marker.
4. With mouth wide open, slowly breathe in as much air as possible.
5. Put the mouthpiece on the tongue and place lips around it.
6. Blow out as hard and fast as you can. Give a short, sharp blast, not a slow blow. The meter measures the fastest puff, not the longest.
7. Repeat steps 1–6 three times. Wait at least 10 seconds between puffs. Move the pointer to zero after each puff.
8. Record the best reading.

GUIDELINES FOR TREATMENT

Each child has a unique pattern of asthma episodes. Most episodes begin gradually, and a drop in peak flow can alert you to start medications before the actual symptoms appear. This early treatment can prevent a flare-up from getting out of hand. One way to look at peak flow scores is to match the scores with three colors:

Green	Yellow	Red
80%–100% personal best	50%–80% personal best	Below 50% personal best
No symptoms	Mild to moderate symptoms	Serious distress
Full breathing reserve	Diminished reserve	Pulmonary function is significantly impaired
Mild trigger may not cause symptoms	A minor trigger produces noticeable symptoms	Any trigger may lead to severe distress
Continue current management	Augment present treatment regimen	Contact physician

Remember, treatment should be adjusted to fit the individual's needs. Your physician will develop a home management plan with you. When in doubt, consult your care provider.

● *Figure 35.5* The child with asthma uses a peak flow meter and keeps track of readings on a daily basis.

control medications to achieve and maintain control of the symptoms. The classifications of drugs used to treat asthma include bronchodilators (sympathomimetics and xanthine derivatives), as well as other antiasthmatic drugs (corticosteroids, leukotriene inhibitors, and mast cell stabilizers). Table 35-2 lists some of the medications used to treat asthma. Many of these drugs can be given either by a **nebulizer** (tube attached to a wall unit or cylinder that delivers moist air via a face mask) or a **metered-dose inhaler** ([MDI]; hand-held plastic device that delivers a premeasured dose). The MDI may have a spacer unit attached that makes it easier for the young child to use (Fig. 35-6).

Bronchodilators

Bronchodilators are used for quick relief of acute exacerbations of asthma symptoms. They are short acting and available in pill, liquid, or inhalant form. These drugs are administered every 6 to 8 hours or every 4 to 6 hours by inhalation, if breathing difficulty continues. In severe attacks, epinephrine by subcutaneous injection often affords quick relief of symptoms. Some bronchodilators such as salmeterol (Serevent) are used in long-term control.

Theophylline preparations have long been used in the treatment of asthma. The drug is available in short-acting and long-acting forms. The short-acting forms are given about every 6 hours. Because they enter the bloodstream quickly, they are most effective when used only as needed for intermittent episodes of asthma. Long-acting preparations of theophylline are given every 8 to 12 hours. Some of these preparations come in sustained release forms. These are helpful in patients who continually need medication because these drugs sustain more consistent theophylline levels in the blood than do short-acting forms. Patients hospitalized for status asthmaticus may receive theophylline intravenously.

Corticosteroids

Corticosteroids are anti-inflammatory drugs used to control severe or chronic cases of asthma. Steroids may be given in inhaled form to decrease the systemic effects that accompany oral steroid administration.

TABLE 35.1	Stepwise Approach to Treating Asthma	
Steps	**Symptoms**
Step One Mild intermittent	Symptoms occur less than 2 times a week No symptoms between exacerbations Exacerbations brief Nighttime symptoms less than 2 times a month
Step Two Mild persistent	Symptoms occur more than 2 times a week but less than 1 time a day Exacerbations may affect activity Nighttime symptoms greater than 2 times a month
Step Three Moderate persistent	Daily symptoms Daily use of inhaled short-acting beta-2 agonist Exacerbations affect activity Exacerbations more than 2 times a week, may last days Nighttime symptoms more than 1 time a week
Step Four Severe persistent	Continual symptoms Limited physical activity Frequent exacerbations Frequent nighttime symptoms

TABLE 35.2	Medications Used in the Treatment of Asthma			
Generic Name	**Trade Name**	**Dose Form**	**Uses**	**Adverse Reactions/Side Effects**
Bronchodilators				
Sympathomimetics (Beta-2-receptor Agonists)				
albuterol sulfate	Proventil, Ventolin	MDI PO Nebulizer	Quick relief	Restlessness, anxiety, fear, palpitations, insomnia, tremors
metaproterenol hydrochloride	Alupent, Metaprel	MDI PO Nebulizer	Quick relief Short-term control	Tremors, anxiety, insomnia, dizziness, tachycardia
terbutaline sulfate	Brethine	MDI PO	MDI—Quick relief PO—Long-term control	Tremors, anxiety, insomnia, dizziness, tachycardia
salmeterol	Serevent	MDI	Long-term control	Headache, tremors, tachycardia
Xanthine Derivative				
Theophylline	Slo-Phyllin, Elixophyllin Theo-Dur	PO Timed-release	Long-term control	Nausea, vomiting, headache, nervousness, irritability, insomnia
Antiasthma Drugs				
Corticosteroids				
beclomethasone	Beclovent	MDI	Long-term control	Throat irritation, cough, nausea, dizziness
triamcinolone	Azamacort	MDI	Long-term control	Throat irritation, cough, nausea, dizziness
Leukotriene Inhibitors				
Montelukast	Singulair	PO	Long-term control	Headache, nausea, abdominal pain, diarrhea
Mast Cell Stabilizers				
Cromolyn	Intal	Intranasal nebulizer	Long-term control	Nasal irritation, unpleasant taste, headache, nausea, dry throat

MDI = metered-dose inhaler

Leukotriene Inhibitors

These are given by mouth along with other asthma medications for long-term control and prevention of mild, persistent asthma. Leukotrienes are bronchoconstrictive substances that are released in the body during the inflammatory process. These drugs inhibit leukotriene production, which helps with bronchodilation and decreases airway edema.

Mast Cell Stabilizers

These help to stabilize the cell membrane by preventing mast cells from releasing the chemical mediators that cause bronchospasm and mucous membrane inflammation They are used to help decrease wheezing and exercise-induced asthma attacks. These are nonsteroidal anti-inflammatory drugs (NSAID) and have relatively few side effects. A bronchodilator often is given to open up the airways just before the mast cell stabilizer is used. Children dislike the taste of the medication, but receiving sips of water after the administration minimizes the distaste.

Chest Physiotherapy

Because asthma has multiple causes, treatment and continued management of the disease require more than medication. Chest physiotherapy includes breathing exercises, physical training, and inhalation therapy. Studies have shown that breathing exercises to improve respiratory function and help control asthma attacks can be an important adjunct to using medications for treatment. These exercises teach children how to help control their own symptoms and thereby build

Check out this tip. For the asthmatic child, if exercises can be taught as part of play activities, children are more likely to find them fun and to practice them more often.

● **Figure 35.6** **(A)** Girl using a nebulizer with a mask. **(B)** Boy using a metered-dose inhaler with spacer.

self-confidence, which is sometimes lacking in asthmatic children.

Nursing Process for the Child With Asthma

ASSESSMENT

Obtain information from the caregiver about the asthma history, the medications the child takes, and the medications taken within the last 24 hours. Ask if the child has vomited, because vomiting would prevent absorption of oral medications. Ask about any history of respiratory infections; possible allergens in the household, such as pets; type of furniture and toys; if there is a damp basement (which could contain mold spores); and a history of breathing problems after exercise.

In the physical examination, include vital signs, observation for diaphoresis and cyanosis, position, type of breathing, alertness, chest movement, intercostal retractions, and breath sounds. Note any wheezing.

If the child is old enough and alert enough to cooperate, involve him or her in gathering the history, and encourage the child to add information. Ask questions that can be answered "yes" or "no" to minimize tiring the distressed child.

SELECTED NURSING DIAGNOSES

- Ineffective Airway Clearance related to bronchospasm and increased pulmonary secretions
- Risk for Deficient Fluid Volume related to water loss from tachypnea and diaphoresis and reduced oral intake
- Fatigue related to dyspnea
- Anxiety related to sudden attacks of breathlessness

- Deficient Knowledge of the caregiver related to disease process, treatment, home care, and control of disease

OUTCOME IDENTIFICATION AND PLANNING

The initial major goals for the child include maintaining a clear airway and an adequate fluid intake, as well as relieving fatigue and anxiety. The family's goals include learning how to manage the child's life with asthma. Base the nursing plan of care on these goals.

IMPLEMENTATION

Monitoring Respiratory Function
Continuously monitor the child while he or she is in acute distress from an asthma attack using pulse oximetry and an electronic monitor. If this equipment is unavailable, take the child's respirations every 15 minutes during an acute attack and every 1 or 2 hours after the crisis is over. Listening to lung sounds should be done to further monitor the respiratory function. Observe for nasal flaring and chest retractions; observe the skin for color and diaphoresis.

Elevate the child's head. An older child may be more comfortable resting forward on a pillow placed on an over-bed table. Monitor the child for response to medications and their side effects, such as restlessness, gastrointestinal upset, and seizures. Use humidified oxygen and suction as needed during periods of acute distress.

Monitoring and Improving Fluid Intake
During an acute attack, the child may lose a great quantity of fluid through the respiratory tract and may have a poor oral intake because of coughing and vomiting. Theophylline administration also has a diuretic effect, which compounds

the problem. Monitor intake and output. Encourage oral fluids that the child likes. IV fluids are administered as ordered. IV fluid intake is monitored, and all precautions for parenteral administration are followed. Note the skin turgor and observe the mucous membranes at least every 8 hours. Weigh the child daily to help determine fluid losses.

Promoting Energy Conservation

The child might become extremely tired from the exertion of trying to breathe. Activities and patient care should be spaced to provide maximum periods of uninterrupted rest. Provide quiet activities when the child needs diversion. Keep visitors to a minimum and maintain a quiet environment.

Reducing Child and Parent Anxiety

The sudden onset of an asthma attack can be frightening to the child and the family caregivers. Respond quickly when the child has an attack. Reassure the child and the family during an episode of dyspnea.

A PERSONAL GLIMPSE

The first time I put Bobbie in the hospital it was very scary. I knew the nurses, but still I was afraid for him. I felt like someone was punishing me. I couldn't leave him for a minute. I was afraid he wouldn't be alive when I came back. I was also afraid he would be frightened. He was so small he needed me to protect him, but I couldn't help him. We were in the hospital every couple of weeks. He would get better then have another attack. It got to the point where I would call the doctor and say that Bobbie was having another attack and they would just send us to admitting. After a few times, I got used to caring for him in the hospital. The nurses taught me how to keep his tent humidified and I could just take care of it myself. Finally I was able to go back to work during the day and care for him on my breaks and time off. It was very difficult each and every time, but we adjusted to hospital life. Although I was afraid for him, I knew he was a fighter and I had to be too. I feel this experience made him a stronger person. He is now 8 years old and has had no severe attacks since he was about 2 years old. He has had a few mild attacks but it doesn't affect him or myself.

Tracee

LEARNING OPPORTUNITY: Give specific examples of what the nurse could do to support this mother and to help decrease the fear she had when her child was hospitalized.

Teach the child and the caregiver the symptoms of an impending attack and the immediate response needed to decrease the threat of an attack. This knowledge will help them to cope with impending attacks and plan how to handle the attacks. When they are prepared with information, the child and family may be less fearful. Give the child examples of sports figures, entertainers, actors and actresses, and political leaders who have or have had asthma; for example, Olympic track and field athlete Jackie Joyner Kersee and President John F. Kennedy. Others include Jerome Bettis, professional football player; Amy Van Dyken, American swimming champion; Nancy Hogshead, Olympic gold medalist in swimming; Dennis Rodman, NBA basketball player; and Diane Keaton, actress.

Nursing judgment is in order. The asthmatic child's fear of attacks can be increased by the caregiver's behavior.

Providing Family Teaching

Child and family caregiver teaching is of primary importance in the care of asthmatic children. Family caregivers might overprotect the child because of the fear that an attack will occur when the child is with a baby-sitter, at school, or anywhere away from the caregiver. Asthma attacks can be prevented or decreased by prompt and adequate intervention. Teach the caregiver and child, within the scope of the child's ability to understand, about the disease process, recognition of symptoms of an impending attack, environmental control, avoidance of infection, exercise, drug therapy, and chest physiotherapy.

Teach the caregiver and the child how to use metered-dose inhaler medications and have them demonstrate correct usage (Family Teaching Tips: How to Use a Metered-Dose Inhaler). Give instructions on home use of a peak flow meter. Urge them to maintain a diary to record the peak flow, as well as asthma symptoms, onset of attacks, action taken, and results. Include instructions about administering premedication before the child is exposed to situations in which an attack may occur.

Inform caregivers of allergens that may be in the child's environment and encourage them to eliminate or control the allergens as needed. Stress the importance of quick response when the child has a respiratory infection. Give instructions for exercise and chest physiotherapy.

FAMILY TEACHING TIPS

How to Use a Metered-Dose Inhaler

- When ready to use, shake the inhaler well with the cap still on. The child should stand, if possible.
- Remove the cap.
- Hold the inhaler with the mouthpiece down, facing the child.
- Be sure the child's mouth is empty.
- Hold the mouthpiece about 1 to 1½ inches from the lips.*
- Breathe out normally. Open mouth wide and begin to breathe in.
- Press top of medication canister firmly while inhaling deeply. Hold breath as long as possible (at least 10 seconds—teach child to count slowly to 10).
- Breathe out *slowly* through nose or pursed lips.
- Relax 2 to 5 minutes and repeat as directed by physician.

*The mouthpiece can also be put between the lips, with the lips forming an airtight seal, or a spacer can be attached to the inhaler and the mouthpiece held between the lips.

Stress to the caregivers the importance of informing the child's classroom teacher, physical education teacher, school nurse, baby-sitter, and others who are responsible for the child about the child's condition. With a physician's order, including directions for use, the child should be permitted to bring medications to school and keep them so they can be used when needed.

Provide information on support groups available in the area. The American Lung Association has many materials available to families and can provide information about support groups, camps, and workshops (website: http://www.lungusa.org). The Asthma and Allergy Foundation of America (website: http://www.aafa.org) and the National Heart, Lung, and Blood Institute (website: http://www.nhlbi.nih.gov) are also resources.

EVALUATION: GOALS AND EXPECTED OUTCOMES

- **Goal:** The child's airway will remain open.
  Expected Outcomes: The child's breath sounds are clear with no wheezing, retractions, or nasal flaring; and the skin color is good.
- **Goal:** The child's fluid intake will be adequate.
  Expected Outcomes: The child's hourly urine output is 30 to 40 mL; mucous membranes are

moist; skin turgor is good; and weight remains stable.
- **Goal:** The child will have increased energy levels.
  Expected Outcomes: The child participates in age-appropriate activities after period of rest; activities are well-spaced.
- **Goal:** The child and caregivers' anxiety and fear related to impending attacks will be minimized.
  Expected Outcomes: The child and the caregiver list the symptoms of an impending attack, describe appropriate responses, and display confidence in their ability to handle an attack.
- **Goal:** The child and the caregiver will gain knowledge of how to live with asthma.
  Expected Outcomes: The child and the caregiver verbalize an understanding of the disease process, treatment, and control. They interact with health care personnel and ask and answer relevant questions. The caregiver obtains information and makes contact with support groups.

Test Yourself

- What is the most important aspect in the treatment of asthma?
- What are the two categories of medications used in the treatment of asthma?
- What are the routes of administration for many of the medications used to treat asthma?
- Why is chest physiotherapy used in the treatment of asthma?

BACTERIAL PNEUMONIA

Pneumococcal pneumonia is the most common form of bacterial pneumonia in infants and children. Its incidence has decreased during the last several years. This disease occurs mainly during the late winter and early spring, principally in children younger than 4 years of age.

In the infant, pneumococcal pneumonia is generally of the bronchial type. In older children, pneumococcal pneumonia is generally of the lobar type. It is usually secondary to an upper respiratory viral infection. The most common finding in infants is a patchy infiltration of one or several lobes of the lung. Pleural effusion is often present. In the older child the pneumonia may localize in a single lobe. Immunization with the pneumococcal vaccine (PCV) is currently recommended beginning at 2 months of age.

H. influenzae pneumonia also occurs in infants and young children. Its clinical manifestations are similar to those of pneumococcal pneumonia, but its onset is more insidious, its clinical course is longer and less acute, and it is usually seen in the lobe of the lung. Complications in the infant are common—usually bacteremia, pericarditis, and empyema (pus in the lungs). The treatment is the same. Immunization with *H. influenzae* type B conjugate vaccine (HIB) is currently recommended beginning at 2 months of age.

Clinical Manifestations

The onset of the pneumonic process is usually abrupt, following a mild upper respiratory illness. Temperature increases rapidly to 103°F to 105°F (39.4°C to 40.6°C). Respiratory distress is marked with obvious air hunger, flaring of the nostrils, **circumoral** (around the mouth) cyanosis, and chest retractions. Tachycardia and tachypnea are present, with a pulse rate frequently as high as 140 to 180 beats per minute and respirations as high as 80 breaths per minute.

Generalized convulsions may occur during the period of high fever. Cough may not be noticeable at the onset but may appear later. Abdominal distention caused by swallowed air or paralytic ileus commonly occurs.

Diagnosis

Diagnosis is made based on clinical symptoms, chest radiograph, and culture of the organism from secretions. The white blood cell count may be elevated. The antistreptolysin titer (ASO titer) is usually elevated in children with staphylococcal pneumonia.

Treatment

The use of anti-infectives early in the disease gives a prompt and favorable response. Penicillin or ampicillin has proved to be the most effective treatment and is generally used unless the child has a penicillin allergy. Cephalosporin anti-infectives are also used. Oxygen started early in the disease process is important. In some instances a croupette or mist tent is used. Some consider the use of mist tents without constant observation unsafe. Children have become cyanotic in mist tents, with subsequent arrest, because of the difficulty of seeing the child; therefore,

a mask or hood is thought to be the better choice. Intravenous fluids are often necessary to supply the needed amount of fluids.

Prognosis for recovery is excellent.

● Nursing Process for the Child With Pneumonia

ASSESSMENT

Conduct a thorough interview with the caregiver. In addition to standard information, include specific data, such as when the symptoms were first noticed, the course of the fever thus far, a description of respiratory difficulties, and the character of any cough. Collect data regarding how well the child has been taking nourishment and fluids. Ask about nausea, vomiting, urinary and bowel output, and history of exposure to other family members with respiratory infections.

Conduct a physical exam, including measurement of temperature, apical pulse, respirations (rate, respiratory effort, retractions [costal, intercostal, sternal, suprasternal, substernal], and flaring of nares) (see Chapter 28). Also note breath and lung sounds (crackles, wheezing), cough (dry, productive, hacking), irritability, restlessness, confusion, skin color (pallor, cyanosis), circumoral (around the mouth) cyanosis, cyanotic nail beds, skin turgor, anterior fontanelle (depressed or bulging), nasal passage congestion (color, consistency), mucous membranes (mouth dry, lips dry or cracked), and eyes (bright, glassy, sunken, moist, crusted). If the child is old enough to communicate verbally, ask questions to determine how the child feels.

SELECTED NURSING DIAGNOSES

- Ineffective Airway Clearance related to obstruction associated with edema, mucous secretions, nasal and chest congestion
- Impaired Gas Exchange related to inflammatory process
- Risk for Deficient Fluid Volume related to respiratory fluid loss, fever, and difficulty swallowing
- Hyperthermia related to infection process
- Risk for Further Infection related to location and anatomic structure of the eustachian tubes
- Activity Intolerance related to inadequate gas exchange

- Anxiety related to dyspnea, invasive procedures, and separation from caregiver
- Compromised Family Coping related to child's respiratory symptoms and child's illness
- Deficient Knowledge of the caregiver related to child's condition and home care

OUTCOME IDENTIFICATION AND PLANNING

The major goals for the child with pneumonia are maintaining respiratory function, preventing fluid deficit, maintaining body temperature, preventing otitis media, conserving energy, and relieving anxiety. Goals for the family include relieving anxiety and improving caregiver knowledge.

The need for immediate intubation is always a possibility; thus, vigilance is essential. The child's energy must be conserved to reduce oxygen requirements. The child may need to be placed on infection control precautions, according to the policy of the health care facility, to prevent nosocomial spread of infection. Many children with a respiratory condition need to be placed in a croupette or mist tent, making additional nursing interventions necessary. If IV fluids are ordered, interventions that promote tissue and skin integrity are needed. To ensure that the child does not interfere with the IV infusion site, it may be necessary to prepare restraints. Intravenous administration and the use of restraints are discussed in Chapter 30. (See Nursing Care Plan 35-1: The Child With Pneumonia).

IMPLEMENTATION

Maintaining Airway Clearance

A humidified atmosphere is provided with an ice-cooled mist tent or cool vaporizer. The moisturized air helps thin the mucus in the respiratory tract to ease respirations. Suction or clear secretions as needed to keep the airway open. Position the child to provide maximum ventilation, and change positions at least every 2 hours. Use pillows and padding to maintain the child's position. Observe frequently for slumping, which causes crowding of the diaphragm. Avoid use of constricting clothes and bedding. Stuffed toys are not recommended in mist tents because they become saturated and provide an environment in which organisms flourish.

Monitoring Respiratory Function

Be continuously alert for warning signs of airway obstruction. Monitor the child at least every hour; uncover the child's chest and observe the child's breathing efforts. Observe for tachypnea (rapid respirations), note the amount of chest movement, shallow breathing, and retractions. Listen with a stethoscope for breath sounds, particularly noting the amount of stridor, which indicates difficult breathing. Oxygen saturation levels are monitored using oximetry. Increasing hoarseness should be reported. In addition, observe for pallor, listlessness, circumoral cyanosis, cyanotic nail beds, and restlessness; these are indications of impaired oxygenation and should be reported at once. Cool, high humidity provides relief. Oxygen may be administered by hood, mist tent, or nasal cannula if the practitioner orders.

Promoting Adequate Fluid Intake

It is important to clear the nasal passages immediately before feeding. For the infant, use a bulb syringe. Administer normal saline nose drops to thin secretions about 10 to 15 minutes before feedings and at bedtime. Feed the child slowly, allowing frequent stops with suctioning during feeding as needed. Avoid overtiring the infant or child during feeding.

Adequate hydration helps reduce thick mucus. Maintaining adequate fluid intake may be a problem for children of any age because the child may be too ill to want to eat. Offer warm, clear fluids to encourage oral intake. Between meals, offer juices and water appropriate for the infant or child's age. For infants, use a relatively small-holed nipple so he does not choke but does not work too hard. Maintain accurate intake and output measurements. Observe carefully for aspiration, especially in severe respiratory distress. The child may need to be kept NPO to prevent this threat. Parenteral fluids may be administered to replace those lost through respiratory loss, fever, and anorexia. Follow all safety measures for administration of parenteral fluids. Observe patency, placement, site integrity, and flow rate at least hourly. Fluid needs are determined by the amount needed to maintain body weight with sufficient amounts added to replace the additional losses. Monitor daily weights and accurately record intake and output. Monitor serum electrolyte levels to ensure they are within normal limits. At least once per shift, observe and record skin turgor and the condition of mucous membranes. Observe the child for dehydration: skin turgor, anterior fontanelle (in infants), and urine output are good indicators. For the infant, maintain diaper counts and weigh

NURSING CARE PLAN 35.1

The Child With Pneumonia

CASE SCENARIO:
CW, a 6-month-old child with pneumonia, has been brought to the hospital from the doctor's office by his mother. He has a copious amount of thick nasal discharge and has rapid, shallow respirations with substernal and intercostal retractions. His temperature is 101.5°F (39.1°C). His young mother appears very anxious.

NURSING DIAGNOSIS
Ineffective Airway Clearance related to infectious process

GOAL: The child's respiratory function will improve and airway will be patent.

EXPECTED OUTCOMES:
• The child no longer uses respiratory accessory muscles to aid in breathing.
• The child's breath sounds are clear and respirations are regular.
• Mucous secretions become thin and scant; nasal passages are clear.

NURSING INTERVENTIONS	*RATIONALE*
Provide moist atmosphere by placing him in ice-cooled mist tent.	Moisture helps liquefy and thin secretions for easier respirations.
Keep nasal passages clear, using bulb syringe.	Open passages increase air flow.
Monitor respiratory function by observing for retractions, respiratory rate, and listening to breath sounds at least every 4 hours. Monitor more frequently if tachypnea or deep retractions are noted.	Changes in the child's breathing may be early indicators of respiratory distress.
Monitor child's bedding and clothing every 4 hours.	Clothing and bedding can become very wet from mist. Dry clothing and bedding help to prevent chilling.

NURSING DIAGNOSIS
Imbalanced Nutrition: Less Than Body Requirements related to inability to suck, drink, or swallow because of congested nasal passages or fatigue from difficulty breathing

GOAL: The child will have adequate food and fluid intake to maintain normal growth and development.

EXPECTED OUTCOMES:
• The child has an adequate caloric intake as evidenced by appropriate weight gain of 1 oz or more a day.
• The child is able to suck, drink, and swallow easily without tiring.
• Skin turgor returns to normal.

NURSING INTERVENTIONS	*RATIONALE*
Clear nasal passages immediately before feeding. Teach family caregiver to use bulb syringe.	Infants are obligatory nasal breathers. Clearing eases child's breathing to permit adequate feeding. Family caregiver can use this technique at home as needed.
Administer normal saline nose drops before feedings and at bedtime.	Normal saline nose drops help thin mucous secretions.
Weigh infant daily in morning before first feeding.	Child will maintain appropriate weight gain.

NURSING DIAGNOSIS
Risk for Further Infection (otitis media) related to current respiratory infection and the size and location of child's eustachian tube

GOAL: The child will remain free from further infection and complications of otitis media.

EXPECTED OUTCOMES:
• The child shows no signs of ear pain, such as irritability, shaking head, pulling on ears.

NURSING CARE PLAN 35.1 continued

The Child With Pneumonia

NURSING INTERVENTIONS	RATIONALE
Change child's position, turning from side to side every hour. Feed child in upright position. Observe for irritability, shaking of head, or pulling at ears.	Turning child prevents mucus from pooling in the eusctachian tubes. Upright position improves drainage and helps open nasal passages. Early recognition of signs of otitis media promotes early diagnosis and treatment.

NURSING DIAGNOSIS
Compromised Family Coping related to child's illness

GOAL: The caregiver's anxiety will be reduced.

EXPECTED OUTCOMES:
- The family caregivers verbalize understanding of the child's condition and treatments.
- The family caregivers reflect confidence in the staff evidenced by cooperation and appropriate questions.

NURSING INTERVENTIONS	RATIONALE
Actively listen to caregivers' concern.	Family members gain confidence when they feel their concerns are being heard.
Provide reassurance and explain what you are doing and why you are doing it when working with the child. Involve caregivers in caring for child. Teach techniques of care that can be used at home.	Understanding the disease and treatment methods helps family to feel that the child's illness is under control. Family caregivers feel valued and benefit from nursing care tips that they can use at home.

diapers to determine the amount of urine output (1 mL urine weighs 1 g).

Maintaining Body Temperature
Monitor the child's temperature frequently, at least every 2 hours if it is higher than 101.3°F (38.6°C). If the child has a fever, remove excess clothing and covering. Antipyretic medications may be ordered.

Promoting Energy Conservation
During an acute stage, allow the child to rest as much as possible. Plan work so that rest and sleep are interrupted no more than necessary.

Preventing Additional Infections
Turn the child from side to side every hour so that mucus is less likely to drain into the eustachian tubes, thereby reducing the risk for development of otitis media. An infant seat may help facilitate breathing and prevent the complication of otitis media in the younger child. Observe the child for irritability, shaking of the head, pulling at the ears, or complaints of ear

pain. Do not give the infant a bottle while he or she is lying in bed. The best position for feeding is upright to avoid excessive drainage into the eustachian tubes.

Reducing the Child's Anxiety
When frightened or upset and crying, the child with a respiratory condition may hyperventilate, which causes additional respiratory distress. For this reason, maintain a calm, soothing manner while caring for the child. When possible, the child should be cared for by a constant caregiver with whom a trusting relationship has been achieved. Offering support to the child during invasive procedures, such as when an IV is being started, will help decrease the child's anxiety. The family can provide the child with a favorite blanket or toy. The family caregiver is encouraged to stay with the child if possible to provide reassurance and avoid separation anxiety in the child. Plan care to minimize interrupting the child's much-needed rest. Give the child age-appropriate explanations of treatment and procedures.

As the child's condition improves, provide age-appropriate diversional activities to help relieve anxiety and boredom. Make extra efforts to relieve the child's feelings of loneliness, especially when infection control precautions are being used.

Promoting Family Coping

Watching a child with severe respiratory symptoms is frightening for the parent or family caregiver. Family caregivers need teaching and reassurance. The parent or caregiver may feel helpless, and these feelings of anxiety and helplessness may be exhibited in a variety of ways. To alleviate these feelings, encourage the caregiver to discuss them. Using easily understood terminology, explain equipment, procedures, treatments, the illness, and the prognosis to the caregiver. Include the caregiver in the child's care as much as possible and encourage him or her to soothe and comfort the child. Actively listen to caregivers and use communication skills to respond to their worries.

Providing Family Teaching

Provide the caregiver with thorough explanations of the condition's signs and symptoms. Teach the use of cool humidifiers or vaporizers, including cleaning methods and safety measures to avoid burns when using a steam vaporizer. Explain the effects, administration, dosage, and side effects of medications. To be certain the information was understood, have the parent relate specific facts to you. Write the information down in a simple way so that it can be clearly understood, and determine that the parent can read and understand the written material. When appropriate, observe the caregiver demonstrate care of equipment and any treatments to be done at home. See Family Teaching Tips: Respiratory Infections.

EVALUATION: GOALS AND EXPECTED OUTCOMES

- **Goal:** The child's airway will remain clear and patent.
  Expected Outcomes: The child's airway is clear with no evidence of retractions, stridor, hoarseness, or cyanosis. The mucous secretions are thin and scant.
- **Goal:** The child's respiratory function will be within normal limits for age.
  Expected Outcomes: The child's respiratory rate is 20 to 35 per minute, normal range for child's age, regular, with breath sounds clear; the infant no longer uses respiratory accessory

FAMILY TEACHING TIPS

Respiratory Infections

- Clear nasal passages with a bulb syringe for the infant.
- Feed the child slowly, allow the infant to breast-feed without tiring.
- Frequently burp the infant to expel swallowed air.
- Offer child extra fluids.
- Leave the child in mist tent except for feeding and bathing (unless otherwise indicated).
- Soothe and comfort child in mist or croup tent.
- Follow respiratory infection control precautions and good handwashing techniques.
- Discourage persons with infections from visiting child.
- Use a humidifier at home after discharge.
- Clean humidifier properly and frequently.

muscles to aid in breathing. Oxygen saturation levels are within established limits.

- **Goal:** The child's fluid intake will be adequate for age and weight.
  Expected Outcomes: The child exhibits good skin turgor and moist, pink mucous membranes. Urine output is 1 to 3 mL/kg/hr.
- **Goal:** The child will maintain a temperature within normal limits.
  Expected Outcomes: The child's temperature is 98.6°F to 100°F (37°C to 37.8°C).
- **Goal:** The child's energy will be conserved.
  Expected Outcomes: The child has extended periods of uninterrupted rest and tolerates increased activity.
- **Goal:** The child will be free from complications of otitis media.
  Expected Outcomes: The child shows no signs of ear pain, such as irritability, shaking of the head, pulling on the ears, or reporting ear pain.
- **Goal:** The child will experience a reduction in anxiety.
  Expected Outcomes: The child rests quietly with no evidence of hyperventilation, cooperates with care, cuddles a favorite toy for reassurance, smiles, and plays contentedly.
- **Goal:** The family caregiver's anxiety will be reduced.
  Expected Outcomes: The caregiver cooperates with and participates in the child's care, appears more relaxed, verbalizes his or her feelings, and soothes the child.
- **Goal:** The family caregivers will verbalize an understanding of the child's condition and how to provide home care for the child.

Expected Outcomes: The family caregivers accurately describe facts about the child's condition; ask appropriate questions; relate signs and symptoms to observe in the child; and name the effects, side effects, dosage, and administration of medications.

CYSTIC FIBROSIS

When first described, cystic fibrosis (CF) was called "fibrocystic disease of the pancreas." Additional research has revealed that this disorder represents a major dysfunction of all exocrine glands. The major organs affected are the lungs, pancreas, and liver. Because about half of all children with CF have pulmonary complications, this disorder is discussed here with other respiratory conditions.

Cystic fibrosis is hereditary and transmitted as an autosomal recessive trait. Both parents must be carriers of the gene for CF to appear. With each pregnancy, the chance is one in four that the child will have the disease. In the United States, the incidence is about 1 in 3,300 in white children and 1 in 16,300 in black children.

The normal gene produces a protein, cystic fibrosis transmembrane conductance regulator, which serves as a channel through which chloride enters and leaves cells. The mutated gene blocks chloride movement, which brings on the apparent signs of CF. The blocking of chloride transport results in a change in sodium transport; this in turn results in abnormal secretions of the exocrine (mucous-producing) glands that produce thick, tenacious mucus, rather than the thin, free-flowing secretion normally produced. This abnormal mucus leads to obstruction of the secretory ducts of the pancreas, liver, and reproductive organs. Thick mucus obstructs the respiratory passages, causing trapped air and overinflation of the lungs. In addition, the sweat and salivary glands excrete excessive electrolytes, specifically sodium and chloride.

Clinical Manifestations

Meconium ileus is the presenting symptom of CF in 5% to 10% of the newborns who later develop additional manifestations. Depletion or absence of pancreatic enzymes before birth results in impaired digestive activity, and the meconium becomes viscid (thick) and mucilaginous (sticky). The inspissated (thickened) meconium fills the small intestine, causing complete obstruction. Clinical manifestations are bile-stained emesis, a distended abdomen, and an absence of stool. Intestinal perforation with symptoms of shock may occur. These newborns taste salty when kissed because of the high sodium chloride concentration in their sweat.

Initial symptoms of CF may occur at varying ages during infancy, childhood, or adolescence. A hard, nonproductive chronic cough may be the first sign. Later, frequent bronchial infections occur. Development of a barrel chest and clubbing of fingers (Fig. 35-7) indicate chronic lack of oxygen.

Don't be misled. Despite an excellent appetite in the child with cystic fibrosis, malnutrition is apparent and becomes increasingly severe.

The abdomen becomes distended, and body muscles become flabby.

Pancreatic Involvement

Thick, tenacious mucus obstructs the pancreatic ducts, causing **hypochylia** (diminished flow of pancreatic enzymes) or **achylia** (absence of pancreatic enzymes). This achylia or hypochylia leads to intestinal malabsorption and severe malnutrition. The deficient pancreatic enzymes are lipase, trypsin, and amylase. Malabsorption of fats causes frequent steatorrhea. Anemia or rectal prolapse is common if the pancreatic condition remains untreated. The inci-

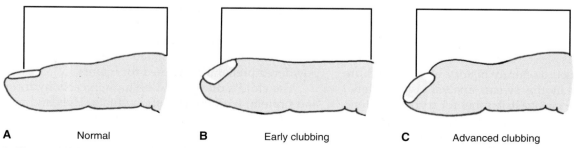

A Normal   **B** Early clubbing   **C** Advanced clubbing

● *Figure 35.7* Clubbing of fingers indicates chronic lack of oxygen. (**A**) Normal angle; (**B**) early clubbing—flattened angle; (**C**) advanced clubbing—the nail is rounded over the end of the finger.

dence of diabetes is greater in these children than in the general population, possibly because of changes in the pancreas. The incidence of diabetes in patients with CF is expected to increase because of their increasing life expectancy.

Pulmonary Involvement

The degree of lung involvement determines the prognosis for survival. The severity of pulmonary involvement differs in individual children, with a few showing only minor involvement. Now more than half of children with CF are expected to live beyond the age of 18 years, with increasing numbers living into adulthood.

Respiratory complications pose the greatest threat to children with CF. Abnormal amounts of thick, viscid mucus clog the bronchioles and provide an ideal medium for bacterial growth. *Staphylococcus aureus* coagulase can be cultured from the nasopharynx and sputum of most patients. *Pseudomonas aeruginosa* and *H. influenzae* also are found frequently. However, the basic infection appears most often to be caused by *S. aureus*.

Numerous complications arise from severe respiratory infections. Atelectasis and small lung abscesses are common early complications. Bronchiectasis and emphysema may develop with pulmonary fibrosis and pneumonitis; this eventually leads to severe ventilatory insufficiency. In advanced disease, pneumothorax, right ventricular hypertrophy, and cor pulmonale are common complications. Cor pulmonale is a common cause of death.

Other Organ Involvement

The tears, saliva, and sweat of children with CF contain abnormally high concentrations of electrolytes, and most such children have enlarged submaxillary salivary glands. In hot weather, the loss of sodium chloride and fluid through sweating produces frequent heat prostration. Additional fluid and salt should be given in the diet as a preventive measure. In addition, males with CF who reach adulthood will most likely be sterile because of the blockage or absence of the vas deferens or other ducts. Females often have thick cervical secretions that prohibit the passage of sperm.

Diagnosis

Diagnosis is based on family history, elevated sodium chloride levels in the sweat, analysis of duodenal secretions (via a nasogastric tube) for trypsin content, a history of failure to thrive, chronic or recurrent respiratory infections, and radiologic findings of hyperinflation and bronchial wall thickening. In the event of a positive sodium chloride sweat test, at least one other criterion must be met to make a conclusive diagnosis.

The principal diagnostic test to confirm CF is a sweat chloride test using the pilocarpine iontophoresis method. This method induces sweating by using a small electric current that carries topically applied pilocarpine into a localized area of the skin. Elevations of 60 mEq/L or more are diagnostic, with values of 50 to 60 mEq/L highly suspect. Although the test itself is fairly simple, conducting the test on an infant is difficult, and false-positive results do occur.

Treatment

In the newborn, meconium ileus is treated with hyperosmolar enemas administered gently. If this does not resolve the blockage of thick, gummy meconium, surgery is necessary. During surgery, a mucolytic such as Mucomyst may be used to liquefy the meconium. If this procedure is successful, resection may not be necessary.

In the older child, treatment is aimed at correcting pancreatic deficiency, improving pulmonary function, and preventing respiratory infections. If bowel obstruction does occur (meconium ileus equivalent), the preferred management includes hyperosmolar enemas and an increase in fluids, dietary fiber, oral mucolytics, lactulose, and mineral oil.

The overall treatment goals are to improve the child's quality of life and to provide for long-term survival. A health care team is needed, including a primary care provider, a nurse, a respiratory therapist, a dietitian, and a social worker, to work together with the child and family. Treatment centers with a staff of specialists are becoming more common, particularly in larger medical centers. With improved treatment, it is not unusual for a child with CF to grow into adulthood.

Dietary Treatment

Commercially prepared pancreatic enzymes given during meals or with snacks aid digestion and absorption of fat and protein. Because pancreatic enzymes are inactivated in the acidic environment of the stomach, microencapsulated capsules are used to deliver the enzymes to the duodenum, where they are activated. These enzymes come in capsules that can be swallowed or opened and sprinkled on the child's food. A powdered preparation is used for infants.

The child's diet should be high in carbohydrates and protein, with no restriction of fats. The child may need 1.5 to 2 times the normal caloric intake to promote growth. These children have large appetites unless they are acutely ill. However, even with their large appetites they can receive little nourishment without a pancreatic supplement. With proper diet and enzyme supplements, these children show evidence of improved nutrition, and their stools become relatively normal. Enteric-coated pancreatic enzymes essentially eliminate the need for dietary restriction of fat.

Because of the increased loss of sodium chloride, these children are allowed to use as much salt as they wish, even though onlookers may think it is too much. During hot weather, additional salt may be provided with pretzels, salted bread sticks, and saltine crackers.

Supplements of fat-soluble vitamins A, D, and E are necessary because of the poor digestion of fats. Vitamin K may be supplemented if the child has coagulation problems or is scheduled for surgery. Water-miscible preparations can be given to provide the needed supplement.

Pulmonary Treatment

The treatment goal is to prevent and treat respiratory infections. Respiratory drainage is provided by thinning the secretions and by mechanical means, such as postural drainage and clapping, to loosen and drain secretions from the lungs. Antibacterial drugs for the treatment of infection are necessary as indicated. Some physicians prescribe a prophylactic antibiotic regimen when the child receives the diagnosis of CF. Antibiotics may be administered orally or parenterally even in the home. With home parenteral administration of antibiotic therapy, a central venous access device is used. Immunization against childhood communicable diseases is extremely important for these chronically ill children. All immunization measures may be used and should be maintained at appropriate intervals.

Physical activity is essential because it improves mucous secretion and helps the child feel good. The child can be encouraged to participate in any aerobic activity he or she enjoys. Activity along with physical therapy should be limited only by the child's endurance.

Inhalation therapy can be preventive or therapeutic. A bronchodilator drug such as theophylline or a beta-adrenergic agonist (metaproterenol, terbutaline, or albuterol) may be administered either orally or through nebulization. Recombinant human DNA (DNase, Pulmozyme) breaks down DNA molecules in sputum, breaking up the thick mucus in the airways. A mucolytic such as Mucomyst may be prescribed during acute infection. Hand-held nebulizers are easy to use and convenient for the ambulatory child.

Humidifiers provide a humidified atmosphere. In summer, a room air conditioner can help provide comfort and controlled humidity.

Chest physical therapy, a combination of postural drainage and chest percussion, is performed routinely at least every morning and evening, even if little drainage is apparent (Fig. 35-8). Performed correctly, chest percussion (clapping and vibrating of the affected areas) helps to loosen and move secretions out of the lungs. The physical therapist usually performs this procedure in the hospital and teaches it to the family. Chest physical therapy, although time consuming, is part of the ongoing, long-term treatment and should be continued at home.

Home Care

The home care for a child with CF places a tremendous burden on the family. This is not a one-time hospital treatment, and there is no prospect of cure to brighten the horizon. Each day, much time is spent performing treatments. Family caregivers must learn to perform chest physical therapy and how to operate respiratory equipment and administer IV antibiotics when necessary. The child's diet must be planned with additional enzymes regulated according to need. Great care is needed to prevent exposure to infections.

Family caregivers must guard against overprotection and against undue limitation of their child's physical activity. Somehow a good family relationship must be preserved, with time and attention given to other members of the family.

Physical activity is an important adjunct to the child's well-being and is necessary to get rid of secretions. Capacity for exercise is soon learned, and the child can be trusted to become self-limiting as necessary, especially if given an opportunity to learn the nature of the disease. The child may find postural drainage fun when a caregiver raises the child's feet in the air and walks the child around "wheelbarrow" fashion.

A little fun can be good. The older child with cystic fibrosis can learn to hang from a monkey bar by the knees, having fun and at the same time increasing postural drainage.

Providing as much normalcy as possible is always desirable. Hot-weather activity should be watched a little more closely, with additional attention to increased salt and fluid intake during exercise.

Caring for a child with CF places great stress on a family's financial resources. The expense of daily medications, frequent clinic or office visits, and sometimes lengthy hospitalizations can be devastating to an ordinary family budget, even with medical insurance coverage. The Cystic Fibrosis Foundation (www.cff.org), with chapters throughout the United States, is helpful in providing education and services. Some assistance may be available through local agencies or community groups.

Upper lobes
apical segment

Upper lobes
posterior segment

Left lingula

Right middle
lobe

Right lateral lobe
anterior segment

Lower lobes
posterior segments

Lower lobes
anterior segments

● *Figure 35.8* Positions for postural drainage.

● Nursing Process for the Child With Cystic Fibrosis

ASSESSMENT

The collection of data on the child with CF varies, depending on the child's age and the circumstances of the admission. Conduct a complete parent interview that includes the standard information, as well as data concerning respiratory infections, the child's appetite and eating habits, stools, noticeable salty perspiration, history of bowel obstruction as an infant, and family history for CF, if known. Also determine the caregiver's knowledge of the condition.

When collecting data about vital signs, include observation of respirations, such as cough, breath sounds, and barrel chest; respiratory effort, such as retractions and nasal flaring; clubbing of the fingers; and signs of pancreatic involvement, such as failure to thrive and steatorrhea. Examine the skin around the rectum for irritation and breakdown from frequent foul stools. Ask the child age-appropriate questions, involve the child in the interview process, and determine the child's perception of the disease and this current illness.

SELECTED NURSING DIAGNOSES

- Ineffective Airway Clearance related to thick, tenacious mucus production
- Ineffective Breathing Pattern related to tracheobronchial obstruction
- Risk for Infection related to bacterial growth medium provided by pulmonary mucus and impaired body defenses
- Imbalanced Nutrition: Less Than Body Requirements related to impaired absorption of nutrients
- Anxiety related to hospitalization
- Compromised Family Coping related to child's chronic illness and its demands on caregivers
- Deficient Knowledge of the caregiver related to illness, treatment, and home care

OUTCOME IDENTIFICATION AND PLANNING

As already stated, much depends on the reason for the specific admission and other factors discussed in Nursing Diagnoses. The child's age and ability for self-expression affect any goal setting the child can do. The major goals for the child include relieving immediate respiratory distress, maintaining adequate oxygenation, remaining free from infection, improving nutritional status, and relieving anxiety. The caregivers' primary goal may include relieving problems related to this admission. However, other goals may include concerns about stress on the family related to the illness, as well as a need for additional information about the disease, treatment, and prevention of complications.

IMPLEMENTATION

Improving Airway Clearance
Mucus causes obstruction of the airways and diminishes gas exchange. Monitor the child for signs of respiratory distress, while observing for dyspnea, tachypnea, labored respirations with or without activity, retractions, nasal flaring, and color of nail beds. Perform aerosol treatments. Teach the child to cough effectively. Examine and document the mucus produced, noting the color, consistency, and odor. Send cultures to the laboratory as appropriate. Increase fluid intake to help thin mucous secretions. Encourage the child to drink extra fluids and ask the child (or the caregiver if the child is too young) what favorite drinks might be appealing. Intravenous fluids may be necessary. Provide humidified air, either in the form of a cool mist humidifier or mist tent as prescribed.

Improving Breathing
Maintain the child in a semi-Fowler's or high Fowler's position to promote maximal lung expansion. Pulse oximetry may be used. Maintain oxygen saturation higher than 90%. Administer oxygen as ordered if the oxygen saturation falls below this level for an extended period. Administer mouth care every 2 to 4 hours, especially when oxygen is administered. Perform chest physical therapy every 2 to 4 hours as ordered. If respiratory therapy technicians or physical therapists do these treatments, observe the child after the treatment to determine effectiveness and if more frequent treatments may be needed. Supervise the child who can self-administer nebulizer treatments to ensure correct use.

Conserve the child's energy. Plan nursing and therapeutic activities so that maximal rest time is provided for the child. Note dyspnea and respiratory distress in relation to any activities. Plan quiet diversional activities as the child's physical condition warrants. Help the child and family to understand that activity is excellent for the child not in an acute situation. Teach them that exercise helps loosen the thick mucus and also improves the child's self-image.

Preventing Infection

The child with CF has low resistance, especially to respiratory infections. For this reason, take care to protect the child from any exposure to infectious organisms. Good handwashing techniques should be practiced by all; teach the child and family the importance of this first line of defense. Practice and teach other good hygiene habits. Carefully follow medical asepsis when caring for the child and the equipment. Monitor vital signs every 4 hours for any indication of an infectious process. Restrict people with an infection, such as staff, family members, other patients, and visitors, from contact with the child. Advise the family to keep the child's immunizations up to date. Administer antibiotics as prescribed, and teach the child or caregiver home administration as needed. Also teach the family the signs and symptoms of an impending infection so they can begin prophylactic measures at once.

Maintaining Adequate Nutrition

Adequate nutrition helps the child resist infections. Greatly increase the child's caloric intake to compensate for impaired absorption of nutrients and to provide adequate growth and development. In addition to increased caloric intake at meals, provide the child with high-calorie, high-protein snacks, such as peanut butter and cheese. Low-fat products can be selected if desired. Administer pancreatic enzymes with all meals and snacks. In addition, multiple vitamins and iron may be prescribed. Reinforce the need for these supplements to both the child and the family. The child also may require additional salt in the diet. Encourage the child to eat salty snacks. If the child has bouts of diarrhea or constipation, the dosage of enzymes may need to be adjusted. Report any change in bowel movements. Weigh and measure the child. Plot growth on a chart so that progress can easily be visualized.

Reducing the Child's Anxiety

Provide age-appropriate activities to help alleviate anxiety and the boredom that can result from enforced hospitalization. Choose activities such as reading or arts and crafts according to age. School work may help ease some anxiety. Some older children may enjoy a video game, if available, but watch the child for overexcitement. Encourage the family caregiver to stay with the child to help diminish some of the child's anxiety. Allow the child to have familiar toys or mementos from home. Stay with the child during acute episodes of coughing and dyspnea to reduce anxiety. Give the child age-appropriate information about CF. Quiz the child in a relaxed, friendly manner to help determine what the child knows and what teaching may be needed. Learning about CF can be turned into a game for some children, making it much more enjoyable.

Providing Family Support

The family is faced with a long-term illness and may have already seen deterioration in the child's health. Give the family and the child opportunities to voice fears and anxieties. Respond with active-listening techniques to help authenticate their feelings. Provide emotional support throughout the entire hospital stay. Demonstrate an interest and willingness to talk to the family; do not make family members feel as though they are intruding on time needed to do other things. The nurse is the person who can best provide overall support.

Providing Family Teaching

Evaluate the family's knowledge about CF to determine their teaching needs. The family may need to have all the information repeated or may have just a few areas of need. Provide information for resources, such as the Cystic Fibrosis Foundation, the American Lung Association (www.lungusa.org), and other local organizations. The family may have questions about genetic counseling and may need referrals for counseling.

EVALUATION: GOALS AND EXPECTED OUTCOMES

- **Goal:** The child's airway will be clear.
  Expected Outcomes: The child effectively clears mucus from the airway and the airway remains patent. The child cooperates with chest physical therapy.
- **Goal:** The child will exhibit adequate respiratory function.
  Expected Outcomes: The child rests quietly with no dyspnea; the respiratory rate is even and appropriate for age. The oxygen saturation remains above 90%.
- **Goal:** The child will remain free of signs and symptoms of infection.
  Expected Outcomes: The child's vital signs are within normal limits for age. The child and family follow infection-control practices.
- **Goal:** The child's nutritional intake will be adequate to compensate for decreased absorption of nutrients and to provide for adequate growth and development.
  Expected Outcomes: The child has weight gain appropriate for age, and the child's growth chart reflects normal growth.

- Goal: The child's anxiety will subside.
  Expected Outcomes: The child engages in age-appropriate activities and appears relaxed.
- Goal: The family caregivers will verbalize feelings related to the child's chronic illness.
  Expected Outcomes: The family caregivers verbalize fears, anxieties, and other feelings related to the child's illness.
- Goal: The family caregivers will verbalize an understanding of the child's illness and treatment.
  Expected Outcomes: The family caregivers can explain CF, describe treatments and possible complications, and become involved in available support groups.

Test Yourself

- What two immunizations have decreased the incidence of bacterial pneumonia in children?

- What major organs are affected by cystic fibrosis?

- What is the dietary treatment for cystic fibrosis?

- For what type of infection is the child with cystic fibrosis most susceptible?

PULMONARY TUBERCULOSIS

Tuberculosis is present in all parts of the world and is the most important chronic infectious disease in terms of illness, death, and cost (Starke, 1999). The incidence of tuberculosis in the United States had declined steadily until about 1985. In the years since, there has been an increase in the number of cases reported in the United States. Several factors contribute to this increase; one factor is the number of people who have human immunodeficiency virus (HIV) and have become infected with tuberculosis.

Tuberculosis is caused by *Mycobacterium tuberculosis*, a bacillus spread by droplets of infected mucus that

CULTURAL SNAPSHOT

In some cultures it is common for many people to live together in one home or in a close living arrangement. Respiratory illness is easily spread from person to person when people live in close contact with each other.

become airborne when the infected person sneezes, coughs, or laughs. The bacilli, when airborne, are inhaled into the respiratory tract of the unsuspecting person and become implanted in lung tissue. This process is the beginning of the formation of a primary lesion.

Clinical Manifestations

Primary tuberculosis is the original infection that goes through various stages and ends with calcification. Primary lesions in children generally are unrecognized. The most common site of a primary lesion is the alveoli of the respiratory tract. Most cases arrest with the calcification of the primary infection. However, in children with poor nutrition or health, the primary infection may invade other tissues of the body, including the bones, joints, kidneys, lymph nodes, and meninges. This is called miliary tuberculosis. In the small number of children with miliary tuberculosis, general symptoms of chronic infection, such as fatigue, loss of weight, and low-grade fever, may occur accompanied by night sweats.

Secondary tuberculosis is a reactivation of a healed primary lesion. It often occurs in adults and contributes to the exposure of children to the organism. Although secondary lesions are more common in adults, they may occur in adolescents. Symptoms resemble those in an adult, including cough with expectoration, fever, weight loss, malaise, and night sweats.

Diagnosis

The tuberculin skin test is the primary means by which tuberculosis is detected. A skin test can be performed using a multipuncture device that deposits purified protein derivative (PPD) intradermally (tine test) or by intradermal injection of 0.1 mL of PPD. Either test is administered on the inner aspect of the forearm. The site is marked and read at 48 and 72 hours. Redness, swelling, induration, and itching of the site indicate a positive reaction. Persons with a positive reaction are further examined by radiographic evaluation. Sputum tests of young children are rarely helpful because children do not produce a good specimen. Screening by means of skin testing is recommended for all children at 12 months, before entering school, and in adolescence. Screening is recommended annually for children in high-risk situations or communities including children in whose family there is an active case, Native Americans, and children who recently immigrated from Central or South America, the Caribbean, Africa, Asia, or the Middle East. Other high-risk children are those infected with HIV, those who are homeless or live in overcrowded conditions, and those immunosuppressed from any reason.

Treatment

Drug therapy for tuberculosis includes administration of isoniazid (INH), often in combination with rifampin. Although INH has been known to cause peripheral neuritis in children with poor nutrition, few problems occur in children whose diets are well balanced. Rifampin is tolerated well by children but causes body fluids such as urine, sweat, tears, and feces to turn orange-red. A possible disadvantage for adolescents is that it may permanently stain contact lenses. Rifamate is a combination of rifampin and INH. Other drugs that may be used are ethambutol, streptomycin, and pyrazinamide.

Drug therapy is continued for 9 to 18 months. After drug therapy has begun, the child or adolescent may return to school and normal activities unless clinical symptoms are evident. An annual chest radiograph is necessary from that time on.

Prevention

Prevention requires improvements in social conditions, such as overcrowding, poverty, and poor health care. Also needed are health education; medical, laboratory, and radiographic facilities for examination; and control of contacts and persons suspected of infection.

A vaccine called bacilli Calmette-Guérin (BCG) is used in countries with a high incidence of tuberculosis. It is given to tuberculin-negative persons and is said to be effective for 12 years or longer. Mass vaccination is not considered necessary in parts of the world where the incidence of tuberculosis is low. After administration of BCG vaccine, the skin test will be positive, so screening is no longer an effective tool. The use of BCG vaccine remains controversial because of the effect it has on screening for the disease, as well as the questionable effectiveness of the vaccine.

KEY POINTS

- An infant or child's respiratory system, because of its small size and underdeveloped anatomic structures, is more prone to respiratory problems. Smaller structures lead to a greater chance of obstruction and respiratory distress. As the child grows, the use of the thoracic muscles takes the place of the use of the diaphragm and abdominal muscles for breathing.

- The most common complication of acute nasopharyngitis (common cold) is otitis media.
- The most common complication of a tonsillectomy is hemorrhage or bleeding. The child must be observed especially in the first 24 hours after surgery and in the 5th to 7th postoperative days for unusual restlessness, anxiety, frequent swallowing, or rapid pulse. Vomiting bright, red-flecked emesis or bright red oozing or bleeding may indicate hemorrhage. If noted, these should be reported immediately.
- Spasmodic laryngitis is treated using humidified air to decrease the laryngospasm. A low dose of an emetic may be used to reduce spasms of the larynx.
- Acute laryngotracheobronchitis is often caused by the staphylococcal bacterium. The child may become hoarse and have a barking cough and elevated temperature. Breathing difficulty, a rapid pulse, and cyanosis may occur. Antibiotics are given, and the child placed in a croupette or mist tent with oxygen.
- An asthma attack can be triggered by a hypersensitive response to allergens; foods such as chocolate, milk, eggs, nuts, and grains; exercise; or exposure to cold or irritants such as wood-burning stoves, cigarette smoke, dust, and pet dander. Infections, stress, or anxiety can also trigger an asthma attack.
- During an asthma attack, the combination of smooth muscle spasms, which cause the lumina of the bronchi and bronchioles to narrow; edema; and increased mucus production causes respiratory obstruction.
- Anti-infectives such as penicillin or ampicillin have proved to be the most effective in the treatment of pneumonia. If the child has a penicillin allergy, cephalosporin anti-infectives are also used.
- Cystic fibrosis causes the exocrine (mucous-producing) glands to produce thick, tenacious mucus, rather than thin, free-flowing secretions. These secretions obstruct the secretory ducts of the pancreas, liver, and reproductive organs.
- The most common and serious complications of cystic fibrosis arise from respiratory infections, which may lead to severe respiratory concerns.
- The sweat chloride test, which shows elevated sodium chloride levels in the sweat, is the principal diagnostic test used to confirm cystic fibrosis. Family history, analysis of duodenal secretions for trypsin content, history of failure to thrive, chronic or recurrent respiratory infections, and radiologic findings also help diagnose the disorder.
- Pancreatic enzymes given with meals and snacks are used in the dietary treatment of children with cystic fibrosis. The child's diet is high in protein and carbohydrates, and salt in large amounts is allowed. The use of chest physiotherapy, antibiotics, and inhalation therapy help in the prevention and treatment of respiratory infections.

◆ Tuberculosis can be detected by doing a tuberculin skin test using purified protein derivative (PPD). When a person has a positive reaction to the skin test, additional evaluation using radiography is done to confirm the disease

REFERENCES AND SELECTED READINGS

Books and Journals

Cooper, K. E. (2001). The effectiveness of ribavirin in the treatment of RSV. *Pediatric Nursing, 27*(1), 95–98.

Davis, P. B. (2001). Cystic fibrosis. *Pediatrics in Review, 22*(8), 257.

Dudek, S. G. (2000). *Nutrition essentials for nursing practice* (4th ed.). Philadelphia: Lippincott Williams & Wilkins.

Eggleston, P. A. (1999). Asthma. In *Oski's pediatrics: Principles and practice* (3rd ed.). Philadelphia: Lippincott Williams & Wilkins.

England, A. C., Dalheim Rydstrom, I., & Astrid, N. (2001) Being the parent of a child with asthma. *Pediatric Nursing, 27*(4), 365.

Herbst, D. D. (2001). Cystic fibrosis and lung transplantation: Ethical concerns. *Pediatric Nursing, 27*(1), 87.

Karch, A. M. (2003). *2004 Lippincott's nursing drug guide.* Philadelphia: Lippincott Williams & Wilkins.

Kline, A. (2003). Pediatric respiratory distress. *Nursing 2003, 33*(9), 58–64.

Malhotra, A., & Krilow, L. (2001). Viral croup. *Pediatrics in Review, 22*(1), 5.

North American Nursing Diagnosis Association (NANDA). (2001). *NANDA nursing diagnoses: Definitions and classification 2001–2002.* Philadelphia: Author.

Palmer EA. (2001) Family caregiver experiences with asthma in school age children. *Pediatric Nursing, 27*(1), 75.

Pillitteri, A. (2003). *Maternal and child health nursing* (4th ed.). Philadelphia: Lippincott Williams & Wilkins.

Schmidt, C. K. (2001). Development of children's body knowledge: Using knowledge of the lungs as an exemplar. *Issues in Comprehensive Pediatric Nursing, 24*(3), 177–191.

Skoner, D. P. (2002). Balancing safety and efficacy in pediatric asthma management. *Pediatrics, 109*(2), 381.

Smeltzer, S. C., & Bare, B. G. (2003). *Textbook of medical–surgical nursing* (10th ed.). Philadelphia: Lippincott Williams & Wilkins.

Sparks, S., & Taylor, C. (2001). *Nursing diagnosis reference manual* (5th ed.). Springhouse, PA: Springhouse Corporation.

Stadtler, A. C., Tronick, E. Z., & Brazelton, T. B. (2001). The Touchpoints pediatric asthma program. *Pediatric Nursing, 27*(5), 459.

Starke, J. R. (1999). Tuberculosis. In *Oski's pediatrics: Principles and practice* (3rd ed.). Philadelphia: Lippincott Williams & Wilkins.

Wong, D. L., Perry, S., & Hockenberry, M. (2002). *Maternal–child nursing care* (2nd ed.). St. Louis: Mosby.

Web Addresses
www.cff.org
www.nhlbi.nih.gov
www.aafa.or
www.lungusa.org
www.aaaai.org

WORKBOOK

NCLEX-STYLE REVIEW QUESTIONS

1. The nurse is doing teaching with the caregivers of a child who has had a tonsillectomy the previous day and is being discharged. The nurse would reinforce that which of the following should be reported *immediately* to the child's physician? The child:

   a. complains of a sore throat on the 3rd postoperative day.

   b. refuses to leave the ice collar on for more than 10 minutes.

   c. vomits dark, old blood within 4 hours after being discharged.

   d. has frequent swallowing around the 6th day after surgery.

2. A toddler with a diagnosis of a respiratory disorder has a fever and decreased urinary output. When planning care for this child, which of the following goals would be *most* appropriate for this toddler? The child's

   a. anxiety will be reduced.

   b. fluid intake will be increased.

   c. caregivers will talk about their concerns.

   d. caloric intake will be adequate for age.

3. The nurse is teaching a group of caregivers of children who have asthma. The caregivers make the following statements. Which of these statements indicates a need for additional teaching?

   a. "We need to identify the things that trigger our child's attacks."

   b. "I always have him use his bronchodilator before he uses his steroid inhaler."

   c. "We will be sure our child does not exercise to prevent attacks."

   d. "She drinks lots of water, which I know helps to thin her secretions."

4. A child with cystic fibrosis will have which of the following interventions included in the child's plan of care?

   a. Maintain a flat lying position when in bed.

   b. Provide low protein snacks between meals.

   c. Perform postural drainage in the morning and evening.

   d. Teach infection control procedures when hospitalized.

5. After discussing the disease with the caregiver of a child with cystic fibrosis, the caregiver makes the following statements. Which of these statements indicates a need for additional teaching?

   a. "It is good to know that my other children won't have the disease."

   b. "I will be sure to give my child the medication every time she eats."

   c. "It is important to let my child play with the other kids when she is at school."

   d. "When she exercises, I will feed her a salty snack."

6. The nurse is completing the intake and output record for a toddler who has a respiratory infection. The dry weight of the child's diaper is 38 grams. The child has had the following intake and output during the shift:

   Intake: 3 oz of apple juice

   ½ serving of pancakes

   5 oz of milk

   4 saltine crackers

   ¼ cup of chicken soup

   2 oz of gelatin

   130 cc of IV fluid

   Output: Diaper with urine weighing 87 grams

   Diaper with stool only weighing 124 grams

   Diaper with urine weighing 138 grams

   Diaper with urine weighing 146 grams

   Diaper with urine weighing 95 grams

   a. How many milliliters should the nurse document as the child's total intake?

   b. How many milliliters should the nurse document as the child's urinary output?

STUDY ACTIVITIES

1. Draw a diagram to explain the heredity pattern of cystic fibrosis.
2. Research your community to find sources of help for families with children who have cystic fibrosis.

What support groups and organizations are available that you might recommend to families of children with CF? Discuss with your peers what you found and make a list of resources to share.

3. Go to the following Internet site:
http://www.lungusa.org/asthma
Scroll down the screen on the right hand side. Click on the section "Asthma in Children." Click on "Early Warning Signals."

a. List six areas covered on this site that you could share with a family of a child with asthma.

b. What five suggestions are given in the area covering "What to Listen For?"

c. Read the section on "How to Listen."

d. Describe how you listen to the breath sounds in a child with asthma.

e. What are five emergency signs that require immediate treatment?

CRITICAL THINKING: What Would You Do?

1. Sandy calls the 24-hour pediatric health line at 10:30 p.m. about her 2½-year-old child Jared. Jared had gone to bed at his usual bedtime of 8:00 p.m. after an uneventful evening. He had awakened with a bark-like cough, respiratory difficulty, and a high-pitched, harsh sound on inspiration.

a. What questions would you ask this mother to further clarify Jared's situation?

b. What would you suggest Sandy should do to decrease Jared's symptoms?

c. What would you tell Sandy to watch for that might indicate Jared needs emergency attention?

2. Rachel, a 6-year-old girl, is brought to the clinic with a dry hacking cough, wheezing, and difficulty breathing. Rachel is coughing up thick mucus. Her parents are with her and are extremely anxious about Rachel's condition. The pediatrician examines Rachel, and a diagnosis of an acute asthma attack is made.

a. What other findings might have been noted during a physical exam of Rachel?

b. What will mostly likely be done to treat Rachel's current condition?

c. What medications might have been given?

d. What would you teach Rachel's parents about prevention of additional attacks?

3. Dosage calculation: A toddler with a diagnosis of cystic fibrosis is being treated with the bronchodilator Theophylline. The child weighs 32 pounds. The usual dosage of this medication is 4 mg/kg/dose every 6 hours. Answer the following:

a. How many kilograms does the child's weigh?

b. How many milligrams per dose will be given?

c. How many doses will the child receive in a day?

d. How much Theophylline will be given in a 24-hour period?

The Child With Cardiovascular/ Hematologic Disorders

36

STUDENT OBJECTIVES

On completion of this chapter, the student should be able to

1. State the signs and symptoms of congestive heart failure.
2. Name the bacterium usually responsible for the infection that leads to the development of rheumatic fever.
3. List the major manifestations of rheumatic fever.
4. State the most serious concern for the child with Kawasaki disease.

KEY TERMS

adenopathy
alopecia
arthralgia
bradycardia

STUDENT OBJECTIVES

5. Identify the common causes of iron deficiency anemia.
6. Explain how (a) sickle cell trait and (b) sickle cell anemia are inherited.
7. Describe the shape of the red blood cell and the effect it has on the circulation in sickle cell anemia.
8. Discuss the common complications and prognosis for the child with thalassemia.
9. Name the most common types of hemophilia and state how they are inherited.
10. State how hemophilia is treated.
11. Describe the symptoms noted in the child with idiopathic thrombocytopenic purpura.
12. State the symptoms usually seen in children with leukemia.
13. List four drugs commonly used in the treatment of acute lymphatic leukemia.

KEY TERMS

carditis
chorea
congestive heart failure
digitalization
granulocytes
hemarthrosis
hirsutism
intrathecal administration
leukemia
lymphoblast
lymphocytes
monocytes
petechiae
polyarthritis
purpura

ardiovascular system disorders and hematologic disorders, which are disorders having to do with the blood and blood-forming tissues, are usually serious and may be chronic or long-term conditions. Many of these conditions are hereditary and often present at birth. The congenital heart disorders are discussed in Chapter 21. The seriousness of disorders related to the cardiovascular system creates fear and concern in the child and family. An understanding of the cardiovascular system and how it functions can be helpful in decreasing the anxiety these families have.

Blood is a fluid composed of many elements, including plasma, red blood cells, white blood cells, and platelets. Each of these elements has a different function. These blood cells are formed in the bone marrow. The diseases and disorders of the circulatory system and the blood forming tissues occur when the heart itself or the blood or blood forming tissues are genetically altered, infection or damage has occurred, the organs or tissues are not shaped or functioning normally, or when the elements in the blood are increased or decreased in amount.

GROWTH AND DEVELOPMENT OF THE CARDIOVASCULAR AND HEMATOLOGIC SYSTEM

All systems of the body depend on the cardiovascular system. It works to carry the needed chemicals to and from the cells in the body so they can function properly. The major organ of the cardiovascular system is the heart, which is the pump that keeps the blood, containing oxygen and nutrients, circulating through the body. It also works to remove the waste products from the cells so they can be excreted from the body. The vessels, which carry the blood to and from the heart and through the body, include the arteries, veins, and capillaries. Arteries carry blood away from the heart to the body, and veins collect the blood and return it to the heart. Capillaries are the exchange vessels for the materials that flow through the body.

DIFFERENCES BETWEEN THE CHILD'S AND ADULT'S CARDIOVASCULAR AND HEMATOLOGIC SYSTEMS

Normal fetal circulation and the changes that occur in the cardiovascular system when the infant is born are covered in Chapter 21. Congenital heart disorders often occur in infants because the heart is not formed properly or the structures do not close at birth. At birth, both the right and left ventricles are about the same size, but by a few months of age, the left ventricle is about two times the size of the right. The infant's heart rate is higher than the older child or adult so that the infant's cardiac output can provide adequate oxygen to the body. If the infant has a fever, respiratory distress, or any increased need for oxygen, the pulse rate goes up to increase the cardiac output. Although the size is smaller, by the time

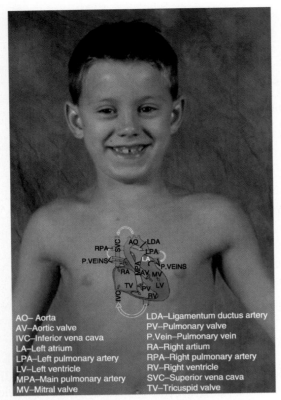

● **Figure 36.1** Anatomy of the normal heart.

AO– Aorta
AV–Aortic valve
IVC–Inferior vena cava
LA–Left atrium
LPA–Left pulmonary artery
LV–Left ventricle
MPA–Main pulmonary artery
MV–Mitral valve

LDA–Ligamentum ductus artery
PV–Pulmonary valve
P.Vein–Pulmonary vein
RA–Right artium
RPA–Right pulmonary artery
RV–Right ventricle
SVC–Superior vena cava
TV–Tricuspid valve

the child is 5 years old, the heart has matured, developed, and functions just as the adults (Fig. 36-1). The blood volume in the body is proportionate to the body weight. The younger the child, the higher the blood volume is per kilogram of body weight.

CONGESTIVE HEART FAILURE

Congestive heart failure (CHF) occurs when blood and fluids accumulate in the organs and body tissues. This happens because the heart is not able to pump and circulate enough blood to supply the oxygen and nutrient needs of the body cells. Manifestations of CHF may appear in children with conditions such as congenital heart disorders (see Chapter 21 for additional discussion), rheumatic fever, or Kawasaki disease. The condition places an increased workload on the ventricles of the heart.

Clinical Manifestations

The indications of CHF vary in children of different ages. Signs in the infant may be hard to detect because they are subtle. These include easy fatigability, which is manifested by feeding problems. The infant tires easily, breathes hard, and may have rapid respirations with an expiratory grunt, flaring of the nares, and sternal retractions. The infant may refuse the bottle after just 1 or 2 ounces but soon becomes hungry again. During feeding the infant may even become diaphoretic from the effort of feeding. Lying flat causes stress for the infant, who may appear more comfortable if held upright over an adult's shoulder. Periorbital edema may be present. A rapid weight gain may also indicate CHF.

In infants and older children, one of the first signs of CHF is tachycardia. The heart beats faster in an attempt to increase the blood flow. Other signs of CHF often seen in the older child include failure to gain weight; weakness; fatigue; restlessness; irritability; and a pale, mottled, or cyanotic color. Rapid respirations or tachypnea, dyspnea, and coughing with bloody sputum also are seen. Edema and enlargement of the liver and heart may be present.

Diagnosis

The clinical symptoms are the primary basis for diagnosis of CHF. Chest radiographs reveal an enlarged heart; electrocardiography may indicate ventricular hypertrophy, and an echocardiogram may be done to note cardiac function.

Treatment

Treatment of CHF includes improving the cardiac function using cardiac glycosides, such as digoxin (Lanoxin), removing excess fluids with the use of diuretics, decreasing the workload on the heart by limiting physical activity, and improving tissue oxygenation. Digoxin is used to improve the cardiac efficiency by slowing the heart rate and strengthening the cardiac contractility. The use of large doses of digoxin, at the beginning of therapy, to build up the blood levels of the drug to a therapeutic level is known as **digitalization**. A maintenance dose is given, usually daily, after digitalization. ACE (angiotensin-converting enzyme) inhibitors, such as captopril (Capoten) and enalapril (Vasotec), are given to increase vasodilatation. Diuretics, such as furosemide (Lasix), thiazide diuretics, or spironolactone (Aldactone), and fluid restriction in the acute stages of CHF help to eliminate excess fluids. The child should be placed with the head elevated, and energy requirements should be minimized to ease the workload of the heart. Often the child is placed on bed rest. Small, frequent feedings improve nutrition with minimal energy output. Oxygen is administered to increase oxygenation of tissues.

● Nursing Process for the Child With Congestive Heart Failure

ASSESSMENT

The interview of the family caregiver of a child with CHF must include the gathering of information about the current illness and any previous episodes. Ask about any problems the child may have during feeding, episodes of rapid or difficult respirations, episodes of turning blue, and difficulty with lying flat. Determine if the child has been gaining weight. Avoid causing any feelings of guilt in the caregiver.

The physical examination of the child includes a complete measurement of vital signs. Note the quality and rhythm of the apical pulse. Observe respiratory status, including any use of accessory muscles, retractions, breath sounds, rate, and type of cry. Examine the skin and extremities for color, skin temperature, and evidence of edema. Observe the child closely for signs of easy fatigability or an increase in symptoms on exertion.

SELECTED NURSING DIAGNOSES

- Decreased Cardiac Output related to structural defects or decreased cardiac functioning
- Ineffective Breathing Pattern related to pulmonary congestion and anxiety
- Risk for Imbalanced Nutrition: Less Than Body Requirements related to fatigue and dyspnea
- Activity Intolerance related to insufficient oxygenation
- Deficient Knowledge of caregivers related to the child's illness

OUTCOME IDENTIFICATION AND PLANNING

The major goals include improving cardiac output and oxygenation, relieving inadequate respirations, maintaining adequate nutritional intake, and conserving energy. The family's goals include increasing understanding of the condition and its prognosis.

IMPLEMENTATION

Monitoring Vital Signs
Monitor vital signs regularly to detect symptoms of decreased cardiac output. Monitor pulse rates closely. If digoxin is ordered, count the apical pulse for a full minute before administering digoxin. Withhold digoxin and notify the physician if the apical rate is lower than the established norms for the child's age and baseline information

(90 to 110 beats per minute for infants, 70 to 85 beats per minute for older children). Always check the dosage of digoxin with another nurse before administering it. Observe closely for any signs of digoxin toxicity, such as anorexia, nausea and vomiting, irregular pulse, or decreased pulse rate (**bradycardia**). Regularly observe the child for evidence of periorbital or peripheral edema. Before the first feeding of the day, weigh the undressed child early in the morning, using the same scale every time. Maintain careful intake and output measurements. If diuretics are administered, monitor serum electrolyte levels, especially potassium levels.

Improving Respiratory Function
Elevate the head of the crib mattress so that it is at a 30-degree to 45-degree angle. Do not allow the child to shift down in the crib and become "scrunched up," which causes decreased expansion room for the chest. Avoid constricting clothing. Administer oxygen as ordered. Monitor respirations at least every 4 hours, paying close attention to breath sounds, dyspnea, tachypnea, and retractions. Observe the child for cyanosis, especially noting the color of the nail beds and around the mouth, lips, hands, and feet. Monitor oxygen saturation levels with pulse oximetry. Respiratory infections can be a concern for the child with CHF. The child has a decreased resistance to these infections, and exposure to people who have respiratory infections should be avoided. Monitor closely for any signs of infection and report any findings.

Maintaining Adequate Nutrition
Give frequent feedings in small amounts to avoid overtiring the child. For the infant, use a soft nipple with a large opening to ease the child's workload. If adequate nutrition cannot be taken during feedings, gavage feedings may be necessary.

Promoting Energy Conservation
Nursing care is planned so that the child has long periods of uninterrupted rest. While carrying out nursing procedures, talk to the child softly and soothingly and handle him or her gently with loving care. Respond to the child's cries quickly to avoid tiring the child.

Providing Family Teaching
The family of this child has reason to be apprehensive and anxious. The nurse needs to be understanding, empathic, and nonjudgmental when communicating with them. Give them information about CHF in a way that they can understand. Repeat information about signs and symptoms and offer explanations as many times as necessary. Include teaching about medication, feeding and care techniques, growth and

development expectations, and future plans for correction of the defect, if known. Involve the family in the child's care as much as possible within the limitations of the child's condition.

EVALUATION: GOALS AND EXPECTED OUTCOMES

- **Goal:** The child's cardiac output will improve and be adequate to meet the child's needs.
  Expected Outcomes: The child's heart rate is within the normal limits for age; no arrhythmia or evidence of edema exists. Peripheral perfusion is adequate.
- **Goal:** The child's respiratory function will improve.
  Expected Outcomes: The child's respirations are regular with no retractions; breath sounds are clear; oxygen saturation is within the acceptable range for the child's status.
- **Goal:** The child's caloric intake will be adequate to maintain nutritional needs for growth.
  Expected Outcomes: The child consumes most of the feeding each time and feeds with minimal tiring. The child has appropriate weight gain for age.
- **Goal:** The child will have increased levels of energy.
  Expected Outcomes: The child rests quietly during uninterrupted periods of rest and does not become overly tired when awake.
- **Goal:** The family caregivers are prepared for the child's home care.
  Expected Outcomes: The family verbalizes anxieties, asks appropriate questions, participates in the child's care, and discusses the child's condition.

RHEUMATIC FEVER

Rheumatic fever is a chronic disease of childhood, affecting the connective tissue of the heart, joints, lungs, and brain. An autoimmune reaction to group A beta-hemolytic streptococcal infections, rheumatic fever occurs throughout the world, particularly in the temperate zones. It has become less common in developed countries, but there have been recent indications of increased occurrences in some areas of the United States.

Rheumatic fever is precipitated by a streptococcal infection, such as strep throat, tonsillitis, scarlet fever, or pharyngitis, which may be undiagnosed or untreated. The resultant rheumatic fever manifestation may be the first indication of trouble. However, an elevation of antistreptococcal antibodies that indicates recent streptococcal infection can be demonstrated in about 95% of the rheumatic fever patients tested within the first 2 months of onset. An antistreptolysin-O titer (ASO titer) measures these antibodies.

Clinical Manifestations

A latent period of 1 to 5 weeks follows the initial infection. The onset is often slow and subtle. The child may be listless, anorectic, and pale. He or she may lose weight and complain of vague muscle, joint, or abdominal pains. Often there is a low-grade late afternoon fever. None of these is diagnostic by itself, but if such signs persist, the child should have a medical examination.

Major manifestations of rheumatic fever are **carditis** (inflammation of the heart), **polyarthritis** (migratory arthritis), and **chorea** (disorder characterized by emotional instability, purposeless movements, and muscular weakness). The onset may be acute, rather than insidious, with severe carditis or arthritis as the presenting symptom. Chorea generally has an insidious onset.

Carditis

Carditis is the major cause of permanent heart damage and disability among children with rheumatic fever. Carditis may occur alone or as a complication of either arthritis or chorea. Presenting symptoms may be vague enough to be missed. The child may have a poor appetite, pallor, a low-grade fever, listlessness, or moderate anemia. Careful observation may reveal slight dyspnea on exertion. Physical examination shows a soft systolic murmur over the apex of the heart. Unfortunately, such a child may have been in poor physical health for some time before the murmur is discovered.

Acute carditis may be the presenting symptom, particularly in young children. An abrupt onset of high fever (perhaps as high as 104°F [40°C]), tachycardia, pallor, poor pulse quality, and a rapid decrease in hemoglobin are characteristic. Weakness, prostration, cyanosis, and intense precordial pain are common. Cardiac dilation usually occurs. The pericardium, myocardium, or endocardium may be affected.

Polyarthritis

Polyarthritis moves from one major joint to another (ankles, knees, hips, wrists, elbows, shoulders). The joint becomes painful to either touch or movement (**arthralgia**) and hot and swollen. Body temperature is moderately elevated; the erythrocyte sedimentation rate (ESR) is increased. Although extremely painful, this type of arthritis does not lead to the disabling deformities that occur in rheumatoid arthritis.

Chorea

The onset of chorea is gradual with increasing incoordination, facial grimaces, and repetitive involuntary movements. Movements may be mild and remain so, or they may become increasingly severe. Active arthritis is rarely present when chorea is the major manifestation. Carditis occurs, although less commonly than when polyarthritis is the major condition. Attacks tend to be recurrent and prolonged but are rare after puberty. It is seldom possible to demonstrate an increase in the antistreptococcal antibody level because of the generally prolonged latency period.

Diagnosis

Rheumatic fever is difficult to diagnose and sometimes impossible to differentiate from other diseases. The possible serious effects of the disease demand early and conscientious medical treatment. However, avoid causing apprehension and disruption of the child's life because the condition could prove to be something less serious. The nurse should not attempt a diagnosis but should understand the criteria on which a presumptive diagnosis is based.

The modified Jones criteria (Fig. 36-2) are generally accepted as a useful rule for guidance when deciding whether or not to treat the patient for rheumatic fever. The criteria are divided into major and minor categories. The presence of two major or one major and two minor criteria indicates a high probability of rheumatic fever if supported by evidence of a preceding streptococcal infection. This system is not infallible, however, because no one criterion is specific to the disease; additional manifestations can help confirm the diagnosis.

Treatment

The chief concern in caring for a child with rheumatic fever is the prevention of residual heart disease. As long as the rheumatic process is active, progressive heart damage is possible, so bed rest is essential for reducing the heart's workload. The length of bed rest is determined by the degree of carditis present. This may be from 2 weeks to several weeks, depending on how long heart failure is present.

Residual heart disease is treated in accordance with its severity and its type with digitalis, restricted activities, diuretics, and a low-sodium diet as indicated.

Laboratory tests, although nonspecific, provide an evaluation of the disease activity to guide treatment. Two commonly used indicators are the ESR and the presence of C-reactive protein. The ESR is elevated in the presence of an inflammatory process and is nearly always increased in the polyarthritis or carditis manifestation of rheumatic fever. It remains elevated until clinical manifestations have ceased and any subclinical activity has subsided. It seldom increases in uncomplicated chorea. Therefore, ESR elevation in a choreic patient may indicate cardiac involvement.

C-reactive protein in the body indicates an inflammatory process is occurring. It appears in the serum of

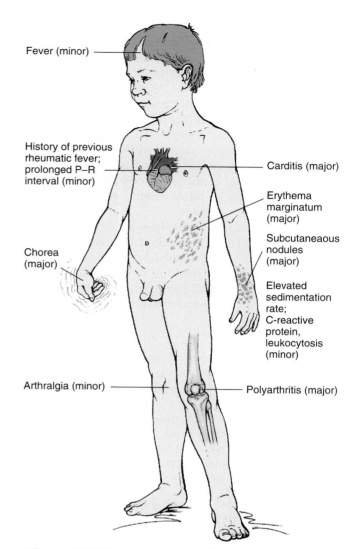

● **Figure 36.2** Major and minor manifestations of rheumatic fever.

acutely ill people, including people ill with rheumatic fever. As the patient improves, C-reactive protein decreases or disappears.

Leukocytosis is also an indication of an inflammatory process. Until the leukocyte count returns to a normal level, the disease probably is still active.

Medications used in the treatment of rheumatic fever include penicillin, salicylates, and corticosteroids. Penicillin is administered to eliminate the hemolytic streptococci. If the child is allergic to penicillin, erythromycin is used. Penicillin administration continues after the acute phase of the illness to prevent the recurrence of rheumatic fever.

Salicylates are given in the form of acetylsalicylic acid (aspirin) to children, with the daily dosage calculated according to the child's weight. Aspirin relieves pain and reduces the inflammation of polyarthritis. It is also used for its antipyretic effect. The continued administration of a relatively large dosage may cause toxic effects; individual tolerance differs greatly.

For mild or severe carditis, corticosteroids appear to be the drug of choice because of their prompt, dramatic action.

Administration of salicylates or corticosteroids is not expected to alter the course of the disease, but the control of the toxic manifestations enhances the child's comfort and sense of well-being and helps reduce the burden on the heart. This is of particular importance in acute carditis with congestive heart failure. Diuretics may be administered when needed in severe carditis.

Corticosteroids and salicylates are of little value in the treatment of uncomplicated chorea. The child may be sedated with phenobarbital, chlorpromazine (Thorazine), haloperidol (Haldol), or diazepam (Valium). Bed rest is necessary, with protection such as padding of the sides of the bed if the movements are severe.

Prevention

Because the peak of onset of rheumatic fever occurs in school-age children, health services for this age group take on added importance. The overall approach is to promote continuous health supervision for all children, including the school-age child. The use of well-child conferences or clinics needs to increase to provide continuity of care for children. The nurse who has contact in any way with school-age children must be aware of the importance of teaching the public about the need to have upper respiratory infections evaluated for group A beta-hemolytic streptococcus and the need for treatment with penicillin.

This is critical to teach. The nurse needs to stress that the child must take the complete prescription of penicillin (usually 10 days' supply), even though the symptoms disappear and the child feels well.

Test Yourself

- What are the common symptoms and treatments for congestive heart failure?
- What type of infection would likely be found in the history of a child who has rheumatic fever?
- Explain the terms carditis, polyarthritis, and chorea.
- What are two important aspects in the prevention of rheumatic fever?

● Nursing Process for the Child With Rheumatic Fever

ASSESSMENT

Conduct a thorough exam of the child. Begin with a careful review of all systems and note the child's physical condition. Observe for any signs that may be classified as major or minor manifestations. In the physical exam, include observation for elevated temperature and pulse and careful examination for erythema marginatum, subcutaneous nodules, swollen or painful joints, or signs of chorea. A throat culture determines if there is an active infection. Obtain a complete, up-to-date history from the child and the caregiver. Ask about a recent sore throat or upper respiratory infection. Find out when the symptoms began, the extent of the illness, and what if any treatment was obtained. Include the school-age child in the nursing interview to help contribute to the history.

SELECTED NURSING DIAGNOSES

- Acute Pain related to joint pain when extremities are touched or moved
- Deficient Diversional Activity related to prescribed bed rest
- Activity Intolerance related to carditis or arthralgia
- Risk for Injury related to chorea
- Risk for Noncompliance with prophylactic drug therapy related to financial or emotional burden of lifelong therapy
- Deficient Knowledge of caregiver related to the condition, need for long-term therapy, and risk factors

OUTCOME IDENTIFICATION AND PLANNING

The goals are determined in cooperation with the child and the caregiver. Goals for the child include reducing pain, providing diversional activities and sensory stimulation, conserving energy, and preventing injury. Goals for the caregiver include complying with drug therapy and increasing knowledge about the long-term care of the child. Throughout planning and implementation, bear in mind the child's developmental stage.

IMPLEMENTATION

Providing Comfort Measures and Reducing Pain

Position the child to relieve joint pain. Large joints, including the knees, ankles, wrists, and elbows, usually are involved. Carefully handle the joints when moving the child to help minimize pain. Warm baths and gentle range-of-motion exercises will help to alleviate some joint discomfort. Use pain indicator scales with children so they are able to express the level of their pain (see Fig. 29-8, Chapter 29).

Salicylates are administered in the form of aspirin to reduce fever and relieve joint inflammation and pain. Because of the risks of long-term administration of salicylates, note any signs of toxicity and record and report them promptly. Tinnitus, nausea, vomiting, and headache are all important signs of toxicity. Administer aspirin after meals or with a glass of milk to lessen gastrointestinal irritation. Enteric-coated aspirin is also available for patients who are sensitive to the effects of aspirin. Large doses may alter the prothrombin time and thus interfere with the clotting mechanism. Salicylate therapy is usually continued until all laboratory findings are normal.

Watch out. Even the weight of blankets may cause pain for the child with rheumatic fever. Be alert to this possibility and improvise covering as needed.

The child whose pain is not controlled with salicylates may be administered corticosteroids. Side effects such as **hirsutism** (abnormal hair growth) and "moon face" may be upsetting to the child and family. Toxic reactions such as euphoria, insomnia, gastric irritation, and growth suppression must be watched for and reported. Because premature withdrawal of a steroid drug is likely to cause a relapse, it is important to discontinue use of the drug gradually by decreasing dosages.

Providing Diversional Activities and Sensory Stimulation

Children vary greatly in how ill they feel during the acute phase of rheumatic fever. For those who do not feel very ill, bed rest can cause distress or resentment. Be creative in finding diversional activities that allow bed rest but prevent restlessness and boredom. This may be a good time to choose a book that involves the child's imagination and that has enough excitement to create ongoing interest. Do not use the television as an all-day baby-sitter. Quiet games can provide some entertainment. Use of a computer can be beneficial because both entertaining and educational games are available, and most children enjoy working with a computer. Simple needlework and model

building are other useful diversional activities. During the school year, make efforts (or encourage the caregiver) to provide the child with a tutor and work from school; this helps relieve boredom and also maintains contact with peers. Plan all activities with the child's developmental age in mind. The pain of arthralgia may be so great that the child will not want to be involved in any kind of activity. Administer analgesics as ordered to help decrease the inflammation of the joints and decrease the pain, so the child will feel like participating in age-appropriate activities.

Promoting Energy Conservation

Provide rest periods between activities to help pace the child's energies and provide for maximum comfort. During times of increased cardiac involvement or exacerbations of joint pain, the child may want to rest and perhaps have someone read a story. Peers may be encouraged to visit, but these visits must be monitored so that the child is not overly tired. The child's classmates could be encouraged to write to the child to provide contact with everyday school activities and keep the child in touch. If the child has chorea, inform visitors that the child cannot control these movements, which are as upsetting to the child as they are to others.

Preventing Injury

The child with chorea may be frustrated with his or her inability to control the movements. Provide an opportunity for the child to express feelings. Protect the child from injury by keeping the side rails up and padding them. Do not leave a child with chorea unattended in a wheelchair. Use all appropriate safety measures.

Promoting Compliance With Drug Therapy

A child does not become immune from future attacks of rheumatic fever after the first illness. Rheumatic fever can recur whenever the child has a group A beta-hemolytic streptococcal infection if the child is not properly treated. For this reason, the child who has had rheumatic fever must be maintained on prophylactic doses of penicillin for 5 years or longer. Whenever the child is to have oral surgery, including dental work, extra prophylactic precautions should be taken, even in adulthood. Because of this long-term therapy, noncompliance can become a problem for both financial and emotional reasons. Oral penicillin is usually prescribed, but if compliance is poor, monthly injections of Bicillin can be substituted. Encourage the family to contact the local chapter of the American Heart Association (website: www.americanheart.org) for help finding economical sources of penicillin. Become informed about other resources that may be available in your community. Emphasize to the child and the family the need to prevent recurrence of the disease because of the danger of heart damage. Follow-up care must be ongoing, even into adulthood.

Providing Family Teaching

Inform the family and child about the importance of having all upper respiratory infections checked by a health care provider to prevent another episode of a streptococcal infection. Be certain that they understand the child can have recurrences and that a future recurrence could have much more serious effects. If the child has had carditis and heart damage has occurred, instruct the caregiver that the child must be regularly followed up to evaluate the damage. The child may need to be maintained on cardiac medications. Instruct the family about these medications. Mitral valve dysfunction is a common aftereffect of severe carditis. A girl who has had mitral valve damage from cardiac involvement may have problems in adulthood during pregnancy. Inform the caregiver that heart failure for such a girl is a possibility during pregnancy and that she should be followed up closely to determine heart problems in the event that a mitral valve replacement is needed.

Teaching time is an excellent opportunity to stress the importance of preventing rheumatic fever. Other children in the family may benefit if caregivers are given this information.

EVALUATION: GOALS AND EXPECTED OUTCOMES

- **Goal:** The child's joint pain will be minimal.
  Expected Outcome: The child verbalizes or indicates, by using a pain scale to express degree of pain, that the pain level is decreased.
- **Goal:** The child will become engaged in activities while on bed rest.
  Expected Outcome: The child displays interest and is actively involved in age-appropriate activities.
- **Goal:** The child will learn when and how to conserve energy.
  Expected Outcomes: The child rests quietly during rest periods, identifies when he or she needs rest, and engages in quiet diversional activities.
- **Goal:** The child remains free of injury from chorea movements and a safe environment is maintained.
  Expected Outcomes: The child has no evidence of injury, and safety measures are followed.

- **Goal:** The family caregivers will comply with follow-up drug therapy, and the child will take prophylactic medications.
  Expected Outcome: The child and family caregivers verbalize an understanding of the importance of prophylactic medication and identify means for obtaining it.
- **Goal:** The family caregivers will verbalize an understanding of the child's condition, need for long-term therapy, and risk factors.
  Expected Outcomes: The caregivers discuss the child's condition and need for follow-up care for the child and indicate how they will obtain it.

KAWASAKI DISEASE

Kawasaki disease (mucocutaneous lymph node syndrome) is an acute, febrile disease that is most often seen in boys younger than 5 years. The etiology is unknown, but the disease appears to be caused by an infectious agent. After an infection, an alteration in the immune system occurs. Most cases are seen in the late winter or early spring. The major concern for the child is development of cardiac involvement.

Clinical Manifestations

An elevated temperature (102°F to 104°F) is noted from the 1st day of the illness and may continue 1 to 3 weeks. Irritability; lethargy; inflammation in the conjunctiva in both eyes; strawberry colored tongue; dry, red, cracked lips; edema in the hands and feet; and red, swollen joints are seen. The skin on the fingers and toes peels in layers, and a rash covers the trunk and extremities. Cervical lymph nodes may be enlarged. Inflammation of the arteries, veins, and capillaries occurs, and this inflammation can lead to serious cardiac concerns, including aneurysms and thrombus. The child may report abdominal pain. The disease is seen in three stages:

- Acute—high fever that does not respond to antibiotics or antipyretics; child is irritable.
- Subacute—fever resolves, irritability continues; greatest risk for aneurysms.
- Convalescent—symptoms are gone; phase continues until lab values are normal and child's energy, appetite, and temperament have returned.

Diagnosis

For Kawasaki disease to be diagnosed, the child must have an elevated temperature and four of the following symptoms: cervical lymphadenopathy; conjunctivitis;

dry, swollen, cracked lips; strawberry tongue; aneurysm; abdominal pain; peeling of hands and feet; trunk rash; or red, swollen joints. The white blood cell count (WBC) and erythrocyte sedimentation rate (ESR) are elevated. During the subacute stage, the platelet count increases, which may lead to blood clotting and cardiac problems. Echocardiograms may show cardiac involvement.

Treatment and Nursing Care

A high dose of intravenous immunoglobulin (IVIG) therapy is given to relieve the symptoms and prevent coronary artery abnormalities. Aspirin is used to control inflammation and fever and is continued for as long as 1 year in lower doses as an antiplatelet. Nursing care for the child with Kawasaki disease focuses on management of the symptoms. Relieving the pain, discomfort, and itching are important. Temperature, cardiac status, intake and output, and daily weight are monitored closely. Extra fluids and soft foods are offered. Mouth and lip care help decrease the soreness. The use of passive range-of-motion exercises increases joint movement. Dealing with the irritability is sometimes difficult for the nurse and the family. Rest and a quiet environment help in decreasing irritability. Encouraging the parents to have times away from the child is essential. Discharge teaching includes information regarding the disease and symptoms, which may persist for a period of time. Follow-up treatments, visits, medication routines, and side effects are covered. Most children recover without long-term effects, but the cardiac involvement may not be seen for a period of time after the child's recovery.

Do you know the why of it?
Immunizations, especially live vaccines such as MMR (measles, mumps, and rubella), should not be given for 3 to 6 months to a child who has been treated with immunoglobulin (IG). The IG prevents the body from building antibodies, so the vaccine will likely be ineffective in preventing the disease it is being given to prevent.

IRON DEFICIENCY ANEMIA

Iron deficiency anemia is a common nutritional deficiency in children. It is a hypochromic, microcytic anemia—in other words, the blood cells are deficient in production of hemoglobin and smaller than normal—and is common between the ages of 9 and 24 months. The full-term newborn has a high hemoglobin level (needed during fetal life to provide adequate oxygenation) that decreases during the first 2 or 3 months of life. Considerable iron is reclaimed and stored, however, usually in sufficient quantity to last for 4 to 9 months of life.

A child needs to absorb 0.8 to 1.5 mg of iron per day. Because only 10% of dietary iron is absorbed, a diet containing 8 to 10 mg of iron is needed for good health. During the 1st years of life, obtaining this quantity of iron from food is often difficult for a child. If the diet is inadequate, anemia quickly results. (In addition, adolescent girls may have iron deficiency anemia because of improper dieting to lose weight.)

Babies with an inordinate fondness for milk can take in an astonishing amount and, with their appetites satisfied, show little interest in solid foods. These babies are prime candidates for iron deficiency anemia. They may have a history of consuming 2 or 3 quarts of milk daily while not accepting any other foods or, at best, only foods with a high carbohydrate content. Many caregivers incorrectly believe that milk is a perfect food and that they should let the baby have all the milk desired. These children are commonly known as milk babies. They have pale, almost translucent (porcelain-like) skin, and are chubby and susceptible to infections.

Many children with iron deficiency anemia, however, are undernourished because of the family's economic problems. Along with the economic factor, a caregiver knowledge deficit about nutrition is often present. The Women, Infants, and Children (WIC) program, discussed in Chapter 23, does much to alleviate this problem.

Clinical Manifestations

The signs of iron deficiency anemia include below-average body weight, pale mucous membranes, anorexia, growth retardation, and listlessness, in addition to the characteristics of milk babies described earlier.

Diagnosis

In blood tests that measure hemoglobin, a level lower than 11 g/dL or a hematocrit lower than 33% is highly suspect. Stool is tested for occult blood to rule out low gastrointestinal bleeding as a cause for the depleted hemoglobin and hematocrit.

Treatment and Nursing Care

Treatment consists of improved nutrition, with ferrous sulfate administered between meals with juice (preferably orange juice, because vitamin C aids in iron absorption). For best results, iron should not be given with meals. Tell the caregivers that ferrous sulfate can cause constipation or turn the child's stools black.

A few children have a hemoglobin level so low or anorexia so acute that they need additional therapy. An iron/dextran mixture (Imferon) for intramuscular use is administered. Because of its irritating nature, this medication should be administered in the vastus lateralis by the Z-track method to avoid leakage into the subcutaneous tissues. For children who are seriously ill, refer to "Nursing Process for the Child With Nutritional Problems" in Chapter 37.

Here's a tip to share with family caregivers. To prevent staining, brush the child's teeth after administering iron preparations such as ferrous sulfate.

For most children with iron deficiency anemia, teaching for home care is needed. When teaching caregivers, remember that attitudes and food choices are often influenced by cultural differences. See Family Teaching Tips: Iron Deficiency Anemia.

FAMILY TEACHING TIPS

Iron Deficiency Anemia

- One of the most important things you can do for your child and family is to learn about the foods that will help them stay healthy.
- Milk is good for your child, but no more than a quart a day (four 8-oz bottles for the infant).
- Liquid iron preparations should be taken through a straw to prevent staining of teeth.

FOODS HIGH IN IRON

- Baby cereals fortified with iron.
- For older children, fortified instant oatmeal and cream of wheat are good sources of iron.
- Some infant formulas are iron fortified.
- Egg yolks are rich in iron. Avoid egg whites for young children because of allergies.
- Green, leafy vegetables are good sources of iron.
- Dried beans, dried peas, canned refried beans, and peanut butter provide good iron sources for toddlers and older children.
- Fruits that are iron-rich include peaches, prune juice, and raisins (don't give to child younger than 3 years of age because of danger of choking).
- Read labels to check for iron content of processed foods.
- Organ meat, poultry, and fish are good iron sources.
- Orange juice helps the body absorb iron.

SICKLE CELL DISEASE

Sickle cell disease is a hereditary trait occurring most commonly in African Americans. It is characterized by the production of abnormal hemoglobin that causes the red blood cells to assume a sickle shape. It appears as an asymptomatic trait when the sickling trait is inherited from one parent alone (heterozygous state). There is a 50% probability that each child born to one parent carrying the sickle cell trait will inherit the trait from that parent. When the trait is inherited from both parents (homozygous state), the child has sickle cell disease, and anemia develops (Fig. 36-3). A rapid breakdown of red blood cells carrying hemoglobin S, the abnormal hemoglobin, causes a severe hemolytic anemia. Persons who inherit the gene for the sickle cell trait from only one parent have no symptoms and normal hemoglobin levels and red blood cell counts.

The sickling trait occurs in about 10% of African Americans; there is a much higher incidence in parts of Africa. In African Americans, the disease itself, sickle cell anemia, has an incidence of 0.3% to 1.3%. The tendency to sickle can be demonstrated by a laboratory test.

Clinical Manifestations

Clinical symptoms of the disease usually do not appear before the latter half of the 1st year of life because sufficient fetal hemoglobin is still present to prevent sickling. Sickle cell disease causes a chronic anemia, with a hemoglobin level of 6 to 9 g/dL (the normal level in an infant is 11 to 15 g/dL). The chronic anemia causes the child to be tired and have a poor appetite and pale mucous membranes.

Sickle cell crisis is the most severe manifestation of the condition. Normal red blood cells, which carry oxygen to the tissues, are disc shaped and normally move through the blood vessels while bending and flexing to flow through smoothly. The smooth, uniform shape of the red blood cells and the low viscosity

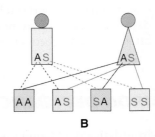

● **Figure 36.3** Inheritance patterns. **(A)** Heterozygous type. One parent carries a hemoglobin S gene, and one does not. Two children will be free of the gene (AA), and two will be carriers (AS). **(B)** Homozygous type. Each parent is carrying one hemoglobin A gene and one hemoglobin S gene. One child is free of the gene (AA), two are carriers (AS), and one has sickle cell disease (SS).

(thickness) of the blood is such that these cells split relatively easily at Y-intersections and go single file through the capillaries with little or no clustering. The affected red blood cells (hemoglobin S) do much the same thing until an episode causes sickling. An episode (sickle cell crises) can be precipitated by low oxygen levels, which can be caused by a respiratory infection or extremely strenuous exercise, dehydration, acidosis, or stress. When sickling occurs, the affected red blood cells become crescent-shaped and, therefore, do not slip through as easily as do the disc-shaped cells. The viscosity of the blood increases (becomes thicker), causing slowdown and sludging of the red blood cells. The impaired circulation results in tissue damage and infarction.

A sickle cell crisis may be the first clinical manifestation of the disease and may recur frequently during early childhood. This disturbance presents a variety of symptoms. The most common symptom is severe, acute abdominal pain (caused by sludging, which leads to enlargement of the spleen) together with muscle spasm, fever, and severe leg pain that may be muscular, osseous (bony), or localized in the joints, which become hot and swollen. The abdomen becomes boardlike with an absence of bowel sounds. This makes it extremely difficult to distinguish the condition from an abdominal condition requiring surgery. Several days after a crisis, the child will be jaundiced, as evidenced by yellow sclera, as a result of the hemolysis. The crisis may have a fatal outcome caused by cerebral, cardiac, or hemolytic complications.

Diagnosis

Screening for the presence of hemoglobin S may be done with a test called Sickledex, a fingerstick screening test that gives results in 3 minutes. Definite diagnosis is made through hemoglobin electrophoresis ("fingerprinting"). If the Sickledex screening results are positive, diagnosis can be done to determine if the child is carrying the trait or has sickle cell disease.

Treatment

Prevention of crises is the goal between episodes. Adequate hydration is vital; fluid intake of 1,500 to 2,000 mL daily is desirable for a child weighing 20 kg and should be increased to 3,000 mL during the crisis. Extremely strenuous activities that may cause oxygen depletion are to be avoided. These children should also avoid visiting areas of high altitude. Small blood transfusions help bring the hemoglobin to a near-normal level temporarily. Iron preparations have no effect in sickle cell disease.

Treatment for a crisis is supportive for each presenting symptom, and bed rest is indicated. Oxygen may be administered. Analgesics are given for pain. Dehydration and acidosis are vigorously treated. Prognosis is guarded, depending on the severity of the disease.

● Nursing Process for the Child With Sickle Cell Crisis

ASSESSMENT

The parents who have a child with sickle cell disease may experience a great deal of guilt for having passed the disease to their child. Take care not to increase this guilt but help them cope with it. During the interview with the family caregivers, ask about activities or events that led to this crisis, obtain a history of the child's health and any previous episodes, and evaluate the caregivers' knowledge about the condition.

Data collection techniques vary somewhat, depending on the child's age. Record vital signs, particularly noting fever, abdominal pain, presence of bowel sounds, pain or swelling and warmth in the joints, and muscle spasms. Observe the young child for dactylitis (hand-foot syndrome), which results from soft-tissue swelling caused by interference with circulation. This swelling further impairs circulation.

SELECTED NURSING DIAGNOSES

- Acute Pain related to disease condition affecting abdominal organs or joints and muscles
- Deficient Fluid Volume related to low fluid intake, impaired renal function, or both
- Activity Intolerance related to oxygen depletion and pain
- Impaired Physical Mobility related to muscle and joint involvement
- Risk for Impaired Skin Integrity related to altered circulation
- Compromised Family Coping related to child's condition
- Deficient Knowledge of caregivers related to understanding of disorder and appropriate care measures

OUTCOME IDENTIFICATION AND PLANNING

Maintaining comfort and relieving pain, increasing fluid intake, and conserving energy are major goals for the child with sickle cell disease. Other goals include improving physical mobility, maintaining skin integrity, and reducing the caregivers' anxiety. Another important goal is decreasing the number of future episodes by increasing the caregiver's knowledge about the causes of crisis episodes. Plan individualized nursing care according to these goals.

IMPLEMENTATION

Relieving Pain

The child in sickle cell crisis often has severe abdominal pain because of enlargement of the spleen (splenomegaly). Joint and muscle pain are also common because of poor perfusion of the tissues. Monitoring the child's pain level, nursing measures to relieve pain, and prompt administration of analgesics are essential. The family caregivers can be involved, if they wish, in helping administer comfort measures to the child. Sometimes diverting activities can help alleviate perceived pain.

This is critical to remember. Be assured that children with sickle cell anemia are in pain and need analgesics promptly.

Maintaining Fluid Intake

The child is prone to dehydration because of the kidneys' inability to concentrate urine. Observe for signs of dehydration, such as dry mucous membranes, weight loss, or in the case of infants, sunken fontanelles. Strict intake and output measurements and daily weights are necessary. In sickle cell crisis, urine specific gravity is not a good indicator of dehydration. Teach the family caregivers that fluid intake is important, and intake should be maintained at 1,500 to 2,000 mL when the child is not in crisis. Offer the child appealing fluids, such as juices, popsicles, non-caffeinated soda, and favorite flavored gelatins. Teach family caregivers that increasing fluid intake as the child ages will help to avoid a crisis during the child's activities, such as hiking, swimming, and sports. The child also needs increased fluids during episodes of infections.

Promoting Energy Conservation

The child may become dyspneic doing any kind of activity. Plan nursing care so that the child is disturbed as little as possible and can rest. Bed rest is necessary to decrease the demands of oxygen supply. Oxygen may be administered by mask or nasal cannula to improve tissue perfusion.

Improving Physical Mobility

Sickling that affects the muscles and joints causes a great deal of pain for the child. The child needs careful handling and should be moved slowly and gently. Joints can be supported with pillows. Warm soaks and massages may help relieve some of the discomfort. Administer analgesics before exercise and as needed. Passive exercises help prevent contractures and wasting of muscles.

Promoting Skin Integrity

Increased fluid intake and improved nutrition are important. Observe the child's skin regularly each shift and provide good skin care consisting of lotion, massage, and skin-toughening agents, especially over bony prominences. Additional padding in the form of foam protectors and egg-crate pads or mattresses may be helpful when there is irritation from bedding.

Promoting Family Coping

Guilt plays an important part in the anxiety that the family caregivers experience. Explain procedures, planned treatments, and care to help the caregivers feel that they are being included in the care. Caregivers need to feel that they have some control over the disease.

Providing Family Teaching

Teach measures that may help alleviate pain or encourage fluid intake. Also, emphasize the importance of protecting the child from situations that may cause over-exhaustion or that may otherwise deplete the child's oxygen supplies or lead to dehydration. This knowledge may give the family caregivers a feeling of control. In addition, caregivers may need more information concerning the disorder. If the child's diagnosis is not new, the caregivers should already have had information presented to them. In this instance, determine their knowledge level and supplement and reinforce that information.

EVALUATION: GOALS AND EXPECTED OUTCOMES

- **Goal:** The child's pain will be reduced or eliminated.
  Expected Outcome: The child rests quietly and, if possible, reports his or her comfort.

CULTURAL SNAPSHOT

In working with children and families of children who have disorders that are passed through genetics, it is important that genetic counseling be done in a sensitive, nonthreatening manner. Some cultures believe that the mother or the parents caused a hereditary disease because of certain behaviors or actions. The parents often feel guilty, so a sensitive, objective approach is essential.

- **Goal:** The child's fluid intake will improve.
  Expected Outcome: The child has an intake of at least 3,000 mL/day.
- **Goal:** The child's energy will be conserved.
  Expected Outcomes: The child's activities are restricted to conserve energy. The oxygen saturation is greater than 90%.
- **Goal:** The child's muscles and joints will remain flexible.
  Expected Outcome: The child cooperates with daily passive exercises.
- **Goal:** The child's skin integrity will be maintained.
  Expected Outcome: The child's skin shows no signs of redness, irritation, or breakdown.
- **Goal:** The family caregivers' anxiety will be reduced.
  Expected Outcome: The family caregivers are more self-confident and cooperate with nursing personnel.
- **Goal:** The family caregivers express understanding of disease process.
  Expected Outcome: The family caregivers verbalize an understanding of the disease process and state ways to prevent a crisis from occurring.

THALASSEMIA

The thalassemia blood disorders are inherited, mild to severe anemias in which the hemoglobin production is abnormal. Thalassemia major (Cooley's anemia) presents in childhood and is the most common. The disorder often occurs in people of Mediterranean descent but may also be seen in other populations.

Clinical Manifestations

Anemia, fatigue, pallor, irritability, and anorexia are noted in children with thalassemia. Bone pain and fractures are seen. Many body systems can be affected, including enlargement of the spleen, overstimulation of bone marrow, and heart failure. The liver, gallbladder, and pancreas can also be involved. The skin may appear bronze-colored or jaundiced. Skeletal changes occur, including deformities of the face and skull. The upper teeth protrude, the nose is broad and flat, and the eyes are slanted.

Treatment and Nursing Care

Blood transfusions maintain the hemoglobin levels; diet and medications are used to prevent heart failure; and splenectomy or bone marrow transplants

may be necessary. Frequent transfusions can lead to complications and additional concerns for the child, including the possibility of iron overload. For these children, iron-chelating drugs such as deferoxamine mesylate (Desferal) may be given. Slowed growth and delayed sexual maturation may cause the child to feel self-conscious. Child and family support is important because of the chronic nature, long-term treatment, and poor outcome of the disease. Even with treatment the prognosis is poor, and the child often dies of cardiac failure.

Test Yourself

- What are some reasons iron deficiency anemias might be seen in infants?
- Explain the shape of the red blood cell and how it affects the child with sickle cell anemia.
- What is the most common symptom in the child with a sickle cell crisis?

HEMOPHILIA

Hemophilia is one of the oldest known hereditary diseases. Recent research has demonstrated that hemophilia is a syndrome of several distinct inborn errors of metabolism; all result in the delayed coagulation of blood. Defects in protein synthesis lead to deficiencies in any of the factors in the blood plasma needed for thromboplastic activity. The principal factors involved are factors VIII, IX, and XI.

Mechanism of Clot Formation

The mechanism of clot formation is complex. In a simplified form, it can best be described as occurring in three stages:

1. Prothrombin is formed through plasma-platelet interaction.
2. Prothrombin is converted to thrombin.
3. Fibrinogen is converted into fibrin by thrombin.

Fibrin forms a mesh that traps red and white blood cells and platelets into a clot, closing the defect in the injured vessel. A deficiency in one of the -thromboplastin precursors may lead to hemophilia. This progression of events is shown in Figure 36-4. Refer to a specialized text on the circulatory system for a detailed discussion of the clot-forming mechanism.

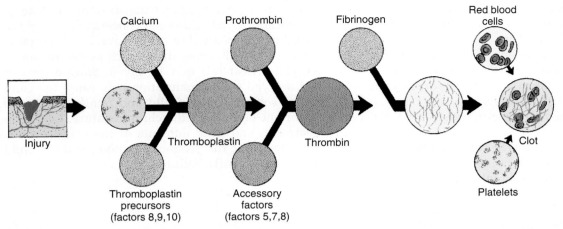

● **Figure 36.4** The mechanism of the formation of a blood clot is complex.

Clinical Manifestations

Hemophilia is characterized by prolonged bleeding, with frequent hemorrhages externally and into the skin, the joint spaces, and the intramuscular tissues. Bleeding from tooth extractions, brain hemorrhages, and crippling disabilities are serious complications. Death during infancy or early childhood is not unusual in severe hemophilia and results from a great loss of blood, intracranial bleeding, or respiratory obstruction caused by bleeding into the neck tissues.

An infant with hemophilia who is beginning to creep or walk bruises easily, and serious hemorrhages may result from minor lacerations. Bleeding often occurs from lip biting or from sharp objects put in the mouth. Tooth eruption seldom causes bleeding, but extractions require specialized handling and should be avoided by preventive care if possible. However, family caregivers must avoid overprotecting the child. The preschooler is active and plays hard, and injuries are practically unavoidable. Clinical manifestations in any type of hemophilia are similar and are treated by administration of the deficient factor and by measures to prevent or treat complications. In severe bleeding, the quantities of fresh blood or frozen plasma needed may easily overload the circulatory system. Administration of factor VIII concentrate eliminates this problem.

Diagnosis

A careful examination of the family history and the type of bleeding present is conducted. Abnormal bleeding beginning in infancy when combined with a positive family history suggests hemophilia. A markedly prolonged clotting time is characteristic of severe factor VIII or IX deficiency, but mild conditions may have only a slightly prolonged clotting time. The partial prothrombin time is the test that most clearly demonstrates that factor VIII is low.

Common Types of Hemophilia

The two most common types of hemophilia are factor VIII deficiency and factor IX deficiency. These two types are briefly presented here.

Factor VIII Deficiency

Factor VIII deficiency includes hemophilia A, antihemophilic globulin deficiency, and classic hemophilia. Classic hemophilia is inherited as a sex-linked recessive Mendelian trait, with transmission to affected males by carrier females. Hemophilia A (classic hemophilia), the most common type, occurs in about 1 in 10,000 people and is also the most severe. It is caused by a deficiency of antihemophilic globulin C, which is the factor VIII necessary for blood clotting.

Factor IX Deficiency

Factor IX deficiency includes hemophilia B; plasma thromboplastin component deficiency; and Christmas disease. Christmas disease was named after a 5-year-old boy who was one of the first patients diagnosed with a deficiency of factor IX. This deficiency constitutes about 15% of the hemophilias. It is a sex-linked recessive trait appearing in male offspring of carrier females and is caused by a deficiency of one of the necessary thromboplastin precursors: factor IX, the plasma thromboplastin component. Hemophilia B is indistinguishable from classic hemophilia in its clinical manifestations, particularly in its severe form. It also may exist in a mild form, probably more commonly than in hemophilia A. In either hemophilia A or B, 25% or more of the affected people can trace no family history of the disease; it is assumed that spontaneous mutations have occurred in some cases.

Treatment

For many years, the only treatment for bleeding in hemophilia was the use of fresh blood or plasma.

When fresh-frozen plasma came into use, it became the mainstay in hemophilia management. It has been particularly helpful in emergencies. Frozen plasma does, however, have several shortcomings. One major problem has been the large volumes needed to control bleeding. Another is the danger that injections of large amounts of plasma may lead to congestive heart failure. In addition, plasma must be given within 30 minutes because factor VIII loses its potency at room temperature.

Commercial preparations now are available that supply higher-potency factor VIII than previous preparations. These concentrates are supplied in dried form together with diluent for reconstitution. Directions for mixing and administration are included with the package. The preparations can be stored for a long time but have the disadvantage of exposing the recipient to a large number of donors. A synthetic preparation, DDAVP (1-deamino-8-D-arginine vasopressin), is used in mild factor VIII deficiencies and von Willebrand disease. Von Willebrand disease (vascular hemophilia; pseudohemophilia) is classified with the hemophilias. It is a Mendelian dominant trait present in both sexes and is characterized by prolonged bleeding times. One of the serious problems with using blood products of any kind has been the risk of exposure to hepatitis B and human immunodeficiency virus (HIV), the causative organism of acquired immunodeficiency syndrome (AIDS). Currently, blood is screened thoroughly for viral contamination, which greatly diminishes the danger of HIV transmission. However, large numbers of hemophiliacs treated before the late 1980s were exposed to HIV and now test positive for HIV antibodies. Researchers continue to explore new ways to replace the missing factor while protecting the recipient from the threat of contracting an unknown illness.

● Nursing Process for the Child With Hemophilia

ASSESSMENT

Begin the nursing data collection by reviewing the child's history with the caregiver. Include previous episodes of bleeding, the usual treatment, medications the child takes, and the current episode of bleeding. Include the child in the interview if he or she is old enough to answer questions. Carefully observe the child for any signs of bleeding. Inspect the mucous membranes, examine the joints for tenderness and swelling, and check the skin for evidence of bruising. Question the child or caregiver about hematuria, hematemesis, headache, or black tarry stools.

SELECTED NURSING DIAGNOSES

- Acute Pain related to joint swelling and limitations secondary to hemarthrosis
- Impaired Physical Mobility related to pain and tenderness of joints
- Risk for Injury related to hemorrhage secondary to trauma
- Deficient Knowledge related to condition, treatments, and hazards
- Compromised Family Coping related to treatment and care of the child

OUTCOME IDENTIFICATION AND PLANNING

Use the information gathered to set goals with the cooperation and input of the caregiver and the child. The major goals for the child include stopping the bleeding, decreasing pain, increasing mobility, and preventing injury. The family goals include increasing knowledge about the child's condition and care and helping the family learn to cope with the disease condition.

IMPLEMENTATION

Relieving Pain
Bleeding into the joint cavities often occurs after some slight injury and seems nearly unavoidable if the child is allowed to lead a normal life. Extreme pain is caused by the pressure of the confined fluid in the narrow joint spaces and requires the use of sedatives or narcotics.

Pay attention to the details. Do not administer aspirin (or drugs containing aspirin) or other nonsteroidal anti-inflammatory drugs (NSAIDs), such as indomethacin, to the child with hemophilia because of the danger of prolonging bleeding.

Promptly immobilize the involved extremity to prevent contractures of soft tissues and the destruction of the bone and joint tissues. Immobilization helps to relieve pain and decrease bleeding. A bivalve plaster cast may be applied in the hospital to immobilize the affected part.

Although aspirin and most nonsteroidal anti-inflammatory drugs (NSAIDs) are not given to children with hemophilia, ibuprofen, also an NSAID, has been proven safe for these children. Use of cold packs to stop bleeding is acceptable. The affected limb may be elevated above the level of the heart to slow blood flow. Use age-appropriate diversionary activities to help the child deal with the pain. Handle the affected joints carefully to prevent additional pain.

Preventing Joint Contractures

Passive range-of-motion exercises help prevent the development of joint contractures. Do not use them, however, after an acute episode because stretching of the joint capsule may cause bleeding. Encourage the child to do active range-of-motion exercises because he or she can recognize his or her own pain tolerance. Many patients who have had repeated episodes of **hemarthrosis** (bleeding into the joints) develop functional impairment of the joints, despite careful treatment. Use splints and devices to position the limb in a functional position. Physical therapy is helpful after the bleeding episode is under control. Joint contractures are a serious risk, so make every effort to avoid them.

Preventing Injury

The child with hemophilia is continuously at risk for additional injury. Protect the child from trauma caused by necessary procedures. Limit invasive procedures as much as possible; if possible, collect blood samples by a fingerstick. Avoid intramuscular injections. When an invasive procedure must be done, compress the site for 5 minutes or longer after the procedure and apply cold compresses.

Remove any sharp objects from the child's environment. If the child is young, pad the crib sides to prevent bumping and bruising. Examine toys for sharp edges and hard surfaces. Soft toys are best for the young child. For mouth care, use a soft toothbrush or sponge-type brush to decrease the danger of bleeding gums. During daily hygiene, trim the nails to prevent scratching and give adequate skin care to prevent irritation.

Providing Family Teaching

Provide the family with a thorough explanation of hemophilia or reinforce information they already have. Review the family's knowledge about the disease and give additional information when needed. A child with hemophilia is healthy between bleeding episodes, but the fact that bleeding may occur as the result of slight trauma or often without any known injury causes considerable anxiety. For an unknown reason, bleeding episodes are more common in the spring and fall. Some evidence indicates that emotional stress can initiate bleeding episodes.

Topical fluoride applications to the teeth are particularly important in these children. Pay particular attention to proper oral hygiene, a well-balanced diet, and proper dental treatment, and teach the family about these considerations.

Advise the family to select a dentist who understands the problems presented and who will set up an appropriate program of preventive dentistry.

Discuss safety measures for the home and the child's lifestyle. When possible, carpeting in the home helps to soften the falls of a toddler just learning to walk. An older child may need to wear protective devices when playing outdoors. Playground areas can be treacherous for these children, but the child can participate in normal play activities within reason.

This advice could be a life-saver. A young child with hemophilia may need a protective helmet and elbow and knee pads for everyday wear, especially when first becoming mobile.

Instruct the family about medications, range-of-motion exercises, emergency measures to stop or limit bleeding, and all aspects of the child's care. Emergency splints should be kept in the home of every person with hemophilia. Ice packs also should be available for instant use. If possible, the bleeding area can be raised above the level of the heart. Before leaving for the health care facility, the caregiver should apply a splint and cold packs and give factor replacement according to the protocol established with the child's physician.

The family experiences continuous anxiety over how much activity to allow their child, how to keep from overprotecting him or her, and how to help the child achieve a healthy mental attitude, all the while preventing mishaps that may cause serious bleeding episodes. They must guide the child toward autonomy and independence within the framework of necessary limitations. At times, the emotional effects of social deprivation and restrained activity must be weighed against possible physical harm.

The financial strain on the family is considerable, as it is with most families with a child who has a chronic condition. Children who have had several episodes of hemarthrosis may be disabled to the extent of needing crutches and braces or wheelchairs. Measures toward rehabilitation require hospitalization, with possible surgery, casts, and other orthopedic appliances.

A hemophiliac child usually loses much school time. Any child who must frequently interrupt schooling for whatever reason experiences a considerable setback. Each child should be considered individually and provided with as normal an environment as possible.

Promoting Family Coping

Both the child and family must accept the limitations and yet realize the importance of having normal social experiences. School, health, and community agencies can offer the family counseling and encouragement and can help them raise the affected child in a healthy manner, both emotionally and physically. The National Hemophilia Foundation is a resource for services and publications (Website: http://www.hemophilia.org). Give the family information about other available support systems.

Review all these concerns with the family. Through discussion, questions, and demonstrations, confirm that the family understands the information provided. Counseling may be required for the family to learn to cope with the child's needs. Encourage family members to express their feelings about the effect the disease has on their lifestyle. The family may fear that the child will die of hemorrhaging. Guilt may play an important part in the family's reactions to the child. Recognizing and validating these feelings are important aspects of active listening. During hospitalization, involve the family in the child's care so they can learn how to help the child without causing additional pain.

EVALUATION: GOALS AND EXPECTED OUTCOMES

- **Goal:** The child will experience diminished pain.
  Expected Outcome: The child rests quietly with minimal pain as evidenced by the child using a pain scale to report decreased pain.
- **Goal:** The child will move freely with minimal pain.
  Expected Outcomes: There is no evidence of new joint contractures. The child maintains range of motion.
- **Goal:** The child will be protected from any new injuries.
  Expected Outcome: The child is free from injuries or bleeding episodes caused as a result of procedures, treatments, or unsafe environment.
- **Goal:** The family caregivers will verbalize an understanding of the disease, injury prevention, and care of the child.
  Expected Outcomes: The family caregivers can list five safety measures to decrease the possibilities of injury to the child. The family can

explain the disease and the child's home care and ask and answer appropriate questions.
- **Goal:** The family caregivers will develop appropriate coping mechanisms.
  Expected Outcome: The family members express their feelings and demonstrate good coping mechanisms, such as seeking help from appropriate support systems.

Test Yourself

- Give examples of where bleeding might be seen in the child with hemophilia.
- Discuss how hemophilia is treated.
- What areas should be covered when teaching a family who has a child with hemophilia?

A PERSONAL GLIMPSE

My 9-year-old son Samuel has hemophilia. When he had a circumcision after he was born, he just kept bleeding. They asked us if anyone in our family had a bleeding disorder, we told them we didn't think so. We found out later my grandfather did have a bleeding problem, we just had never known that. When Sam was little, he had bruises a lot, and finally they told us he had hemophilia. I felt so guilty because it came from my side of the family. We were so afraid and tried to protect him from any little accident, but he was such an active boy, it was so hard. I would get so nervous and upset whenever he got any kind of cut or even a little scratch. Now that he is older, he understands better, but he is disappointed when he can't ride a bike or skateboard like his friends do. We had to learn all about how to stop the bleeding and giving him Factor VIII. I still always worry that he could get AIDS—they say it would be unlikely, but I know it has happened. Sam's sisters are both younger than he is; they love their big brother so much and always try to protect him, too. I have learned to relax a little more, and he really handles it well, but every day I still worry that some day he will have something serious happen to him and we won't be able to stop the bleeding.

Theresa

LEARNING OPPORTUNITY: What are some resources and information you could offer to this mother? What would you say in response to the mother's statement regarding her child getting AIDS?

IDIOPATHIC THROMBOCYTOPENIC PURPURA

Purpura is a blood disorder associated with a deficit of platelets in the circulatory system. The most common type of purpura is idiopathic thrombocytopenic purpura (ITP). Purpura is preceded by a viral infection in about half the diagnosed cases.

Clinical Manifestations and Diagnosis

The onset of ITP is often acute. Bruising and a generalized rash occur. In severe cases, hemorrhage may occur in the mucous membranes; hematuria or difficult-to-control epistaxis may be present. Rarely, the serious complication of intracranial hemorrhage occurs. In most cases, symptoms disappear in a few weeks without serious hemorrhage. A few cases may continue in a chronic form of the disease.

In ITP, the platelet count may be $20,000/mm^3$ (normal, 150,000 to $300,000/mm^3$) or lower. The bleeding time is prolonged, and the clot retraction time is abnormal. The white blood cell count remains normal, and anemia is not present unless excessive bleeding has occurred.

Treatment and Nursing Care

Corticosteroids are useful in reducing the severity and shortening the duration of the disease in some, but not all, cases of ITP. Intravenous immunoglobulin (IVIG) has been used to increase the production of platelets until recovery occurs spontaneously. If the platelet count is higher than $20,000/mm^3$, treatment may be delayed to see if a spontaneous remission will occur.

Nursing care consists of protecting the child from falls and trauma, observing for signs of external or internal bleeding, and providing a regular diet and general supportive care.

ACUTE LEUKEMIA

Leukemia, the most common type of cancer in children, accounts for about 30% of all childhood cancers. Acute lymphatic leukemia (ALL) is responsible for about 70% to 75% of the childhood leukemias and acute myeloid leukemia (AML) for almost all the rest. Fortunately, ALL is also the most curable of all major forms of leukemia. The cure rate for AML is about 40%. The incidence of ALL is greatest between the ages of 2 and 6 years and is higher in boys; ALL is more common in white children than in African-American children. This discussion focuses on ALL.

Pathophysiology

Leukemia is the uncontrolled reproduction of deformed white blood cells. Despite intensive research, its cause is unknown. Mature leukocytes (white blood cells) are made up of three types of cells:

- **Monocytes** (5% to 10% of white blood cells) defend the body against infection.
- **Granulocytes** are divided into eosinophils, basophils, and neutrophils. Neutrophils (60% of the white blood cells) can pass through capillary walls to surround and destroy bacteria.
- **Lymphocytes** (30% of white blood cells) are divided into T cells that attack and destroy virus-infected cells, foreign tissue, and cancer cells, and B cells that produce antibodies (proteins that help destroy foreign matter). An immature lymphocyte is called a **lymphoblast**. Leukemia occurs when lymphocytes reproduce so quickly that they are mostly in the blast, or immature, stage. This rapid increase in lymphocytes causes crowding, which in turn decreases the production of red blood cells and platelets. The decrease in red blood cells, platelets, and normal white blood cells causes the child to become easily fatigued and susceptible to infection and increased bleeding.

Clinical Manifestations

Clinical manifestations of leukemia appear with surprising abruptness in many affected children with few, if any, warning signs. The symptoms result from the proliferation of lymphoblasts. Presenting manifestations are often fatigue, pallor, and low-grade fever caused by anemia. Other early or presenting symptoms are bone and joint pain caused by invasion of the periosteum by lymphocytes, widespread **petechiae** (pinpoint hemorrhages beneath the skin), and **purpura** (hemorrhages into the skin or mucous membranes) as a result of a low thrombocyte count. The lymph nodes often are enlarged.

Although they are seldom presenting signs, anorexia, nausea and vomiting, headache, diarrhea, and abdominal pain often occur during the course of the disease as a result of enlargement of the liver and spleen. Easy bruising is a constant problem. Ulceration of the gums and throat develops as a result of bacterial invasion and contributes to anorexia. Intracranial hemorrhages are not uncommon. Anemia becomes increasingly severe.

Diagnosis

In addition to the history, symptoms, and laboratory blood studies, a bone marrow aspiration must be done to confirm the diagnosis of leukemia. The preferred site for bone marrow aspiration in children is the iliac crest. Radiographs of the long bones demonstrate changes caused by the invasion of the lymphoblasts.

Treatment

The advances in the treatment of ALL have dramatically improved long-term survival. In children whose initial prognosis is good, about 90% have long-term survival. For children who have a relapse, survival rates are greatly reduced. Each succeeding relapse reduces the probability of survival.

Intensive chemotherapy is initially divided into three phases:

- Induction—geared to achieving a complete remission with no leukemia cells
- Sanctuary—preventing invasion of the central nervous system by leukemia cells (no sanctuary is given to the leukemia cells)
- Maintenance—maintaining the remission. A combination of drugs is used during the induction phase to bring about remission; among the drugs used are vincristine, prednisone, and asparaginase. During the sanctuary phase, **intrathecal administration** (drugs injected into the cerebrospinal fluid by lumbar puncture) of methotrexate is used to eradicate leukemia cells in the central nervous system. The maintenance phase may last 2 or 3 years and includes treatment with methotrexate, vincristine, prednisone, and 6-mercaptopurine. The drugs are often administered through a double-lumen catheter (Broviac) placed in the subclavian vein.

Two additional phases are instituted for children who experience relapse.

- Reinduction—administration of the drugs previously used plus additional drugs
- Bone marrow transplant—usually recommended after the second remission in children with ALL

● Nursing Process for the Child With Leukemia

ASSESSMENT

The process of collecting data on the child with leukemia varies according to the stage of the illness. Conduct the admission interview with both the family caregiver and the child. Do not allow the caregiver to monopolize the interview; give the child an opportunity to express feelings and fears and answer the questions. The physical examination should include observing for **adenopathy** (enlarged lymph glands), abnormal vital signs (especially a low-grade fever), signs of

bruising, petechiae, bleeding from or ulcerations of mucous membranes, abdominal pain or tenderness, and bone or joint pain. Observe the child for lethargic behavior, and question the caregiver about this. Note signs of local infection, including edema, redness, and swelling, or any indication of systemic infection. The diagnosis of leukemia is devastating. Observe and note the child and family's emotional states so that the nursing care plan can include helping them to discuss and resolve their feelings and fears.

SELECTED NURSING DIAGNOSES

- Risk for Infection related to increased susceptibility secondary to leukemic process and side effects of chemotherapy
- Risk for Injury related to bleeding tendencies
- Acute Pain related to the effects of chemotherapy and the disease process
- Fatigue related to disease, decreased energy, and anxiety
- Delayed Growth and Development related to impaired ability to achieve developmental tasks secondary to limitations of disease and treatment
- Disturbed Body Image related to alopecia and weight loss
- Anticipatory Grieving by the family related to the prognosis

OUTCOME IDENTIFICATION AND PLANNING

Goals for the child with leukemia vary depending on individual circumstances. Preventing infection, preventing injury, relieving pain, and reducing fatigue are major goals. Other important goals for the child may be promoting normal growth and development and improving body image. The goal for the family may be to verbalize feelings and to increase coping abilities.

IMPLEMENTATION

Preventing Infection

The immune system is weakened by the uncontrolled growth of lymphoblasts that overpower the normal production of granulocytes (particularly neutrophils) and monocytes. In addition, the chemotherapy necessary to inhibit this proliferation of lymphoblasts causes immunosuppression. Thus, these children are susceptible to infection, especially during chemotherapy. Infections such as meningitis, septicemia, and pneumonia are the most common causes of death. The organism most often responsible is Pseudomonas. Other organisms that can be dangerous for the child are

Escherichia coli, Staphylococcus aureus, Klebsiella, *Pneumocystis carinii, Candida albicans,* and Histoplasmosis. These infectious organisms can threaten the child's life. To protect the child from infectious organisms, follow standard guidelines for protective isolation. Carefully screen staff, family, and visitors to eliminate any known infection. Enforce handwashing, gowning, and masking. The social isolation that this imposes on the child can be difficult for the child to understand and tolerate, so spend additional time with the child beyond that necessary for direct care. Playing games, coloring, reading stories, and doing puzzles are all good activities the child will enjoy. This also provides a much-needed break for the caregiver staying with the child.

Preventing Bleeding and Injury

The mucous membranes bleed easily, so be gentle when doing oral hygiene. Use a soft, sponge-type brush or gauze strips wrapped around your finger. Mouthwash composed of one part hydrogen peroxide to four parts saline solution or normal saline solution may be used. Epistaxis (nosebleed) is a common problem that can usually be handled by applying external pressure to the nose. Apply pressure to sites of injections or venipunctures to prevent excessive bleeding. At least every 4 hours, monitor the child for other signs of bleeding, such as petechiae, ecchymosis, hematemesis (bloody emesis), tarry stools, and swelling and tenderness of the joints. Protect the child from injury by external forces to prevent the possibility of hemorrhage from the injury. Take extra caution when the child's platelet count is especially low.

Reducing Pain

Pain from the invasion of lymphoblasts into the periosteum and bleeding into the joints can be excruciating. Use gentle handling: place sheepskin pads under bony prominences and position the child to help relieve discomfort and skin breakdown. Many times painful procedures must be done that add to the child's discomfort. Explain to the child that these procedures are necessary to help and are not in any way a form of punishment. Provide a pain scale to help the child rate the pain and communicate its intensity. The numeric and the faces pain rating scales are useful with children 3 years of age and older (Fig. 29-8, Chapter 29). Administer analgesics as ordered to achieve maximum comfort.

Promoting Energy Conservation and Relieving Anxiety

As a result of anemia, the child is fatigued. Pace procedures so that the child has as much uninterrupted rest as possible. Stress adds to the child's feelings of exhaustion; to decrease fatigue, help the child deal with the stress caused by the illness and treatments. To help relieve anxiety, encourage the child to talk about feelings and acknowledge the child's feelings as valid.

Promoting Normal Growth and Development

During treatment, the child frequently may be prevented from participating in normal activity. The social isolation that accompanies reverse isolation often interferes with normal development. Physical activities often are limited simply because of the child's lack of energy. Knowledge of normal growth and development expectations is important to consider when planning developmental activities. Stimulate growth and development within the child's physical capabilities.

Think about this. Even when working with the sick child, always stress positive developmental tasks; for example, the school-age child can practice or improve reading skills and learn or increase computer skills.

Encourage the family to help the child return to normal activities as much as possible during the treatment's maintenance phase when the child has been discharged from the hospital.

Promoting a Positive Body Image

The drugs administered in chemotherapy cause **alopecia** (loss of hair) (Fig. 36-5). Prepare the child and the family psychologically for this change in appearance. The child may want to wear a wig,

● *Figure 36.5* The child with alopecia needs support and encouragement.

especially when returning to school. Encourage the family to choose the wig before chemotherapy is started so that it matches the child's hair and the child has time to get used to it. A cap or scarf often is appealing to a child, particularly if it carries a special meaning for him or her. Reassure the child and family that the hair will grow back in about 3 to 6 months. Wash the scalp regularly to avoid scaling. Prednisone therapy may cause the child to have a moon-faced appearance, which may be upsetting to the child or the family. Reassure them that this is temporary and will disappear when the drug is no longer needed. The child may be hesitant for peers to see these changes. Encourage visits from peers before discharge, if possible, so that the child can be prepared to handle their reactions and questions.

Acceptance is not as hard as you think. A schoolteacher can be invaluable in preparing classmates to welcome the child with leukemia back to school, with minimal reaction to the child's physical changes.

Encourage the family to enlist the assistance of the child's teacher, school nurse, and pediatrician to ease the transition. Meeting other children who are undergoing chemotherapy and are in various stages of recovery often is helpful to the child and helps to relieve the feeling that no one else has ever looked like this. Provide the child and the family opportunities to express their feelings and apprehensions.

Promoting Family Coping

Family members often are devastated when they first learn that their child has leukemia. Provide support from the moment of the first diagnosis, through the hospitalization, and continuing through the maintenance phase. Family members live one day at a time, hoping that the remission will not end and that their child will be one who does not have a relapse and is finally considered cured. Provide opportunities for family members to freely express their feelings about the illness and treatment. The family will find comfort and stability in having one nurse caring for the child consistently. Involve the caregivers in the care of the child during hospitalization, and give them complete information about what to expect when caring for the child at home during the maintenance phase. Identify a contact person for the family

to call to answer questions during this phase. Help the family work through feelings of over-protectiveness toward the child so that the child can lead as normal a life as possible. Encourage the family to consider how siblings can fit into the child's return home. Siblings may have many questions about the seriousness of the illness and about the possible death of their brother or sister. Provide support for families to deal with these concerns. Most hospitals that provide care for pediatric oncology patients have caregiver support groups that meet regularly. Candlelighters is a national organization for parents of young cancer patients (Website: http://www.candlelighters.org).

EVALUATION: GOALS AND EXPECTED OUTCOMES

- **Goal:** The child will remain free of signs and symptoms of infection.
  Expected Outcomes: The child's temperature does not exceed 100°F (37.9°C), and there is no inflammation, discharge, or other signs of infection.
- **Goal:** The child will remain free from injury related to bleeding.
  Expected Outcomes: The child has no signs of petechiae, ecchymosis, hematemesis, tarry stools, or swelling and tenderness of the joints.
- **Goal:** The child will show signs of being comfortable.
  Expected Outcomes: The child rests quietly and uses a pain scale to indicate that the pain is at a tolerable level.
- **Goal:** The child's energy level will be maintained or will increase.
  Expected Outcomes: The child participates in activities and procedures paced so that the child has adequate rest periods. The child expresses anxieties.
- **Goal:** The child will accomplish appropriate growth and development milestones within the limits of the condition.
  Expected Outcome: The child is involved in age-appropriate activities provided by staff and family.
- **Goal:** The child will accept changes in physical appearance.
  Expected Outcome: The child shows pride and adjustment in changes in body image and shares feelings about body image changes.
- **Goal:** The family will verbalize feelings and develops coping mechanisms.

Expected Outcome: The family expresses feelings and fears about the child's prognosis and accepts counseling and support as needed.

Test Yourself

- What symptoms are usually seen in the child with leukemia?

- Give some examples of how infection can be prevented in the child with leukemia.

- Define alopecia and discuss ways the nurse can support the child who has alopecia.

KEY POINTS

- The signs and symptoms seen in the child with congestive heart failure often include fatigue; feeding problems; failure to gain weight; pale, mottled, or cyanotic color; tachycardia; rapid respiration; dyspnea; flaring of the nares; and use of accessory muscles with retractions. Such children may also have edema and heart and liver enlargement.

- Group A beta-hemolytic streptococcus is the bacterium usually responsible for rheumatic fever.

- Major manifestations of rheumatic fever include carditis (inflammation of the heart), polyarthritis (migratory arthritis), and chorea (disorder characterized by emotional instability, purposeless movements, and muscular weakness).

- The most serious concern for a child with Kawasaki disease is development of cardiac involvement, which may not be seen for a period of time after the child's recovery.

- Iron deficiency anemia is a common nutritional deficiency in children. It is difficult to get enough iron from food the child eats, and if the iron intake is inadequate, anemia quickly results.

- If the sickle cell trait is inherited from one parent, a child can inherit the trait and carry the sickle cell trait. If both parents carry the trait, the child can inherit the trait from each parent and have sickle cell disease.

- In sickle cell anemia, the abnormal hemoglobin causes the red blood cells to assume a sickle shape. When sickling occurs, the affected red blood cells become crescent-shaped and the blood viscosity increases (blood becomes thicker), causing slowdown and sludging of the red blood cells. The impaired circulation results in tissue damage and infarction.

- Complications, including enlargement of the spleen, overstimulation of bone marrow, and heart failure, occur frequently in the child with thalassemia. Even with blood transfusions to maintain the hemoglobin levels, diet and medications to prevent heart failure, and splenectomy or bone marrow transplants, the prognosis is poor, and the child often dies of cardiac failure.

- The most common types of hemophilia are factor VIII deficiency and factor IX deficiency, which are inherited as a sex-linked recessive trait, with transmission to male offspring by carrier females.

- Hemophilia used to be treated by the use of fresh blood or plasma, but newer commercial preparations are now available that supply higher-potency factor VIII. These concentrates are supplied in dried form together with diluent for reconstitution. The preparations can be stored for a long time. A synthetic preparation, DDAVP (1-deamino-8-D-arginine vasopressin), is used in mild factor VIII deficiencies.

- Symptoms of idiopathic thrombocytopenic purpura include bruising, a generalized rash and, in severe cases, hemorrhage in the mucous membranes, hematuria, or difficult-to-control epistaxis. Rarely the serious complication of intracranial hemorrhage is seen.

- The child with leukemia often has fatigue, pallor, low-grade fever, bone and joint pain, petechiae (pinpoint hemorrhages beneath the skin), and purpura (hemorrhages into the skin or mucous membranes). The lymph nodes may be enlarged, and bruising is a constant problem.

- Four drugs commonly used in the treatment of acute lymphatic leukemia are methotrexate, vincristine, prednisone, and 6-mercaptopurine.

REFERENCES AND SELECTED READINGS

Books and Journals

Bryant, R. (2003). Managing side effects of childhood cancer treatment. *Journal of Pediatric Nursing, 18*(2), 113.

Colby-Graham, M. F., & Chordas, C. (2003). The childhood leukemias. *Journal of Pediatric Nursing, 18*(2), 87.

Hockenberry, M. J., Wilson, D., Winkelstein, M. L., & Kline, N. E. (2003). *Wong's nursing care of infants and children* (7th ed.). St. Louis: Mosby.

North American Nursing Diagnosis Association (NANDA). (2001). *NANDA nursing diagnoses: Definitions and classification 2001–2002.* Philadelphia: Author.

Pillitteri, A. (2003). *Maternal and child health nursing* (4th ed.). Philadelphia: Lippincott Williams & Wilkins.

Sparks, S., & Taylor, C. (2001). *Nursing diagnosis reference manual* (5th ed.). Springhouse, PA: Springhouse Corporation.

Wong, D. L., Perry, S., & Hockenberry, M. (2002). *Maternal–child nursing care* (2nd ed.). St. Louis: Mosby.

Web Addresses

Sickle Cell Disease
www.sicklecelldisease.org

Hemophilia
www.hemophilia.org

Kawasaki Disease
www.kdfoundation.org

Leukemia
www.leukemiafoundation.org

WORKBOOK

NCLEX-STYLE REVIEW QUESTIONS

1. A child with rheumatic fever will *most* likely have a history of which of the following?

    a. A sibling diagnosed with the disease

    b. A recent strep throat infection

    c. Bruising easily

    d. Increased urinary output

2. When developing a plan of care for a child with sickle cell disease, which of the following nursing interventions would be *most* important to include?

    a. Provide support for family caregivers.

    b. Observe skin for any breakdown.

    c. Move the extremities gently.

    d. Administer analgesics promptly.

3. After discussing measures used to stop bleeding with the caregiver of a child diagnosed with hemophilia, the caregiver makes the following statements. Which of these statements indicates a need for further teaching?

    a. "I always have ice and cold packs in our freezer."

    b. "Keeping pressure on an injury usually helps stop the bleeding."

    c. "Whenever my child gets hurt, I have him sit up with his head elevated and his feet down."

    d. "I know how to keep his arm from moving by using splints."

4. A nurse admits a child with a diagnosis of possible leukemia. Of the following signs and symptoms, which would *most* likely be seen in the child with leukemia?

    a. Low grade fever, bone and joint pain

    b. High fever, sore throat

    c. Swelling around eyes, ankles, and abdomen

    d. Upward and outward slanted eyes

5. In planning care for a child with leukemia, which of the following goals would be *most* important for this child? The child will

    a. remain free of signs and symptoms of infection.

    b. participate in age-appropriate activities.

    c. eat at least 60% of each meal.

    d. share feelings about changes in body image.

6. The nurse is caring for a client who has leukemia. Which of the following nursing interventions should the nurse implement to decrease the likelihood of bleeding or injury? Select all that apply:

    a. Use a soft, sponge-type brush or gauze strips to give oral care.

    b. Maintain reverse isolation.

    c. Use mouthwash composed of hydrogen peroxide and saline solution.

    d. Wear gloves when delivering the client's meal tray.

    e. Have the child wear a cap or scarf.

    f. Apply pressure to sites of injections or venipunctures.

STUDY ACTIVITIES

1. Using the table below, make a list of safety measures to help protect the child with hemophilia. Include measures to be taken at home, school, and in the hospital settings. Explain the reasons that these measures are important.

Setting	Safety Measure	Reasons Measures Are Important
Home School Hospital		

2. Missy is a 6-year-old girl with leukemia. Her single mother is unable to be away from her job to stay with Missy. Because of Missy's increased risk for infection, she has been placed in protective isolation. Create an age-appropriate game or list of activities that could be used in caring for Missy.

3. Go to the following Internet site: http://www.emory.edu/PEDS/SICKLE This is a site for the Sickle Cell Information Center. Go to section "How May We Serve You." Click on "Patients and Families Online Resources."

a. What are some of the topics available that you might share with your peers?

b. What are some of the topics available that you might suggest to a family who has a child with sickle cell anemia?

CRITICAL THINKING: What Would You Do?

1. The family of Sean, a 3-year-old boy with hemophilia, is concerned that Sean might get AIDS from his treatments.

   a. What is the likelihood of Sean being HIV positive or of contracting AIDS from his treatments?

   b. What explanation will you give this family to reassure them?

   c. What are your thoughts and feelings about children who are HIV positive because of a transfusion they received?

2. Andrew is an 18-month-old boy who has been admitted in a sickle cell crisis. His mother Jessica is 4 months pregnant with the family's second child. Tyrone, Andrew's father, tells you that they don't know much about sickle cell anemia, but they have heard their second child may also have the disease.

   a. What information would you share about sickle cell disease?

   b. What would you teach this family about the genetic factors related to sickle cell anemia?

   c. What is the likelihood that their second child will also have the disease?

   d. What organizations would you refer this family to?

3. Dosage calculation: The nurse is caring for a newborn who has symptoms of congestive heart failure and is being treated with Digoxin. The child weighs 6.5 pounds. The usual dosage range of this medication is 4 to 8 μg/kg/day in divided doses every 12 hours. Answer the following:

   a. How many micrograms (mcg) are in a milligram (mg)?

   b. How many kilograms (kg) does the child weigh?

   c. What is the lowest dose of Digoxin (in mcg) that this child could be given in a 24-hour time period?

   d. What is the highest dose of Digoxin (in mcg) that this child could be given in a 24-hour time period?

   e. How many doses will the child receive in a day?

4. Dosage calculation: A 5-year-old boy with a diagnosis of Kawasaki disease is being treated with aspirin. His initial dose is 90 mg/kg in divided doses every 6 hours. After his symptoms have subsided, he will be given a dose of 5 mg/kg a day for the antiplatelet effect of the drug. The child weighs 39 pounds. The medication comes in 80-mg tablets. Answer the following:

   a. How many kilograms (kg) does the child's weigh?

   b. How many milligrams (mg) per day will be given for the initial dose?

   c. How many milligrams (mg) per dose will be given for the initial dose?

   d. How many tablets will be given for each of the initial doses?

   e. How many milligrams (mg) per day will be given for the antiplatelet dose?

The Child With Gastrointestinal/ Endocrine Disorders

STUDENT OBJECTIVES

On completion of this chapter, the student should be able to

1. Discuss ways the child's gastrointestinal system differs from the adult's system.
2. Discuss ways the child's endocrine system differs from the adult's system.
3. Identify the symptoms of pyloric stenosis.
4. Explain the diagnosis of celiac disease.
5. State another name for congenital megacolon and list its common symptoms.
6. Describe the diagnosis and treatment of intussusception.
7. Discuss the cause of gastroesophageal reflux in the child.
8. Differentiate between mild diarrhea and severe diarrhea.
9. List the symptoms of appendicitis; differentiate symptoms of the older and the younger child.
10. Identify three intestinal parasites common to children and state the route of entry for each.
11. State the most common cause of poisoning in toddlers.
12. List five common substances that children ingest.
13. List seven sources of lead that may cause chronic lead poisoning.
14. Describe the symptoms, diagnosis, treatment, and prognosis of lead poisoning.
15. Describe the treatment of a child who has swallowed a foreign object.
16. Discuss the importance of good skin care, correct insulin administration, and exercise in the diabetic child.

KEY TERMS

anthelmintic
celiac syndrome
chelating agent
craniotabes
currant jelly stools
diabetic ketoacidosis
encephalopathy
gastroenteritis
insulin reaction
invagination
Kussmaul breathing
kwashiorkor
lactose
lactose intolerance
marasmus
pica
polydipsia
polyphagia
polyuria
pruritus
steatorrhea
urticaria

The gastrointestinal (GI) system is responsible for taking in and processing nutrients that nourish all parts of the body. As a result, any problem of the GI system, whether a lack of nutrients, an infectious disease, or a congenital disorder, can quickly affect other parts of the body and ultimately affect general health, growth, and development. The endocrine system consists of a number of ductless glands throughout the body that secrete hormones. All of the body systems overlap with the working of the endocrine glands.

GROWTH AND DEVELOPMENT OF THE GASTROINTESTINAL AND ENDOCRINE SYSTEMS

Gastrointestinal System

The main organs of the gastrointestinal or digestive system are the mouth, pharynx (throat), esophagus, stomach, small intestine, large intestine, rectum, and anal canal. Other organs, called accessory organs, include structures that aid in the digestive process, as well as

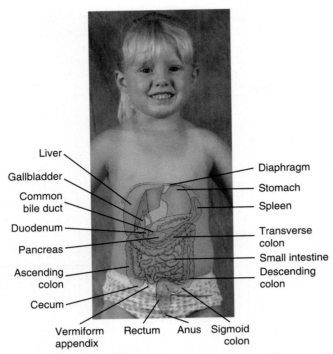

● *Figure 37.1* Anatomy of a child's gastrointestinal system.

glands that secrete substances that further aid in digestion. These accessory organs include the teeth, tongue, gallbladder, appendix, the salivary glands, liver, and pancreas. Each of these organs and accessory organs plays a part in the process of digestion (Fig. 37-1).

The child takes in food and fluids through the GI tract, where they are broken down and absorbed to promote growth and maintain life. Food enters the mouth, and the digestive process begins. Digestion takes place by mechanical and chemical mechanisms. Chewing, muscular action, and peristalsis are physical or mechanical actions that break down food. Chemicals secreted along the GI tract by accessory organs further help the breakdown of food so that absorption can take place. As food is processed, nutrients are absorbed and distributed to the body cells. The large intestine is the organ of elimination that collects wastes and pushes them to the anus so the waste materials can be excreted.

The functioning of the gastrointestinal system begins at birth. The GI tract of the newborn works in the same manner as that of the adult but with some limitations. For example, the enzymes secreted by the liver and pancreas are reduced. Thus, complex carbohydrates cannot be broken down and used by the infant. As a result, the newborn diet must be adjusted to allow for this immaturity. By the age of 4 to 6 months, the needed enzymes are usually sufficient in amount.

The capacity of the infant's stomach and the increased speed at which food moves through the GI tract require feeding smaller amounts at more frequent intervals. In addition, the small capacity of the colon leads to a bowel movement after each feeding. Reflexes are present in infants that allow for swallowing and prevention of aspiration when swallowing. The cardiac sphincter at the end of the esophagus may be lax in the infant, and food may be regurgitated from the stomach back into the esophagus. As the child grows, the muscles of the sphincter work more effectively and prevent food from going back into the esophagus. With continued growth, the GI tract matures and the capacity of the GI tract increases, but the digestive functioning throughout childhood into adulthood is the same.

Disorders and disruptions in the GI tract can cause a change in the functioning of the system. Most of these disorders stem from congenital defects, diseases, or infections in the GI tract. If any of these occur and the body does not get the needed nutrients to the cells, health and normal growth and development can be altered in children.

Endocrine System and Hormonal Function

The hormones secreted by the endocrine system are circulated through the bloodstream to control and regulate most of the activities and functions in the body. Regulating metabolism, growth, development, and reproduction are all functions of hormones. The endocrine system of the infant is adequately developed, although the functions are immature. As the child grows, the endocrine system matures in function.

Various disorders are caused by decreases, increases, or the absence of hormone secretions by the endocrine glands. The pancreas is the gland that secretes the hormone insulin. Type 1 diabetes mellitus occurs in children when an insufficient amount of insulin is produced.

GASTROINTESTINAL DISORDERS

PYLORIC STENOSIS

The pylorus is the muscle that controls the flow of food from the stomach to the duodenum. Pyloric stenosis is characterized by hypertrophy of the circular muscle fibers of the pylorus, with a severe narrowing of its lumen. The pylorus is thickened to as much as twice its size, is elongated, and has a consistency resembling cartilage. As a result of this obstruction at the distal end of the stomach, the stomach becomes dilated (Fig. 37-2).

● **Figure 37.2** Pyloric stenosis (narrowed lumen of the pylorus).

Pyloric stenosis is rarely symptomatic during the 1st days of life. It has occasionally been recognized shortly after birth, but the average affected infant does not show symptoms until about the 3rd week of life. Symptoms rarely appear after the 2nd month. Although symptoms appear late, pyloric stenosis is classified as a congenital defect. Its cause is unknown, but it occurs more frequently in white males and has a familial tendency.

Clinical Manifestations

During the 1st weeks of life, the infant with pyloric stenosis often eats well and gains weight, then starts vomiting occasionally after meals. Within a few days, the vomiting increases in frequency and force, becoming projectile. The vomited material is sour, undigested food; it may contain mucus but never bile because it has not progressed beyond the stomach.

Because the obstruction is a mechanical one, the baby does not feel ill, is ravenously hungry, and is eager to try again and again, but the food invariably comes back. As the condition progresses, the baby becomes irritable, loses weight rapidly, and becomes dehydrated. Alkalosis develops from the loss of potassium and hydrochloric acid, and the baby becomes seriously ill.

Constipation becomes progressive because little food gets into the intestine, and urine is scanty. Gastric peristaltic waves passing from left to right across the abdomen usually can be seen during or after feedings.

Diagnosis

Diagnosis is usually made on the clinical evidence. The nature, type, and times of vomiting are documented. When the infant drinks, gastric peristaltic waves are observed. The infant may have a history of weight loss with hunger and irritability.

Ultrasonographic or radiographic studies with barium swallow show an abnormal retention of barium in the stomach and increased peristalsis.

Treatment

A surgical procedure called a pyloromyotomy (also known as a Fredet-Ramstedt operation) is the treatment of choice. This procedure simply splits the hypertrophic pyloric muscle down to the submucosa, allowing the pylorus to expand so that food may pass. Prognosis is excellent if surgery is performed before the infant is severely dehydrated.

● Nursing Process for the Child With Pyloric Stenosis

ASSESSMENT

When the infant of 1 or 2 months of age has a history of projectile vomiting, pyloric stenosis is suspected. Carefully interview the family caregivers. Ask when the vomiting started and determine the character of the vomiting (undigested formula with no bile, vomitus progressively more projectile). The caregiver will relate a story of a baby who is an eager eater but cannot retain food. Ask the caregiver about constipation and scanty urine.

Physical exam reveals an infant who may show signs of dehydration. Obtain the infant's weight and observe skin turgor and skin condition (including excoriated diaper area), anterior fontanelle (depressed, normal, or bulging), temperature, apical pulse rate (observing for weak pulse and tachycardia), irritability, lethargy, urine (amount and concentration), lips and mucous membranes of the mouth (dry, cracked), and eyes (bright, glassy, sunken, dark circles). Observe for visible gastric peristalsis when the infant is eating. Document and report signs of severe dehydration to help determine the need for fluid and electrolyte replacement.

Do you know the why of it? An experienced practitioner often can feel an olive-sized mass through deep palpation in the infant with pyloric stenosis.

SELECTED NURSING DIAGNOSES: PREOPERATIVE PHASE

● Imbalanced Nutrition: Less Than Body Requirements related to inability to retain food

- Deficient Fluid Volume related to frequent vomiting
- Impaired Oral Mucous Membrane related to NPO status
- Risk for Impaired Skin Integrity related to fluid and nutritional deficit
- Compromised Family Coping related to seriousness of illness and impending surgery

OUTCOME IDENTIFICATION AND PLANNING: PREOPERATIVE PHASE

Before surgery, the major goals for the infant with pyloric stenosis include improving nutrition and hydration, maintaining mouth and skin integrity, and relieving family anxiety. Plan individualized nursing care according to these goals, including interventions to prepare the infant for surgery.

IMPLEMENTATION: PREOPERATIVE PHASE

Maintaining Adequate Nutrition and Fluid Intake

Hypertrophy of the pylorus narrows the passage from the stomach into the duodenum. As a result, food (breast milk or formula) cannot pass. The infant loses weight and becomes dehydrated. If the infant is severely dehydrated and malnourished, rehydration with intravenous (IV) fluids and electrolytes is necessary to correct hypokalemia and alkalosis and prepare the infant for surgery. Carefully monitor the IV site for redness and induration. Improved skin turgor, weight gain, correction of hypokalemia and alkalosis, adequate intake of fluids, and no evidence of gastric distention are signs of improved nutrition and hydration.

Feedings of formula thickened with infant cereal and fed through a large-holed nipple may be given to improve nutrition before surgery. A smooth muscle relaxant may be ordered before feedings. Feed the infant slowly while he or she is sitting in an infant seat or being held upright. During the feeding, burp the infant frequently to avoid gastric distention. Document the feeding given and the approximate amount retained. Also record the frequency and type of emesis.

In preparation for surgery, fluid and electrolyte balance must be restored and the stomach must be empty. Typically, oral fluids are omitted for a specified time before the procedure, and the infant receives IV fluids. After the infant undergoes a barium swallow x-ray for diagnosis, the physician may order placement of a nasogastric (NG) tube with saline lavage to empty the stomach. The NG tube is left in place when the infant goes to surgery.

Providing Mouth Care

The infant needs good mouth care because the mucous membranes of the mouth may be dry because of dehydration and the omission of oral fluids before surgery. A pacifier can satisfy the baby's need for sucking because of the interruption in normal feeding and sucking habits.

Promoting Skin Integrity

Depending on the severity of dehydration, the skin may easily crack or break down and become irritated. The infant is repositioned, the diaper is changed, and lanolin or A and D Ointment is applied to dry skin areas. Intravenous therapy may also affect skin integrity. Monitor the IV insertion site for redness and inflammation. Closely observe and document the infant's skin condition.

Promoting Family Coping

The family caregivers are anxious because their infant is obviously seriously ill, and when they learn that the infant is to undergo surgery, their apprehensions increase. Include the caregivers in the preparation for surgery and explain:

- The importance of added IV fluids preoperatively to improve electrolyte balance and rehydrate the infant.
- The reason for ultrasonographic or barium swallow examination.
- The function of the NG tube and saline lavage.

Explain the location of the pylorus (at the distal end of the stomach) and what happens when the circular muscle fibers hypertrophy. You can liken it to a doughnut that thickens, so that the opening closes and very little food gets through. Describe the surgical procedure to be performed. During the procedure, the muscle is simply split down to, but not through, the submucosa, allowing it to balloon and let food pass.

Direct the family caregivers to the appropriate waiting area during surgery so that the surgeon can find them immediately after surgery. Explain to the caregivers what to expect and about how long the operation will last. Describe the procedure for the postanesthesia care unit so that the caregivers know the infant will be under close observation after surgery until fully recovered.

EVALUATION: GOALS AND EXPECTED OUTCOMES—PREOPERATIVE PHASE

- **Goal:** The infant's nutritional status will be adequate for normal growth.
  Expected Outcomes: The infant maintains weight.
- **Goal:** The infant will be hydrated.

Expected Outcomes: The infant's skin turgor improves, mucous membranes are moist and pink, and the hourly urine output is 2 to 3 mL/kg.

- Goal: The infant's IV infusion site will remain intact.

  Expected Outcome: The infant's skin shows no signs of redness or induration.

- Goal: The infant's oral mucous membranes will remain intact.

  Expected Outcomes: The infant's mucous membranes are moist and pink and saliva is sufficient, as evidenced by typical drooling; the infant uses a pacifier sufficiently to meet sucking needs.

- Goal: The infant's skin integrity will be maintained.

  Expected Outcome: The infant shows no signs of skin irritation or breakdown.

- Goal: The family caregivers' anxiety will be reduced.

  Expected Outcomes: The family caregivers verbalize an understanding of the procedures and treatments, cooperate with the nursing staff, ask appropriate questions, and express confidence in the treatment plan.

SELECTED NURSING DIAGNOSES: POSTOPERATIVE PHASE

- Risk for Aspiration related to postoperative vomiting
- Acute Pain related to surgical trauma
- Imbalanced Nutrition: Less Than Body Requirements related to postoperative condition
- Risk for Impaired Skin Integrity related to surgical incision
- Compromised Family Coping related to postoperative condition

OUTCOME IDENTIFICATION AND PLANNING: POSTOPERATIVE PHASE

After surgery, the major goals for the infant include keeping the airway clear, maintaining comfort, improving nutrition status, preserving skin integrity, and reducing family anxiety. Individualize the nursing plan of care according to these goals.

IMPLEMENTATION: POSTOPERATIVE PHASE

Maintaining a Patent Airway
After surgery, position the infant on his side and prevent aspiration of mucus or vomitus, particularly during the anesthesia recovery period. After fully waking from surgery, the infant may be held by a family caregiver. Help the caregiver find a position that does not interfere with IV infusions and that is comforting to both the caregiver and child.

Promoting Comfort
Observe the infant's behavior to evaluate discomfort and pain. Excessive crying, restlessness, listlessness, resistance to being held and cuddled, rigidity, and increased pulse and respiratory rates can indicate pain. Administer analgesics as ordered. Nursing interventions that may provide comfort include rocking, holding, cuddling, and offering a pacifier. Include the family caregivers in helping to comfort the infant.

Providing Nutrition
The first feeding, given 4 to 6 hours after surgery, is usually an electrolyte replacement solution, such as Lytren or Pedialyte. Give feedings slowly, in small amounts, with frequent burping. Intravenous fluid is necessary until the infant is taking sufficient oral feedings. Continue to use all nursing measures for IV care that were followed before surgery. Accurate intake and output and daily weight determinations are required.

Promoting Skin Integrity
Closely observe the surgical site for blood, drainage, and secretions. Make observations at least every 4 hours. Record and report any odor. Care for the incision and dressings as ordered by the physician.

Promoting Family Coping
The family caregivers will be anxious if the infant vomits after surgery, but reassure them that this is not uncommon during the first 24 hours after surgery. The caregivers should be involved in postoperative care. Reassure them that the care they gave at home did not cause the condition. Offer them support and understanding and encourage them in feeding and providing for the infant's needs. They can be told that the likelihood of a satisfactory recovery in a few weeks, with steady progression to complete recovery, is excellent. The operative fatality rate under these conditions has become less than 1%.

EVALUATION: GOALS AND EXPECTED OUTCOMES—POSTOPERATIVE PHASE

- Goal: The infant will not aspirate vomitus or mucus.

  Expected Outcome: The infant rests quietly in a side-lying position without choking or coughing.

- **Goal:** The infant will show signs of being comfortable.

    Expected Outcomes: The infant sleeps and rests in a relaxed manner, cuddles with caregivers and nurses, and does not cry excessively.

- **Goal:** The infant's nutrition status and fluid intake will improve.

    Expected Outcomes: The infant's daily weight gain is 0.75 to 1 oz (22 to 30 g). Oral fluids are retained with minimal vomiting. Hourly urine output is 2 to 3 mL/kg.

- **Goal:** The infant's skin integrity will be maintained.

    Expected Outcome: The infant's surgical site shows no signs of infection, as evidenced by absence of redness, foul odor, or drainage.

- **Goal:** The family caregivers' anxiety will be reduced.

    Expected Outcomes: The family caregivers are involved in the postoperative feeding of the infant and demonstrate an understanding of feeding technique.

Test Yourself

- What type of vomiting is seen in the child with pyloric stenosis?

- What is done to treat a child with pyloric stenosis?

- Explain the reason it is important to monitor accurate intake and output in the child with pyloric stenosis.

CELIAC SYNDROME

The term **celiac syndrome** is used to designate the complex of malabsorptive disorders. Intestinal malabsorption with **steatorrhea** (fatty stools) is a condition brought about by various causes, the most common being cystic fibrosis and gluten-induced enteropathy, the so-called idiopathic celiac disease. Cystic fibrosis is described in Chapter 35. Gluten-induced enteropathy is presented here.

Idiopathic celiac disease is a basic defect of metabolism precipitated by the ingestion of wheat gluten or rye gluten, which leads to impaired fat absorption. The exact cause is not known; the most acceptable theory is that of an inborn error of metabolism with an allergic reaction to the gliadin fraction of gluten (a protein factor in wheat) as a contributing or possibly the sole factor.

Severe manifestations of the disorder have become rare in the United States and in western Europe, but mild disturbances in intestinal absorption of rye, wheat, and sometimes oat gluten are common, occurring in about 1 in 2,000 children in the United States.

Clinical Manifestations

Signs generally do not appear before the age of 6 months and may be delayed until age 1 year or later. Manifestations include chronic diarrhea with foul, bulky, greasy stools and progressive malnutrition. Anorexia and a fretful, unhappy disposition are typical. The onset is generally insidious, with failure to thrive, bouts of diarrhea, and frequent respiratory infections. If the condition becomes severe, the effects of malnutrition are prominent. Retarded growth and development, a distended abdomen, and thin, wasted buttocks and legs are characteristic signs (Fig. 37-3).

The chronic course of this disease may be interrupted by a celiac crisis, an emergency situation. Frequently this is triggered by an upper respiratory infection. The child vomits copious amounts, has large, watery stools, and becomes severely dehydrated. As the child becomes drowsy and prostrate, an acute medical emergency develops. Parenteral fluid therapy is essential to combat acidosis and to achieve normal fluid balance.

Diagnosis and Treatment

One way to determine if a small child's failure to thrive is caused by celiac disease is to initiate a trial

● *Figure 37.3* A child with celiac disease. Notice the protruding abdomen and wasted buttocks.

gluten-free diet and observe the results. Improvement in the nature of the stools and general well-being with a gain in weight should follow, although several weeks may elapse before clear-cut manifestations can be confirmed. Conclusive diagnosis can be made by a biopsy of the jejunum through endoscopy that shows changes in the villi. Serum screening of IgG and IgA antigliadin antibodies shows the presence of the condition and also aids in monitoring the progress of therapy.

Response to a diet from which rye, wheat, and oats are excluded is generally good, although probably no cure can be expected, and dietary indiscretions or respiratory infections may bring relapses. The omission of wheat products in particular should continue through adolescence because the ingestion of wheat appears to inhibit growth in these children.

Dietary Program

The young child is usually started on a starch-free, low-fat diet. If the condition is severe, this diet consists of skim milk, glucose, and banana flakes. Bananas contain invert sugar and are usually well tolerated. Lean meats, puréed vegetables, and fruits are gradually added to the diet. Eventually fats may be added, and the child can be maintained on a regular diet, with the exception of all wheat, rye, and oat products.

The forbidden list of foods include wheat products, as well as malted milk drinks, some candies, many baby foods, and breads, cakes, pastries, and biscuits, unless they are made from corn flour or cornmeal. Vitamins A and D in water-miscible (able to be mixed with water) solutions are needed in double amounts to supplement the deficient diet.

Watch out. Commercially canned creamed soups, cold cuts, frankfurters, and pudding mixes generally contain wheat products.

Nursing Care

The primary focus of nursing care is to help caregivers maintain a restrictive diet for the child. Family teaching should include information regarding the disease and the need for long-term management, as well as guidelines for a gluten-free diet. Caregivers must learn to read the list of ingredients on packaged foods carefully before purchasing anything. The diet of the young child may be monitored fairly easily, but when the child goes to school, monitoring becomes a much greater challenge. As the child grows, caregivers and children might need additional nursing support to help them make dietary modifications.

CONGENITAL AGANGLIONIC MEGACOLON

Congenital aganglionic megacolon, also called Hirschsprung disease, is characterized by persistent constipation resulting from partial or complete intestinal obstruction of mechanical origin. In some cases, the condition may be severe enough to be recognized during the neonatal period; in other cases the blockage may not be diagnosed until later infancy or early childhood.

Parasympathetic nerve cells regulate peristalsis in the intestine. The name aganglionic megacolon actually describes the condition because there is an absence of parasympathetic ganglion cells within the muscular wall of the distal colon and the rectum. As a result, the affected portion of the lower bowel has no peristaltic action. Thus, it narrows, and the portion directly proximal to (above) the affected area becomes greatly dilated and filled with feces and gas (Fig. 37-4).

Clinical Manifestations

Accurate reporting of the first meconium stool in the newborn is vital. Failure of the newborn to have a stool in the first 24 hours may indicate a number of conditions, one of which is megacolon.

Other neonatal symptoms are suggestive of complete or partial intestinal obstruction, such as bile-stained emesis and generalized abdominal distention. Gastroenteritis with diarrheal stools may be present, and ulceration of the colon may occur.

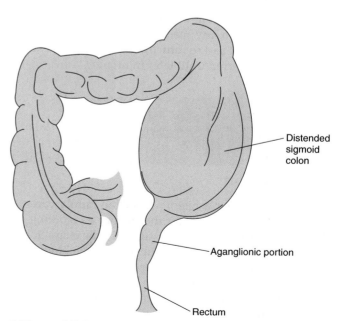

● **Figure 37.4** Dilated colon in Hirschsprung disease.

This is critical to remember. If a newborn does not have a stool within the first 24 hours, this must be documented and reported.

The affected older infant or child has obstinate, severe constipation dating back to early infancy. Stools are ribbon-like or consist of hard pellets. Formed bowel movements do not occur, except with the use of enemas, and soiling does not occur. The rectum is usually empty because the impaction occurs above the aganglionic segment.

As the child grows older, the abdomen becomes progressively enlarged and hard. General debilitation and chronic anemia are usually present. Differentiation must be made between this condition and psychogenic megacolon because of coercive toileting or other emotional problems. The child with aganglionic megacolon does not withhold stools or defecate in inappropriate places, and no soiling occurs.

Diagnosis

In the newborn, the absence of a meconium stool within the first 24 hours, and in the older infant or child, a history of obstinate, severe constipation may indicate the need for further evaluation. Definitive diagnosis is made through barium studies and must be confirmed by rectal biopsy.

Treatment

Treatment involves surgery with the ultimate resection of the aganglionic portion of the bowel. A colostomy is often performed to relieve the obstruction. This allows the child to regain any weight lost and also gives the bowel a period of rest to return to a more normal state. Resection is deferred until later in infancy.

● Nursing Process for the Child Undergoing Surgery for Congenital Aganglionic Megacolon

ASSESSMENT

Carefully gather a history from the family caregivers, noting especially the history of stooling. Ask about the onset of constipation, the character and odor of stools, the frequency of bowel movements, and the presence of poor feeding habits, anorexia, and irritability.

During the physical exam, observe for a distended abdomen and signs of poor nutrition (see "Nursing Process for the Child With Nutritional Problems"). Record weight and vital signs. Observe the child for developmental milestones.

SELECTED NURSING DIAGNOSES: PREOPERATIVE PHASE

- Constipation related to decreased bowel motility
- Imbalanced Nutrition: Less Than Body Requirements related to anorexia
- Fear (in the older child) related to impending surgery
- Compromised Family Coping related to the serious condition of the child and lack of knowledge about impending surgery

OUTCOME IDENTIFICATION AND PLANNING: PREOPERATIVE PHASE

The preoperative goals for the child undergoing surgery for congenital aganglionic megacolon include preventing constipation, improving nutritional status, and relieving fear (in the older child). The major goal for the family is reducing anxiety. Base the preoperative nursing plan of care on these goals. Plan interventions that prepare the child for surgery.

IMPLEMENTATION: PREOPERATIVE PHASE

Preventing Constipation
Decreased bowel motility may lead to constipation, which in turn may result in injury. Enemas may be given to achieve bowel elimination. They also may be ordered before diagnostic and surgical procedures are performed. Administer colonic irrigations with saline solutions. Neomycin or other antibiotic solutions are used to cleanse the bowel and prepare the GI tract.

Don't! Never administer soap suds or tap water enemas to a child with Hirschsprung disease. The lack of peristaltic action causes the enemas to be retained and absorbed into the tissues, causing water intoxication. This could cause syncope, shock, or even death after only one or two irrigations.

Maintaining Adequate Nutrition
Parenteral nutrition may be needed to improve nutritional status because the constipation and distended abdomen cause loss of appetite. IV fluid therapy may be necessary. The child does not want to eat and has a poor nutritional status. In older children a low residue diet is given.

Reducing Fear

Children who are preschool-age and older are more aware of the approaching surgery and have a number of fears reflective of the developmental stage. Preschoolers are still in the age of magical thinking. They may overhear a word or two that they misinterpret and exaggerate; this can lead to imagined pain and danger. Careful explanations must be provided for the preschooler to reduce any fears about mutilation. Talk about the surgery; reassure the child that the "insides won't come out," and answer questions seriously and sincerely. Encourage family caregivers to stay with the child if possible to increase the child's feelings of security.

The older school-age child may have a more realistic view of what is going to happen but may still fear the impending surgery. Peer contact may help comfort the school-age child. For more information on reducing preoperative fears and anxiety, see Chapter 29.

Promoting Family Coping

Family caregivers are apprehensive about the preliminary procedures and the impending surgery. Explain all aspects of the preoperative care, including examinations, colonic irrigations, and IV fluid therapy. As with other surgical procedures, inform the caregivers about the waiting area, the postanesthesia care unit, and the approximate length of the operation, and answer any questions. Building good rapport before surgery is an essential aspect of good nursing care. Answer the family caregivers' questions about the later resection of the aganglionic portion. With successful surgery, these children will grow and develop normally.

EVALUATION: GOALS AND EXPECTED OUTCOMES—PREOPERATIVE PHASE

- **Goal:** The child will have adequate bowel elimination with episodes of constipation.
  Expected Outcomes: The child has bowel elimination daily, and the colon is clean and well prepared for surgery.
- **Goal:** The child's nutritional status will be maintained preoperatively.
  Expected Outcomes: The child ingests diet adequate to maintain weight and promote growth.
- **Goal:** The older child will display minimal fear of bodily injury.
  Expected Outcomes: The older child realistically describes what will happen in surgery and interacts with family, peers, and nursing staff in a positive manner.

- **Goal:** The family caregivers will demonstrate an understanding of preoperative procedures.
  Expected Outcomes: The family caregivers cooperate with care, ask relevant questions, and accurately explain procedures when asked to repeat information.

SELECTED NURSING DIAGNOSES: POSTOPERATIVE PHASE

- Risk for Impaired Skin Integrity related to irritation from the colostomy
- Acute Pain related to the surgical procedure
- Deficient Fluid Volume related to postoperative condition
- Impaired Oral and Nasal Mucous Membranes related to NPO status and irritation from NG tube
- Deficient Knowledge of caregivers related to understanding of postoperative care of the colostomy

OUTCOME IDENTIFICATION AND PLANNING: POSTOPERATIVE PHASE

The major postoperative goals for the child include maintaining skin integrity, promoting comfort, maintaining fluid balance, and maintaining moist, clean nasal and oral mucous membranes. Goals for the family include reducing caregiver anxiety and preparing for home care of the child. Develop the individualized nursing plan of care according to these goals.

IMPLEMENTATION: POSTOPERATIVE PHASE

Promoting Skin Integrity

Maintaining skin integrity of the surgical site, especially around the colostomy stoma, is very important. When routine colostomy care is performed, give careful attention to the area around the colostomy. Record and report redness, irritation, and rashy appearances of the skin around the stoma. Prepare the skin with skin-toughening preparations that strengthen it and provide better adhesion of the appliance.

Promoting Comfort

The child may have abdominal pain after surgery. Observe for signs of pain, such as crying, pulse and respiration rate increases, restlessness, guarding of the abdomen, or drawing up the legs. Administer analgesics promptly as ordered. Additional nursing measures that can be used are changing the child's position, holding the child when possible, stroking, cuddling, and engaging in age-appropriate activities. Observe for abdominal distention, which must be documented and reported promptly.

Maintaining Fluid Balance

The NG tube is left in place after surgery and IV fluids are given until bowel function is established. Accurate intake and output determinations and reporting the character, amount, and consistency of stools help determine when the child may have oral feedings. To monitor fluid loss, record and report the drainage from the NG tube every 8 hours. Immediately report any unusual drainage, such as bright-red bleeding.

Providing Oral and Nasal Care

Perform good mouth care at least every 4 hours. At the same time, gently clean the nares to relieve any irritation from the NG tube. If the child is young, sucking needs can be satisfied with a pacifier.

Providing Family Teaching

Show the family caregiver how to care for the colostomy at home. If available, a wound, continence, and ostomy nurse (WOCN) may be consulted to help teach the family caregivers. Discuss topics such as devices and their use, daily irrigation, and skin care. The caregivers should demonstrate their understanding by caring for the colostomy under the supervision of nursing personnel several days before discharge. Family caregivers also need referrals to support personnel.

EVALUATION: GOALS AND EXPECTED OUTCOMES: POSTOPERATIVE PHASE

- **Goal:** The child's skin integrity will be maintained.
  Expected Outcomes: The child has no skin irritation at the colostomy site; no redness, foul odor, or purulent drainage is noted at the surgical site.
- **Goal:** The child's behavior will indicate minimal pain.
  Expected Outcomes: The child rests quietly without signs of restlessness; he or she verbalizes comfort if old enough to communicate verbally.
- **Goal:** The child's fluid intake will be adequate.
  Expected Outcomes: The child's hourly urine output is 2 to 3 mL/kg, indicating adequate hydration.
- **Goal:** The child's oral and nasal mucous membranes will remain intact.
  Expected Outcomes: The child's oral and nasal mucous membranes are moist and pink; the infant uses a pacifier to meet sucking needs.

- **Goal:** The family caregivers will demonstrate skill and knowledge in caring for the colostomy.
  Expected Outcome: The family caregivers irrigate the colostomy and clean the surrounding skin under the supervision of nursing personnel.

INTUSSUSCEPTION

Intussusception is the **invagination**, or telescoping, of one portion of the bowel into a distal portion. It occurs most commonly at the juncture of the ileum and the colon, although it can appear elsewhere in the intestinal tract. The invagination is from above downward, the upper portion slipping over the lower portion and pulling the mesentery along with it (Fig. 37-5).

This condition occurs more often in boys than in girls and is the most common cause of intestinal obstruction in childhood. The highest incidence occurs in infants between the ages of 4 and 10 months. The condition usually appears in healthy babies without any

A PERSONAL GLIMPSE

When our son was born my wife and I were thrilled; we were so happy to be parents. My wife was breast-feeding, and I would get up at night and bring him to her so she could feed him; it was just like we had thought it would be. He started growing and getting bigger, so at first we weren't worried about his big belly. It was my job to change the "dirty" diapers when I was home. We started noticing the baby seemed constipated at times and had little hard stools but then had diarrhea. The pediatrician used the word "obstruction," and that was hard for us to really understand. They did a barium test and other tests; we felt so bad for our baby. My wife was so upset, she cried all the time. He had to have IVs and TPN, and then they told us he would have to have surgery and a colostomy. Seeing him with all those tubes and bags after surgery was heartbreaking. We took him home with the colostomy, and my job was still the "diaper" duty, but now it was taking care of the colostomy. I have gotten so good, now I can change the colostomy bag pretty fast. We know he has to go back for more surgery, but for now we are just glad we can take care of him at home and love and enjoy him.

David

LEARNING OPPORTUNITY: In what ways do you think this father was supportive of his wife and his son? What would be important to teach these parents about care of the colostomy? What community support might be available for this family?

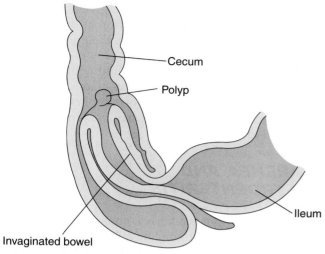

● *Figure 37.5* In this drawing of intussusception, note the telescoping of a portion of the bowel into the distal portion.

demonstrable cause. Possible contributing factors may be the hyperperistalsis and unusual mobility of the cecum and ileum normally present in early life. Occasionally a lesion such as Meckel's diverticulum or a polyp is present.

Clinical Manifestations

The infant who previously appeared healthy and happy suddenly becomes pale, cries out sharply, and draws up the legs in a severe colicky spasm of pain. This spasm may last for several minutes, after which the infant relaxes and appears well until the next episode, which may occur 5, 10, or 20 minutes later.

Most of these infants start vomiting early. Vomiting becomes progressively more severe and eventually is bile-stained. The infant strains with each paroxysm, emptying the bowels of fecal contents. The stools consist of blood and mucus, thereby earning the name **currant jelly stools**.

> **Observation skills are critical.**
> Currant jelly stools are an important clue in the child with intussusception.

Signs of shock appear quickly and characteristically include a rapid, weak pulse; increased temperature; shallow, grunting respirations; pallor; and marked sweating. Shock, vomiting, and currant jelly stools are the cardinal symptoms of this condition. Because these signs coupled with the paroxysmal pain are quite severe, professional health care is often initiated early.

The nurse, who is often consulted by neighbors, friends, and relatives when things go wrong, needs to be informed and alert; therefore, a word of caution is

needed. The nurse needs to be aware that on rare occasions a more chronic form of the condition appears, particularly during an episode of severe diarrheal disturbance. The onset is more gradual, and the infant may not show all the classic symptoms, but the danger of sudden, complete strangulation is present. Such an infant should already be in the care of a physician because of the diarrhea.

Diagnosis

The care provider usually can make a diagnosis from the clinical symptoms, rectal examination, and palpation of the abdomen during a calm interval when it is soft. A baby is often unwilling to tolerate this palpation, and sedation may be ordered. A sausage-shaped mass can often be felt through the abdominal wall.

Treatment and Nursing Care

Unlike pyloric stenosis, this condition is an emergency in the sense that prolonged delay is dangerous. The telescoped bowel rapidly becomes gangrenous, thus markedly reducing the possibility of a simple reduction. Adequate treatment during the first 12 to 24 hours should have a good outcome with complete recovery. The outcome becomes more uncertain as the bowel deteriorates, making resection necessary.

Immediate treatment consists of IV fluids, NPO status, and a diagnostic barium enema. The barium enema can often reduce the invagination simply by the pressure of the barium fluid pushing against the telescoped portion. The barium enema should not be done if signs of bowel perforation or peritonitis are evident. Abdominal surgery is performed if the barium enema does not correct the problem. Surgery may consist of manual reduction of the invagination, resection with anastomosis, or possible colostomy if the intestine is gangrenous.

If the invagination was reduced, the infant is returned to normal feedings within 24 hours and discharged in about 48 hours. Carefully observe for recurrence during this period. If surgery is necessary, many of the same preoperative and postoperative nursing diagnoses used for congenital aganglionic megacolon also can be used when surgery is required for this condition.

Test Yourself

- How is celiac disease diagnosed and treated?

- Explain what happens in the gastrointestinal tract of the child who has Hirschsprung disease.

- Explain the cause of intussusception and describe the symptoms seen in the child with the diagnosis.

GASTROESOPHAGEAL REFLUX

Gastroesophageal reflux (GER) occurs when the sphincter in the lower portion of the esophagus, which leads into the stomach, is relaxed and allows gastric contents to be regurgitated back into the esophagus. GER is usually noted within the 1st week of the infant's life and is resolved within the first 18 months. The condition may correct itself as the esophageal sphincter matures, the child eats solid foods, and the child is more often in a sitting or standing position. Premature infants and children with neurologic conditions frequently have diagnoses of GER.

Clinical Manifestations

Almost immediately after feeding, the child vomits the contents of the stomach. The vomiting is effortless, not projectile in nature. The child with GER is irritable and hungry. Aspiration after vomiting may lead to respiratory concerns, such as apnea and pneumonia. Although the child may take in adequate nutrition, because of the vomiting, failure to thrive and lack of normal weight gain occurs.

Diagnosis and Treatment

A complete history will offer information regarding feeding, vomiting, and weight patterns. An endoscopy will confirm the relaxed esophageal sphincter. Correcting the nutritional status of the child includes giving formula thickened with rice cereal, placing the child in an upright position during and after feeding, and nasogastric or gastrostomy feedings if necessary. A histamine-2 (H2) receptor antagonist such as ranitidine (Zantac) may be given to reduce the acid secretion, lessening the complications gastric acid may have on the esophageal tissue. Other medications such as omeprazole (Prilosec) may also be given to reduce the gastric acid. In severe cases, a surgical procedure known as Nissen fundoplication may be done to create a valve-like structure to prevent the regurgitation of stomach contents.

Nursing Care

Feedings thickened with rice cereal decrease the likelihood of aspiration in the child with GER. Any signs of respiratory distress are immediately reported. The child is offered small, frequent feedings; burped frequently; and kept upright during and after feeding. In the past, an infant car seat was used to keep the child positioned after feedings, but studies now suggest keeping the child in a prone position with the head elevated. Intake and output, daily weight, and observing emesis for amount and character are monitored and documented. If a nasogastric or gastrostomy tube is inserted, good skin care will help to maintain skin integrity. Teaching the family caregivers regarding feeding, positioning, and medication administration and working with them to decrease their anxiety is an important role of the nurse.

The prone positioning of the child with GER is an exception to the recommendation that children be placed in the supine position for sleeping. This may create concern for the family caregiver, and explanations need to be offered.

DIARRHEA AND GASTROENTERITIS

Diarrhea in children is a fairly common symptom of a variety of conditions. It may be mild, accompanied by slight dehydration, or it may be extremely severe, requiring prompt and effective treatment. Simple diarrhea that does not respond to treatment can quickly turn into severe, life-threatening diarrhea.

Chronically malnourished children with diarrheal symptoms are a common problem in many areas of the world. This condition is prevalent in areas where adequate clean water and sanitary facilities are lacking. Certain metabolic diseases, such as cystic fibrosis, have diarrhea as a symptom. Diarrhea also may be caused by antibiotic therapy.

Some conditions that cause diarrhea require readjustment of the child's diet. Allergic reactions to food are not uncommon and can be controlled by avoiding the offending food.

Adjusting the child's diet, adding less sugar to formula, or reducing bulk or fat in the diet may be necessary.

Did you know? Overfeeding as well as underfeeding or an unbalanced diet may be the cause of diarrhea in a child.

Many diarrheal disturbances in children are caused by contaminated food or human or animal fecal waste through the oral-fecal route. Infectious diarrhea is commonly referred to as **gastroenteritis**. The infectious organisms may be salmonella, *Escherichia coli*, dysentery bacilli, and various viruses, most notably rotaviruses. It is difficult to determine the causative factor in many instances. Because of the seriousness of infectious diarrhea in children and the danger of spreading diarrhea, the child with moderate or severe diarrhea is often isolated until the causative factor has been proved to be noninfectious.

Clinical Manifestations

Mild diarrhea may present as little more than loose stools; the frequency of defecation may be 2 to 12 per day. The child may be irritable and have a loss of

Watch closely. A child with diarrhea can rapidly become severely dehydrated and gravely ill.

appetite. Vomiting and gastric distention are not significant factors, and dehydration is minimal.

Mild or moderate diarrhea can rather quickly become severe diarrhea in a child. Vomiting usually accompanies the diarrhea; together, they cause large losses of body water and electrolytes.

The skin becomes extremely dry and loses its turgor. The fontanelle becomes sunken, and the pulse is weak and rapid. The stools become greenish liquid and may be tinged with blood.

Diagnosis

Stool specimens may be collected for culture and sensitivity testing to determine the causative infectious organism, if there is one. Subsequently, effective antibiotics can be prescribed as indicated.

Treatment

Treatment to stop the diarrhea must be initiated immediately. Establishing normal fluid and electrolyte balance is the primary concern in treating gastroenteritis. The child with acute dehydration may be given oral feedings of commercial electrolyte solutions, such as Pedialyte, Rehydralyte, and Infalyte unless there is shock or severe dehydration. This treatment is called oral rehydration therapy. As the diarrhea clears, food may be offered. Once commonly used, the BRAT diet (ripe banana, rice cereal, applesauce, and toast) has become somewhat controversial because it is high in calories, low in energy and protein, and does not provide adequate nutrition. Salty broths should be avoided. Infants can return to breast-feeding if they have been NPO; formula-fed infants are given their formula. Foods can be added as the child's condition improves, returning to a regular diet. Early return to the usual diet has been shown to reduce the number of stools and to decrease weight loss and the length of the illness.

In severe diarrhea with shock and severe dehydration, oral feedings are discontinued completely. Fluids to be given IV must be carefully calculated to replace the lost electrolytes. Frequent laboratory determinations of the child's blood chemistries are necessary to guide the physician in this replacement therapy. For the child who has had a serious bout of diarrhea, the care provider may prescribe soybean formula for a few weeks to avoid a possible reaction to milk proteins.

CULTURAL SNAPSHOT

Diarrhea, constipation, and vomiting are symptoms that may be embarrassing to the child and family. In some cultures the embarrassment of discussing these symptoms may lead to attempts to control or manage the symptom by using home remedies. Sometimes serious concerns may be missed or ignored. Exploration of these symptoms with the family caregiver and child during the interview and ongoing assessment process is necessary.

● Nursing Process for the Child With Diarrhea and Gastroenteritis

ASSESSMENT

In addition to basic information about the child, the interview with the family caregiver must include specific information about the history of bowel patterns and the onset of diarrheal stools, with details on number and type of stools per day. Suggest terms to describe the color and odor of stools to assist the caregiver with descriptions. Inquire about recent feeding patterns, nausea, and vomiting. Ask the caregiver about fever and other signs of illness in the child and signs of illness in any other family members.

The physical exam of the child includes observation of skin turgor and condition, including excoriated diaper area, temperature, anterior fontanelle (depressed, normal, or bulging), apical pulse rate (observing for weak pulse), stools (character, frequency, amount, color and presence of blood), irritability, lethargy, vomiting, urine (amount and concentration), lips and mucous membranes of the mouth (dry, cracked), eyes (bright, glassy, sunken, dark circles), and any other notable physical signs.

SELECTED NURSING DIAGNOSES

A primary nursing diagnosis is "Diarrhea related to (whatever the cause is)." Other nursing diagnoses vary with the intensity of the diarrhea (mild or severe) as determined by the physical exam and caregiver interview and may include the following:

- Risk for Infection related to inadequate secondary defenses or insufficient knowledge to avoid exposure to pathogens

- Impaired Skin Integrity related to constant presence of diarrheal stools
- Deficient Fluid Volume related to diarrheal stools
- Imbalanced Nutrition: Less Than Body Requirements related to malabsorption of nutrients
- Hyperthermia related to dehydration
- Risk for Delayed Development related to decreased sucking when infant is NPO
- Compromised Family Coping related to the seriousness of the child's illness
- Deficient Knowledge of caregivers related to understanding of treatment for diarrhea

OUTCOME IDENTIFICATION AND PLANNING

The major goal for the ill child is to control and stop the diarrhea while minimizing the risk for infection transmission. Other important goals for the ill child include maintaining good skin condition, improving hydration and nutritional intake, and satisfying sucking needs in the infant. A major goal for the family with a child who has diarrhea or gastroenteritis is eliminating the risk of infection transmission. The family should also be supported and educated regarding the disease and treatment for the child. Plan individualized nursing care according to these goals.

IMPLEMENTATION

Controlling Diarrhea and Reducing the Risk of Infection Transmission

Measures to control and stop the diarrhea are instituted as ordered. To prevent the spread of possibly infectious organisms to other pediatric patients, follow standard precautions issued by the Centers for Disease Control. All caregivers must wear gowns, and measures to control and stop the diarrhea are instituted. Gloves are used when handling articles contaminated with feces, but masks are unnecessary. Place contaminated linens and clothing in specially marked containers to be processed according to the policy of the health care facility. Place disposable diapers and other disposable items in specially marked bags and dispose of them according to policy. Visitors are limited to family only.

Teach the family caregivers the principles of aseptic technique and observe them to ensure understanding and compliance. Good handwashing must be carried out and also taught to the family caregivers. Stress that gloves are needed for added protection, but careful handwashing is also necessary.

Promoting Skin Integrity

To reduce irritation and excoriation of the buttocks and genital area, cleanse those areas frequently and apply a soothing protective preparation such as lanolin or A and D Ointment. Change diapers as quickly as possible after soiling. Some infants may be sensitive to disposable diapers, and others may be sensitive to cloth diapers, so it may be necessary to try both types. Leaving the diaper off and exposing the buttocks and genital area to the air is often helpful. Placing disposable pads under the infant can facilitate easy and frequent changing. Teach caregivers that waterproof diaper covers hold moisture in and do not allow air circulation, which increases irritation and excoriation of the diaper area.

Preventing Dehydration

A child can dehydrate quickly and can get into serious trouble after less than 3 days of diarrhea. Carefully count diapers and weigh them to determine the infant's output accurately. Measure each voiding in the older child. Closely observe all stools. Document the number and character of the stools, as well as the amount and character of any vomitus.

Maintaining Adequate Nutrition

Weigh the child daily on the same scale. Take measurements in the early morning before the morning feeding if the child is on oral feedings. Maintain precautions to prevent contamination of equipment while the child is weighed. Monitor intake and output strictly.

In severe dehydration, IV fluids are given to rest the GI tract, restore hydration, and maintain nutritional requirements. Monitor the placement, patency, and site of the IV infusion at least every 2 hours. The use of restraints, with relevant nursing interventions, may be necessary. Good mouth care is essential while the child is NPO.

When oral fluids are started, the child is given oral replacement solutions, such as those listed earlier. After the infant tolerates these solutions, half-strength formula may be introduced. After the infant tolerates this formula for several days, full-strength formula is given (possibly lactose-free or soy formula to avoid disaccharide intolerance or reaction to milk proteins). The breast-fed infant can continue breastfeeding. Give the mother of a breast-fed infant access to a breast pump if her infant is NPO. Breast milk may be frozen for later use, if desired. The infant who is NPO needs to have his or her sucking needs fulfilled. To accomplish this, offer the infant a pacifier.

Maintaining Body Temperature

Monitor vital signs at least every 2 hours if there is fever. Do not take the temperature rectally because insertion of a thermometer into the rectum can cause stimulation of stools, as well as trauma and tissue injury to sensitive mucosa. Follow the appropriate procedures for fever reduction, and administer antipyretics and antibiotics as prescribed. Take the temperature with a thermometer that is used only for that child.

Supporting Family Coping

Being the family caregiver of a child who has become so ill in such a short time is frightening. Meeting the child's emotional needs is difficult but very important. Suggest to the caregiver ways that the child might be consoled without interfering with care. Soothing, gentle stroking of the head, and speaking softly help the child bear the frustrations of the illness and its treatment. The child can be picked up and rocked, as long as this can be done without jeopardizing the IV infusion site. Threading a needle into the small veins of a dehydrated child is difficult, and replacement may be nearly impossible. The child's life may depend on receiving the proper parenteral fluids. Help fulfill the child's emotional needs, and encourage the family caregiver to have some time away from the child's room without feeling guilty about leaving.

Promoting Family Teaching

Explain to the family caregivers the importance of GI rest for the child. The family caregivers (especially if young or poorly educated) may not understand the necessity for NPO status. Cooperation of the caregiver is improved with increased understanding. See Family Teaching Tips: Diarrhea and Family Teaching Tips: Vomiting.

EVALUATION: GOALS AND EXPECTED OUTCOMES

- **Goal:** The child's bowel elimination will return to pre-illness level.
  Expected Outcomes: The child passes stool with decreasing frequency; stool is soft; consistency is appropriate for age.
- **Goal:** The family caregivers will follow infection control measures.
  Expected Outcomes: The family caregivers verbalize standard precautions for infection control and follow those measures.
- **Goal:** The child's skin integrity will be maintained.
  Expected Outcomes: The infant's diaper area shows no evidence of redness or excoriation.

FAMILY TEACHING TIPS

Diarrhea

The danger in diarrhea is dehydration (drying out). If the child becomes dehydrated, he or she can become very sick. Increasing the amount of liquid the child drinks is helpful. Solid foods may need to be decreased so the child will drink more.

SUGGESTIONS

- Give liquids in small amounts (3 or 4 tbsp) about every half hour. If this goes well, increase the amount a little each half hour. Don't force the child to drink, because he or she may vomit.
- Give solid foods in small amounts. Do not give milk for a day or two, because this can make diarrhea worse.
- Give only nonsalty soups or broths.
- Liquids recommended for vomiting also may be given for diarrhea.
- Soft foods to give in small amounts: applesauce, fine chopped or scraped apple without peel, bananas, toast, rice cereal, plain unsalted crackers or cookies, any meats.

CALL THE CARE PROVIDER IF

- Child develops sudden high fever.
- Stomach pain becomes severe.
- Diarrhea becomes bloody (more than a streak of blood).
- Diarrhea becomes more frequent or severe.
- Child becomes dehydrated (dried out).

SIGNS OF DEHYDRATION

- Child has not urinated for 6 hours or more.
- Child has no tears when crying.
- Child's mouth is dry or sticky to touch.
- Child's eyes are sunken.
- Child is less active than usual.
- Child has dark circles under eyes.

WARNING

Do not use medicines to stop diarrhea for children younger than 6 years of age unless specifically directed by the physician. These medicines can be dangerous if not used properly.

DIAPER AREA SKIN CARE

- Change diaper as soon as it is soiled.
- Wash area with mild soap, rinse, and dry well.
- Use soothing, protective lotion recommended by your physician or hospital.
- Do not use waterproof diapers or diaper covers; they increase diaper area irritation.
- Wash hands with soap and water after changing diapers or wiping the child.

FAMILY TEACHING TIPS

Vomiting

Vomiting will usually stop in a couple days and can be treated at home as long as the child is getting some fluids.

WARNING

Some medications used to stop vomiting in older children or adults are dangerous in infants or young children. DO NOT use any medicine unless your physician has told you to use it for this child.
    Give child clear liquids to drink in small amounts.

SUGGESTIONS

- Pedialyte, Lytren, Rehydralyte, Infalyte
- Flat soda (no fizz). Use caffeine-free type; do not use diet soda.
- Jell–O water—double the amount of water, let stand to room temperature.
- Ice popsicles
- Gatorade
- Tea
- Solid Jell-O
- Broth (not salty)

HOW TO GIVE

Give small amounts often. One tbsp every 20 minutes for the first few hours is a good rule of thumb. If this is kept down without vomiting, increase to 2 tbsp every 20 minutes for the next couple of hours. If there is no vomiting, increase the amount the child may have. If the child vomits, wait for 1 hour before offering more liquids.

The older child's skin is clean and dry with no redness or irritation.
- **Goal:** The child will be well hydrated.
  Expected Outcomes: The child's intake is sufficient to produce hourly urine output of 2 to 3 mL/kg; skin turgor is good; mucous membranes are moist and pink; and fontanelles in the infant exhibit normal tension.
- **Goal:** The child will consume adequate caloric intake.
  Expected Outcomes: The child consumes an age-appropriate amount of full-strength formula, breast milk, or other fluids 3 days after therapy with oral replacement solution.
- **Goal:** The infant will satisfy nonnutritive sucking needs.
  Expected Outcomes: The infant uses a pacifier to satisfy sucking needs.
- **Goal:** The child will maintain a temperature within normal limits.

Expected Outcomes: The child's temperature is 98.6°F to 100°F (37°C to 37.8°C).
- **Goal:** The family caregivers' anxiety will be reduced.
  Expected Outcomes: The family caregivers participate in the care and soothing of the child.
- **Goal:** The family caregivers will verbalize an understanding of the child's treatment.
  Expected Outcomes: The family caregivers describe three methods to increase hydration and list the warning signs of dehydration.

Test Yourself

- What is the major concern in the child who has diarrhea and vomiting?
- How is the child with diarrhea treated? What is this treatment called?
- What do the health care providers do when caring for a child with diarrhea to prevent the spread of infection from one child to another?

COLIC

Colic consists of recurrent paroxysmal bouts of abdominal pain and is fairly common in young infants. Although many theories have been proposed, none has been accepted as the causative factor.

Clinical Manifestations and Diagnosis

Attacks occur suddenly, usually late in the day or evening. The infant cries loudly and continuously. The infant appears to be in considerable pain but otherwise seems healthy, breastfeeds or takes formula well, and gains weight as expected. The baby may be momentarily soothed only by rocking or holding but eventually falls asleep, exhausted from crying. The infant with colic is often considered a "difficult" baby.

A little sensitivity is in order. Colic often disappears around the age of 3 months, but this is small comfort to the caregiver vainly trying to soothe a colicky infant.

Differential diagnosis should be made to rule out an allergic reaction to milk or certain foods. Changing to a nonallergenic formula helps determine if there is an allergic factor or if the infant has lactose intolerance. If the baby is breast-fed, the mother's diet should be studied to determine if anything she is eating might be affecting the baby. Intestinal obstruction or infection also must be ruled out.

Treatment and Nursing Care

No single treatment is consistently successful. A number of measures may be employed, one or more of which might work. Medications such as sedatives, antispasmodics, and antiflatulents are sometimes prescribed, but their effectiveness is inconsistent. The family must remember that the condition will pass, even though at the time it seems it will last forever. Family caregivers need to be reassured that their parenting skills are not inadequate. The nurse can support the family and promote coping skills by providing family teaching. See Family Teaching Tips: Colic.

APPENDICITIS

Appendicitis refers to an inflammation of the appendix. The appendix is a blind pouch located in the cecum near the ileocecal junction. Obstruction of the lumen of the appendix is the primary cause of appendicitis. The obstruction usually is caused by hardened

---

FAMILY TEACHING TIPS

Colic

- Pick up and rock the baby in a rocker or, with baby's tummy down across your knees, swing your legs side to side. (Be sure baby's head is supported.)
- Walk around the room while rocking baby in your arms or in a front carrier. Hum or sing to baby.
- Try a bottle, but don't overfeed. Give a pacifier if baby has eaten well within 2 hours.
- Baby may like the rhythmic movements of a baby swing.
- Try taking baby outside or for a car ride.
- When feeding baby, try methods to decrease gas formation: frequent burping, giving smaller feedings more frequently; position baby in infant seat after eating.
- Try doing something to entertain but not overexcite baby.
- Gently rub baby's abdomen if it is rigid.
- Sit with baby resting on your lap with legs toward you; gently move baby's legs in pumping motion.
- Try putting baby down to sleep in a darkened room.
- Keep remembering that it's temporary. Try to stay as calm and relaxed as possible.

---

fecal matter or a foreign body. This obstruction causes circulation to be slowed or interrupted, resulting in pain and necrosis of the appendix. The necrotic area can rupture, causing escape of fecal matter and bacteria into the peritoneal cavity and resulting in the complication of peritonitis. Most cases of appendicitis in childhood occur in the school-age child.

Clinical Manifestations

In young children, the symptoms may be difficult to evaluate. Symptoms in the older child may be the same as in an adult: pain and tenderness in the right lower quadrant of the abdomen, nausea and vomiting, fever, and constipation. However, these symptoms are uncommon in young children; many children already have a ruptured appendix when first seen by the physician. The young child has difficulty localizing the pain, may act restless and irritable, and may have a slight fever, a flushed face, and a rapid pulse. Usually the white blood cell count is slightly elevated. It may take several hours to rule out other conditions and make a positive diagnosis.

Do you know the why of it?
When appendicitis is suspected, laxatives and enemas are contraindicated because they increase peristalsis, which increases the possibility of rupturing an inflamed appendix.

Treatment

Surgical removal of the appendix is necessary and should be performed as soon as possible after diagnosis. If the appendix has not ruptured before surgery, the operative risk is nearly negligible. Even after perforation has occurred, the mortality rate is less than 1%.

Food and fluids by mouth are withheld before surgery. If the child is dehydrated, IV fluids are ordered. If fever is present, the temperature should be reduced to below 102°F (38.9°C).

Recovery is rapid and usually uneventful. The child is ambulated early and can leave the hospital a few days after surgery. If peritonitis or a localized abscess occurs, gastric suction, parenteral fluids, and antibiotics may be ordered.

● Nursing Process for the Child With Appendicitis

ASSESSMENT

When a child is admitted with a diagnosis of possible appendicitis, an emergency situation exists. The family caregiver who brings the child to the hospital often is upset and anxious. The admission exam and assessment must be performed quickly and skillfully. Obtain information about the child's condition for the last several days to formulate a picture of how the condition has developed. Emphasize GI complaints, appetite, bowel movements for the last few days, and general activity level. During the physical exam, include vital signs, especially noting any elevation of temperature, presence of bowel sounds, abdominal guarding, and nausea or vomiting. Report immediately diminished or absent bowel sounds. Provide the child and caregiver with careful explanations about all procedures to be performed. Use special empathy and understanding to alleviate the child's and family's anxieties.

SELECTED NURSING DIAGNOSES

- Fear of child and family caregiver related to emergency surgery
- Acute Pain related to necrosis of appendix and surgical procedure
- Risk for Deficient Fluid Volume related to decreased intake
- Deficient Knowledge of caregiver related to postoperative and home care needs

OUTCOME IDENTIFICATION AND PLANNING

Because of the urgent nature of the child's admission and preparation for surgery, great efforts must be taken to provide calm, reassuring care to both the child and the caregivers. A major goal for both the child and the caregivers is relieving fear. Additional goals for the child are relieving pain and maintaining fluid balance. Another goal for the family is increasing knowledge of the postoperative and home care needs of the child.

IMPLEMENTATION

Reducing Fear

Although procedures must be performed quickly, consider both the child's and the family's fear. The child may be extremely frightened by the sudden change of events and also may be in considerable pain. The family caregiver may be apprehensive about impending surgery. Introduce various health care team members by name and title as they come into the child's room to perform procedures. Explain to the child and the family what is happening and why. Explain the postanesthesia care unit (recovery room) to the child and the family. Encourage the family and child to verbalize fears and try to allay these

fears as much as possible. Let family members know where to wait during surgery, how long the surgery will last, where dining facilities are located, and where the surgeon will expect to find them after surgery. If possible, demonstrate deep breathing, coughing, and abdominal splinting to the child and have her or him practice it. Throughout the preoperative care, be sensitive to verbalized or nonverbalized fears and provide understanding care.

Promoting Comfort

Analgesics are not given before surgery because they may conceal signs of tenderness that are important for diagnosis. Provide comfort through positioning and gentle care while performing preoperative procedures. Heat to the abdomen is contraindicated because of the danger of rupture of the appendix. After surgery, observe the child hourly for indications of pain and administer analgesics as ordered. Provide quiet activities to help divert the child's attention from the pain. The child may fear postoperative ambulation because of pain. Many children (and adults, too) are worried that the stitches will pull out. Reassure the child that this worry is understood but that the sutures (or staples) are intended to withstand the strain of walking and moving. Activity is essential to the child's recovery but should be as pain free as possible. Help the child understand that as activity increases, the pain will decrease. The child whose appendix ruptured before surgery may also have pain related to the nasogastric tube, abdominal distention, or constipation.

Monitoring Fluid Balance

Dehydration can be a concern, especially if the child has had preoperative nausea and vomiting. On admission to the hospital, the child is maintained NPO until after surgery. Accurately measure and record intake and output. IV fluids are administered as ordered. After surgery, check dressings to detect evidence of excessive drainage or bleeding that indicate loss of fluids. Clear oral fluids are usually ordered soon after surgery. After the child takes and retains fluids successfully, a progressive diet is ordered. Monitor, record, and report bowel sounds at least every 4 hours because the physician may use this as a gauge to determine when the child can have solid food.

Providing Family Teaching

The child who has had an uncomplicated appendectomy usually convalesces quickly and can return to school within 1 or 2 weeks. Teach the caregiver to keep the incision clean and dry. Activities are limited according to the physician's recommendations. The child whose appendix ruptured may be hospitalized for as long as a week and is more limited in activities after surgery. Instruct the family to observe for signs and symptoms of postoperative complications, including fever, abdominal distention, and pain. Emphasize the need for making and keeping follow-up appointments.

EVALUATION: GOALS AND EXPECTED OUTCOMES

- **Goal:** The child and family caregivers will have reduced or alleviated fear.
  Expected Outcomes: The child and family verbalize fears and ask questions before surgery; the child cooperates with health care personnel.
- **Goal:** The child's pain will be controlled.
  Expected Outcomes: The child's pain is at an acceptable level, as evidenced by the child's verbalization of pain according to a pain scale.
- **Goal:** The child will have adequate fluid intake.
  Expected Outcomes: The child's skin turgor is good, vital signs are within normal limits, and hourly urine output is at least 30 to 40 mL.
- **Goal:** The family caregivers will verbalize an understanding of postoperative and home care needs of the child.
  Expected Outcomes: The family caregivers discuss recovery expectations, demonstrate wound care as needed, and list signs and symptoms to report.

MALNUTRITION AND NUTRITIONAL PROBLEMS

The World Health Organization has widely publicized the malnutrition and hunger that affect more than half the world's population. In the United States, malnutrition contributes to the high death rate of the children of migrant workers and Native Americans. Malnourished children grow at a slower rate, have a higher rate of illness and infection, and have more difficulty concentrating and achieving in school. Appendix D lists foods that are good sources of the nutrients that a child needs for healthy growth.

Protein Malnutrition

Protein malnutrition results from an insufficient intake of high-quality protein or from conditions in which protein absorption is impaired or a loss of protein increases.

Clinical evidence of protein malnutrition may not be apparent until the condition is well advanced.

Kwashiorkor

Kwashiorkor results from severe deficiency of protein with an adequate caloric intake. It accounts for most of the malnutrition in the world's children today. The highest incidence is in children 4 months to 5 years of age. The affected child develops a swollen abdomen, edema, and GI changes; the hair is thin and dry with patchy alopecia; and the child becomes apathetic and irritable and has retarded growth with muscle wasting. In untreated patients, mortality rates are 30% or higher. Although strenuous efforts are being made around the world to prevent this condition, its causes are complex.

Did you know? The term kwashiorkor means "the sickness the older baby gets when the new baby comes."

Traditionally these babies have been breast-fed until the age of 2 or 3 years. The child is weaned abruptly when the next child in the family is born.

The older child is then given the regular family diet, which consists mostly of starchy foods with little meat or vegetable protein. Cow's milk generally is unavailable; in many places where goats are kept, their milk is not considered fit for human consumption (Fig. 37-6).

Marasmus

Marasmus is a deficiency in calories as well as protein. The child with marasmus is seriously ill. The condition is common in children in Third World countries

● ***Figure 37.6*** A child with kwashiorkor often has been abruptly weaned and may have a distended abdomen and muscle wasting.

because of severe drought conditions. Not enough food is available to supply everyone in these countries, and the children are not fed until adults are fed. The child is severely malnourished and highly susceptible to disease. This syndrome may be seen in the child with nonorganic failure to thrive (NFTT).

Vitamin Deficiency Diseases

Vitamin D Deficiency

Rickets, a disease affecting the growth and calcification of bones, is caused by a lack of vitamin D. The absorption of calcium and phosphorus is diminished because of the lack of vitamin D, which is needed to regulate the use of these minerals. Early manifestations include **craniotabes** (softening of the occipital bones) and delayed closure of the fontanelles. There is delayed dentition, with defects in tooth enamel and a tendency to develop caries. As the disease advances, thoracic deformities, softening of the shafts of long bones, and spinal and pelvic bone deformities develop. The muscles are poorly developed and lacking in tone, so standing and walking are delayed. Deformities occur during periods of rapid growth. Although rickets itself is not a fatal disease, complications such as tetany, pneumonia, and enteritis are more likely to cause death in children with rickets than in healthy children.

Infants and children require an estimated 400 U of vitamin D daily to prevent rickets. Because a child living in a temperate climate may not receive sufficient exposure to ultraviolet light, vitamin D is administered orally in the form of fish liver oil or synthetic vitamin. Whole milk and evaporated milk fortified with 400 U of vitamin D per quart are available throughout the United States. Breast-fed infants should receive vitamin D supplements, especially if the mother's intake of vitamin D is poor.

Vitamin C Deficiency

Scurvy is caused by inadequate dietary intake of vitamin C (ascorbic acid). Early inclusion of vitamin C in the diet, in the form of orange or tomato juice or a vitamin preparation, prevents the development of this disease. Febrile diseases seem to increase the need for vitamin C. A variety of fresh vegetables and fruits supply vitamin C for the older infant and child. Because much of the vitamin C content is destroyed by boiling or by exposure to air for long periods, the family caregivers should be taught to cook vegetables with minimal water in a covered pot and to store juices in a tightly covered opaque container. Vegetables cooked in a microwave oven retain more vitamin C because little water is added in the cooking process.

Early clinical manifestations of scurvy are irritability, loss of appetite, and digestive disturbances. A general tenderness in the legs severe enough to cause a

pseudoparalysis develops. The child is apprehensive about being handled and assumes a frog position, with the hips and knees semiflexed and the feet rotated outward. The gums become red and swollen, and hemorrhage occurs in various tissues. Characteristic hemorrhages in the long bones are subperiosteal, especially at the ends of the femur and tibia.

Recovery is rapid with adequate treatment, but death may occur from malnutrition or exhaustion in untreated cases. Treatment consists of therapeutic daily doses of ascorbic acid.

Thiamine Deficiency

Thiamine is one of the major components of the vitamin B complex. Children whose diets are deficient in thiamine exhibit irritability, listlessness, loss of appetite, and vomiting. A severe lack of thiamine in the diet causes beriberi, a disease characterized by cardiac and neurologic symptoms. Beriberi does not occur when balanced diets that include whole grains are eaten.

Riboflavin Deficiency

Riboflavin deficiency usually occurs in association with thiamine and niacin deficiencies. It is mainly manifested by skin lesions. The primary source of riboflavin is milk. Riboflavin is destroyed by ultraviolet light; thus, opaque milk cartons are best for storage. Whole grains are also a good source of riboflavin.

Niacin Insufficiency

Niacin insufficiency in the diet causes a disease known as pellagra, which presents with GI and neurologic symptoms. Pellagra does not occur in children who ingest adequate whole milk or who eat a well-balanced diet.

Mineral Insufficiencies

Iron deficiency results in anemia. This condition is the most common cause of nutritional deficiency in children older than 4 to 6 months of age whose diets lack iron-rich foods. Anemia is often found in poor children younger than 6 years of age in the United States. Iron deficiency anemia is discussed more fully in Chapter 36.

Calcium is necessary for bone and tooth formation and is also needed for proper nerve and muscle function. Hypocalcemia (insufficient calcium) causes neurologic damage, including mental retardation. Rich sources of calcium include milk and milk products. Children with milk allergies are at an increased risk for hypocalcemia.

Food Allergies

The symptoms of food allergies vary from one child to another. Common symptoms are **urticaria** (hives),

pruritus (itching), stomach pains, and respiratory symptoms. Some of the symptoms may appear quickly after the child has eaten the offending food, but other foods may cause a delayed reaction. Thus, the investigation needed to find the cause can be frustrating.

Foods should be introduced to the child one at a time, with an interval of 4 or 5 days between each new food. If any GI or respiratory reaction occurs, the food should be eliminated. Among the foods most likely to cause allergic reactions are milk, eggs, wheat, corn, legumes (including peanuts and soybeans), oranges, strawberries, and chocolate (Table 37-1). If a food has been eliminated because of a suspected allergy or reaction, it can be reintroduced at a later time in small amounts to test again for the child's response. This testing should be done in a carefully controlled manner to avoid serious or life-threatening reactions. Many allergies disappear as the child's GI tract matures.

Milk Allergy

Milk allergy is the most common food allergy in the young child. Symptoms that may indicate an allergy to milk are diarrhea, vomiting, colic, irritability, respiratory symptoms, or eczema. Infants who are breast-fed for the first 6 months or more may avoid developing milk allergies entirely unless a strong family history of allergies exists. Children with severe allergic reactions to milk are given commercial formulas that are soybean or meat-based and formulated to be similar in nutrients to other infant formulas.

Here's a teaching tip for you.
If the child has a severe milk allergy, the caregiver must learn to carefully read the labels on prepared foods to avoid lactose or lactic acid ingredients.

Lactose Intolerance

Children with **lactose intolerance** cannot digest **lactose**, the primary carbohydrate in milk, because of an inborn deficiency of the enzyme lactase. Congenital lactose intolerance is seen in some children of African-American, Native American, Eskimo, Asian, and Mediterranean heritage. Symptoms include cramping, abdominal distention, flatus, and diarrhea after ingesting milk. Commercially available formulas such as Isomil, Nursoy, Nutramigen, and ProSobee are made from soybean, meat-based, or protein mixtures and contain no lactose. The child needs supplemental vitamin D. Yogurt is tolerated by these children.

● Nursing Process for the Child With Nutritional Problems

ASSESSMENT

Carefully interview the family caregiver to determine the underlying cause. If the difficulty lies in the caregiver's inability to give proper care, try to determine if this can be attributed to lack of information, financial problems, indifference, or other reasons. Do not make assumptions until the interview is completed. Cases of malnutrition have been reported in children of families who believed it was better for their child to eat vegetables only; this severely limits fat intake, which the child needs. If food allergies are suspected as the cause of malnourishment, include a careful history of food intake. Obtain a history of stools and voiding from the caregiver.

The physical exam of the child includes observing skin turgor and skin condition, the anterior fontanelle, signs of emaciation, weight,

TABLE 37.1	Some Foods That May Cause Allergies and Possible Sources
Food	Sources
Milk	Yogurt, cheese, ice cream, puddings, butter, hot dogs, foods made with nonfat dry milk, lunch meat, chocolate candies
Eggs	Baked goods, ice cream, puddings, meringues, candies, mayonnaise, salad dressings, custards
Wheat	Breads, baked goods, hot dogs, lunch meats, cereals, cream soups. Oat, rye, and cornmeal products may have wheat added.
Corn	Products made with cornstarch, corn syrup, or vegetable starch; many children's juices, popcorn, cornbreads or muffins, tortillas
Legumes	Soybean products, peanut butter and peanut products
Citrus fruits	Oranges, lemons, limes, grapefruit, gelatins, children's juices, some pediatric suspensions (medications)
Strawberries	Gelatins, some pediatric suspensions
Chocolate	Cocoa, candies, chocolate drinks or desserts, colas

temperature, apical pulse, respirations, responsiveness, listlessness, and irritability.

SELECTED NURSING DIAGNOSES

- Imbalanced Nutrition: Less Than Body Requirements related to inadequate intake of nutrients secondary to poor sucking ability, lack of interest in food, lack of adequate food sources, or lack of knowledge of caregiver
- Deficient Fluid Volume related to insufficient fluid intake
- Constipation related to insufficient fluid intake
- Impaired Skin Integrity related to malnourishment
- Deficient Knowledge of caregivers related to understanding of the child's nutritional requirements

OUTCOME IDENTIFICATION AND PLANNING

The major goals for the nutritionally deprived child focus on increasing nutritional intake, improving hydration, monitoring elimination, and maintaining skin integrity. Other goals concentrate on improving caregiver knowledge and understanding of nutrition and facilitating the infant's ability to suck. Even with focused and individualized goals, developing a plan of care for the malnourished child may be challenging. It may be necessary to try a variety of tactics to feed the child successfully. Include the family caregiver in the plan of care because this is in the best interest of both the child and the caregiver.

IMPLEMENTATION

Promoting Adequate Nutrition
One primary nursing care problem may be persuading the child to take more nourishment than he or she wants. Inexperienced nurses may find it difficult to persuade an uninterested child to take formula or food, and this can become frustrating. Perhaps the nurse's insecurity and uncertainty communicate themselves to the child in the way he or she handles the child. An experienced nurse may succeed in feeding an infant 3 or 4 oz in a short period, whereas the inexperienced nurse who seems to be going through the same motions persuades the child to take only 1 oz or less. As the nurse and the child become accustomed to each other, however, they both relax, and feeding becomes easier. In addition to having a lack of interest, the child often is weak and debilitated with little strength to suck.

The baby who is held snugly, wrapped closely, and rocked gently finds it easier to relax and take in a little more feeding. An impatient, hurried attitude nearly always communicates tension to the child. Ask for help if the need to attend to other feedings causes tension. Never prop the bottle in the crib.

Gavage feedings or intravenous (IV) fluids may be needed to improve the child's nutritional status, but it is important for the child to develop an interest in food and in the process of sucking. A hard or small-holed nipple may completely discourage the child. The nipple should be soft with holes large enough to allow the formula to drip without pressure. However, it should not be so soft that it offers no resistance and collapses when sucked on. The holes should not be so large that milk pours out, causing the child to choke. This situation can frustrate a weak child, who then no longer attempts to nurse.

Scheduling feedings every 2 or 3 hours is best because most weak babies can handle frequent, small feedings better than feedings every 4 hours. With more frequent feedings, promptness is important. Feedings should be limited to 20 to 30 minutes so that the child does not tire. Demand schedules are not wise because the child has probably lost the power to regulate the supply-and-demand schedule.

Improving Fluid Intake
Improved nutritional status is evidenced by improved hydration, which is noted by monitoring skin turgor, fontanelle tension, and intake and output. Check the fontanelles each shift and weigh the child daily in the early morning. Oral mucous membranes should be moist and pink. Intravenous fluids may be needed initially to build up the child's energy so that he or she can take more oral nourishment and to correct the fluid and electrolyte imbalance. During IV therapy, restraints should be adequate but kept to a minimum. Accurately document intake and output. At least every 2 hours, monitor the IV infusion placement, its patency, and the site for redness and induration. Report any unusual signs immediately.

Monitoring Elimination Patterns
Carefully document intake and output, as well as the character, frequency, and amount of stools. Report any unusual characteristics of the stools or urine at once.

Promoting Skin Integrity
Closely observe the skin condition. Use A and D Ointment or lanolin for dry or reddened skin, and promptly change soiled diapers to prevent skin breakdown in the weakened child.

Providing Family Teaching

If malnutrition is related to economic factors or inadequate caregiver knowledge of the child's needs, teach the family caregivers the essential facts of infant and child nutrition and make referrals for social services. Be alert to the possibility that the caregiver cannot read or understand English, and be certain that the teaching materials used are understood. Simply asking the family caregivers if they have questions is not sufficient to determine if the material has been understood.

Family caregivers may need information regarding assistance in obtaining nutritious food for the child. Infant formulas and baby food can be expensive, and economic factors may be the actual cause of the child's malnutrition. A referral to social services or the Women, Infant, and Children (WIC) program may be appropriate (see Chapter 23).

EVALUATION: GOALS AND EXPECTED OUTCOMES

- **Goal:** The child's nutritional intake will be adequate for normal growth.
  Expected Outcomes: The child gains 0.75 to 1 oz (22 to 30 g) per day if younger than 6 months of age and 0.5 to 0.75 oz (13 to 22 g) per day if older than 6 months of age.
- **Goal:** The child will show interest in feedings.
  Expected Outcomes: The child shows evidence of adequate sucking and the ability to extend the amount of time feeding without showing signs of tiring. The older child eats meals and snacks.
- **Goal:** The child's fluid intake will improve.
  Expected Outcomes: The child's fontanelles are of normal tension, skin turgor is good, and mucous membranes are pink and moist.
- **Goal:** The child's urine and bowel outputs will be normal for age.
  Expected Outcomes: The child's hourly urine output is 2 to 3 mL/kg; stool is soft and of normal character.
- **Goal:** The child's skin will remain intact.
  Expected Outcomes: The child's skin shows no signs of redness or breakdown. The child's skin at the IV infusion site shows no signs of redness or induration.
- **Goal:** The family caregivers will verbalize a beginning knowledge of appropriate nutrition for a growing child.
  Expected Outcomes: The family caregivers state five essential facts about child nutrition.

Test Yourself
- What is the appendix and where is it located?
- Give some examples of vitamin and mineral deficiencies that can cause malnutrition in children.
- What are examples of foods to which children often are allergic?

Intestinal Parasites

A few intestinal parasites are common in the United States, especially in young and school-age children. Hand-to-mouth practices contribute to infestations.

ENTEROBIASIS (PINWORM INFECTION)

The pinworm (Enterobius vermicularis) is a white, threadlike worm that invades the cecum and may enter the appendix. Articles contaminated with pinworm eggs spread pinworms from person to person. The infestation is common in children and occurs when the pinworm eggs are swallowed. The eggs hatch in the intestinal tract and grow to maturity in the cecum. The female worm, when ready to lay her eggs, crawls out of the anus and lays the eggs on the perineum.

Itching around the anus causes the child to scratch and trap new eggs under the fingernails, which often causes reinfection when the child's fingers go into the mouth. Clothing, bedding, food, toilet seats, and other articles become infected, and the infestation spreads to other members of the family. Pinworm eggs also can float in the air and be inhaled.

The life cycle of these worms is 6 to 8 weeks, after which reinfestation commonly occurs without treatment. The incidence is highest in school-age children and next highest in preschoolers. All members of the family are susceptible.

Clinical Manifestations and Diagnosis

Intense perianal itching is the primary symptom of pinworms. Young children who cannot clearly verbalize their feelings may be restless, sleep poorly, or have episodes of bed-wetting.

The usual method of diagnosis is to use cellophane tape to capture the eggs from around the anus and to examine them under a microscope. Adult worms also may be seen as they emerge from the anus when the child is lying quietly or sleeping. The cellophane tape test for identifying worms is performed in the early morning, just before or as soon as the child wakens. The test is performed in the following manner:

1. Wind clear cellophane tape around the end of a tongue blade, sticky side outward.
2. Spread the child's buttocks and press the tape against the anus, rolling the tape from side to side.
3. Transfer the tape to a microscope slide and cover with a clean slide to send to the laboratory. If the caregiver does not have slides or a commercially prepared kit, advise the caregiver to place the tongue blade in a plastic bag and bring to the agency.

The tape then is examined microscopically for eggs in the laboratory.

Treatment and Nursing Care

Treatment consists of the use of an **anthelmintic** (or vermifugal, a medication that expels intestinal worms). Mebendazole (Vermox) is the most commonly used product. The medication should be repeated in 2 or 3 weeks to eliminate any parasites that hatch after the initial treatment. Because pinworms are easily transmitted, the nurse should encourage all family members to be treated.

It is often disturbing to children and caregivers for the child to be found to have pinworms. They may need reassurance from the nurse that pinworm infestation is as common as an infection or a cold. This support is important when caring for a child with any type of intestinal parasite.

As a preventive measure, the nurse should teach the child to wash the hands after bowel movements and before eating. The child should also be encouraged to observe other hygiene measures, such as regular bathing and daily change of underclothing. The nurse must teach caregivers to keep the child's fingernails short and clean. Caregivers also need to know that bedding should be changed frequently to avoid reinfestation. All bedding and clothing, especially underclothing, should be washed in hot water.

ROUNDWORMS

Ascaris lumbricoides is a large intestinal worm found only in humans. Infestation is from the feces of people with infestation. It is usually found in areas where sanitary facilities are lacking and human excreta are deposited on the ground.

The adult worm is pink and 9 to 12 inches long. The eggs hatch in the intestinal tract, and the larvae migrate to the liver and lungs. The larvae reaching the lungs ascend up through the bronchi, are swallowed, and reach the intestine, where they grow to maturity and mate. Eggs are then discharged into the feces. Full development requires about 2 months. In tropical countries where infestation may be heavy, bowel obstructions may present serious problems.

Generally, no symptoms are present in ordinary infestations. Identification is made by means of microscopic examination of feces for eggs. Pyrantel pamoate (Antiminth) is the medication commonly used. Caregivers require education about improved hygiene practices, with sanitary disposal of feces, including diapers as necessary to prevent infestation.

HOOKWORMS

The hookworm lives in the human intestinal tract, where it attaches itself to the wall of the small intestine. Eggs are discharged in the feces of the host. These parasites are prevalent in areas where infected human excreta is deposited on the ground and where the soil, moisture, and temperature are favorable for the development of infective larvae of the worm. In the southeastern United States and tropical West Africa, the prevailing species is Necator americanus.

Clinical Manifestations and Diagnosis

After feces containing eggs are deposited on the ground, larvae hatch. They can survive there as long as 6 weeks and usually penetrate the skin of barefoot people. They produce an itching dermatitis on the feet (ground itch). The larvae pass through the bloodstream to the lungs and into the pharynx, where they are swallowed and reach the small intestine. In the small intestine, they attach themselves to the intestinal wall, where they feed on blood. Heavy infestation may cause anemia through loss of blood. Chronic infestation produces listlessness, fatigue, and malnutrition. Identification is made by examination of the stool under the microscope.

Treatment and Nursing Care

Pyrantel pamoate or mebendazole may be used in the treatment of hookworms. The nurse must stress the need for the affected child to receive a well-balanced diet with additional protein and iron. Transfusions are rarely necessary. To prevent hookworm infestation, the nurse should instruct caregivers to keep children from running barefoot where there is any possibility of ground contamination with feces.

GIARDIASIS

Giardiasis is not caused by a worm but by the protozoan parasite Giardia lamblia. It is a common cause of diarrhea in world travelers and is also prevalent in children who attend day care centers and other types of residential facilities; it may be found in contaminated mountain streams or pools frequented by diapered infants. The child ingests the cyst containing the protozoa. The cyst is activated by stomach acid and passes into the duodenum, where it matures and causes signs and symptoms.

Clinical Manifestations and Treatment

Maturation of the cyst leads to diarrhea, weight loss, and abdominal cramps. Identification and diagnosis are made through examination of stool under the microscope.

Metronidazole (Flagyl) or quinacrine (Atabrine) is effective in treating the infestation.

Nursing Care

The nurse should alert the caregiver that quinacrine causes a yellow discoloration of the skin. To prevent infestations, the nurse should stress to caregivers the importance of careful handling of soiled diapers, especially in a childcare facility. Handwashing, avoiding pools and streams used by diapered infants, and avoiding contact with infected persons are also important.

INGESTION OF TOXIC SUBSTANCES

One way in which toddlers find out about their environment is to taste the world around them. Toddlers and preschoolers are developing autonomy and initiative, which add to their tendency to examine their environment on their own. Because their senses of

Be careful. Young children ingest substances that would repel an adult because of the taste or smell of the substance.

taste and smell are not yet refined, these age groups are prime targets for ingestion of poisonous substances.

The ordinary household has an abundance of poisonous substances in almost every room. The kitchen, bathroom, bedroom, and garage are the most common sites harboring substances that are poisonous when ingested. Although most poisonings occur in the child's home, grandparents' homes offer many temptations to the young child as well. Grandparents tend to be less concerned about placing dangerous substances out of children's reach simply because the children are not part of the household, or the grandparents may place supplies where they are convenient, while never considering the young grandchild's developmental stage and exploratory nature (see Family Teaching Tips: Poison Prevention in the Home).

When a child is found with a container whose contents he or she has obviously sampled, action should be taken immediately. When a child manifests symptoms that are difficult to pinpoint or that do not appear to relate specifically to any known cause, the possibility of poisoning should be suspected. Ingestion of a poisonous substance can produce symptoms that simulate an attack of an acute disease: vomiting, abdominal pain, diarrhea, shock, cyanosis, coma, and convulsions. If evidence of such a disease is lacking, acute poisoning should be suspected.

In instances of apparent poisoning where the substance is unknown, family caregivers are asked to consider all medications in their home. Is it possible that any medication could have been available to the child, or did an older child or other person possibly give the child the container to play with? Is it possible that a parent inadvertently gave a wrong dose or wrong medication to a child? All such possibilities need to be considered. In the meantime, the most important priority is treatment for the child who shows symptoms of poisoning.

The rate of deaths caused by poisoning has dramatically decreased in the recent years (American Academy of Pediatrics [AAP], 2003). Child-resistant closures, safer products, education, public awareness, poison control centers, and antidotes available are factors that have helped to decrease the number of poisoning deaths.

FAMILY TEACHING TIPS

Poison Prevention in the Home

- Keep potential poisons out of sight and out of reach
- Use safety latches or locks on drawers and cabinets
- Replace child-resistant closures immediately after using product
- Never transfer a substance from its original container to an alternate container
- Safely dispose of unused or no-longer-needed medications
- Do not refer to medicines as candy
- Post the Poison Control Center number near each telephone: (800) 222-1222

Adapted from the American Academy of Pediatrics, "Protect Your Child . . . Prevent Poisoning." Retrieved August 28, 2004, from http://www.aap.org/healthtopics/safety.cfm

Emergency Treatment

If the child has collapsed or is not breathing, 911 should be called for emergency help. In cases in which the child is conscious and alert and the caregiver suspects poison ingestion, the Poison Control Center should be called. The universal telephone number in the United States is (800) 222-1222. All homes with young children should have the Poison Control Center number posted by every telephone for quick reference. The caregiver should remove any obvious poison from the child's mouth before calling. The poison control center evaluates the situation and tells the caller whether the child can be treated at home or needs to be transported to a hospital or treatment center.

Except when corrosive or highly irritant poisons have been swallowed, the accepted treatment for many years has been to induce vomiting. The AAP now believes that inducing vomiting has not been shown to prevent poisoning and should no longer be recommended. In addition, the AAP recommends that syrup of ipecac, recommended for many years to be kept in the home in case of poisoning, should no longer be used in the home for treatment of poisoning. The Academy further suggests that because of the potential of misuse, existing ipecac in homes be disposed of safely (AAP, 2003).

In the emergency care setting, gastric lavage may be used to empty the stomach of the toxic substances. Activated charcoal, which absorbs many types of materials, may be used to reduce the dangers of ingested substances. The charcoal is a black, fine powder that is mixed with water. A dose of 5 to 10 g per gram of ingested poison is given by mouth in 6 to 8 ounces of water or may be given through a nasogastric (NG) tube if necessary.

If the substance the child has swallowed is known, the ingredients can be found on the label and the Poison Control Center can suggest an antidote. If the substance is a prescription drug, the pharmacist who filled the prescription or who is familiar with the drug also can be contacted for information. In some instances, it is necessary to analyze the stomach contents.

Specific antidotes are available for certain poisons but not for all. Some antidotes react chemically with the poison to render it harmless, whereas others prevent absorption of the poison.

Treatment Steps in Order of Importance

The treatment steps in order of importance are:

1. Remove the obvious remnants of the poison.
2. Call 911 for emergency help if child has collapsed or stopped breathing.
3. Call the Poison Control Center if child is conscious and alert. The universal poison control number is (800) 222-1222.
4. Follow instructions given by the Poison Control Center.
5. Administer appropriate antidote if recommended.
6. Administer general supportive and symptomatic care.

Further specific treatment is given according to the kind and amount of the toxic substance ingested.

Common types of poisoning and general treatment are described in Table 37-2. Complete listings of poisonous substances with the specific treatment for each are available from the Poison Control Center, clinics, and pharmacies.

LEAD POISONING (PLUMBISM)

Chronic lead poisoning has been a serious problem among children for many years. It is responsible for neurologic handicaps, including mental retardation, because of its effect on the central nervous system. Infants and toddlers are potential victims because of their tendency to put any object within their reach into their mouths. In some children, this habit leads to **pica** (the ingestion of nonfood substances, such as laundry starch, clay, paper, and paint). The unborn fetus of a pregnant mother who is exposed to lead (such as lead dust from renovation of an older home) also can be affected by lead contamination. Screening for lead poisoning is part of a complete well-child checkup between ages 6 months and 6 years.

Sources of Chronic Lead Poisoning

The most common sources of lead poisoning are:

- Lead-containing paint used on the outside or the inside of older houses
- Furniture and toys painted with lead-containing paint; vinyl miniblinds
- Drinking water contaminated by lead pipes or copper pipes with lead-soldered joints
- Dust containing lead salts from lead paint; emission from lead smelters
- Storage of fruit juices or other food in improperly glazed earthenware
- Inhalation of fumes from engines containing lead or from burning batteries
- Exposure to industrial areas with smelteries or chemical plants
- Exposure to hobby materials containing lead (e.g., stained glass, solder, fishing sinkers, bullets)

Lead poisoning has other causes, but the most common cause has been the lead in paint. Children tend to nibble on fallen plaster, painted wooden furniture (including cribs), and painted toys because they have a sweet taste. Fine dust that results from removing lead

TABLE 37.2	Commonly Ingested Toxic Substances	
Agent	**Symptoms**	**Treatment**
acetaminophen	Under 6 y—vomiting is the earliest sign. Adolescents—vomiting, diaphoresis, general malaise. Liver damage can result in 48–96 h if not treated.	Gastric lavage may be necessary. Administer acetylcysteine (Mucomyst) diluted with cola, fruit juice, or water if plasma level elevated. Mucomyst may be administered by gavage, especially because its odor of rotten eggs makes it objectionable.
acetylsalicyclic acid (aspirin)	Hyperpnea (abnormal increase in depth and rate of breathing), metabolic acidosis, hyperventilation, tinnitus, and vertigo are initial symptoms. Dehydration, coma, convulsions, and death follow untreated heavy dosage.	Gastric lavage may be necessary. Activated charcoal may be administered. IV fluids, sodium bicarbonate to combat acidosis, and dialysis for renal failure may be necessary when large amounts are ingested.
ibuprofen (Motrin, Advil)	Similar to aspirin; metabolic acidosis, GI bleeding, renal damage	Activated charcoal is administered in emergency department. Observe for and treat GI bleeding. Electrolyte determination is done to detect acidosis. IV fluids are given.
ferrous sulfate (iron)	Vomiting, lethargy, diarrhea, weak rapid pulse, hypotension are common symptoms. Massive dose may produce shock; erosion of small intestine; black, tarry stools; bronchial pneumonia.	Deferoxamine, a chelating agent that combines with iron, may be used when child has ingested a toxic dose.
barbiturates	Respiratory, circulatory, and renal depression may occur. Child may become comatose.	Establish airway; administer oxygen if needed; perform gastric lavage. Close observation of level of consciousness is needed.
corrosives alkali: lye, bleaches acid: drain cleaners, toilet bowl cleaners, iodine, silver nitrate	Intense burning and pain with first mouthful; severe burns of mouth and esophageal tract; shock, possible death.	*Never have child vomit.* Alkali corrosives are treated initially with quantities of water, diluted acid fruit juices, or diluted vinegar. Acid corrosives are treated with alkaline drinks such as milk, olive oil, mineral oil, or egg white. *Lavage or emetics are never used.* Continuing treatment includes antidotes, gastrostomy or IV feedings, and specialized care. A tracheostomy may be needed.
hydrocarbons kerosene, gasoline, furniture polish, lighter fluid, turpentine	Damage to the respiratory system is the primary concern. Vomiting often occurs spontaneously, possibly causing additional damage to the respiratory system. Pneumonia, bronchopneumonia, or lipoid pneumonia may occur.	Emergency treatment and assessment are necessary. Vital signs are monitored; oxygen is administered as needed. Gastric lavage is performed only if the ingested substance contains other toxic chemicals that may threaten another body system such as the liver, kidneys, or cardiovascular system.

paint in remodeling also can cause harm to the children in the household without parents being aware of exposure. When the danger of lead poisoning became apparent, attempts were made to control the sale of lead-based paint. In 1973, federal regulations banned the sale of paint containing more than 0.5% lead for interior residential use or use on toys. However, this has not eliminated the problem because many homes built before the 1960s were painted with lead-based paint, and they still exist in inner-city areas, as well as small towns and suburbs. Older mansions where upper-income families may live also may have lead paint because of the building's age. Only contractors experienced in lead-based paint removal should do renovations.

Clinical Manifestations

The onset of chronic lead poisoning is insidious. Some early indications may be irritability, hyperactivity, aggression, impulsiveness, or disinterest in play. Short attention span, lethargy, learning difficulties, and distractibility also are signs of poisoning.

The condition may progress to **encephalopathy** (degenerative disease of the brain) because of intracranial pressure. Manifestations may include convulsions, mental retardation, blindness, paralysis, coma, and death. Acute episodes sometimes develop sporadically and early in the condition.

Diagnosis

The nonspecific nature of the presenting symptoms makes it important to examine the child's environmental history. Testing blood lead levels is used as a screening method. Target screening is done in areas where the risk of lead poisoning is high. Fingersticks, or heelsticks for infants, can be used to collect samples for lead level screening. In 1997, the Centers for Disease Control (CDC) in Atlanta modified the guidelines related to lead screening. The CDC continues to define elevated blood levels of lead as equal to or greater than 10 μg/dL. The CDC's emphasis is on primary prevention and screening.

Treatment and Nursing Care

The most important aspect of treatment of a child with lead poisoning is to remove the lead from the child's system and environment. The use of a **chelating agent** (an agent that binds with metal) increases the urinary excretion of lead. Several chelating agents are available; individual circumstances and the physician's choice determine the particular drug used. Edetate calcium disodium, known as EDTA, is usually given IV because intramuscular administration is painful. Renal failure can occur with inappropriate dosage. Dimercaprol, also known as BAL, causes excretion of lead through bile and urine; it may be administered intramuscularly. Because of its peanut oil base, BAL should not be used in children allergic to peanuts. These two drugs may be used together in children with extremely high levels of lead.

The oral drug penicillamine can be used to treat children with blood lead levels lower than 45 μg/dL. The capsules can be opened and sprinkled on food or mixed in liquid for administration. This drug should not be administered to children who are allergic to penicillin. The drug succimer (Chemet) is an oral drug used for treating children with blood lead levels higher than 45 μg/dL. Succimer comes in capsules that can be opened and mixed with applesauce or other soft foods or can be taken from a spoon, followed by a flavored beverage.

All the chelating drugs may have toxic side effects, and children being treated must be carefully monitored with frequent urinalysis, blood cell counts, and renal function tests. Any child receiving chelation therapy should be under the care of an experienced health care team.

Prognosis

The prognosis after lead poisoning is uncertain. Early detection of the condition and removal of the child from the lead-containing surroundings offer the best hope. Follow-up should include routine examinations to prevent recurrence and to observe for signs of any residual brain damage not immediately apparent.

Although the incidence of lead poisoning has decreased, it is still prevalent. Measures to educate the public on the importance of preventing this disorder are essential if the problem is to be eliminated. Education of the family caregivers is an essential aspect of the treatment (see Family Teaching Tips: Preventing Lead Poisoning).

FAMILY TEACHING TIPS

Preventing Lead Poisoning

- If you live in an older home, make sure your child does not have access to any chips of paint or chew any surface painted with lead-based paint. Look for paint dust on window sills, and clean with a high-phosphate sodium cleaner (the phosphate content of automatic dishwashing detergent is usually high enough).
- Wet-mop hard-surfaced floors and woodwork with cleaner at least once a week. Vacuuming hard surfaces scatters dust.
- Wash child's hands and face before eating.
- Wash toys and pacifiers frequently.
- Prevent child from playing in dust near an old lead-painted house.
- Prevent child from playing in soil or dust near a major highway.
- If your water supply has a high lead content, fully flush faucets before using for cooking, drinking, or making formula.
- Avoid contamination from hobbies or work.
- Make sure your child eats regular meals. Food slows absorption of lead.
- Encourage your child to eat foods high in iron and calcium.

From Centers for Disease Control and Prevention. *Preventing lead poisoning in young children: a statement by The Centers for Disease Control.* Atlanta, 2002. *http://www.cdc.gov*

INGESTION OF FOREIGN OBJECTS

Young children are apt to put any small objects into their mouths; they often swallow these objects. Normally many of these objects pass smoothly through the digestive tract and are expelled in the feces. Occasionally, however, something such as an open safety pin, a coin, a button, or a marble may lodge in the esophagus and need to be extracted. Foods such as hot dogs, peanuts, carrots, popcorn kernels, apple pieces, grapes, and round candy are frequent offenders.

Unless symptoms of choking, gagging, or pain are present, waiting and watching the feces carefully for 3 or 4 days is usually safe. Any object, however, may pass safely through the esophagus and stomach only to become fixed in one of the curves of the intestine, causing an obstruction or fever due to infection. Sharp objects also present the danger of perforation somewhere in the digestive tract.

Diagnosis of a swallowed solid object is often, but not always, made from the history. If a foreign object in the digestive tract is suspected, fluoroscopic and radiographic studies may be required.

Treatment and Nursing Care

If a caregiver has seen a child swallow an object and begin choking, the caregiver should hold the child along the rescuer's forearm with the child's head lower than his chest and give the child several back blows. After delivering the back blows, the caregiver should support the child's back and head and turn the child over onto the opposite thigh. The caregiver should deliver as many as five quick downward chest thrusts and remove the foreign body if visualized. A child older than age 1 year can be encouraged to continue to cough as long as the cough remains forceful. If the cough becomes ineffective (no sound with cough) or respirations become more difficult and stridor is present, the caregiver can attempt the Heimlich maneuver (Fig. 37-7).

If the child is not having respiratory problems and coughing has not resulted in removal of the object, the child needs to be transported to an emergency department to be assessed by a physician. Objects in the esophagus are removed by direct vision through an esophagoscope. Attempts to push the object down into the stomach or to extract it blindly can be dangerous. Some objects may need to be removed surgically. If the object is small and the physician believes that there is little danger to the gastrointestinal tract, the caregiver may be advised to take the child home and watch the child's bowel movements over the next several days to confirm that the object has passed through the system.

Increasing respiratory difficulties indicate that the object has been aspirated, rather than swallowed. Foreign objects aspirated into the larynx or bronchial tree may become lodged in the trachea or larynx. Back blows and chest thrusts or the Heimlich maneuver should be delivered as described. The child's airway should be opened and rescue breathing attempted. If the child's chest does not rise, the child should be repositioned and rescue breathing tried again. If the airway is still obstructed, these steps should be repeated until the object is removed and respirations are established. The child should be transported to the emergency department as quickly as possible. The caregiver should get emergency assistance while continuing to try to remove the offending object.

Adults must be aware of the power of example. A child who sees an adult holding pins or nails in his or her mouth may follow this example with disastrous, and often fatal, results.

Test Yourself

- What are some indications that a child may have lead poisoning?
- How is lead poisoning treated?

ENDOCRINE DISORDERS

Type 1 diabetes mellitus is the most significant endocrine disorder that affects children. Other conditions that may affect children are disorders of the pituitary gland that alter growth and diabetes insipidus. The incidence of these latter conditions is low.

TYPE 1 DIABETES MELLITUS

At least 15 million Americans have received the diagnosis of diabetes. A significant number of them are children: type 1 diabetes mellitus is estimated to affect about 1 in 600 children between the ages of 5 and 15 years. The incidence of this condition continues to increase.

Diabetes is often considered an adult disease, but at least 5% of cases begin in childhood, usually at about 6 years of age or around the time of puberty. Management of diabetes in children is different from that in adults and requires conscientious care geared to the child's developmental stage.

Diabetes is classified into two major types: Type 1 diabetes, formerly called insulin-dependent diabetes

● **Figure 37.7** (**A**) Back blows (*top*) and chest thrusts (*bottom*) to relieve foreign-body airway obstruction in infant. Hold infant over arm as illustrated, supporting head by firmly holding jaw. Deliver up to five back blows. Turn infant over while supporting head, neck, jaw, and chest with one hand and back with other hand. Keep head lower than trunk. Give five quick chest thrusts with one finger below intermammary line. If foreign body not removed and airway remains obstructed, attempt rescue breathing. Repeat these 2 steps until successful. (**B**) Abdominal thrusts with child standing or sitting can be performed when child is conscious. Standing behind child, place thumb side of one fist against child's abdomen in midline slightly above navel and well below xiphoid process. Grab fist with other hand and deliver five quick upward thrusts. Continue until successful or child loses consciousness. (**C**) Abdominal thrusts with child lying can be performed on a conscious or unconscious child. Place heel of hand on child's abdomen slightly above the navel and below the xiphoid process and rib cage. Place other hand on top of first hand. Deliver five separate, distinct thrusts. Open airway and attempt rescue breathing if object is not removed. Repeat until successful. (**D**) Combined jaw thrust–spine stabilization maneuver for a child trauma victim with possible head or neck injury. To protect from damage to cervical spine, the neck is maintained in a neutral position and traction on or movement of neck is avoided.

mellitus (IDDM) or juvenile diabetes; and type 2 diabetes, formerly called noninsulin-dependent diabetes mellitus. As noted in Table 37-3, diabetes in children is type 1.

Pathogenesis

The exact pathophysiology of diabetes is not completely understood; however, it is known to result from dysfunction of the beta (insulin-secreting) cells of the islets of Langerhans in the pancreas. Some researchers believe that the presence of an acute infection during childhood may trigger a mechanism in genetically susceptible children, activating beta-cell dysfunction and disrupting insulin secretion. Other conditions that may contribute to type 1 diabetes are pancreatic tumors, pancreatitis, and long-term corticosteroid use.

Normally the sugar derived from digestion and assimilation of foods is burned to provide energy for the body's activities. Excess sugar is converted into fat or glycogen and stored in the body tissues. Insulin, a hormone secreted by the pancreas, is responsible for the burning and storage of sugar. In diabetes, the secretion of insulin is inadequate or nonexistent, allowing sugar to accumulate in the bloodstream and spill over into the urine. In children, diabetes causes an abrupt, pronounced decrease in insulin production, resulting in decreased ability to derive energy from the food eaten. Large amounts of protein and fat are used to supply the child's energy needs, causing loss of weight and slowed growth. This combination of failure to gain weight and lack of energy may be the initial reason the child is brought to the health care provider's attention. However, a health care provider may not see the child until symptoms of ketoacidosis are evident.

Clinical Manifestations

Classic symptoms of type 1 diabetes mellitus are **polyuria** (dramatic increase in urinary output proba-

TABLE 37.3	Comparison of Type 1 and Type 2 Diabetes	
Assessment	Type 1 Diabetes	Type 2 Diabetes
Age of onset	5–7 y or at puberty	40–65 y
Type of onset	Abrupt	Gradual
Weight changes	Marked weight loss is often initial sign	Associated with obesity
Other symptoms	Polydipsia	Polydipsia
	Polyuria (often begins as bed-wetting)	Polyuria
	Fatigue (marks fall in school)	Fatigue
	Blurred vision (marks fall in school)	Blurred vision
	Glycosuria	Glycosuria
	Polyphagia	Pruritus
	Pruritus	Mood changes
	Mood changes (may cause behavior problems in school)	
Therapy	Hypoglycemic agents never effective; insulin needed	Managed by diet, oral hypoglycemic agents, or insulin
	Diet only moderately restricted; no dietary foods used	Diet tends to be strict
	Common-sense foot care for growing children	Good skin and foot care necessary
Period of remission	Period of remission for 1–12 mo generally follows initial diagnosis	Not demonstrable

Adapted from Pillitteri, A. (2003). *Maternal and child health nursing* (4th ed). Philadelphia: Lippincott Williams & Wilkins.

bly with enuresis), **polydipsia** (increased thirst), and **polyphagia** (increased hunger and food consumption). These symptoms are usually accompanied by weight loss or failure to gain weight and lack of energy, even though the child has increased food consumption. Symptoms of diabetes in children often have an abrupt onset.

If the child's symptoms are not noted and referred for diagnosis, the disorder is likely to progress to diabetic ketoacidosis. Because of inadequate insulin production, carbohydrates are not converted into fuel for energy production. Fats are then mobilized for energy but are incompletely oxidized in the absence of glucose. Ketone bodies (acetone, diacetic acid, and oxybutyric acid) accumulate. They are readily excreted in the urine, but the acid–base balance of body fluids excreted is upset and results in acidosis.

Diabetic ketoacidosis is characterized by drowsiness, dry skin, flushed cheeks and cherry-red lips, acetone breath with a fruity smell, and **Kussmaul breathing** (abnormal increase in the depth and rate of the respiratory movements). Nausea and vomiting may occur. If untreated, the child lapses into coma and exhibits dehydration, electrolyte imbalance, rapid pulse, and subnormal temperature and blood pressure.

Diagnosis

Early detection and control are critical in postponing or minimizing later complications of diabetes. The nurse should observe carefully for any signs or symptoms in all members of a family with a history of diabetes. The family also should be taught to observe the children for frequent thirst, urination, and weight loss. All relatives of diabetics are considered a high-risk group and should have periodic testing.

At each visit to a health care provider, children with a family history of diabetes should be monitored for glucose using a fingerstick glucose test and for ketones in the urine using a urine dipstick test. If the blood glucose level is elevated or ketonuria is present, a fasting blood sugar (FBS) is performed. An FBS result of 200 mg/dL or higher almost certainly is diagnostic for diabetes when other signs such as polyuria and weight loss, despite polyphagia, are present.

Although glucose tolerance tests are performed in adults to confirm diabetes, they are not commonly used in children. The traditional oral glucose tolerance test is often unsuccessful in children because they may vomit the concentrated glucose that must be swallowed.

Treatment

Management of diabetes in children includes insulin therapy and a meal and exercise plan. Treatment of the diabetic child involves the family and child and a number of health team members, such as the nurse, the pediatrician, the nutritionist, and the diabetic nurse educator. After diabetes is diagnosed, the child may be hospitalized for a period of time. This allows the condition to be stabilized under supervision. This is a trying time, and the nurse must plan care with an understanding of the emotional impact of the diagnosis. The child's teacher, the school nurse, and others who supervise the child during daily activities must be informed of the diagnosis.

Insulin Therapy

Insulin therapy is an essential part of the treatment of diabetes in children. The dosage of insulin is adjusted according to blood glucose levels so that the levels are maintained near normal. Two kinds of insulin are often combined for the best results. Insulin can be grouped into rapid-acting, short-acting, intermediate-acting, and long-acting (Table 37-4).

The introduction of the rapid acting insulin Lispro or Humalog has greatly changed insulin administration in children (Selekman, Scofield, & Swenson-Brousell, 1999).

The onset of action of Lispro is less than 15 minutes. An intermediate-acting and a short-acting insulin often are given together. Some preparations come in a premixed proportion of 70% intermediate-acting and 30% short-acting insulin, eliminating the need for mixing.

Good news. Lispro or Humalog insulin can be administered immediately *after* the child has eaten, so the amount of food eaten can be taken into consideration when determining the dosage.

Many children are prescribed an insulin regimen in which a dose containing a short-acting insulin and an intermediate-acting insulin are given at two times during the day: one before breakfast and the second before the evening meal. Children's insulin doses have to be individually regulated to keep their blood glucose levels as close to normal as possible.

Insulin Reaction. Insulin reaction (insulin shock, hypoglycemia) is caused by insulin overload, resulting in too-rapid metabolism of the body's glucose. This may be attributable to a change in the body's requirement, carelessness in diet (such as failure to eat proper amounts of food), an error in insulin measurement, or excessive exercise. Because diabetes in children is very labile (unstable, fluctuating), the child is subject to insulin reactions.

Some symptoms of impending insulin reaction in children are any type of odd, unusual, or antisocial behavior; weakness; nervousness; lethargy; headache; blurred vision and dizziness; and undue fatigue or hunger. Other symptoms might include pallor, sweating, convulsions, and coma. Children often have hypoglycemic reactions in the early morning.

This advice could be a life-saver: Treatment of an insulin reaction should be immediate.

The nurse must observe the child at least every 2 hours during the night. Note tossed bedding, which would indicate restlessness, and any excessive perspiration. If necessary, try to arouse the child. As the child becomes regulated and observes a careful diet at home, parents need not watch so closely but should have a thorough understanding of all aspects of this condition. Blood glucose monitoring often is scheduled for this early morning time in an effort to detect abnormal glucose levels.

To treat an insulin reaction, give the child sugar, candy, orange juice, or one of the commercial products designed for this emergency. Repeated or impending reactions require consultation with the physician.

If the child cannot take a sugar source orally, glucagon should be administered subcutaneously to bring about a prompt increase in the blood glucose level. Every adult responsible for a diabetic child should clearly understand the procedure for administering this drug and should have easy access to it. Glucagon is a hormone produced by alpha cells of the pancreatic islets. An elevation in the blood glucose level results in insulin release in a normal person, but a decrease in the blood glucose level stimulates glucagon

TABLE 37.4	Types of Insulin: Onset, Peak, and Duration			
Action	Preparation	Onset (hrs)	Peak (hrs)	Duration (hrs)
Rapid-acting	Lispro Humalog	0.25	0.5–1	3–4
Short-acting	Regular	0.5–1	2–4	5–7
Intermediate-acting	NPH	1.5–2	6–12	18–24
	Lente	1.5–2	6–12	18–24
Long-acting	Ultralente	4–6	18–24	36–48

*References may vary slightly on these figures.

release. The released glucagon in the bloodstream acts on the liver to promote glycogen breakdown and glucose release. Glucagon is available as a pharmaceutical product and is packaged in prefilled syringes for immediate use. It is administered in the same manner as insulin.

Glucagon acts within minutes to restore consciousness, after which the child can take candy or sugar. This treatment prevents the long delay while waiting for a physician to administer glucose IV or for an ambulance to reach the child. However, it is not a substitute for proper medical supervision.

Insulin Regimen. Most children with newly diagnosed diabetes show a decreased need for insulin during the 1st weeks or months after control is established. This is often referred to as the "honeymoon period," and it should be explained to the family in advance to avoid false hope. As the child grows, the need for insulin increases and continues to do so until the child reaches full growth. Again, family caregivers need to know that this is normal and that the child's condition is not getting worse.

Insulin Administration Methods. Insulin often is administered subcutaneously at different times of the day or it may be administered continuously via a pump.

The child may not be able to take over management of the insulin injection as early as blood glucose monitoring, but he or she can watch the preparation of the syringe and learn the technique for drawing up the dosage. It may be helpful to encourage the child to watch the process until it becomes routine. By 8 or 9 years of age, the child should be encouraged to talk with the caregiver about the dose and to practice working with the syringe. The child also may draw up the dose and prepare for self-administration. The age at which this is possible varies. No two children mature at the same rate; some may be able to do this much earlier than others. Automatic injection devices can help the child self-administer insulin at a younger age. The child should be encouraged to take over the management of the therapy when ready. If included in decision making, the child can learn the importance of the routine and accept the restrictions the disease imposes.

The insulin pump is a method of continuous insulin administration useful for some diabetics. The pump is about the size of a transistor radio and can be worn strapped to the waist or on a shoulder strap. It delivers a steady low dose of insulin through a syringe housed in the pump and connected by polyethylene tubing to a small-gauge subcutaneous needle implanted in the abdomen. Extra insulin is released at mealtimes and other times when needed by pressing a button. The pump does not sense the blood glucose level; therefore, careful blood glucose monitoring at least four times a day is necessary to adjust the dosage as needed. The pump must be removed to bathe, swim, or shower. The child may want to wear loose clothing that will hide the pump. The needle site must be regularly observed for redness and irritation. The site is changed every 24 to 48 hours using aseptic technique.

Unique Needs of the Adolescent. Adolescence is an extremely trying period for many diabetics, as it is for other young people. Diabetics, like healthy adolescents, must work from dependence to independence. Even when an adolescent has accepted responsibility for self-care, it is not unusual for him or her to rebel against the control that this condition demands, become impatient, and appear to ignore future health. The adolescent may skip meals, drop diet controls, or neglect glucose monitoring. Going barefoot and neglecting proper foot care also can cause problems for the diabetic adolescent. It can be a difficult time for both the family and the adolescent. The caregivers naturally become concerned and are apt to give the adolescent more controls to rebel against. Special care should be taken by the family, teachers, nurses, and physicians to see that these young people find enough maturing satisfaction in other areas and do not need to rebel in this vital area.

The adolescent who completely understands all aspects of the condition (especially if allowed to assume control of treatment previously) should be allowed to continue managing her or his own treatment. Should the adolescent run into difficulty, an adolescent clinic can be of great value. There the adolescent can discuss problems with understanding people who respond with care and provide dignity and attentive listening.

Treatment of Diabetic Ketoacidosis

Treatment for ketoacidosis requires skilled nursing care, and the child may be admitted to a pediatric intensive care unit. Fluid depletion is corrected; blood and urine glucose levels and other blood studies are monitored closely to evaluate the degree of ketoacidosis and electrolyte imbalance. If the child cannot urinate, a catheter is inserted. Regular insulin is given intravenously along with IV electrolyte fluids.

● Nursing Process for the Child With Type 1 Diabetes Mellitus

ASSESSMENT

When collecting data, ask the caregiver about the child's symptoms leading up to the present illness. Ask about the child's appetite, weight loss or gain, evidence of polyuria or enuresis in a previously toilet-trained child, polydipsia, dehydration (which may include constipation), irritability, and fatigue. Include the child in the interview and encourage him or her to contribute information. Observe for evidence of the child's developmental stage to help to determine appropriate nursing diagnoses and planning effective care. If the child is first seen in diabetic ketoacidosis, adjust the initial nursing interview accordingly.

In the physical exam, measure the height and weight and examine the skin for evidence of dryness or slowly healing sores. Note signs of hyperglycemia, record vital signs, and collect a urine specimen. Perform a blood glucose level determination using a bedside glucose monitor.

SELECTED NURSING DIAGNOSES

- Imbalanced Nutrition: Less Than Body Requirements related to insufficient caloric intake to meet growth and development needs and the inability of the body to use nutrients
- Risk for Impaired Skin Integrity related to slow healing process and decreased circulation
- Risk for Infection related to elevated glucose levels
- Readiness for Enhanced Management of Therapeutic Regimen related to blood glucose levels
- Deficient Knowledge related to complications of hypoglycemia and hyperglycemia
- Deficient Knowledge related to insulin administration
- Deficient Knowledge related to appropriate exercise and activity
- Compromised Family Coping related to the effect of the disease on the child and family's life
- Risk for Impaired Adjustment related to long-term management of chronic disease

OUTCOME IDENTIFICATION AND PLANNING

The major goals for the child include maintaining adequate nutrition, promoting skin integrity, preventing infection, regulating glucose levels, and learning to adjust to having a chronic disease. Goals for the child and family include learning about and managing hypoglycemia and hyperglycemia, insulin administration, and exercise needs for the child. An additional goal is for family members to express their concerns about coping with the child's illness.

IMPLEMENTATION

Ensuring Adequate and Appropriate Nutrition

The child with diabetes needs a sound nutritional program that provides adequate nutrition for normal growth while it maintains the blood glucose at near-normal levels. The food plan should be well balanced with foods that take into consideration the child's food preferences, cultural customs, and lifestyle (see Family Teaching Tips: Child's Diabetic Food Plan).

Help the child and caregiver to understand the importance of eating regularly scheduled meals. Special occasions can be planned so that the child does not feel left out of celebrations. If a particular meal is going to be late, the child should have a complex carbohydrate and protein snack. Children should be included in meal planning when possible so that they learn what is permissible and what is not. In this way, they will be able to handle eating when they are on their own in school and in social situations.

Preventing Skin Breakdown

Skin breakdowns, such as blisters and minor cuts, can become major problems for the diabetic

FAMILY TEACHING TIPS

Child's Diabetic Food Plan

- Plan well-balanced meals that are appealing to child.
- Be positive with child when talking about foods that he or she can eat; downplay the negatives.
- Space three meals and three snacks throughout the day. Daily caloric intake is divided to provide 20% at breakfast, 20% at lunch, 30% at dinner, and 10% at each of the snacks.
- Calories should be made up of 50% to 60% carbohydrates, 15% to 20% protein, and no more than 30% fat.
- Avoid concentrated sweets such as jelly, syrup, pie, candy bars, and soda pop.
- Artificial sweeteners may be used.
- Child must not skip meals. Make every effort to plan meals with foods that the child likes.
- Include foods that contain dietary fiber such as whole grains, cereals, fruits and vegetables, nuts, seeds, and legumes. Fiber helps prevent hyperglycemia.
- Dietetic food is expensive and unnecessary.
- Keep complex carbohydrates available to be eaten before exercise and sports activities to provide sustained carbohydrate energy sources.
- Teach child day by day about the food plan to encourage independence in food selections when at school or away from home.

child. Teach the caregiver and child to inspect the skin daily and promptly treat even small breaks in the skin. Encourage daily bathing. Teach the child and caregiver to dry the skin well after bathing, and give careful attention to any area where skin touches skin, such as the groin, axilla, or other skin folds. Emphasize good foot care. This includes wearing well-fitting shoes, inspecting between toes for cracks, trimming nails straight across, wearing clean socks, and not going barefoot. Establishing these habits early will help the child prepare for lifelong care of diabetes.

Preventing Infection
Diabetic children may be more susceptible to urinary tract and upper respiratory infections. Teach the child and caregiver to be alert for signs of urinary tract infection, such as itching and burning on urination. Instruct them to report signs of urinary tract or upper respiratory infections to the care provider promptly.

Many children are subject to minor infections and illnesses during the school years with little long-term effect. However, the diabetic child is more susceptible to long-term complications. When the diabetic child has an infection and fever, the temperature and metabolic rate increase and the body needs more sugar and, therefore, more insulin to make the sugar available to the body. Although the child may not be eating because of vomiting or anorexia, the body still needs insulin. Insulin should never be skipped during illness. Blood glucose levels should be checked every 2 to 4 hours during this time. Fluids need to be increased. Instruct the caregivers to contact the care provider when the child becomes ill, especially if the child is vomiting, cannot eat, or has diarrhea, so that close supervision can be maintained. Give the caregiver guidelines for care of an ill child with the initial diabetic instructions.

It is extremely important for the child to wear a MedicAlert identification medal or a bracelet with information about diabetic status. Identification cards, such as those carried by many adult diabetics, are seldom practical for a child.

Regulating Glucose Levels
The child who is seen in the health care facility with diabetes may have a new diagnosis or may be experiencing an unstable episode as a result of illness or changing needs. The child's blood glucose level must be monitored to maintain it within normal limits. Determine the blood glucose level at least twice a day, before breakfast and before the evening meal, by means of bedside glucose monitoring.

● **Figure 37.8** Child uses an automatic lancet to get blood sample (*left*) and blood glucose monitor to determine blood glucose level (*right*).

On initial diagnosis of diabetes, the blood glucose level should be checked as often as every 4 hours until some stability is achieved. Because regular monitoring of the blood glucose level is necessary, teach the child and the caregiver how to perform monitoring (Fig. 37-8).

Because this procedure involves a fingerstick, the child may object and resist it. Offer encouragement and support, helping the child to express fears and acknowledging that the fingerstick does hurt and it is acceptable to dislike it. Consider the child's developmental stage when performing the testing. Table 37-5 provides some guidelines for diabetic care and teaching based on developmental stage. School-age children can be involved in much of the process. Encourage the child to choose the finger to be used and clean it with soap and water. Automatic-release instruments make it easier for the child to do the fingerstick. Teach the child to read the results and learn the desired level. School-age children, in the stage of industry versus inferiority, are usually interested in learning new information. Appeal to this developmental characteristic to gain the cooperation of a child this age.

Providing Child and Family Teaching in the Management of Hypoglycemia and Hyperglycemia
The child is monitored closely for signs of hypoglycemia or hyperglycemia. If the blood glucose level is higher than 240 mg/dL, the urine may be tested for ketones. In addition, during an illness, the urine ketones are monitored. Be aware of the most likely times for an increase or decrease in the blood glucose level in relation to the insulin the child is receiving. Teach the child and family

TABLE 37.5	Developmental Guidelines for Diabetic Child Responsibilities*					
Issue	**Age (yr)**					
	Under 4	4–5	6–7	8–10	11–13	14+
Food	Teaching focuses on parents	Knows likes and dislikes	Can begin to tell sugar content of food and know foods he or she should not have	Has more ability to select foods according to criteria like exchange lists	Knows if foods fit own diet plan	Helps plan meals and snacks
Insulin	Parents take responsibility for care	Can tell where injection should be Can pinch the skin	Can begin to help with aspects of injections	Gives own injections with supervision	Can learn to measure insulin	Can mix two insulins
Testing		Can choose finger for finger stick Can wash finger with soap and water Collects urine; should watch caregiver do testing; helps with recording	Can do own finger stick using automatic puncture device. Can help with some aspects of blood test Can do own urine test and record results	Can do blood tests with supervision	Can see test results forming a pattern	Can begin to use test results to adjust insulin
Psychological		Identifies with being "bad" or "good"; these words should be avoided. A child this age may think he or she is bad if the test is said to be "bad."	Needs many reminders and supervision	Needs reminders and supervision Understands only immediate consequences, not long-term consequences, of diabetes control. "Scientific" mind developing; intrigued by tests	May be somewhat rebellious Concerned with being "different"	Understands long-term consequences of actions including diabetes control Independence and self-image are important. Rebellion continues and some supervision and continued support are still needed.

*These are only guidelines. Each child is an individual. Talk to your health care provider about any concerns you may have.

the signs of both hypoglycemia and hyperglycemia (Family Teaching Tips: Signs of Hypoglycemia and Hyperglycemia) and how to be prepared to take the appropriate action if necessary. They must be alert to signs of hypoglycemia, especially when insulin is at peak action (see Table 37-4).

Teach them to treat blood glucose levels lower than 60 mg/dL with juice, sugar, or nondiet soda.

If the blood glucose level cannot be checked promptly, the child should still consume a simple carbohydrate if there are any signs of hypoglycemia.

If the child cannot swallow, glucagon or dextrose should be administered following the physician's orders. Glucagon is commercially available and can be administered intramuscularly or

Signs of Hypoglycemia and Hyperglycemia

HYPOGLYCEMIA

- Shaking
- Irritability
- Hunger
- Diaphoresis
- Dizziness
- Drowsiness
- Pallor
- Changed level of consciousness
- Feeling "strange"

HYPERGLYCEMIA

- Polyphagia (excessive hunger)
- Polyuria (excessive urination)
- Dry mucous membranes
- Poor skin turgor
- Lethargy
- Change in level of consciousness

subcutaneously. Teach the caregiver how to mix and administer it.

Instruct the child to get help immediately when signs of hypoglycemia occur and to carry and take sugar cubes, Lifesavers, gumdrops, or a small tube of cake frosting. The reaction should be followed with a snack of a complex carbohydrate, such as crackers, and a protein such as cheese, peanut butter, or half of a meat sandwich. The snack is needed to maintain the increase in blood glucose level created by the simple carbohydrates and to prevent another hypoglycemic reaction.

Reassure the caregiver and the child that hypoglycemia is much more likely to occur than hyperglycemia. If there is any doubt as to whether the child is having a hypoglycemic or a hyperglycemic reaction, treat it like hypoglycemia. Instruct caregivers to keep a record of the hypoglycemic reactions to determine if there is a pattern and if the insulin schedule or food plan needs adjustment.

Providing Child and Family Teaching on Insulin Administration

Teach the family caregiver and the child the correct way to give insulin. Disposable syringes make caring for equipment relatively easy. A doll may be used to practice the actual administration until the caregiver (and child, if old enough) is comfortable and confident. Provide direct supervision until proficiency is demonstrated.

This part of the treatment is probably the most threatening aspect of the illness. Remember your feelings when you gave your first injection in nursing school. The child and family need a great deal of empathy and warm support. Increasing their confidence and skills of insulin administration will reduce their fear.

Give clear instructions concerning the importance of rotating injection sites (Fig. 37-9). If used too frequently, a site is apt to become indurated and eventually fibrosed, which hinders proper insulin absorption. The atrophic hollows in the skin, or the lumps of hypertrophied tissue, are unsightly as well. Some people appear to have greater skin sensitivity than do others. Areas on the upper arms, upper thighs, abdomen, and buttocks can be used.

Use of a careful plan allows several weeks to elapse before a site is used again. Usually four to six injections are given in one area before going on to the next area. Starting from the inner, upper corner of the area, each injection is given ½ inches below the preceding one, going down in a vertical line. The next series of injections in this area would start ½ inch outward at the upper level. If there is any sign of induration, the local site should be avoided for a few weeks until all

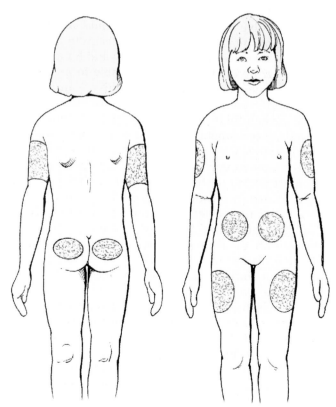

● **Figure 37.9** Subcutaneous injection sites.

signs of irritation have disappeared. A chart recording the sites used and the rotation schedule is recommended.

Providing Child and Family Teaching About Exercise and Activity

Exercise decreases the blood glucose level because carbohydrates are being burned for energy. The therapeutic program should be adjusted to allow for this increase in energy requirements to avoid hypoglycemia. Adjustments also may be needed in the child's school schedule. For instance, physical education should never be scheduled right before lunch for a diabetic child. Also, the diabetic child should not be scheduled for a late lunch period.

Promoting Family Coping

When the diagnosis of diabetes is confirmed, the family caregiver may feel devastated. A young child will not understand the implications, but the school-age or adolescent child will experience a great amount of fear and anxiety. The caregiver may have feelings of guilt, resentment, or denial. Other family members also may experience strong feelings about the illness. All these feelings and concerns must be recognized and resolved to work successfully with the diabetic child. Encourage the family to express these feelings and fears. To help him or her deal with feelings, involve the caregiver in the child's caring during hospitalization. Carefully listen to questions and answer them completely and honestly. Many written materials are available to give to the caregiver, but be sure the caregiver can read and understand them. Videos are also available that are helpful in educating the diabetic and the family. Recommend available community support groups. Cover home care in detail. Provide the family caregiver with a support person to contact when questions arise after discharge.

Because so much information must be absorbed in a brief time, the caregivers may seem forgetful or confused. Careful, patient repetition of all aspects of diabetes and the child's care is necessary. When anxiety levels are high, information is often heard but not digested. Provide written material in an understandable form. Have caregivers repeat information, and question them to confirm that they understand. Demonstrate warmth and caring throughout the teaching to increase the family's comfort; this also will develop their confidence in nursing responses to their questions and apprehensions.

Promoting Self-care and Positive Self-esteem

The school-age or older child may experience some strong feelings of inadequacy or being "sick." These feelings must be expressed and handled. To help allay fear, teach the child as much as is appropriate for his or her age. Tell the child about athletes and other famous people who are diabetic. When possible, another child who is diabetic may visit so that the child does not feel so alone. Encourage the child to become active in helping with self-care. Answer questions about how diabetes will affect the child's activities. Summer camps for children with diabetes are available in many areas and can help develop the child's self-assurance.

The diabetic child can participate in normal activities. However, at least one friend should be told about the diabetic condition, and the child should not go swimming or hiking without a responsible person nearby who knows what to look for and what to do if the child should have a reaction.

Some children are sensitive about their condition and fear that they seem different from their friends. Even with the best instruction and preparation, they may feel this way and wish to keep their condition secret. They must understand that a teacher or some other adult in their environment must be acquainted with their condition. Classroom teachers need to know which of their students have such a condition and should understand the signs of an impending reaction.

Diabetic children with their glucose levels under good control need not be kept from activities such as camp-outs, overnight trips with the school band, or other similar activities away from home. Of course, these children must first be capable of measuring their insulin and giving their own injections. Some young people may find that a desire to participate in such an activity can be the factor that helps them overcome reluctance to measure and administer their own insulin.

EVALUATION: GOALS AND EXPECTED OUTCOMES

- **Goal:** The child's caloric intake will be adequate to meet nutritional needs and to maintain appropriate growth.
  Expected Outcomes: The child eats food at meals and snack times, maintains normal weight for age and height, and the child and caregiver demonstrate understanding of meal planning by making appropriate menu selections.

- **Goal:** The child's skin integrity will be maintained.

  Expected Outcomes: The child's skin is intact with no signs of breakdown; the child and caregiver describe skin inspection and care.

- **Goal:** The child will be free from signs and symptoms of infection.

  Expected Outcomes: The child shows no signs of infection; temperature is within normal range; the child and caregiver discuss the importance of promptly reporting infections.

- **Goal:** The child will maintain normal glucose levels.

  Expected Outcomes: The child's blood glucose level is 60 to 100 mg/dL; the urine is negative for ketones; and there are no signs of hypoglycemia or hyperglycemia.

- **Goal:** The child and caregiver will verbalize an understanding of the signs, symptoms, and management of hypoglycemia and hyperglycemia.

  Expected Outcomes: The child and caregiver list the signs of hypoglycemia and hyperglycemia and discuss how to handle each; they ask questions to clarify information.

- **Goal:** The child and caregiver will verbalize an understanding of insulin administration.

  Expected Outcomes: The child and caregiver demonstrate insulin injection, describe various types of insulin and their reaction and peak times, and develop a site rotation schedule.

- **Goal:** The child and caregiver will verbalize an understanding of exercise and activity for a diabetic child.

  Expected Outcomes: The child and caregiver describe the effects of exercise on the blood glucose levels.

- **Goal:** The child and caregiver will express their concerns about coping with the child's illness.

  Expected Outcomes: As appropriate for age, the child discusses necessary adjustments to the daily schedule and activities and names several people to inform about the diabetic condition. The caregiver demonstrates support of the child in managing daily and long-term care of diabetes.

- **Goal:** The child will show adjustment and have a positive attitude about the condition.

  Expected Outcomes: The child expresses feelings about having diabetes and participates in age-appropriate activities and realistic goal planning.

Test Yourself

- What do the terms polyuria, polydipsia, and polyphagia mean?

- What causes diabetic ketoacidosis to occur?

- How is diabetes in the child treated?

- Describe the symptoms of hypoglycemia and hyperglycemia.

KEY POINTS

- The child with pyloric stenosis eats initially but then starts vomiting after meals. The vomiting increases in frequency and force, becoming projectile. The child is irritable, loses weight rapidly, and becomes dehydrated.

- Celiac disease is a malabsorptive disorder. Ingestion of wheat gluten or rye gluten leads to impaired fat absorption. It is often caused by an allergic reaction to the gliadin fraction of gluten (a protein factor in wheat).

- Congenital aganglionic megacolon is also called Hirschsprung disease. The common symptoms include failure of the newborn to have a stool in the first 24 hours, bile-stained emesis, and generalized abdominal distention. Gastroenteritis with diarrheal stools, ulceration of the colon, and severe constipation with ribbon-like or hard pellet stools are also seen.

- Intussusception is the invagination, or telescoping, of one portion of the bowel into a distal portion. It occurs most commonly at the juncture of the ileum and the colon. Immediate treatment consists of a barium enema to attempt to correct the telescoping or abdominal surgery if the barium enema does not correct the problem.

- Mild diarrhea is loose stools, with the frequency of defecation 2 to 12 times per day. Severe diarrhea is usually accompanied by vomiting, and together they cause large losses of body water and electrolytes. The child is severely dehydrated and gravely ill.

- Symptoms of appendicitis in the older child may be pain and tenderness in the right lower quadrant of the abdomen, nausea and vomiting, fever, and constipation. The young child has difficulty localizing the pain, may act restless and irritable, and may have a slight fever, a flushed face, and a rapid pulse. Usually the white blood cell count is slightly elevated.

- Pinworms invade the cecum and may enter the appendix. The infestation occurs when the pinworm eggs are swallowed. Roundworms are spread from the feces of infested people. It is usually found in areas where sanitary facilities are lacking and human excreta are deposited on the ground. The hookworm lives in the human intestinal tract and is prevalent in areas where infected human excreta is deposited on the ground; the hookworms penetrate the skin of barefoot people.

- The toddler and preschool age children find out about their environment often by tasting the world around them. Because their senses of taste and smell are not yet refined, young children ingest substances that would repel an adult because of their taste or smell and often are poisoned by the substance.

- Common substances children ingest include drugs such as acetaminophen, acetylsalicylic acid (aspirin), ibuprofen, ferrous sulfate, and barbiturates. They also ingest corrosives such as lye, bleach, and other cleaners and hydrocarbons, such as gasoline and kerosene.

- Chronic lead poisoning may be caused when children ingest lead from lead-containing paint, furniture, toys, and vinyl miniblinds. Drinking water contaminated by lead pipes; storage of food in improperly glazed earthenware; inhalation of engine fumes; and exposure to industrial areas and materials such as stained glass, solder, fishing sinkers, and bullets can also cause lead poisoning.

- Children with lead poisoning may have irritability, hyperactivity, aggression, impulsiveness, or disinterest in play. Short attention span, lethargy, learning difficulties, and distractibility also are signs of poisoning. Acute manifestations include convulsions, mental retardation, blindness, paralysis, coma, and death.

- Blood lead levels are used to diagnose lead poisoning; the best treatment for lead poisoning is to remove the lead from the child's system by using chelating agents. Early detection of the condition and removal of the child from the lead-containing surroundings offer the best prognosis.

- If a child who has swallowed a foreign object is having respiratory distress, the Heimlich maneuver should be used and cardiopulmonary resuscitation started if necessary. If the child is not having respiratory problems and coughing has not resulted in removal of the object, the child should

be taken to an emergency department to be assessed.

- Good skin care in the child with diabetes is important because even small breaks in the skin can become major problems for the diabetic child. Correct insulin administration and rotating of sites will help insulin absorption. Exercise is important in the diabetic because it decreases the blood glucose level by burning carbohydrates for energy.

REFERENCES AND SELECTED READINGS

Books and Journals

American Academy of Pediatrics, Committee on Injury, Violence, and Poison Prevention. (2003). Poison treatment in the home. *Pediatrics, 112*(5), 1182–1185. Retrieved November 3, 2003, from http://www.aap.org/policy/s010120.html

Azar, R., & Solomon, C. R. (2001). Coping strategies of parents facing child diabetes mellitus. *Journal of Pediatric Nursing, 16*(6), 418.

Centers for Disease Control and Prevention. (2002). *Preventing lead poisoning in young children: A statement by The Centers for Disease Control.* Atlanta. http://www.cdc.gov

Cohen, S. M. (2001). Lead poisoning: A summary of treatment and prevention. *Pediatric Nursing, 27*(2), 125.

Hockenberry, M. J., Wilson, D., Winkelstein, M. L., & Kline, N. E. (2003). *Wong's nursing care of infants and children* (7th ed.). St. Louis: Mosby.

Karch, A. M. (2003). *2004 Lippincott's nursing drug guide.* Philadelphia: Lippincott Williams & Wilkins.

Lawless, M. R., & McElderry, D. H. (2001). Nocturnal enuresis: Current concepts. *Pediatrics in Review, 22*(12), 399–407.

Lifschitz, C. H. (1999). Celiac disease. In *Oski's pediatrics: Principles and practice* (3rd ed.). Philadelphia: Lippincott Williams & Wilkins.

Maniatis, A. K., Klingensmith, G. J., Slover, R. H., Mowry, C. J., & Chase, H. P. (2001). Continuous subcutaneous insulin infusion therapy for children and adolescents: An option for routine diabetes care. *Pediatrics, 107*(2), 351–356.

North American Nursing Diagnosis Association (NANDA). (2001). *NANDA nursing diagnoses: Definitions and classification 2001–2002.* Philadelphia: Author.

Pillitteri, A. (2003). *Maternal and child health nursing* (4th ed.). Philadelphia: Lippincott Williams & Wilkins.

Putman, H. (2002) Food allergies—keeping kids safe. *RN, 65*(6), 26–30.

Selekman, J., Scofield, S., & Swenson-Brousell, C. (1999). Diabetes update in the pediatric population. *Pediatric Nursing, 25*(6), 666–669.

Smeltzer, S. C., & Bare, B. G. (2003). *Textbook of medical–surgical nursing* (10th ed.). Philadelphia: Lippincott Williams & Wilkins.

Sparks, S., & Taylor, C. (2001). *Nursing diagnosis reference manual* (5th ed.). Springhouse, PA: Springhouse Corporation.

Wolfe, C. A. (2000). Pediatric alert: Assess for lead. *RN*, 63(8), 27–31.

Wong, D. L., Perry, S., & Hockenberry, M. (2002). *Maternal–child nursing care* (2nd ed.). St. Louis: Mosby.

Web Addresses

Allergies
Allergicchild.com
www.allergicchild.com

Celiac Disease
www.celiac.com

Diabetes
www.jdf.org
www.childrenwithdiabetes.com

Food Allergies
www.foodallergy.org

WORKBOOK

NCLEX-STYLE REVIEW QUESTIONS

1. If an infant has a diagnosis of pyloric stenosis, the child will likely have a history of which of the following?

   a. Iron deficiency

   b. Projectile vomiting

   c. Muscle spasms

   d. Nasal congestion

2. A nurse admits a child with a diagnosis of possible appendicitis. Of the following signs and symptoms, which would *most* likely be seen in the child with appendicitis?

   a. Sore throat, bone and joint pain

   b. Itching, swelling around eyes and ankles

   c. Convulsions, weight gain or loss

   d. Fever, nausea and vomiting

3. The nurse is teaching a group of parents of toddlers about what to do in cases of poisoning. If a toddler has swallowed an unknown substance, which of the following should be the *first* action of the caregiver? The caregiver should

   a. administer a recommended antidote.

   b. call the Poison Control Center.

   c. encourage the child to drink water.

   d. place the child on a flat surface.

4. The nurse is working with a 12-year-old child with type 1 diabetes mellitus. The child asks the nurse why she can't take pills instead of shots like her grandmother does. Which of the following would be the *best* response by the nurse?

   a. "The pills correct a different type of diabetes than you have."

   b. "When your blood glucose levels are better controlled, you can take the pills too."

   c. "Your body does not make its own insulin so the insulin injections help replace it."

   d. "The pills only work for adults who have diabetes. Maybe when you are older, you can take the pills."

5. A child with a diagnosis of failure to thrive because of malnutrition has had an inadequate intake of calories. In planning care, all of the following goals would be appropriate for this child and or family caregiver. Which two goals would be the *highest* priority for this child or family? The child and/or family caregiver will

   a. maintain good mouth and skin integrity.

   b. improve knowledge and understanding of nutrition.

   c. maintain current weight.

   d. increase amount of daily exercise.

   e. have decreased anxiety.

   f. satisfy sucking needs.

   g. increase daily fluid intake.

   h. increase intake for appropriate weight gain.

STUDY ACTIVITIES

1. Develop a teaching aid or poster to use in teaching diabetic children how to administer their own insulin injections. Include how you will help this child make an insulin site rotation chart. Present your project to your peers.

2. Survey your house (or a house you select) and list the hazards for ingestion of poisonous substances, drowning, and burns. Include all types of burns. After the hazards are identified, formulate a plan to correct or lessen the hazards.

3. Carmella has idiopathic celiac disease. Using the foods listed in the table below, identify the foods that would be recommended and those that would not be recommended in her meal plan. With the help of a nutrition text or by reading labels, state why each of those foods is either recommended or not recommended.

Food	Recommended	Not Recommended	Explanation of Why Food Would or Would Not Be Recommended
Ice cream			
Corn flakes			
Grits			
Rice pudding			
Whole-wheat bread			
Baked beans			
Hamburger			
Hot dog			
French fries			
Fresh vegetables			
Yogurt			
Oatmeal			
Rice Krispies			
Orange juice			
Graham crackers			
Corn chips			
Peanut butter			
Baked potato			
Tuna salad			
Pizza			

4. Go to the Internet site: http://www.diabetes.org/wizdom

    Scroll down the screen on the right-hand side. Click on "Click here for More Cool Stuff." Click on "If You Are a Kid or Teen." Click on "School and Discrimination."

    After reading about the diabetic child at school, answer the following:

   a. What does this site suggest be included in a school packet?

   b. What would be important for the diabetic child to be allowed to do at school in order to follow his diabetic plan?

   c. What are some ideas suggested to prevent discrimination of a child with diabetes?

CRITICAL THINKING: What Would You Do?

1. Five-year-old Malcolm has been sent home from kindergarten with a note advising of an outbreak of pinworms. There are five children between 2 and 8 years of age in the household where he lives, including cousins. Malcolm's aunt is the person who cares for the children.

   a. What would you explain to Malcolm's aunt when she asks you what pinworms are and how children get them?

   b. What symptoms will you teach her to observe for in the children?

   c. How will the diagnosis of pinworms be made?

   d. What is the treatment for pinworms?

2. Your next-door neighbor has found their 18-month-old child with an empty bottle of chil-

dren's acetaminophen. She brings the child to your house.

   a. What immediate actions should you take?

   b. What is the specific antidote used in acetaminophen overdose? (Use a drug reference.)

   c. What organ can be damaged with an overdose of acetaminophen?

3. Nine-month-old Tina has severe diarrhea. She has been admitted to your unit and you have been assigned to be her nurse.

   a. What symptoms would you expect Tina to exhibit?

   b. What physical characteristics will you observe her for?

   c. What documentation is especially important in her care?

4. Dosage calculation: After an appendectomy an 8-year-old child is being medicated with meperidine (Demerol) for postoperative pain. The dosage range for this child is 1.0 to 1.8 mg per kg. The child weighs 55 pounds. The Demerol comes in a prefilled syringe with 50 mg per 1 mL. Answer the following:

   a. How many kilograms (kg) does the child weigh?

   b. What is the low dose for this child?

   c. What is the high dose for this child?

   d. How many milliliters (mL) will be given for the low dose of the medication?

   e. How many milliliters (mL) will be given for the high dose of the medication?

The Child With Genitourinary Disorders

38

STUDENT OBJECTIVES

On completion of this chapter, the student should be able to

1. Discuss ways the child's genitourinary system differs from the adult's system.
2. Describe the usual treatment for urinary tract infections.
3. Identify the physiologic causes of enuresis.
4. Describe the symptoms of nephrotic syndrome.
5. Identify the cause of acute glomerulonephritis.
6. Name the most common presenting symptom of acute glomerulonephritis.
7. Compare nephrotic syndrome with acute glomerulonephritis.
8. Describe the structural defects that occur with hydrocele and cryptorchidism.
9. Compare premenstrual syndrome, dysmenorrhea, and amenorrhea.

KEY TERMS

amenorrhea
ascites
dysmenorrhea
enuresis
intercurrent infections
leukopenia
menarche
mittelschmerz
oliguria
orchiopexy
premenstrual syndrome (PMS)
pyelonephritis
striae
vaginitis

Adequate functioning of the genitourinary (urinary and reproductive) system is affected by structural problems or defects, infections, disorders, and conditions. Although the symptoms seen in these conditions may be vague or seemingly not serious, they can be chronic, long term, or serious in their effect on the genitourinary system.

GROWTH AND DEVELOPMENT OF THE GENITOURINARY SYSTEM

The genitourinary system is made up of the kidneys, ureters, urinary bladder, and the urethra (Fig. 38-1). There are two kidneys and two ureters, located on each side of the body, just above the waistline. Functions of the kidney include excreting excess water and waste products and maintaining a balance of electrolytes and acid–base. Other functions of the kidney are regulating blood pressure by making the enzyme renin and making erythropoietin, which helps stimulate the production of red blood cells. Waste products are removed from the blood and excreted from the body through the urinary system.

The urine formed in the kidneys travels down the ureters and collects in the urinary bladder. When the bladder fills, there is an urge to empty the bladder. Urine passes through the urethra to be excreted from the body. In infants and children, the emptying of the bladder is a reflex action. Between ages 2 and 3 years, the child is able to hold the urine in the bladder and

TABLE 38.1	Child's Average Urine Output in 24 Hours
Age	**Amount of Urine (mL)**
6 months–2 years	540–600
2–5 years	500–780
5–8 years	600–1,200
8–14 years	1,000–1,500
Over 14 years	1,500

Taken from Pillitteri, A. (2003). *Material and child health nursing*, (4th ed., p. 1404). Philadelphia: Lippincott Williams & Wilkins.

learns to urinate voluntarily, thus developing the control of urination.

The kidneys in children are located lower in relationship to the ribs than in adults. This and the fact that the child has less of a fat cushion around the kidneys makes the child at greater risk for trauma to the kidneys. As the child grows, the kidneys also grow, especially during the first 2 years of life. The kidneys reach their full size and function by the time the child is an adolescent.

In the newborn, the bladder empties when only about 15 mL of urine is present, so the newborn voids as many as 20 times a day. As the child gets older, the bladder has more capacity to hold larger amounts of urine before the child feels the urge to void. The child at different ages voids average amounts, depending on fluid intake and kidney health (Table 38-1). The urethra in females is much shorter than in males at all ages, making the female more susceptible to urinary tract infections.

The reproductive portion of the genitourinary system in males and females matures at the time of puberty. The systems are made up of organs with the primary function being to produce cells necessary for reproduction. The organs also provide the mechanism for conception to occur. Males and females have different structures in the reproductive systems. In the male, the reproductive structures include the testes, located in the scrotum, which produce sperm, the ducts that aid in the passage of sperm, the glands that secrete necessary fluids, and the external genitalia, including the penis. In the female the reproductive organs include the ovaries, fallopian tubes, uterus, vagina, and the external genitalia. The genitals gradually increase in size during childhood. The hormone changes in both males and females during puberty cause the reproductive system to more fully develop during adolescence.

URINARY TRACT INFECTIONS

Urinary tract infections (UTIs) are fairly common in the "diaper age," in infancy, and again between the ages of 2 and 6 years. The condition is more common in

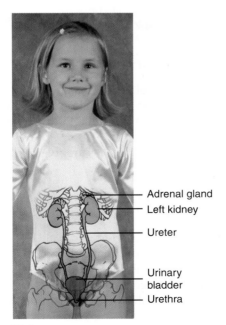

— Adrenal gland
— Left kidney

— Ureter

— Urinary bladder
— Urethra

● *Figure 38.1* The urinary tract.

girls than in boys, except in the first 4 months of life, when it is more common in boys. Although many different bacteria may infect the urinary tract, intestinal bacteria, particularly *Escherichia coli,* account for about 80% of acute episodes. The female urethra is shorter and straighter than the male urethra, so it is more easily contaminated with feces. Inflammation may extend into the bladder, ureters, and kidney.

Clinical Manifestations

In children, the symptoms may be fever, nausea, vomiting, foul-smelling urine, weight loss, and increased urination. Occasionally there is little or no fever. Vomiting is common, and diarrhea may occur. The child is irritable. In acute **pyelonephritis** (inflammation of the kidney and renal pelvis), the onset is abrupt, with a high fever for 1 or 2 days. Convulsions may occur during the period of high fever. In younger children, bedwetting may be a symptom.

Diagnosis

Diagnosis is based on the finding of pus in the urine under microscopic examination. The urine specimen must be fresh and uncontaminated. A "clean catch" voided urine, properly performed, is essential for microscopic examination (see Chapter 30). If a culture is needed, the child may be catheterized, but this is usually avoided if possible. A suprapubic aspiration also may be done to obtain a sterile specimen. In the cooperative, toilet-trained child, a clean midstream urine may be used successfully.

Treatment

Simple UTIs may be treated with antibiotics (usually sulfisoxazole or ampicillin) at home. The child with acute pyelonephritis is hospitalized. Fluids are given freely. The symptoms usually subside within a few days after antibiotic therapy has been initiated, but this is not an indication that the infection is completely cleared. Medication must be continued after symptoms disappear. An intravenous pyelogram or ultrasonographic study may be performed to assess the possibility of structural defects if the child has recurring infections.

● Nursing Process for the Child With a Urinary Tract Infection

ASSESSMENT

During the interview with the family caregiver, include basic information about the child, such as

feeding and sleeping patterns and history of other illnesses. Gather information about the current illness: when the fever started and its course thus far, signs of pain or discomfort on voiding, recent change in feeding pattern, presence of vomiting or diarrhea, irritability, lethargy, abdominal pain, unusual odor to urine, chronic diaper rash, and signs of febrile convulsions. If the child is toilet-trained, ask the caregivers about toileting habits (how does the child wipe? does the child wash the hands when toileting?). Also ask about the use of bubble baths and the type of soap used, especially for girls.

Collecting data regarding the child includes temperature; pulse (be alert for tachycardia) and respiration rates; weight and height; observation of a wet diaper or the urine in an older child; inspection of the perineal area for rash; presence of irritability and lethargy; and general skin condition, color, and turgor. A urine specimen is needed on admission. A midstream urine collection method is desirable, and catheterization is avoided if possible. Record and report any indications of urinary burning, frequency, urgency, or pain.

In the child who has repeated UTIs, observe the interaction between the child and the family caregivers to detect any indications that the infection may be caused by sexual abuse. Look for possible indications of sexual abuse.

Pay attention. Bruising, bleeding, or lacerations on the external genitalia, especially in the child who is extremely shy and frightened, may be a sign of child abuse and should be further explored.

SELECTED NURSING DIAGNOSES

- Hyperthermia related to infection
- Impaired Urinary Elimination related to pain and burning on urination and decreased fluid intake
- Deficient Knowledge of caregivers related to understanding of UTI

OUTCOME IDENTIFICATION AND PLANNING

Major goals for the child with a UTI include reducing temperature, maintaining normal urinary elimination, and increasing fluid intake. An important family goal is improving knowledge about infection control to help prevent recurrent infections. Base the nursing plan of care on these goals, with adjustments appropriate for the child's age. To promote normal elimination, plan nursing care that helps relieve pain and increase fluid intake. Be sure to include family teaching that focuses on infection prevention at home.

IMPLEMENTATION

Maintaining Body Temperature
Monitor the child's temperature frequently, at least every 2 hours if it is higher than 101.3°F (38.5°C). If the child has a fever, follow the procedures to reduce elevated temperatures. Administer antibiotics as ordered and observe the child for signs of any reactions to the antibiotics. Antipyretic medications may be ordered. Increasing oral fluids also will help to reduce body temperature.

Promoting Normal Elimination
Because of pain and burning on urination, the toilet-trained child may try to hold urine and not void. Encourage the child to void every 3 or 4 hours to prevent recurrent infection. Observe the child for signs of burning, pain, and frequency. If possible, observe the voiding pattern to note trickling or other signs that the bladder is not being emptied completely. Carefully monitor and measure urine output. An infant's diaper should be weighed for accuracy. Accurate intake and output measurements are important.

Increasing the child's fluid intake is necessary to help dilute the urine and flush the bladder. An increase in fluid intake also helps decrease the pain experienced on urination. Although getting the child to accept fluids often is difficult, frequent, small amounts of glucose water or liquid gelatin may be accepted. Enlisting the aid of family caregivers may be helpful, but if they are unsuccessful, the nurse must persevere. Most infants and children like apple juice, which helps acidify the urine. Cranberry juice is a good choice for the older child, if he or she tolerates it. Administer analgesics and antispasmodics as ordered.

Providing Family Teaching
The family caregivers are the key people in helping prevent recurring infections. See Family Teaching Tips: Urinary Tract Infection. Prepare the family caregivers and the child for any other procedures that may be ordered and give appropriate explanations.

EVALUATION: GOALS AND EXPECTED OUTCOMES

● **Goal:** The child will maintain a temperature within normal limits.
   Expected Outcome: The child's temperature is 98.6°F to 100°F (37°C to 37.8°C).

FAMILY TEACHING TIPS

Urinary Tract Infection

* Change infant's diaper when soiled, and clean baby with mild soap and water. Dry completely.
* Teach girls to wipe from front to back.
* Teach child to wash hands before and after going to the toilet.
* Avoid using bubble baths, which create a climate that encourages bacteria to grow, especially in young girls.
* Teach young girls to take showers. Avoid using water softeners in tub baths.
* Encourage child to try to urinate every 3 or 4 hours and to empty the bladder.
* Have girls wear cotton underpants to provide air circulation to perineal area.
* Encourage child to drink fluids, especially cranberry juice.
* Have older girls avoid whirlpools or hot tubs.

● **Goal:** The child's normal urinary elimination will be maintained.
   Expected Outcomes: The infant produces 2 to 3 mL/kg of urine per hour; the older child voids every 3 to 4 hours, emptying the bladder each time without apprehension.
● **Goal:** The family caregivers will verbalize an understanding of the genitourinary system and good hygiene habits.
   Expected Outcomes: The family caregivers list signs and symptoms of a UTI, methods to prevent a recurrence, and state when to contact a health practitioner.

Test Yourself

* What bacterium is the most common cause of urinary tract infections?

* How are urinary tract infections detected and treated?

* Explain the reason a child with a urinary tract infection may try to hold her urine.

ENURESIS

Enuresis, or bed-wetting, is involuntary urination beyond the age when control of urination commonly is acquired. Many children do not acquire complete nighttime control before 5 to 7 years of age, and occasional bed-wetting may be seen in children as late as

9 or 10 years of age. Boys have more difficulty than girls do, and in some instances enuresis may persist into the adult years.

Enuresis may have a physiologic or psychological cause and may indicate a need for additional exploration and treatment. Physiologic causes may include a small bladder capacity, urinary tract infection, and lack of awareness of the signal to empty the bladder because of sleeping too soundly. Persistent bed-wetting in a 5- or 6-year-old child may be a result of rigorous toilet training before the child was physically or psychologically ready. Enuresis in the older child may express resentment toward family caregivers or a desire to regress to an earlier level of development to receive more care and attention. Emotional stress can be a precipitating factor. The health care team also needs to consider the possibility that enuresis can be a symptom of sexual abuse.

Here's a tip for you to share.

An upcoming event the child is excited about attending, such as going to camp or visiting friends overnight, might be a motivator in helping the child with enuresis to achieve bladder control.

If a physiologic cause has been ruled out, efforts should be made to discover possible causes, including emotional stress. If the child is interested in achieving control, waking the child during the night to go to the toilet or limiting fluids before retiring may be helpful.

However, these measures should not be used as a replacement for searching for the cause. Help from a pediatric mental health professional may be needed.

The family caregiver may become extremely frustrated about having to deal with smelly, wet bedding every morning. The child may go to great efforts to hide the fact that the bed is wet. Health care personnel must take a supportive, understanding attitude toward the problems of the caregiver and the child, allowing each of them to ventilate feelings and providing a place where emotions can be freely expressed.

NEPHROTIC SYNDROME

Several different types of nephrosis have been identified in the nephrotic syndrome. The most common type in children is called lipoid nephrosis, idiopathic nephrotic syndrome, or minimal change nephrotic syndrome (MCNS). All forms of nephrosis have early characteristics of edema and proteinuria; therefore, definite clinical differentiation cannot be made early in the disease.

Nephrotic syndrome has a course of remissions and exacerbations that usually lasts for months. The recovery rate generally is good with the use of inten-

---

A PERSONAL GLIMPSE

My 9-year-old daughter was potty trained when she was just barely 2 years old. I was so proud of her and happy that she was out of diapers and that she had so quickly been trained. When she was almost 4, I had her little brother. She occasionally had an accident and wet pants, but I wasn't concerned. I just thought she wanted some attention. It was quite upsetting to me when shortly after she started the second grade she started wetting the bed. At first she was wet a few times a week, then every night. One day I got a call from the school saying I needed to bring her some dry clothes because she had wet her pants at school. That is when the worst part began. Now at 9 years old she wets her pants everyday. She takes dry clothes to school, but sometimes she just stays in her wet ones. She smells like urine all the time. It is so upsetting to me. I feel frustrated and sometimes angry. Most of all I just feel so bad for my daughter. Her friends make fun of her; she never wants to spend the night anywhere except at home, and now she doesn't even seem to care. About 3 weeks ago I started taking her to a counselor the school nurse recommended. I hope she can help my daughter and me understand and change what is going on for her. It is painful to watch this happen.

Angela

LEARNING OPPORTUNITY: What are some of the possible causes of this child's enuresis? What could you suggest to this mother to help her deal with her feelings regarding her child's situation?

---

sive steroid therapy and protection against infection. The cause of MCNS is unknown. In rare cases, it is associated with other specific diseases. Nephrotic syndrome is present in as many as seven children per 100,000 population younger than 9 years of age. The average age of onset is 2.5 years, with most cases occurring between the ages of 2 and 6 years.

Clinical Manifestations

Edema is usually the presenting symptom, appearing first around the eyes and ankles (Fig. 38-2). As the swelling advances, the edema becomes generalized, with a pendulous abdomen full of fluid. Respiratory embarrassment may be severe, and edema of the scrotum on the male is characteristic. The edema shifts when the child changes position when lying quietly or walking about. Anorexia, irritability, and loss of appetite develop. Malnutrition may become severe. However, the generalized edema masks the loss of body tissue, causing the child to present a chubby appearance and to double his or her weight. After

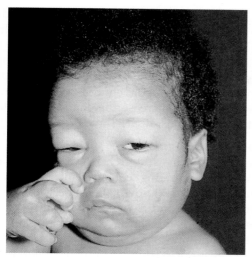

● *Figure 38.2* A child with nephrotic syndrome. Note the edema around the eyes.

diuresis, the malnutrition becomes quite apparent. These children are usually susceptible to infection, and repeated acute respiratory conditions are the usual pattern. This is intensified by the immunosuppression caused by the administration of prednisone.

Diagnosis

Laboratory findings include marked proteinuria, especially albumin, with large numbers of hyaline and granular casts in the urine. Hematuria is not usually present, although a few red blood cells may appear in the urine. The blood serum protein level is reduced, and there is an increase in the level of cholesterol in the blood (hyperlipidemia).

Treatment

The management of nephrotic syndrome is a long process with remissions and recurrence of symptoms common. The use of corticosteroids has induced remissions in most cases and has reduced recurrences. Corticosteroid therapy usually produces diuresis in about 7 to 14 days, but use of the drug is continued until a remission occurs. Prednisone is the drug most commonly used. After the diuresis occurs, intermittent therapy is continued every other day or for 3 days a week. Daily urine testing for protein is continued whether the child is at home or in the hospital. It is important that accurate documentation be kept to track patterns of protein loss in the child.

Diuretics may not be necessary when diuresis can be induced with steroids. Diuretics have not been effective in reducing the edema of nephrotic syndrome, although a loop diuretic (furosemide) may be administered if the edema causes respiratory compromise.

Immunosuppressant therapy may be used to reduce symptoms and prevent further relapses in children who do not respond adequately to corticosteroids. Cyclophosphamide (Cytoxan) is the drug most commonly used. Because cyclophosphamide has serious side effects, the family caregivers must be fully informed before therapy is started. **Leukopenia** (leukocyte count less than $5,000/mm^3$) can be expected, as well as the other common side effects of immunosuppressant therapy, such as gastrointestinal symptoms, hematuria, and alopecia. The length of therapy is usually a brief period of 2 or 3 months.

> **Maybe this will jog your memory on an exam.** Including foods high in potassium, such as bananas, oranges, and raisins, in the diet of a child taking a loop diuretic is helpful in maintaining adequate potassium levels.

A general diet is recommended that appeals to the child's poor appetite with frequent, small feedings if necessary. The addition of salt is discouraged, and sometimes the child is put on a low sodium diet. Family caregivers need encouragement and support for the long months ahead. Relapses usually become less frequent as the child gets older.

● Nursing Process for the Child With Nephrotic Syndrome

ASSESSMENT

Observe for edema when performing the physical examination of the child with nephrotic syndrome. Weigh the child and record the abdominal measurements to serve as a baseline. Obtain vital signs, including blood pressure. Note any swelling about the eyes or the ankles and other dependent parts, and record the degree of pitting. Inspect the skin for pallor, irritation, or breakdown. Examine the scrotal area of the male child for swelling, redness, and irritation. Question the caregiver about the onset of symptoms, the child's appetite, urine output, and signs of fatigue or irritability.

SELECTED NURSING DIAGNOSES

- Excess Fluid Volume related to fluid accumulation in tissues and third spaces
- Risk for Imbalanced Nutrition: Less Than Body Requirements related to anorexia
- Risk for Impaired Skin Integrity related to edema
- Fatigue related to edema and disease process

- Risk for Infection related to immunosuppression
- Deficient Knowledge of the caregiver related to disease process, treatment, and home care
- Compromised Family Coping related to care of a child with chronic illness

OUTCOME IDENTIFICATION AND PLANNING

The major goals for the child with nephrotic syndrome are relieving edema, improving nutritional status, maintaining skin integrity, conserving energy, and preventing infection. The family goals include learning about the disease and treatments, as well as learning ways to cope with the child's long-term care. Design the nursing care plan to include all these goals.

IMPLEMENTATION

Monitoring Fluid Intake and Output

Accurately monitor and document intake and output. Weigh the child at the same time every day on the same scale in the same clothing. Measure the child's abdomen daily at the level of the umbilicus, and make certain that all staff personnel measure at the same level.

The abdomen may be greatly enlarged with **ascites** (edema in the peritoneal cavity). The abdomen can even become marked with striae (stretch marks). Test the urine regularly for albumin and specific gravity. Albumin can be tested with reagent strips dipped into the urine and read by comparison with a color chart on the container.

This advice will be useful.
Note the desired location for measuring the abdomen of the child with nephrotic syndrome on the nursing care plan so that everyone follows the same practice.

Improving Nutritional Intake

Although the child may look plump, underneath the edema is a thin, possibly malnourished child. The child's appetite is poor for several reasons:

- The ascites diminishes the appetite because of the full feeling in the abdomen.
- The child may be lethargic, apathetic, and simply not interested in eating.
- A no-added-salt diet may be unappealing to the child.
- Corticosteroid therapy may decrease the appetite.

Offer a visually appealing and nutritious diet. Consult the child and the family to learn which foods are appealing to the child. Cater to the child's wishes as much as possible to perk up a lagging appetite. A dietitian can help to plan appealing meals for the child. Serving six small meals may help increase the child's total intake better than the customary three meals a day.

Promoting Skin Integrity

The child's skin is stretched with edema and becomes thin and fragile. Inspect all skin surfaces regularly for breakdown. Because the child is lethargic, turn and position the child every 2 hours. Protect skin surfaces from pressure by means of pillows and padding. Protect overlapping skin surfaces from rubbing by careful placement of cotton gauze. Bathe the child regularly. Thoroughly wash the skin surfaces that touch each other with soap and water and dry them completely. A sheer dusting of cornstarch may be soothing. If the scrotum is edematous, use a soft cotton support to provide comfort.

Promoting Energy Conservation

Bed rest is common during the edema stage of the condition. The child rarely protests because of his or her fatigue. The sheer bulk of the edema makes movement difficult. When diuresis occurs several days after beginning prednisone, the child may be allowed more activity, but balance the activity with rest periods and encourage the child to rest when fatigued. Plan quiet, age-appropriate activities that interest the child. Most children love having someone read to them. Coloring books, dominoes, puzzles, and some kinds of computer and board games are quiet activities that many children enjoy. Involve the family in providing some of these activities. Avoid using television excessively as a diversion.

Preventing Infection

The child with nephrotic syndrome is especially at risk for respiratory infections because the edema and the corticosteroid therapy lower the body's defenses. Protect the child from anyone with an infection: staff, family, visitors, and other children. Handwashing and strict medical asepsis are essential. Monitor vital signs every 4 hours and observe for any early signs of infection.

Providing Family Teaching and Support

Children with nephrotic syndrome are usually hospitalized for diagnosis, thorough evaluation of their general health and specific condition, and institution of therapy. If the child has an infection, a course of antibiotic therapy may be given; unless unforeseen complications develop, the child is discharged with complete instructions for management. Provide a written plan to help family caregivers follow the program successfully. They must keep a careful record of home treatment for the health care provider to review at regular intervals. Teach the family caregivers about reactions that may occur with the use of steroids and the adverse effects of abruptly discontinuing use of these drugs. If the family understands these aspects well, the incidence of forgetting to give the medication or of neglecting to refill the prescription may be reduced or eliminated. Encourage the family caregivers to report promptly any symptoms that they think are caused by the medication. Teach the family that the necessary special care is important to keep the child in optimum health, and that **intercurrent infections** (those occurring during the course of an already existing disease) must be reported promptly. Also teach the family that exacerbations are common and that they need to understand these will probably occur. Stress the information that they should report, including rapidly increasing weight, increased proteinuria, or signs of infections. Any of these may be a reason for altering the therapeutic regimen or changing the specific antibiotic agents used.

Provide the family caregivers with home care information appropriate for any chronically ill child. Bed rest is indicated during an intercurrent illness. Activity is restricted only by edema, which may slow the child down considerably; otherwise, normal activity is beneficial. Sufficient food intake may be a problem, as in other types of chronic illness. Fortunately there are usually no food restrictions, and the appetite can be tempted by attractive, appealing foods. As the name implies, MCNS causes few changes in the kidneys; these children have a good prognosis. Complications from kidney damage alter the course of treatment. Failure to achieve satisfactory diuresis or the need to discontinue steroids because of adverse reactions requires a reevaluation of treatment. The presence of gross hematuria suggests renal damage. In a few children, the persistence of abnormal urinary findings after diuresis presents a less hopeful outlook. A child who has frequent relapses lasting

into adolescence or adulthood may develop renal failure and eventually be a candidate for a kidney transplant.

EVALUATION: GOALS AND EXPECTED OUTCOMES

- **Goal:** The child's edema will be decreased.
  Expected Outcome: The child has appropriate weight loss and decreased abdominal girth.
- **Goal:** The child will have an adequate nutritional intake to meet normal growth needs.
  Expected Outcome: The child eats 80% or more of his or her meals.
- **Goal:** The child's skin integrity will be maintained.
  Expected Outcome: The child's skin remains free of breakdown with no redness or irritation.
- **Goal:** The child's energy will be conserved.
  Expected Outcome: The child rests as needed and engages in quiet diversional activities.
- **Goal:** The child will be free from signs and symptoms of infection.
  Expected Outcome: The child has normal vital signs with no respiratory or gastrointestinal symptoms.
- **Goal:** The family caregivers will verbalize an understanding of the disease process, treatment and the child's home care needs.
  Expected Outcomes: The family can explain nephrotic syndrome and can describe aspects of medications given. They state signs and symptoms of infection, discuss home care, and ask and answer appropriate questions.
- **Goal:** The family caregivers will verbalize feelings and concerns.
  Expected Outcomes: The family verbalizes feelings and concerns related to caring for a child with a chronic illness; the family receives adequate support.

Here's a hint. Help the family caregivers of the child with nephrotic syndrome develop a method for keeping accurate records—charts or calendars might work well.

Test Yourself

- Give examples of physiologic and psychological causes of enuresis.

- What is the presenting symptom in the child with nephrotic syndrome and where is this symptom noted?

- Why is the abdomen measured daily for the child with nephrotic syndrome? What might be detected with this measurement?

ACUTE GLOMERULONEPHRITIS

Acute glomerulonephritis is a condition that appears to be an allergic reaction to a specific infection, most often group A beta-hemolytic streptococcal infection, as in rheumatic fever. The antigen-antibody reaction causes a response that blocks the glomeruli, permitting red blood cells and protein to escape into the urine. Acute glomerulonephritis has a peak incidence in children 6 to 7 years of age and occurs twice as often in boys. The disease is similar in some ways to nephrotic syndrome (Table 38-2). The prognosis is usually excellent, but a few children develop chronic nephritis.

Clinical Manifestations

Presenting symptoms appear 1 to 3 weeks after the onset of a streptococcal infection, such as strep throat, otitis media, tonsillitis, or impetigo. Usually the presenting symptom is grossly bloody urine. The caregiver may describe the urine as smoky or bloody. Periorbital edema may accompany or precede hematuria. Fever may be 103°F to 104°F (39.4°C to 40°C) at the onset but decreases in a few days to about 100°F (37.8°C). Slight headache and malaise are usual, and vomiting may occur. Hypertension appears in 60% to 70% of patients during the first 4 or 5 days. Both hematuria and hypertension disappear within 3 weeks.

Oliguria (production of a subnormal volume of urine) is usually present, and the urine has a high specific gravity and contains albumin, red and white blood cells, and casts. The blood urea nitrogen and serum creatinine levels and the sedimentation rates are elevated. Cerebral symptoms consisting mainly of headache, drowsiness, convulsions, and vomiting occur in connection with hypertension in a few cases. When the blood pressure is reduced, these symptoms disappear. Cardiovascular disturbance may be revealed in electrocardiogram tracings, but few children have clinical signs. In most children, this condition is short-term; in some children, it progresses to congestive heart failure.

Treatment

Although the child usually feels well in a few days, activities should be limited until the clinical manifestations subside, generally 2 to 4 weeks after the onset. Penicillin may be given during the acute stage to eradicate any existing infection; however, it does not affect the recovery from the disease because the condition is an immunologic response. The diet is generally not restricted, but additional salt may be limited if edema is excessive. Treatment of complications is symptomatic.

Nursing Care

Bed rest should be maintained until acute symptoms and gross hematuria have disappeared. The child must be protected from chilling and contact with people with infections. When the child is allowed out of bed, he or she must not become fatigued.

Urinary output should be monitored closely and recorded.

TABLE 38.2	Comparison of Features of Acute Glomerulonephritis and Nephrotic Syndrome	
Assessment Factor	**Acute Glomerulonephritis**	**Nephrotic Syndrome**
Cause	Immune reaction to group A β-hemolytic streptococcal infection	Idiopathic; possibly a hypersensitivity reaction
Onset	Abrupt	Insidious
Hematuria	Grossly bloody	Rare
Proteinuria	3+ or 4+ but not massive	Massive
Edema	Mild	Extreme
Hypertension	Marked	Mild
Hyperlipidemia	Rare or mild	Marked
Peak age frequency	5–10 y	2–3 y
Interventions	Limited activity; antihypertensives as needed; symptomatic therapy if congestive heart failure occurs	Bed rest during edema stage Corticosteroid administration Possible cyclophosphamide administration
Diet	Normal for age; no added salt if child is hypertensive	Nutritious for age; no added salt; small, frequent meals may be desirable
Prevention	Prevention through treatment of group A β-hemolytic streptococcal infections	None known
Course	Acute: up to 2–3 weeks	Chronic: may have relapses

Adapted from Pillitteri, A. (2003). *Maternal and child health nursing* (4th ed.). Philadelphia: Lippincott Williams & Wilkins.

The amount of fluid the child is allowed may be based on output, as well as on evidence of continued hypertension and oliguria. Fluid intake should be carefully recorded; special attention is needed to keep the intake within prescribed limits. Blood pressure should be monitored regularly using the same arm and a properly fitting cuff. If hypertension develops, a diuretic may help reduce the blood pressure to normal levels. An antihypertensive drug may be added if the diastolic pressure is 90 mm Hg or higher. The urine must be tested regularly for protein and hematuria using dipstick tests. Traces of protein in the urine may persist for months after the acute symptoms disappear, and an elevated Addis count indicating red blood cells in the urine persists as well. Family caregivers must learn to test for urinary protein routinely. If the urinary signs persist for more than 1 year, the disease has probably assumed a chronic form.

Pay attention to the details. Weigh the child with acute glomerulonephritis daily, at the same time, on the same scale, and in the same clothes.

WILMS' TUMOR (NEPHROBLASTOMA)

Wilms' tumor, an adenosarcoma in the kidney region, is one of the most common abdominal neoplasms of early childhood. The tumor arises from bits of embryonic tissue that remain after birth. This tissue can spark rapid cancerous growth in the area of the kidney. The tumor is rarely discovered until it is large enough to be palpated through the abdominal wall. As the tumor grows, it invades the kidney or the renal vein and disseminates to other parts of the body. When the child is being evaluated and treated, a sign must be visibly posted stating that abdominal palpation should be avoided because cells may break loose and spread the tumor. Treatment consists of surgical removal as soon as possible after the growth is discovered, combined with radiation and chemotherapy.

Prognosis is best for the child younger than 2 years of age but has improved markedly for others with improved chemotherapy. Follow-up consists of regular evaluation for metastasis to the lungs or other sites. All long-term implications for chemotherapy apply to this child.

HYDROCELE

Hydrocele is a collection of peritoneal fluid that accumulates in the scrotum through a small passage called the processus vaginalis. This processus is a finger-like projection in the inguinal canal through which the testes descend. Usually the processus closes soon after birth; if the processus does not close, fluid from the peritoneal cavity passes through, causing hydrocele. This is the same passage through which intestines may slip, causing an inguinal hernia. If the hydrocele remains by the end of the 1st year, corrective surgery is performed.

CRYPTORCHIDISM

Shortly before or soon after birth, the male gonads (testes) descend from the abdominal cavity into their normal position in the scrotum. Occasionally one or both of the testes do not descend, which is a condition called cryptorchidism. The testes are usually normal in size; the cause for failure to descend is not clearly understood.

In most infants with cryptorchidism, the testes descend by the time the infant is 1 year old. If one or both testes have not descended by this age, treatment is recommended. If both testes remain undescended, the male will be sterile.

A surgical procedure called **orchiopexy** is used to bring the testis down into the scrotum and anchor it there. Some physicians prefer to try medical treatment—injections of human chorionic gonadotropic hormone—before doing surgery. If this is unsuccessful in bringing the testis down, orchiopexy is performed. Surgery usually is performed when the child is 1 to 2 years of age. Prognosis for a normal functioning testicle is good when the surgery is performed at this young age and no degenerative action has taken place before treatment.

MENSTRUAL DISORDERS

The beginning of menstruation, called **menarche,** normally occurs between the ages of 9 and 16 years. For many girls, this is a joyous affirmation of their womanhood, but others may have negative feelings about the event, depending on how they have been prepared for menarche and for their roles as women. Irregular menstruation is common during the 1st year until a regular cycle is established.

Some adolescent girls experience **mittelschmerz**, a dull, aching abdominal pain at the time of ovulation (hence the name, which means "midcycle"). The cause is not completely understood but the discomfort usually lasts only a few hours and is relieved by analgesics, a heating pad, or a warm bath.

Premenstrual Syndrome

Women of all ages are subject to the discomfort of **premenstrual syndrome (PMS),** but the symptoms may

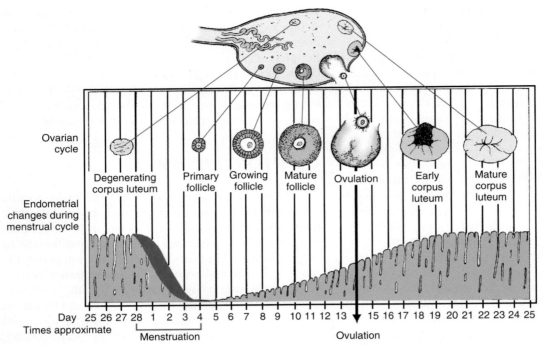

● **Figure 38.3** Schematic representation of a 28-day ovarian cycle. Menstruation occurs with shedding of the endometrium. The follicular phase is associated with the rapidly growing ovarian follicle and the production of estrogen. Ovulation occurs midcycle, and mittelschmerz may occur. The secretory phase follows in preparation for the fertilized ovum. If fertilization does not occur, the corpus luteum begins to degenerate, estrogen and progesterone levels decline, and menstruation again occurs.

be alarming to the adolescent. Symptoms include edema (resulting in weight gain), headache, increased anxiety, mild depression, and mood swings. The major cause of PMS is thought to be water retention after progesterone production after ovulation (Fig. 38-3).

Generally the discomforts of PMS are minor and can be relieved by reducing salt intake during the week before menstruation, taking mild analgesics, and applying local heat. When symptoms are more severe, the physician may prescribe a mild diuretic to be taken the week before menstruation to relieve edema; occasionally oral contraceptive pills are prescribed to prevent ovulation.

Dysmenorrhea

Dysmenorrhea (painful menstruation) is classified as primary or secondary. Many adolescent girls experience pain associated with menstruation, including cramping abdominal pain, leg pain, and backache. Primary dysmenorrhea occurs as part of the normal menstrual cycle without any associated pelvic disease. The increased secretion of prostaglandins, which occurs in the last few days of the menstrual cycle, is thought to be a contributing factor in primary dysmenorrhea. Nonsteroidal anti-inflammatory drugs (NSAIDs), such as ibuprofen (Advil, Motrin), inhibit prostaglandins

and are the treatment of choice for primary dysmenorrhea. These drugs are most effective when taken before cramps become too severe. Because NSAIDs are irritating to the gastric mucosa, they always should be taken with food and discontinued if epigastric burning occurs.

Secondary dysmenorrhea is the result of pelvic pathologic changes, most often pelvic inflammatory disease (PID) or endometriosis. The adolescent girl who has severe menstrual pain should be examined by a physician to determine if any pelvic pathologic changes are present. Treatment of the underlying condition helps relieve severe dysmenorrhea.

Amenorrhea

The absence of menstruation, or **amenorrhea,** can be primary (no previous menstruation) or secondary (missing three or more periods after menstrual flow has begun). Primary amenorrhea after 16 years of age warrants a diagnostic survey for genetic abnormalities, tumors, or other problems. Secondary amenorrhea can be the result of discontinuing contraceptives, a sign of pregnancy, the result of physical or emotional stressors, or a symptom of an underlying medical condition. A complete physical examination, including gynecologic screening is necessary to help determine the cause.

TABLE 38.3	Infectious Causes of Vaginitis		
Organism/Incidence	Symptoms	Sexual Transmission	Treatment
Candida albicans First episodes occur in adolescence, especially in sexually active girls	Severe itching, exacerbated just before menstruation Odor not present Milky "cottage cheese"–like discharge may be noted on examination	Normally present in vagina; most often results from glycosuria, antibiotic therapy, birth control pills, steroid therapy, or other factor that alters normal pH of vagina May result from oral–genital sex	Nystatin, miconazole (Monistat), or clotrimazole (Gyne-Lotrimin) vaginal suppositories or creams
Bacterial Vaginosis (multiple organisms) Common among adolescent girls; sexual partner will probably also be infected	About half of patients have no symptoms Fishy odor after intercourse Discharge, if present, grayish and thin	Sexually transmitted	Metronidazole (Flagyl)* or ampicillin; sexual partners may be treated
Trichomoniasis Most frequently diagnosed STD	Itching with severe infection, especially after menstruation Discharge has foul odor and may be frothy, gray or green	Sexually transmitted	Metronidazole (Flagyl)*, sexual partners also should be treated

* Flagyl is not ordered for the pregnant patient due to possible danger to fetus.

Test Yourself

- Acute glomerulonephritis may be an allergic reaction to what bacterium?

- If the testes remain undescended, what is the long-term complication for the male?

- When are the symptoms of glomerulonephritis seen and what is the most common symptom?

- How do premenstrual syndrome, dysmenorrhea, and amenorrhea differ?

VAGINITIS

Vaginitis (inflammation of the vagina) can result from a number of causes, such as diaphragms or tampons left in place too long, irritating douches or sprays, estrogen changes caused by birth-control pills, and antibiotic therapy. Actually these causes are precursors that provide an opportunity for the organisms to become active. The most common causes of vaginitis are *Candida albicans*, bacterial vaginosis (caused by *Gardnerella vaginalis*

and other organisms), and Trichomonas. Trichomonas is the only one of these organisms transmitted solely by sexual contact. (Table 38-3).

KEY POINTS

▶ Urinary tract infections are usually treated with antibiotics such as ampicillin or sulfisoxazole. The entire course of the medication should be taken, even if the symptoms subside after a few days.

▶ Physiologic causes of enuresis may include a small bladder capacity, urinary tract infection, and lack of awareness of the signal to empty the bladder because of sleeping too soundly.

▶ Edema is usually the presenting symptom in nephrotic syndrome, appearing first around the eyes and ankles. The edema becomes generalized with an abdomen full of fluid. Respiratory problems and edema of the scrotum on the male is characteristic. Anorexia, irritability, and loss of appetite develop.

▶ Acute glomerulonephritis is a condition that appears to be an allergic reaction to a specific infection, most often group A beta-hemolytic streptococcal infection, as in rheumatic fever.

- Presenting symptoms of acute glomerulonephritis appear 1 to 3 weeks after the onset of a streptococcal infection, with the most common symptom being grossly bloody urine. The urine may be described as smoky or bloody. Periorbital edema may accompany or precede hematuria.
- Nephrotic syndrome has an insidious onset and a course of remissions and exacerbations that usually last for months. Acute glomerulonephritis has an abrupt onset and usually last for 2 to 3 weeks.
- Hydrocele is a collection of peritoneal fluid that accumulates in the scrotum through a small finger-like projection in the inguinal canal through which the testes descend. Usually the processus closes soon after birth; if the processus does not close, fluid from the peritoneal cavity passes through, causing hydrocele.
- The condition called cryptorchidism occurs when the male gonads (testes) do not descend from the abdominal cavity into their normal position in the scrotum.
- Premenstrual syndrome (PMS) symptoms include edema (resulting in weight gain), headache, increased anxiety, mild depression, and mood swings. The major cause of PMS is thought to be water retention. Dysmenorrhea (painful menstruation) has symptoms of pain associated with menstruation, including cramping abdominal pain, leg pain, and backache. The absence of menstruation is called amenorrhea.

REFERENCES AND SELECTED READINGS

Books and Journals

Hockenberry, M. J., Wilson, D., Winkelstein, M. L., & Kline, N. E. (2003). *Wong's nursing care of infants and children* (7th ed.). St. Louis: Mosby.

Karch, A. M. (2003). *2004 Lippincott's nursing drug guide*. Philadelphia: Lippincott Williams & Wilkins.

Lawless, M. R., & McElderry, D. H. (2001). Nocturnal enuresis: Current concepts. *Pediatrics in Review, 22*(12), 399–407.

McEvoy, M., Chang, J., & Coupey, S. (2004). Common menstrual disorders in adolescence: Nursing interventions. *The American Journal of Maternal/Child Nursing, 29*, 41–49.

North American Nursing Diagnosis Association (NANDA). (2001). *NANDA nursing diagnoses: Definitions and classification 2001–2002*. Philadelphia: Author.

Pillitteri, A. (2003). *Maternal and child health nursing* (4th ed.). Philadelphia: Lippincott Williams & Wilkins.

Smeltzer, S. C., & Bare, B. G. (2003). *Textbook of medical–surgical nursing* (10th ed.). Philadelphia: Lippincott Williams & Wilkins.

Sparks, S., & Taylor, C. (2001). *Nursing diagnosis reference manual* (5th ed.). Springhouse, PA: Springhouse Corporation.

Wong, D. L., Perry, S., & Hockenberry, M. (2002). *Maternal–child nursing care* (2nd ed.). St. Louis: Mosby.

Web Addresses

www.kidney.org

www.enuresis.org

http://nephrologychannel.com

WORKBOOK

NCLEX-STYLE REVIEW QUESTIONS

1. After discussing ways to lower a fever with the caregiver of an infant who has a urinary tract infection, the caregiver makes the following statements. Which statement requires further teaching?

   a. "I won't give my child baby aspirin when she has a fever."

   b. "I know I need to dress my baby lightly if she has a fever."

   c. "When my baby has a fever, I will sponge her in cool water for 20 minutes."

   d. "I need to recheck my baby's temperature until it is below 101°F."

2. In caring for a child with nephrotic syndrome, which of the following interventions will be included in the child's plan of care?

   a. Ambulating three to four times a day

   b. Weighing on the same scale each day

   c. Increasing fluid intake by 50 cc an hour

   d. Testing the urine for glucose levels regularly

3. A child diagnosed acute glomerulonephritis will *most* likely have a history of which of the following?

   a. Sibling diagnosed with the same disease

   b. Recent illness such as strep throat

   c. Hemorrhage or history of bruising easily

   d. Hearing loss with impaired speech development

4. The nurse is teaching the caregiver of a 5-year-old child diagnosed with nephrotic syndrome regarding the no-added salt diet the child has been placed on. In addition to not adding salt to foods, the nurse has discussed with the caregiver that helping the child avoid foods high in sodium is also recommended. The caregiver marks the following foods on the child's menu selection for the next day. The nurse recognizes the caregiver needs further teaching when which of the following foods high in sodium were selected?
   Select all that apply.

   a. Cheddar cheese omelet

   b. Apple juice

   c. Blueberry muffin

   d. Hot dog in bun

   e. Fresh green beans

   f. Canned peaches

5. In caring for a child with a urinary tract infection, the nurse would do all of the following nursing interventions. Which two interventions would be the priority for the nurse? The nurse will

   a. collect a "clean catch" voided urine.

   b. record and report any indications of urinary burning, frequency, or urgency.

   c. observe for possible indications of sexual abuse.

   d. instruct caregivers to avoid bubble baths, especially in young girls.

   e. observe the child for signs of any reactions to the antibiotics.

   f. teach girls to wipe from front to back.

STUDY ACTIVITIES

1. Create a poster to use as a teaching aid for a group of family caregivers of a child with nephrotic syndrome. Include information regarding the use of steroids and the adverse effects of abruptly discontinuing use of the drug, as well as symptoms that might be caused by the medication.

2. Develop a method to help the caregivers of a child with nephrotic syndrome record information to be shared with their provider. Include information such as the child's weight, protein in the urine, and signs of infection.

3. Go to the following Internet site: http://www.pediatriconcall.com
   Click on "Childhood Diseases" under the "Parent Corner." On the left side of screen, click on "Childhood Ailments." Under "Kidney Problems in Children," click on "Nephrotic Syndrome." After reading the questions and answers, answer the following:

   a. What organ is involved in nephrotic syndrome?

   b. How is the child with nephrotic syndrome monitored?

c. What precautions should the caregivers of a child with nephrotic syndrome take for their child?

CRITICAL THINKING: What Would You Do?

1. Bradley is a 6-year-old boy who is in a play group with your child. Bradley's mother is talking with you and tells you she is concerned about Bradley because he has been potty trained, but now he is wetting the bed every night and sometimes has accidents during the day. She asks you if you think she should take her child to see their pediatrician.

   a. What would you suggest to Bradley's mother about seeing his pediatrician?

   b. What questions do you think the pediatrician might ask Bradley's mother?

   c. What are the possible physiologic causes of enuresis in children?

   d. What are frequent psychological causes of enuresis in children?

2. A classmate of yours has asked you to help give a presentation to a group of 12-year-old girls. The topic is human reproduction and sexuality.

During the discussion, one of the girls tells you she has heard of PMS (premenstrual syndrome) but doesn't know what it means.

   a. What will you explain to this group of girls regarding what PMS is?

   b. What is the physiologic cause of PMS?

   c. What symptoms might be seen when a woman is experiencing PMS?

   d. What will you explain to this group regarding the treatments that may be done when a woman experiences PMS?

3. Dosage calculation: A preschool child with a diagnosis of nephrotic syndrome is being treated with Prednisolone. The child is being given a dose of 40 mg a day. The child weighs 44 pounds. Answer the following:

   a. How many kilograms (kg) does the child's weigh?

   b. How many milligrams (mg) per kilogram is this child's dose?

   c. If the dose is decreased to 30 mg a day, how many milligrams per kilogram will this dose be?

The Child With Musculoskeletal Disorders

STUDENT OBJECTIVES

On completion of this chapter, the student should be able to

1. Discuss ways the child's musculoskeletal system differs from the adult's system.
2. Discuss four types of fractures seen in children.
3. Describe the purpose of doing neurovascular checks in a child with a musculoskeletal disorder.
4. List and define the five Ps to observe, record, and report when caring for a child in a cast.
5. Name the bacterium that usually causes osteomyelitis.
6. Identify the most common form of muscular dystrophy and describe its characteristics.
7. Identify the treatment for the child with osteosarcoma and Ewing's sarcoma.
8. Name the drugs of choice in the treatment of juvenile rheumatoid arthritis and state the primary purpose of these drugs.
9. Describe scoliosis and identify three methods of correction.

KEY TERMS

ankylosis
compartment syndrome
halo traction
kyphosis
lordosis
scoliosis
skeletal traction
skin traction
traction

As children explore the environment around them, they often cause injury to their musculoskeletal system. Physical activities including play and team sports create situations in which minor skeletal injuries, such as sprains and minor fractures, occur. However, some disorders of the musculoskeletal system can have lifelong effects.

GROWTH AND DEVELOPMENT OF THE MUSCULOSKELETAL SYSTEM

The musculoskeletal system provides the structure and framework to support, protect, and permit movement of the body. Bones are attached to each other by connecting links called joints, which allows for movement of the body parts. Skeletal muscles attach to the bones, with a moveable joint between them. Tendons and ligaments hold the bones together. Contraction of the muscles causes movement to take place. The heat produced as the muscles contract maintains the body temperature at a stable level. Minerals such as calcium, phosphorus, magnesium, and fluoride are stored in the bones. Blood cells are produced in the bone marrow.

The skeletal system is made up of four types of bone, each having a different function. Each of these types of bones has a specific shape—long, short, flat, irregular. During fetal life, tissue called cartilage, a type of connective tissue consisting of cells implanted in a gel-like substance, gradually calcifies and becomes bone. This calcification process develops the cartilage tissue into the major bones of the body.

Long bones grow from the long central shaft of the bone called the diaphysis to the rounded end part of the bone called the epiphysis. Cartilage makes up the epiphyseal plate that is between the epiphysis and the diaphysis. As long as cartilage remains, the child's bones continue to grow. Bones grow in width at the same time they are growing in length. When the epiphyseal plate becomes an epiphyseal line and cartilage no longer is present, this marks the end of the growth of that bone in the child. Bone growth takes place between birth and puberty, with most growth being complete by age 20 years.

During childhood the bones are more sponge-like and can bend and break more easily than in adults. In addition, because the bones are still in the process of growing, breaks in the bone heal more quickly than do breaks in adults.

The bones of the skull give shape to the head. The areas where these bones meet are called suture lines. These suture lines do not ossify or harden into bone during fetal life. Because these suture lines are not

● **Figure 39.1** Bones and muscles of the body.

fused, during delivery the bones of the skull can move and overlap, allowing for the head to pass through the birth canal. Within the first 2 years of life, these suture lines or fontanels fuse together.

The spine or vertebral column is made up of a series of separate bones connected in a way that allows for flexibility. There are four distinct curves in the adult spine. At birth the spine is a continuous rounded convex curve. As the infant learns to hold up the head, the neck develops into a reverse curve. When the child begins to stand, another reverse curve is formed in the lower part of the back. The curves in the spine give support, strength, and balance to the body.

As the child grows, the muscles become stronger and the child has more muscle tone, strength, and coordination (Fig. 39-1).

FRACTURES

A fracture, a break in a bone that is usually accompanied by vascular and soft tissue damage, is characterized by pain, swelling, and tenderness. Children's fractures differ from those of adults in that generally they are less complicated, heal more quickly, and usually occur from different causes. The child has an urge to explore the environment but lacks the experience and judgment to recognize possible hazards. In some instances, caregivers may be negligent in their supervision, but often the child uses immature judgment or is simply too fast for them.

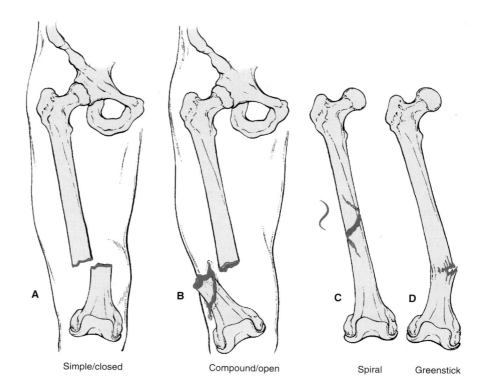

● *Figure 39.2* Types of fractures. All are examples of complete fractures except *D*, which is an incomplete fracture.

Simple/closed   Compound/open   Spiral   Greenstick

The bones most commonly fractured in childhood are the clavicle, femur, tibia, humerus, wrist, and fingers. The classification of a fracture reflects the kind of bone injury sustained (Fig. 39-2). If the fragments of fractured bone are separated, the fracture is said to be complete. If fragments remain partially joined, the fracture is termed incomplete. Greenstick fractures are one kind of incomplete fracture, caused by incomplete ossification, common in children.

Did you know? When a child has a greenstick fracture, the bone bends and often just partially breaks, just as a green tree stick does when one tries to break it, thus the name "greenstick" fracture.

When a broken bone penetrates the skin, the fracture is called compound, or open. A simple, or closed, fracture is a single break in the bone without penetration of the skin. Spiral fractures, which twist around the bone, are frequently associated with child abuse and are caused by a wrenching force. Fractures in the area of the epiphyseal plate (growth plate) can cause permanent damage and severely impair growth (Fig. 39-3).

Be aware. Fractures occurring in the epiphyseal plate (growth plate) can cause permanent damage.

Treatment and Nursing Care

Most childhood fractures are treated by realignment and immobilization using either traction or closed manipulation and casting. A few patients with

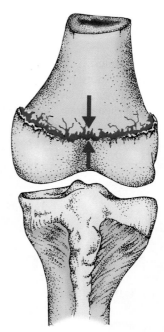

● *Figure 39.3* One form of epiphyseal injury; a crushing injury (as might occur in a fall from a height) can destroy the layer of germinal cells of the epiphysis, resulting in disturbance of growth.

severe fractures or additional injuries, such as burns and other soft tissue damage, may require surgical reduction, internal or external fixation, or both. Internal fixation devices include rods, pins, screws, and plates made of inert materials that will not trigger an immune reaction. They allow early mobilization of the child to a wheelchair, crutches, or a walker.

External fixation devices are used primarily in complex fractures often with other injuries or complications. These devices are applied under sterile conditions in the operating room and may be augmented by soft dressings and elevated by means of an overhead traction rope. External fixation devices rarely are used on young children.

Casts

The kind of cast used is determined by the age of the child, the severity of the fracture, the type of bone involved, and the amount of weight bearing the child is allowed to have on the extremity. Most casts are formed from gauze strips impregnated with plaster of Paris or other synthetic material, such as fiberglass or polyurethane resin, which is pliable when wet but hardens when dry. Synthetic materials are lighter in weight and present a cleaner appearance because they can be sponged with water when soiled.

Have some fun with this. Casts made of synthetic material are available in many colors. Children enjoy choosing a color that is a favorite, a school color, or a color associated with a specific holiday, such as red for Valentine's Day.

Synthetic casts dry more rapidly than do plaster of Paris casts. The lightweight casts tend to be used as arm casts and hip spica casts that are used to treat infants with congenital hip conditions. The hip spica cast covers the lower part of the body, usually from the waist down, and either one or both legs while leaving the feet open. The cast maintains the legs in a frog-like position. Usually there is a bar placed between the legs to help support the cast.

The child and the family should be taught what to expect after the cast is applied and how to care for the casted area. A stockinette is applied over the area to be casted, and the bony prominences are padded before the wet gauze-impregnated rolls are applied. Although the wet plaster of Paris feels cool on the skin when applied, evaporation soon causes a temporary sensation of warmth. The cast will feel heavy and cumbersome (Fig. 39-4).

A wet plaster cast should be handled only with open palms because fingertips can cause indentations and result in pressure points. If the cast has no protective edge, it should be petaled (see Figure 22B in Chapter 21) with adhesive tape strips. If the cast is near the genital area, plastic should be taped around the edge to prevent wetting and soiling of the cast.

After the fracture has been immobilized, any reports of pain signal possible complications, such as **compartment syndrome,** and should be recorded and reported immediately. Compartment syndrome is a serious neurovascular concern that occurs when increasing pressure within the muscle compartment causes decreased circulation. It is important for the nurse to monitor the child's neurovascular status frequently because of the risk of tissue and nerve damage.

This is critical to remember. *Any* complaint of pain in a child with a new cast or immobilized extremity needs to be explored and monitored closely for the possibility of compartment syndrome.

● *Figure 39.4* (**A**) Fiberglass cast is being applied (**B**) Following cast application, nurse checks the circulation in the hand.

Monitoring the neurovascular status is sometimes referred to as CMS (circulation, movement, sensation) checks and includes observing, documenting, and reporting the five Ps:

- Pain: Any sign of pain should be noted and the exact area determined.
- Pulse: If an upper extremity is involved, brachial, radial, ulnar, and digital pulses should be checked. If a lower extremity is involved, femoral, popliteal, posterior tibial, and dorsalis pedis pulses should be monitored.
- Paresthesia: Check for any diminished or absent sensation or for numbness or tingling.
- Paralysis: Check hand function by having the child try to hyperextend the thumb or wrist, oppose the thumb and little finger, and adduct all fingers. Check function of the foot by having the child try to dorsiflex and plantarflex the ankles and flex and extend the toes.
- Pallor: Check the extremity and the nail beds distal to the site of the fracture for color. Pallor, discoloration, and coldness indicate circulatory impairment.

In addition to the five Ps, any foul odor or drainage on or under the cast, "hot spots" on the cast (areas warm to touch), looseness or tightness, or any elevation of temperature must be noted, documented, and reported. Family caregivers should be instructed to watch carefully for these same danger signals.

A PERSONAL GLIMPSE

One day I was jumping on my bed, trying to do a flip, but instead I fell on my arm. It hurt really bad and I cried. I told my mom, and she put ice on it. But then I went to soccer camp the next day, and I fell on it again. It hurt even worse. My mom took me to the doctor's office. I could wiggle my fingers, but it only kind of hurt at the doctor's. So they took an x-ray. It was fun to see the picture of my arm. The next day I fell again at soccer camp; I was standing on my ball. This time my mom was sure it was broken. We went to get a cast. I chose a blue cast. My arm felt better, but I felt bad because it was my big sister's birthday. Everyone signed it. I had my cast on for 4 weeks. I couldn't wait to get it off. I finally got my cast off. I was excited! The girl used a saw to take it off. I wasn't scared. My arm really smelled bad! They took another x-ray to make sure my arm was better. It was!! Then we left and my mom washed my arm and put sunscreen on it. After that everyone had trouble telling me and my twin apart.

Cassey, age 8

LEARNING OPPORTUNITY: What explanations would you give this child regarding the reason the x-rays were taken, the process of putting the cast on, and what to expect when the cast was removed? Which actions carried out by this mother would be important for the nurse to reinforce as appropriate actions for this situation?

Here's a helpful hint. Blowing cool air through a cast with a hair dryer set on a cool temperature or using a fan may help to relieve discomfort under a cast.

Children and caregivers should be cautioned not to put anything inside the cast, no matter how much the casted area itches. Small toys and sticks or stick-like objects should be kept out of reach until the cast has been removed.

When the fracture has healed, the cast is removed with a cast cutter. This can be frightening for the child unless the person using the cast cutter explains and demonstrates that the device will not cut flesh but only the hard surface of the cast. The child should be told that there will be vibration from the cast cutter, but it will not burn.

After cast removal, the casted area should be soaked in warm water to help remove the crusty layer of accumulated skin. Application of oil or lotion may prove comforting. Family caregivers and the child must be cautioned against scrubbing or scraping this area because the tender layer of new skin underneath the crust may bleed. Sunscreen should be applied to the previously casted area when the child will have sun exposure.

Traction

Traction is a pulling force applied to an extremity or other part of the body. A body part is pulled in one direction against a counter-pull or countertraction exerted in the opposite direction. A system of weights, ropes, and pulleys is used to realign and immobilize fractures, reduce or eliminate muscle spasm, and prevent fracture deformity and joint contractures.

Two basic types of traction are used: skin traction and skeletal traction. **Skin traction** applies pull on tape, rubber, or a plastic material attached to the skin, which indirectly exerts pull on the musculoskeletal system. Examples of skin traction are Bryant's traction, Buck extension traction, and Russell traction. **Skeletal traction** exerts pull directly on skeletal structures by means of a pin, wire, tongs, or other device surgically inserted through a bone. Examples of skeletal traction are 90-degree traction and balanced suspension traction. Dunlop's traction, sometimes used for fractures of the

● *Figure 39.5* Types of traction. (**A**) Buck extension, skin traction. (**B**) Russell traction, skin traction. Two lines of traction (one horizontal and one vertical) allow for good bone alignment for healing. (**C**) 90°–90° (skeletal) traction; a wire pin is inserted into the distal femur. (**D**) Balanced suspension traction. (**E**) Dunlop's traction (skeletal).

humerus or the elbow, can be either skin or skeletal traction. It is skeletal traction if a pin is inserted into the bone to immobilize the extremity (Fig. 39-5).

Bryant's traction (Fig. 39-6) is often used for the treatment of a fractured femur in children younger

than 2 years of age. These fractures are often transverse (crosswise to the long axis of the bone) or spiral fractures. The child's legs are wrapped with elastic bandages that should be removed at least daily to observe the skin, then rewrapped. Skin temperature and the color of the legs and feet must be checked frequently to detect any circulatory impairment. The use of Bryant's traction entails some risk of compromised circulation and may result in contractures of the foot and lower leg, particularly in an older child. Severe pain may indicate circulatory difficulty and should be reported immediately. When a child is in Bryant's traction, the hips should not rest on the bed; a hand should be able to pass between the child's buttocks and the sheet.

Buck extension traction, in which the child's body provides the countertraction to the weights, is used for short-term immobilization. It is used to correct contractures and bone deformities such as Legg-Calvé-Perthes disease. For older children, Russell traction seems to be more effective.

● *Figure 39.6* An infant in Bryant's traction is being fed.

However, a child in either type of traction tends to slide down until the weights rest on the bed or the floor. The child should be pulled up to keep the weights free, the ropes must be in alignment with the pulleys, and the alignment should be checked frequently. An older child may try to coax a roommate to remove the weights or the sandbags used as weights.

Pay attention to the details. When a child is in traction the weights must be hanging freely, not touching the bed or floor.

Children in any kind of traction must be carefully monitored to detect any signs of neurovascular complications. Skin temperature and color, presence or absence of edema, peripheral pulse, sensation, and motion must be monitored every hour for the first 24 hours after traction has been applied and every 4 hours after the first 24 hours unless ordered otherwise. Skin care must be meticulous. Skin preparation (Skin-Prep) should be used to toughen the skin, rather than lotions or oils that soften the skin and contribute to tissue breakdown.

Children in skeletal traction require special attention to pin sites. Pin care should be performed every 8 hours. The provider may order that povidone-iodine or a hydrogen peroxide solution be used to clean the pin sites. Standard precautions and aseptic technique reduce the risk for infection. Any sign of infection (odor, local inflammation, or elevated temperature) must be recorded and reported at once. (See the Nursing Care Plan 39-1: The Child in Traction.)

External Fixation Devices

In children who have severe fractures or conditions such as having one extremity shorter than the other, external fixation devices are used to correct the condition (Fig. 39-7). When an external fixation device is used, special skin care at the pin sites is also necessary. The sites are left open to the air and should be inspected and cleansed every 8 hours. The appearance of the pins puncturing the skin and the unusual appearance of the device can be upsetting to the child, so be sensitive to any anxiety the child expresses.

As early as possible, the child (if old enough) or family caregivers should be taught to care for the pin sites. External fixation devices are sometimes left in place for as long as 1 year; therefore, it is important that the child accepts this temporary change in body image and learns to care for the affected site. Children with these devices probably will work with a physical therapist during the rehabilitation period and will have specific exercises to perform. Before discharge from the hospital, the child should feel comfortable

● **Figure 39.7** External fixation device.

moving about and should be able to recognize the signs of infection at the pin sites.

Crutches

Children with fractures of the lower extremities and other lower leg injuries often must learn to use crutches to avoid weight bearing on the injured area. Several types of crutches are available. The most common are axillary crutches, which are principally used for temporary situations. Forearm, or Canadian, crutches usually are recommended for children who need crutches permanently, such as paraplegic children with braces. Trough, or platform, crutches are more suitable for children with limited strength or function in the arms and hands.

The use of crutches is generally taught by a physical therapist, but it can be the responsibility of nurses. The type of crutch gait taught is determined by the amount of weight bearing permitted, the child's degree of stability, whether or not the knees can be flexed, and the specific treatment goal.

NURSING CARE PLAN 39.1

The Child in Traction

TD is a 9-year-old boy who has been hospitalized following a serious bicycle accident in which he was struck by a motor vehicle. In the accident he sustained a fractured right femur and several cuts and abrasions. He has been placed in balanced suspension traction and will be in traction for several weeks before the extremity can be cast. He is in the 4th grade at school and plays soccer and basketball.

NURSING DIAGNOSIS
Risk for Peripheral Neurovascular Dysfunction related to fracture or effects of traction

GOAL: The child will maintain circulation and normal neurovascular status in extremities.

EXPECTED OUTCOMES
- The child's pulse rate is within a normal range with adequate pulses and capillary refill in all extremities.
- The child has good skin color and temperature, appropriate movement and sensation in all extremities.

NURSING INTERVENTIONS	RATIONALE
Maintain proper body alignment with traction weights and pulleys hanging free of bed and off the floor.	Body alignment must be maintained to prevent permanent injury or disalignment and decreased range of motion in effected extremity.
Monitor pulses in right leg and compare to pulses in other extremity.	Comparison helps to determine if circulation is adequate in affected extremity.
Monitor skin in extremities for color, temperature, sensation, and movement.	Any change in neurovascular status could indicate impaired nerve function.
Record and report any change in neurovascular status.	Immediate reporting leads to rapid treatment and decreases likelihood of long-term damage.

NURSING DIAGNOSIS
Impaired Skin Integrity related to abrasions
High Risk for Impaired Skin Integrity related to immobility

GOAL: The child will exhibit healed skin abrasions and no further skin breakdown.

EXPECTED OUTCOMES
- The child's skin abrasions heal without signs or symptoms of infection.
- The child's skin remains intact without redness or irritation.

NURSING INTERVENTIONS	RATIONALE
Wash and thoroughly dry skin every day.	Stimulates circulation and keeps skin clean
Inspect skin at least every 4 hours for evidence of redness or broken skin.	Allows early detection and treatment of skin breakdown, which can prevent long-term complications
Change position every 2 hours within restraints of traction.	Relieves pressure and decreases likelihood of skin breakdown and decreased circulation
Clean pin sites as ordered following standard precautions.	Decreases risk of infection
Observe for redness, drainage at pin sites, and elevated temperature.	Identifies signs and symptoms of possible infection

NURSING DIAGNOSIS
Activity Intolerance related to skeletal traction and bed rest

GOAL: The child will maintain adequate range of motion.

EXPECTED OUTCOMES
- The child performs range of motion within limits of traction.
- The child does own self-care activities.
- The child participates in age-appropriate activities within restrictions of traction.

NURSING CARE PLAN 39.1 continued

The Child in Traction

NURSING INTERVENTIONS	RATIONALE
Teach child active and passive range-of-motion exercises.	Maintains joint function and exercises circulation
Encourage child to become active in self-care.	Provides a feeling of control over hospitalization; increases use of parts of body not immobilized to allow normal muscle function

NURSING DIAGNOSIS
Deficient Diversional Activity related to lengthy hospitalization

GOAL: The child will achieve developmental tasks appropriate for age.

EXPECTED OUTCOMES
- The child selects and participates in age-appropriate activities and play.
- The child shows enjoyment in participating in activities.
- The child communicates and interacts with peers.

NURSING INTERVENTIONS	RATIONALE
Provide age-appropriate games, supplies, and activities that the child can do while in traction such as books, puzzles, computer games.	Permits access to age-appropriate activities to help the child develop and achieve milestones of growth and development.
Encourage child to communicate with peers by telephone, letter, computer.	Allows for normal growth and development opportunities
Move child's bed to hallway or playroom to enable participation in activities.	Increases interaction with other children; decreases boredom

Test Yourself

- Explain the difference between a simple or closed fracture and a compound or open fracture.

- What is a greenstick fracture? What is a spiral fracture?

- How are fractures usually treated?

- What is monitored when doing neurovascular checks on a child with a fracture?

OSTEOMYELITIS

Osteomyelitis is an infection of the bone usually caused by *Staphylococcus aureus*. Acute osteomyelitis is twice as common in boys and results from a primary infection, such as a staphylococcal skin infection (impetigo), burns, a furuncle (boil), a penetrating wound, or a fracture. The bacteria enter the bloodstream and are carried to the metaphysis of a bone, where an abscess forms, ruptures, and spreads the infection along the bone under the periosteum.

Clinical Manifestations and Diagnosis

Symptoms usually begin abruptly with fever, malaise, and pain and localized tenderness over the metaphysis of the affected bone. Joint motion is limited. Diagnosis is based on laboratory findings of leukocytosis (15,000 to 25,000 cells or more), an increased erythrocyte sedimentation rate, and positive blood cultures. Radiographic examination does not reveal the process until 5 to 10 days after the onset.

Treatment

Treatment for acute osteomyelitis must be immediate. Intravenous antibiotic therapy is started at once and continued for at least 6 weeks. Depending on the physician and the compliance of the child and family, a short course of intravenous (IV) antibiotics may be followed by administration of oral antibiotics to complete treatment. Surgical drainage of the involved metaphysis may be performed. If the abscess has ruptured into the subperiosteal space, chronic osteomyelitis follows.

If prompt, specific antibiotic treatment is vigorously employed, acute osteomyelitis may be brought under control rapidly and extensive bone destruction of chronic osteomyelitis is prevented. If extensive destruction of bone has occurred before treatment, surgical removal of necrotic bone becomes necessary.

Nursing Care

During the acute stage, nursing care includes reducing pain by positioning the affected limb, minimizing movement of the limb, and administering medication.

Nursing judgment is in order.
In children with osteomyelitis, transmission-based precautions may be required if a wound is open and draining.

Follow the usual procedure for IV antibiotic therapy, including careful observance of the venipuncture site and monitoring of the rate, dosage, and time of antibiotic administration. An intermittent infusion device or peripherally inserted central catheter may be used for long-term IV therapy.

Monitor oral nutrition and fluids because the child's appetite may be poor during the acute phase and may improve in later stages. Weight bearing on the affected limb must be avoided until healing has occurred because pathologic fractures occur very easily in the weakened stage. Physical therapy helps restore limb function.

MUSCULAR DYSTROPHY

Muscular dystrophy is a hereditary, progressive, degenerative disease of the muscles. The most common form of muscular dystrophy is Duchenne (pseudohypertrophic) muscular dystrophy. Duchenne muscular dystrophy, an X-linked recessive hereditary disease, occurs almost exclusively in males. Females usually are carriers of the disease. When muscular dystrophy has been diagnosed in a child, the mother and the siblings should be tested to see if they have the disease or are carriers.

Clinical Manifestations and Diagnosis

The first signs are noted in infancy or childhood, usually within the first 3 to 4 years of life. The child has difficulty standing and walking, and later trunk muscle weakness develops. Mild mental retardation often accompanies this disease. The child cannot rise easily to an upright position from a sitting position on the floor; instead, he or she rises by climbing up the lower extremities with the hands (Fig. 39-8). Weakness of leg, arm, and shoulder muscles progresses gradually. Increasing abnormalities in gait and posture appear by

● **Figure 39.8** Child "climbing up" lower extremities.

● **Figure 39.9** Characteristic posture of a child with Duchenne muscular dystrophy. Along with the typical toe gait, the child develops a lordotic posture as Duchenne dystrophy causes further deterioration.

school age, with **lordosis** (forward curvature of the lumbar spine or swayback), pelvic waddling, and frequent falling (Fig. 39-9). The child becomes progressively weaker, usually becoming wheelchair-bound by 10 to 12 years of age (middle school or junior high school age). The disease continues into adolescence and young adulthood, when the patient usually succumbs to respiratory or heart failure.

In addition to symptoms in the first 2 years of life, highly increased serum creatinine phosphokinase levels, as well as a decrease in muscle fibers seen in a muscle biopsy, can confirm the diagnosis.

Treatment and Nursing Care

No effective treatment for the disease has been found, but research is rapidly closing in on genetic identification, which promises exciting changes in treatment in the future. The child is encouraged to be as active as possible to delay muscle atrophy and contractures. To help keep the child active, physiotherapy, diet to avoid obesity, and parental encouragement are important.

When a child becomes wheelchair-bound, **kyphosis** (hunchback) develops and causes a decrease in respiratory function and an increase in the incidence of infections. Breathing exercises are a daily necessity for these children.

The nurse should advise the family to keep the child's life as normal as possible, which may be difficult. This disease can drain the emotional and financial reserves of the entire family. The nurse might suggest assistance through the Muscular Dystrophy Association—USA (National Headquarters, 3300 E. Sunrise Drive, Tucson, AZ 85718; 800-572-1717; website: http://www.mdausa.org), through local chapters of this organization, and by talking with other parents who face the same problem.

LEGG-CALVÉ-PERTHES DISEASE (COXA PLANA)

Legg-Calvé-Perthes disease is an aseptic necrosis of the head of the femur. It occurs four to five times more often in boys than in girls and 10 times more often in whites than in other ethnic groups. It can be caused by trauma to the hip, but generally the cause is unknown.

Clinical Manifestations and Diagnosis

Symptoms first noticed are pain in the hip or groin and a limp accompanied by muscle spasms and limitation of motion. These symptoms mimic synovitis (inflammation of a joint, which is most commonly the hip in children), which makes immediate diagnosis difficult. Radiographic examination may need to be repeated several weeks after the initial visit to demonstrate vascular necrosis for a definitive diagnosis.

There are three stages of the disease; each lasts 9 months to 1 year. In the first stage, radiographic studies show opacity of the epiphysis. In the second stage, the epiphysis becomes mottled and fragmented; during the third stage, reossification occurs.

Treatment and Nursing Care

In the past, immobilization of the hip through the use of braces and crutches and bed rest with traction or casting was considered essential for recovery without deformity. However, restricting a child's activity for 2 years or more was extremely difficult. Current treatment focuses on containing the femoral head within the acetabulum during the revascularization process so that the new femoral head will form to make a smoothly functioning joint. The method of containment varies with the portion of the head affected. Use of a brace that holds the necrotic portions of the head in place during healing is considered an effective method of containment. Reconstructive surgery is now possible, enabling the child to return to normal activities within 3 to 4 months.

The prognosis for complete recovery without difficulty later in life depends on the child's age at the time of onset, the amount of involvement, and the cooperation of the child and the family caregivers.

Nursing care focuses on helping the child and caregivers to manage the corrective device and the importance of compliance to promote healing and avoid long-term disability.

OSTEOSARCOMA

Osteosarcoma is a malignant tumor seen in the long bones, such as the femur, thigh, and humerus. It is more frequently seen in boys than in girls. Children who have had exposure to radiation or retinoblastoma are more prone to the malignancy.

Clinical Manifestations and Diagnosis

An injury such as a sports injury may draw attention to the pain and swelling at the sight of the tumor, but the injury itself did not cause the tumor. It is important to explain this to the child and caregiver to decrease their possible feelings of guilt. Pathologic fractures of the bone can occur.

A biopsy, as well as radiography, bone scan, computed tomography (CT), and magnetic resonance imaging (MRI), confirm the diagnosis. Metastasis to the lungs can occur.

Treatment and Nursing Care

Surgical removal of the bone or the limb followed by chemotherapy is the treatment for the tumor. A prosthesis is fitted, often soon after the surgery.

A cancer diagnosis is frightening to the child and family, and honest answers and support are helpful. After an amputation, phantom pain in the amputated extremity can be relentless. Learning to live with a prosthesis may be a long and challenging process. Support groups with other children living with a prosthetic device can be helpful. With early diagnosis and treatment, many children survive this diagnosis and live into adulthood.

EWING'S SARCOMA

Ewing's sarcoma is a malignant tumor found in the bone marrow of the long bones. It is often seen in older school-age or adolescent boys.

Clinical Manifestations and Diagnosis

As with osteosarcoma, many times an injury draws attention to the pain at the site of the tumor. The pain may be sporadic for a period of time but continues and becomes severe enough to keep the child awake at nighttime. Metastasis to the lung and other bones may already have taken place by the time of diagnosis.

A biopsy, bone scan, and bone marrow aspiration are done to further diagnose the tumor.

Treatment and Nursing Care

The tumor is removed and radiation as well as chemotherapy is given. In many cases the limb does not have to be amputated, although this may be part of the treatment.

About half of the children with Ewing's sarcoma achieve a 5-year survival rate, especially if there is no metastasis at the time of diagnosis. Adjusting to the course and effects of chemotherapy, such as hair loss, nausea, and vomiting, is difficult and offering support and encouragement is an important role of the nurse.

JUVENILE RHEUMATOID ARTHRITIS

Juvenile rheumatoid arthritis (JRA) is the most common connective tissue disease of childhood. Connective tissues are those that provide a supportive framework and protective covering for the body, such as the musculoskeletal system and skin and mucous membranes. The occurrence of JRA appears to peak at two age levels: 1 to 3 years and 8 to 12 years. This disease has a long duration, but 85% of children with JRA reach adulthood without serious disability (Cassidy, 1999).

Clinical Manifestations

Joint inflammation occurs first; if untreated, inflammation leads to irreversible changes in joint cartilage, ligaments, and menisci (the crescent-shaped fibrocartilage in the knee joints), eventually causing complete immobility. It can be subdivided into three different types: systemic; polyarticular, involving five or more joints; and oligoarthritis (pauciarticular), involving four or fewer joints, most often the knees and the ankles (Table 39-1).

Treatment and Nursing Care

The treatment goal is to maintain mobility and preserve joint function. Treatment can include drugs,

TABLE 39.1	Characteristics of Different Types of Juvenile Rheumatoid Arthritis		
Sign/Symptom of Onset	Polyarthritis	Oligoarthritis (Pauciarticular)	Systemic
Frequency of cases	30%–40%	50%–60%	10%–15%
Number of joints involved	5 or more	4 or fewer	Variable
Sex ratio (F:M)	3:1	5:1	1:1
Systemic involvement	Moderate	Not present	Prominent
Uveitis*	5%	20%	Rare
Sensitivity Rheumatoid factors Antinuclear bodies	10% 40%–50%	Rare 75%–85%	Rare 10%
Course	Systemic disease is generally mild; articular involvement may be unremitting	Systemic disease is absent; major cause of morbidity is uveitis	Systemic disease is often self-limited; arthritis is chronic and destructive in 50%
Prognosis	Guarded to moderately good	Excellent except for eyesight	Moderate to poor

*Uveitis–an inflammation of the middle (vascular) tunic of the eye: includes the iris, cilliary body, and choroide.

Adapted from Cassidy, J. T. (1999). Rheumatic disease of childhood. In J. A. McMillan, C. D. DeAngelis, R. D. Feigin, & J. W. Warghaw (Eds.), *Oski's pediatrics: Principles and practice* (3rd ed.). Philadelphia: Lippincott Williams & Wilkins.

physical therapy, and surgery. Early diagnosis and drug therapy to control inflammation and other systemic changes can reduce the need for other types of treatment.

Drug Therapy

Enteric-coated aspirin has long been the drug of choice for JRA, but because of the concern of aspirin therapy and Reye syndrome (see Chapter 34), NSAIDs (nonsteroidal anti-inflammatory drugs) are being used frequently to replace aspirin in treatment of JRA. Aspirin may still be used because it is an effective anti-inflammatory drug, inexpensive, easily administered, and has few side effects when carefully regulated. Both aspirin and NSAIDs such as naproxen and ibuprofen may cause gastrointestinal irritation and bleeding.

Don't forget. Administer aspirin and NSAIDs with food or milk to decrease the side effects of gastrointestinal irritation and bleeding.

Acetaminophen is not an appropriate substitute because it lacks anti-inflammatory properties. Teach family caregivers the importance of regular administration of the medications, even when the child is not experiencing pain. The primary purpose of aspirin or NSAIDs is not to relieve pain but to decrease joint inflammation.

When aspirin or NSAIDs are no longer effective, gold preparations, steroids, D-penicillamine, or immunosuppressives may be used. All these are toxic, and their use must be closely monitored.

Physical Therapy

Physical therapy includes exercise, application of splints, and heat. Implementing this program at home requires the cooperation of the nurse, physical therapist, and care provider. Joints must be immobilized by splinting during active disease, but gentle daily exercise is necessary to prevent **ankylosis** (immobility of a joint). Stress to the caregivers the importance of encouraging the child to perform independent activities of daily living to maintain function and independence. The family caregiver must be patient, allowing the child time to accomplish necessary tasks.

Depending on the degree of disease, activity, range-of-motion exercises, isometric exercises, swimming, and riding a tricycle or bicycle may be part of the treatment plan. Inform caregivers that these exercises should not increase pain; if exercise does trigger increased pain, the amount of exercise should be decreased.

SCOLIOSIS

Scoliosis, a lateral curvature of the spine, occurs in two forms: structural and functional (postural). Structural scoliosis involves rotated and malformed vertebrae. Functional scoliosis, the more common type, can have several causes: poor posture, muscle spasm caused by trauma, or unequal length of legs. When the primary problem is corrected, elimination of the functional scoliosis begins.

Most cases of structural scoliosis are idiopathic (no cause is known); a few are caused by congenital deformities or infection. Idiopathic scoliosis is seen in school-age children at 10 years of age and older. Although mild curves occur as often in boys as in girls, idiopathic scoliosis requiring treatment occurs eight times more frequently in girls than in boys (Sponseller, 1999).

Diagnosis

Diagnosis is based on a screening exam. Many states require regular examination of students for scoliosis, beginning in the 5th or 6th grade. Scoliosis screening should last through at least 8th grade. Nurses play an important role in screening for this disorder. School nurses and others who work in health care settings with children aged 10 years and older should conduct or assist with screening programs. A school nurse often does the initial screening. Nurses in other health care settings are responsible for further screening of these children during regular well-child visits.

During examination, observe the undressed child from the back and note any lateral curvature of the spinal column, asymmetry of the shoulders, shoulder blades, or hips, and an unequal distance between the arms and waist (Fig. 39-10). The examiner then asks the child to bend at the hips (touch the toes) and observes for prominence of the scapula on one side and curvature of the spinal column (see Chapter 26).

● *Figure 39.10* (**A**) Posterior view of child's back with lateral curvature. (**B**) View of child bending over with prominence of scapular area and asymmetry of flank demonstrated.

Treatment

Treatment depends on many factors and is either nonsurgical or surgical. Treatment is long term and often lasts through the rest of the child's growth cycle.

Curvatures of less than 25 degrees are observed but not treated. Electrical stimulation, a type of nonsurgical treatment, may be used for mild curvatures, but its effectiveness is unclear. Other nonsurgical treatment includes the use of braces or traction.

Curvatures between 25 degrees and 40 degrees are usually corrected with a brace. The Milwaukee brace was the first used for treatment and is still used to treat some spinal curvatures, such as kyphosis, but is not used as frequently now. The Boston brace or thoracic-lumbar-sacral orthotic (TLSO) braces are commonly used.

Curvatures of more than 40 degrees are usually corrected surgically. Surgical treatment includes the use of rods, screws, hooks, and spinal fusion.

Electrical Stimulation

Electrical stimulation may be used as an alternative to bracing for the child with a mild to moderate curvature. Electrodes are applied to the skin or surgically implanted. Treatment occurs at night while the child is asleep. The leads are placed to stimulate muscles on the convex side of the curvature to contract as impulses are transmitted. This causes the spine to straighten. If external electrodes are used, the skin under the leads must be checked regularly for irritation. This treatment is the least disruptive to the child's life, but there is some controversy about its effectiveness.

Braces

The Milwaukee brace was the first type of brace used for scoliosis but is now more commonly used to treat kyphosis, an abnormal rounded curvature of the spine that is also called humpback. Either the Boston brace or the TLSO brace is used to treat scoliosis (Fig. 39-11).

The Boston brace and the TLSO brace are made of plastic and are customized to fit the child.

The brace should be worn constantly, except during bathing or swimming, to achieve the greatest benefit. It is worn over a T-shirt or undershirt to protect the skin. The fit of the device is monitored closely, and the child and caregiver should be taught to notify the health care provider if there is any rubbing. During the first couple weeks of wearing the brace, the child can be given a mild analgesic for discomfort and aching. The child's provider may also prescribe certain exercises to be done several times a day. These are taught before the brace is applied but are done while the brace is in place.

Traction

When a child has a severe spinal curvature or cervical instability, a form of traction known as **halo traction** (Fig. 39-12) may be used to reduce spinal curves and straighten the spine. Halo traction is achieved by using stainless steel pins inserted into the skull while countertraction is applied by using pins inserted into the femur. Weights are increased gradually to promote correction. When the curvature has been corrected, spinal fusion is performed. In some cases, halo traction might be used after surgery if there is cervical instability.

The strange appearance of the halo traction apparatus magnifies the problems of body image; in addition, the head may need to be shaved. The child needs a thorough explanation of what will occur during the procedure and should be given the opportunity to talk about his or her feelings. Frequent shampooing, cleansing of the pin sites, and observation for signs of complications are critical for the child in halo traction.

Surgical Treatment

Various types of instruments such as rods, screws, and hooks may be placed along the spinal column to

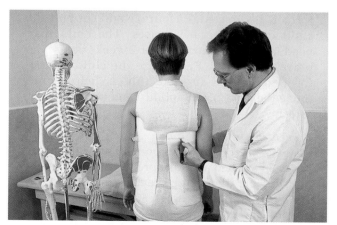

● *Figure 39.11* A girl with scoliosis being fitted with a TLSO brace for treatment.

● *Figure 39.12* A 9-year-old girl in halo traction.

● *Figure 39.13* Two nurses use a draw-sheet to logroll the child to a side-lying position.

realign the spine, then spinal fusion is performed to maintain the corrected position. This procedure, which is done in cases of severe curvatures, is frightening to the child and family. It is major surgery, and the child and family must be well prepared for it. Because this is an elective procedure, thorough preoperative teaching can be carried out for the child and the family. The child can expect to have postoperative pain and will have to endure days of remaining flat in bed, being turned only in a logrolling fashion (Fig. 39-13). After surgery, the neurovascular status of the extremities is monitored closely. The child may be given a patient-controlled analgesia pump to control pain. An indwelling urinary (Foley) catheter is usually inserted because of the need for the patient to remain flat. The rods remain in place permanently. In some cases, the child may be placed in a body cast for a period of time to ensure fusion of the spine. About 6 months after surgery, the child will be able to take part in most activities, except contact sports (such as tackle football, gymnastics, and wrestling). Because the bones are fused and rods are implanted, this procedure arrests the child's growth in height, which contributes to the emotional adjustment that the child and family must make.

● Nursing Process for the Child With Scoliosis Requiring a Brace

ASSESSMENT

The child with scoliosis must be reassessed every 4 to 6 months. Document the degree of curvature and related impairments. Scoliosis often is diagnosed in late school age or early adolescence. This is a sensitive age for children,

when privacy and the importance of being like everyone else are top priorities. Keep this in mind when interviewing and during examination of the child. Provide privacy and protect the child's modesty.

The child who is admitted to a health care facility for application of a brace or other instrumentation may be carrying a lot of unseen emotional baggage. Be sensitive to this emotional state. The family caregivers also may be upset but trying to hide it for the child's sake. In addition to routine observations, look for clues to the emotional state of both the child and family caregivers.

SELECTED NURSING DIAGNOSES

- Impaired Physical Mobility related to restricted movement
- Risk for Injury related to decreased mobility
- Risk for Impaired Skin Integrity related to irritation of brace
- Risk for Disturbed Body Image related to wearing a brace continuously
- Risk for Noncompliance related to long-term treatment

OUTCOME IDENTIFICATION AND PLANNING

Consult the child and caregiver when establishing nursing goals. Be especially sensitive to the child's needs. Goals for the child may include minimizing the disruption of activities, preventing injury, and maintaining skin integrity and self-image. Goals for the child and caregiver include complying with long-term care.

IMPLEMENTATION

Promoting Mobility
Prescribed exercises must be practiced and performed as directed. Encourage and support the child during these exercises. The child may need to be in traction for 1 or 2 weeks before the brace is applied. Encourage the child to perform exercises as directed. This can help to minimize the risks of immobility and promote self-esteem.

Preventing Injury
Evaluate the child's environment after the brace has been applied and take precautions to prevent injury. Help the child practice moving about safely: going up and down stairs; getting in and out of vehicles, chairs, and desks; and getting out of bed. Teach the child to avoid hazardous surfaces. Listen carefully to the child and the family

caregiver to determine any other hazards in the home or school environment. Advise the family caregiver to contact school personnel to ensure that the child has comfortable, supportive seating at school and that adjustments are made in the physical education program.

Preventing Skin Irritation

When the brace is first applied, check the child regularly to confirm proper fit. Observe for any areas of rubbing, discomfort, or skin irritation and adjust the brace as necessary. Teach the child how to inspect all areas under the brace daily. Instruct the child and caregiver that reddened areas should be reported to the care provider so that adjustments can be made. Skin under the pads should be massaged daily. Daily bathing is essential, and clean cotton underwear or a T-shirt should be worn under the brace to provide protection.

Promoting Positive Body Image

The child should be involved in all aspects of care planning. Self-image and the need to be like others are very important at this age. Wearing a brace creates a distinct change in body image, especially in the older school-age child or adolescent at a time when body consciousness is at an all-time high. Clothing choices are a challenge when wearing a brace.

Acceptance is important. Wearing clothing similar to what peers are wearing helps the child with scoliosis to feel more accepted.

The need to wear the brace and deal with the limitations it involves may cause anger; the change in body image can cause a grief reaction. Handling these feelings successfully requires understanding support from the nurse, family, and peers. It is important for the child to have an opportunity to talk about his or her feelings. Sometimes it is helpful for the patient in a brace to talk with other scoliosis patients and learn how they have coped. Understanding the disorder itself and the important benefits of treatment also can ease the adjustment.

Learning to be confident enough to handle the comments of peers can be difficult for the child. Give the child frequent opportunities to ventilate feelings about being different. Help the child select clothing that blends with current styles but is loose enough to hide the brace. Encourage the child to find extracurricular activities with which the brace will not interfere. Active sports are not permitted, but many other activities are available. Help the child focus and enhance a positive attribute about characteristics such as hair or complexion. Encourage the child and caregiver to discuss accommodations with school personnel together.

Promoting Compliance With Therapy

The child must wear the brace for years until the spinal growth is completed. Then the child needs to be weaned from it gradually for another 1 or 2 years by wearing it only at night. During this period, the caregivers and the child need emotional support from health care personnel. Be certain that the child and caregivers have a complete understanding of the importance of wearing the brace continually. To encourage compliance, teach them about possible complications of spinal instability and possible further deformity if correction is unsuccessful. Inform the caregiver about the need to monitor the child for compliance. Help the caregiver understand the importance of being empathic to the child's need to be like others during this period of development. Offer ways in which the caregiver can help the child deal with adjustment to the therapy.

EVALUATION: GOALS AND EXPECTED OUTCOMES

- **Goal:** The child will move effectively within the limits of the brace.
  Expected Outcome: The child ambulates and participates in daily activities.
- **Goal:** The child will remain free from injury while in the brace.
  Expected Outcome: The child demonstrates safe practices related to everyday activities at home and in the school environment.
- **Goal:** The child's skin will remain intact.
  Expected Outcome: The child uses methods to reduce skin irritation and bathes regularly. Skin remains free from irritation and breakdown.
- **Goal:** The child will exhibit positive coping behaviors.
  Expected Outcome: The child is self-confident, has an attractive, well-groomed appearance, and verbalizes feelings about the need to wear the brace.
- **Goal:** The child will comply with therapy.
  Expected Outcome: The child wears the brace as directed. Caregivers report compliance, and the child's condition shows evidence of compliance.

Test Yourself

- Explain the difference between structural and functional scoliosis.

- When should screening for scoliosis be started? What is the procedure for scoliosis screening?

- What are the ways scoliosis can be treated?

KEY POINTS

- In a complete fracture, the fragments of the bone are separated. In an incomplete fracture the fragments remain partially joined. The types of fractures seen in children are simple or closed; compound or open, where the bone penetrates the skin; spiral fractures, which twist around the bone; or greenstick fractures.

- Neurovascular checks are done in a child with a musculoskeletal disorder to monitor the child's neurovascular status to detect and prevent tissue and nerve damage.

- Monitoring the neurovascular status is sometimes referred to as CMS (circulation, movement, sensation) checks and includes observing, documenting, and reporting pain, pulses, paresthesia, paralysis, or pallor.

- Osteomyelitis is an infection of the bone usually caused by *Staphylococcus aureus*.

- The most common form of muscular dystrophy is Duchenne (pseudohypertrophic) muscular dystrophy. The characteristics include difficulty standing or walking, trunk muscle weakness, and often mild mental retardation. Weakness of leg, arm, and shoulder muscles progresses gradually, with the child usually becoming wheelchair-bound.

- The treatment for osteosarcoma is to remove the bone or the limb where the tumor is found. For Ewing's sarcoma, the tumor must be removed, and radiation is done. In both disorders chemotherapy is given.

- Enteric-coated aspirin has long been the drug of choice for JRA, but because of the concern of aspirin therapy and Reye syndrome, NSAIDs (nonsteroidal anti-inflammatory drugs) such as naproxen and ibuprofen are being used. The primary purpose of using these drugs is because of their anti-inflammatory effects. To decrease the side effects, the drugs should be administered with food or milk.

- Scoliosis is a lateral curvature of the spine, either structural or functional. Nonsurgical treatment includes electrical stimulation or the use of braces, such as the Boston brace or TLSO brace, or traction. Surgical treatment includes the use of rods, screws, hooks, and spinal fusion.

REFERENCES AND SELECTED READINGS

Books and Journals

Cassidy, J. T. (1999). Rheumatic diseases of childhood. In J. A. McMillan, C. D. DeAngelis, R. D. Feigin, & J. W. Warshaw (Eds.), *Oski's pediatrics: Principles and practice* (3rd ed.). Philadelphia: Lippincott Williams & Wilkins.

Chin, K. R., Price, J. S., Zimbler, S. (2001). A guide to early detection of scoliosis. *Contemporary Pediatrics, 18*(9), 77.

Hockenberry, M. J., Wilson, D., Winkelstein, M. L., & Kline, N. E. (2003). *Wong's nursing care of infants and children* (7th ed.). St. Louis: Mosby.

Karch, A. M. (2003). *2004 Lippincott's nursing drug guide*. Philadelphia: Lippincott Williams & Wilkins.

Katz, D. R. (2001). Adolescent idiopathic scoliosis: The effect of brace treatment on the incidence of surgery. *Physical Therapy, 81*(9), 1591.

National Institute of Arthritis and Musculoskeletal and Skin Diseases, National Institutes of Health. (2001). *Questions and answers about scoliosis in children and adolescents.* Available: www.niams.nih.gov/hi/index.htm

North American Nursing Diagnosis Association (NANDA). (2001). *NANDA nursing diagnoses: Definitions and classification 2001–2002.* Philadelphia: Author.

Pillitteri, A. (2003). *Maternal and child health nursing* (4th ed.). Philadelphia: Lippincott Williams & Wilkins.

Smeltzer, S. C., & Bare, B. G. (2003). *Textbook of medical–surgical nursing* (10th ed.). Philadelphia: Lippincott Williams & Wilkins.

Sparks, S., & Taylor, C. (2001). *Nursing diagnosis reference manual* (5th ed.). Springhouse, PA: Springhouse Corporation.

Splete, H. (2001). Catch curves like scoliosis in time for bracing. *Pediatric News, 35*(11), 42.

Sponseller, P. D. (1999). Bone, joint, and muscle problems. In *Oski's pediatrics: Principles and practice* (3rd ed.). Philadelphia: Lippincott Williams & Wilkins.

Wong, D. L., Perry, S., & Hockenberry, M. (2002). *Maternal–child nursing care* (2nd ed.). St. Louis: Mosby.

Websites
Scoliosis
www.scoliosis-assoc.org

Muscular Dystrophy
www.mdausa.org

Juvenile Rheumatoid Arthritis
www.arthritis.org

WORKBOOK

NCLEX-STYLE REVIEW QUESTIONS

1. The nurse is teaching a group of peers regarding different types of fractures. Which of the following best describes an open fracture? A fracture in which

   a. the fragments of the bone are separated.

   b. the broken bone penetrates the skin.

   c. there is a single break in the bone without penetration of the skin.

   d. the fragments of the bone remain partially joined.

2. In caring for a child in traction, of the following interventions, which is the *highest* priority for the nurse? The nurse should

   a. monitor for decreased circulation every 4 hours.

   b. clean the pin sites at least once every 8 hours.

   c. provide age-appropriate activities for the child.

   d. record accurate intake and output.

3. The nurse is doing patient teaching with a child who has been placed in a brace to treat scoliosis. Which of the following statements made by the child indicates an understanding of the treatment?

   a. "I am so glad I can take this brace off for the school dance."

   b. "At least when I take a shower I have a few minutes out of this brace."

   c. "Wearing this brace only during the night won't be so embarrassing."

   d. "When I start feeling tired, I can just take my brace off for a few minutes."

4. The nurse is caring for a child after an accident in which the child fractured his arm. A cast has been applied to the child's right arm. Which of the following actions should the nurse implement? Select all that apply.

   a. Wear a protective gown when moving the child's arm.

   b. Document any signs of pain.

   c. Check radial pulse in the both arms.

   d. Wear sterile gloves when removing or touching the cast.

   e. Monitor the color of the nail beds in the right hand.

STUDY ACTIVITIES

1. Using the table below, list the areas that must be checked and monitored when doing a neurovascular status check (CMS check) on a child with a fracture. Include the area to be monitored, the definition or explanation, observations, and documentation.

Area to Be Monitored (the 5 Ps)	Definition or Explanation	Observations (What Signs to Look for)	Documentation

2. Develop a list of games and activities that would be appropriate to use for a 10-year-old girl in skeletal traction. Keep in mind the child's age and stage of growth and development. Share your list with your peers.

3. Call the Muscular Dystrophy Association national headquarters or your local Muscular Dystrophy Association chapter. Ask what is available in your community to help and support children and families of children with muscular dystrophy.

4. Go to the following Internet site: http://www.arthritis.org/conditions On the left side of the screen, click on "Juvenile Arthritis." On the right side of screen, click on "Exercise Tips." After reading the section on exercise and juvenile arthritis, answer the following:

   a. What does this site say about the importance of exercise for the child with juvenile arthritis?

   b. Read the section "Exercise Countdown." What are the 10 things suggested to remember before exercising?

   c. What are some examples of books or videos available for children and parents of children who have juvenile arthritis?

CRITICAL THINKING: What Would You Do?

1. Twelve-year-old Carrie has scoliosis and must wear a TLSO brace. She says she thinks it's really ugly. Carrie tells you she doesn't want to go to school because she can't wear clothes similar to those of her friends.

   a. What feelings do you think Carrie might be going through in this situation?

   b. What would you say in response to Carrie?

   c. What are some ideas you could share with Carrie regarding clothing she might wear?

2. You are caring for 2-year-old Cole, who has muscular dystrophy. Cole's family begins asking you questions about the disease. How would you answer the following questions?

   a. What caused Cole to have muscular dystrophy?

   b. What will happen to Cole physically as he gets older and the disease progresses?

   c. What is the long-term prognosis for Cole?

   d. Where can we find other families who have a child with muscular dystrophy?

3. Dosage calculation: After a course of IV antibiotics for treatment of osteomyelitis, a child has been prescribed a regimen of nafcillin (Unipen) by mouth. The child weighs 17.6 pounds. The usual dosage range of this medication is 6.25 mg to 12.5 mg per kg every 6 hours. Answer the following:

   a. How many kilograms does the child weigh?

   b. What is the low dose of nafcillin for this child every 6 hours?

   c. What is the high dose of nafcillin for this child every 6 hours?

   d. If the child is given the high dose, how much nafcillin will be given in a 24-hour period?

The Child With Integumentary Disorders/Communicable Diseases

On completion of this chapter, the student should be able to

1. Discuss ways the child's integumentary and immune systems differ from the adult's system.
2. Identify the causative organism of thrush.
3. Discuss the factors that cause acne vulgaris.
4. List the drugs commonly used for mild acne, inflammatory acne, and severe acne.
5. Describe the treatment for pediculosis of the scalp, and state the protection the nurse must use when treating a child with this condition in the hospital.
6. Discuss how allergens that produce a positive reaction on skin testing are commonly treated.
7. Discuss how skin allergies are commonly treated.
8. State the three major causes of burns in small children.
9. Differentiate between first-, second-, and third-degree burns.
10. Describe emergency treatment of a minor burn and of a moderate or severe burn.
11. List the reasons hypovolemic shock occurs in the first 48 hours after a burn.
12. List the organisms that cause and the drug of choice to treat gonorrhea, chlamydia, genital herpes, and syphilis.
13. Identify the only certain way to prevent sexually transmitted diseases.
14. Identify how the human immunodeficiency virus is transmitted.
15. Describe infectious mononucleosis.
16. Describe modes of transmission for communicable diseases.
17. Discuss ways to prevent children from getting communicable diseases.
18. Differentiate among active, natural, and passive immunity.
19. Identify nursing interventions that might be done in the care of a child with a communicable disease.

KEY TERMS

allergen
allograft
autograft
comedones
contractures
débridement
eschar
heterograft
homograft
hydrotherapy
hypervolemic
hyposensitization
tinea

GROWTH AND DEVELOPMENT OF THE INTEGUMENTARY AND IMMUNE SYSTEM

The skin is the major organ of the integumentary system and is the largest organ of the body. Accessory structures such as the hair and nails also make up the integumentary system. The major role of the skin is to protect the organs and structures of the body against bacteria, chemicals, and injury. The skin helps regulate the body temperature by heating and cooling. Excretion in the form of perspiration is also a function of the skin glands, called the sweat glands. Sebaceous glands in the skin secrete oils to lubricate the skin and hair. These oils help in preventing dryness of the skin. As a sensory organ, the skin has nerve endings that respond to pain, pressure, heat, and cold. When the skin is exposed to sunlight (ultraviolet light), synthesis of vitamin D occurs.

The integumentary system, including the accessory structures, is in place at birth, but the system is immature. The newborn's skin is thin and has less subcutaneous fat between the layers of skin. Regulating temperature is more difficult in the newborn because

of these factors. As the child grows, the sweat glands mature and increase the capability of the skin to help in the regulation of the temperature. The sebaceous secretions in the infant and young child are less than those in the older child and adult, causing the skin of children to dry and crack more easily. In addition, the infant is more susceptible to bacteria, which might cause infection, and to irritants that might have an effect on the skin. Injury and some disorders can cause bruising to the skin, especially in the child.

Protecting the body from attacks from microorganisms and helping the body get rid of or resist invasion by foreign materials are the major roles of the immune system. Unlike other systems in the body that are made up of organs, the immune system is made up of cells and tissues that work to protect the body. Protective barriers such as the skin and mucous membranes help to prevent pathogens from entering the body. When a pathogen enters the body, the immune system works to destroy the pathogen. This occurs when white blood cells known as macrophages surround, ingest, or neutralize the pathogen. The inflammatory process further helps to get rid of the foreign substances. Another process of the immune system occurs when substances called antibodies destroy antigens, foreign protein substances. When the body is exposed to certain bacteria or viruses, the immune system fights to destroy the substance. In addition, immunity to that disease is developed, so if the person has an exposure in the future, the immune system immediately responds and symptoms do not occur. The use of immunizations creates an artificial exposure to a certain agent and helps the body create immunity to that agent.

During fetal life, the mother's antibodies cross the placenta, giving the fetus a temporary immunity against certain diseases. This immunity is present at birth and decreases during the 1st year of life. In the meantime, the infant begins developing antibodies to fight against pathogens and disease. In addition, during the 1st year of life immunizations are started to help the infant develop protection against certain diseases. As the child grows and develops, the immune system also develops. The antibodies in the child increase as the child progresses through childhood.

SEBORRHEIC DERMATITIS

Seborrheic dermatitis is commonly known as cradle cap. It can usually be prevented by daily washing of the child's hair and scalp. Characterized by yellowish, scaly, or crusted patches on the scalp, it occurs in newborns and older infants, possibly as a result of excessive sebaceous gland activity. Family caregivers may be afraid to wash vigorously over the "soft spot." However, they need to understand that this is where cradle cap often begins and that careful but vigorous washing of the area with a washcloth can prevent this disorder. Using a fine-toothed baby comb after shampooing is also a helpful preventive measure. These principles are stressed during teaching about care of the newborn.

Once the condition exists, daily application of mineral oil helps loosen the crust. However, no attempt should be made to loosen it all at once because the delicate skin on the scalp may break and bleed and can easily become infected.

MILIARIA RUBRA

Miliaria rubra, often called prickly heat, is common in children who are exposed to summer heat or are overdressed. It also may appear in febrile illnesses and may be mistaken for the rash of one of the communicable diseases.

Clinical Manifestations

The rash appears as pinhead-sized erythematous (reddened) papules. It is most noticeable in areas where sweat glands are concentrated, such as folds of the skin, the chest, and about the neck. It usually causes itching, making the child uncomfortable and fretful.

Treatment and Nursing Care

Treatment primarily should be preventive. Family caregivers should be taught that a diaper might be all the child needs to wear.

Here's a tip to share. Caregivers are often concerned that their baby is going to be cold; it is important they avoid bundling their child in layers of clothing in hot weather.

Tepid baths without soap help control the itching. A small amount of baking soda may be added to the bath water to help relieve discomfort.

DIAPER RASH

Diaper rash is common in infancy, causing the baby discomfort and fretfulness. Bacterial decomposition of urine produces ammonia, which is irritating to a child's tender skin. Diarrheal stools also produce a burning erythematous area in the anal region. Some children seem to be more susceptible than others, possibly because of inherited sensitive skin. Prolonged exposure to wet or soiled diapers, use of plastic or rubber pants, infrequently changed disposable diapers, inadequate cleansing of the diaper area (especially after bowel movements), sensitivity to some soaps or disposable diaper perfumes, and the use of strong laundry detergents without thorough rinsing are considered to be causes. Yeast infections, notably candidiasis, are also causative factors.

Treatment and Nursing Care

Caregivers should be taught that the primary treatment is prevention. Diapers must be changed frequently without waiting for obvious leaking. Regular checking is necessary. Manufacturers of disposable diapers are constantly trying to improve the ability of disposable diapers to wick the wetness away from the child's skin. Diapers washed at commercial laundries are sterilized, preventing the growth of ammonia-forming bacteria. However, caregivers may be unable to afford disposable diapers or a commercial diaper service. Diapers washed at home should be presoaked (good commercial products are available), washed in hot water with a mild soap, and rinsed thoroughly with an antiseptic added to the final rinse. Drying diapers in the sun or in a dryer also helps destroy bacteria.

Exposing the diaper area to the air helps clear up the dermatitis.

Did you know. The use of baby powder when diapering is discouraged because caked powder helps create an environment in which organisms thrive.

Cleaning the diaper area from front to back with warm water and drying thoroughly with each diaper change helps improve or prevent the condition. If soap is necessary when cleaning stool from the child's buttocks and rectal area, be certain that the soap is completely rinsed before diapering. The use of commercial wet wipes may aggravate the condition. If the area becomes excoriated and sore, the health care provider may prescribe an ointment. See Family Teaching Tips: Preventing and Treating Diaper Rash.

FAMILY TEACHING TIPS

Preventing and Treating Diaper Rash

- Rinse all baby's clothes thoroughly to eliminate soap or detergent residue that may irritate baby's skin.
- Rinse cloth diapers in clear water. Do not use fabric softeners because they can cause a skin reaction.
- Use plastic or rubber diaper covers only when necessary. They hold moisture, which makes rash worse.
- Change diapers as soon as wet or soiled. Disposable diapers hold moisture the same as plastic or rubber covers.
- Avoid fastening diaper too tightly, which irritates baby's skin.
- Expose baby's bottom to air without diapers as much as possible to help rash heal.
- Do not overdress or overcover baby. Sweating makes rash worse.
- Wash baby's bottom with lukewarm water only, using wet cotton balls or pouring over bath basin or sink. Pat dry with soft cloth. Do not use commercial baby wipes. Do not rub rash.
- Use a cool, wet cloth placed over red diaper rash, which can be very soothing. Try this for 5 minutes three or four times a day.
- Use ointment only as recommended by health care provider. Apply very thin layer only. Wash off at each diaper change.
- Dry diaper area thoroughly before rediapering. A hair dryer on low warm setting used after patting dry may help.

CANDIDIASIS

Candidiasis is caused by *Candida albicans*, the organism responsible for thrush and some cases of diaper rash. Newborns can be exposed to a candidiasis vaginal infection in the mother during delivery. Thrush appears in the child's mouth as a white coating that looks like milk curds. Poor handwashing practices and inadequate washing of bottles and nipples are contributing factors. In addition, infants and toddlers may experience episodes of thrush or diaper rash after antibiotic therapy, which may upset the balance of normal intestinal flora, leading to candidal overgrowth.

Treatment and Nursing Care

Treatment for diaper rash caused by *Candida albicans* (Fig. 40-1) is the application of nystatin ointment or cream to the affected area. Application of nystatin (Mycostatin, Nilstat) to the oral lesions every 6 hours is an effective treatment. In all cases, good hygiene practices should be reinforced.

Test Yourself

- How can seborrheic dermatitis (cradle cap) be prevented?
- What causes diaper rash?
- What is the causative agent for thrush? How might a newborn be exposed to this, and how is it treated?

IMPETIGO

Impetigo is a superficial bacterial skin infection (Fig. 40-2). In the newborn, the primary causative organism is *Staphylococcus aureus*. In the older child, the most common causative organism is group A beta-hemolytic streptococci. Impetigo in the newborn is usually bullous (blister-like); in the older child, the lesions are nonbullous.

Warning. Impetigo is highly contagious and can spread quickly.

Impetigo in the newborn nursery is cause for immediate concern.

Nursing Care

The nurse caring for a young child who has impetigo and is hospitalized must follow contact (skin and wound) precautions, including wearing a cover gown

● **Figure 40.1** Diaper rash caused by *Candida*.

and gloves. The child should be segregated from other children to deter spread of the disease. Crusts can be soaked off with warm water, followed by an application of topical antibiotics such as Bacitracin and Neosporin. The child's hands must be covered or elbow restraints applied to prevent scratching of lesions. Careful handwashing by nursing personnel and family members is essential.

The older child with impetigo is treated at home. The family caregivers must be taught hygiene practices to prevent the spread of impetigo to other children in

● **Figure 40.2** Typical lesions of impetigo.

the household or other contacts of the child in the day care center, nursery school, or elementary school. Lesions occur primarily on the face but may spread to any part of the body. The crusts and drainage are contagious. Because the lesions are pruritic (itchy), the child must learn to keep his or her fingers and hands away from the lesions. Nails should be trimmed to prevent scratching of lesions. Family members should be taught not to share towels and washcloths. Medical treatment includes oral penicillin or erythromycin for 10 days. Daily washing of the crusts helps speed the healing process. Mupirocin (Bactroban) ointment may be used.

Because this is commonly a streptococcal infection in the older child, rheumatic fever or acute glomerulonephritis may follow. Family caregivers should be alerted to this rare possibility.

ACNE VULGARIS

Acne, one of the most common health problems of adolescence, may be only a mild case of oily skin and a few blackheads or it may be a severe type with ropelike cystic lesions that leave deep scars, both physical and emotional. To adolescents who want to be attractive and popular, even a mild case of acne (often called "zits") can cause great anxiety, shyness, and social withdrawal.

Clinical Manifestations

Characterized by the appearance of **comedones** (blackheads and whiteheads), papules, and pustules on the face and the back and chest to some extent, acne is caused by a variety of factors, including

- Increased hormonal levels, especially androgens
- Hereditary factors
- Irritation and irritating substances, such as vigorous scrubbing and cosmetics with a greasy base
- Growth of anaerobic bacteria

Each hair follicle has an associated sebaceous gland that in adolescents produces increased sebum (oily secretion). The sebum is blocked by epithelial cells and becomes trapped in the follicle. When anaerobic organisms infect this collection, inflammation occurs, which causes papules, pustules, and nodules (Fig. 40-3). Several types of acne lesions are often present at one time.

Treatment and Nursing Care

The topical medications benzoyl peroxide (Clearasil, Benoxyl) and tretinoin (Retin-A) come in a variety of forms, such as topical cleansers, lotions, creams, sticks, pads, gels, and bars. The usual treatment plan for mild acne is topical application of one of these

● *Figure 40.3* Facial acne in an adolescent.

medications once or twice a day. These medications should not be applied to normal skin or allowed to get into the eyes or nose or on other mucous membranes. Antibiotics such as erythromycin and tetracycline may be administered for inflammatory acne. Antibiotic therapy requires an extended treatment course of at least 6 to 12 months, followed by tapering of the dosage.

Isotretinoin (Accutane) may be used for severe inflammatory acne. This potent, effective oral medication is used for hard-to-treat cystic acne. Side effects are common but often diminish when the drug dosage is reduced. Warn the adolescent about some of the side effects, including dry lips and skin, eye irritation, temporary worsening of acne, epistaxis (nosebleed), bleeding and inflammation of the gums, itching, photosensitivity (sensitivity to the sun), and joint and muscle pain.

This is critical to remember. Isotretinoin is a pregnancy category X drug: it must not be used at all during pregnancy because of serious risk of fetal abnormalities.

To rule out pregnancy, a urine test is done before treatment is begun. For the sexually active adolescent girl, an effective form of contraception must be used for a month before beginning and during isotretinoin therapy. The risk to the fetus should pregnancy occur should be discussed with the girl, whether or not she is sexually active.

Although the adolescent's perception of the disfigurement caused by acne may seem out of proportion to the actual severity of the condition, acknowledge and accept his or her feelings. Teach the adolescent and the family caregiver to wash the lesions gently with soap and water; do not scrub vigorously. Comedones should be removed gently by fol-lowing the physician's recommendations and using careful aseptic techniques. Careful removal produces no scarring—a goal for every teen.

Understanding and support by the nurse and family caregiver are the most important aspects of caring for the adolescent with acne. Reassure the teen that eating chocolate and fatty foods does not cause acne, but a well-balanced, nutritious diet does promote healing.

FUNGAL INFECTIONS

Fungi that live in the outer (dead) layers of the skin, hair, and nails can develop into superficial infections. **Tinea** (ringworm) is the term commonly applied to these infections, which are further differentiated by the part of the body infected.

Tinea Capitis (Ringworm of the Scalp)

Ringworm of the scalp is called tinea capitis or tinea tonsurans. The most common cause is *Microsporum audouinii*, which is transmitted from person to person through combs, towels, hats, barber scissors, or direct contact. A less common type, *Microsporum canis*, is transmitted from animal to child.

Clinical Manifestations

Tinea capitis begins as a small papule on the scalp and spreads, leaving scaly patches of baldness. The hairs become brittle and break off easily.

Treatment and Nursing Care

Griseofulvin, an oral antifungal, is the medication of choice. Because treatment may be prolonged (3 months or more), compliance must be reinforced. Be sure that parents and children understand the medication therapy. Children who are being properly treated may attend school. Advise the child and parents that hair loss is not permanent.

Tinea Corporis (Ringworm of the Body)

Tinea corporis is ringworm of the body that affects the epidermal skin layer. The child usually contracts tinea corporis from contact with an infected dog or cat.

The lesions appear as a scaly ring with clearing in the center, occurring on any part of the body. They resemble the lesions of scalp ringworm. Topical anti-fungal agents, such as clotrimazole, econazole nitrate, tolnaftate, and miconazole, are effective. Griseofulvin also is used in this condition.

Tinea Pedis

Tinea pedis, ringworm of the feet, is more commonly known as athlete's foot. It is evidenced by the scaling or cracking of the skin between the toes. Transmission is by direct or indirect contact with skin lesions from infected people. Contaminated sidewalks, floors, pool decks, and shower stalls spread the condition to those who walk barefoot. Tinea pedis, usually found in ado-lescents and adults, is becoming more prevalent among school-age children because of the popularity of plastic shoes. Examination under a microscope of scrapings from the lesions is necessary for definite diagnosis.

Care includes washing the feet with soap and water, then gently removing scabs and crusts and applying a topical agent such as tolnaftate. Griseoful-vin by mouth is also useful. During the chronic phase, the use of ointment, scrupulous foot hygiene, frequent changing of white cotton socks, and avoidance of plas-tic footwear are helpful. Continuing application of a topical agent for as long as 6 weeks is recommended.

Tinea Cruris

Tinea cruris, more commonly known as jock itch, or ringworm of the inner thighs and inguinal area, is caused by the same organisms that cause tinea cor-poris. It is more common in athletes and is uncommon in preadolescent children. Tinea cruris is pruritic and localized to the area. Treatment is the same as for tinea corporis. Sitz baths also may be soothing.

Test Yourself

- Why is impetigo a concern in the newborn nursery? What procedures should the nurse follow when caring for a child with impetigo?

- Why should comedones, seen in acne vul-garis, be removed carefully?

- How is ringworm of the scalp, tinea capitis, usually transmitted?

- Which classification of medication is given to treat ringworm?

PARASITIC INFECTIONS

Parasites are organisms that live on or within another living organism from which they obtain their food supply. Lice and the scabies mite live by sucking the blood of the host.

Pediculosis

Pediculosis (lice infestation) may be caused by Pedicu-lus humanus capitis (head lice), Pediculus humanus corporis (body lice), or Pthirus pubis (pubic lice). Head lice are the most common infestation in children. Ani-mal lice are not transferred to humans.

Head lice are passed from child to child by direct contact or indirectly by contact with combs, headgear, or bed linen.

Clinical Manifestations

Lice, which are rarely seen, lay their eggs, called nits, on the head where they attach to hair strands. The nits can be seen as tiny pearly white flecks attached to the hair shafts. They look much like dandruff, but dandruff flakes can be flicked off easily, whereas the nits are tightly attached and not easily removed. The nits hatch in about 1 week, and the lice become sexually mature in about 2 weeks.

Don't forget the importance of your observation skills. Severe itching of the scalp is the most obvious symp-tom in cases of head lice.

Treatment and Nursing Care

Nonprescription medications are available to treat cases of head lice. Products such as Pronto, RID, and A-200 contain pyrethrins, which are extracts from the chrysanthemum flower. Permethrin (Nix) may also be used. These medications are safe and usually effective in killing the lice. A second treatment is suggested in 7 to 10 days to kill the nits after they have hatched. If over-the-counter preparations do not effectively kill the lice, prescription medications may be used. Malathion (Ovide) is effective in treating lice and nits. Few side effects have been reported, but if used on open sores, it may cause the skin to sting, so it should not be used if the head has been scratched. Lindane (Kwell) shampoo has been one of the most commonly used treatments for many years and is usually safe. Overuse, misuse, or accidentally swallowing of Lindane can be toxic to the brain and nervous system, so its use is suggested only in cases that do not respond to other treatments.

After the hair is wet with warm water, the medication is applied like any ordinary shampoo; about 1 oz is used. The head should be lathered for several minutes, following the directions on the label for each specific medication, then rinsed thoroughly and dried. After the hair is dry, it should be combed with a combing tool such as a LiceMeister or a fine-toothed comb dipped in warm white vinegar to remove remaining nits and nit shells. Shampooing may be repeated in 2 weeks to remove any lice that may have been missed as nits and since hatched. Avoid getting medication into the eyes or on mucous membranes. When treating a child in the hospital for pediculosis, wear a disposable gown, gloves, and head cover for protection.

Family caregivers are often embarrassed when the school nurse sends word that the child has head lice. They can be reassured that lice infestation is common and can happen to any child; it is not a reflection on the caregiver's housekeeping. All family members should be inspected and treated as needed. See Family Teaching Tips: Eliminating Pediculi Infestations for other useful information.

Scabies

Scabies is a skin infestation caused by the scabies mite Sarcoptes scabiei. The female mite burrows in areas between the fingers and toes and in warm folds of the body, such as the axilla and groin, to lay eggs.

Clinical Manifestations

Burrows are visible as dark lines, and the mite is seen as a black dot at the end of the burrow. Severe itching occurs, causing scratching with resulting secondary infection.

Treatment and Nursing Care

The body, except for the face, is treated with permethrin cream (Elimite) or lindane lotion. The directions for each medication should be followed closely. The body is first scrubbed with soap and water, then the lotion is applied on all areas of the body except the face. Permethrin is the preferred treatment because of the decreased risk of neurologic problems. It is usually left on the skin for 8 to 14 hours. With lindane, the medication is left on for 8 to 12 hours and then completely washed off with warm water.

Caregivers should follow the tips recommended for pediculosis. All who had close contact with the child within a 30- to 60-day period should be treated. The rash and itch may continue for several weeks even though the mites have been successfully eliminated.

Test Yourself

- Explain what pediculosis is and at what sites it is frequently found in children.
- How is pediculosis treated?
- Why is it important for the child with scabies to avoid scratching involved areas?

FAMILY TEACHING TIPS

Eliminating Pediculi Infestations

- Wash all child's bedding and clothing in hot water and dry in hot dryer.
- Vacuum carpets, car seats, mattresses, and upholstered furniture very thoroughly. Discard vacuum dust bag.
- Wash pillows, stuffed animals, and other washable items the same way clothing is washed.
- Dry clean nonwashable items.
- If items cannot be washed or dry cleaned, seal in plastic bag for 2 weeks to break the reproductive cycle of lice.
- Wash combs, brushes, and other hair items (rollers, curlers, barrettes, etc.) in shampoo and soak for 1 hour.
- If you discover the infestation, report to child's school or day care.
- Have school personnel disinfect headphones.

ALLERGIC DISORDERS

Millions of Americans have allergic diseases, most of which begin in childhood. Children with allergies are hampered because of poor appetites, poor sleep, and restricted physical activity in play and at school, all of which often result in altered physical and personality development. Children whose parents or grandparents have allergies are more likely to become allergic than are other children. An allergic condition is caused by sensitivity to a substance called an **allergen** (an antigen that causes an allergy). Thousands of allergens exist. Some of the most common are

- Pollen
- Mold
- Dust
- Animal dander
- Insect bites

- Tobacco smoke
- Nuts
- Chocolate
- Milk
- Fish
- Shellfish

Drugs, particularly aspirin and penicillin, can be allergens as well. Some plants and chemicals cause allergic reactions on the skin. Allergens may enter the body through various routes, the most common being the nose, throat, eyes, skin, digestive tract, and bronchial tissues in the lungs. The first time the child comes in contact with an allergen, no reaction may be evident, but an immune response is stimulated—helper lymphocytes stimulate B lymphocytes to make immunoglobulin E (IgE) antibody. The IgE antibody attaches to mast cells and macrophages. When contacted again, the allergen attaches to the IgE receptor sites, and a response occurs in which certain substances, such as histamine, are released; these substances produce the symptoms known as allergy.

Diagnosis of an allergy requires a careful history and physical examination and possibly skin and blood tests, including a complete blood count, serum protein electrophoresis, and immunoelectrophoresis. Skin testing is generally done when removal of obvious allergens is impossible or has not brought relief. If a food allergy is suspected, an elimination diet may help identify the allergen. Eliminating the food suspected is sometimes difficult because there are often "hidden" ingredients in food products.

Be careful. The caregivers of a child allergic to peanuts must always read labels of food products. They will find many unsuspecting products contain peanuts or peanut oil.

When specific allergens have been identified, patients can either avoid them or, if this is impossible, undergo immunization therapy by injection. This process is called **hyposensitization** or immunotherapy.

Hyposensitization is performed for the allergens that produce a positive reaction on skin testing. The allergist sets up a schedule for injections in gradually increasing doses until a maintenance dose is reached. The patient should remain in the physician's office for 20 to 30 minutes after the injection in case any reaction occurs. Reactions are treated with epinephrine. Severe reactions in children are uncommon, and hyposensitization is considered a safe procedure with considerable benefit for some children.

Symptomatic relief in allergic reactions can be gained through antihistamine or steroid therapy, but the best treatment is prevention.

Atopic Dermatitis (Infantile Eczema)

Atopic dermatitis or infantile eczema is considered at least in part an allergic reaction to an irritant. It is fairly common during the 1st year of life after the age of 3 months. It is uncommon in breast-fed babies before they are given additional foods.

Infantile eczema is characterized by three factors:

- Hereditary predisposition
- Hypersensitivity of the deeper layers of the skin to protein or protein-like allergens
- Allergens to which the child is sensitive that may be inhaled, ingested, or absorbed through direct contact, such as house dust, egg white, and wool. Infants who have eczema tend to have allergic rhinitis or asthma later in life.

Clinical Manifestations

Infantile eczema usually starts on the cheeks and spreads to the extensor surfaces of the arms and legs (Fig. 40-4). Eventually the entire trunk may become affected. The initial reddening of the skin is quickly followed by papule and vesicle formation. Itching is intense, and the child's scratching makes the skin weep and crust. The areas easily become infected by hemolytic streptococci or by staphylococci.

Diagnosis

The most common allergens involved in eczema are

- Foods: egg white, cow's milk, wheat products, orange juice, tomato juice
- Inhalants: house dust, pollens, animal dander
- Materials: wool, nylon, plastic

However, diagnosis is not simple. Often trial by elimination is as effective as any other diagnostic tool.

● *Figure 40.4* Infant with infantile eczema (atopic dermatitis).

Skin testing on a young child generally is not considered valid, so it is discouraged as a means of diagnosis.

An elimination diet may be helpful in ruling out offending foods. A hypoallergenic diet consisting of a milk substitute such as soy formula, vitamin supplement, and other foods known to be hypoallergenic is given. If the skin condition shows improvement, other foods are added one at a time at an interval of about 1 week; the effects are noted and any foods that cause a reaction are eliminated. The protein of egg white is such a common offender that most pediatricians advise against feeding whole eggs to infants until late in the 1st year of life (see Chapter 37, Table 37-1 for a list of foods that may cause allergies).

Great care must be taken to prevent the child from becoming undernourished. An elimination program must always be initiated under the supervision of a competent pediatric nurse practitioner, dietitian, or physician.

Treatment

Smallpox vaccination is definitely contraindicated for the child with eczema. In fact, such a child must be kept away from anyone who has recently been vaccinated. A serious condition called eczema vaccinatum results when a child with eczema is vaccinated or is exposed to the vaccination of another person. The child becomes seriously ill, and mortality rates have been high. Fortunately, because smallpox vaccination is no longer required, this is not a major concern; the reaction could occur if the child is exposed to someone who's been vaccinated in preparation for travel.

Of greater current concern is protecting the child from anyone with a herpes simplex infection (cold sore). If the lesions become infected with herpes simplex, a generalized reaction may occur. In the child with severe eczema with many lesions, body fluid loss from oozing through the lesions can be serious. The child may have severe pain and be gravely ill with this complication.

Oral antibiotics may be ordered for a coexistent infection such as a staphylococcal or streptococcal infection. Oral antihistamines and sedatives may help relieve the itching and allow rest. If no infection exists, topical hydrocortisone ointments may be used to relieve inflammation. Wet soaks or colloidal baths also may be prescribed for their soothing effects. The water should be tepid for further soothing, and soap may not be used because of its drying effect. Some physicians recommend the use of a mild soap, such as Dove or Neutrogena, or a soap substitute. Lubrication is essential to retain moisture and prevent evaporation after the bath. Emollients containing lanolin or petrolatum, such as Eucerin, may be prescribed.

Inhalant and contact allergens should be avoided as far as possible. In the child's bedroom, window drapes or curtains, dresser scarves, and rugs should be removed or made of washable fabric that can be frequently laundered. Furniture should be washed frequently. The crib mattress should have a nonallergenic covering and be washed frequently with careful cleaning along the binding. Feather pillows must be eliminated, and stuffed toys should be washable. It may be necessary to provide new homes for household pets. However, dander from the pets can remain in carpets, crevices, and overstuffed furniture for a long time. Carpets and area rugs may need to be removed. A home, especially an older one with a damp basement, may be harboring molds that shed allergenic spores. Bathrooms are also places for molds and mildews to hide, especially in warm, humid climates.

● Nursing Process for the Child With Infantile Eczema

ASSESSMENT

The family caregivers of the child with eczema are often frustrated and exhausted. Although the caregiver can be assured that most cases of eczema clear up by the age of 2 years, this does little to relieve the current situation. Hospitalization is avoided when possible because these children are highly susceptible to infections. Sometimes, however, admission seems to be the only answer to provide more intensive therapy or to relieve an exhausted caregiver.

During the interview with the family caregivers, cover the history of the condition, including treatments that have been tried and foods that have been ruled out as allergens. Include a thorough review of the home environment. Evaluate the caregivers' knowledge of the condition.

The data collection about the child includes obtaining vital signs, observing general nutritional state, and doing a complete examination of all body parts with careful documentation of the eruptions and their location and size. Unaffected areas as well as those that are weeping and crusted should be indicated.

SELECTED NURSING DIAGNOSES

- Impaired Skin Integrity related to lesions and inflammatory process
- Acute Pain related to intense itching and irritation
- Disturbed Sleep Pattern related to itching and discomfort
- Imbalanced Nutrition: Less Than Body Requirements related to elimination diet

- Risk for Infection related to broken skin and lesions
- Deficient Knowledge of caregivers related to disease condition and treatment

OUTCOME IDENTIFICATION AND PLANNING

The major goals for the child with infantile eczema are preserving skin integrity, maintaining comfort, improving sleep patterns, maintaining good nutrition (within the constraints of allergens), and preventing infection of skin lesions. A family goal is increasing knowledge about the disease process. Base the nursing plan of care on these goals.

IMPLEMENTATION

Maintaining Skin Integrity

Cover the lesions with light clothing. Especially appropriate are the one-piece, loose-fitting terry pajamas, or one-piece cotton underwear known as "onesies."

Check out this tip. "Onesies," one-piece outfits for children, come in many colors, patterns, and designs and can be helpful in keeping a child from scratching.

The child's nails must be kept closely cut, and mitten-like hand coverings can be used. Use restraints only if necessary. Elbow restraints may sometimes be used. Remove restraints at least every 4 hours—more often, if feasible—but do not allow the child to rub or scratch while the restraints are off. If ointments or wet dressings must be kept in place on the child's face, a mask may be made by cutting holes into a cotton stockinette-type material to correspond to eyes, nose, and mouth. Wet dressings on the rest of the body can be kept in place by wrapping the child "mummy" fashion. Dressings may be left on for an extended period but should not be allowed to dry, because that can create open areas when they are removed.

Providing Comfort Measures

Plan soothing baths, such as a colloidal bath (Aveeno), just before naptime or bedtime. Time medications such as sedatives or antihistamines so that they will be effective immediately after the bath, when the child is most relaxed.

Maintaining Adequate Nutrition

Weigh the child on admission and daily thereafter. This procedure gives some indication of weight gain. If an elimination diet is being used, the diet should be carefully balanced within the framework of the foods permitted and supplemented with vitamin and mineral preparations as needed. The drinking of fluids is encouraged to prevent dehydration.

Preventing Infection

As stated, usually these children are kept out of the health care facility because of the concern about infection. However, they can also become infected at home. Whether in the health care facility or at home, the child should be placed in a room alone or in a room where there is no other child with any type of infection. Administer antibiotics as ordered. For open lesions, aseptic techniques are necessary to prevent infection.

Providing Family Teaching

Help the family caregivers understand the condition and possible food, contact, or inhalant allergens. Teach them ways to soothe the child. They should avoid overdressing and overheating the child because perspiration causes itching. Explain that they should use a mild detergent to launder the child's clothing and bedding. Help them determine ways to encourage normal growth and development. Teach them to read labels of prepared foods, watching carefully for hidden allergens. Family caregivers may feel apprehensive or repulsed by this unsightly child. Support them in expressing their feelings, and help them view this as a distressing but temporary skin condition.

Children with eczema are frequently active and "behaviorally itchy." Assist caregivers in handling challenging behavior. Help caregivers develop a strong self-image in the child to protect against strangers' openly negative reactions.

EVALUATION: GOALS AND EXPECTED OUTCOMES

- **Goal:** The child's skin integrity will be maintained or will improve.
  Expected Outcome: The child has decreased scratching and the skin will have fewer breakdowns.
- **Goal:** The child will report less itching.
  Expected Outcome: The child states itching is lessened.
- **Goal:** The child's sleep pattern will not be disturbed.
  Expected Outcome: The child sleeps an adequate amount for his or her age after comfort measures are provided.
- **Goal:** The child's nutritional intake will meet the needs for growth and development.

Expected Outcome: The child has no weight loss and has weight gain appropriate for age.
- **Goal:** The child will be free of infected skin lesions.
    Expected Outcome: The child does not scratch lesions; lesions do not become infected.
- **Goal:** The family caregivers understand the disease and its treatment.
    Expected Outcome: The family caregivers demonstrate an acceptance of the child and the condition by interacting in a positive fashion with the child.

● *Figure 40.5* Poison ivy on a child's hand.

Skin Allergies

Skin disorders of allergic origin include hives (urticaria) and giant swellings (angioedema) and rashes caused by poison ivy, poison oak, and other plants or drug reactions. Skin rashes are common in children. Infectious diseases cause some, and allergies cause others. Whatever the cause, rashes are usually treated with topical preparations, such as lotions, ointments, and greases, plus cool soaks. The itching must be relieved as much as possible because scratching can introduce additional pathogens to the affected area.

Clinical Manifestations

Hives appear in different sizes on many different parts of the body and are usually caused by foods or drugs. They are bright red and itchy and can occur on the eyelids, tongue, mouth, hands, feet, or in the brain or stomach. When affecting the mouth or tongue, hives can cause difficulty in breathing; in the stomach, the swelling can produce pain, nausea, and vomiting. Swelling in brain tissue causes headache and other neurologic symptoms.

Foods such as chocolate, nuts, shellfish, berries or other raw fruit, fish, and highly seasoned foods are likely to cause hives. Possible drug allergens include aspirin and related drugs, laxatives, anti-inflammatory drugs, tranquilizers, and antibiotics (penicillin is the most common allergen of this group). Sometimes it is impossible to identify the cause.

Treatment

Treatment is aimed at reducing the swelling and relieving the itching. If the allergen can be identified, it can be removed from the child's environment and hyposensitization can be performed. If the allergen is a certain food, that food must be eliminated from the child's diet. Antihistamines (topical or systemic) are used to relieve itching and reduce swelling. Cool soaks also help to relieve itching. Fingernails should be kept short and clean. In severe cases, corticosteroids may be necessary.

Plant Allergies

Poison ivy, oak, and sumac are common causes of contact dermatitis. Of these, poison ivy is the worst offender, particularly during the summer (Fig. 40-5). The cause of the allergy is the extremely potent oil, urushiol, which is present in all parts of these plants.

Clinical Manifestations

Its effects vary from slight inflammation and itching to severe, extensive swelling that can virtually immobilize the child. This disorder causes intense itching (pruritus) and forms tiny blisters that weep and continue to spread the inflammation.

Treatment

Antihistamines or oral corticosteroids help to relieve itching and prevent scratching. Cool soaks, Aveeno baths, calamine lotion, or topical corticosteroids help minimize discomfort. The child should be taught to recognize and avoid the poisonous plants. The plants also should be removed from the environment when possible.

BITES

Because children are active, inquisitive, and not completely inhibited in their actions, they commonly experience animal and human bites, as well as insect stings and bites. Many of these are minor, particularly if the skin is not broken.

Animal Bites

Children enjoy pets, but often they are not alert to possibly dangerous encounters with pets or wild animals. Dog bites are common. Fortunately because of rabies vaccination programs for dogs, few dog bites cause rabies; in fact, cats are the domestic animal most likely to carry rabies.

Pay attention. Some bites can have life-threatening implications if proper care is not given.

Any pet that bites should be held until it can be determined if the animal has been vaccinated against rabies. If not, the child must undergo a series of injections to prevent this potentially fatal disease. The series consists of both active and passive immunizations. Active immunity is established with five injections of human diploid cell vaccine beginning on the day of the bite and on days 3, 7, 14, and 28. Human rabies immune globulin is given on the 1st day, along with the diploid cell vaccine.

All animal and human bites should be thoroughly washed with soap and water. An antiseptic such as 70% alcohol or povidone-iodine should be applied after the wound has been thoroughly rinsed. The wound must be observed for signs of infection until well healed. Animal bites should be promptly reported to the proper authorities.

Children should be taught at an early age about the danger of animal bites, particularly of strange or wild animals such as skunks, raccoons, bats, and squirrels.

Spider Bites

Spider bites can cause serious illness if untreated. Bites of black widow spiders, brown recluse spiders, and scorpions demand medical attention. Applying ice to the affected area until medical care is obtained can slow absorption of the poison.

Tick Bites

Wood ticks carried by chipmunks, ground squirrels, weasels, and wood rats can cause Rocky Mountain spotted fever. Most cases are found in the South Atlantic, South Central, and Southeastern United States. Dogs are often the carriers to humans. People living in areas where ticks are common can be immunized against this disease.

Deer ticks, carried by white-footed mice and white-tailed deer, can carry the organism that causes Lyme disease. Most cases of Lyme disease in the United States have been seen in northeastern, mid-Atlantic, and upper north central regions, and in some northwestern counties of California. The first stage of the disease begins with a lesion at the site of the bite. The lesion appears as a macule with a clear center. The second stage occurs several weeks to months later if the patient is not treated. The symptoms of this stage may affect the central nervous system and the heart. If untreated, the third stage may occur months to years later, causing arthritis, neurologic disorders, and bone and joint disease.

Children and adults should wear long pants, long-sleeved shirts, and insect repellent when walking in the woods. Pant legs should be tucked into socks. If a tick is found on the body, alcohol may be applied and the tick carefully removed with tweezers. To prevent the release of pathogenic organisms, care should be taken not to crush the tick. A health care provider must be consulted if there is any suspicion that a deer tick has bitten a child or an adult.

Snake Bites

Snake bites demand immediate medical intervention. The wound should be washed, ice applied, and the involved body part immobilized. Prompt transport to the nearest medical facility is essential.

Insect Stings or Bites

Insect stings or bites can prove fatal to children who are sensitized. Swelling may be localized or may include an entire extremity. Circulatory collapse, airway obstruction, and anaphylactic shock can cause death within 30 minutes if the child is untreated. Immediate treatment is necessary and may include injection of epinephrine, antihistamines, or steroids. These children should wear a MedicAlert bracelet and carry an anaphylaxis kit that includes a plastic syringe of epinephrine and an antihistamine. The teacher, school nurse, and anyone who cares for the child should be alerted to the child's allergy and should know where the anaphylaxis kit is and how to use it when necessary.

BURNS

Among the many accidents that occur in children's lives, burns are the most frightening. More than 70% of burn accidents happen to children younger than age 5 years. Nearly all childhood burns are preventable, and this causes considerable guilt for families and the child. Adult carelessness, the child's exploring and curious nature, and failure to supervise the child adequately all contribute to the high incidence of burns in children. In addition, burns are a common form of child abuse.

Burns may result from various causes, including:

- Scalds from hot liquids, which are common in small children and result from a dangling electric coffee-maker cord, pans of hot liquid on the stove with handles turned out, cups of hot tea or coffee, bowls of soup or other hot liquids, or small children left alone in bathtubs. Dangerous, sometimes fatal, burns can occur from these conditions.
- Burns from fire are the second most common kind of burn, resulting from children playing with matches or being left alone in buildings that catch fire. Careless use of smoking materials is a common cause of house fires. Although cigarette lighters are currently being produced with a "child-safe" lighting mechanism, they should still be kept away from children.

Caution! Children are fascinated by fires and must be carefully supervised around fireplaces, campfires, room heaters, and outside barbecues.

- Electricity can cause severe facial or mouth burns in infants and toddlers who bite on electrical cords plugged into a socket; such burns may require extensive plastic surgery. These burns may be more serious than they first appear because of the damage to underlying tissues.

Types of Burns

Burns are divided into types according to the depth of tissue involvement: superficial, partial thickness, or full thickness (Fig. 40-6, Table 40-1).

Superficial or First-Degree Burns

The epidermis is injured, but there is no destruction of tissue or nerve endings. Thus, there is erythema, edema, and pain but prompt regeneration.

Partial-Thickness or Second-Degree Burns

The epidermis and underlying dermis are both injured and devitalized or destroyed. Blistering usually occurs with an escape of body plasma but regeneration of the skin occurs from the remaining viable epithelial cells in the dermis (Fig. 40-7).

Full-Thickness or Third-Degree Burns

The epidermis, dermis, and nerve endings are all destroyed (Fig. 40-8). Pain is minimal, and there is no longer any barrier to infection or any remaining viable epithelial cells. Fourth, fifth, and sixth degree burns have been described that are extensions of full-thickness burns with involvement of fat, muscle, and bone, respectively.

Depths of burns

Superficial (1st degree)

Partial thickness (2nd degree)

Full thickness (3rd degree)

Skin grafts

Epidermis

Dermis

Subcutaneous tissue

● **Figure 40.6** Cross-section of the skin showing the relative depths of the types of burn injuries.

TABLE 40.1	Characteristics of Burns					

Degree	Cause	Surface Appearance	Color	Pain Level	Histologic Depth	Healing Time
First (superficial) All are considered minor unless under 18 mo, over 65 yrs, or with severe loss of fluids	Flash, flame, ultraviolet (sunburn)	Dry, no blisters, edema	Erythematous	Painful	Epidermal layers only	2 to 5 days with peeling, no scarring, may have discoloration
Second (partial thickness) Minor—less than 15% in adults, less than 10% in children Moderate—15% to 30% in adults or less than 15% with involvement of face, hands, feet, or perineum; minor chemical or electrical; in children, 10% to 30% Severe—more than 30%	Contact with hot liquids or solids, flash flame to clothing, direct flame, chemical	Moist blebs, blisters	Mottled white to pink, cherry red	Very painful	Epidermis, papillary, and reticular layers of dermis; may include fat domes of subcutaneous layer	Superficial—5 to 21 days with no grafting Deep with no infection—21 to 35 days If infected, convert to full thickness.
Third (full thickness) Minor—less than 2% Moderate—2% to 10%, any involvement of face, hands, feet, or perineum Severe—more than 10% and major chemical or electrical	Contact with hot liquids or solids, flame, chemical, electricity	Dry with leathery eschar until débridement; charred blood vessels visible under eschar	Mixed white (waxy or pearly), dark (khaki or mahogany), charred	Little or no pain; hair pulls out easily	Down to and including subcutaneous tissue; may include fascia, muscle, and bone	Large areas require grafting that may take many months. Small areas may heal from the edges after weeks.

Adapted from Wiebelhaus, P. (2001). Managing burn emergencies. *Nursing Management*, 32(7), 29–36.

Emergency Treatment

Cool water is an excellent emergency treatment for burns involving small areas. The immediate application of cool compresses or cool water to burn areas appears to inhibit capillary permeability and thus suppress edema, blister formation, and tissue destruction. Ice water or ice packs must not be used because of the danger of increased tissue damage. Immersing a burned extremity in cool water alleviates pain and may prevent further thermal injury. This can be done after the airway, breathing, and circulation have been observed and restored if necessary. This action should not be done when large areas are involved because of the danger of hypothermia.

● *Figure 40.7* Partial-thickness burns. **(A)** Infant with first-degree burn on arm and chest caused by scalding. **(B)** Toddler with second-degree burn caused by scalding.

In the case of a fire victim, special attention should be given to the airway to observe for signs of smoke inhalation and respiratory passage burns. Clothing should be removed to inspect the whole body for burned areas; in addition, clothing may retain heat, which can cause additional tissue damage. The child should be transported to a medical facility for assessment. If transported to a special burn unit, the child may be wrapped in a sterile sheet and the burn treated on arrival.

Superficial Burns

Superficial burns can usually be treated on an outpatient basis because they heal readily unless infected. The area is cleaned, an anesthetic ointment is applied, and the burn is covered with a sterile gauze bandage or dressing. An analgesic may be needed to relieve pain. Blisters should not be intentionally broken because of the risk of infection, but blisters that are already broken may be débrided (cut away). The child is seen again in 2 days to inspect for infection. The caregiver is instructed to keep the area clean and dry (no

bathing the area) until the burn is healed, usually in about a week to 10 days.

Partial and Full-Thickness Burns

Distinguishing between partial and full-thickness burns is not always possible. In the presence of infection, a partial-thickness burn may be converted into a full-thickness one, and with extensive burns, a greater amount of full-thickness burn often exists than had been estimated.

Full-thickness burns require the attention, skill, and conscientious care of a team of specialists. Children with mixed second- and third-degree burns or with third-degree burns involving 15% or more of the body surface require hospitalization. Burns are classified according to criteria of the American Burn Association (Fig. 40-8, Table 40-2).

Treatment of Moderate to Severe Burns: First Phase—48 to 72 Hours

Hypovolemic shock is the major manifestation in the first 48 hours in massive burns. As extracellular fluid pours into the burned area, it collects in enormous quantities, which dehydrates the body. Edema becomes noticeable, and symptoms of severe shock appear. Intense pain is seldom a major factor. Symptoms of shock are low blood pressure, rapid pulse, pallor, and often considerable apprehension.

Airway

The adequacy of the airway must be determined in case an endotracheal tube needs to be inserted or (rarely) a tracheostomy performed. Inhalation injury is a leading cause of complications in burns. If there are burns around the face and neck or if the burns occurred in a small enclosed space, inhalation injury should be suspected. In fires, toxic substances and the

● *Figure 40.8* Full-thickness (third-degree) burn of the foot.

TABLE 40.2	Classification of Burns
Classification	Description
Minor	First-degree burn or second degree <10% of body surface or third degree <2% of body surface; no area of the face, feet, hand, or genitalia is burned
Moderate	Second-degree burn 10% to 20% body surface or on the face, hands, feet, or genitalia, or third-degree burn <10% body surface or if smoke inhalation has occurred
Severe	Second-degree burn >20% body surface or third-degree burn >10% body surface

Oral Fluids

The administration of oral fluids should be omitted or minimized for 1 or 2 days. Delayed gastric emptying causing acute gastric dilatation is a common complication of burns and can become a serious problem resulting in vomiting and anorexia. A nasogastric tube may be inserted and attached to low suction to prevent vomiting. IV fluids should relieve the child's thirst, which is usually severe, and sips of water may be allowed.

Oral feedings can be started when bowel sounds are heard. Nasogastric feedings may be needed to supplement intake. The child's caloric and nutritional requirements are two or three times those needed for normal growth; thus, nutritional supplements will most likely be needed.

Urine Output and Diuresis

Urinary output, which may be decreased because of the decrease in blood volume, must be monitored closely. Renal shutdown may be a threat. An output of

heat produced can cause damage to the respiratory tract. All these possibilities must be considered and the child should be observed for them.

Intravenous Fluids

The primary concern is to replace body fluids that have been lost or immobilized at the burn areas. Because there is a distinct relationship between the extent of the surface area burned and the amount of fluid lost, the percentage of affected skin area, as well as the classification of the burns, must be estimated to determine the medical treatment (Fig. 40-9). The extent and depth of the burn and the expertise available within the hospital determine whether the child is treated at the general hospital or immediately transported to a burn unit.

An intravenous (IV) infusion site must be selected and fluids started; most often lactated Ringer's solution, isotonic saline, or plasma is used with a large-bore catheter to administer replacement fluids and maintain total parenteral nutrition (TPN). Intravenous fluids for maintenance and replacement of lost body fluids are estimated for the first 24 hours, with half of this calculated requirement given during the first 8 hours.

However, the patient's needs may change rapidly, necessitating a change in the rate of flow or the amount or type of fluid. The patient's urinary output, vital signs, and general appearance are all part of the information that the physician needs to determine the fluid requirements. With TPN, fluids can be administered to provide needed amino acids, glucose, fats, vitamins, and minerals so that large amounts of food do not need to be consumed orally. This nutrition is essential for tissue repair and healing.

Relative Percentages of Areas Affected by Growth			
Area	Age 0	1	5
A = $\frac{1}{2}$ of head	$9\frac{1}{2}$	$8\frac{1}{2}$	$6\frac{1}{2}$
B = $\frac{1}{2}$ of one thigh	$2\frac{3}{4}$	$3\frac{1}{4}$	4
C = $\frac{1}{2}$ of one leg	$2\frac{1}{2}$	$2\frac{1}{2}$	$2\frac{3}{4}$

● **Figure 40.9** Determination of extent of burns in children.

1 to 2 mL/kg/hr for children weighing 30 kg (66 lb) or less or 30 to 50 mL/hr for those weighing more than 30 kg is desirable. An indwelling catheter facilitates the accurate measurement of urine and specific gravity. After the 1st hour, the volume of urine should be relatively constant. Any change in volume or specific gravity should be reported.

After the initial fluid therapy has brought the burn shock under control and the extracellular fluid deficit has been compensated, the patient faces another hazard with the onset of the diuretic phase. This occurs within 24 to 96 hours after the accident. The plasma-like fluid is picked up and reabsorbed from the third space in the burn areas, and the patient may rapidly become **hypervolemic** (exhibit an abnormal increase in the blood volume in the circulatory system) even to the point of pulmonary edema. This is the principal reason for the extremely close check on all vital signs and for the close monitoring of IV fluids that must now be slowed or stopped entirely.

Notifying the physician immediately is necessary if any of the following signs of the onset of this phase occur:

- Rapid rise in urinary output; may increase to 250 mL/hr or higher
- Tachypnea followed by dyspnea
- Increase in pulse pressure; mean blood pressure also may increase. Central venous pressure, if measured, is elevated.

Infection Control

The child has lost a portion of the integumentary system, which is a primary defense against infection. For this reason, measures must be taken to protect the child from infection. Antibiotics are not considered very effective in controlling infection of this type, most likely because the injured capillaries cannot carry the antibiotic to the site. If used, antibiotics are usually added to the IV fluids. Tetanus antitoxin or toxoid should be ordered, according to the status of the child's previous immunization. If inoculations are up to date, a booster dose of tetanus toxoid is all that is required.

To protect the child from infection introduced into the burn, sterile equipment must be used in the child's care. Everyone who cares for the child must wear a gown, a mask, and a head cover. Visitors also are required to scrub, gown, and mask.

Burn units are designed to be self-contained with treatment and operating areas, hydrotherapy units, and patient care areas. In hospitals where there is no specific burn unit, a private room with a door that can be closed should be set up as a burn unit. The strictest aseptic technique must be observed.

Wound Care

Two types of burn care are generally used: the open method and the closed method. The open method of burn care is most often used for superficial burns, burns of the face, and burns of the perineum. In open burn care, the wound is not covered but antimicrobial ointment is applied topically. This type of care requires strict aseptic technique.

In the closed burn method of burn care, nonadherent gauze is used to cover the burn. The child can be moved more easily, and the danger of added injury or pain is decreased. However, in the closed method dressing changes are very painful, and infection may occur under the dressings. Occlusive dressings help minimize pain because of the reduced exposure to air.

In both methods, daily **débridement** (removal of necrotic tissue) usually preceded by **hydrotherapy** (use of water in treatment) is performed. Débridement is extremely painful, and the child must have an analgesic administered before the therapy. The child is placed in the tub of water to soak the dressings; this helps to remove any sloughing tissue, **eschar** (hard crust or scab), exudate, and old medication. Often the tissue is trapped in the mesh gauze of the dressing, so soaking eases necrotic tissue removal. Loose tissue is trimmed before the burn is redressed. Hosing instead of tub soaking is used in some centers to reduce the risk of infection. Débridement is difficult emotionally for both the child and the nurse (Fig. 40-10). Diversionary activities may be used to help distract the child. Researchers also have found that children who are encouraged to participate actively in their burn care, even to help change dressings, experience healthy control over their situation and often experience less anxiety than do

● **Figure 40.10** The nurse gives support to the child during débridement.

those who are completely dependent on the nurse. The child should never be scolded or reprimanded for uncooperative behavior.

Remember this. Praise for cooperation should be used generously in the child who has to undergo débridement for a burn.

Topical medications that may be used to reduce invading organisms are silver sulfadiazine (Silvadene), silver nitrate, mafenide acetate (Sulfamylon), Bacitracin, and povidone-iodine (Betadine). Each of these agents has advantages and disadvantages. The choice of agent is made by the physician and is determined, at least partially, by the organisms found in cultures of the burn area.

Grafting

Grafts may be **homografts**, **heterografts** (xenografts), or **autografts**. Homografts and heterografts are temporary grafts. A homograft consists of skin taken from another person, which is eventually rejected by the recipient tissue and sloughed off after 3 to 6 weeks. Skin from cadavers is often used in a procedure called an **allograft**; this skin can be stored and used up to several weeks, and permission for this use is seldom refused.

A heterograft is skin obtained from animals, usually pigs (porcine). Both homografts and heterografts provide a temporary dressing after débridement and have been proven to be lifesaving measures for children with extensive burns.

An autograft, consisting of skin taken from the child's own body, is the only kind of skin accepted permanently by recipient tissues, except for the skin from an identical twin. Obtaining enough healthy skin to cover a large area is usually impossible; therefore, homografts are of great value for immediate covering. If the donor site is kept free from infection and grafts of sufficient thinness are taken, the site should be ready for use again in 10 to 12 days.

After grafting, the donor and the graft sites are kept covered with sterile dressings.

Complications

Curling's ulcer (also called a stress ulcer) is a gastric or duodenal ulcer that often occurs after serious skin burns. It can easily be overlooked when attention is directed toward the treatment of the burn area and the prevention of infection. Symptoms are those of any gastric ulcer but usually are vague, concerned with abdominal discomfort, with or without localization, or related to eating. Ulcers appear during the first 6 weeks. Blood in the stools combined with abdominal discomfort may be the basis for diagnosis. If desired, roentgenograms can confirm the diagnosis. Treatment consists of a bland diet and the use of antacids and antispasmodics.

The health care team must guard carefully against the complication of **contractures**. If the burn extends over a movable body part, fibrous scarring that forms in the healing process can cause serious deformities and limit movement. Joints must be positioned, possibly in overextension, so that maximal flexibility is maintained. Splinting, exercise, and pressure also are used to prevent contractures. When burns are severe, pressure garments may be used. These garments help decrease hypertrophy of scar tissue. However, they may need to be worn for 12 to 18 months. The child must wear these garments continuously, except when bathing.

Long-term Care

The rehabilitative phase of care for the child is often long and difficult. Even after discharge from the health care facility, the child needs to return for additional treatment or plastic surgery to release contractures and revise scar tissue. The emotional scars of the family and the child must be evaluated, and therapy must be initiated or continued. The impact of scarring and disfigurement may need to be resolved by both the child and members of the family. If the child is of school age, school work and social interaction must be considered. (See Nursing Care Plan 40-1: The Child With a Burn.)

● Nursing Process for the Child With a Burn

ASSESSMENT

Assessment of the child with a burn is complex and varies with the extent and depth of the burn, the stage of healing, and the age and general condition of the child. Initially the primary concerns are the cardiac and respiratory state, the assessment of shock, and an evaluation of the burns.

After the first phase (the first 24 to 48 hours), the healing of the child's burns must be evaluated and the child's nutrition, signs of infection, and pain level must be monitored. The emotional conditions of the child and the family also must be evaluated.

SELECTED NURSING DIAGNOSES

- Risk for Infection related to the loss of protective layer (skin) secondary to burn injury

Read these

NURSING CARE PLAN 40.1

The Child With a Burn

Two-year-old JW was watching his mother fix dinner. She turned away from the stove where she had vegetables cooking. JW climbed on his chair and grabbed the handle of the pan. Before his mother could react, the boiling liquid from the vegetables poured down over his right arm, the right side of his torso, and his right groin and leg. He is now in the pediatric unit for care of second- and third-degree burns of his right arm, right torso and groin, and right leg.

NURSING DIAGNOSIS
Risk for Infection related to the loss of a protective layer secondary to burn injury

GOAL: The child will be free from signs and symptoms of infection.

EXPECTED OUTCOMES
• The child's burns show no signs of foul-smelling drainage.
• The child's vital signs remain within normal limits: pulse ranging between 80 and 110 bpm, respirations 20–30/minute, and temperature ranging between 98.6° and 101°F (37°–38.4°C).

NURSING INTERVENTIONS	RATIONALE
Carry out conscientious handwashing and follow other infection control precautions including the use of sterile equipment and supplies. Wear sterile gown, mask, and cap; use sterile gloves when giving direct care to the burned area.	Sterile technique decreases the introduction of microorganisms. Handwashing is the foundation of good medical asepsis. These procedures reduce the risk of infection.
Teach family and visitors handwashing and sterile techniques.	Infection control procedures must include all who enter the child's room in order to be effective.
Screen visitors for signs of upper respiratory or skin infections.	The child with severe burns may be easily susceptible to upper respiratory and skin infections.
Note and document all drainage and any unusual odor; take regular cultures as ordered.	Early detection and prompt treatment of infection are essential as severe infection places an additional burden on the child's already stressed system.

NURSING DIAGNOSIS
Imbalanced Nutrition: Less than Body Requirements related to increased caloric needs secondary to burns and anorexia

GOAL: The child's caloric intake will be adequate to meet needs for tissue repair and growth.

EXPECTED OUTCOMES
• The child will consume at least 80% of diet high in calories and protein.
• The child will maintains his preburn weight or will have weight gain appropriate for age.

NURSING INTERVENTIONS	RATIONALE
Offer a high-calorie, high-protein, bland diet.	Increased calories and high-protein diet are required to promote wound healing.
Plan appealing meals offered in small servings catering to the child's food likes and dislikes. Give choices when appropriate.	Small servings are more appealing to a child. Allowing JW to make choices gives him some feeling of control and encourages his cooperation.
Weigh daily in the morning with only underwear on.	Daily or weekly weights provide information to determine nutritional status.

NURSING DIAGNOSIS
Acute Pain related to tissue destruction and painful procedures

GOAL: The child will show signs of being comfortable and pain will be kept at an acceptable level.

EXPECTED OUTCOMES
• The child rests quietly with pulse between 80 and 110 bpm and respirations 20–30/minute and regular.
• The child uses the faces pain rating scale to indicate his pain level as appropriate for age.
• Analgesics are administered before dressing changes and débridement procedures.

NURSING CARE PLAN 40.1 continued

The Child With a Burn

NURSING INTERVENTIONS	RATIONALE
Monitor every 2 to 4 hours to determine the child's comfort level, vital signs and if the child is restless.	Each individual reacts differently to pain and analgesics. Learning child's responses helps to effectively plan to reduce his pain.
Administer analgesics 20 to 30 minutes before dressing changes and débridement.	This gives the analgesics time to reach optimum effectiveness for pain relief during procedures.
Support and comfort during procedures. Plan a favorite activity after procedures to give child something pleasant to anticipate.	Acknowledging that the procedures are painful and his cooperation deserves a reward may help the child accept the inevitable.
Give opportunities to exercise some control when possible over timing, what gets done first, or other details.	A feeling of control over some aspects of his care and situation helps offset feelings of powerlessness.

NURSING DIAGNOSIS
Risk for Impaired Physical Mobility related to pain and scarring

GOAL: The child will have increased mobility and contractures will be minimal.

EXPECTED OUTCOMES
- The child participates in range-of-motion activities and uses both arms and legs.
- The child's splints, pressure suit, and positions are maintained.
- The child has no evidence of contractures.
- The child participates in ambulatory activities.

NURSING INTERVENTIONS	RATIONALE
Position so that no two skin surfaces touch; give special attention to right armpit, right elbow, wrist and hand, right groin, and right knee.	When any two skin surfaces touch, scarring will occur that results in contractures and limited movement.
Maintain splints and pressure dressings to hyperextend joints.	Hyperextension limits the formation of contractures.
Plan self-care activities that give child some control and also will encourage movement of affected joints.	Encouraging child to do small activities to help himself promotes movement and decreases contractures.
Encourage active play and ambulation.	A child is more likely to cooperate in exercise and movement that is fun.

NURSING DIAGNOSIS
Deficient Knowledge of the Caregiver related to optimizing the child's healing process and to the long-term care required by the child

GOAL: The child's family caregivers will verbalize an understanding of the child's long-term home care.

EXPECTED OUTCOMES
- Family caregivers demonstrate wound care and dressing changes.
- Family caregivers verbalize an understanding of the long-term management of child's care and needed treatment.
- The child's family secures the home care equipment needed for his care.
- The family caregivers plan for follow-up care and utilize social service assistance.

NURSING INTERVENTIONS	RATIONALE
Explain to mother and other family caregivers what you are doing and why as you give care and perform procedures for child.	Having a child with a burn is an overwhelming experience. Providing explanations as you give care helps the family to begin to grasp the care process.
Provide information to the child's mother and other family caregivers in small amounts, repeating information from one time to another. Allow ample opportunity for questions.	Family caregivers can absorb only so much information at a time. Repetition and patient, careful answering of questions helps the family to understand the long-term view.

(nursing care plan continues on page 966)

NURSING CARE PLAN 40.1 continued

The Child With a Burn

NURSING INTERVENTIONS	RATIONAL
Teach the child's family about the importance of diet, infection control, exercise, rest, activity, pressure suit, and all aspects of child's care.	The child's family needs to understand all aspects of care including how the pressure suit is worn, the care of the suit, and the need to change the suit as the child grows.
Teach signs and symptoms that are important to note and what may need to be reported promptly.	Learning what to observe for and which signs or symptoms need to be reported promptly gives the family caregivers confidence in their ability and improves the level of home care that they give.
Provide family with information and contacts for social services, which will help in the care for the child.	Long-term care is improved and aided by contact and interaction with appropriate social services.

- Imbalanced Nutrition: Less Than Body Requirements related to increased caloric needs secondary to burns and anorexia
- Acute Pain related to tissue destruction and painful procedures
- Risk for Impaired Physical Mobility related to pain and scarring
- Anxiety related to changes in body image caused by thermal injury
- Compromised Family Coping related to the effect of the injury on the child and family's life
- Deficient Knowledge of caregivers related to optimizing the child's healing process and to the long-term care required by the child

OUTCOME IDENTIFICATION AND PLANNING

During the first phase of care, the major goals relate to cardiopulmonary stabilization, fluid and electrolyte balance, and infection control. After the first 72 hours in the phase, sometimes called the management or subacute phase, more long-term goals are developed. The child's goals are limited by his or her age and ability to communicate. Goals related to the child include preventing infection, maintaining adequate nutrition, reducing pain, increasing mobility, and relieving anxiety. The family caregiver goals include concerns about stress on the family related to the child's injury. Other goals relate to optimizing healing and decreasing complications to minimize permanent disability and gaining an understanding of the long-term implications of care.

IMPLEMENTATION

Preventing Infection

The immaturity of the child's immune system, the destruction of the skin layer, and the presence of necrotic tissue (an ideal medium for bacterial growth) contribute to a significant danger of infection. Conscientious handwashing is necessary by anyone who has contact with the child. Observe rigid infection control precautions and use only sterile equipment and supplies. Monitor vital signs, including temperature, on a 1-, 2-, or 4-hour schedule. Screen all people who have any contact with the child, including visitors, family, or staff caregivers for any signs of upper respiratory or skin infection.

When caring for the burn, wear a sterile gown, mask, and cap. Wear sterile gloves or use a sterile tongue blade to apply ointment to the burn. Maintain the room temperature at around 80°F because water evaporates quickly through the denuded areas and even through the leathery burn eschar, with thermal loss resulting. Note and document all drainage. Report immediately and document any unusual odor. Cultures are done regularly, usually several times a week. Avoid injury to the eschar and the donor site. Hair on the tissue adjacent to the burn area is usually shaved.

Ensuring Adequate Nutrition

The child who has received extensive burns requires special attention regarding nutritional needs. The nutritional problem is much more complex than simply getting a seriously ill child to eat. The child is in negative caloric balance from a number of causes, including

- Poor intake because of anorexia, ileus, Curling's ulcer, or diarrhea
- External loss caused by exudative losses of protein through the burn wound
- Hypermetabolism caused by fever, infection, and the state of toxicity

A bland diet high in protein (for healing and replacement) and calories is an essential component of therapy. Use every effort possible to interest the child in foods essential for tissue building and repair. Do not serve large servings because the child often experiences anorexia. In addition, the child's physical condition often interferes with his or her ability to eat. Foods are of no value if the child refuses to eat them. Try using colorful trays, foods with eye appeal, and any special touches to spur a child's appetite. Allow the child to have some control to encourage cooperation. Foods that may appeal are flavored milk shakes, ice cream shakes, high-protein drinks containing eggs with the addition of dried protein milk, ice cream, milk and egg desserts, and puréed meats and vegetables.

Even with the best efforts of nurses, dietitians, and the child, the burn patient seldom can eat enough food to meet the increased needs. Total parenteral nutrition (TPN) or tube feedings often are necessary as supplements to the oral intake. Commercial high-calorie formulas are available for tube feedings that meet the child's needs. Avoid using TPN or tube feedings as a threat to the child. Explain carefully to the child what is to be done and why and make sure the child understands. Try demonstrating the feeding process with a doll to help the child grasp the idea.

Weigh the child daily at the same time and with the child wearing the same amount of clothing or covering. Carefully monitor intake and output.

Relieving Pain and Providing Comfort Measures

The pain of a thermal injury can be severe. As a result of the pain or the fear and anxiety that pain causes, the child may not sleep well, may experience anorexia, and may be apprehensive and uncooperative during treatments and care. Analgesics must be administered to provide the most relief possible. Administer analgesics at least 20 to 30 minutes before dressing changes and débridement. Avoid scheduling the administration of pain medications close to mealtimes. Otherwise the child may be too sedated to eat.

Monitor the child's physiologic response to the pain and analgesics. Document the child's pupil reaction, heart and respiratory rates, and behavior in response to pain and analgesics.

Provide support and comfort during painful procedures. Use diversionary activities to help the child focus on something other than the pain. Promising a favorite activity after the dreaded procedure is acceptable. Television may be helpful, but be cautious not to overuse it. The younger child may enjoy learning new songs, playing age-appropriate games, or listening to someone reading stories. The older child may enjoy video or computer games, tape recordings, books, and board or card games. The child should never be admonished for crying or behaving "like a baby." Acknowledge the child's pain, give the child as much control as possible, and work with the child and the family to minimize the pain and to bring about the greatest rewards for all involved.

Promoting Mobility and Preventing Contractures

Care must be taken to avoid contractures and scarring that limit movement. Never permit two burned body surfaces, such as fingers, to touch. If the neck is involved, the child may have to be kept with the neck hyperextended; the arms may need to be placed in a brace to prevent underarm contractures; joints of the knee or elbow must be extended to prevent scar formation from causing contractures that limit movement. Pressure dressings and pressure suits may be used for this purpose and may need to be worn for more than a year. Physical therapy may be needed, and splints may be used to position the body part to prevent contractures. All these measures can add to the child's discomfort.

Encourage range of motion, early ambulation, and self-help activities as additional means of promoting mobility and preventing contractures. Use creativity to devise ways to involve the child in enjoyable activities that encourage movement of the affected part.

Reducing Anxiety

The child's age and level of understanding influence the amount of anxiety that he or she has about scarring and disability related to the burn. If the child is in a burn unit with other children, seeing others may cause unrealistic fears. Encourage the child to explore his or her feelings about changes, especially those involving body image. Use therapeutic play with puppets or dolls if possible. Encourage both the family and the nursing staff to provide the child with continuous support.

Promoting Family Coping

The family may feel guilty about the injury; one member may feel especially responsible. These feelings affect the family's coping abilities. Give both the family and the child opportunities to discuss and express their feelings. Suggest counseling if necessary to help family members handle their feelings. Put the family in touch with support groups if available to help the family work through problems. Explain the child's care to family members and involve them in the care when possible. Avoid saying anything that might add to the guilt or anxiety that the family members are feeling.

Providing Family Teaching

Provide the family caregivers with explanations about the whole process of burns, the care, the healing process, and the long-term implications. Give information to the family as they are ready for it; do not thrust it on them all at once. To prepare for home care, teach the family about wound care, dressing changes, signs and symptoms to observe and report, and the importance of diet, rest, and activity. Help the family to find resources for any necessary supplies and equipment. Make a referral to social services to assist them in home care planning.

EVALUATION: GOALS AND EXPECTED OUTCOMES

- **Goal:** The child will be free from signs or symptoms of infection.
  Expected Outcome: The child's pulse and respirations are within normal limits for age; temperature is 98.6° to 101°F (37° to 38.4°C); there is no malodorous drainage.
- **Goal:** The child's caloric intake will be adequate to meet his needs for tissue repair and growth.
  Expected Outcome: The child consumes at least 80% of diet high in calories and protein and maintains weight or has weight gain appropriate for age.
- **Goal:** The child will show signs of being comfortable.
  Expected Outcome: The child rests quietly and does not cry or moan excessively; the pulse and respiratory rates are regular and normal for age.
- **Goal:** The child will have increased mobility and contractures will be minimal.

Expected Outcome: The child participates in range-of-motion activities; splints, pressure dressings and suits, and positions are maintained; there is no evidence of contractures.
- **Goal:** The older child will express feelings related to changes associated with burns.
  Expected Outcome: The child expresses feelings and fears about body image and demonstrates a positive attitude of acceptance.
- **Goal:** The family caregivers will verbalize feelings related to the child's injury and take steps to develop coping skills.
  Expected Outcome: The family caregivers verbalize fears, anxieties, and other feelings related to the child's injury; discuss the impact of the injury on the child and family's life; cooperate with counseling; and become involved in support groups.
- **Goal:** The family caregivers will verbalize an understanding of the child's long-term home care management.
  Expected Outcome: Family members demonstrate wound care and dressing changes, list signs and symptoms to observe for and report, secure needed home care equipment, and use social service assistance if appropriate.

Test Yourself

- What causes an allergic reaction? What are some of the common allergens?
- Explain ways to keep a child from scratching the skin when he has eczema.
- What are the major causes of burns in children?
- Explain the differences among first-, second-, and third-degree burns.

SEXUALLY TRANSMITTED DISEASES

The incidence of sexually transmitted diseases (STDs) is higher in adolescents than in any other age group. The diseases range from infections that can be easily treated to life-threatening diseases such as infection with human immunodeficiency virus (HIV; Table 40-3). Although communicable diseases, STDs are addressed separately here because of their high incidence.

TABLE 40.3 | Major Sexually Transmitted Diseases

Infection and Agent	Transmission	Symptoms	Possible Complications	Prevention
Gonorrhea— gonococcus: *Neisseria gonorrhoeae*	Sexual contact; mother to fetus during vaginal delivery	Yellow mucopurulent discharge of the genital area, painful or frequent urination, pain in the genital area; may be asymptomatic Frequent cause of pelvic inflammatory disease	Sterility, cystitis, arthritis, endocarditis	Public should be educated on safe sex practices; mother should be tested before delivery. Newborn's eyes should be treated with tetracycline ointment, erythromycin ointment, or silver nitrate. All contacts should be treated with antibiotics.
Chlamydia— bacteria: *Chlamydia trachomatis*	Sexual contact; mother to fetus during vaginal delivery	Mucopurulent genital discharge, genital pain, dysuria Frequent cause of pelvic inflammatory disease, often in combination with gonorrhea	Sterility	Public should be educated about safe sex practices. Sexual contact should be avoided when lesions are present. Infected mothers should have a cesarean delivery.
Genital herpes virus: herpes simplex type 2	Sexual contact; mother to fetus during vaginal delivery	Genital soreness, pruritus, and erythema; vesicles appear that usually last for about 10 days during which time transmission of virus is likely		Public should be educated about safe sex practices. Sexual contact should be avoided when lesions are present. Infected mother should have a cesarean delivery.
Syphilis— spirochete: *Treponema pallidum*	Sexual contact; mother to fetus via placenta; blood transfusions if undiagnosed donor is in early stage of disease	Primary stage: genital lesion, enlarged lymph nodes Secondary stage (6 weeks later): lesions of skin and mucous membrane with generalized symptoms of headache and fever	Tertiary stage: central nervous system and cardiovascular damage, paralysis, psychosis	Public should be educated about safe sex practices. Screen blood donors; do serologic testing before and during pregnancy. Contact with body secretions from infected patients should be avoided.
Acquired immunodeficiency syndrome (AIDS)—virus: human immunodeficiency virus	Sexual contact; exposure to blood or blood products; mother to fetus or infant	Primary infection: rash, fever, cough, malaise, lymphadenopathy Mildly symptomatic: HIV-positive, enlarged lymph nodes, liver, spleen, persistent upper respiratory infections, otitis media Moderately symptomatic: HIV positive, candidiasis, meningitis, pneumonia, sepsis, herpes infections Severely symptomatic: HIV positive, serious infections, opportunistic infections	Neurologic impairment	Public, especially high-risk groups, should be educated about safe sex practices. Blood or blood products used for transfusion should be carefully screened. Intravenous drug abusers should not share needles. Standard precautions should be used consistently in all health care settings. Measures to avoid needlesticks among health care workers should be instituted.

Infants infected with STDs usually are infected prenatally or during birth. Children infected after the neonatal period must be considered victims of sexual abuse until disproved. Severe or repeated cases of pelvic inflammatory disease (PID) or severe genital warts are warning signs that a girl should be tested for HIV.

Prevention is the most effective tool in the campaign against STDs. The only certain way to avoid contracting an STD is sexual abstinence. However, sexual activity in adolescents indicates that this is often not a practical solution. Condoms with spermicide (discussed in Chapter 27) provide protection, although they are not fail-safe. Adolescents must be educated about all aspects of the consequences of sexual activity.

Gonorrhea

An estimated 800,000 cases of gonorrhea are reported annually, and an equal number of cases are believed to be undiagnosed. It is one of the most commonly reported communicable diseases in the United States. Also called "the clap," "the drips," or "the dose," gonorrhea has mild primary symptoms, particularly in females, and often goes undetected and thus untreated until it progresses to a serious pelvic disorder. This disease can cause sterility in males.

Several drugs may be used to treat gonorrhea, but the current drug of choice is ceftriaxone (Rocephin) followed by a week of oral doxycycline (Vibramycin) to prevent an accompanying chlamydial infection. Adolescents are asked to name their sexual contacts so that they also may be treated. Penicillin-resistant strains of the organism have developed, so penicillin is no longer an effective method of treatment. Adolescents must learn that their bodies will not develop immunity to the organism and they might become infected again if they continue to expose themselves by engaging in sexual activity, especially high-risk sexual behavior.

Chlamydial Infection

Chlamydial infections have replaced gonorrhea as the most common and fastest spreading STD in the United States. Symptoms may be mild, causing a delay in diagnosis and treatment until serious complications and transmission to others have occurred.

Adolescents must be made aware of the seriousness of PID, a common result of a chlamydial infection. Pelvic inflammatory disease can cause sterility in the female, primarily by causing scarring in the fallopian tubes that prohibits the passage of the fertilized ovum into the uterus. A tubal pregnancy may be the consequence of a chlamydial infection. In the male, sterility may result from epididymitis caused by a chlamydial infection.

Doxycycline or azithromycin is used to treat chlamydial infection. In the pregnant adolescent, erythromycin or amoxicillin can be used to avoid the teratogenic effects of these drugs. All sexual partners must be treated.

Genital Herpes

Genital herpes has reached epidemic proportions in the United States. The disease begins as a vesicle that ruptures to form a painful ulcer on the genitalia. The initial ulcer lasts 10 to 12 days. Recurrent episodes occur intermittently and last 4 to 5 days. No cure is available, but acyclovir (Zovirax) is useful in relieving or suppressing the symptoms.

Genital herpes is associated with a much higher than average risk for cervical cancer; therefore, the female who has genital herpes should have an annual Pap smear. Genital herpes is not transmitted to the fetus in utero. However, if the mother has an active case of genital herpes at the time of delivery, cesarean birth is indicated to reduce the risk of infection as the fetus passes through the vagina. In newborns, the infection can become systemic and cause death.

Syphilis

Caused by the spirochete *Treponema pallidum*, syphilis is a destructive disease that can involve every part of the body. Untreated, it can have devastating long-term effects. Infected mothers are highly likely to transmit the infection to their unborn infants.

Syphilis is spread primarily by sexual contact. Symptoms of the primary stage usually appear about 3 weeks after exposure. If allowed to progress without treatment, syphilis has a secondary stage, a latent stage, and a tertiary stage.

Clinical Manifestations

The cardinal sign of the primary stage is the chancre, which is a hard, red, painless lesion at the point of entry of the spirochete. This can appear on the penis, the vulva, or the cervix. It also can appear on the mouth, the lips, or the rectal area as a result of oral-genital or anal-genital contact. The secondary stage, marked by rash, sore throat, and fever, appears 2 to 6 months after the original infection. Signs of both the first and second stages disappear without treatment, but the spirochete remains in the body. The latent period can persist for as long as 20 years without symptoms; however, blood tests are still positive. In the tertiary stage, syphilis causes severe neurologic and cardiovascular damage, mental illness, and gastrointestinal disorders.

Treatment

Syphilis responds to one intramuscular injection of penicillin G benzathine; if the child is sensitive to penicillin, oral doxycycline, tetracycline, or erythromycin can be administered as alternative treatment. If treatment is not obtained before the tertiary stage, the neurologic and cardiovascular complications can lead to death.

Acquired Immunodeficiency Syndrome

Acquired immunodeficiency syndrome (AIDS) is caused by the human immunodeficiency virus (HIV), which attacks and destroys the T-helper lymphocytes (CD4+). The T-helper lymphocytes are cells that direct the immune response to viral, bacterial, and fungal infections and remove some malignant cells from the body.

Because not all persons who test positive for HIV develop AIDS immediately, the Centers for Disease Control and Prevention (CDC) have established criteria for a classification system for HIV infection and AIDS surveillance. The most significant of these criteria for children and adults is the CD4+ T-lymphocyte count. Normal CD4 cell counts vary in children, depending on the age of the child. As the disease progresses, the CD4 count drops and puts the child at risk for developing life-threatening infections. The CDC classifies HIV/AIDS in three categories:

- Category A: Mildly symptomatic: HIV positive as well as two or more symptoms, such as enlarged spleen, liver, or lymph nodes, frequent respiratory or ear infections.
- Category B: Moderately symptomatic: HIV positive as well as illnesses such as candidiasis, bacterial pneumonia or meningitis, chronic diarrhea, herpes simplex virus or herpes zoster, persistent fever.
- Category C: Severely symptomatic: HIV positive as well as serious bacterial infections, encephalopathy, lymphoma, tuberculosis, severe failure to thrive, or an opportunistic infection.

Transmission of HIV occurs through contact with infected blood or blood products during transfusions or sharing of infected needles, exposure to infected body secretions through sexual contact, as well as from an HIV-positive woman to her unborn fetus or new-born infant. The virus cannot be transmitted through casual contact. The diagnosis of any STD increases the statistical risk of HIV infection by 300%.

Infants usually are infected through the placenta during prenatal life, in the birth process when contaminated by the mother's blood, or through breast-feeding. Children and teens also can be infected through sexual abuse. Adolescents are most often infected through intimate heterosexual or homosexual relations and through intravenous drug use. Hemophiliacs who received blood products before 1985 were infected in some cases, but safeguards are now in place, and the blood supply has become much safer.

Although most children with AIDS are between the ages of 1 and 4 years, the alarming increase occurring among adolescents is causing great concern in those who work with adolescents. African-American adolescents have a disproportionately high rate of AIDS. The numbers of adolescent girls with HIV continues to rise.

Teenagers' attitude of impunity (the belief that nothing can hurt them) and the increasing rate of sexual activity in this age group, often involving multiple partners, contribute to the fear that this group will experience widespread illness from HIV. The incubation period for HIV can vary from 3 to 10 years; thus many who contract the disease in adolescence will not have symptoms until they are in their 20s, when they are at their reproductive peak. The proper use of a condom with spermicide (see Chapter 27) during any type of sexual contact is essential to prevent the spread of HIV. Adolescent girls may have sexual experiences with older men who have had many previous sexual partners. This increases the risk for the girl and, in turn, can increase the risk for any adolescent boy with whom she is sexually intimate. Adolescent boys also are at increased risk if they engage in unprotected homosexual relations, use intravenous drugs, have multiple partners, or have sex with a prostitute.

CULTURAL SNAPSHOT

Cultural influences may play an important role in the spread of HIV. The adolescent girl often finds it difficult to insist that her partner use a condom. If the partner refuses and claims to be "safe" (uninfected) or protests that the condom decreases his pleasure, she might give in for fear of breaking up the relationship. In addition, in some cultures the more sexual conquests a boy has, the more manly he is considered.

About 20% to 30% of the infants born to HIV-infected mothers develop AIDS. Although the infants may test positive in the 1st year of life, testing is not reliable until 18 months of age because the infant may retain antibodies from the mother for this length of time. However, for affected infants younger than 1 year of age, the disease can move rapidly to AIDS and serious complications. Failure to thrive, *Pneumocystis carinii* pneumonia, recurrent bacterial infections, progressive encephalopathy, and malignancy often develop in affected infants. Some of these children progress quickly to terminal illness and death, but with aggressive chemotherapy some of them are living long enough to enter school.

Clinical Manifestations and Treatment

Children and adolescents manifest the symptoms of HIV in much the same way as adults. Females rarely have Kaposi sarcoma, a cancer often seen in homosexual men. Many women including adolescents present with a chronic infection of vaginitis caused by *C. albicans* that has not responded to local antifungal treatments. These infections may be controlled by oral systemic medications. The female who tests positive for HIV should have a pelvic examination every 6 months to detect early STDs and institute vigorous treatment as needed.

● Nursing Process for the Child With AIDS

ASSESSMENT

When seeking data from the child with AIDS, gather a complete history, including chief complaint, presenting symptoms, past medical history, immunization status, family history, and social history. Interview the family caregiver if present, but be certain to provide the adolescent with a private interview. The adolescent may be extremely reluctant to reveal either social or sexual history, especially in the presence of a family member. Review carefully the teen girl's history of vaginal candidiasis, PID, and sexual activity. Review the teen boy's sexual activity, including partners who are of the same sex or who are intravenous drug users. The adolescent may have various emotions, including anger, denial, guilt, and rebelliousness; the nurse should accept all these emotions as legitimate reactions to the illness.

During the physical exam, maintain strict standard precautions. Include vital signs and especially observe for fever, which may indicate infection, and perform a thorough survey of all body systems. Observe for poor skin turgor, rashes or lesions, alopecia, mucous membrane lesions or thrush, weight loss, mental or neurologic changes, respiratory infections or signs of tuberculosis, diarrhea or abdominal pain, vaginal discharge, perineal lesions, or genital warts. Help prepare the child for diagnostic tests that must be performed.

SELECTED NURSING DIAGNOSES

- Risk for Infection related to increased susceptibility secondary to a compromised immune system
- Risk for Injury related to the possible transmission of the virus
- Risk for Impaired Skin Integrity related to perineal and anal tissue excoriation secondary to genital candidiasis or genital warts
- Acute Pain related to symptoms of the disease
- Imbalanced Nutrition: Less Than Body Requirements related to anorexia, oral or esophageal lesions, or diarrhea
- Social Isolation related to rejection by others secondary to the diagnosis of AIDS
- Hopelessness related to the diagnosis and prognosis
- Compromised Family Coping related to the diagnosis of AIDS

OUTCOME IDENTIFICATION AND PLANNING

Planning the nursing care of a child with AIDS can be challenging. The child needs support to accept the diagnosis and move in a positive direction to follow the treatment plan to the best of his or her ability. The nurse can play a critical role in helping the child understand the treatment and prognosis and their impact on his or her life. Major goals for the child include maintaining the highest level of wellness possible by preventing infection and the spread of the infection, maintaining skin integrity, minimizing pain, improving nutrition, alleviating social isolation, and diminishing a feeling of hopelessness. The primary goal for the family is improving coping skills and helping the teen cope with the illness.

IMPLEMENTATION

Preventing Infection

In the health care facility, strict adherence to appropriate infection control measures is extremely important. A primary goal is to teach the child to prevent infections. Teach good handwashing technique; the patient should take care to wash between the fingers and under rings and should use a pump-type soap. He or she should keep nails trimmed to avoid harboring microorganisms under the nails. Teach the teen that skin care includes showering (not a tub bath) with a mild soap (no strong, perfumed soaps), using an emollient cream, and patting the skin dry while avoiding vigorous rubbing.

Raw fruits and vegetables should be washed and peeled or cooked to avoid the danger of bacteria; meats must be well cooked. The child must avoid unpasteurized dairy products and foods grown in organic fertilizer.

Instruct the child to brush the teeth at least three times a day using a soft toothbrush and nonabrasive toothpaste. Routine dental care is vital.

The household where the child lives must be cleaned carefully and regularly. A household bleach solution of one part bleach to 10 parts of water is a good solution to use. Particular attention should be paid to the refrigerator, the stove, the oven, and the microwave to prevent contamination of foods during preparation or storage. Household items that may be contaminated should be discarded in double plastic bags to prevent spread to others. Laundry bleach should be used when washing the child's clothing, especially underwear.

Teach the child that someone else should care for pets. Cleaning an aquarium or birdcage or emptying a cat's litter box can expose the child to opportunistic organisms that will attack the compromised immune system. Help the child learn to avoid persons who have any infectious disease. Advise him or her that prompt attention to an apparently minor infection helps avoid more serious illness. The child with AIDS should not receive any live vaccine immunizations but should continue to receive other immunizations as indicated.

Preventing Infection Transmission

The good hygienic practices necessary to protect the child from an acquired or opportunistic infection also help to prevent transmission of the virus to others. In addition, the adolescent needs counseling about sexual practices. One of the most emotionally difficult tasks for the adolescent may be to list sexual contacts. This is a delicate matter that must be approached in a nonjudgmental, sympathetic manner, but the teen needs to understand that anyone with whom he or she has been sexually intimate may be infected and must be identified. The teen may find that the sexual partner from whom he or she contracted the virus already knew that he or she

was infected. Infection with HIV does not necessarily mean that the child was promiscuous. The adolescent may have been sexually intimate with only one person, and that person may have assured the teen that he or she was not infected. The adolescent may be extremely angry about exposure by a trusted person.

Teach the adolescent about safe sex practices. The adolescent needs to understand that he or she is protecting not only future sexual partners from contracting the disease but also himself or herself from contracting other strains of the virus. Both boys and girls need to have complete instructions on the use of condoms and spermicide (see Chapter 27). The adolescent must not be sexually intimate with anyone without using a condom, no matter what kind of argument the other person uses. Also the teen needs to learn how HIV is transmitted, including vaginal intercourse, oral-genital contact, anal intercourse, or any contact with blood or body fluids, including menstrual discharge. The teen who practices oral-genital sex must learn to use a dental dam (a square of latex worn in the mouth to prevent contact of body fluids with mucous membranes of the mouth).

The adolescent girl needs counseling about pregnancy. The probability of transmitting the virus to her unborn child may be as high as 30%, and no way currently exists to determine if she will pass the virus to her child. She must consider that even if her child is not infected, there is a possibility that she may not live to see the child reach adulthood. All these considerations are overwhelming, and the adolescent needs continuous support to understand, accept, and deal with them.

A discussion of the use of illicit, injectable drugs is important. Counsel the child and adolescent about the importance of stopping drug use. However, the reality is that he or she may not quit, so explain how to sterilize needles using chlorine bleach. A mixture of one part bleach to five parts water should be drawn through the needle into the syringe, flushed two or three times, and finally rinsed with water. Remember that the adolescent has the right to decide how to conduct his or her life, and remain nonjudgmental through all contacts with the teen.

Promoting Skin Integrity

Skin lesions are common symptoms of many STDs. The child must report any new skin lesion to the health care provider for diagnosis and immediate treatment. The best preventive measure is to follow careful infection control measures, including careful handwashing and to protect skin integrity by using skin emollients to guard against dryness; avoiding harsh, perfumed soaps; and guarding against injury to the skin. In advanced disease, nursing measures are implemented to protect and pad pressure points and improve peripheral circulation.

Promoting Comfort

Pain is caused by several manifestations of AIDS. Skin and mucous membrane lesions may be very painful. Topical anesthetic solutions, such as viscous lidocaine, and meticulous mouth care can relieve pain caused by oral mucous membrane infections. Smoking, alcohol, and spicy or acidic foods irritate the oral mucous membranes and often cause additional pain. Pelvic inflammatory disease, a common complication of STDs, is usually accompanied by abdominal pain. The child with respiratory complications also has bouts of chest pain. Administer analgesics to relieve pain and use all appropriate nursing measures to help the child feel more comfortable. As the disease develops, the pain may be greater, so every effort must be made to provide comfort.

Improving Nutrition

Anorexia, or a poor appetite, is a common problem of the patient with AIDS. Dehydration, diarrhea, infection, malabsorption, oral candidiasis, and some drugs also can contribute to the child's poor state of nutrition. Malnutrition can cause additional problems with increased and more serious infections. The child's diet must be more nutritious and higher in calories than normal. Several small meals supplemented by high-calorie, high-protein snacks may be desirable. Dietary supplements, such as Ensure and Isocal, also may be useful. Explore the child's food likes and dislikes and develop a meal plan using this information. If malnutrition becomes severe, the child may need tube feedings or parenteral nutrition.

Easing Social Isolation and Hopelessness

The child may fear having others know about the illness because he or she anticipates a negative reaction from peers and family. Provide the child with supportive counseling and guidance to help him or her deal with these fears. The child may not feel that he or she can tell the family for fear of rejection. In fact, many families have rejected their children who have AIDS. Many others have risen to the challenge; although family members may tell the teenager they do not like his or her behavior, they continue to offer love and support. The child may need support to help tell social acquaintances as

well. Refer the child or adolescent to an HIV support group if one is available through the hospital or community. Adolescents often find that adult support groups are not as helpful because the adults' needs are different from those of adolescents.

Because the child is facing life with a serious, chronic illness that requires frequent treatment and lifelong medication and has an unknown outcome, the child may feel a special sense of purpose to "spread the word" to others. The child needs support and guidance to set priorities. School officials may need to be told, but families have the legal right to decide whether or not they share the diagnosis with others. If the family is not supportive, the child needs even more support from health care providers.

Promoting Family Coping

The adolescent must be involved in telling family members about the diagnosis if they do not already know. The sexual activity of adolescent children is a topic that many families find difficult to deal with, especially if the activity is homosexual or promiscuous.

The family caregivers usually need support as much as the child does. They often are devastated by the prospect of their child's illness. If the adolescent is pregnant or has a child, the family also must consider the future of that child. For the family who plays a supportive role in the child's life, the period after diagnosis is a difficult one.

Teach the family as much about the disease as possible. They must learn how to prevent the spread of the virus among family members, as well as how to prevent opportunistic infections in the child who is HIV positive. It is important to teach the family about treatments, medications, nutrition guidelines, and signs and symptoms of opportunistic infections. Stress the importance of reporting even minor complications to the health care provider, and suggest ways to help support the child (Family Teaching Tips: Supporting the Child or Adolescent With HIV/AIDS).

A little sensitivity is in order. When working with children and families of children diagnosed with HIV or AIDS, be aware of possible unspoken feelings and questions and carefully bring them into the discussion.

Although teaching the child and the family all this information is necessary, remember that a person can absorb only so much detail at

Read this

one time. To teach them successfully and to be sure they understand the information, do not present too much information at one time. Give the family and the child written materials that repeat the information, and review it verbally with them by asking questions and clarifying material until they show evidence of clear understanding of the concepts they need to know. It is important to provide the entire family with the best possible support and information.

EVALUATION: GOALS AND EXPECTED OUTCOMES

- **Goal:** The child will experience minimal risk of infection.

Expected Outcome: The child practices good hygiene measures and identifies ways to prevent infection and ways to protect his or her health at home.

- **Goal:** The child will not spread the disease to others.

Expected Outcome: The child practices infection control measures and identifies sexual partners and safer sexual practices.

- **Goal:** The child's skin integrity will remain intact.

Expected Outcome: The child protects the skin and mucous membranes and promptly reports skin lesions or infections.

- **Goal:** The child will experience minimal pain from complications of the disease.

Expected Outcome: The child learns to manage pain and rests comfortably with minimal discomfort.

- **Goal:** The child's food intake will meet his or her nutritional needs.

Expected Outcome: The child eats nutritionally sound meals, includes frequent small meals in the food plan, and maintains his or her weight.

- **Goal:** The child will not experience social isolation.

Expected Outcome: The child voices fears about social isolation and makes and carries out plans to maintain relationships.

- **Goal:** The adolescent will make adjustments to his or her future expectations.

Expected Outcome: The child or adolescent expresses feelings about his or her future, seeks support from others, and begins to make realistic future plans.

- **Goal:** The family will show evidence of coping with the illness and supporting the child.

Expected Outcome: The family expresses anxieties, voices understanding of the illness, and supports the child in future plans.

INFECTIOUS MONONUCLEOSIS

Common in the adolescent population and sometimes called the "kissing disease," infectious mononucleosis ("mono") is caused by the Epstein-Barr virus, one of the herpes virus groups. The organism is transmitted through saliva. No immunization is available, and treatment is symptomatic. Adolescents and young adults seem to be most susceptible to this disorder, although sometimes it also is seen in younger children.

Clinical Manifestations

Infectious mononucleosis can present a variety of symptoms, ranging from mild to severe, and including symptoms that mimic hepatitis. Symptoms include fever; sore throat with enlarged tonsils; thick, white membrane covering the tonsils; palatine petechiae (red spots on the soft palate) (Fig. 40-11); swollen lymph nodes; and enlargement of the spleen accompanied by extreme fatigue and lack of energy. In some instances, headache, abdominal pain, and epistaxis are also present.

Diagnosis

Diagnosis of infectious mononucleosis is based on clinical symptoms, laboratory evidence of lymphocytes in the peripheral blood (with 10% or more abnormal lymphocytes present in a peripheral blood smear), and a positive heterophil agglutination test. Monospot is a valuable diagnostic test—rapid, sensitive, inexpensive, and simple to perform. Monospot can detect significant agglutinins at lower levels, thus allowing earlier diagnosis. Infectious mononucleosis often is confused with streptococcal infections because of the fever and the appearance of the throat and tonsils.

Treatment and Nursing Care

No cure exists for infectious mononucleosis; treatment is based on symptoms. An analgesic-antipyretic, such as acetaminophen, usually is recommended for the fever and headaches. Fluids and a soft, bland diet are encouraged to reduce throat irritation. Corticosteroids sometimes are used to relieve the severe sore throat and fever. Bed rest is suggested to relieve fatigue but is not imposed for a specific

● *Figure 40.11* Tonsils of an adolescent who has infectious mononucleosis; note the red, enlarged tonsils with the thick white covering.

amount of time. If the spleen is enlarged, the child is cautioned to avoid contact sports that might cause a ruptured spleen. Because the immune system is weakened, the child must take precautions to avoid secondary infections.

The course of mononucleosis is usually uncomplicated. Fever and sore throat may last from 1 week to 10 days. Fatigue generally disappears 2 to 4 weeks after the appearance of acute symptoms but may last as long as 1 year. The limitations that this disorder imposes on the teenager's school and social life may cause depression. However, in most instances the child can resume normal activities within 1 month after symptoms present.

Nursing care includes encouraging the child to express feelings about the interruptions the illness is causing in school, social, and work plans. Long-term effects rarely are seen.

Test Yourself

- List the most common sexually transmitted diseases in adolescents and explain how each of these is treated.

- Discuss what you could talk to an adolescent about regarding sexually transmitted diseases.

- How is mononucleosis treated?

COMMUNICABLE DISEASES OF CHILDHOOD

Half a century ago, growing up meant being able to survive measles, mumps, whooping cough, diphtheria, and often poliomyelitis. These diseases were expected almost as routinely as the loss of the deciduous teeth. Immunization has changed that outcome so drastically that some caregivers have become less conscientious about having their children immunized until the immunization is required for entrance to school. Nevertheless, the incidence of childhood diseases has decreased with only an occasional outbreak in certain communities where many children are not immunized.

Understanding the various communicable diseases and their prevention, symptoms, and treatment (Table 40-4) requires knowledge of specific terms (Box 40-1). Some communicable diseases require specific precautions to prevent spreading of the infection. Specific transmission precaution procedures

TABLE 40.4	Communicable Diseases of Childhood				
Disease	Period of Communicability When/How Long Contagious	Prevention Immunization Immunity	Clinical Manifestations	Treatment Nursing Care Implementation	Complications
Hepatitis B Causative agent: A *Hepadnavirus; hepatitis B virus* Mode of transmission: body fluids, transfusion of contaminated blood, use of contaminated needle, to fetus via mother Incubation period: average 60–90 days	End of incubation time and during acute stage	Use of standard precautions Vaccine for hepatitis B After exposure— HBIG (hepatitis B immune globulin)	Anorexia, abdominal discomfort, nausea, vomiting, jaundice	Rest, nutrition with good caloric intake	Possibly fatal, liver problems, in some cases possibly leading to chronic hepatitis
Diphtheria Causative agent: *Corynebacterium diphtheriae* Mode of transmission: droplet, direct contact with infected person, carrier, or contaminated article Incubation period: 2–7 days	2–4 weeks in untreated person 1–2 days with antibiotic therapy	Active immunity from diphtheria toxin in DTaP vaccine Passive immunity with diphtheria antitoxin	Mucous membranes of nose and throat covered by gray membrane; purulent nasal discharge; brassy cough; toxin from organism passes through bloodstream to heart and nervous system	Strict droplet precautions; intravenous antitoxin and antibiotics; bed rest; liquid to soft diet; analgesics for throat pain; immunization for nonimmunized contacts	Neuritis, carditis, heart failure, respiratory failure
Tetanus (lockjaw) Causative agent: *Clostridium tetani* Mode of transmission: direct or indirect contamination of a closed wound Incubation period: 3–21 days	None—not transmitted from person to person	Active immunity from tetanus toxoid in DTaP vaccine	Stiffness of neck and jaw, muscle rigidity of trunk and extremities, arched back, abdominal muscle stiffness, unusual facial appearance, pain due to muscle spasms	Quiet room, wound cleaning and débridement, penicillin G or erythromycin, muscle relaxants	Serious, fatal if untreated, possible respiratory complications
Pertussis (whooping cough) Causative agent: *Bordetella pertussis* Mode of transmission: droplet, direct contact with respiratory discharges Incubation period: 5–21 days	About 4–6 weeks, greatest in respiratory stage	Active immunity from pertussis vaccine in DTaP vaccine; Disease gives natural immunity	Begins with mild upper respiratory symptoms; in 2nd week progresses to severe paroxysmal cough with inspiratory whoop, sometimes followed by vomiting; especially dangerous for young infants, may last 4–6 weeks	Bed rest; infants hospitalized; oxygen therapy possible, observation for airway obstruction; provision of high humidity; protection from secondary infections, increased fluid intake; refeeding if vomiting occurs	Pneumonia (can cause death of infant); otitis media; hemorrhage; convulsions

(table continues on page 978)

TABLE 40.4 (continued)	Communicable Diseases of Childhood					
Disease	Period of Communicability When/How Long Contagious	Prevention Immunization Immunity	Clinical Manifestations	Treatment Nursing Care Implementation	Complications
Haemophilus influenzae type B Causative agent: *Coccobacilli H. influenzae bacteria* Mode of transmission: droplet, discharge from nose and throat Incubation period: 2–4 days	As long as organisms are present; noncommunicable after antibiotic therapy for 24–48 hours	Vaccine *haemophilus influenzae* type b (HIB)	Fever, vomiting, lethargy, meningeal irritation with bulging fontanel or stiff neck and back, stupor, coma	Antibiotics	Meningitis, epiglottitis, pneumonia
Poliomyelitis (infantile paralysis) Causative agent: *poliovirus* Mode of transmission: Direct and indirect contact, fecal-oral route Incubation period: 7–14 days	Greatest just before onset and just after onset of symptoms, when virus is present in throat and feces, 1–6 weeks	Inactivated polio vaccine (IPV) Disease causes active immunity against specific strain	Fever, headache, nausea, vomiting, abdominal pain; stiff neck, pain, and tenderness in lower extremities that proceeds to paralysis	Bed rest; moist hot packs to extremities; range-of-motion exercises; supportive care; long-term ventilation if respiratory muscles involved	Permanent paralysis; respiratory arrest
Rubeola (measles) Causative agent: *measles virus* Mode of transmission: Direct or indirect contact with droplets, nasal, and throat secretions Incubation period: 10–12 days	5th incubation day through first few days after rash erupts	Attenuated live vaccine (part of MMR vaccine) Disease gives lasting natural immunity	High fever, sore throat, coryza (runny nose), cough, enlarged lymph nodes (head and neck), Koplik spots (small red spots with blue-white centers on oral mucosa, specific to rubeola), conjunctivitis, photophobia, maculopapular rash starts at hairline and spreads to entire body	Antipyretics, comfort measures for rash including tepid baths, soothing lotion, maintenance of dry skin; dimly lighted room for comfort, fluids	Otitis media, pneumonia, encephalitis, airway obstruction
Parotitis (mumps) Causative agent: *Paramyxovirus* Mode of transmission: airborne, droplet, direct contact with saliva of infected person Incubation period: 14–21 days	Shortly before swelling appears until after it disappears	Attenuated live mumps vaccine (part of MMR vaccine) Disease gives natural immunity	Parotid glands swollen, unilaterally or bilaterally; may have fever, headache, malaise, and complain of earache before swelling appears; angle of jaw obliterated on affected side	Liquids and soft foods because chewing is painful; avoidance of sour foods, which cause discomfort; analgesics for pain; antipyretics for fever; local compresses of heat or cold	In males past puberty orchitis (inflammation of the testes); meninoencephalitis; possible severe hearing impairment (rare)

TABLE 40.4 (continued)	Communicable Diseases of Childhood				
Disease	**Period of Communicability When/How Long Contagious**	**Prevention Immunization Immunity**	**Clinical Manifestations**	**Treatment Nursing Care Implementation**	**Complications**
Rubella (German measles) Causative agent: Rubella virus Mode of transmission: direct or indirect contact with droplets, nasopharyngeal secretions Incubation period: 14–21 days	5–7 days before until about 5 days after rash appears	Attenuated live vaccine (part of MMR vaccine) Disease gives lasting natural immunity Immune serum globulin may be given to pregnant women	Low-grade fever; headache, malaise, anorexia, sore throat, lymph glands of neck and head enlarged; pink-red rash begins on face, spreads downward, disappears in 3 days, may have joint pain	Comfort measures for rash, antipyretics for fever and joint pain	Severe birth defects possible if mother is exposed and nonimmunized (especially in 1st trimester)
Varicella (chickenpox) Causative agent: *Varicella zoster* virus Mode of transmission: airborne, direct or indirect contact with saliva or uncrusted vesicles Incubation period: 10–21 days	1 day before rash appears to about 5–6 days after it appears (until all vesicles crusted)	Attenuated live varicella virus vaccine gives active immunity Disease causes lasting natural immunity; may reactivate in adult as herpes zoster	Low-grade fever; malaise; successive crops of macules, papules, vesicles, and crusts, all present at the same time; itching is intense; scarring may occur when scabs are removed before ready to fall off	Antihistamines, soothing baths and lotions to reduce itching; prevention of scratching with short fingernails or use of mittens; acyclovir to shorten the course of the disease; **no aspirin** should be given	Reye syndrome possible if child has had aspirin during illness; secondary infection of lesions if scratched; pneumonia, encephalitis
Hepatitis A Causative agent: *A picornavirus*; *hepatitis A virus* Mode of transmission: Ingestion of fecal contaminated food or water or contaminated surfaces Incubation period: Average 25–30 days	Highest during 2 weeks before onset of symptoms	Good handwashing, sanitary disposal of feces Vaccine for hepatitis A After exposure— immune globulin	Fever, malaise, anorexia, nausea, abdominal discomfort, jaundice	Enteric precautions, rest, nutritious diet	
Erythema infectiosum (fifth disease) Causative agent: *Human parvovirus B19* Mode of transmission: droplet, contact with respiratory secretions Incubation period: 6–14 days	Uncertain, child may return to school when rash appears, no longer infectious at that point	No immunity	Fever, headache, malaise; a week later, red rash appears on face, called a "slapped face" rash; rash appears on extremities, then on trunk; rash can reappear with heat, sunlight, cold	Supportive treatment with antipyretics, analgesics, droplet precautions (when hospitalized)	Arthritis possible; dangerous for fetus (keep infected child away from pregnant women)

(table continues on page 980)

TABLE 40.4 (continued)	Communicable Diseases of Childhood				
Disease	Period of Communicability When/How Long Contagious	Prevention Immunization Immunity	Clinical Manifestations	Treatment Nursing Care Implementation	Complications
Roseola (exanthema subitum) Causative agent: Human *herpesvirus* type 6 Mode of transmission: Unknown Incubation period: about 10 days	During febrile period	Contracting disease gives lasting immunity	High fever; irritability; anorexia; lymph nodes enlarged; decreased WBC; rash appears just after sharp decline in temperature; rash is rose-pink, mostly on trunk, lasts 1–2 days	Symptomatic for rash and fever; standard precautions (if hospitalized)	
Lyme disease Causative agent: *Borrelia burgdorferi* Mode of transmission: deer tick bite Incubation period: 3–30 days	Not communicable from one person to another	Avoid tick-infected areas; inspect skin after being in wooded areas Active immunity from Lyme disease vaccine	Starts as a red papule that spreads and becomes a large, round red ring; fever; malaise; headache; mild neck stiffness with rash; leads to systemic symptoms and chronic problems	Antibiotics	Cardiac, musculoskeletal and neurologic involvement
Scarlet Fever Causative agent: *Beta-hemolytic streptococci group A* Mode of transmission: direct contact, droplet Incubation period: 2–5 days	During acute respiratory phase, 1–7 days	Lasting immunity after having disease	Begins abruptly; fever; sore throat; headache; chills; malaise; red rash on skin and mucous membranes; tonsils inflamed; enlarged; white exudate; tongue—differentiates from other rashes, by day 4–5 "red strawberry" appearance	Soft or liquid diet, antipyretics, analgesics, comfort measures for itching rash; penicillin for streptococcal infection	Glomerulonephritis or rheumatic fever if untreated

can be found in the procedure manuals of individual institutions.

Prevention

The recommended schedule of childhood immunization is found in Chapter 23. Parents of children whose immunizations are incomplete must be urged to have the immunizations brought up to date. For families of limited means, free immunizations are usually available at clinics.

Nursing Care

Many times the child who develops a communicable disease is at home. However, in some cases the child may develop the disease while hospitalized. For the child who develops a communicable disease and is hospitalized, the nurse should explain to the child and the caregivers the reason for the transmission precautions. Precautions are done to protect the child from the threat of infection or to protect others from the infection the child has. Otherwise, the child may feel

BOX 40.1	Common Terms in Communicable Disease Nursing

Active immunity: stimulates development of antibodies to destroy infective agent without causing disease; occurs when vaccine is given

Antibody: a protective substance in the body produced in response to the introduction of an antigen

Antigen: a foreign protein that stimulates the formation of antibodies

Antitoxin: an antibody that unites with and neutralizes a specific toxin

Carrier: a person in apparently good health whose body harbors the specific organisms of a disease

Causative agent: pathogen that causes disease

Enanthem: an eruption on a mucous surface

Endemic: habitual presence of a disease within a given area

Epidemic: an outbreak in a community of a group of illnesses of similar nature in excess of the normal expectancy

Erythema: redness of the skin produced by congestion of the capillaries

Exanthem: an eruption appearing on the skin during an eruptive disease

Host: a human, animal, or plant that harbors or nourishes another organism

Incubation period: the time interval between the infection and the appearance of the first symptoms of the disease

Macule: a discolored skin spot not elevated above the surface

Mode of transmission: mechanism by which infectious agent is spread or transferred to humans

Natural immunity: resistance to pathogen or infection, genetically determined

Pandemic: a worldwide epidemic

Papule: a small, circumscribed, solid elevation of the skin

Passive immunity: antibodies obtained from an immune person, given to someone exposed to disease to prevent him or her from getting disease

Period of communicability: time that infectious agent can be transmitted or passed from an infected person or animal to another person

Pustule: a small elevation of epidermis filled with pus

Toxin: a poisonous substance produced by certain organisms such as bacteria

Toxoid: a toxin that has been treated to destroy its toxicity but that retains its antigenic properties

Vaccine: a suspension of attenuated or killed microorganisms administered for the prevention of a specific infection

that the precautions are a form of punishment. Families are more likely to follow the correct procedures if they understand the need for them. Transmission precautions may intensify the normal loneliness of being ill, so the child needs extra attention and stimulation during this time

A PERSONAL GLIMPSE

One time last year when I was in kindergarten I felt so sick. I had a red spot on my face, and when I woke up my tummy was covered with spots. I was so hot, and I itched all over. My mom called the nurse at my doctor's office to see if she should take me and they said, "No way. She's got the chickenpox." It was like Halloween at school, but it was really called the Fall Fiesta. I was going to be Bruce the shark from Finding Nemo because I watch it all the time on DVD. My sister and all my friends walked to school in their costumes, but I couldn't go, and I itched a lot. I was so sad. To keep me from being sad my mom said I could draw pictures and I drew pictures of me making a soccer goal and of my slingshot. I decided when I was better I could use my costume to play Shark Attack. I would pretend I was swimming in the ocean and if I catch other people, they turn into friendly sharks. I was crying and I was so itchy and my mom put lotion on, but it didn't help. My mom said she could give me a bath in oatmeal and it would feel better. I was kind of grossed out because I don't usually take a bath in food, but she said we could put it in a special cloth instead of a bowl. She was right; I stopped itching a little. When my sister came home with candy and treats I felt a little better, but I still had the chickenpox.

Jocie, age 6

LEARNING OPPORTUNITY: What questions do you think the nurse in the pediatrician's office asked to determine this child should be cared for at home, rather than be seen in the office? For what reason would this mother give her child an "oatmeal" bath?

KEY POINTS

◗ The integumentary system including the accessory structures are in place at birth and mature as the child grows. Protecting the body from attacks from microorganisms and helping the body get rid of or resist invasion by foreign materials are the major roles of the immune system. The immune system matures and develops as the child progresses through childhood.

◗ *C. albicans* is the causative agent for thrush and some cases of diaper rash.

◗ Acne vulgaris is caused by a variety of factors, including increased hormonal levels, hereditary factors, irritation and irritating substances, and growth of anaerobic bacteria.

- Mild acne is treated using topical medications such as benzoyl peroxide (Clearasil, Benoxyl) and tretinoin (Retin-A) once or twice a day. Antibiotics such as erythromycin and tetracycline may be administered for inflammatory acne. Isotretinoin (Accutane) may be used for severe inflammatory acne.
- Pediculosis of the scalp is treated using nonprescription medications such as Pronto, RID, A-200, and permethrin (Nix). After the hair is shampooed thoroughly and dried, it is combed with a fine-toothed comb dipped in warm white vinegar to remove remaining nits and nit shells. For protection when treating a child in the hospital, wear a disposable gown, gloves, and head cover.
- Hyposensitization is performed for the allergens that produce a positive reaction on skin testing. The allergist sets up a schedule for injections in gradually increasing doses until a maintenance dose is reached.
- Skin allergies and rashes are usually treated with topical preparations, such as lotions, ointments, and greases, plus cool soaks.
- Major causes of burns in children include hot liquids, fire, and electricity.
- Superficial or first-degree burns occur when the epidermis is injured but there is no destruction of tissue or nerve endings. Partial-thickness or second-degree burns occur when the epidermis and underlying dermis are both injured and devitalized or destroyed. Blistering usually occurs, as does an escape of body plasma. With full-thickness or third-degree burns, the epidermis, dermis, and nerve endings are all destroyed. Pain is minimal, and there is no longer any barrier to infection or any remaining viable epithelial cells.
- Emergency treatment for burns involving small areas is the immediate application of cool compresses or cool water to burn areas to inhibit capillary permeability and thus suppress edema, blister formation, and tissue destruction. For moderate burns, immersing a burned extremity in cool water alleviates pain and may prevent additional thermal injury. In severe burns, the airway, breathing, and circulation must be observed and restored if necessary and the child transported to a medical facility for assessment.
- Gonorrhea is caused by the organism *Neisseria gonorrhoeae*, Chlamydia by *Chlamydia trachomatis*, genital herpes by herpes simplex type 2, and syphilis by *Treponema pallidum*.
- The only certain way to avoid contracting an STD is sexual abstinence.
- The drug of choice to treat gonorrhea is ceftriaxone (Rocephin) followed by a week of oral doxycycline (Vibramycin) to prevent an accompanying chlamy-

dial infection. Doxycycline or azithromycin is used to treat chlamydial infection. Acyclovir (Zovirax) is useful in relieving or suppressing the symptoms of genital herpes. Syphilis responds to one intramuscular injection of penicillin G benzathine; if the individual is sensitive to penicillin, oral doxycycline, tetracycline, or erythromycin can be administered.
- The human immunodeficiency virus (HIV) is transmitted by contact with infected blood or sexual contact with an infected person.
- Infectious mononucleosis ("mono") is caused by the Epstein-Barr virus, which is one of the herpes virus groups. The organism is transmitted through saliva and treatment is symptomatic.
- Active immunity occurs when antibodies are formed after immunization with a vaccine. Natural immunity often is genetically determined and gives a person a resistance to a pathogen. Passive immunity occurs when a person who has been exposed to a certain disease is given antibodies that have been obtained from an immune person.
- Modes of transmission of communicable diseases include droplet, direct or indirect contact with body fluids and discharges, and contaminated blood, food, or water. Many communicable diseases can be prevented by immunization with vaccinations and the use of standard precautions.
- Nursing interventions for the child with a communicable disease are usually supportive. Depending on the disease symptoms, the implementations might include providing rest, adequate nutrition and fluids, following standard precautions, giving medications as appropriate, and offering comfort measures

REFERENCES AND SELECTED READINGS

Books and Journals

Adger, H. (1999). Sexually transmitted diseases. In J. A. McMillan, C. D. DeAngelis, R. D. Feigin, & J. W. Warshaw (Eds.), *Oski's pediatrics: Principles and practice* (3rd ed.). Philadelphia: Lippincott Williams & Wilkins.

Butensky, E. A. (2001). The role of nutrition in pediatric HIV/AIDS: A review of micronutrient research. *Journal of Pediatric Nursing, 16*(6), 402.

Centers for Disease Control. (2001). *Fact Sheet: Treating Head Lice, Centers for Disease Control*. Retrieved from www.cdc.gov/ncidod/dpd/parasites/headlice/factsht_head_lice_treating.htm

Centers for Disease Control. (1999). Guidelines for national human immunodeficiency virus case surveillance, including monitoring for human immunodeficiency virus infection and acquired immunodeficiency syndrome. *MMWR,*

48(RR13), 1–28. Retrieved from www.cdc.gov/mmwr/preview/mmwrhtml/rr4813a1.htm

Chin, J. (2000). *Control of communicable diseases manual* (17th ed.). Washington, DC: American Public Health Association (APHA).

Corrarino, J., Walsh, P., & Nadel, E. (2001). Does teaching scald burn prevention to families of young children make a difference. *Journal of Pediatric Nursing, 16*(4), 256.

Feroli, K. L., & Burstein, G. (2003). Adolescent sexually transmitted diseases: New recommendations for diagnosis, treatment, and prevention. *The American Journal of Maternal Child Nursing, 28,* 113–118.

Hockenberry, M. J., Wilson, D., Winkelstein, M. L., & Kline, N. E. (2003). *Wong's nursing care of infants and children* (7th ed.). St. Louis: Mosby.

Holzemer, W. L. (2002). HIV and AIDS: The symptom experience. *American Journal of Nursing, 102*(4), 48.

Karch, A. M. (2003). *2004 Lippincott's Nursing Drug Guide.* Philadelphia: Lippincott Williams & Wilkins.

North American Nursing Diagnosis Association (NANDA). (2001). *NANDA nursing diagnoses: Definitions and classification 2001–2002.* Philadelphia: NANDA.

Novatnack, E., & Schweon, S. (2002). What's causing that itch? *RN, 65*(8), 43–47.

Pickering, L. K., Ed. (2003). *Red Book: 2003 report of the Committee on Infectious Diseases* (26th ed.). Elk Grove Village, IL: American Academy of Pediatrics.

Pillitteri, A. (2003). *Maternal and child health nursing* (4th ed.). Philadelphia: Lippincott Williams & Wilkins.

Smeltzer, S. C., & Bare, B. G. (2003). *Textbook of medical–surgical nursing* (10th ed.). Philadelphia: Lippincott Williams & Wilkins.

Sparks, S., & Taylor, C. (2001). *Nursing diagnosis reference manual* (5th ed.). Springhouse, PA: Springhouse Corporation.

Wiebelhaus, P. (2001). Managing burn emergencies. *Nursing Management, 32*(7), 29–36.

Wong, D. L., Perry, S., & Hockenberry, M. (2002). *Maternal–child nursing care* (2nd ed.). St. Louis: Mosby.

Worf, N. (2000). Tetanus—still a problem. *RN, 63*(6), 44–49.

Websites
Burns
www.ameriburn.org

Sexually Transmitted Diseases
www.ashastd.org

WORKBOOK

NCLEX-STYLE REVIEW QUESTIONS

1. In caring for a 3 ½-year-old child admitted after being severely burned, the nurse collects the following data. Which of the following would be *most* important for the nurse to report immediately? The child's

   a. respiratory rate is 32 breaths a minute.

   b. temperature is 38.4°C.

   c. hourly urinary output is 150 cc.

   d. pain level is an 8 on the pain scale.

2. The nurse is discussing sexually transmitted diseases with a group of adolescents. If the adolescents make the following statements, which statement indicates a need for further teaching?

   a. "Even though guys don't like to use condoms, at least they protect a person from most STDs."

   b. "My girlfriend has never had sex with anyone except me, so I don't have to worry about STDs."

   c. "It is a relief to know that other than HIV, most STDs can be treated with antibiotics."

   d. "My girlfriend is pregnant, but since she does not have an STD, our baby most likely won't either."

3. In caring for a child with atopic dermatitis (infantile eczema), which of the following nursing interventions would be included in this child's care? Select all that apply in completing this sentence: The nurse will

   a. keep child's fingernails cut short.

   b. dress the child in several layers of clothing at all times.

   c. monitor for symptoms of infection.

   d. give soothing baths just before bedtime.

   e. encourage the child to drink fluids frequently.

   f. use a bleach solution to launder the child's clothing.

4. After an outbreak of pediculosis in the school, the nurse is doing teaching with a group of parents and teachers about ways to help prevent the spread of head lice in the classroom and at home. Which of the following actions would the nurse recommend to this group? Select all that apply.

   a. Wash all bedding and clothing in hot water and dry in a hot dryer.

   b. Apply medicated lotion to all areas of the body except the face.

   c. Wash combs and brushes in medicated shampoo and soak for at least an hour.

   d. Report any evidence of infestation immediately to the school officials.

   e. Vacuum carpets, car seats, mattresses, and upholstered furniture thoroughly.

   f. Wear gloves when preparing food or snacks.

STUDY ACTIVITIES

1. Using the table below, compare the five most common sexually transmitted diseases (STDs) seen in adolescents. Describe the symptoms, treatment, and complications or long-term concerns seen with these diseases.

Sexually Transmitted Disease (STD)	Symptoms	Treatment	Complications or Long-term Concerns

2. Using the table below, make a list of substances that may cause allergies in infants and children. List some sources of these substances that may cause allergies.

Substance That May Cause Allergies	Sources of Substances That May Cause Allergies

3. Identify the relation between *Candida albicans* and some cases of diaper rash. Detail the teaching that you would provide for a mother about diaper rash.

4. Go to the following Internet site:
   http://www.cooltheburn.com
   Click on "Learn about burns." Click on "The Burn Center." Click on "Bandages."

   a. How could you use this site to help explain a dressing change to a child with a burn?

   b. Click on "fun things." Explain the activities available to use with a hospitalized child.

   c. What is available on this site for caregivers of a child with a burn?

CRITICAL THINKING: What Would You Do?

1. Brian is HIV positive and lives with his family. The family is frightened that other members may get the virus.

   a. What will you tell the family to reassure them?

   b. What will you teach them in regard to prevention of the spread of the virus in their home?

   c. What guidelines will you give the family caregivers to help them protect Brian from infectious or opportunistic diseases?

2. Two-year-old Omar has partial and total thickness burns from a wood stove accident. You are helping develop a teaching plan covering the importance of infection control for Omar during his convalescence.

   a. What is the most important action that can be taken to prevent infection?

   b. Who should be included in teaching regarding infection control?

   c. What are signs that might indicate an infection?

   d. Why is it important to detect signs and symptoms of an infection early?

3. Dosage calculation: An adolescent with a diagnosis of gonorrhea is being treated with Rocephin. The dose to be given is 250 mg IM. The medication is available in a preparation of l gram/10 mL. Answer the following:

   a. How many milligrams (mg) are in 1 gram?

   b. How many milliliters will be given in this 250 mg dose to this adolescent?

   After the administration of the Rocephin, the adolescent will be given doxycycline 100 mg BID by mouth for 7 days. Answer the following:

   c. How many milligrams (mg) will be given in a 24-hour period?

   d. How many total milligrams (mg) will be given in the 7 days?

The Child With Psychosocial Disorders

41

STUDENT OBJECTIVES

On completion of this chapter, the student should be able to

1. Describe four characteristics of autism.
2. Identify four goals of treatment of autism.
3. Discuss the warning signs seen in children who are considering suicide.
4. List substances commonly abused by children.
5. State the negative effects of commonly abused substances.
6. Describe the unpredictable behavior of an addicted parent and its effect on the child.
7. List six behaviors that suggest there is an addiction problem in the child's family.
8. Identify 10 characteristics that may be seen in a child with attention deficit hyperactivity disorder.
9. Describe the characteristics of the child with nonorganic failure to thrive.
10. State two goals of treatment for the hospitalized anorexic patient.

KEY TERMS

anorexia nervosa
bulimia nervosa
child neglect
co-dependent parent
dependence
dysfunctional family
echolalia
encopresis
gynecomastia
incest
obesity
overweight

STUDENT OBJECTIVES

11. Describe the signs and symptoms often seen in the child with bulimia.
12. Discuss the goal of health care professionals who work with obese children.
13. State the cause of the symptoms seen in children with school phobia.
14. Identify how poor parenting skills may lead to child abuse.
15. Identify the circumstances under which physical punishment can be classified as abusive.
16. Describe the differences between bruises that occur accidentally to a child and those that have been inflicted in an abusive manner.
17. Identify the injuries that occur with shaken baby syndrome.
18. Define Munchausen syndrome by proxy.
19. Identify ways that a child may be emotionally abused.

KEY TERMS

polyphagia
rumination
sexual abuse
sexual assault
substance abuse
tolerance
withdrawal symptoms

AUTISM

Although often called infantile autism because it is thought to be present from birth, autism usually is not conclusively diagnosed until after 12 months of age. The word *autism* comes from the Greek word auto meaning "self" and was first used by Dr. Leo Kanner in 1943 to describe a group of behavioral symptoms in children. The term *pervasive developmental disorder* was introduced in 1980 when the American Psychiatric Association revised the terminology. Disorders in this category are characterized by severe behavioral disturbance that affects the practical use of language as a means of communication, interpersonal interaction, attention, perception, and motor activity. Autistic children are totally self-centered and unable to relate to others; they often exhibit bizarre behaviors and often are destructive to themselves and others.

Autism occurs in about 2 to 5 of 10,000 births and four times as often in males as in females. Several theories exist about its cause, as well as its treatment or management. Originally thought to result from an unsatisfactory early mother–child relationship (with emotionally cold, detached mothers sometimes described as "refrigerator mothers"), autism now appears to have organic and perhaps genetic causes instead. Researchers suggest that autism may result from a disturbance in language comprehension, a biochemical problem involving neurotransmitters or abnormalities in the central nervous system and probably brain metabolism. These children score poorly on intelligence tests but may have good memories and good intellectual potential.

Because the cause of autism is not understood, treatment attempts have met with limited success. These children experience the normal health problems of childhood in addition to those that result from their behaviors. Therefore, it is important that nurses understand this unexplained disorder and how it affects children and families.

Clinical Manifestations

The characteristics of autism are divided into three categories: inability to relate to others, inability to communicate with others, and obviously limited activities and interests. Children with autism do not develop a smiling response to others or an interest in being touched or cuddled. In fact, they can react violently to attempts to hold them. Their blank expressions and lack of response to verbal stimulation can suggest deafness. They do not show the normal fear of separation from parents that most toddlers exhibit. Often they seem not to notice when family caregivers are present.

During their 2nd year, autistic children become completely absorbed in strange repetitive behaviors such as spinning an object, flipping an electrical switch on and off, or walking around the room feeling the walls. Their bodily movements are bizarre: rocking, twirling, flapping arms and hands, walking on tiptoe, twisting and turning fingers. If these movements are interrupted or if objects in the environment are moved, a violent temper tantrum may result. These tantrums may include self-destructive acts such as hand biting and head banging. Although infants and toddlers normally are self-centered, ritualistic, and prone to displays of temper, autistic children show these characteristics to an extreme degree coupled with an almost total lack of response to other people.

The autistic child is slow to develop speech, and any speech that develops is primitive and ineffective in its ability to communicate. **Echolalia** ("parrot speech") is typical of autistic children; they echo words they have heard,

Think about this. Although autistic children are self-centered, their speech indicates that they seem to have no sense of self because they never use the pronouns "I" or "me."

such as a television commercial, but offer no indication that they understand the words.

Standard intelligence tests that count on verbal ability usually indicate that these children test in the mentally retarded range of intelligence. However, many of these children also demonstrate unusual memory and mathematic, artistic, and musical abilities.

Diagnosis

To confirm a diagnosis of autism, at least 8 of 16 identified characteristics must be present, and all three categories of characteristics must be represented. The symptoms of autism can suggest other disorders, such as lead poisoning, phenylketonuria, congenital rubella, and measles encephalitis. Therefore, a complete pediatric physical and neurologic examination is necessary, including vision and hearing testing, electroencephalography, radiographic studies of the skull, urine screening, and other laboratory studies. In addition, a complete prenatal, natal, and postnatal history, including development, nutrition, and family dynamics, is taken. Other members of the health team may be involved in the evaluation and treatment of the autistic child, including audiologists, psychiatrists, psychologists, special education teachers, speech and language therapists, and social workers.

Treatment

The treatment of an autistic child is extremely challenging. The child is mentally retarded but may demonstrate exceptional talent in areas such as factual memory and art or music. Treatment is geared to four goals:

- Promotion of normal development
- Specific language development
- Social interaction
- Learning

Behavioral modification, pharmacotherapeutics, and other techniques are used. These treatments must be individually planned and highly structured. Mixed results occur, and no one technique has met with resounding success. The family needs therapy to help relieve guilt and help them understand this puzzling child. The overall long-term prognosis for these children is not optimistic; however, the long-term outlook is better the earlier treatment is started. Facilitated communication involves working with language development of autistic children by helping them express themselves in language through use of a computer keyboard. However, this method is viewed as controversial and is not totally supported by the American Psychological Association.

Nursing Care

Caring for the autistic child requires recognizing that autism creates great stresses for the entire family. The problems that cause family caregivers to seek diagnosis are difficult to live with; diagnosis itself is usually a lengthy and expensive process, and the hope for successful treatment is slight. Most caregivers of autistic children feel guilty, despite the fact that current theories accept organic, rather than psychological, causes for this disorder. The possibility of genetic factors adds to this guilt. Often other children in the family who are normal suffer from a lack of attention because the caregivers' energies are almost totally directed to solving the autistic youngster's problems.

Nurses who care for these children should consider the family caregivers as their most valuable source of information about the child's habits and communication skills. To gain the child's cooperation, the nurse must learn which techniques the caregivers use to communicate with the child. Establishing a relationship of trust between the child and the nurse is essential. To provide consistency, this child should be cared for by a constant primary nurse.

In the hospital setting, a private or semiprivate room is generally preferred; visual and auditory stimulation should be minimized. Familiar toys or other valued objects from home reduce the child's anxiety about the strange environment.

Test Yourself

- Into what three categories are the characteristics of autism divided?
- When a child with autism is said to have echolalia, what does this mean?
- Explain the goals in the treatment of autism.

SUICIDE

Suicide is one of the leading causes of death in children 10 to 19 years of age, falling just short of the death rate for homicide. Because some deaths reported as accidents, particularly one-car accidents, are thought to be suicides, the rate actually may be higher. Adolescent males commit suicide four times more often than do girls, but girls attempt suicide five times more often than do boys. Boys use more violent means of committing suicide than do girls and thus are successful more often.

Children who have attempted suicide once have a high risk of attempting it again, perhaps more effectively. Attempted suicide rarely occurs without warning and usually is preceded by a long history of emotional problems, difficulty forming relationships, feelings of rejection, and low self-esteem. Loss of one or both parents through death or divorce, a family history that includes suicide of one or more members, and lack of success in academic or athletic performance are other common contributing factors. To this history is added one or more of the normal developmental crises of adolescence:

- Difficulty establishing independence
- Identity crisis
- Lack of intimate relationships
- Breakdown in family communication
- A sense of alienation
- A conflict that interferes with problem solving

The child's situation may be further complicated by an unwanted or unplanned pregnancy, alcohol or drug addiction, or physical or sexual abuse that leads to depression and a feeling of total hopelessness.

Clinical Manifestations

Health professionals involved with children and family caregivers must be aware of factors that place a child at risk for suicide, as well as hints that signal an impending suicide attempt (Family Teaching Tips: Suicide Warning Signs for Caregivers). Some of these desperate young people will verbalize their hopelessness with statements such as "I won't be around much longer" or

Never, never! Don't ignore behaviors or statements of hopelessness in children and teenagers. Make an effort to ensure the child's safety until counseling and treatment resources are in place.

"After Monday, it won't matter anyhow." They may begin giving away prized possessions or appear suddenly elated after a long period of acting dejected.

During the initial interview with the child, include questions that draw out feelings of alienation, depression, and hopelessness. If any of these indications are present, report and document

FAMILY TEACHING TIPS

Suicide Warning Signs for Caregivers

WARNING SIGNS IN CHILDREN'S BEHAVIOR

- Previous suicide attempt
- Thoughts of wishing to kill self
- Plans for self-destructive acts
- Feeling "down in the dumps"
- Withdrawal from social activities
- Loss of pleasure in daily activities
- Change in activity—increase or decrease
- Poor concentration
- Complaints of headaches, upset stomach, joint pains, frequent colds
- Change in eating or sleeping patterns
- Strong feelings of guilt, inadequacy, hopelessness
- Preoccupation with thoughts of people dying, getting sick, or being injured
- Substance abuse
- Violence, truancy, stealing, or lying
- Lack of judgment
- Poor impulse control
- Rapid swing in appropriateness of expressed emotions, sudden lift in mood
- Pessimistic view of self and world
- Saying goodbye
- Giving things away

CHANGES IN CHILD'S INTERPERSONAL RELATIONSHIPS

- Conflicts with peers
- Loss of boyfriend or girlfriend
- School problems—behavioral or academic
- Feelings of great frustration, being misunderstood, or not being part of the group
- Lack of positive support from family, peers, or other
- Earlier suicide of family member, friend, or classmate
- Separations, deaths, births, moves, or serious illnesses in the family

these findings immediately. Question the family caregiver about any such signs and follow through with seeking additional help for the child.

Treatment and Nursing Care

It is important that counseling and treatment resources be found to help these children. Strive to help the child understand that although suicide is an option in problem solving, it is a final option, and other options exist that are not so final. Be aware of the community resources such as hotlines and counselors that specialize in working with persons who are contemplating or have attempted suicide.

CULTURAL SNAPSHOT

Depression and other psychological concerns in some cultures may be disregarded or not expressed because of the fear of social stigma or shame. A confidential and compassionate approach by the nurse may encourage the child to express his or her feelings or the family to share the worry they have about symptoms in their child.

SUBSTANCE ABUSE

Substance abuse is the misuse of an addictive substance that changes the user's mental state. The addictive substances commonly abused are tobacco, alcohol, and controlled or illicit drugs. Children influenced by peers and in some instances adults in their family use drugs and alcohol to avoid facing their problems, escape and forget the pain of life as they see it, add excitement to social events, or bow to peer pressure. Throughout history, people have used alcohol and other mood-altering drugs as a means of relieving the tensions and pressures of their lives. Many cultures still sanction use of some of these substances but object to their abuse (excessive use or use in a way that is medically, socially, or culturally unacceptable).

Unfortunately, frequent use or abuse of these substances can lead to addiction or **dependence** (a compulsive need to use a substance for its satisfying or pleasurable effects). Dependence may be psychological, physical, or both. Psychological dependence means that the substance is desired for the effects or sensations it produces: alertness, euphoria, relaxation, a sense of well-being, and a false sense of control over problems. Physical dependence results from drug-induced changes in body tissue functions that require the drug for normal activity. The magnitude of physical dependence determines the severity of **withdrawal symptoms** (physical and psychological symptoms that occur when the drug is no longer being used), such as vomiting, chills, tremors, and hallucinations. The symptoms vary with the amount, type, frequency, and duration of drug use. Continued use of an addictive substance can result in **tolerance** (the ability of body tissues to endure and adapt to continued or increased use of a substance); this dynamic means the drug user requires larger doses of the drug to produce the desired effect.

Four stages of use have been identified that help describe the progression of substance abuse (Table 41-1). Using the clues from these stages, the nurse who works in any capacity with children can be more alert to signs of possible substance abuse.

The children at greatest risk of becoming substance abusers are those who

- Have families in which alcohol or drug abuse is or has been present
- Suffer from abuse, neglect, loss, or have no close relationships as a result of a dysfunctional family
- Have behavior problems, such as aggressiveness, or are excessively rebellious
- Are slow learners or have learning disabilities or attention deficit disorder
- Have problems with depression and low self-esteem

In some instances, early identification of these factors by family, teachers, counselors, or other caregivers and prompt referral for treatment can help avoid the potential tragedy of substance abuse.

Prevention and Treatment

The most effective and least expensive treatment for substance abuse is prevention, beginning with education in the early school years. Information about drugs and about how to cope with problems without using drugs should be provided.

Balance is the order of the day. "Scare" techniques are completely ineffective in trying to persuade children to refrain from using substances. These techniques arouse disbelief and often add the tempting thrill of danger.

The impact of educational programs may be diluted if the child comes from a home where alcohol or other drugs are used by family caregivers.

When prevention is ineffective, emergency care and long-term treatment become necessary. An overdose or a "bad trip" may force the child to seek treatment. Emergency measures may even require artificial ventilation and oxygenation to restore normal respiration.

Long-term treatment involves many health professionals such as psychiatric nurses, psychologists or psychiatrists, social workers, drug rehabilitation counselors, and community health nurses. The child is an important member of the treatment team and must admit the problem and the need for help and be willing to take an active part in treatment. Both outpatient and inpatient treatment programs are available. Many of these programs are geared specifically to adolescents. The human services section of the local telephone directory provides specific listings.

Alcohol Abuse

In many parts of American culture, drinking alcoholic beverages is considered acceptable and desirable social behavior. Although the purchase of alcohol is legally restricted to adults 21 years of age and older in all states and the District of Columbia, it is available in many homes and consequently is the first drug most children try. It is also the most commonly abused drug among children and adolescents. Alcohol abuse occurs when a person ingests a quantity sufficient to cause intoxication (drunkenness). Alcoholism (chronic alcohol abuse or dependence) has reached epidemic proportions in America.

TABLE 41.1	Progression of Substance Abuse in Children		
Stage	Predisposition	Behavior	Family Reaction

Stage 1. Experimentation, Learning the Mood Swing

Infrequent use of alcohol/ marijuana	Curiosity	Learning the mood	Often unaware
No consequences	Peer pressure	Feels good	Denial
Some fear of use	Attempt to assume adult role	Positive reinforcement	
Low tolerance		Can return to normal	

Stage 2. Seeking the Mood Swing

Increasing frequency in use of various drugs	Impress others	Using to get high	Attempts at elimination
Minimal defensiveness	Social function	Pride in amount consumed	Blaming others
Tolerance	Modeling adult behavior	Using to relieve feelings (i.e., anxieties of dating)	
		Denial of problem	

Stage 3. Preoccupation With the Mood Swing

Peer group activities revolve around use	Using to get loaded, not just high	Begins to violate values and rules	Conspiracy of silence
Steady supply		Use before and during school	Confrontation
Possible dealing		Use despite consequences	Reorganization with or without affected person
Few or no straight friends		Solitary use	
Consequences frequent		Trouble with school	
		Overdoses, "bad trips," blackouts	
		Promises to cut down or attempts to quit	
		Protection of supply, hides use from peers	
		Deterioration in physical condition	

Stage 4. Using to Feel Normal

Continue to use despite adverse outcomes	Use to feel normal	Daily use	Frustration
Loss of control		Failure to meet expectations	Anger
Inability to stop		Loss of control	May give up
Compulsion		Paranoia	
		Suicide gestures, self-hate	
		Physical deterioration (poor eating and sleep habits)	

Adger, H. (1999). Adolescent drug abuse. In J. A. McMillan, C. D. DeAngelis, R. D. Feigin, & J. W. Warshaw (Eds.) *Oski's pediatrics: Principles and practice* (3rd ed.). Philadelphia: Lippincott Williams & Wilkins.

Drinking often begins in the late school-age years and increases in frequency throughout adolescence. Some children use alcohol in combination with marijuana and other drugs, potentiating the effects of both substances and increasing the probability of intoxication.

Alcoholism is costly in dollars and in damage to the lives of alcohol abusers and their families. During adolescence, alcohol abuse is closely linked to automobile accidents. A car is another symbol of adult status and a means to escape adult supervision. Drinking with friends before or while driving often has tragic results. Most states determine charges of driving under the influence using a standard of 0.1% blood alcohol content. However, many states have lowered the limit to 0.08%. Many children do not realize that fine motor control and judgment are affected at even lower levels, and driving ability may be decreased. Although the number of fatal alcohol-related accidents involving children has decreased because all states have set 21 years as the legal age for drinking, the fatality rate remains high.

Children and adolescents who receive treatment and counseling for problem drinking are more likely to recover than are adults who have been problem drinkers for a long period. However, children, especially adolescents, are difficult to treat because of their feelings of immortality and the rapid progression of the disease in adolescents.

Alcoholism is not a weakness of character but a major chronic, progressive, and potentially fatal disease process that affects every organ of the body, mental health, and social competence. Alcoholism tendencies appear to be inherited, so children with a family history of alcoholism may be prone to problems with alcohol. Treatment is lengthy and expensive and has no chance of success until the alcoholic acknowledges the problem and his or her helplessness to deal with it.

Treatment begins with detoxification ("drying out") and management of withdrawal symptoms. After that, a well-balanced diet, high-potency vitamins (especially vitamin B), and plenty of rest help to eliminate the disease's harmful side effects.

Counseling to identify and address the problems that led to compulsive drinking is an essential part of treatment. Many counselors who work with alcoholic patients are people who are recovering from a drinking problem themselves. This experience gives the counselor additional insight and empathy for the problem and the victim and adds credibility to the counseling offered.

Alcoholics Anonymous (AA), the best known of all self-help groups, offers fellowship and understanding to the compulsive drinker (website: http://www.alcoholics-anonymous.org). Chapters are available in every sizable community, and many have special programs for children, as well as for families of alcoholics (Alateen, Al-Anon, ACOA—Adult Children of Alcoholics). Anyone who has a desire to stop drinking is welcomed into AA and is helped to stay sober by taking it "one day at a time." Recovery from alcoholism is a lifetime matter. The earlier the problem is diagnosed, the better the person's chances to respond to treatment. Ongoing support from health professionals, peers, family, and community is essential to successful treatment.

Tobacco Abuse

Tobacco is a commonly abused drug among preadolescents and adolescents. Any use of tobacco is abuse. A high percentage of young people try tobacco, by smoking or chewing. Many children smoke because it gives them a feeling of maturity. Threats of long-term physical illnesses are far enough in the future that the child tends to ignore them. Many elementary and secondary schools have developed programs that warn children of the dangers of smoking, but the danger seems distant, and children believe that they can quit any time they want to quit. The more immediate result of smoking that may stir interest in adolescents is the fact that their hair, breath, and clothes smell bad.

Adolescents also have strong feelings of fairness and justice, so they may respond to the fact that children who are around persons who smoke are at increased risk for respiratory illness and cancer.

The use of "smokeless tobacco" (snuff or chewing tobacco) has increased steadily among adolescent males in the last several years. These children believe that they are not damaging their lungs. However, this type of tobacco use can cause mouth, lip, and throat cancers that are disfiguring and life threatening.

Children whose family caregivers smoke are at increased risk for smoking. They have difficulty accepting that they are seriously endangering themselves by smoking. Most hospitals, schools, and public buildings have adopted no-smoking policies. Perhaps the pressure of society will help deter smoking in the future. There is an effort at the federal level to discourage children and adolescents from beginning to smoke, but children do not seem to be responding to the warnings. This may be attributable in part to the previously mentioned attitude among adolescents that nothing can hurt them.

Marijuana Abuse

The most frequently used illicit drug among adolescents is marijuana. The reported use of marijuana among children has decreased somewhat, but smoking marijuana at a younger age appears to be a current trend. Many children believe that marijuana smoking is not risky.

The effects of marijuana are mostly behavioral. It affects judgment, sense of time, and motivation. These effects make driving hazardous and may even cause hallucinations at higher doses. In addition, marijuana smoke is three to five times more carcinogenic than cigarette smoke. The marijuana available today may be three to five times more potent than that smoked in the 1960s. Because marijuana is illegal, no manufacturing control over it exists, and the user has no idea where it came from or what additives may have been used. Nurses must make every effort to inform children about the dangers of marijuana and to discourage them from using it.

Cocaine Abuse

Although cocaine may not rank among the first three drugs most commonly used by children, it is an extremely dangerous drug. Use of cocaine and its derivative, "crack," had decreased among adolescents, but statistics indicate that cocaine use is no longer decreasing. Cocaine and crack use can be found everywhere from inner cities to rural neighborhoods.

Cocaine is a fine, white, powdery substance that directly affects the brain cells and causes physical and psychological effects. It usually is inhaled or smoked and is absorbed through the mucous membranes into the bloodstream. The physical results are an increase in pulse, respirations, blood pressure, and temperature. The psychological effect is a feeling of euphoria and increased sociability. The high is reached in about 20 minutes and lasts 20 to 30 minutes. In contrast, crack enters the bloodstream in about 30 seconds with a fast, powerful but short high that lasts only about 5 minutes. As a result of the rapid, short high from crack, users tend to seek repeated highs over a short period, decreasing the time it takes to become addicted. Because of the rapid absorption of crack, immediate cardiac arrest can occur from its use. After smoking crack, the user may experience a "crash" that causes depression. To relieve this depression, crack users turn to alcohol and marijuana. This multiple use further complicates the drug's effects. Some cocaine users inject cocaine to obtain a faster high, which adds to their risk of contracting HIV from contaminated needles.

This is important. A drug-education program should include activities that help the students increase their feeling of self-worth.

Nurses must stress to children the danger of using cocaine and crack. School education programs should start at the elementary level. Nurses can perform a community service by volunteering to present programs to local schoolchildren. Children and adolescents must be alerted to the dangers of these drugs and taught ways to refuse offers of drugs.

Narcotic Abuse

The most commonly abused narcotics are morphine and heroin. These drugs decrease anger, sex drive, and hunger by producing a dreamlike, euphoric state. Narcotics are highly addictive and extremely expensive, and narcotic abuse results in teenage prostitution, pushing (selling) drugs, and robbery as a means to support the drug habit. As mentioned, any drugs that are injected subject adolescents to the added risk of contracting HIV from using contaminated needles.

Although heroin use in actual numbers is lower than that of other illicit drugs, adolescents' use of heroin has increased because of several factors. In general, there is a decrease among children in the perceived danger of drug use. This trend seems to be evident across the entire scope of illicit drug use. Because heroin is now available in forms that can be smoked or snorted, the threat of HIV infection is no longer a deterrent.

Other Abused Drugs

Other mood-altering drugs commonly abused by children include hallucinogens (psychedelic drugs), depressants, amphetamines, and analgesics. Anabolic steroids, although not mood altering, are also abused by adolescents.

Hallucinogens (psychedelic drugs), although not addictive in a physical sense, can create a psychological dependence from the resulting hallucinations. This category of drugs includes LSD, PCP ("angel dust"), psilocybin (derived from mushrooms), mescaline, DMT (derived from plants), and airplane glue. These drugs cause distortions in vision, smell, or hearing. Effects can include intoxication, "bad trips," and flashbacks, and overdoses are common.

The drug known as Ecstasy is similar to amphetamines in chemical makeup, but has the effect of elevating mood and increasing tactile sensations similar to the use of hallucinogens. Use of Ecstasy has increased dramatically in the adolescent population. The drug releases large amounts of serotonin, the neurotransmitter that regulates mood and emotion, and does not have the unpredictable effects of the other psychedelics. The drug is used in party and club settings, where the users dance and party for extended periods of time; the drug suppresses their needs to eat, drink, or sleep.

Depressants, sometimes referred to as hypnotics, are as addictive as narcotics, and withdrawal from them must be carefully controlled to prevent delirium, seizures, or death. Barbiturates, glutethimide (Doriden), ethchlorvynol (Placidyl), and methaqualone (Quaalude) are the most commonly abused drugs in this group; they are sometimes used with alcohol, which increases the intoxicating effects, such as sleepiness, slurred speech, and impaired cognitive and motor functions.

Amphetamines ("uppers" or "speed") produce increased alertness, wakefulness, reduced awareness of fatigue, and increased confidence and energy. Although not physically addicting, they encourage psychological dependence and are abused by millions of Americans, many of whom become trapped in a destructive cycle of uppers and "downers" (barbiturates). The amphetamines are often manufactured in methamphetamine ("meth") labs in people's homes, which increases the potential dangers to the child who uses these substances.

Children abuse analgesics, particularly those that are combinations of narcotic and non-narcotics such as Percocet and Darvon. Chronic abuse can result in blood and kidney disorders. These drugs may be prescribed to a family member, which makes them easy for the child to obtain.

Anabolic steroids are not mood-altering drugs, but their abuse among athletes is a cause for great concern.

Adolescent athletes take anabolic steroids to build up muscle mass in the belief that the drug will increase their athletic ability. These athletes take megadoses of illegally obtained drugs. Other adolescents may take them to build muscles and to achieve a "manly" appearance that they believe will make them more attractive. The side effects of euphoria and decreased fatigue make these drugs even more inviting to adolescents. Some use also has been reported in high-school female athletes.

The use of excessively large doses of steroids may cause **gynecomastia** (excessive development of mammary glands in the male) or premature fusion of the long bones, which stunts growth in the adolescent who has not yet completed growth. Liver damage, predisposition to atherosclerosis, acne, hypertension, aggressiveness, and psychotic and manic symptoms also may result (National Institute of Drug Abuse/National Institutes of Health, 2002). School programs about drug abuse should include the topic of anabolic steroid abuse.

Test Yourself

- What warning signs are often seen in children who are contemplating committing suicide?
- What are the reasons children use alcohol and other substances?
- Explain the difference between psychological and physical dependence in substance use.
- Name common substances children might use.

Parents Addicted to Drugs or Alcohol

More than 10% of children come from a home affected by the alcoholism of one or both parents. Alcoholism exacts a terrible toll on the functioning of the family. Children of alcoholics are four times more likely to become alcoholics. When other substances are included, the number of affected homes increases substantially. Many women who abuse drugs and alcohol were themselves victims of physical, emotional, or sexual abuse as children (Hall, 2000).

Effects on the Family

Developmental delays occur in young children of substance abusers. Infants of cocaine abusers avoid the caregiver's gaze, which contributes further to bonding delays. The parent who is addicted may be so involved in procuring the drug that any parenting is forgotten. The parent, caught in the ups and downs of addiction, is not dependable and cannot provide any stability for the child. The parent may waver between overindulgence—smothering the child with attention, leniency, and gifts—and the opposite behavior of irritability, unreasonable accusations, threats, and anger. This unpredictable behavior has a severe impact on the relationships in the family.

Children of substance-abusing parents often become loners and avoid relationships with others for fear that the substance-abusing parent might do or say something to embarrass them in front of their peers.

As the parent's substance abuse worsens, the family's dysfunction and social isolation increase. The **co-dependent parent** supports, directly or indirectly, the addictive behavior of the other parent. This behavior usually involves making excuses for the addict's actions and expecting others (i.e., the children) to overlook the parent's moodiness, erratic behavior, and consumption of alcohol or drugs. Co-dependency adds to the dilemma of children living with an addicted parent.

Children Coping With Parental Addiction

Children react in a variety of ways. Children rarely talk about the parent's problem even to the other parent. These children often experience guilt, anxiety, confusion, anger, depression, and addictive behavior. An older child, often a girl, may take on the responsibility of running the household, taking care of the younger children, making meals, and performing the tasks that the parent normally should do. These children may become overachievers in school but remain isolated emotionally from their peers and teachers. Another child in the family may try to deflect the embarrassment and anger of the other siblings by trying to make everyone feel good. As these children become adolescents or young adults, they may have problems such as substance abuse or eating disorders. The child in the family who "acts out" and engages in delinquent behavior is most likely to come to the attention of social services and be identified as a child who needs help.

Behaviors that may alert nurses and other health care personnel to an addiction problem in the family include:

- The loner child who avoids interaction with classmates
- The child who is failing in school or has numerous episodes of unexcused absences or truancy
- The child with frequent minor physical complaints, such as headaches or stomachaches

- The child who steals or commits acts of violence
- The aggressive child
- The child who abuses drugs or alcohol

Nurses and others who work with children must be alert to these signals for help. Children can benefit from programs that support them and help them understand what is happening in the home. Such a program may include group therapy sessions at school in which the child learns that others have the same problems; this reduces his or her feelings of isolation. Other programs may include the whole family, perhaps as part of the program for the addicted parent who is trying to break the addiction. Professional help is necessary to prevent the child from developing more serious problems. The earlier the child can be identified and treatment begun, the better the prognosis. Box 41-1 provides a list of resources for information and help with drug and alcohol problems.

ATTENTION DEFICIT HYPERACTIVITY DISORDER

Attention deficit hyperactivity disorder (ADHD), or attention deficit disorder (ADD), is a syndrome characterized by degrees of inattention, impulsive behavior, and hyperactivity. About 3% to 5% of all American school-age children have ADHD; boys are more commonly affected than are girls. The cause of the disorder is unclear: developmental lag, biochemical disorder, and food sensitivities are all theories under consideration. The disorder affects every part of the child's life.

Clinical Manifestations

The child with ADHD may have these characteristics:

- Impulsiveness
- Easy distractibility
- Frequent fidgeting or squirming
- Difficulty sitting still
- Problems following through on instructions, despite being able to understand them
- Inattentiveness when being spoken to
- Frequent losing of things
- Going from one uncompleted activity to another
- Difficulty taking turns
- Frequent excessive talking
- Engaging in dangerous activities without considering the consequences

These children also often demonstrate signs of clumsiness or poor coordination, such as the inability to use a pencil or scissors in a child who is older than 3 or 4 years of age. No one child has all these

BOX 41.1	Resources for Information and Help With Drug and Alcohol Problems

If you suspect your child may be using alcohol or drugs, you must confront the situation directly. Your doctor, local hospital, school social worker, or county mental health society may be able to refer you to a treatment facility.

A number of helpful national organizations are just a phone call away. If you have a computer and access to the Internet, several groups also offer valuable information at their World Wide Web sites.

Center for Substance Abuse Treatment: For drug and alcohol information and referral, call 1-800-662-HELP. Web site: *www.samhsa.gov/centers/csat2002*

The National Clearinghouse for Alcohol and Drug Information: For pamphlets, publications, and materials for schools, call 1-800-SAY-NOTO. Web site: *www.health.org*

American Council for Drug Education: Call 1-800-488-DRUG.

National Families in Action: Call 404-248-9676. Web site: *www.emory.edu/NFIA*

National Family Partnership: Call 1-800-705-8897. Web site: *www.nfp.org*

PRIDE (Parents' Resource Institute for Drug Education): Call 770-458-9900. Web site: *www.prideusa.org*

Community Anti-Drug Coalitions of America: For information on current issues or legislation, call 1-800-54 CADCA. Web site: *www.cadca.org*

Al-Anon/Alateen Family Group Headquarters, Inc.: Call 1-800-356-9996. Web site: *www.al-anon.org*

Alcoholics Anonymous World Services: Check the phone directory for your local AA chapter or call 212-870-3400. Web site: *www.aa.org*

Nar-Anon Family Group Headquarters, Inc.: Call 310-547-5800. Web site: *www.naranon.com*

Partnership for a Drug-Free America: Web site: *www.drugfreeamerica.org*

U.S. Department of Education: Call 1-800-624-0010. Web site: *www.ed.gov*

National Criminal Justice Reference Service: Web site: *www.ncjrs.org*

Drug Free Kids: *www.drugfreeusa.net*

symptoms. Although it was believed that these symptoms were resolved by late adolescence, it is now apparent that they continue into adulthood, at least for some people.

Although these children may have poor success in the classroom because of their inability to pay attention, they are not intellectually impaired. The child's poor impulse control also contributes to disciplinary problems in the classroom. Some children with ADHD may have learning disorders, such as dyslexia and perceptual deficits. The child's self-confidence can suffer from feeling inferior to the other children in the class. Special arrangements can be made to provide an educational atmosphere that is supportive for the child without the need for the child to leave the classroom.

Diagnosis

Diagnosis can be made after the child is 3 years old but often is not made until the child reaches school age and has trouble settling into the routine of being in the classroom setting. Diagnosis can be difficult and also may be controversial because many of the symptoms are subjective and rely on the assessment of caregivers and teachers. Some authorities have expressed concern that teachers incorrectly label children as hyperactive. The symptoms may be a result of environmental factors that can include broken homes, stress, and non-supportive caregivers.

The multidisciplinary approach is most effective for diagnosis, i.e., one involving pediatric and education specialists, a psychologist, the classroom teacher, family caregivers, and others. A careful, detailed history, including school and social functioning, psychological testing, and physical and neurologic examinations, can help in making the diagnosis.

Treatment and Nursing Care

Treatment is also multidisciplinary. Learning situations should be structured so that the child has minimal distractions and a supportive teacher. Home support is necessary and requires structured, consistent guidance from the caregivers. Medication is used for some children. Stimulant medications, such as methylphenidate (Ritalin, Concerta) and dextroamphetamine (Dexedrine), have often been used. When given in large amounts, these medications may suppress the appetite and affect the child's growth. Pemoline (Cylert) has been used but generally with less success than methylphenidate and dextroamphetamine. Using stimulants for a hyperactive child seems paradoxical, but these drugs apparently stimulate the area of the child's brain that aids in concentration, thus enabling the child to have better control.

In the health care setting, the nurse should maintain a calm, patient attitude toward the child with ADHD. The child should be given only one simple instruction at a time. Limiting distractions, using consistency, and offering praise for accomplishments are invaluable methods of working with these children. The families of children with ADHD need a great deal of support. Primary family caregivers in particular can become frustrated and upset by the constant challenge of dealing with a child with ADHD. Building the child's self-esteem, confidence, and academic success

A PERSONAL GLIMPSE

I don't really mind it. When I don't take my meds. I go crazy or bonkers (sometimes). I'm on my pills cause of my behavior. And also to control the ways I talk (like so I won't blurt out in class). I was taught to control my actions, don't let my actions control me.

Eddie, a 9-year-old who takes medication for ADHD.

LEARNING OPPORTUNITY: What feelings do you think this child experiences in those times when he is not able to control his behavior? What would you say to this child to encourage him to talk about his disorder and his feelings?

must be the primary goal of all who work with these children.

ENURESIS AND ENCOPRESIS

Enuresis, or bed-wetting, is involuntary urination beyond the age when control of urination commonly is acquired. Enuresis may have a physiologic or psychological cause and may indicate a need for further exploration and treatment (see Chapter 38 for further discussion).

Encopresis is chronic involuntary fecal soiling beyond the age when control is expected (about 3 years of age). Speech and learning disabilities may accompany this problem. If no organic causes (e.g., worms, megacolon) exist, encopresis indicates a serious emotional problem and a need for counseling for the child and the family caregivers. Some experts believe that overcontrol or undercontrol by a caregiver can cause encopresis. Recommendations for treatment differ; however, the most important goal is recognition of the problem and referral for treatment and counseling.

NONORGANIC FAILURE TO THRIVE

Four principal factors are necessary for human growth: food; rest and activity; adequate secretions of hormones; and a satisfactory relationship with a caregiver or nurturing person who provides consistent, loving human contact and stimulation. Growth is disturbed and development can be delayed when one of these four factors is missing or when the infant has a major birth defect, such as congenital heart disease or a metabolic disorder.

Infants who fail to gain weight and who show signs of delayed development are classified as failure-to-thrive infants. Failure to thrive can be divided into two classifications: organic failure to thrive, which is a result of a disease condition, and nonorganic failure to thrive (NFTT), which has no apparent physical cause. The section below discusses NFTT. Organic failure to thrive is covered under specific diseases, including congenital heart disease, gastrointestinal reflux, celiac syndrome, and cystic fibrosis.

Clinical Manifestations

Infants with NFTT often are listless and seriously below average weight and height; have poor muscle tone and a loss of subcutaneous fat; and are immobile for long periods of time (Fig. 41-1). They may be unresponsive to (or actually try to avoid) cuddling and vocalization. Examination of the child is likely to reveal no organic cause for this condition. However, examination of the family relationship, particularly the mother–child relationship, often provides important insights into the problem.

The family relationships of these children are often so disrupted that there is no warm, close relationship with a family caregiver. For some reason, proper attachment has not occurred. Often the father is absent or emotionally unavailable, adding to the mother's feelings of isolation and inadequacy and leading to an atmosphere of additional stress and conflict.

The problem is not with the caregiver alone or with the child but instead with their interaction and mutual lack of responsiveness. They are not in harmony. The caregiver does not stimulate the child; therefore, the child has no one to respond to and fails to do the "cute baby" things that would gain attention and stimulation. The child cannot accomplish the developmental task of establishing basic trust.

Children with NFTT often fall into the classification of "difficult" or irritable babies, but others may be listless and passive and do not seem to care about feedings. A common characteristic is **rumination** (voluntary regurgitation), perhaps as a means of self-satisfaction when the desired response is not received from the caregiver. When rumination occurs, a chain of events is activated that further strains the caregiver–child relationship. The child loses weight, sometimes becomes severely emaciated, grows listless and irritable, and smells "sour" because of frequent vomiting. None of this makes for an attractive baby to love, cuddle, and show off.

Diagnosis

The child must be thoroughly evaluated by the physician to rule out a systemic or congenital disorder. Signs of deprivation are important elements in the diagnosis. When the child begins to improve in a nurturing atmosphere, the diagnosis is confirmed.

Treatment

Treatment initially depends almost entirely on good nursing care. By teaching child care skills, acting as a role model, and supporting caregiver–child interactions, the nurse can help reverse the child's growth failure and begin an improved caregiver–child relationship.

Prognosis is uncertain; much depends on the support and counseling the family receives. Long-term care is almost certainly necessary and may require several members of the health care team, such as a family therapist, clergy, social worker, and public health nurse. Avoid judgmental, stereotyped feelings when dealing with the family of such a child.

You can make a difference. A positive, nonjudgmental attitude when working with family caregivers of children with failure to thrive can have a direct and lasting effect on the family's interaction with their child.

● **Figure 41.1** The child with failure to thrive is often seriously below average weight.

● Nursing Process for the Child With Nonorganic Failure to Thrive

ASSESSMENT

Conduct a careful physical exam of the child, including observing skin turgor, anterior fontanel, signs of emaciation, weight, temperature, apical pulse, respirations, responsiveness, listlessness, and irritability. Observe for rumination or odor of vomitus.

When interviewing the family caregiver, carefully observe the interaction between the caregiver and the child and note the caregiver's responsiveness to the child's needs and the child's response to the caregiver. Listen carefully for underlying problems while talking with the family caregivers. Note if other supportive, involved people are present or if the caregiver is a single parent with no support system. Take a careful history of feeding and sleeping patterns or problems. Determine the caregiver's confidence in handling the child and note any apparent indication of feelings of stress or inadequacy.

SELECTED NURSING DIAGNOSES

- Disturbed Sensory Perception related to insufficient nurturing
- Imbalanced Nutrition: Less Than Body Requirements related to inadequate intake of calories
- Deficient Fluid Volume related to inadequate oral intake
- Impaired Urinary Elimination related to decreased fluid intake
- Constipation related to dehydration
- Risk for Impaired Skin Integrity related to malnourishment
- Impaired Parenting related to lack of knowledge and confidence in parenting skills

OUTCOME IDENTIFICATION AND PLANNING

The major goals for the NFTT child focus on improving alertness and responsiveness, increasing caloric and oral fluid intake, maintaining normal urinary and bowel elimination, and maintaining skin integrity. Other goals for the child and family include improving parenting skills and building parental confidence. The caregiver's participation in the child's care is essential. Plan individualized nursing according to these goals.

IMPLEMENTATION

Providing Sensory Stimulation

The nurse plays a critical role in reversing the child's growth failure and improving the caregiver–child relationship. Providing sensory stimulation is vital in the care of the NFTT child. Attempt to cuddle the child and talk to him or her in a warm, soothing tone. Allow for play activities appropriate for the child's age. Family caregivers should be provided with information about normal growth and developmental activities appropriate for the child.

Maintaining Adequate Nutrition and Fluid Intake

Feed the child slowly and carefully in a quiet environment. During feeding, the child might be closely snuggled and gently rocked. It may be necessary to feed the child every 2 or 3 hours initially. Burp the child frequently during and at the end of each feeding, then place him or her on the side with the head slightly elevated or held in a chest-to-chest position. Feed the child until good eating habits are established. Extra fluids of unsweetened juices are encouraged. If a family caregiver is present, encourage him or her to become involved in the child's feedings. Demonstrate the importance of talking encouragingly as the baby eats. An older child can sit at a low table facing the feeder while eating. Make the feeding time pleasant and comforting. Carefully document food intake with caloric intake and strict intake and output records.

Monitoring Elimination Patterns

As food and fluids are gradually increased and the child becomes hydrated, bowel activity and urine production return to normal. Daily stools are of a soft consistency, and the hourly urinary output is 2 to 3 mL/kg.

Promoting Skin Integrity

Protect the child's skin to prevent irritation. Lanolin or A and D Ointment can be used to lubricate dry skin. Apply the ointment at least once each shift and turn the child at least every 2 hours.

Providing Family Teaching

While caring for the child, point out to the caregiver the child's development and responsiveness, noting and praising any positive parenting behaviors the caregiver displays. The caregiver who has not had a close, warm childhood relationship may not understand the child's needs for cuddling and stimulation. Teaching about these needs must be done carefully and in a manner that doesn't further damage the caregiver's self-esteem. Many of these family caregivers are overly concerned about spoiling the child: it is important to dispel these fears. Explain the need for the child to develop trust, and teach the caregiver about the developmental tasks appropriate for children. Involve other health care team members as needed.

EVALUATION: GOALS AND EXPECTED OUTCOMES

- **Goal:** The child will be more alert and responsive.
  Expected Outcome: The child visually follows the caregiver around the room.
- **Goal:** The child's caloric intake will be adequate for age.
  Expected Outcome: The child's weight increases at a predetermined goal of 1 oz or more per day.
- **Goal:** The child will have adequate fluid intake and urine output for age.
  Expected Outcome: The child's urine output will be 2 to 3 mL/kg/hr.
- **Goal:** The child will have normal bowel elimination.
  Expected Outcome: The child will have a bowel elimination pattern and the stools will be soft.
- **Goal:** The child's skin integrity will be maintained.
  Expected Outcome: The child's skin shows no signs of redness or irritation and remains intact.
- **Goal:** The family caregivers will demonstrate positive signs of good parenting.
  Expected Outcome: The family caregivers feed the child successfully and exhibit an appropriate response to the child.

EATING DISORDERS

Anorexia Nervosa

Preoccupation with reducing diets and the quest for the "perfect" (i.e., thin) figure sometimes leads to **anorexia nervosa**, or self-inflicted starvation. This disorder occurs most commonly in adolescent white females, although there are reported cases among males and among African-American, Hispanic, and Asian adolescents. First described more than 100 years ago, anorexia has increased in incidence in recent years and is currently estimated to affect as many as 1% of adolescent girls. Anorexia is found in all the developed countries. Two age ranges are identified as the usual age of onset: 11 to 13 years and 19 to 20 years. Although considered a psychiatric problem, it causes severe physiologic damage and even death.

Characteristics

These children often are described as successful students who tend to be perfectionists and are always trying to please parents, teachers, and other adults. The families of anorexic children characteristically show little emotion and display no evidence of conflict within the family. An adolescent in a controlled family environment, in which the parents do not freely express emotions, may try to establish independence and identity by controlling his or her own appetite and body weight. Depression is common in these adolescents. Anorexic persons deny weight loss and actually see themselves as fat, even when they look skeletal to others. They often adhere to a rigid program of exercise to further their efforts in weight reduction. They may make demands on themselves for cleanliness and order in their environment, or they may engage in rigid schedules for studying and other ritualistic behavior. These adolescents deny hunger but often suffer from fatigue.

Clinical Manifestations and Diagnosis

Persons with anorexia are visibly emaciated, with an almost skeleton-like appearance. They appear sexually immature, have dry skin and brittle nails, and often have lanugo (downy hair) over their backs and extremities. Other symptoms include amenorrhea (absence of menstruation), constipation, hypothermia, bradycardia, low blood pressure, and anemia.

The American Psychiatric Association (2000) identifies the following criteria for the diagnosis of anorexia nervosa:

- Weight loss leading to maintenance of body weight less than 85% of that expected for age and height; or failure to make expected weight gain during a period of growth, leading to body weight less than 85% of that expected
- Intense fear of gaining weight or becoming fat even though underweight
- Disturbance in how one's body weight or shape is experienced; undue influence of body weight or shape on self-evaluation; denial of seriousness of the current low body weight (e.g., feeling fat even when emaciated or, although underweight, perceiving one part of the body as being too fat)
- Amenorrhea as evidenced by absence of three consecutive menstrual cycles

Treatment and Nursing Care

Children with anorexia nervosa may be hospitalized to achieve the two goals of treatment: correction of malnutrition and identification and treatment of the psychological cause. An approach involving several disciplines is necessary. Therapy is required to help the child gain insight into the problem. In addition, family therapy, nutritional therapy, and behavior modification are used. Affected children fear they will gain too much weight; therefore, a compromise between what the physician prefers and what the adolescent desires may be necessary.

Adolescents with anorexia have become experts in manipulating others and their environment. Once treatment begins, they may try to avoid gaining weight by ordering only low-calorie foods; by disposing of their meals in plants, trash, toilets, or dirty linen; or by exercising in the hall or jogging in place in their rooms. In some instances, nasogastric tube feedings or total parenteral nutrition (TPN) is necessary to provide nutritional support.

Treatment based on behavior modification may deprive the patient of all privileges, such as visitors, television, and telephone, until the child begins to gain weight. Privileges are then gradually restored. These techniques are effective only when the patient and the caregivers understand the program and its purpose and have agreed on individualized goals and rewards.

Warning. Death may occur from suicide, infection, or the effects of starvation in the child with anorexia.

Group therapy may be used to rely on peer support and provide the opportunity to associate with other patients with the same diagnosis in a nonthreatening setting.

The long-term outlook for the child with anorexia is unclear.

Some children recover completely; others have eating problems into adulthood; still others have problems with social adjustment that are not related to eating. Predicting the outcome is difficult, and more studies are needed before a definitive answer is available (Fig. 41-2).

Bulimia

Bulimia nervosa (usually referred to simply as bulimia) is characterized by binge eating followed by purging. The typical bulimic person is a white female in late adolescence. Most often, the bulimic person is of normal weight or slightly overweight. Those who are underweight usually fulfill the criteria for anorexia nervosa, although some anorexic persons periodically

● **Figure 41.2** This anorexic teen, who is in the later stages of treatment, continues to meet with the counselor to discuss her food choices, exercise program, and overall well-being.

practice binging and purging. Bulimia is seen increasingly in young adult women as well.

The binging often occurs late in the day when the child is alone. Secrecy is an important aspect of the process. The child eats large quantities of food within 1 or 2 hours. This binging is followed by guilt, fear, shame, and self-condemnation. To avoid weight gain from the food eaten, the child follows the binging with purging by means of self-induced vomiting, laxatives, diuretics, and excessive exercise.

Clinical Manifestations and Diagnosis

The clues to bulimia may be few but include dental caries and erosion from frequent exposure to stomach acid, throat irritation, and endocrine and electrolyte imbalances that may cause cardiac irregularities and menstrual problems. Calluses or abrasions may be noted on the back of the hand from frequent contact with the teeth while inducing vomiting. Possible complications are esophageal tears and acute gastric dilation. Hypokalemia also may occur, especially if the child abuses diuretics to prevent weight gain. Other behavior problems seen in many bulimic persons include drug abuse, alcoholism, stealing (especially food), promiscuity, and other impulsive activities.

According to the American Psychiatric Association, the diagnostic criteria for bulimia include

- Recurrent episodes of binge eating
- A feeling of lack of control over behavior during binges
- Self-induced purging; use of laxatives or diuretics, enemas, or other medications; and strict dieting, fasting, or vigorous exercise to prevent weight gain
- Average of at least two binge-eating episodes a week during a 3-month period
- Obsessiveness regarding body weight and shape

Treatment

Treatment of bulimia is varied. Many aspects of the treatment are similar to treatment for the child with anorexia. Food diaries often are used as a tool to assess the child's eating patterns. In some instances, antidepressant drugs may be useful. The nurse can refer the child to a support group that may prove helpful.

● Nursing Process for the Child With Anorexia Nervosa or Bulimia

ASSESSMENT

Data collection of the child with an eating disorder begins with a complete interview and history, including previous illnesses, allergies, a dietary history, and a description of eating habits. The child may not give an accurate dietary history or description of eating habits. Question the family caregiver in a separate interview to gain added information. In the physical exam include height, weight, blood pressure, temperature, pulse, and respirations. Carefully inspect and observe the skin, mucous membranes, state of nutrition, and state of alertness and cooperation. Complete documentation of what is found is necessary.

SELECTED NURSING DIAGNOSES

- Imbalanced Nutrition: Less Than Body Requirements related to self-induced vomiting and use of laxatives or diuretics
- Disturbed Body Image related to fear of obesity and potential rejection
- Risk for Activity Intolerance related to fatigue secondary to malnutrition
- Risk for Constipation related to decreased food and fluid intake
- Risk for Diarrhea related to use of laxatives
- Risk for Impaired Skin Integrity related to loss of subcutaneous fat and dry skin secondary to malnutrition
- Noncompliance with treatment regimen related to unresolved conflicts over food and eating
- Compromised Family Coping related to eating disorders, treatment regimen, and dangers associated with an eating disorder

OUTCOME IDENTIFICATION AND PLANNING

The major goals for the child with an eating disorder relate to meeting nutritional needs and improving body image, self-concept, and self-esteem. Other goals include establishing appropriate activity levels, maintaining normal bowel activity, maintaining skin integrity, and complying with the treatment program. The goals for the family include understanding the condition, learning how to manage the condition and its treatment, and reinforcing the child's self-esteem.

IMPLEMENTATION

Improving Nutrition

The child with bulimia or anorexia nervosa does not receive the nutrients needed to achieve adequate growth during this period of development. Supervise food intake. Weigh the child at the same time each day, but do not make an issue of weight fluctuation. Be observant when weighing the patient: the child may try to add weight by putting heavy objects in pockets, shoes, or other hiding places. While being weighed, the patient should wear minimal clothing (preferably a patient gown with no pockets) and have bare feet.

The care provider and a dietitian work with the child to devise a food plan to meet the child's nutrition requirements. The goal of the food plan is not a sudden weight gain, but a slow, steady gain with an established goal that has been agreed on by the health care team and the child. Often the child keeps a food diary that is reviewed daily with the health team.

Patients with eating disorders are often manipulative and deceptive. Observe the patient during and after eating to make certain the child eats the required food and does not get rid of it after apparently consuming it.

Contract agreements are often recommended for patients with eating disorders. These agreements, which are usually part of a behavioral modification plan, specify the child's and the staff's responsibilities for the diet, activity expectations for the child, and other aspects of the child's behavior. The contract also may spell out specific privileges that can be gained by meeting the contract goals. This places the child in greater control of the outcome.

In addition to daily weights, test urine for ketones and regularly evaluate the skin turgor and mucous membranes to gather further information about nutritional status. Report and document immediately any evidence of deteriorating physical condition. If weight loss continues, nasogastric tube feedings may need to be implemented. This possibility also can be included in the contract.

If the child's condition is at a critical stage with fluid and electrolyte deficiencies, parenteral fluids are necessary immediately to hydrate the patient before additional treatment can be implemented. Observe the child continuously to prevent any attempt to remove intravenous lines or otherwise disrupt the treatment. Closely monitor serum electrolytes, cardiac and respiratory status, and renal complications. During administration of parenteral fluids, continue to encourage the child to maintain an oral intake.

Reinforcing Positive Body Image and Self-concept

The nurse must function as an active, nonjudgmental listener to the child. Consistent assignment of the same nursing personnel to care for the child helps to establish a climate in which the child can relate to the nurse and begin to build a positive self-concept. Report and document without delay any signs of depression. Also report and document any negative feelings expressed by the child. Do not minimize or ignore these feelings. Reinforce positive behavior. Psychotherapy and counseling groups are necessary to help the child work through feelings of negative self-worth. Encourage the child to express fears, anger, and frustrations and help the patient recognize that everyone has these feelings from time to time. Never ridicule or belittle these feelings. Encourage the child to explore ways in which destructive feelings may be changed. These are feelings that can be dealt with in counseling sessions; therefore, report and document them carefully.

Balancing Rest and Activity

Exercise and activity are important parts of the contract negotiated with the child. Explain to the child that fatigue is a result of the extreme depletion of energy reserves related to nutritional deficits. Encourage the child to become involved in all activities of daily living. Provide ample rest periods when the child's energy reserves are depleted. Discourage the child from pushing beyond endurance and closely observe for secretive excessive activity.

Monitoring Bowel Habits

Make a careful record of bowel movements. The child may not be reliable as a reporter of bowel habits, so devise methods to prevent the child from using the bathroom without supervision. Report at once and document constipation or diarrhea. Watch carefully to prevent the child from obtaining and taking a laxative. These patients are devious and may go to great lengths to obtain a laxative to purge themselves of food. Report immediately any evidence or suspicions of this type of behavior.

Promoting Skin Integrity

Good skin care is essential in the care of the child with a severely restricted nutritional intake. The skin may be dry and tend to break down easily because of the lack of a subcutaneous fat cushion. Inspect daily for redness, irritation, or signs of decubitus ulcer formation. Observe specifically the bony prominences. Encourage the child to be out of bed most of the day. When the child is in bed, encourage regular position changes so that no pressure areas develop.

Promoting Compliance

The long-term outcome for child with eating disorders is precarious. Children with severe eating disorders often have multiple inpatient admissions. During inpatient treatment, goals should be set and plans made for discharge. Specific consequences must be established for noncompliance. Counseling must continue after discharge. A support group referral may be helpful in encouraging compliance. Family involvement is necessary. The child must recognize that discharge from the health care facility does not mean that he or she is "cured."

Improving Family Coping

The family of the child needs counseling along with the child. Some families may deny that the child has a problem or that the problem is as severe as perceived by health care team members. Family therapy meets with varied success. Usually the earlier family therapy is initiated, the better the results. Family members must be able to identify behaviors of their own that contribute to the child's problem. Family members also must learn to cooperate with behavior modification programs and with guidance carry them out at home when necessary. Ongoing contact between the family, the child, and consistent health team members is essential (see Nursing Care Plan 41-1: The Child With Anorexia Nervosa).

EVALUATION: GOALS AND EXPECTED OUTCOMES

The evaluation of a child with anorexia or bulimia is an ongoing process that continues throughout the hospital stay as well as in outpatient settings. Goals and expected outcomes include

- **Goal:** The child will gain a predetermined amount of weight per week.
  Expected Outcome: The child eats at least 80% of each meal, gains 1 to 2 lb (450 to 900 g) a week, keeps a food diary, and signs a contract agreement.
- **Goal:** The child will show evidence of improved self-esteem.

NURSING CARE PLAN 41.1

The Child With Anorexia Nervosa

FW is a 15-year-old girl who has had a complete physical examination to determine why she has lost weight. After her examination and testing was completed, a diagnosis of anorexia nervosa was made. The child denies that she is underweight. She has been hospitalized to initiate treatment because her weight has dropped to 87 pounds (39.5 kg).

NURSING DIAGNOSIS

Imbalanced Nutrition: Less Than Body Requirements related to self-inflicted starvation and excessive exercise

GOAL: The child's nutritional status will improve, reaching a goal weight of 100 pounds, and an adequate fluid intake will be maintained.

EXPECTED OUTCOMES
- The child gains at least 1.5 pounds (680 grams) per week.
- The child eats 80% of her meals.
- The child is involved in plans to improve her nutrition.
- The child does not interrupt parenteral fluid administration.
- The child's mucous membranes are moist; her skin turgor is good.
- The child's electrolytes, cardiac and respiratory status, and renal function are within normal limits.

NURSING INTERVENTIONS	RATIONALE
Supervise intake by observing her during and after meals.	A child with an eating disorder may go to any length to avoid eating.
Weigh daily at the same time wearing the same type of clothes. Make certain nothing can be secreted in pockets or other hiding places that could add to her weight.	A child can be very innovative in finding ways to hide heavy objects on her to increase her weight gain.
Include the child with other health care providers to establish a mutually agreed upon, long-term weight goal and food plan that provide her with a slow, steady, weekly weight gain. Make a contract agreement to clearly state expectations and privileges that she can gain or lose.	The child is central to the planning process and cannot be made to meet goals set by others. Her participation and agreement to specific plans give her a feeling of more control of the overall outcome and encourage her to stick to the plan.
Observe continuously when parenteral fluids are being administered to prevent any attempts to disrupt the IV line. Also encourage her to take oral fluids at the same time.	The anorectic child may deprive herself so much that the fluid and electrolyte deficiencies become life-threatening. A balance must be restored before any further treatment can begin.
Test urine for ketones and regularly evaluate her skin turgor and mucous membranes.	These tests provide further indication of nutritional status.

NURSING DIAGNOSIS

Disturbed Body Image related to fear of obesity and potential rejection

GOAL: The child will express positive feelings about self.

EXPECTED OUTCOMES
- The child verbally expresses positive attitudes about herself.
- The child expresses insight into reasons behind eating patterns and self-destructive behavior.
- The child expresses feelings about food, exercise, weight loss, and medical condition.

NURSING INTERVENTIONS	RATIONALE
Be a nonjudgmental, active listener; never minimize or ignore feelings expressed.	This is a first step in establishing and maintaining a climate of trust.
Report any negative feelings or any signs of depression expressed.	The child's negative feelings and expression of depression are important to the therapeutic treatment plan. All health care providers need to know about signs of depression to alert them to take appropriate precautions.
Maintain continuity of care throughout treatment.	The same person working with the child will help foster trust and a relationship will be developed.

(nursing care plan continues on page 1004)

NURSING CARE PLAN 41.1 continued

The Child With Anorexia Nervosa

NURSING DIAGNOSIS
Risk for Activity Intolerance related to fatigue secondary to malnutrition

GOAL: The child will balance rest and activity.

EXPECTED OUTCOMES
- The child follows her contract for activity.
- The child is not excessively active.
- The child paces her activity to avoid fatigue.

NURSING INTERVENTIONS	*RATIONALE*
Teach the child that a nutritional deficit depletes energy reserves and results in fatigue; encourage her to engage in activities of daily living, but provide for rest periods when her energy is low.	The child needs to understand that activity and rest are related to her nutritional status and that a healthy balance is crucial to overall health.
Discourage the child from pushing herself beyond her physical limits, and observe closely for secretive excessive exercise.	The child with an eating disorder may attempt to burn off excess calories with exercise.

NURSING DIAGNOSIS
Risk for Constipation related to decreased food and fluid intake
Risk for Diarrhea related to use of laxatives

GOAL: The child will maintain normal bowel habits.

EXPECTED OUTCOMES
- The child has bowel movements every day or every other day.
- The child's stools are soft-formed.
- The child's fluid and electrolyte balances are maintained.

NURSING INTERVENTIONS	*RATIONALE*
Observe the child's trips to the bathroom and keep a careful record of bowel habits; report and document any occurrence of diarrhea or constipation at once.	Typically the child may not be a reliable reporter of her bowel habits. A nurse observer is necessary to validate her stools.
Observe carefully to be certain that she does not have opportunity for purging or taking a laxative.	These children can be devious and will go to almost any length to prevent weight gain.
Monitor fluid intake and output and electrolyte levels.	Loss of fluids and electrolytes can cause long-term health conditions.

NURSING DIAGNOSIS
Risk for Impaired Skin Integrity related to loss of subcutaneous fat and dry skin secondary to malnutrition.

GOAL: The child's skin integrity will be maintained.

EXPECTED OUTCOMES
- The child has no areas of red, dry, irritated skin.
- The child has no pressure ulcer formations.
- The child expresses feelings about body image and skin changes.

NURSING INTERVENTIONS	*RATIONALE*
Inspect skin daily for redness, irritation, or dryness. Provide good skin care.	Signs of redness, irritation, and dryness are preliminary signs for skin breakdown and formation of pressure ulcers.
Protect any bony prominences that may break down. Encourage position changes for child in bed to prevent decubiti formation.	Protection of pressure on bony surfaces and frequent changes of position improve circulation and prevent formation of pressure ulcers.

NURSING CARE PLAN 41.1 continued

The Child With Anorexia Nervosa

NURSING DIAGNOSIS
Noncompliance with treatment regimen related to unresolved conflicts over food and eating

GOAL: The child will comply with treatment regimen.

EXPECTED OUTCOMES
- The child keeps counseling appointments.
- The child joins a support group.
- The child continues to gain weight as per her contract agreement.
- The child participates in decisions about care and treatment.

NURSING INTERVENTIONS	*RATIONALE*
Make plans for discharge while she is still in the hospital. Include counseling plans in the contract.	Eating disorders are not cured with one hospitalization. Counseling is necessary to continue after discharge.
Encourage the child to make and maintain contact with a support group after discharge.	A support group may strengthen her desire to comply with the treatment regimen.
Make clear the established consequences for noncompliance with the program.	Consequences for noncompliance are important to reinforce the need to follow the program. Consequences set out a disciplinary action that will occur if the child fails to follow the program.
Encourage child to make decisions about care.	When the child makes decisions about care and treatment and complies with those plans, appropriate decision-making skills are fostered.

NURSING DIAGNOSIS
Compromised Family Coping related to eating disorders, treatment regimen, and dangers associated with an eating disorder

GOAL: The family's understanding of illness and treatment goals will improve.

EXPECTED OUTCOMES
- The family attends counseling sessions.
- The family identifies behaviors that impact negatively on child behavior.

NURSING INTERVENTIONS	*RATIONALE*
Provide for family counseling as well as counseling for the child.	It is important for the family to understand the dynamics of the problem and to face their possible contributions to the disorder.
Teach family members about the behavior modification program the child is using. Provide guidance on how to carry out the program at home.	Eating disorders are not cured simply because the child is discharged. Counseling, a continuation of the treatment program, and adherence to the signed contact agreement are essential. For these reasons, the family must become involved.

Expected Outcome: The child verbally expresses positive attitudes, maintains peer relationships, and improves grooming.
- **Goal:** The child will pace activity to avoid fatigue.
  Expected Outcome: The child is involved in activity as prescribed in a contract; no excessive activity is detected.
- **Goal:** The child's bowel elimination will be normal.

Expected Outcome: The child experiences no episodes of diarrhea or constipation. The child will not attempt deceit to obtain laxatives.
- **Goal:** The child's skin will show no evidence of breakdown.
  Expected Outcome: The child's skin is intact with no signs of redness, irritation, or excessive pressure; skin turgor is good.
- **Goal:** The child will show signs of compliance.

Expected Outcome: The child agrees to, signs, and adheres to a contract agreement; keeps counseling appointments; joins a support group; and continues to gain or maintain weight as per contract agreement.

- **Goal:** The family will show evidence of improved coping.

   Expected Outcome: The family attends counseling sessions and identifies behaviors that aggravate the child's condition.

Test Yourself

- What characteristics are seen in the child with attention deficit hyperactivity disorder (ADHD)?

- How is ADHD treated?

- What symptoms are seen in the child with nonorganic failure to thrive?

- Explain the difference between anorexia nervosa and bulimia.

OBESITY

Obesity is a national problem in the United States, largely as a result of an overabundance of food and too little exercise. The thin figure, particularly for women, has become so idealized that being fat can handicap a person socially and professionally and severely damage self-esteem. **Obesity** generally is defined as an excessive accumulation of fat that increases body weight by 20% or more over ideal weight (see Appendix G). **Overweight**, although not necessarily signifying obesity, means that a person's weight is more than average for height and body build.

Obesity often begins in childhood and, if not treated successfully, leads to chronic obesity in adult life. The obese child often feels isolated from the peer group that is normally a source of support and friendship. Because of the obesity, the child often is embarrassed to participate in sports, thus eliminating one method of burning excess calories.

Many children use food as a means of satisfying emotional needs, which establishes a vicious cycle. Children's eating habits include skipping meals, especially breakfast, and indulging in late-night eating. This behavior compounds the problem because calories consumed before a person goes to bed are not used for energy but are stored as fat. Snacking while watching television also contributes to the overindulgence in caloric intake.

Some children experience **polyphagia** (compulsive overeating). They lack control of their food intake, cannot postpone their urge to eat, hide food for later secret consumption, eat when not hungry or to escape from worries, and expend a great deal of energy thinking about securing and eating food. However, not all compulsive eaters are overweight, and in some ways this disorder resembles anorexia nervosa.

Many factors, including genetic, social, cultural, metabolic, and psychological ones, contribute to the development of obesity. Children of obese parents are likely to share this problem, not only because of some inherited predisposition toward obesity but also because of family eating patterns and the emotional climate surrounding food. Certain cultures equate obesity with being loved and being prosperous. If these values carry over into a modern family, the child is torn between the standards of the peer group and those of the family.

Obesity is difficult to treat in any age group but especially difficult in adolescence. Much of teenage life centers on food: after-school snacks, the ice cream shop, late-night diners, the pizza parlor, and fast-food restaurants serving high-fat, high-calorie foods with little nutritional value. Diets that emphasize nutritionally sound meals and reduced caloric intake produce results too slowly for impatient teenagers. Thus, the many quick–weight-loss programs, diet pills, and diet books find a ready market among children.

Treatment must include a thorough exploration of the obese child's food attitudes. A team approach using the skills of a psychiatrist or psychologist, nutritionist, nurse, or other counselor is often useful in developing a complete treatment plan. Summer camps that center on weight reduction with nutritious, calorie-controlled food, exercise, and activity are successful for some children but are too costly for many families. In addition, many children may fall back into old habits after summer camp is over unless there is a continuing support system.

Caregivers who work with obese children should try to make them feel like worthwhile persons, stressing that obesity does not automatically make them unacceptable. Finding the support of a caring adult who will help the child gain control of this aspect of his or her life can help give the necessary incentive to lose weight (see Family Teaching Tips: Tips for Caregivers of Obese Children).

SCHOOL PHOBIA

School absenteeism is a national problem. Children are absent from school for a variety of reasons, one of which may be school phobia. Children who develop

FAMILY TEACHING TIPS

Tips for Caregivers of Obese Children

- Have child keep a food diary for a week. Include food eaten, time eaten, what child was doing, and how child felt before and after eating; identify what stimulates urge to eat.
- Study diary with child to look for eating triggers.
- Set a reasonable goal of no more than 1 or 2 lbs of weight loss a week or perhaps maintaining weight with no gain.
- Advise child to eat only at specific, regular mealtimes.
- Recommend that child eat only at dining or kitchen table (not in front of TV or on the run).
- Have child use small plates to make amount of food seem larger.
- Teach child to eat slowly: count and chew each bite (25 to 30 is a good goal).
- Suggest that the child try to leave a little on the plate when done.
- Have child survey home and get rid of tempting high-calorie foods.
- Stock up on low-calorie snacks: carrot sticks, celery sticks, and other raw vegetables.
- Help child get involved in an active project that occupies time and also helps burn calories: any active team sport; bicycling, walking, hiking, swimming, skating.
- Promote walking instead of riding whenever possible.
- Encourage the child to attend a support group or develop a buddy system for support.
- Weigh only once a week on the same scale at the same time of day in the same clothing.
- Make a chart to keep track of child weight.
- Help child to focus on a positive asset and make the most of it to help build self-concept.
- Encourage good grooming. A group could put on a "mini" fashion show, choosing with guidance clothes that help maximize best features, or simply using magazine illustrations if actual clothing is not available.
- Reward each small success with positive reinforcement.
- Enlist cooperation of all family members to support the child with encouragement and a positive atmosphere.

school phobia may be good students, with girls being affected more often than boys. Teachers and nurses can help detect school phobia by paying close attention to absence patterns.

Clinical Manifestations

School-phobic children may have a strong attachment to one parent; usually the mother, and they fear separation from that parent, perhaps because of anxiety about losing her or him while away from home. School phobia may be the child's unconscious reaction to a seemingly overwhelming problem at school. The parent can unwittingly reinforce school phobia by permitting the child to stay home. The symptoms—vomiting, diarrhea, abdominal or other pain, and even a low-grade fever—are genuine and are caused by anxiety that may approach panic. They disappear with relief of the immediate anxiety after the child has been given permission to stay home.

Treatment and Nursing Care

Treatment includes a complete medical examination to rule out any organic cause for the symptoms and school–family conferences to help the child return to school. Those working with these children must recognize that they really do want to go to school but for whatever reason cannot make themselves go; these children are not delinquents. The school nurse and teacher along with other professionals, such as a social worker, psychologist, or psychiatrist, all may contribute to resolving the problem. If the child fears a specific factor at school, such as an overly critical teacher, the child may need to be moved to another class or school.

CHILD ABUSE

Every family faces many types of stress at one time or another. In addition to substance abuse, events that create stress for a family include illness, job loss, economic crisis or poverty, relocation, birth, death, and trauma. How the family handles these stresses affects greatly the emotional, social, and physical health of each member of the family. A **dysfunctional family** is one that cannot resolve these stresses and work through them in a positive, socially acceptable manner. The atmosphere in such a family creates additional stress for all family members. Because of the lack of support within the family for individual members, these members respond negatively to real or perceived problems. This may set the stage for child abuse, runaway children, substance abuse, and other unhealthy coping behaviors. Single-parent families often face multiple pressures at the same time; this dynamic creates additional stress and adds to the risk of dysfunctional coping.

Although child abuse has occurred throughout history, the evolution of cultural practices in the United States during the last few decades of the 20th century has emphasized the rights of children. Thus, any sort of mistreatment and abuse of children is regarded as unacceptable. The term child abuse has come to mean any intentional act of physical, emotional, or sexual abuse, including acts of negligence, committed by a person responsible for the care of the child.

Each year, increasing numbers of child abuse cases are brought to the attention of authorities. Estimates of the number of children treated in emergency departments after an episode of abuse range from 500,000 to 1 million annually. However, the actual number of abused children may be much higher because many more cases may go undetected.

Child abuse is not limited to one age group and can be detected at any age. The courts have even viewed fetal exposure to drugs and alcohol as child abuse. Surprisingly, adolescents have the greatest incidence of abuse. For children younger than 2 years of age, the rate is estimated at 6 per 1,000; the rate for children 15 to 17 years of age escalates to more than 14 per 1,000 (Wissow, 1999).

Child abuse has long-term as well as immediate effects. The abused child may be hyperactive; may exhibit angry, antisocial behavior; or may be especially withdrawn. Abusive parents often were abused themselves as children; thus, the problem of child abuse continues in a cyclical fashion from generation to generation. Abusive parents can be found at all socioeconomic levels, but families with greater financial means may be able to evade detection more easily. Low-income families show greater evidence of violence, neglect, and sexual abuse according to some studies. Commonly, abusive parents have inadequate parenting skills; therefore, they have unrealistic expectations of the child and do not respond appropriately to the child's behavior.

State laws require health care personnel to report suspected child abuse. This requirement overrides the concern for confidentiality. Laws have been enacted that protect the nurse who reports suspected child abuse from reprisal by a caregiver (e.g., being sued for slander), even if it is found that the child's situation is not a result of abuse. If the nurse does not report suspected child abuse, the penalty for the nurse can be loss of the nursing license.

This is critical to remember. Usually a health care facility can hold a child for 72 hours after suspected abuse has been reported so that a caseworker can investigate the charge.

After the time period a child suspected of being abused can be held by a health care facility, a hearing is held to determine if the charges are true and to decide where the child should be placed.

Physical Abuse

Physical abuse often occurs when the caregiver is unfamiliar with normal child behavior. Inexperienced caregivers do not know what is normal behavior for a child and become frustrated when the child does not respond in the way they expect. Some young women become pregnant to have a child to love, and they expect that love to be returned in full measure. When the child resists the caregiver's control or seems to do the opposite of what is expected, the caregiver takes it as a personal affront and becomes angry, possibly responding with physical punishment. Some cultures support physical punishment for children, citing the principle "spare the rod, spoil the child." Despite evidence that physical punishment often results in negative behavior and that other forms of punishment are more effective, corporal punishment continues to be approved occasionally, even in some schools. However, physical punishment that leaves marks, causes injury, or threatens the child's physical or emotional well-being is considered abusive.

An important role of the health care team is to identify abusive or potentially abusive situations as early as possible. When a child is brought to a physician or hospital because of physical injuries, family caregivers may attribute the injury to some action of the child's that is not in keeping with the child's age or level of development. The caregiver may also attribute the injury to an action of a sibling. When the child's symptoms do not match the injury the caregiver describes, be alert for possible abuse. However, do not accuse the caregiver before a complete investigation takes place.

Young, active children often have a number of bruises that occur from their usual activities. Most of these bruises occur over bony areas, such as the knees, elbows, shins, and forehead. Bruises that occur in areas of soft tissue, such as the abdomen, buttocks, genitalia, thighs, and mouth, may be suspect (Fig. 41-3). Bruises in the inner aspect of the upper arms may indicate that the child raised the arms to protect the face and head from blows.

● *Figure 41.3* Bruises on a child's body may be caused by physical abuse.

● ***Figure 41.4*** **(A)** Cigarette burn on child's foot. **(B)** Imprint from a radiator cover. **(C)** Rope burn from being tied to crib rail. **(D)** Imprint from a looped electrical cord.

Bruises may be distinctive in outline, clearly indicating the instrument that was used. Cigarettes, hangers, belt buckles, electrical cords, hand prints, teeth (from biting), and sticks leave identifiable marks (Fig. 41-4). The injuries may be in varying stages of healing, which indicate that not all the injuries occurred during one episode.

Signs or possible evidence of child abuse can be further evaluated by the use of technology. On a radiograph, bone fractures in various stages of healing may be noted. Spiral fractures of the long bones of a young child are not common, and their presence might indicate possible abuse. Children who have been harshly shaken may not show a clear picture of abuse, but computed tomography scanning may demonstrate cerebral edema or cerebral hemorrhage.

Burns are another common type of injury seen in the abused child (Fig. 41-5). Although burns may be accidental in young children, certain types of burns are highly suspicious. Cigarette burns, for example, are common abuse injuries. Burns from immersion of a hand in hot liquid, a hot register (as evidenced by the grid pattern), a steam iron, or a curling iron are not uncommon. Caregivers have been known to immerse the buttocks of a child in hot water if they thought the child was uncooperative in toilet training. Caregivers are often unaware of how quickly a child can be seriously burned. A burn that is neglected or not reported immediately must be considered suspicious until all the facts can be gathered and examined.

Shaken Baby Syndrome

Shaken baby syndrome occurs when a small child is shaken by the arms or shoulders in a repetitive, violent manner. When the child is shaken, a whiplash type injury occurs to the neck. In addition, the child may

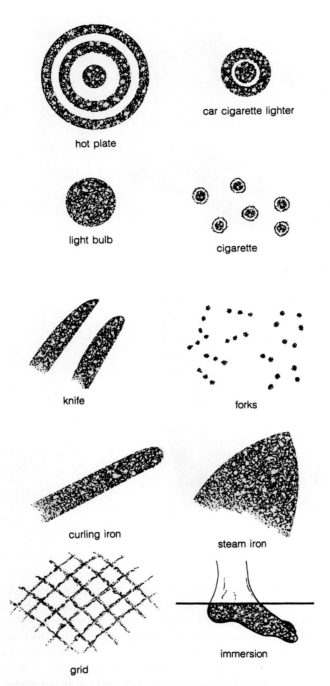

● **Figure 41.5** Burn patterns from objects used for inflicting burns in child abuse.

have edema to the brain stem and retinal or brain hemorrhages. Loss of vision, mental retardation, or even death may occur in these children. Clinical manifestations may include lethargy, irritability, vomiting, and seizures, but often this form of child abuse does not have easily noted signs and can be missed on examination of the child. Internal symptoms are detected by the use of computed tomography (CT) and magnetic resonance imaging (MRI) scans.

Munchausen Syndrome by Proxy

In Munchausen syndrome by proxy, one person either fabricates or induces illness in another to get attention. The child is frequently brought to a health care facility and symptoms of illness reported when the child is actually well. When injury to a child is involved, the mother is most often the person who has the syndrome. Often the mother injures the child to get the attention of medical personnel. She may slowly poison the child with prescription drugs, alcohol, or other drugs, or she may suffocate the child to cause apnea. Many times the symptoms, such as seizures or abdominal pain, are not easy to find on physical exam but are reported as history. The mother appears very attentive to the child and often is familiar with medical terminology. This situation is frustrating for health care personnel because it is difficult to catch the suspect in the act of endangering the child. Close observation of the caregiver's interactions with the child is necessary. For instance, if episodes of apnea occur only in the presence of the caregiver, be alert for this syndrome. The caregiver who suffers from this syndrome must receive psychiatric help.

Emotional Abuse and Neglect

Injury from emotional abuse can be just as serious and lasting as that from physical abuse, but it is much more difficult to identify. Several types of emotional abuse can occur, including

- Verbal abuse, such as humiliation, scapegoating, unrealistic expectations with belittling, and erratic discipline
- Emotional unavailability when caregivers are absorbed in their own problems
- Insufficient or poor nurturing, or threatening to leave the child or otherwise end the relationship
- Role reversal in which the child must take on the role of parenting the parent and is blamed for the parent's problems

Children may show evidence of emotional abuse by appearing worried or fearful or having vague complaints of illness or nightmares. Caregivers may display signs of inappropriate expectations of the child when in the health care facility by sometimes mocking or belittling the child for age-appropriate behavior. In young children, failure to thrive may be a sign of emotional abuse. In the older child, poor school performance and attendance, poor self-esteem, and poor peer relationships may be clues.

Child neglect is failure to provide adequate hygiene, health care, nutrition, love, nurturing, and supervision needed for growth and development. If a child is not given adequate care for a serious medical condition, the caregivers are considered neglectful. For example, if a child is seriously burned, even accidentally, and the caregivers do not take the child for evaluation and treatment until several days later, they may be judged to be neglectful. Often the child with failure to thrive as a result of being underfed, deprived of love, or constantly criticized can be classified as neglected; however, be careful not to make an unsubstantiated accusation of neglect.

Sexual Abuse

Sexual abuse of children has existed in all ages and cultures, but it seldom has been admitted when perpetrated by parents or other relatives in the home. **Incest** (sexually arousing physical contact between family members not married to each other) occurs in an estimated 240,000 to 1 million American families annually, and that number is growing each year. As with other types of child abuse, sexual abuse knows no socioeconomic, racial, religious, or ethnic boundaries. However, substance abuse, job loss, and poverty are contributing factors. Like other forms of child abuse, sexual abuse is being recognized and reported more often. The Federal Child Abuse Prevention and Treatment Act defines **sexual abuse** as "the employment, use, persuasion, inducement, enticement, or coercion of any child to engage in, or assist any other person to engage in, any sexually explicit conduct" (retrieved October 18, 2003, from http://nccanch.acf.hhs.gov/pubs/factsheet/childmal.cfm). When a person has power or control over a child, that person, even if a child, can be a sexual abuser.

Several terms are commonly used when sexual abuse is discussed. From a legal viewpoint, sexual contact between a child and another person in a caregiving position, such as a parent, babysitter, or teacher, is classified as sexual abuse. A sexual contact made by someone who is not functioning in a caregiver role is classified as **sexual assault**. Incest includes fondling of breasts or genitalia, intercourse (vaginal or anal), oral–genital contact, exhibitionism, and voyeurism.

Did you know? Someone who is the same age but bigger or stronger could sexually abuse a child his or her own age.

Regardless of the relationship of the perpetrator to the child, the outcome of the abuse is devastating. Episodes of sexual abuse that involve a person whom the child trusts seem to be the most damaging. Incest often goes unreported because the person committing the act uses intimidation by means of threats, appeals to the child's desire to be loved and to please, and convinces the child of the importance of keeping the act secret.

When a child is sexually assaulted by a stranger, the caregivers usually become aware of the incident, promptly report it, and take the child for a physical examination. However, in the case of incest, the child rarely tells another person what is happening. The child may exhibit physical complaints, such as various aches and pains, gastrointestinal upsets, changes in bowel and bladder habits (including enuresis), nightmares, and acts of aggression or hostility. Some of these complaints or behaviors may be the presenting problem when a health care provider sees the child.

Test Yourself

- What are the different types of child abuse often seen?
- What differentiates punishment for inappropriate behavior from child abuse?
- Who is the person who usually has the disease in Munchausen syndrome by proxy?

● Nursing Process for the Child Who Is Abused

ASSESSMENT

When assessing a child who may have been abused or neglected, the health care provider must be thorough and complete in observation and documentation. The child should have a complete physical exam; all bruises, blemishes, lacerations, areas of redness and irritation, and marks of any kind on the child's body must be carefully described and accurately documented. It may be necessary to request that photographs be taken.

Observe the interaction between the child and the caregiver, and carefully document your observations using nonjudgmental terms. The child's body language may be revealing, so be alert for significant information. For example, if the child shrinks away from contact by the caregiver or health care practitioner or, on the other hand, is especially clinging to the caregiver, watch for other signs of inappropriate behavior. These assessments vary with the child's age (Table 41-2).

Perhaps the most difficult part may be to maintain a nonjudgmental attitude throughout the interview and examination. Be calm and

TABLE 41.2   Signs of Abuse in Children

Physical Signs	Behavioral Signs
Physical Abuse Bruises and welts: may be on multiple body surfaces or soft tissue; may form regular pattern (e.g., belt buckle) Burns: cigar or cigarette, immersion (stocking/glovelike on extremities or doughnut-shaped on buttocks or genitals), or patterned as an electrical appliance (e.g., iron) Fractures: single or multiple; may be in various stages of healing Lacerations or abrasions: rope burns; tears in and around mouth, eyes, ears, genitalia Abdominal injuries: ruptured or injured internal organs Central nervous system injuries: subdural hematoma, retinal or subarachnoid hemorrhage	Less compliant than average Signs of negativism, unhappiness Anger, isolation Destructive Abusive toward others Difficulty developing relationships Either excessive or absent separation anxiety Inappropriate caregiving concern for parent Constantly in search of attention, favors, food, etc. Various developmental delays (cognitive, language, motor)
Physical Neglect Malnutrition Repeated episodes of pica Constant fatigue of listlessness Poor hygiene Inadequate clothing for circumstances Inadequate medical or dental care	Lack of appropriate adult supervision Repeated ingestions of harmful substances Poor school attendance Exploitation (forced to beg or steal; excessive household work) Role reversal with parent Drug or alcohol use
Sexual Abuse Difficulty walking or sitting Thickening or hyperpigmentation of labial skin Vaginal opening measures >4 mm horizontally in preadolescence Torn, stained, or bloody underclothing Bruises or bleeding of genitalia or perianal area Lax rectal tone Vaginal discharge Recurrent urinary tract infections Nonspecific vaginitis Venereal disease Sperm or acid phosphatase on body or clothes Pregnancy	Direct or indirect disclosure to relative, friend, or teacher Withdrawal with excessive dependency Poor peer relationships Poor self-esteem Frightened or phobic of adults Sudden decline in academic performance Pseudomature personality development Suicide attempts Regressive behavior Enuresis or encopresis Excessive masturbation Highly sexualized play Sexual promiscuity
Emotional Abuse Delays in physical development Failure to thrive	Distinct emotional symptoms or functional limitations Deteriorating conduct Increased anxiety Apathy or depression Developmental lags

reassuring with the child; let the child lead the way when possible.

SELECTED NURSING DIAGNOSES

- Anxiety, Fear by child related to history of abuse and fear of abuse from others
- Ineffective Coping by the nonabusive parent related to fear of violence from abusive partner or feelings of powerlessness
- Impaired Parenting related to situational stressors or poor coping skills

- Disabled Family Coping related to unrealistic expectations of the child by the parent

OUTCOME IDENTIFICATION AND PLANNING

Major goals for the abused child include caring for any injuries the child has sustained, as well as relieving anxiety and fear. An important family goal is to improve parenting and coping skills of the caregiver or family.

IMPLEMENTATION

Relieving the Child's Anxiety and Fear

Observe the child for behavior that indicates anxiety or fear, such as withdrawal, ducking or shying away from the nurse or caregivers, and avoiding eye contact. Assign one nurse to care for the child so that the child can relate to one person consistently. Provide physical contact, such as hugging, rocking, and caressing, only if the child accepts it. Identify nursing actions that seem to comfort the child and use them consistently. Use a calm, reassuring, and kind manner, and provide a safe atmosphere in which the child has an opportunity to express feelings and fears. Use play to help the child express some of these emotions. Be careful not to do anything that might alarm or upset the child. Psychological support is provided through social services or an abuse team.

Supporting the Nonabusive Caregiver

In some cases, one caregiver in the family may be an abuser while the other is not. The nonabusive caregiver is a victim, as is the child. Give the nonabusive caregiver an opportunity to express fears and anxieties. He or she may feel powerless in the situation. Help the passive caregiver decide whether to continue the relationship or leave it. Try to preserve the caregiver's self-esteem because this is not an easy decision to make. Remember that confidentiality is essential when discussing such problems.

Observing Interaction Between the Caregiver and Child

While caring for the abused child when the caregiver is present, take the opportunity to observe how the caregiver relates to the child and how the child reacts to the caregiver. Give the caregiver the same courtesy extended to all caregivers. Offer a compliment when the caregiver does something well in caring for the child. Give the caregiver an opportunity to discuss in private any concerns; during this time, you may be able to gain his or her confidence.

Promoting Parenting Skills and Coping

Often abuse occurs when a caregiver is unfamiliar with normal growth and development and the behaviors common to a particular stage of development. Help the caregiver develop realistic expectations of the child. To help accomplish this goal, design a teaching plan and include the caregiver in caring for the child. Teach the caregiver the child's expected responses and help him or her learn about normal development. Praise the caregiver for displaying positive behaviors. Point out specific behaviors of the child and explain them to the caregiver. Explore the reasons for the caregiver's absence when he or she does not visit regularly. Discuss specific behaviors of the child that are upsetting to the caregiver and explain that these are common for the child's age.

The caregiver may be facing temporary or permanent placement of the child in another home. Help the caregiver and the child accept this change. Emotions that a caregiver has had for a long period cannot be easily eliminated. The assistance of social services and a child life specialist is beneficial in these situations. Act as a member of the team to aid in the transition. The foster parents may need support from the nursing staff to help ease the child's transition to the new home. Abused children must be followed up carefully after discharge from the health care facility to ensure that their well-being is protected.

EVALUATION: GOALS AND EXPECTED OUTCOMES

- **Goal:** The child will exhibit decreased signs of anxiety and fear.
  Expected Outcome: The child's play, facial expressions, and posture are relaxed; the child displays no withdrawal or guarding during contacts with the nursing staff.
- **Goal:** The nonabusive caregiver will begin to cope with fears and feelings of powerlessness.
  Expected Outcome: The nonabusive caregiver expresses fears and concerns and makes plans to resolve problems.
- **Goal:** The caregiver will exhibit positive interaction with the child.
  Expected Outcome: The caregiver talks with the child, is sensitive to his or her needs, and refrains from making unreasonable demands on the child.
- **Goal:** The caregiver will be involved in the child's care and will verbalize examples of normal growth and development and ways to handle the child's misbehavior.
  Expected Outcome: The caregiver states age-appropriate behavior for the child, discusses ways to handle the child's irritating behavior, and is involved in counseling or other discharge plans.

KEY POINTS

♦ The characteristics of autism include a lack of development of a smiling response to others or an interest in being touched or cuddled, blank expressions, and lack of response to verbal stimulation.

These children do not show the normal fear of separation from parents.

- Four goals in the treatment of autism include promotion of normal development, language development, social interaction, and learning.
- Children who are considering suicide often have previous suicide attempts, withdraw from or change participation in activities, have physical complaints and a preoccupation with dying, change moods, say goodbye, or give away personal items.
- Substances often abused by children include alcohol, tobacco, marijuana, cocaine, morphine, heroin, hallucinogens, depressants, amphetamines, analgesics, anabolic steroids, hallucinogens, and Ecstasy.
- The use of substances can lead to addiction or dependence, which may be psychological, physical, or both. Tobacco or smokeless tobacco damages the lungs and can cause mouth, lip, and throat cancers. Marijuana affects judgment, sense of time, and motivation. The physical results of using cocaine are an increase in pulse, respirations, blood pressure, and temperature. Narcotics are highly addictive and extremely expensive, which can result in teenage prostitution, pushing (selling) drugs, and robbery as a means to support the drug habit. Hallucinogens (psychedelic drugs), although not addictive in a physical sense, can create a psychological dependence, as well as the effects of intoxication, "bad trips," and flashbacks, and often are associated with overdoses. Withdrawal from barbiturates must be carefully controlled to prevent delirium, seizures, or death.
- The addicted parent is not dependable and cannot provide stability for the child. The parent may waver between overindulgence and the opposite— unreasonable and unpredictable behavior toward the child.
- Behaviors seen in children who have an addiction problem in the family include avoidance of interaction with classmates, failing in school, unexcused absences or truancy, frequent minor physical complaints, stealing or committing acts of violence, aggressive behavior, and abuse of drugs or alcohol.
- Characteristics seen in the child with attention deficit hyperactivity disorder (ADHD) include impulsive behavior, ease in being distracted, fidgeting or squirming, difficulty sitting still, problems following through on instructions despite being able to understand them, inattentiveness when spoken to, losing of things, going from one uncompleted activity to another, difficulty taking turns, and talking excessively. The child often engages in dangerous activities without considering the consequences.
- Children with NFTT are often listless and below average in weight and height; have poor muscle tone

and a loss of subcutaneous fat; and are immobile for long periods of time. They may be unresponsive or try to avoid cuddling and vocalization. A common characteristic is rumination (voluntary regurgitation), perhaps as a means of self-satisfaction.
- Two goals of treatment for the hospitalized anorexic are correction of malnutrition and identification and treatment of the psychological cause.
- The child with bulimia may have dental caries and erosion from frequent exposure to stomach acid. She or he may also have throat irritation, endocrine and electrolyte imbalances, cardiac irregularities, and menstrual problems. Calluses or abrasions may be noted on the back of the hand from frequent contact with the teeth while inducing vomiting. Possible complications are esophageal tears, acute gastric dilation, and hypokalemia.
- Professionals who work with obese children should try to make them feel like worthwhile persons, stressing that obesity does not automatically make them unacceptable. Finding the support of a caring adult who will help the child gain control of this aspect of his or her life can help give the necessary incentive to lose weight.
- The symptoms seen in the child with school phobia are caused by anxiety that may approach panic.
- Poor parenting skills may lead to child abuse because the parent has unrealistic expectations of the child, thereby responding inappropriately to the child's behavior.
- Physical punishment can be classified as abusive if it leaves marks, causes injury, or threatens the child's physical or emotional well-being.
- Bruises that occur accidentally to a child occur over bony areas such as the knees, elbows, shin, and forehead. Those that have been inflicted in an abusive manner are found in soft tissue, such as the abdomen, buttocks, genitalia, thighs, and mouth.
- Munchausen syndrome by proxy occurs when one person, commonly the mother, either fabricates or induces illness in another to get attention.
- A child may be emotionally abused verbally, or by emotional unavailability of the caregiver, poor nurturing, threats involving leaving the child, or role reversal in which the child must take on the role of parenting or is blamed for the parent's problems.

REFERENCES AND SELECTED READINGS

Books and Journals

Adger, H. (1999). Adolescent drug abuse. In J. A. McMillan, C. D. DeAngelis, R. D. Feigin, & J. W. Warshaw (Eds.), *Oski's pediatrics: Principles and practice* (3rd ed.). Philadelphia: Lippincott Williams & Wilkins.

Nonorganic failure to thrive

American Psychiatric Association (APA). (2000). *Diagnostic and statistical manual of mental disorders, text revision* (4th ed.). Washington, DC: Author.

Andrist, L. C. (2003). Media images, body dissatisfaction, and disordered eating in adolescent women. *The American Journal of Maternal Child Nursing, 28*(2), 119–123.

Broadwater, H. (2002). Reshaping the future for overweight kids. *RN, 65*(11), 36–42.

Guevara, J., Lozano, P., Wickizer, T., Mell, L., & Gephart, H. (2001). Utilization and cost of health care services for children with attention-deficit/hyperactivity disorder. *Pediatrics, 108*(1), 71–78.

Hall, J. M. (2000). Core issues for female child abuse survivors in recovery from substance misuse. *Qualitative Health Research, 10*(5), 612–631.

Hess, D., & DeBoer, S. (2002). Emergency: Ecstasy. *American Journal of Nursing, 102*(4), 45.

Hockenberry, M. J., Wilson, D., Winkelstein, M. L., & Kline, N. E. (2003). *Wong's nursing care of infants and children* (7th ed.). St. Louis: Mosby.

Karch, A. M. (2003). 2004 *Lippincott's nursing drug guide.* Philadelphia: Lippincott Williams & Wilkins.

Kirkland, R. T. (1999). Failure to thrive. In *Oski's pediatrics: Principles and practice* (3rd ed.). Philadelphia: Lippincott Williams & Wilkins.

Meaux, J. B. (2000). Stop, look, listen: The challenge for children with ADHD. *Issues in Comprehensive Pediatric Nursing, 23*(1), 1–13.

National Institute of Drug Abuse/National Institutes of Health (NIDA/NIH). (2002). *Anabolic steroids: A threat to mind and body.* National Institute of Drug Abuse research report, National Institutes of Health, retrieved from http://www.thebody.com/nih/steroids

North American Nursing Diagnosis Association (NANDA). (2001). *NANDA nursing diagnoses: Definitions and classification 2001–2002.* Philadelphia: Author.

Pillitteri, A. (2003). *Maternal and child health* nursing (4th ed.). Philadelphia: Lippincott Williams & Wilkins.

Rew, L., Taylor-Seehafer, M., & Fitzgerald, M. L. (2001). Sexual abuse, alcohol and other drug use, and suicidal behaviors in homeless adolescents. *Issues in Comprehensive Pediatric Nursing, 24*(4), 225–240.

Smeltzer, S. C., & Bare, B. G. (2003). *Textbook of medical–surgical nursing* (10th ed.). Philadelphia: Lippincott Williams & Wilkins.

Sparks, S., & Taylor, C. (2001). *Nursing diagnosis reference manual* (5th ed.). Springhouse, PA: Springhouse Corporation.

Wissow, L. (1999). Child maltreatment. In J. A. McMillan, C. D. DeAngelis, R. D. Feigin, & J. W. Warshaw (Eds.), *Oski's pediatrics: Principles and practice* (3rd ed.). Philadelphia: Lippincott Williams & Wilkins.

Wong, D. L., Perry, S., & Hockenberry, M. (2002). *Maternal–child nursing care* (2nd ed.). St. Louis: Mosby.

Websites
Tobacco
www.tobaccofreekids.org

Alcohol
www.ncadd.org

Suicide
www.suicidology.org

Substance Abuse
www.clubdrugs.org

WORKBOOK

NCLEX-STYLE REVIEW QUESTIONS

1. A nurse admits an adolescent girl with a diagnosis of possible anorexia nervosa. Of the following characteristics, which would *most* likely be seen in the adolescent with anorexia? The adolescent

   a. gets low grades in school.

   b. has a sedentary lifestyle.

   c. freely express emotions.

   d. follows a strict routine.

2. The nurse is assisting with a physical exam on an adolescent with bulimia. Of the following signs and symptoms, which would *most* likely be seen in the adolescent with bulimia?

   a. Dry skin

   b. Dental caries

   c. Low body weight

   d. Amenorrhea

3. In planning care for an adolescent with an eating disorder, which of the following goals would be *most* important for the adolescent? The adolescent will

   a. verbally express positive attitudes and feelings.

   b. plan and participate in age-appropriate activities.

   c. maintain a fluid and electrolyte balance.

   d. have normal bowel and bladder patterns.

4. The nurse is discussing teenage depression and suicide with a group of caregivers of adolescent-age children. If the caregivers make the following statements, which statement would require further data collection?

   a. "My child has so many ideas about how she can fix all the problems in the world."

   b. "She told me she is happy that she broke up with her long-time boyfriend."

   c. "My son enjoys spending all his time playing his CD player alone in his room."

   d. "My child eats all the time but never seems to want to go to sleep."

5. The nurse is caring for an infant with failure to thrive. The infant took in 2 ounces of formula every 2 hours during the 12-hour shift, with the first 2 ounces being at 0700 and the last feeding at 1900. She vomited three times: 20 cc the first time, 36 cc the second, and 28 cc the third. The infant had four wet diapers during the shift. After subtracting the dry weight of the diapers, the diapers weighed 20 grams, 18 grams, 25 grams, and 22 grams. She had one medium size stool during the shift. What was the infant's total intake and output during the 12-hour shift?

STUDY ACTIVITIES

1. A co-worker says to you, "That Jeff in room 204 is bouncing off the walls." You are assigned to this child, who has a diagnosis of attention deficit hyperactivity disorder (ADHD). Make a list of behavior techniques to use with the child who has ADHD. Develop a plan of care you could use to care for Jeff.

2. Go to the following Internet site: http://www.add.org
   Under the Information section, click on "Kids Area."

   a. List seven areas available on this site that you could share with a child who has ADD.
   Click on "School and me with ADD."

   b. What suggestions could you offer to a child who has ADD to help him/her be more successful in school?

   Click on the back arrow. Click on "Medicine, Me, and ADD."

   c. Share this story with a school-age child with ADD. What was this child's reaction?

3. Go to the following Internet site: http://www.dancesafe.org/parents
   Click on the section "Communicating with Your Teenagers About Drugs." Read down to and including the section "Communication Approaches."

   a. What are four important communication methods suggested for parents to use in communicating with their teens?

b. List seven barriers that parents should be aware of when communicating with their teenage children.

CRITICAL THINKING: What Would You Do?

1. Tanya, 16 years old, is 65 inches (165 cm) tall and weighs 98 lb (44.5 kg). She moans about how fat her thighs are. You believe she is anorexic. A diagnosis of anorexia is confirmed and she is hospitalized.

   a. What symptoms will you observe for in addition to her weight loss?

   b. What are the characteristics often seen in the anorexic child's personality?

   c. What will be included in Tanya's nursing care plan?

2. Your best friend shares with you that she thinks her teenage son might have a problem with alcohol and drugs. She tells you that her son has behaviors that make her think he is drinking every day and using drugs every weekend.

   a. Why do you think alcohol is the most commonly abused drug among adolescents?

   b. What factors do you think put adolescents at greatest risk of becoming substance abusers?

   c. What do you think could be helpful in reducing each of the above risk factors?

3. Dosage calculation: A child with a diagnosis of attention deficit hyperactivity disorder (ADHD) is being treated with methylphenidate (Ritalin). The child weighs 75 pounds. The usual dosage of this medication is 0.3 mg/kg/dose to 2.0 mg/kg/day, not to exceed 60 mg/day. The medication is given two times a day (BID). Answer the following:

   a. How many kilograms (kg) does the child weigh?

   b. How many milligrams (mg) would be given for the low dose?

   c. How many milligrams (mg) would be given for the high dose?

   d. Would the high dose of the medication be an appropriate dose for this child? Explain your answer.

Glossary

abruptio placentae, or placental abruption the premature separation of a normally implanted placenta.

absence seizure seizure in which there is a sudden, brief loss of awareness, then a return to an alert state.

abstinence (as related to birth control); refraining from vaginal sexual intercourse.

abuse misuse, excessive use, rough or bad treatment; used to refer to misuse of alcohol or drugs (substance abuse) and mistreatment of children or family members (child abuse, domestic abuse).

accelerations spontaneous elevations of the fetal heart rate (FHR).

achylia absence of pancreatic enzymes in gastric secretions.

acid–base balance state of equilibrium between the acidity and the alkalinity of body fluids.

acidosis excessive acidity of body fluids.

acrocyanosis cyanosis of the hands and feet seen periodically in the newborn.

actual nursing diagnoses diagnoses that identify existing health problems.

adenoids mass of lymphoid tissue in the nasal pharynx; extends from the roof of the nasal pharynx to the free edge of the soft palate.

adenopathy enlarged lymph glands.

akinetic seizure that causes a sudden, momentary loss of consciousness and muscle tone; also called atonic.

alcohol abuse drinking sufficient alcoholic beverages to induce intoxication.

alcoholism chronic alcohol abuse.

alkalosis excessive alkalinity of body fluids.

allergen antigen that causes an allergic reaction.

allograft skin graft taken from a genetically different person for temporary coverage during burn healing. Skin from a cadaver sometimes is used.

alopecia loss of hair.

amblyopia dimness of vision from disuse of the eye; sometimes called "lazy eye."

amenorrhea absence of menstruation.

amniocentesis a diagnostic procedure whereby a needle is inserted into the amniotic sac and a small amount of fluid is withdrawn and used for biochemical, chromosomal, and genetic studies.

amnioinfusion infusion of normal saline into the uterus.

amnion a thick fibrous lining, made up of several layers, that helps to protect the fetus and forms the inner part of the sac in which the fetus grows.

amniotic fluid the specialized fluid that fills the amniotic cavity and serves to protect the fetus.

amniotomy artificial rupture of membranes (AROM).

analgesia the use of medication to reduce the sensation of pain.

android pelvis the typical male pelvis; in the woman, the heart shape of the android pelvis is not favorable to a vaginal delivery.

anesthesia the use of medication to partially or totally block all sensation to an area of the body.

ankylosis immobility of a joint.

anorexia nervosa eating disorder characterized by loss of appetite due to emotional causes, e.g., usually excessive fear of becoming (or being) fat.

anthelmintic medication that expels intestinal worms; vermifuge.

anthropoid pelvis woman's pelvis that is elongated in its dimensions and is sometimes referred to as apelike.

anticipatory grief preparatory grieving that often helps caregivers mourn the loss of their child when death actually comes.

antigen protein substance found on the surface of red blood cells capable of inducing a specific immune response and reacting with the products of that response.

antigen-antibody response response of the body to an antigen causing the formation of antibodies that protect the body from an invading antigen.

anuria absence of urine.

apnea temporary interruption of the breathing impulse.

appropriate for gestational age (AGA) a newborn whose weight, length, and/or head circumference falls between the 10th and 90th percentiles for gestational age

archetypes predetermined patterns of human development, which according to Carl Jung, replace instinctive behavior of other animals; prototype.

areola darkened area around the nipple.

arthralgia painful joints.

artificial nutrition infant formula.

ascites edema in the peritoneal cavity.

asphyxia suffocation caused by interference with the oxygen supply of the blood.

aspiration breathing fluid into the lungs.

associative play being engaged in a common activity without any sense of belonging or fixed rules.

astigmatism error in light refraction on the retina caused by unequal curvature in the eye's cornea; light rays bend in different directions to produce a blurred image.

ataxia lack of coordination caused by disturbances in the kinesthetic and balance senses.

atonic seizure that causes a sudden, momentary loss of consciousness and muscle tone; also called akinetic.

atresia absence of a normal body opening or the abnormal closure of a body passage.

attachment the enduring emotional bond that develops between the parent and infant.

aura a sensation that signals an impending epileptic attack; may be visual, aromatic, or other sensation.

autistic totally self-centered and unable to relate to others, often exhibiting bizarre behaviors. Autistic children can sometimes be destructive to themselves and others.

autograft skin taken from an individual's own body. Except for the skin of an identical twin, autograft is the only kind of skin accepted permanently by recipient tissues.

autonomy ability to function in an independent manner.

autosomal dominant trait trait or condition appearing in a heterozygous person resulting from a dominant gene within a pair.

autosomal recessive trait trait or condition that is not expressed unless both parents carry the gene for that trait.

autosomes 22 pairs of chromosomes that are alike in the male and female. The sex chromosomes are not autosomes.

azotemia nitrogen-containing compounds in the blood.

Babinski reflex the flaring open of the infant's toes when the lateral plantar surface is stroked. Also called the plantar reflex, this reaction usually disappears by the end of the first year.

ballottement a probable sign of pregnancy that occurs when the examiner pushes up on the uterine wall during a pelvic examination, then feels the fetus bounce back against the examiner's fingers.

bilateral pertaining to both sides; e.g., bilateral cleft lip involves both sides of the lip.

binocular vision normal vision maintained through the muscular coordination of eye movements of both eyes. A single vision results.

biophysical profile (BPP) a method that uses a combination of factors to determine fetal well-being.

Bishop score one commonly used scoring method to determine cervical readiness that evaluates five factors: cervical consistency, position, dilation, effacement, and fetal station.

blastocyst the structure that forms about 5 days after fertilization when the dividing cell mass develops a hollow, fluid-filled core.

blended family both partners in a marriage bring children from a previous marriage into the household: his, hers, and theirs.

body surface area (BSA) formula used to calculate dosages. Using a West nomogram, the child's weight is marked on the right scale and the height is marked on the left scale. A straightedge is used to draw a line between the two marks. The point at which the line crosses the column labeled SA (surface area) is the BSA expressed in square meters (m^2).

boggy uterus a uterus that feels soft and spongy, rather than firm and well contracted.

bonding development of a close emotional tie between the newborn and the parent or parents.

bottle mouth (nursing bottle) caries condition caused by the erosion of enamel on the infant's deciduous teeth from sugar in formula or sweetened juice that coats the teeth for long periods. This condition also can occur in infants who sleep with their mothers and nurse intermittently throughout the night.

brachycephaly shortness of the head.

bradycardia decreased pulse rate

Braxton Hicks contractions the painless, intermittent, "practice" contractions of pregnancy.

breakthrough pain pain that occurs when the basal dose of analgesia does not control the pain adequately.

bronchodilators medications used for quick relief of acute exacerbations of asthma symptoms.

brown fat a specialized form of heat-producing tissue found only in fetuses and newborns.

bulimia eating disorder characterized by episodes of binge eating, followed by purging by self-induced vomiting or use of laxatives.

capitation a method that managed care plans use to reduce costs by paying a fixed amount per person to the health care provider to provide services for enrollees.

caput succedaneum edematous swelling of the soft tissues of the scalp caused by prolonged pressure of the occiput against the cervix during labor and delivery. The edema disappears within a few days.

cardinal movements the turns and movements made during the journey of the fetus; referred to as the mechanisms of delivery.

carditis inflammation of the heart.

case management a systematic process to ensure that a client's health and service needs are met.

cataract development of opacity in the crystalline lens that prevents light rays from entering the eye.

cavernous hemangiomas congenital malformations that are subcutaneous collections of blood vessels with bluish overlying skin. Although these lesions are benign tumors, they may become so extensive as to interfere with the functions of the body part on which they appear.

celiac syndrome term used to designate the complex of malabsorptive disorders.

cephalhematoma collection of blood between the periosteum and the skull caused by excessive pressure on the head during birth.

cephalocaudal the pattern of growth of the child that follows an orderly pattern, starting with the head and moving downward.

cerclage procedure that involves placing a purse string type suture in the cervix to keep it from dilating.

cesarean birth the delivery of a fetus through abdominal and uterine incisions: laparotomy and hysterotomy, respectively. Cesarean comes from the Latin word "caedere," meaning "to cut."

Chadwick's sign the bluish-purplish color of the cervix, vagina, and perineum during pregnancy.

chancre hard, red, painless primary lesion of syphilis at the point of entry of the spirochete.

chelating agent agent that binds with metal.

child advocacy speaking or acting on behalf of a child to ensure that her or his needs are recognized.

child neglect failing to provide adequate hygiene, health care, nutrition, love, nurturing, and supervision as needed for a child's growth and development.

child-life program program to make hospitalization less threatening for children and their parents. These programs are usually under the direction of a child-life specialist whose background is in psychology and early childhood development.

chloasma or mask of pregnancy; brown blotchy areas on the forehead, cheeks, and nose of the pregnant woman.

chordee chordlike anomaly that extends from the scrotum to the penis; pulls the penis downward in an arc.

chorea continuous, rapid, jerky involuntary movements.

chorioamnionitis bacterial or viral infection of the amniotic fluid and membranes.

choriocarcinoma malignancy of the uterine lining.

chorion a second layer of thick fibrous tissue that surrounds the amnion.

chorionic villi finger-like projections that extend out from the chorion giving it a rough appearance.

chorionic villus sampling (CVS) a newer procedure that can provide chromosomal studies of fetal cells similar to that of amniocentesis.

chromosomes thread-like structures that occur in pairs and carry genetic information.

chronic illness condition that interferes with daily functioning, progresses slowly, and shows little change over a long duration of time.

circumcision surgical removal of all or part of the foreskin (prepuce) of the penis.

circumoral pallor a white area around the mouth.

classification ability to group objects by rank, grade, or class.

cleavage the process of mitotic division performed by the zygote.

client advocacy speaking or acting on behalf of others to help them gain greater independence and to make the health care delivery system more responsive and relevant to their needs.

climacteric the interlude surrounding menopause in which changes in reproductive functioning take place.

clonus rapid involuntary muscle contraction and relaxation.

clove hitch restraints restraints used to secure an arm or leg; used most often when a child is receiving an intravenous infusion. The restraint is made of soft cloth formed in a figure eight.

co-dependent parent parent who supports, directly or indirectly, the other parent's addictive behavior.

cognitive development progressive change in the intellectual process, including perception, memory, and judgment.

cohabitation family a living situation in which a man and woman live together but are not legally married.

coitus interruptus or withdrawal; requires the man to pull the penis out of the vagina before ejaculation to avoid depositing sperm in or near the vagina.

cold stress a body temperature of less than 97.6°F (36.5°C) in the newborn.

colic recurrent paroxysmal bouts of abdominal pain that are fairly common among young infants and that usually disappear around the age of 3 months.

colostomy a surgical procedure in which a part of the colon is brought through the abdominal wall to create an outlet for elimination of fecal material.

colostrum thin, yellowish, milky fluid secreted by the woman's breasts during pregnancy or just after delivery (before the secretion of milk).

comedones collection of keratin and sebum in the hair follicle; blackhead; whitehead.

communal family alternative family in which members share responsibility for homemaking and child rearing. All children are the collective responsibility of adult members.

community-based nursing a type of nursing practice focused on wellness and a holistic approach to caring for the child in a community setting.

compartment syndrome a serious neurovascular concern that occurs when increasing pressure within the muscle compartment causes decreased circulation.

congenital hip dysplasia abnormal fetal development of the acetabulum that may or may not cause dislocation of the hip. If the malformed acetabulum permits dislocation, the head of the femur displaces upward and backward. This may be difficult to recognize in early infancy.

congestive heart failure (CHF) result of impaired pumping capability of the heart. It may appear in the 1st year of life in infants with conditions such as large ventricular septal defects, coarctation of the aorta, and other defects that place an increased workload on the ventricles.

conjunctivitis acute inflammation of the conjunctiva that may be caused by a virus, bacteria, allergy, or foreign body.

conservation ability to recognize that change in shape does not necessarily mean change in amount or mass.

contracture fibrous scarring that forms over a burned movable body part. This part of the healing process can cause serious deformities and limit movement.

cooperative play children play with each other, as in team sports.

cordocentesis or **percutaneous umbilical blood sampling (PUBS)**, a procedure similar to amniocentesis whereby fetal blood is withdrawn from the umbilical cord.

corpus luteum a yellow body that forms after ovulation from the remnants of the follicle.

coryza runny nose.

couplet care postpartum care in which the mother and newborn remain together and receive care from one nurse.

couvade syndrome phenomenon in which some fathers actually experience some of the physical symptoms of pregnancy, such as nausea and vomiting, along with their partner.

cradle cap accumulation of oil and dirt that often forms on an infant's scalp; seborrheic dermatitis.

craniotabes softening of the occipital bones caused by a reduction of mineralization of the skull.

cretinism a congenital condition marked by stunted growth and mental retardation.

critical pathways standard plans of care used to organize and monitor the care provided.

croup general term that typically includes symptoms of a barking cough, hoarseness, and inspiratory stridor.

cultural competency the capacity of the nurse to work with people by integrating their cultural needs into their nursing care.

currant jelly stools stools that consist of blood and mucus.

cyanotic heart disease congenital heart disease that causes right-to-left shunting of blood in the heart; results in a depletion of oxygen to such an extent that the oxygen saturation of the peripheral arterial blood is 85% or less. Defects that permit right-to-left shunting may occur at the atrial, ventricular, or aortic level.

cystitis infection of the bladder.

dawdling wasting time; whiling away time; being idle.

débridement removal of necrotic tissue.

decentration ability to see several aspects of a problem at the same time and understand the relationships of various parts to the whole situation.

decidua the endometrium that has changed to support a pregnancy.

deciduous teeth primary teeth that usually erupt between 6 and 8 months of age.

deliriants inhalants that contain chemicals whose fumes can produce confusion, disorientation, excitement, and hallucinations.

denial defense mechanism in which the existence of unpleasant actions or ideas is unconsciously repressed; in the grieving process, one of the stages many people go through; also a type of response by caregivers when caring for chronically ill children in which the caregivers deny the condition's existence and encourage the child to overcompensate for any disabilities.

dependence compulsive need to use a substance for its satisfying or pleasurable effects.

dependent nursing actions nursing actions that the nurse performs as a result of a physician's orders, such as administering analgesics for pain.

dermatome an area on the body surface supplied by a particular sensory nerve.

development progressive change in the child's maturation.

developmental tasks basic achievements associated with each stage of development. Basic tasks must be mastered to move on to the next developmental stage. To achieve maturity, a person must successfully complete developmental tasks at each stage.

diabetic ketoacidosis characterized by drowsiness, dry skin, flushed cheeks, cherry-red lips, and acetone breath with a fruity smell as a result of excessive ketones in the blood in uncontrolled diabetes.

diabetogenic effect of pregnancy the normal state during pregnancy in which blood glucose levels are lower than normal (mild hypoglycemia) when fasting, blood glucose levels are higher than normal (mild hyperglycemia) after meals, and insulin levels are increased (hyperinsulinemia) after meals.

diagonal conjugate area that extends from the symphysis pubis to the sacral promontory, which is measured to provide an estimate of the size of the obstetric conjugate.

diastasis recti abdominis separation of the rectus abdominis muscle that supports the abdomen.

digitalization the use of large doses of digoxin, at the beginning of therapy, to build up the blood levels of the drug to a therapeutic level.

diplopia double vision.

discipline to train or instruct to produce self-control and a particular behavior pattern, especially moral or mental improvement.

dizygotic fraternal twins that develop from separate egg and sperm fertilizations.

doula Greek for servant; birth assistants who are trained to provide the highest quality emotional, physical, and educational support to women and their families during childbirth and the postpartum period.

dramatic play a type of play that allows a child to act out troubling situations and to control the solution to the problem.

ductus arteriosus prenatal blood vessel between the pulmonary artery and the aorta that closes functionally within the first 3 or 4 days of life.

ductus venosus prenatal blood vessel between the umbilical vein and the inferior vena cava; does not achieve complete closure until the end of the 2nd month of life.

dysarthria poor speech articulation.

dysfunctional family family that cannot resolve routine stresses in a positive, socially acceptable manner.

dysmenorrhea painful menstruation.

dyspareunia painful intercourse.

dysphagia difficulty swallowing.

early adolescence begins at about age 10 years in girls and about age 12 years in boys with a dramatic growth spurt that signals the advent of puberty; preadolescence; pubescence.

early deceleration the dip in the fetal heart rate (FHR) tracing that occurs in conjunction with and mirrors a uterine contraction.

echolalia "parrot speech" typical of autistic children. They echo words they hear, such as a television commercial, but do not appear to understand the words.

eclampsia condition in which the woman with severe preeclampsia experiences a convulsion or a coma.

ectopic pregnancy a pregnancy that occurs outside of the uterus.

effacement softening and shortening of the cervix during labor.

effleurage a form of touch that involves light circular fingertip movements on the abdomen; a technique a woman can use in early labor.

ego in psychoanalytic theory, the conscious self that controls the pleasure principle of the id by delaying the instincts until an appropriate time.

egocentric concerned only with one's own activities or needs; unable to put oneself in another's place or to see another's point of view.

elbow restraints restraints made of muslin with two layers. Pockets wide enough to enclose tongue depressors are placed vertically along the width of the fabric. The restraints are wrapped around the arm to prevent the infant from bending the arm.

elective abortion an abortion performed at the woman's request that does not involve preservation of health.

elective induction induction of labor in which the physician and woman decide to end the pregnancy in the absence of a medical reason to do so.

electrolytes chemical compounds (minerals) that break down into ions when placed in water.

embryo the developing conceptus, from weeks 2 through 8.

emetic agent that causes vomiting.

en face position establishment of eye contact in the same plane between the caregiver and infant; extremely important to parent–infant bonding; also called mutual gazing.

encephalopathy degenerative disease of the brain.

encopresis chronic involuntary fecal soiling with no medical cause.

endometriosis a painful reproductive and immunologic disorder in which tissue implants resembling endometrium grow outside of the uterus.

endometritis an infection of the uterine lining.

endometrium the vascular mucosal inner layer of walls of the corpus and fundus that changes under hormonal influence every month in preparation for possible pregnancy.

engagement occurs when the presenting part of the fetus has settled into the true pelvis at the level of the ischial spines.

engorgement occurs when the milk comes in and the woman's body responds with increasing the blood supply to the breast tissues.

enuresis involuntary urination, especially at night; bed-wetting beyond the usual age of control.

epididymis an intricate network of coiled ducts on the posterior portion of each testis that is approximately 6 meters (20 feet) in length.

epiphyses growth centers at the ends of long bones and at the wrists.

episiotomy a surgical incision made into the perineum to enlarge the vaginal opening just before the baby is born.

epispadias condition in which the opening of the urinary meatus is located abnormally on the dorsal (upper) surface of the glans penis.

epistaxis nosebleed.

Epstein's pearls small white cysts found on the midline portion of the hard palate of some newborns.

Erb's palsy a facial paralysis resulting from injury to the cervical nerves.

erythema toxicum fine rash of the newborn that may appear over the trunk, back, abdomen, and buttocks. It appears about 24 hours after birth and disappears in several days.

erythroblastosis fetalis a condition in which the infant's red blood cells are broken down (hemolyzed) and destroyed, producing severe anemia and hyperbilirubinemia.

eschar hard crust or scab.

esotropia eye deviation toward the other eye.

estimated date of confinement (EDC) the estimated date that the baby will be born.

estimated date of delivery (EDD) the estimated date that the baby will be born.

exotropia eye deviation away from the other eye.

extended family consists of one or more nuclear families plus other relatives; often crosses generations to include grandparents, aunts, uncles, and cousins. The needs of individual members are subordinate to the needs of the group, and the children are considered an economic asset.

external hordeolum purulent infection of the follicle of an eyelash; generally caused by *Staphylococcus aureus*. Localized swelling, tenderness, and pain are present with a reddened lid edge; a stye.

extracellular fluid fluid situated outside a cell or cells.

extravasation escape of fluid into surrounding tissue.

extrusion reflex infant's way of taking food by thrusting the tongue forward as if to suck; has the effect of pushing solid food out of the mouth.

exudate drainage; fluid accumulation.

false pelvis the flared upper portion of the bony pelvis.

febrile seizure seizure occurring in infants and young children commonly associated with a fever of 102°F to 106°F (38.9°C to 41.1°C).

fertilization process by which the male's sperm unites with the female's ovum.

fetal alcohol syndrome (FAS) syndrome seen in an infant born to a woman who abused alcohol during pregnancy, including shorter stature, lower birth weight, possible microcephaly, facial deformities, hearing disorders, poor coordination, minor joint and limb abnormalities, heart defects, delayed development, and mental retardation.

fetal attitude the relationship of the fetal parts to one another.

fetal fibronectin a protein found in fetal membranes and amniotic fluid.

fetal lie the long axis of the fetus in relation to the long axis of the pregnant woman.

fetal mortality rate perinatal mortality rate calculated by dividing the number of deaths that occur in utero at 20 or more weeks of gestation by the number of live births plus fetal deaths.

fetal presentation the foremost part of the fetus that enters the pelvic inlet.

fetus term for the organism after it has reached the 8th week of life and acquires a human likeness.

fontanel "soft spot" covered by a tough membrane at the junctures of the six bones of a newborn's skull. At birth, two fontanels can be detected—the anterior fontanel at the junction of the frontal and parietal bones and the posterior fontanel at the junction of the parietal and occipital bones. They are ossified (filled in by bone) during the normal growth process.

foramen ovale opening between the left and right atria of the fetal heart that closes with the first breath.

forceps metal instruments with curved, blunted blades (somewhat like large hollowed-out spoons) that are placed around the head of the fetus by the birth attendant to facilitate delivery.

forceps marks noticeable marks on the infant's face that may occur if delivery was assisted with forceps; usually disappear within a day or two.

foremilk breast milk that is very watery and thin and may have a bluish tint. This is what the infant receives first during the breast-feeding session.

gag reflex reaction to any stimulation of the posterior pharynx by food, suction, or passage of a tube that causes elevation of the soft palate and a strong involuntary effort to vomit; continues throughout life.

galactosemia recessive hereditary metabolic disorder in which the enzyme necessary for converting galactose into glucose is missing. The infant generally appears normal at birth but experiences difficulties after the ingestion of milk.

gametes sex cells.

gametogenesis the formation and development of gametes or germ cells by the process of meiosis.

gastroenteritis infectious diarrhea caused by infectious organisms, including salmonella, *Escherichia coli,* dysentery bacilli, and various viruses, most notably rotaviruses.

gastrostomy tube tube surgically inserted through the abdominal wall into the stomach under general anesthesia. Used in children who have obstructions or surgical repairs in the mouth, pharynx, esophagus, or cardiac sphincter of the stomach or who are respirator dependent.

gavage feeding nourishment provided directly through a tube passed into the stomach.

genes units threaded along chromosomes that carry genetic instructions from one generation to another. Like chromosomes, genes also occur in pairs. There are thousands of genes in the chromosomes of each cell nucleus.

genetic counseling study of the family history and tissue analysis of both partners to determine chromosome patterns for couples concerned about transmitting a specific disease to their unborn children.

gestational age the length of time between fertilization of the egg and birth of the infant.

gestational diabetes mellitus (GDM) a type of diabetes mellitus (DM) that is unique to pregnancy but in many respects mimics type 2 DM.

gestational hypertension (formerly called pregnancy-induced hypertension or PIH) the current term used to describe elevated blood pressure (greater than or equal to 140/90 mm Hg) that develops for the first time during pregnancy without the presence of protein in the urine.

gestational surrogate or surrogate mother; a woman who donates the use of her uterus, or she may also donate her ovum and agree to be inseminated with the male partner's sperm.

glycosuria glucose in the urine.

goniotomy surgical opening into Schlemm's canal that allows drainage of aqueous humor; performed to relieve intraocular pressure in glaucoma.

Goodell's sign softening of the cervix during pregnancy.

gradual acceptance type of response by caregivers when caring for a chronically ill child in which caregivers adopt a common-sense approach to the child's condition and encourage the child to function within his or her capabilities.

grand multiparity five or more pregnancies.

granulocytes type of white blood cell; divided into eosinophils, basophils, and neutrophils.

gravida the number of pregnancies the woman has had (regardless of the outcome).

growth result of cell division and marked by an increase in size and weight; physical increase in body size and appearance caused by increasing numbers of new cells.

gynecoid pelvis categorized as a typical female pelvis (although only about half of all women have this type of pelvis); the rounded shape of the gynecoid inlet allows the fetus room to negotiate the dimensions of the bony passageway.

gynecomastia excessive growth of the mammary glands in the male.

halo traction metal ring attached to the skull that is added to a body cast using stainless steel pins inserted into the skull and into the femurs or iliac wings.

Harlequin sign or Harlequin coloring characterized by a clown-suit–like appearance of the newborn. The newborn's skin is dark red on one side of the body while the other side of the body is pale. The dark red color is caused by dilation of blood vessels, and the pallor is caused by contraction of blood vessels.

health maintenance organizations (HMOs) professional groups of physicians, laboratory service personnel, nurse practitioners, nurses, and consultants who care for the family's health on a continuing basis and are geared to health care and disease prevention. The family pays a set fee for total care; that fee covers any necessary hospitalization. The emphasis is on health and prevention.

Hegar's sign softening of the uterine isthmus during pregnancy.

hemarthrosis bleeding into the joints.

hematoma a clot of blood that collects within tissues and leads to concealed blood loss.

hemolysis destruction of red blood cells with the release of hemoglobin into the plasma.

hernia abnormal protrusion of part of an organ through a weak spot or other abnormal opening in a body wall.

heterograft graft of tissue obtained from an animal. For burn patients, pig skin (porcine) is often used.

heterosexual relationship intimate relationship between two people of the opposite sex.

hierarchical arrangement grouping by some common system, such as rank, grade, or class.

hind milk breast milk that is thicker and whiter. It contains a higher quantity of fat than foremilk and therefore has a higher caloric content than foremilk.

hip dysplasia see congenital hip dysplasia.

hirsutism abnormal body and facial hair growth.

homeostasis uniform state; signifies biologically the dynamic equilibrium of the healthy organism.

homograft graft of tissue, including organs, from a member of one's own species.

homosexual relationship intimate relationship between two people of the same sex.

homozygous term used to describe a particular trait of an individual when any two members of a pair of genes carry the same genetic instructions for that trait.

hospice provides comforting and supportive care to terminally ill patients and their families. There are few hospice programs for children in the United States.

hyaline membrane disease also known as respiratory distress syndrome (RDS); occurs because of immature lungs that lack sufficient surfactant to decrease the surface tension of the alveoli; affects about half of all preterm newborns.

hydatidiform mole, also referred to as a molar pregnancy and gestational trophoblastic disease; a condition characterized by benign growth of placental tissue.

hydramnios excessive amniotic fluid.

hydrotherapy use of water in a treatment.

hyperbilirubinemia high blood bilirubin levels.

hyperemesis gravidarum a disorder of early pregnancy that is characterized by severe nausea and vomiting.

hyperglycemia elevated blood glucose levels.

hyperinsulinemia increased insulin levels.

hyperlipidemia increase in the level of cholesterol in the blood.

hyperopia refractive condition in which the person can see objects better at a distance; farsightedness.

hyperpnea increase in depth and rate of breathing.

hyperthermia overheating.

hypervolemia increased volume of circulating plasma.

hypocholia diminished flow of pancreatic enzymes.

hypoglycemia low blood sugar levels.

hyposensitization immunization therapy by injection; immunotherapy.

hypospadias condition that occurs when the opening to the urethra is on the ventral (under) surface of the glans.

hypothermia low body temperature; may be a symptom of a disease or dysfunction of the temperature-regulating mechanism of the body, or it may be deliberately induced, such as during open-heart surgery, to reduce oxygen needs and provide a longer time for the surgeon to complete the operation without the patient experiencing brain damage. When caring for the newborn, it is important to remember that heat loss can lead to hypothermia because of the infant's immature temperature-regulating system.

hypovolemia decreased volume of circulating plasma.

hypovolemic shock condition characterized by a weak, thready, rapid pulse; drop in blood pressure; cool, clammy skin; and changes in level of consciousness.

id in psychoanalytic theory, part of the personality that controls physical needs and instincts of the body; dominated by the pleasure principle.

ileostomy a surgical procedure in which a part of the ileum is brought through the abdominal wall to create an outlet to drain fecal material.

immunologic properties properties from the woman that help protect the newborn from infections and strengthen the newborn's immune system.

imperforate anus congenital disorder in which the rectal pouch ends blindly above the anus and there is no anal orifice.

impunity belief, common among adolescents, that nothing can hurt them.

incest sexually arousing physical contact between family members not married to each other.

incompetent cervix painless cervical dilation that occurs with bulging of fetal membranes and parts through the external os.

independent nursing actions nursing actions that may be performed based on the nurse's own clinical judgment.

induced abortion the purposeful interruption of pregnancy before 20 weeks' gestation.

induration hardness.

infant mortality rate the number of deaths during the first 12 months of life, which includes neonatal mortality.

infantile spasms a type of seizure activity that occurs in an infant between 3 and 12 months and usually indicates a cerebral defect with a poor prognosis.

infertility the inability to conceive after a year or more of regular and unprotected intercourse, or the inability to carry a pregnancy to term.

inhalant substance that may be taken into the body through inhaling; substance whose volatile vapors can be abused.

insulin reaction excessively low blood sugar caused by insulin overload; results in too-rapid metabolism of the body's glucose; insulin shock; hypoglycemia.

intercurrent infection infection that occurs during the course of an already existing disease.

interdependent nursing actions nursing actions that the nurse must work with other health team members to accomplish, such as meal planning with a dietary therapist and teaching breathing exercises with a respiratory therapist.

intermittent infusion device a type of device that is used for administering medications by the intravenous route and can be left in place and used at intervals.

interstitial fluid also called intracellular or tissue fluid; has a composition similar to plasma but contains almost no protein. This reservoir of fluid outside the body cells decreases or increases easily in response to disease.

interstitial keratitis inflammation of the cornea; often caused by congenital syphilis and usually accompanied by lacrimation, photophobia, and opacity of the lens; may lead to blindness.

intracellular fluid fluid contained within the cell membranes; constitutes about two thirds of total body fluids.

intrathecal administration injection into the cerebrospinal fluid by lumbar puncture.

intrauterine growth restriction (IUGR) condition in which babies are small because of circumstances that occurred during the pregnancy, causing limited fetal growth.

intravascular fluid fluid situated within the blood vessels or blood plasma.

intraventricular hemorrhage (IVH) bleeding within a ventricle of the heart or brain.

invagination telescoping; infolding of one part of a structure into another.

involution the shrinking or returning to normal size of the uterus, cervix, and vagina.

isoimmunization development of antibodies against Rh$_o$(D) positive blood in the pregnant woman.

jacket restraint used to secure the child from climbing out of bed or a chair or to keep the child in a horizontal position; must be the correct size for the child.

jaundice a yellow staining of the skin that occurs when a large amount of unconjugated bilirubin is present (serum levels of 4 to 6 mg/dL and greater)

kangaroo care a way to maintain the newborn's temperature and promote early bonding; the nurse dries the newborn quickly, places a diaper or blanket over the genital area and a cap on the head, then places the newborn in skin-to-skin contact with the mother or father and covers them both with blankets.

kernicterus neurologic complication of unconjugated hyperbilirubinemia in the infant.

Kussmaul breathing abnormal increase in the depth and rate of the respiratory movements.

kwashiorkor syndrome occurring in infants and young children soon after weaning; results from severe deficiency of protein. Symptoms include a swollen abdomen, retarded growth with muscle wasting, edema, gastrointestinal changes, thin dry hair with patchy alopecia, apathy, and irritability.

kyphosis backward and lateral curvature of the cervical spine; hunchback.

labor dystocia an abnormal progression of labor.

lacrimation secretion of tears.

lactation consultant a nurse or layperson who has received special training to assist and support the breast-feeding woman.

lactose intolerance inability to digest lactose because of an inborn deficiency of the enzyme lactase.

lactose a sugar found in milk that, when hydrolyzed, yields glucose and galactose.

laminaria cervical dilators.

lanugo fine, downy hair that covers the skin of the fetus.

large for gestational age (LGA) an infant whose weight, length, and/or head circumference is above the 90th percentile for gestational age.

latchkey child child who comes home to an empty house after school each day because family caregivers are at work.

late decelerations decelerations that are offset from the labor contraction. Late decelerations begin late in the contraction and recover after the contraction has ended.

lecithin major component of surfactant.

leukemia uncontrolled reproduction of deformed white blood cells.

leukopenia leukocyte count less than 5,000 mm^3.

libido sexual drive.

linea nigra a darkened line that develops on the skin in the middle of the abdomen of pregnant women.

lochia vaginal discharge after birth.

long-term variability (LTV) the wider fluctuations that make the electronic fetal monitoring (EFM) tracing look wavy over time.

lordosis forward curvature of the lumbar spine; swayback.

low birth weight (LBW) newborns that weigh less than 2,500 g.

lymphoblast lymphocyte that has been changed by antigenic stimulation to a structurally immature lymphocyte.

lymphocytes single-nucleus, nonphagocytic leukocytes that are instrumental in the body's immune response.

macroglossia abnormally large tongue.

macrosomia condition that is diagnosed if the birth weight exceeds 4,500 grams (9.9 pounds) or the birth weight is greater than the 90th percentile for gestational age.

magical thinking child's belief that thoughts are powerful and can cause something to happen (e.g., illness or death of a loved one occurs because the child wished it in a moment of anger).

malattachment emotional distancing in the maternal–infant relationship.

malocclusion the improper alignment of the teeth.

marasmus deficiency in calories as well as protein. The child suffers growth retardation and wasting of subcutaneous fat and muscle.

mastitis infection of the breast tissue.

maternal mortality rate the number of maternal deaths per 100,000 live births caused by a pregnancy-related complication that occurs during pregnancy or during the 42 days after pregnancy.

maturation completed growth and development.

meconium first stools of the newborn.

meconium aspiration occurs when the fetus inhales some meconium along with amniotic fluid.

menarche beginning of menstruation.

menorrhagia heavy or prolonged uterine bleeding.

metered-dose inhaler hand-held plastic device that delivers a premeasured dose of medicine.

metrorrhagia menstrual bleeding that is normal in amount but occurs at irregular intervals between menstrual periods.

microcephaly a very small cranium.

micrognathia abnormal smallness of the lower jaw.

milia pearly white cysts usually seen over the bridge of the nose, chin, and cheeks of a newborn. They are usually retention cysts of sebaceous glands or hair follicles and disappear within a few weeks without treatment.

mittelschmerz pain experienced midcycle in the menstrual cycle at the time of ovulation.

molding elongation of the fetal skull to accommodate the birth canal.

mongolian spots areas of bluish-black pigmentation resembling bruises; most often seen over the sacral or gluteal regions of infants of African, Mediterranean, Native American, or Asian descent; usually fade within 1 or 2 years.

monocytes 5% to 10% of white blood cells that defend the body against infection.

monozygotic identical twins that are derived from one zygote; one egg and one sperm divide into two zygotes shortly after fertilization.

mons pubis or mons; a rounded fatty pad located atop the symphysis pubis.

Montgomery's tubercles sebaceous glands on the areolas that produce secretions that lubricate the nipple. Montgomery's tubercles become more prominent during pregnancy.

morbidity the number of persons afflicted with the same disease condition per a certain number of population.

Moro reflex abduction of the arms and legs and flexion of the elbows in response to a sudden loud noise, jarring, or abrupt change in equilibrium: fingers flare, except the forefinger and thumb, which are clenched to form a C shape. Occurs in the normal newborn to the end of the 4th or 5th month.

mortality rate statistics recorded as the ratio of deaths in a given category to the number of individuals in that category of the population.

morula the solid cell cluster that forms about 3 days after fertilization, when the total cell count has reached 32.

mottling a red and white lacy pattern sometimes seen on the skin of newborns who have fair complexions.

multigravida a woman who has had more than one pregnancy.

mummy restraint used to restrain an infant or small child during procedures that involve only the head or neck.

mutation fundamental change that takes place in the structure of a gene; results in the transmission of a trait different from that normally carried by that particular gene.

mutual gazing see *en face position*.

myoclonic seizure characterized by sudden jerking of a muscle or group of muscles often in the arms or legs. There is no loss of consciousness.

myometrium the muscular middle layer of the walls of the corpus and fundus that is responsible for the contractions of labor.

myopia ability to see objects clearly at close range but not at a distance; nearsightedness.

myringotomy incision of the eardrum performed to establish drainage and to insert tiny tubes into the tympanic membrane to facilitate drainage of serous or purulent fluid in the middle ear.

nadir the lowest point of the deceleration of the fetal heart rate (FHR).

Nagele's rule a formula used to determine the pregnancy due date by adding 7 days to the date of the first day of the last menstrual period (LMP), then subtracting 3 months.

nebulizer tube attached to a wall unit or cylinder that delivers moist air via a face mask.

necrotizing enterocolitis an acute inflammatory disease of the intestine.

negativism opposition to suggestion or advice; associated with the toddler age group because the toddler, in search of autonomy, frequently responds "no" to almost everything.

neonatal abstinence syndrome (NAS) symptoms seen in the newborn of the woman who has abused substances during pregnancy; withdrawal symptoms.

neonatal adjective used to describe the time period from birth through the first 28 days or 1 month of life.

neonatal mortality rate the number of infant deaths during the first 28 days of life for every 1,000 live births.

neonate term used to describe a newborn in the first 28 days of life.

nocturnal emissions involuntary discharge of semen during sleep; also known as wet dreams.

noncommunicative language egocentric speech exhibited by children who talk to themselves, toys, or pets without any purpose other than the pleasure of using words.

nuchal rigidity stiff neck.

nuclear family family structure that consists of only the father, the mother, and the children living in one household.

nulligravida a woman who has never been pregnant.

nursing process proven form of problem solving based on the scientific method. The nursing process consists of five components: assessment, nursing diagnosis, planning, implementation, and evaluation.

nutrition history information regarding the child's eating habits and preferences.

obesity excessive accumulation of fat that increases body weight by 20% or more over ideal weight.

objective data in the nursing assessment, the data gained by the nurse's direct observation.

obstetric conjugate the smallest diameter of the inlet through which the fetus must pass.

oliguria decreased production of urine, especially in relation to fluid intake.

onlooker play interest in the observation of an activity without participation.

open-glottis pushing method of expelling the fetus that is characterized by pushing with contractions using an open glottis so that air is released during the pushing effort.

opioids medications with opium-like properties (also known as narcotic analgesics); the most frequently administered medications to provide analgesia during labor.

opisthotonos arching of the back so that the head and the heels are bent backward and the body is forward.

ophthalmia neonatorum a severe eye infection contracted in the birth canal of a woman with gonorrhea or Chlamydia.

orchiopexy surgical procedure used to bring an undescended testis down into the scrotum and anchor it there.

orthodontia a type of dentistry dealing with prevention and correction of incorrectly positioned or aligned teeth.

orthoptics therapeutic exercises to improve the quality of vision.

outcomes goals that are specific, stated in measurable terms, and have a time frame for accomplishment.

overprotection type of response by caregivers when caring for chronically ill children in which the caregivers protect the child at all costs, prevent the child from achieving new skills by hovering, avoid the use of discipline, and use every means to prevent the child from suffering any frustration.

overriding aorta in tetralogy of Fallot; the aorta shifts to the right over the opening in the ventricular septum so that blood from both right and left ventricles is pumped into the aorta.

overweight more than 10% over ideal weight.

ovulation releasing the mature ovum into the abdominal cavity, which occurs on day 14 of a 28-day cycle.

palmar grasp reflex phenomenon that results when pressure is placed on the palm of the hand near the base of the digits causing flexion or curling of the fingers.

palpebral fissures opening between the eyes.

papoose board commercial restraint board for use with toddlers or preschool-age children that uses canvas strips to secure the child's body and extremities. One extremity can be released to allow treatment to be performed on that extremity.

parallel play one child plays alongside another child or children involved in the same type of activity, but the children do not interact with each other.

parity or para, communicates the outcome of previous pregnancies in the obstetric history.

partial seizure a type of seizure with manifestations that vary depending on the area of the brain where they arise.

patient-controlled analgesia (PCA) programmed intravenous infusion of narcotic analgesia that the patient can control within set limits.

pediatric nurse practitioner (PNP) professional nurse prepared at the postbaccalaureate level to give primary health care to children and families. These nurses use pediatricians or family physicians as consultants but offer day-to-day assessment and care.

pedodontist dentist who specializes in the care and treatment of children's teeth.

pelvic rest a physician's order requiring the woman to refrain from inserting anything into the vagina, such as tampons or the practitioner's fingers to perform a cervical examination; this order includes sexual abstinence.

percutaneous umbilical blood sampling (PUBS) or cordocentesis a procedure similar to amniocentesis whereby fetal blood is withdrawn from the umbilical cord.

perimenopause the time before menopause when vasomotor symptoms (hot flashes, night sweats) and irregular menses begin.

perimetrium the tough outer layer of the walls of the corpus and fundus, which is made of connective tissues and supports the uterus.

perinatal the period surrounding birth, from conception throughout pregnancy and birth.

perinatal mortality rate the number of fetal/neonatal deaths that occur from 28 weeks of gestation through the first 7 days of life.

perinatologist a maternal–fetal medicine specialist.

periodic changes variations in the fetal heart rate (FHR) pattern that occur in conjunction with uterine contractions.

personal history data collected about a client's personal habits, such as hygiene, sleeping, and elimination patterns, as well as activities, exercise, special interests, and favorite objects (toys).

petechiae a small hemorrhage appearing as a nonraised, purplish-red spot of the skin, nail beds, or mucous membranes.

phenylketonuria (PKU) recessive hereditary defect of metabolism that results in a congenital disease caused by a defect in the enzyme that normally changes the essential amino acid, phenylalanine, into tyrosine. If untreated, PKU results in severe mental retardation.

philtrum vertical groove in the middle of the upper lip.

phimosis adherence of the foreskin to the glans penis.

photophobia intolerance to light.

photosensitivity sensitivity to sunlight.

physiologic jaundice icterus neonatorum; jaundice that occurs in a large number of newborns but has no medical significance; result of the breakdown of fetal red blood cells.

pica compulsive eating of nonfood substances.

pinna the upper, external, protruding part of the ear.

placenta previa a condition in which the placenta is implanted close to, or covers, the cervical os.

plantar grasp reflex phenomenon that results when pressure is placed on the sole of the foot at the base of the toes; causes the toes to curl downward.

platypelloid pelvis pelvis that is flat in its dimensions with a very narrow anterior-posterior diameter and a wide transverse diameter; this shape makes it extremely difficult for the fetus to pass through the bony pelvis.

play therapy technique of psychoanalysis that psychiatrists or psychiatric nurse clinicians use to uncover a disturbed child's underlying thoughts, feelings, and motivations, to better help him/her.

point of maximum impulse (PMI) the point over the heart on the chest wall where the heart beat can be heard the best using a stethoscope.

polyarthritis inflammation of several joints.

polycythemia excess number of red blood cells.

polydipsia abnormal thirst.

polyphagia increased food consumption.

polyuria dramatic increase in urinary output, often with enuresis.

postcoital test evaluates the interaction of the man's sperm with the woman's cervical mucus.

postpartum blues, sometimes called the "baby blues," a temporary depression that usually begins on the 3rd day after delivery and lasts for 2 or 3 days, in which the woman may be tearful, have difficulty sleeping and eating, and feel generally let down.

postterm or postmature, a newborn born at 42 weeks' or more gestation.

precipitous labor labor that lasts less than 3 hours from the start of uterine contractions to birth.

preeclampsia a serious condition of pregnancy in which the blood pressure rises to 140/90 mm Hg or higher accompanied by proteinuria, the presence of protein in the urine.

pregestational diabetes condition in which a woman enters pregnancy with either type 1 or type 2 diabetes mellitus.

premenstrual syndrome (PMS) symptoms occurring before menstruation, including edema (resulting in weight gain), headache, increased anxiety, mild depression, or mood swings; premenstrual tension.

prepuce or foreskin; a layer of tissue that covers the glans of the penis.

preterm, or premature, a newborn born at 37 weeks' gestation or less; commonly called premature.

priapism prolonged, abnormal erection of the penis.

primary circular reactions a stage of development named by Piaget in which infants explore objects by touching or putting them in their mouths; the infant is unaware of actions that he or she can cause.

primary nursing system whereby one nurse plans the total care for a child and directs the efforts of nurses on the other shifts.

primary prevention limiting the spread of illness or disease by teaching, especially regarding safety, diet, rest, and exercise.

prospective payment system predetermined rates to be paid to the health care provider to care for patients with certain classifications of diseases.

proteinuria the presence of protein in the urine.

proximodistal pattern of growth in which growth starts in the center and progresses toward the periphery or outside.

pruritus itching.

pseudomenses (pseudomenstruation) false menstruation; a slight red-tinged vaginal discharge in female infants resulting from a decline in the hormonal level after birth compared with the higher concentration in the maternal hormone environment before birth.

pseudostrabismus the cross-eyed look found in infants caused by incomplete development of the nerves and muscles that control focusing and coordination; begins to disappear in the 6th month.

puberty period during which secondary sexual characteristics begin to develop and reproductive maturity is attained.

puerperal fever an illness marked by high fever caused by infection of the reproductive tract after the birth of a child.

puerperium the postpartum period.

pulmonary stenosis narrowing of the opening between the right ventricle and the pulmonary artery that decreases blood flow to the lungs.

pulse oximeter photoelectric device used to measure oxygen saturation in an artery; can be attached to an infant's finger, toe, or heel.

punishment penalty given for wrongdoing.

purpura hemorrhages into the skin or mucous membranes.

purpuric rash rash consisting of ecchymoses (bruises) and petechiae caused by bleeding under the skin.

pyelonephritis infection of the kidneys.

pyrosis heartburn caused by acid reflux through the relaxed lower esophageal sphincter (LES).

recessive gene gene carrying different information for a trait within a pair that is not expressed (e.g., blue eyes versus brown eyes). A recessive gene is detectable only when present on both chromosomes.

refraction the way light rays bend as they pass through the lens of the eye to the retina.

regurgitation spitting up of small quantities of milk; occurs rather easily in the young infant.

rejection type of response by caregivers when caring for a chronically ill child in which the caregivers distance themselves emotionally from the child and, although they provide physical care, tend to scold and correct the child continuously.

respiratory distress syndrome (RDS) see *hyaline membrane disease.*

respite care care of the child by someone other than the usual caregiver so that the caregiver can get temporary relief and rest.

retinopathy of prematurity (ROP) a complication commonly associated with the preterm newborn that results from the growth of abnormal immature retinal blood vessels.

reversibility ability to think in either direction.

right ventricular hypertrophy increase in thickness of the myocardium of the right ventricle.

risk nursing diagnoses category of diagnoses that identifies health problems to which the patient is especially vulnerable.

ritual a routine; in labor, a repeated series of actions that the woman uses as an individualized way of dealing with the discomfort of labor.

ritualism practice employed by the young child to help develop security; consists of following a certain routine; makes rituals of simple tasks.

rooming-in arrangement in which the health care facility permits a family caregiver to stay with a child. A cot or sleeping chair is provided for the caregiver.

rooting reflex infant's response of turning the head when the cheek is stroked toward the stroked side.

rumination voluntary regurgitation.

runaway child child who is absent from home for overnight or longer without the permission of the caregiver.

salpingectomy removal of the fallopian tube.

salpingitis infection of the fallopian tube.

school history information regarding the child's grade level in school and his or her academic performance.

school phobia child's fear resulting in dread of a school situation or fear of leaving home; can be a combination of both.

scoliosis lateral curvature of the spine.

scurvy a disease that results from severe vitamin C deficiency and is characterized by spongy gums, loosened teeth, and bleeding into the skin and mucous membrane.

seborrhea a scalp condition characterized by yellow, crusty patches; also called cradle cap.

sebum oily secretion of the sebaceous glands.

secondary circular reactions a stage of development named by Piaget in which the infant realizes that his or her actions cause pleasurable sensations.

secondary prevention limiting the impact or reoccurrence of disease by focusing on early diagnosis and treatment.

seizure series of involuntary contractions of voluntary muscles; convulsion.

seminiferous tubules tiny coils of tissue in the lobes of the testis in which spermatogenesis occurs.

sexual abuse sexual contact between a child and someone in a caregiving position, such as a parent, baby-sitter, or teacher.

sexual assault sexual contact made by someone who is not functioning in the role of the child's caregiver.

short-term variability (STV) the moment-to-moment changes in fetal heart rate (FHR) that result in roughness of the electronic fetal monitor (EFM) tracing.

simian crease a single straight palmar crease; an abnormal finding that is associated with Down syndrome.

single-parent family household headed by one adult of either sex. There may be one or more children in the family.

skeletal traction pull exerted directly on skeletal structures by means of pins, wire, tongs, or another device surgically inserted through the bone.

skin traction pull on tape, rubber, or plastic materials attached to the skin that indirectly exerts pull on the musculoskeletal system.

small for gestational age (SGA) a newborn whose weight, length, and/or head circumference falls below the 10th percentile for gestational age.

smegma the cheeselike secretion of the sebaceous glands found under the foreskin.

social history information about the environment in which the child lives.

socialization process by which a child learns the rules of the society and culture in which the family lives, its language, values, ethics, and acceptable behaviors.

solitary independent play playing apart from others without making an effort to be part of the group or group activity.

spermatogenesis production of sperm.

spina bifida failure of the posterior lamina of the vertebrae to close; leaves an opening through which the spinal meninges and spinal cord may protrude.

spinnbarkeit an elastic quality of cervical mucus that allows it to be stretched 5 centimeters or more between the thumb and forefinger.

spontaneous abortion loss of a pregnancy before the age of viability (less than 20 weeks of gestation or fetal size of less than 500 grams). The common name for early pregnancy loss is miscarriage.

startle reflex follows any loud noise; similar to the Moro reflex, but the hands remain clenched. This reflex is never lost.

station the relationship of the presenting part of a fetus to the ischial spines.

status asthmaticus a potentially fatal complication of an acute asthma attack involving severe asthma symptoms that do not respond after 30 to 60 minutes of treatment.

status epilepticus an emergency complication of epilepsy whereby seizure activity continues for 30 minutes or more after treatment is initiated or when three or more seizures occur without full recovery between seizures.

steatorrhea fatty stools.

step reflex also called the dance reflex; tendency of infants to make stepping movements when held upright.

stepfamily consists of custodial parent, children, and a new spouse.

stigma negative perception of a person because he or she is believed to be different from the general population; may cause embarrassment or shame in the person being stigmatized.

strabismus failure of the two eyes to direct their gaze at the same object simultaneously; squint; crossed eyes.

striae stretch marks.

stridor shrill, harsh respiratory sound, usually on inspiration.

subjective data in the nursing assessment, data spoken by the child or family.

sublimation process of directing a desire or impulse into more acceptable behaviors.

substance abuse the misuse of an addictive substance, such as alcohol or drugs, that changes the user's mental state.

sucking reflex infant's response of strong, vigorous sucking when a nipple, finger, or tongue blade is put in his or her mouth.

superego in psychoanalytic theory, the conscience or parental value system; acts primarily as a monitor over the ego.

supernumerary excessive in number (e.g., more than the usual number of teeth).

supine hypotensive syndrome condition that occurs during late pregnancy in which the gravid uterus can compress the woman's vena cava and aorta, causing the blood pressure to fall when the woman is in the supine position.

surfactant a substance found in the lungs of mature fetuses that keeps the alveoli from collapsing after they first expand.

suture narrow band of connective tissue that divides the six nonunited bones of a newborn's skull.

symmetry a balance in shape, size, and position from one side of the body to the other; a mirror image.

sympathetic ophthalmia inflammatory reaction of the uninjured eye. Symptoms can include photophobia, lacrimation, and some dimness of vision.

synovitis inflammation of a joint; most commonly the hip in children.

tachypnea rapid respirations.

talipes equinovarus clubfoot with plantar flexion.

temper tantrum behavior in children that springs from frustrations caused by their urge for independence; a violent display of temper. The child reacts with enthusiastic rebellion against the wishes of the caregiver.

temperament the combination of all of an individual's characteristics, the way the person thinks, behaves, and reacts.

teratogens from the Greek *terato,* meaning monster, and *genesis,* meaning birth; an agent or influence that causes a defect or disruption in the prenatal growth process. The effect of a teratogen depends on when it enters the fetal system and the stage of differentiation of the organs or organ systems at that time. Generally the fetus is most vulnerable to teratogens during the 1st trimester.

term a newborn who is born between the beginning of week 38 and the end of week 41 of gestation.

tertiary prevention a focus on rehabilitation and teaching to prevent additional injury or illness.

thanatologist person, sometimes a nurse, trained especially to work with the dying and their families.

therapeutic abortion a pregnancy termination performed for reasons related to maternal or fetal health or disease.

therapeutic play play technique that may be used by play therapists, nurses, child-life specialists, and trained volunteers.

thermoneutral environment an environment in which heat is neither lost nor gained.

thermoregulation regulation of temperature.

throwaway child child (often a teenager) who has been forced to leave home and is not wanted back by the adults in the home.

thrush A fungal infection (caused by *Candida albicans*) in the oral cavity.

tinea ringworm.

tissue perfusion circulation of blood through the capillaries carrying nutrients and oxygen to the cells.

tocolytic a substance that relaxes the uterine muscle.

tolerance in substance abuse, ability of body tissues to endure and adapt to continued or increased use of a substance.

tonic neck reflex also called the fencing reflex; seen when the infant lies on the back with the head turned to one side, the arm and leg on that side extended, and the opposite arm flexed as if in a fencing position.

tonic-clonic a type of seizure characterized by muscular contractions and rigidity changing to generalized jerking movements of the muscles followed by a state of relaxation.

tonsils two oval masses attached to the side walls of the back of the mouth between the anterior and posterior pillars (folds of mucous membranes at the sides of the passage from the mouth to the pharynx).

TORCH an acronym for a special group of infections that can be acquired during pregnancy and transmitted through the placenta to the fetus. The "T" stands for toxoplasmosis, the "O" for other infections (Hepatitis B, syphilis, varicella and herpes zoster), the "R" is for rubella, the "C" is for cytomegalovirus (CMV), and the "H" stands for herpes simplex virus (HSV).

total parenteral nutrition (TPN) the administration of dextrose, lipids, amino acids, electrolytes, vitamins, minerals, and trace elements into the circulatory system to meet the nutritional needs of the child whose needs cannot be met through the gastrointestinal tract.

tracheostomy surgical opening into the trachea to provide an open airway in emergency situations or when there is a blocked airway.

traction force applied to an extremity or other part of the body to maintain proper alignment and to facilitate healing of a fractured bone or dislocated joint.

true pelvis the portion of the pelvis below the linea terminalis.

tympanic membrane sensor device used to determine the temperature of the tympanic membrane by rapidly sensing infrared radiation from the membrane. The tympanic thermometer offers the advantage of recording the temperature rapidly with little disturbance to the child.

unfinished business completing matters that will help ease the death of a loved one; saying the unsaid and doing the undone acts of love and caring that may seem difficult to express; recognizing time is limited and filling that time with the important issues that need to be taken care of.

unilateral one side (e.g., in cleft lip, only one side of the lip is cleft).

unoccupied behavior daydreaming; fingering clothing or a toy without any apparent purpose.

urge-to-push method method of expelling the fetus in which the woman bears down only when she feels the urge to do so using any technique that feels right for her.

urostomy a surgical opening created to help with the elimination of urine.

urticaria hives.

uterine atony inability of the uterus to contract effectively.

uterine subinvolution a condition in which the uterus returns to its prepregnancy shape and size at a rate that is slower than expected (usually the result of retained placental fragments or an infection).

uteroplacental insufficiency diminished or deficient blood flow to the uterus and placenta.

utilization review a systematic evaluation of services delivered by a health care provider to determine appropriateness and quality of care, as well as medical necessity of the services provided.

vaginitis inflammation of the vagina.

variability fluctuations in fetal heart rate (FHR).

variable deceleration a change in the FHR that may occur at any point during a contraction and has a jagged, erratic shape on the electronic fetal monitor (EFM) tracing.

vas deferens the muscular tube in which sperm begin their journey out of the man's body.

vascular nevus commonly known as a strawberry mark; a slightly raised, bright-red collection of hypertrophied skin capillaries that does not blanch completely on pressure.

vasectomy male sterilization.

vasospasm spasm of the arteries.

ventricular septal defect abnormal opening in the septum of the heart between the ventricles; allows blood to pass directly from the left to the right side of the heart; the most common intracardiac defect.

ventriculoatrial shunting plastic tubing implanted into the cerebral ventricle passing under the skin to the cardiac atrium; provides drainage for excessive cerebrospinal fluid.

ventriculoperitoneal shunting plastic tubing implanted into the cerebral ventricle passing under the skin to the peritoneal cavity, providing drainage for excessive cerebrospinal fluid. Excessive tubing can be inserted to accommodate the child's growth.

vernix caseosa greasy, cheeselike substance that protects the skin during fetal life; consists of sebum and desquamated epithelial cells.

version a process of manipulating the position of the fetus while in utero.

very low birth weight (VLBW) newborns weighing less than 1,500 g.

vestibule the area within the boundaries of the labia minora, which includes the urethral meatus, vaginal opening, and Bartholin glands.

viable able to live outside of the uterus (fetus).

vigorous pushing method of expelling the fetus in which the woman is told to take a deep breath, hold the breath, and push while counting to 10. She is encouraged to complete three "good" pushes in this manner with each contraction.

vulva the external genitalia of the female reproductive system.

wellness nursing diagnoses diagnoses that identify the potential of an individual, family, or community to move to a higher level of wellness.

West nomogram graph with several scales arranged so that when two values are known, the third can be plotted by drawing a line with a straightedge; commonly used to calculate body surface area (BSA).

Wharton's jelly a clear gelatinous substance that gives support to the cord and helps prevent compression of the cord, which could impair blood flow to the fetus.

wheezing sound of expired air being pushed through obstructed bronchioles.

withdrawal symptoms in substance abuse, physical and psychological symptoms that occur when the drug is no longer being used.

zygote or conceptus, results when an ovum and a spermatozoon unite. The zygote has the full complement of 46 chromosomes, arranged in 23 pairs.

English–Spanish Glossary

Helpful Explanatory Phrases

Both the tu (informal for younger people) and the usted (more formal for people, not known, older than one) forms are offered. In each case the informal is stated first.

Hello. My name is _____.	*Hola. Me llamo _____.*
I am your nurse.	*Soy tu enfermera.*
I don't understand much Spanish. When I ask you questions, please answer with one or two words.	*No entiendo mucho español. Por favor contesta con una o dos palabras.* *Por favor conteste con una o dos palabras.*
Please speak more slowly.	*Habla más despacio, por favor.* *Hable más despacio, por favor.*
I'm sorry, but I don't understand.	*Lo siento, pero no entiendo.*

Obstetric Phrases

Admission Questions

What is your name, including your last name?	*¿Cómo te llamas? Incluye tu apellido.* *¿Cómo se llama? Incluya su apellido.*
How many times have you been pregnant?	*¿Cuántas veces has estado embarazada?* *¿Cuántas veces ha estado embarazada?*
When did your contractions begin?	*¿Cuándo empezaron los dolores?*
Did your water bag break?	*¿Se te rompió la bolsa?* *¿Se le rompió la bolsa?*
Is the baby moving normally?	*¿Está moviéndose normalmente el bebé?*
Have you had any problems with this pregnancy?	*¿Has tenido problemas con este embarazo?* *¿Ha tenido problemas con este embarazo?*
Do you have any chronic illnesses, such as asthma, diabetes, tuberculosis, heart disease?	*¿Tienes alguna enfermedad crónica, como asma, diabetes, tuberculosis, enfermedades del corazón?* *¿Tiene alguna enfermedad crónica, como asma, diabetes, tuberculosis, enfermedades del corazón?*
Are you taking any medications?	*¿Estás tomando alguna medicina?* *¿Está tomando usted alguna medicina?*
How much alcohol do you drink?	*¿Tomas bebidas alcohólicas? ¿Cuánto tomas?* *¿Toma bebidas alcohólicas? ¿Cuánto toma?*
How many cigarettes do you smoke per day?	*¿Fumas cigarillos? ¿Cuántos fumas por día?* *¿Fuma cigarillos? ¿Cuántos fuma por día?*
What plans do you have for pain management?	*¿Qué planes tienes para manejar los dolores?* *¿Qué planes tiene para manejar los dolores?*
Do you want an epidural?	*¿Quieres una inyección epidural?* *¿Quiere una inyección epidural?*

Obstetric Phrases

Do you plan to breast-feed?

¿Piensas dar pecho? ¿Piensas amamantar?
¿Piensa dar pecho? ¿Piensa amamantar?

Do you want the baby circumcised?

¿Deseas circuncisión para el bebé?
¿Desea circuncisión para el bebé?

Admission Procedures
Please put on this gown.

Por favor, ponte esta bata.
Por favor, póngase esta bata.

Wipe with these, then urinate in this cup.

Límpiate con éstas. Luego orina en este vaso.
Límpiese con éstas. Luego orine en este vaso.

Press this button when you need the nurse.

Empuja este botón cuando necesitas a la enfermera.
Empuje este botón cuando necesite a la enfermera.

This is a fetal monitor.

Esta máquina es para checar al bebé.

This part monitors the contractions.

Esta parte es para checar los dolores.

This part monitors the baby's heartbeat.

Este es para checar el latido del corazón del bebé.

Intrapartum Procedures
I am going to check your labor progress.

Voy a checar como esta progresando el parto.

Put your heels together and let your legs relax outward to each side.

Pon juntos los talones y deja relajar las piernas hacia fuera para cada lado.
Ponga juntos los talones y deje relajar las piernas hacia fuera para cada lado.

Take a deep breath in, exhale, and then breathe with me.

Respira profundo, exhala, y luego respira conmigo.
Respire profundo, exhale, y luego respire conmigo.

Please turn to your left (right) side.

Por favor, voltéate a tu lado izquierdo (derecho).
Por favor, voltéese a su lado izquierdo (derecho).

I am going to insert a catheter into your vein.

Voy a meterte una aguja a la vena.
Voy a meterle una aguja a la vena.

I am going to put a catheter into your bladder to drain the urine, and then I will remove the catheter.

Voy a meterte(le) un catéter (un tubo) en la vejiga para vaciarla (sacar la orina), y después voy a quitar el catéter.

Don't push. Blow out, like this.

No empujes. Sopla, así.
No empuje. Sople, así.

Push!

¡Empuja!
¡Empuje!

It's a boy (girl)!

¡Es varón!
¡Es mujer!

Congratulations!

¡Felicidades!

Cesarean Delivery
You need a cesarean section.

Usted necesita una sección cesariana

I am going to shave your abdomen and your upper thighs.

Voy a rasurar el abdomen (estomago) y los muslos.

I am going to put a catheter into your bladder. The urine will drain into the bag. The nurses will take the catheter out 24 hours after your surgery.

Voy a insertarte(le) un catéter en la vejiga. La orina va a drenarse en la bolsa. Las enfermeras te(le) sacaran el catéter unas veinticuatro horas después de tu(su) cirugía.

Hold the pillow over your incision, and then cough.

Pon (ponga) la almohada sobre la incisión (cortada) y luego tose (tosa).

What kind of pain do you have? Is it your incision? Is it cramping? Is it gas pains?

¿Qué clase de dolor tienes (tiene)?
¿Es tu (su) incisión (cortada)?
¿Son calambres (espasmos)?
¿Son dolores de gas?

Are you having any nausea?

¿Tienes (tiene) nausea?

Obstetric Phrases

Have you vomited?	*¿Has (Ha) vomitado?*
Are you passing gas?	*¿Estás (Está) pasando gas?*
Have you had a bowel movement?	*¿Has (Ha) defecado?* *¿Has (Ha) hecho del baño?*

Pediatric Phrases

Interviewing the Caregiver

What is your name, including your last name?	*¿Cómo te llamas? Incluye tu apellido.* *¿Cómo se llama? Incluya su apellido.*
What is your child's name?	*¿Cómo se llama tu niño? ¿niña?* *¿Cómo se llama su niño? ¿niña?*
How old is he/she?	*¿Cuántos años tiene?*
What is the reason your child is being seen today?	*¿Por qué lo/la han traído hoy?*
How long has he/she been sick?	*¿Por cuánto tiempo ha estado enfermo/enferma?*

Has he/she had
- fever
- diarrhea
- constipation
- coughing
- sneezing
- nasal drainage
- drooling
- trouble breathing
- pain
- rash
- bruising
- convulsions

¿Ha tenido . . .?
- *fiebre*
- *diarrea*
- *constipación*
- *tos*
- *estornudos*
- *drenaje nasal*
- *babas*
- *dificultades para respirar*
- *dolor*
- *erupciones, ronchas (hives), urticaria, comezón*
- *morotones*
- *convulsions, ataques*

Has he/she vomited?	*¿Ha vomitado?*
Has he/she cried unusually?	*¿Ha llorado fuera de lo normal?*
When did these symptoms begin?	*¿Cuándo empezaron estos síntomas?*
Can you describe the symptoms?	*¿Puedes (puede) describir los síntomas?*
What have you done to treat these symptoms?	*¿Qué has (ha) hecho para tratar estos síntomas?*
Has he/she ever had these symptoms before?	*¿Ha tenido estos síntomas antes de ahora?*
Is anyone else in your family sick?	*¿Está enfermo cualquier otro miembro de tu (su) familia?*
Has he/she been around anyone who was sick?	*¿Ha estado alrededor de (cerca de) alguien que estaba enfermo?*
Is he/she allergic to any medications?	*¿Tiene alergias a cualquier medicina?*
What medications is he/she taking?	*¿Qué medicina está tomando?*
Is he/she breast-fed?	*¿Amamanta? Está criado(a) con pecho?*
Does he/she drink from a bottle?	*¿Bebe de una botella?*
What does your child eat? Drink?	*¿Qué come tu (su) niño? ¿Qué bebe?*
How often does he/she eat?	*¿Con qué frecuencia come?*
When was the last time he/she ate?	*¿Cuándo fue la última vez que comió?*
When was the last time he/she had something to drink?	*¿Cuándo fue la última vez que bebió algo?*
Is he/she allergic to any foods?	*¿Tiene alergias a alguna comida?*

Pediatric Phrases

Does he/she feed himself/herself?	¿El mismo se da de comer? ¿Ella misma se da de comer? ¿Come sin ayuda?
When was the last time he/she urinated?	¿Cuándo fue la última vez que orino?
How many wet diapers has he/she had today?	¿Cuántos panales ha mojado hoy?
When is the last time he/she had a bowel movement?	¿Cuándo fue la última vez que defecó? (. . . que hizo del baño?)
How often does he/she have a bowel movement?	¿Con qué frecuencia defeca? (hace del baño?)
Is he/she toilet trained?	¿Puede usar el baño sin ayuda?
What word does your child use to say he/she needs to urinate?	¿Qué palabra usa tu (su) niño para decir que tiene que orinar?
What word does your child use to say he/she needs to have a bowel movement?	¿Qué palabra usa tu (su) niño para decir que tiene que ir al excusado?
How long does your child sleep at night?	¿Cuánto tiempo duerme tu (su) niño cada noche?
Does he/she wake up during the night?	¿Se despierta durante la noche?
Does he/she take a nap?	¿Toma una siesta?
Have you noticed anything unusual about his/her sleeping?	¿Has (Ha) notado algo raro de su dormir?
Is he/she sleeping more than usual? Less than usual?	¿Está durmiendo más de lo normal? ¿Menos de lo normal?
Has he/she had any unusual behavior?	¿Se ha portado de una manera rara?
Does your child suck his/her thumb?	¿Se chupa el pulgar?
Does your child bite his/her nails?	¿Se come las uñas?
Has he/she ever been hospitalized?	¿Ha sido hospitalizado? ¿Lo han internado?
Why was he/she hospitalized?	¿Por qué fue hospitalizado? ¿Por qué lo internaron?

Working with the Child

What is your name?	¿Cómo te llamas?
How old are you?	¿Cuántos años tienes?
I am your nurse.	Soy tu enfermera.
I am going to • take your temperature • take your blood pressure • listen to your heart • look in your ears • measure how tall you are • measure how much you weigh • give you your medicine	Voy a • tomarte la temperatura • tomarte la presión de sangre • escuchar el latido de tu corazón • mirarte en las orejas • medir qué tan alto eres • medir cuánto pesas • darte medicina
This is going to hurt a little.	Esto va a dolerte un poco.
Point to where it hurts.	Muéstrame donde te duele.
Tell me how it feels.	Dime cómo se siente.
Are you hungry?	¿Tienes hambre?
Are you thirsty?	¿Tienes sed?
Do you feel tired?	¿Te sientes cansado/cansada?
Do you have trouble seeing? Hearing?	¿Tienes dificultad de ver? ¿de oír?
Do you wear glasses?	¿Usas anteojos?

Answers to Workbook Questions

CHAPTER 1

NCLEX-Style Review Questions

1. d
   Rationale. Treatment advances for preterm infants have done the most to improve neonatal mortality statistics. Control of puerperal fever has helped improve maternal morbidity and mortality. Use of anesthesia during labor has led to the most births occurring in hospitals. Enforcement of strict rules in hospitals is generally not a helpful technique. If you had trouble with this question, review the section on Maternal–Infant Health Status.

2. b
   Rationale. The nursing process is a form of problem solving. Although using the nursing process may help contain costs, this is not a primary benefit. Oral communication and health teaching are two tools used in carrying out the nursing process, but these methods do not describe the entire process. If you had trouble answering this question, review the introductory material on the nursing process.

3. a
   Rationale. Data collection and physical assessment are all part of assessment. Planning includes goal setting and planning appropriate interventions. Implementation is the step in which the plan is carried out. Evaluation is the step in which the nurse determines whether or not goals and outcomes were achieved and whether or not the problem has been solved or the care plan needs to be revised. If you answered this question incorrectly, review the section on the steps of the nursing process.

4. c
   Rationale. Nursing care is carried out in the implementation step of the nursing process. Assessment includes data collection and establishing rapport with the patient. Planning includes goal setting and planning appropriate interventions. Evaluation is the step in which the nurse determines whether or not goals and outcomes were achieved and whether or not the problem has been solved, or the care plan needs to be revised. If you

answered this question incorrectly, review the section on the steps of the nursing process.

5. a, c, d, e
   Rationale. The critical pathway decreases cost, is followed by all members of the team, provides organization, and includes all treatments and procedures. It has no relevance on establishing a trusting relationship.

Critical Thinking: What Would You Do?

1. *Suggested answers:*
   a. Explain the CHIP program to the woman. She may not realize that there is a state-sponsored insurance program that charges her for her child's insurance on a sliding scale basis (based on family income). Although her child may not qualify for Medicaid, she will likely be able to purchase affordable insurance for the child's health care needs.
   b. Yes. She does have options. See answer above.

2. *Suggested answers:*
   Sociologic changes that have affected child health concepts and attitudes include the women's movement, with more women working outside the home, high divorce rates, leaving many children to be raised in single parent homes, and scientific and technological advances.

3. *Suggested answers:*
   Care of children in the 19th and early 20th century was usually in the home. Many times children did not survive into adulthood. Institutional care of children during this time period often was in unsanitary conditions; children were neglected, and they had poor nutrition. Children were in the same units, sometimes the same beds as adults. After World War I, in an effort to prevent infection, children were not picked up, were left in cribs draped with plain white sheets, and were not given toys or any environmental stimulus.

4. *Suggested answers:*
   Children are more secure and as a result usually happier and recover more quickly when they are in the presence of the individuals in their lives with

whom they have developed a sense of trust; in most cases these individuals are the child's caregivers. The presence of the caregivers also gives the nurse an opportunity to provide teaching that will benefit the child after discharge. Caregivers can give the child support in a threatening or uncomfortable situation.

CHAPTER 2

NCLEX-Style Review Questions

1. b
   Rationale. In a stepfamily a parent brings children from a previous relationship into a relationship with a new partner. If both partners in this new relationship bring children to this relationship, the family is known as a blended family. This often occurs with the increasing rate of divorce.
2. b
   Rationale. Primary prevention is a health-promoting activity that helps prevent the development of illness or injury. Teaching and disease prevention are major components of primary prevention.
3. a
   Rationale. Secondary prevention includes health-screening activities that aid in early diagnosis and encourage prompt treatment in an effort to reduce long-term negative effects. Secondary prevention might include working with a family or group of individuals to correct or prevent spread of a disease or continuation of a health issue or concern.
4. d
   Rationale. Tertiary prevention includes health-promoting activities that focus on rehabilitation and teaching to prevent additional injury or illness. Financial concerns and resources may be explored as a part of tertiary prevention for long-term health needs.
5. b
   Rationale. One positive aspect of caring for a family member, especially a child, in the home is that the child feels more comfortable in a familiar setting with a familiar person caring for him or her. The caregiver is more comfortable in the home setting as well. A home nurse often teaches and supports the family providing home care.
6. d
   Rationale. When doing teaching in a community-based setting, the nurse must know the needs of the audience to best be able to convey the information to the particular group of individuals. The nurse can then use appropriate teaching strategies and resources to teach the group.

Critical Thinking: What Would You Do?

1. *Suggested answers:*
   a. Caregivers are understandably concerned when the school behavior or emotional state of their child changes. They may feel guilty and responsible for these behaviors, especially in cases of divorce. In addition when a child has physical complaints, the caregivers may have anxiety regarding the cause of these concerns and often are fearful that something is seriously wrong with their child.
   b. The nurse would offer support to the parents; give them options and referrals to community resources, such as counseling services and support groups to help them explore the emotional effects of divorce on children. A complete physical exam would be important to rule out a physical cause for the symptoms the child is experiencing.
   c. To help a child adjust to divorce it is important that each parent spend individual time with the child, reassure the child that the divorce was not caused by the child or the child's behavior, and encourage the child to share his or her feelings about the situation.
2. *Suggested answers:*
   In teaching this family, it would be important to include information regarding phototherapy treatment for the infant, including purpose of treatment; safety factors involved with the treatment; procedure for carrying out the treatment; and follow-up appointments and care for the infant. You should also provide information about the illness of the 6-year-old child, including reviewing what has been done for this child to this point; recommendations for having the child seen by a care provider if she has not been seen; clarification of information and treatments this child's care provider has given the family if a provider has seen the child; follow-up needed for this child; preventive measures to reduce possibilities of further infection; and teaching regarding smoking in the home, including exploration with the parents about their understanding of the effects of smoking on their children and themselves, teaching regarding the effects of smoking on their children and themselves, and recommending community resources and support regarding smoking cessation.
3. *Suggested answers:*
   a. In teaching any group of individuals it is important for the nurse to know the age, educational level, ethnic and gender mix, language barriers, and previous teaching the group has had regarding the subject.

b. In presenting the lesson to these children, the nurse would review growth and development principles of this age child and plan the lesson to be at the appropriate level of understanding, as well as to include activities to enhance learning at their level of development. Keeping in mind the attention span of this age child when presenting the lesson would also be important.

CHAPTER 3

NCLEX-Style Review Questions

1. d

Rationale. The seminal vesicles contribute alkaline fluid and fructose to semen. The fructose is a simple sugar that provides energy for sperm movement. Bartholin glands provide lubrication to the vestibule in the female. Bulbourethral glands provide lubrication to the male urethra and add to the volume of semen. The epididymis is a coiled structure on top of each testis in which sperm mature. If this question was difficult for you, review the section on semen formation.

2. b

Rationale. The vagina has an acidic pH, an environment that is hostile to sperm. Therefore, semen has an alkaline pH, which protects sperm from the acid of the vagina. Testosterone is a testicular hormone that influences sperm development and maturation. The seminiferous tubules are the site within the testes in which male gametes are formed. If you had difficulty with this question, review the section on semen formation.

3. d

Rationale. The urinary meatus is found below the clitoris and is one of the structures of the vestibule. It is located above the vaginal opening (between the clitoris and vaginal opening). The true perineum is the structure found between the vestibule and anus.

4. d

Rationale. The isthmus is called the lower uterine segment during pregnancy. This is the thinnest area of the uterus, making it the most vulnerable site for uterine rupture.

5. c

Rationale. Estrogen stimulates regeneration and growth of the endometrial lining by stimulating blood vessel development. This is the hormone that most influences the proliferative phase of the endometrial cycle. FSH and LH are both anterior pituitary hormones that govern the hormone production of the ovaries. Progesterone is an ovarian hormone that most influences the secretory phase of the endometrial cycle.

Critical Thinking: What Would You Do?

1. *Suggested answers:*
   a. Because Doug wears tight jeans and works in a hot environment, his sperm count might be decreased. The formation and maturation of sperm require a temperature that is a little lower than body temperature. Tight clothing keeps the testes close to the body and increases the temperature.
   b. It would be helpful for Doug to find some looser clothing to wear during the hot days when he is working outside. His tight jeans could be saved for other occasions and for when the weather is cool.
2. *Suggested answers:*
   a. It would be helpful to know if Nancy is taking antibiotics for any reason. It would also be helpful to know if she uses tampons, deodorant-style sanitary napkins, or any type of highly perfumed substances near the vulva.
   b. The practice of douching and using products with deodorant on the external genitalia can change the pH of the vagina. Normally the pH is acidic, but if it becomes more alkaline, the protective function is lost. Nancy would be well advised to discuss the use of these products with her physician. Together they can come up with a plan to meet her hygiene objectives without compromising her reproductive health.

CHAPTER 4

NCLEX-Style Review Questions

1. d

Rationale. Female health screening recommends that the woman should have her first Pap smear 3 years after first intercourse or age 21 years, whichever comes first.

2. d

Rationale. The nurse would document that the woman reports menorrhagia, which refers to heavy or prolonged menstrual bleeding. Dysmenorrhea refers to difficult or painful menses. Metrorrhagia is irregular bleeding. Amenorrhea is absence of menses.

3. d

Rationale. Although medications can be helpful, other measures, including stress reduction and regular exercise, may have the most overall effect.

Prostaglandins, not infection, cause the symptoms of PMS, so antibiotics are not appropriate therapy for this disorder. Diuretics may be used to treat the bloating associated with PMS but are not necessarily the most helpful overall medications.

4. a

Rationale. Cloudy urine may indicate a bladder infection. This condition would need immediate evaluation and treatment by a physician to prevent complications. If she forgot to do Kegel exercises, the appropriate reply would be to go ahead and do them now. Urine escaping during coughing is a symptom associated with a cystocele but does not require immediate intervention. Pessaries should be removed periodically and washed. If the woman forgets to reapply it, then she should reinsert it when she remembers.

Critical Thinking: What Would You Do?

1. *Suggested answers:*
   a. Amanda can expect a detailed history and thorough physical examination to include a pelvic examination and Pap smear.
   b. Amanda is experiencing primary infertility. She and her husband have been trying for 2 years without success. One year of unprotected intercourse is enough to qualify for the diagnosis of infertility. It is primary infertility because Amanda has never before been pregnant.
   c. It may be helpful to point out to Amanda that many women wait until their late 30s to begin having children. This is a normal phenomenon of our culture. It may also help to explain that guilt feelings are a very normal response to initial infertility. Explain that the physician will work with Amanda and her husband to try to determine what the problem is and to do everything possible to help her have a child.

2. *Suggested answers:*
   a. A semen analysis requires that her husband obtain a sperm sample, usually by masturbation. If this is unacceptable to either of them, they may use a special condom to collect the sample during intercourse. It is important that all of the ejaculate be collected and placed into the sterile specimen cup provided for that purpose. The specimen must be delivered to the lab within 30 minutes of collection. The postcoital test involves determination of ovulation by using FAM techniques. Just before ovulation the couple should have intercourse without using lubricants. Amanda must go to the clinic 8 to 12 hours after intercourse; at the clinic, a sample of her cervical mucus will be collected for testing.
   b. ICSI is an advanced reproductive therapy used to treat infertile couples in whom the man has a low sperm count. A sperm sample is obtained through masturbation or testicular biopsy. One sperm is paralyzed by stroking the distal portion of its tail. An ovum is harvested from the woman, then the sperm is injected into the ovum, and the fertilized cell is placed into the woman's uterus.

3. *Suggested answers:*
   a. Hot flashes are caused by low estrogen levels and periodic surges of luteinizing hormone, but the physiology is not completely understood.
   b. The physician may recommend low dose HRT; although this is a controversial therapy. Other options include treatment with a progestin, certain antihypertensives, anticonvulsants, and antidepressants.
   c. Cindy should be careful to get adequate weight-bearing exercise. She may also increase her comfort by lowering the temperature in her house, wearing comfortable lightweight clothing in layers, and avoiding spicy foods, alcohol, and caffeine. She should continue taking calcium and vitamin D supplements. Vaginal estrogen creams and lotions can be used to treat vaginal dryness and decrease sexual discomfort. She should continue having mammograms annually.

CHAPTER 5

NCLEX-Style Review Questions

1. c

Rationale. A teratogen will have the most damage upon the developing embryo. During the pre-embryonic stage a teratogen will have an all-or-nothing effect. A teratogen can affect the developing fetus, but the effect will not be as damaging as a teratogen ingested during the embryonic stage. During the embryonic stage there is tissue differentiation and development of all the organ systems.

2. c

Rationale. The embryonic stage begins at the end of the 2nd week after fertilization and is complete at the end of the 8th week after fertilization. Before this time frame is the pre-embryonic stage, and after this time frame is the fetal stage.

3. d

Rationale. The chorionic villi project into the intervillous spaces, where they are surrounded by maternal blood that enters the spaces from the endometrial arteries. Nutrients from the maternal blood are transferred into the chorionic villi to be taken to the fetus, and waste products from the fetus are transferred into the maternal blood to be removed by the woman's body. They are anchoring villi that help to adhere the placenta to the decidua basalis, but their primary function is to exchange wastes for nutrients.

4. b
Rationale. The foramen ovale is a fetal shunt. The foramen primum and the septum secundum are cardiac structures but are not involved in fetal circulation. The ductus deferens is another name for the vas deferens located in the male. The two other fetal shunts are the ductus venosus and ductus arteriosus.

5. a
Rationale. Identical twins are also known as monozygotic and share the same chromosomal material. Fraternal twins are classified as dizygotic. Trizygotic refers to three zygotes.

Critical Thinking: What Would You Do?

1. *Suggested answers:*
   a. Rebecca is approximately 8 weeks' gestation. The fetus is approximately 1 inch long. All of the organs are formed. The heart is beating, extremities have developed, and facial features are discernible.
   b. Tylenol is generally not considered to be teratogenic and is safe to use during pregnancy in moderation. Explain that she is right to be concerned about substances that she ingests or is exposed to in the environment. Encourage her to consult with her physician before taking any type of over-the-counter medication.

2. *Suggested answers:*
   a. The fetus is 7 to 8 centimeters in length and weighs approximately 45 grams. It is possible to tell the sex of the fetus by looking at it. The heart beat should be audible with a Doppler. Offer to find the heart beat and let Rebecca listen to it.
   b. Explain to Rebecca that it may be difficult to tell if the twins are identical or fraternal until they are born. The physician may be able to give her an idea after looking at the sonogram. If there is only one amniotic sac and one placenta, then the twins probably are identical. If the sonogram shows that one is a boy and one is a girl, then it is clear the twins are fraternal. If an amniocentesis is done, it is possible to tell whether or not the twins are identical because identical twins share the same genetic material.

CHAPTER 6

NCLEX-Style Review Questions

1. b
   Rationale. Amenorrhea, nausea, and fatigue are all presumptive signs of pregnancy because they can be caused by many conditions other than pregnancy. Positive signs of pregnancy, such as sonographic evidence of a fetal outline, audible fetal heart sounds, and fetal movement felt by the examiner, confirm pregnancy because they cannot be attributed to other conditions. Probable signs of pregnancy, such as positive laboratory tests, ballottement, and Braxton Hicks contractions strongly suggest pregnancy.

2. d
   Rationale. Softening of the uterine isthmus is called Hegar's sign and is a probable sign of pregnancy. It is more objective than the presumptive signs; however, there are conditions, other than pregnancy, that can cause this sign, so it is considered probable, rather than positive. Chadwick's sign is a bluish/purple color to the vagina and cervix due to pelvic congestion. Goodell's sign is a softening of the cervix. All of these are probable signs.

3. b
   Rationale. At 16 weeks the uterine fundus should measure halfway between the pubic bone and umbilicus. At approximately 12 weeks the fundus is just above the pubic bone. At 20 weeks, it should be at the umbilicus.

4. a
   Rationale. During pregnancy a woman's caloric needs increase by approximately 300 calories per day. Five hundred extra calories are needed during lactation. Eating for two does not mean that the caloric intake should be doubled. This practice would result in too much weight gain and possibly lead to fetal macrosomia. The pregnant woman should not restrict calories during pregnancy.

Critical Thinking: What Would You Do?

1. *Suggested answers:*
   a. You should find Carla's fundus at the umbilicus.
   b. Yes. You should be able to easily find the heart beat with a Doppler device. In fact the heart beat should be detectable with a Doppler by 10 to 12 weeks.
   c. Carla is adapting well to her pregnancy. The 2nd trimester is generally a time when the woman enjoys being pregnant. The psychological task of this trimester is to accept the baby. She is progressing well toward that goal as evidenced by her preparations of the nursery.

2. *Suggested answers:*
   a. Carla is experiencing supine hypotensive syndrome.
   b. Immediately assist Carla to turn to her left side. Advise her not to lie flat on her back because this compresses the major blood vessels.
   c. Carla's weight gain is on track for a healthy pregnancy. Advise her to continue eating healthy, well-balanced meals.

3. *Suggested answers:*
   a. Vegans can get sufficient protein by paying careful attention to combining foods. Advise Monica to combine legumes with grains each day to meet her needs for complete protein. She can add fortified soy or rice milk to her diet, as well. Seeds and nuts are additional important sources of protein for Monica.
   b. Iron is necessary to build red blood cells. It is difficult for pregnant women to get enough iron from diet alone to meet the requirements. In addition, because Monica is a vegan, all her food sources of iron are from plant sources, which are less well absorbed than are animal sources of iron. Monica should continue to take her iron pills, or she is at risk for developing anemia.
   c. Carrot juice will not likely be harmful for her baby, even in fairly large amounts. Vitamin A from plant sources is in the form of beta carotene. The body converts this substance to vitamin A. Beta carotene is not as likely to be toxic as are megadoses of pre-formed vitamin A.

CHAPTER 7

NCLEX-Style Review Questions

1. a
   Rationale. Nagele's rule states to first add 7 days to the date of the LMP, then subtract 3 months, which would give a due date of October 17 of the current year.
2. d
   Rationale. The woman has been pregnant five times (current pregnancy, three living children, and one abortion). She had two children at term (T2), one preterm child (P1), one abortion (A1), and three living children (L3).
3. b
   Rationale. The woman is larger than expected for her dates. Normally the fundal height should measure 28 centimeters at 28 weeks. A sonogram is the best method to determine the likely cause of the discrepancy. A multiple marker screening test is a variation of the MSAFP test that is routinely offered to all women between 16 and 18 weeks' gestation. It is possible that the woman will need more frequent prenatal visits; however, before this plan is carried out, the cause of the discrepancy must be identified.
4. b
   Rationale. Group B streptococcus is a bacterium that often colonizes the vagina and rectum. It can cause serious neonatal infection if contracted during labor. All women are routinely screened for group B streptococcus after 35 weeks' gestation and before delivery, so that women who are positive can be treated with antibiotics during labor. It is no longer recommended that only women with risk factors be checked for group B streptococcus. If this question was difficult for you, review the section Subsequent Prenatal Visits.
5. d
   Rationale. Telling the woman to think it over and discuss it with her family and then providing support regardless of her decision is the most supportive answer. It also allows the woman time to discuss her options with her family before she makes a decision. It is not dangerous to the mother to carry a child with a chromosomal abnormality to term. Giving the mother advice one way or the other is not therapeutic. It is better to explain options and give information regarding the likely outcome for each available option.

Critical Thinking: What Would You Do?

1. *Suggested answers:*
   a. It is important to get a thorough history from Theresa. First explore with her the chief complaint. What symptoms is she having that lead her to believe that she is pregnant? In addition to the chief complaint, a history includes reproductive, medical–surgical, family, and social histories.
   b. Explain to Theresa that this is important information because the primary care provider will want to follow up more closely because she is at higher risk for gestational diabetes. Be certain to make the RN and the primary care provider aware of this information. Any part of the history that varies from expected should be reported.
   c. You will need to place the patient in a room with an examination table. You will need drapes, sterile gloves, speculum, a swab for the Pap test, a glass slide, fixative, and sterile lubricant.
2. *Suggested answers:*
   a. First you should instruct Amanda to do a fetal kick count. This is an objective way to measure if the baby is moving less than normal. If the baby

moves less than 10 times in 2 hours, instruct Amanda to come to the clinic to be checked.

b. The priority nursing assessment is to take the fetal heart rate (FHR). This assessment will give immediate feedback as to the status of the fetus. A normal FHR is between 110 and 160 bpm.

c. The BPP combines the NST and ultrasound measurements to predict fetal well-being. Instruct her that it is best for her to have a full bladder for the ultrasound examination. Tell her that the examiner will estimate the amount of amniotic fluid, count fetal movements, and observe fetal tone and respiratory movements. An NST will be done to determine if the fetal heart is reactive. A total score will be assigned, which will give the primary care provider information upon which to make treatment decisions. The NST is normally done by the nurse. The ultrasound portion of the examination is done by a trained radiology technician, the physician, or a specially trained nurse.

3. *Suggested answers:*
a. Both tests are invasive and carry risks. The advantage to CVS is that it can be performed earlier in the pregnancy (10 to 12 weeks versus 15 to 20 weeks for amniocentesis). Early diagnosis allows for treatment decisions to be made earlier in the pregnancy. Results are back within 7 to 10 days for CVS; whereas, amniocentesis results may not be available for 2 to 3 weeks. One disadvantage of CVS is that some authorities report a higher rate of spontaneous abortion after CVS than after amniocentesis. Another disadvantage is that because no amniotic fluid is withdrawn, neural tube defects might be missed; whereas, amniocentesis shows increased alpha-fetoprotein levels if a neural tube defect were present. Another disadvantage of CVS is that there is a small risk of placental mosaicism, which could indicate an abnormal fetus, even if the fetus were normal.

b. Explain to Rebecca that some women decide to proceed with genetic testing even if they will not consider abortion. The information gained can be used to research the disorder so that the parents can be better prepared to deal with it after birth. It also allows the primary care provider to determine treatment options other than abortion.

c. The fetus with thrombocytopenia can receive platelet transfusions via cordocentesis if the disorder is severe enough to warrant this therapy. Rebecca will be prepared as for an amniocentesis. Ultrasound will be used to locate the umbilical cord vessels. A needle is used to pierce the blood vessel and infuse platelets. This therapy will likely be done every week until delivery.

CHAPTER 8

NCLEX-Style Review Questions

1. c
Rationale. The powers are the only component that is unexpected at this time. Because she is dilated 4 centimeters, she is considered to be in active labor. In active labor the contractions are generally closer together and are of at least moderate intensity. The contraction pattern described in this scenario is likely to be inefficient, causing the labor process to slow. All of the other components are favorable to the progress of labor. The passageway is roomy. The passenger is in a good position, and the maternal psyche is relaxed, a state that makes coping with contractions less difficult.

2. b
Rationale. The most accurate answer is the one that explains that several factors work together to cause labor to begin. Telling the woman that it is a mystery is not entirely accurate because, although we don't have all the answers, scientists do have a partial understanding of the forces that affect labor. If there is a special hormone that signals labor to begin, it has not been discovered. Telling the woman not to worry about it is not therapeutic and dismisses her concern unnecessarily.

3. c
Rationale. The description fits that of a fetus in the right occiput anterior (ROA) position.

4. c
Rationale. This scenario describes the third stage of labor. The third stage begins just after the baby is born and lasts through delivery of the placenta. The first stage is from the beginning of cervical dilation to full dilation at 10 centimeters. The second stage begins with full dilation and ends with birth of the baby.

Critical Thinking: What Would You Do?

1. *Suggested answers:*
a. Although the bony passageway (the pelvis) is adequate to accommodate a vaginal delivery, if the soft tissue of the passageway (the cervix, in this instance) does not dilate, the fetus cannot travel through. If the cervix does not eventually begin to dilate, the baby will have to be delivered by cesarean section.

b. Because uterine contractions are the power that causes cervical dilation, an ineffective contraction pattern can be one cause of failure to dilate. Perhaps the contractions are too far apart, or they are not strong enough. Another possible explanation for failure to dilate is that the fetus is unusually large, so even if the pelvis is adequate for a normal size fetus, an abnormally large fetus may be too big to fit or may be in an unusual position. This situation could result in failure of the cervix to dilate. Another possible factor is that Anna might be tense, and she might be "fighting" the contractions. The fear-tension-pain cycle also can interfere with labor progress.

2. *Suggested answers:*
   a. Normally, the fetus starts out with the back of his head (his occiput) facing to one side of the maternal pelvis (either right or left occiput transverse). If he starts in an occiput transverse position, he must rotate so that the back of his head (the occiput) faces toward the front of the maternal pelvis, an anterior position. Because Anna's fetus is occiput posterior, the back of his head is positioned toward the back of Anna's pelvis. This means the fetus will have to rotate 180° or deliver face up.
   b. The labor likely will be longer and involve more back pain than would be the case if the fetus were occiput transverse or occiput anterior.

3. *Suggested answers:*
   a. From the description, it sounds as if Anna is entering the transition phase of labor, so the nurse will probably find that she is dilated between 8 and 9 centimeters.
   b. It would be helpful to explain to Anna's partner that her outburst is normal at this time because she is entering the most intense, but fortunately, the shortest phase of labor. The partner can continue to be supportive if he or she knows that Anna's behavior is expected and not to be taken personally.

4. *Suggested answers:*
   a. When a baby is delivered face up, the condition is recorded as "persistent occiput posterior."
   b. He will likely have molding and overriding sutures. Many lay people describe this condition as the baby having a "cone head." He may also have some soft tissue swelling known as caput succedaneum.
   c. Anna will probably be excited and want to hold the baby. She will likely explore his body with her fingertips and count his fingers and toes. The pain of contractions will be forgotten quickly.

CHAPTER 9

NCLEX-Style Review Questions

1. b
   Rationale. Rarely is there a pain-free labor. This woman needs to know that she will likely have some pain before she is far enough dilated to receive an epidural. Discussing pain relief options with the physician and childbirth educator indicates that the woman is taking responsibility for pain relief during labor. It would be appropriate to ask this woman if she has any additional questions about any of the options discussed. Practicing relaxation techniques and asking for IV pain medications are both appropriate actions.

2. a
   Rationale. Caregivers often underrate the woman's pain. Although observing for nonverbal indicators, taking the vital signs, and observing interactions with visitors may give clues as to whether or not the woman is experiencing pain, the only way to know for sure is for the nurse to directly ask the woman to describe her pain and to rate it. The nurse should not wait until the woman complains of pain before doing a thorough pain assessment because some women will attempt to endure the pain without complaining.

3. c
   Rationale. Each woman experiences labor pain in a unique way. The "best" method is the method that coincides with the woman's belief system and works for the woman. It is best to learn several methods because it is difficult to predict which method will be most beneficial for the woman until she actually experiences labor. Stating that an epidural is the best or that natural childbirth is best attempts to impose the nurse's beliefs about labor pain management on the woman. Stating that most women require some type of IV pain medication during labor is incorrect. Many women go through labor without IV pain medications.

4. b
   Rationale. Counter-pressure on the lower back and intradermal water injections are interventions that are specifically indicated for intense back labor. Intermittent labor support and reassurance that the pain is temporary are not particularly helpful for any type of labor pain. Effleurage and ambulation generally are more helpful in early labor and are not specific to back labor. Hypnosis and imagery require special training and are not specific to back labor.

5. d
   Rationale. An IV fluid bolus is given before epidural anesthesia to help prevent hypotension. Telling the woman that it is a routine procedure in preparation for an epidural does not adequately answer the question. It would be inappropriate for the nurse to slow the IV fluids simply because the woman complained that the fluids felt cold. IV hydration is not

given to prevent spinal headaches. If you had trouble with this question, review the section Epidural Anesthesia.

Critical Thinking: What Would You Do?

1. *Suggested answers:*
   a. You should advise Betty to take childbirth classes. It will be best if she chooses an instructor who teaches and has the woman practice relaxation techniques. She may want to attend a Lamaze or Bradley method class. Suggest that she ask about the use of a birthing ball. Recommend a doula. Research has shown that women are more successful with natural childbirth if they have continuous labor support, which a doula provides. Encourage her to pack lip balm and hard candy to treat and prevent dry lips and mouth. Suggest that she explore water therapy options.
   b. Explain to Betty that she may change her mind once she is in labor. Tell her that changing her mind is OK and does not represent a failure on her part. Many women attempt natural childbirth and then elect to use some type of analgesia or anesthesia. If her labor is prolonged or she requires oxytocin augmentation, she may need additional methods of pain relief.

2. *Suggested answers:*
   a. It may be helpful for Betty to ambulate or at least change positions frequently at this point in labor. Engaging in activities that distract her from the contractions may also be helpful. Slow chest breathing and effleurage probably will be helpful in coping with contractions. Using a focal point that she practiced in childbirth classes is often helpful at this stage of labor. Water therapy may be used, although many experts recommend waiting until a more advanced stage of labor to use this method.
   b. Your reply should be supportive of Betty's request. Give her encouragement about the progress she has made thus far. Remind her that IV analgesia won't completely relieve the pain, but it should take the edge off the pain and help her to relax between contractions, which may help her progress. Encourage her to use the call bell before attempting to ambulate after you administer the medication. Explain to her coach/partner that it is normal for her to sleep between contractions after IV analgesia.
   c. Again, your reply should be supportive of Betty's request. Explain that it is OK to change her mind and that you will contact the physician about her request. When you give report to the anesthesiologist, inform him or her that Betty

initially desired natural childbirth and that this is a change of plans for her. This information will be useful when the anesthesiologist interviews Betty for the epidural.

CHAPTER 10

NCLEX-Style Review Questions

1. b
   Rationale. The water running down the woman's legs is an indication that the membranes have ruptured. The fern test would confirm that the fluid is amniotic fluid versus urine.
2. c
   Rationale. The woman should not push until the cervix is dilated completely. Otherwise her cervix may swell, a condition that will slow the progress of labor. Blowing at the peak of contractions (when the urge to push is most intense) helps the woman not to push.
3. c
   Rationale. The woman is low risk, in active labor, and the monitor tracing is reassuring; therefore, her monitor strip should be evaluated every 30 minutes.
4. a
   Rationale. Intermittent auscultation is within the standard of care for low-risk laboring women, so it is appropriate to comply with the woman's request. She will need to be on the monitor for an initial 20-minute period to obtain a baseline recording of the FHR. Although many labor units prefer continuous EFM because intermittent auscultation takes more of the staff member's time, it would not be appropriate to deny the woman her request solely for this reason.
5. d
   Rationale. Amnioinfusion is done in an attempt to relieve cord compression when persistent variables are present, particularly if they are worrisome. The pattern described in answer d is worrisome because the fetal heart tones fall significantly (the variables are "deep") and they are occurring with each contraction.

Critical Thinking: What Would You Do?

1. *Suggested answers:*
   a. All admission assessments should be completed. This includes an evaluation of current labor status, an obstetric, medical–surgical, and social history, and determining desires/plans for labor and birth and for care of the newborn. Current

weight and vital signs should be obtained, and a vaginal examination should be done. A urine specimen is collected, and the EFM applied.

b. Because she is excited and talkative, it appears that Priscilla is in the latent phase of labor (early labor).

c. The cervix will most likely be dilated 1 to 3 cm and be partially effaced with a vertex at −1 to +1 station.

d. Breathing and relaxation techniques and the stages of labor can be reviewed with Priscilla and her husband. Once it is determined that the fetus is doing well per the monitor tracing, the nurse encourages Priscilla to ambulate. Distraction techniques work best during early labor. The nurse could suggest that Priscilla watch a favorite TV show, do crossword puzzles, or talk with friends on the telephone.

e. If the couple had not attended childbirth preparation classes, education about the birth process and what to expect would be appropriate. The nurse could teach a few breathing and relaxation techniques to the woman and her partner. Throughout labor, education and support are a priority. If the woman is extremely anxious, interventions would focus on helping her to cope with the particular phase/stage of labor that she is in. Explanations should be simple and to the point. Overly detailed explanations and instructions might increase her anxiety.

2. *Suggested answers:*
   a. Because Priscilla is dilated 5 cm, she is in the active phase of the first stage of labor. A woman is in active labor when the cervix is dilated from 4 to 8 cm.
   b. The nurse takes vital signs every 30 to 60 minutes. It is important for the nurse to evaluate hydration status by assessing the mucous membranes and intake and output. The nurse evaluates FHR and contraction pattern every 15 to 30 minutes.
   c. Priscilla and her husband are using a ritual to cope with contractions. It appears that the ritual is helping.
   d. The nurse offers comfort measures, such as ice chips and lip balm; a cool, damp washcloth for the forehead; back rubs; effleurage; and frequent perineal care and change of absorbent pads. It is important for the nurse to encourage Priscilla to void at least every 2 hours. Because the ritual is working, the nurse encourages the couple to continue using it. The nurse ensures privacy for the couple and keeps the environment quiet and nonstimulating. The nurse also periodically offers to take over the role of the coach for a few minutes so that Priscilla's husband can take a break.

3. *Suggested answers:*
   a. The practical nurse assists the RN to perform a vaginal examination. Priscilla's behavior indicates that she has probably reached the transition phase of labor.
   b. The nurse informs the couple of the results of the vaginal examination. The focus of interventions should be to help Priscilla relax between contractions. The nurse encourages the husband in his role as coach and reminds him that Priscilla's behavior is normal during the transition phase. It is important for the nurse and the husband to work together to help find the breathing and relaxation techniques that will help Priscilla cope with her labor. The nurse assists Priscilla to change positions and changes the under-buttocks pad frequently to keep her as dry and comfortable as possible.
   c. If Priscilla is able to relax between contractions, and her husband continues to be supportive, the nursing interventions have been effective.

4. *Suggested answers:*
   a. Take in a general overview of the situation, noting in particular the coping status of the woman and her partner. Assess the EFM tracing for FHR pattern and uterine contraction pattern. Palpate the uterine contractions. Check the IV infusion and site. Take the vital signs. Listen to lung and bowel sounds (remember this is your initial assessment). Determine time and amount of last voiding. Palpate the bladder for distention. Observe the perineum for bloody show, bleeding, and/or leaking of fluid.
   b. First note the frequency and duration of the pattern on the fetal monitor tracing. Then stand at Martha's side and place your hand on the fundus. Leave your hand on the fundus through at least two contractions. Note the intensity at the acme (peak) of the contraction (mild feels like tip of your nose, moderate feels like your chin, strong feels like your forehead). Determine if the uterus is completely relaxing between uterine contractions. Chart your findings in the labor record.

5. *Suggested answers:*
   a. The baseline is within the normal range and is reassuring. Early decelerations are occurring with each contraction. This pattern is benign. Therefore, the overall pattern is reassuring because there are no nonreassuring patterns.
   b. Report your findings to the charge nurse and ask if he wants to do a vaginal examination. Martha is showing signs that her labor is progressing (increased restlessness and bloody show); therefore, it is important to determine if she is close to delivery so that preparations can be made.

CHAPTER 11

NCLEX-Style Review Questions

1. d
   Rationale. Sutures used to repair an episiotomy are absorbable and do not need to be removed.
2. a
   Rationale. Providing a general explanation of the procedure is the only response that accurately represents the truth to the woman. Asking the doctor is not appropriate. It is not *always* better to have a vaginal delivery. There are times when a cesarean is preferred, but feeling tired of being pregnant is not one of those instances. Using "why" questions and saying "don't you know" are not usually therapeutic.
3. b
   Rationale. Although the procedure can be uncomfortable, it should not be outright painful. If the woman is experiencing too much pain, the physician will stop the procedure. Stating that the woman wants what is best for the baby and telling her that she will be fine with holding the nurse's hand are nontherapeutic responses.
4. b
   Rationale. The cervix must be dilated fully before forceps can be applied. Forceps are not necessarily dangerous. The physician will determine which instrument (forceps versus vacuum extractor) is best indicated for the situation, if any. In this case it is better to give some information rather than to make a blanket statement of "I don't know." The water bag must be ruptured before forceps can be applied.

Critical Thinking: What Would You Do?

1. *Suggested answers:*
   Amy needs to know that although a vaginal delivery is planned and expected, it cannot be guaranteed. There are many conditions that endanger the life of the woman, her fetus, or both that cannot always be anticipated and for which a cesarean delivery might become necessary. Amy needs encouragement to attend the class because she will be much better prepared to cope if she is prepared versus going into the situation completely uninformed.
2. *Suggested answers:*
   a. A Bishop score of 4 means that her cervix is unripe. It is unlikely that she will go into labor spontaneously within the next few days. It is also unlikely that her body would respond to an induction of labor unless cervical ripening procedures were used first.

   b. The physician would likely recommend that a cervical ripening procedure be used before induction of labor. Mechanical means include membrane stripping, and artificial dilation of the cervix using a balloon catheter or laminaria. Pharmacologic means include prostaglandins such as dinoprostone and misoprostol. Labor induction is more likely to be successful when cervical ripening is done first.
3. *Suggested answers:*
   You will need sterile gloves for the physician, a sterile swab, and a speculum. The test involves collecting a cervical secretion sample during a speculum exam and sending the sample to the lab for testing.
4. *Suggested answers:*
   You should notify the RN and/or the physician immediately and prepare for a cesarean delivery because it is likely Ellen has experienced a uterine rupture. It is imperative that the cesarean be done as quickly as possible to save the baby, as well as Ellen's life.

CHAPTER 12

NCLEX-Style Review Questions

1. c
   Rationale. Suture used to repair episiotomy is absorbable. It is helpful to let the woman know that she is not alone in her fear. This response helps build trust. Because sutures are not removed, telling the woman that she will feel pulling is incorrect information. Although emphasizing the importance of a follow-up checkup, this response is not the best answer because it could be construed as condescending and it does not take into account the woman's feelings. Telling the woman not to worry dismisses the woman's concerns and doesn't give her complete information.
2. c
   Rationale. A shaking chill shortly after delivery is a common occurrence. Placing pre-warmed blankets usually remedies the problem. Finishing vital sign measurement and then making a decision indicates that the nurse doesn't really know what to do. Notifying the RN immediately or summoning assistance is unnecessary because the woman is most likely experiencing a normal postpartum sensation. This is not an emergency situation.
3. a
   Rationale. The woman is experiencing respiratory depression from the narcotic that was given in the spinal anesthesia. It is appropriate to administer

naloxone (Narcan), which should be readily available. This medication is usually part of the preprinted or routine orders after this type of anesthesia. It is not appropriate to instruct her to breathe more rapidly because her respiratory drive is being suppressed artificially by the narcotic. Calling the anesthesiologist would be appropriate only if there were no orders, which is unlikely. Performing rescue breathing is too aggressive. The woman likely will have a good response to the Narcan.

4. c

   Rationale. Itching is common after spinal anesthesia in which a narcotic was administered. This is the likely cause of the itching. It is most appropriate for the nurse to inquire first to make sure the woman wants treatment. Benadryl would be the most appropriate first choice. Narcan is reserved for cases of severe itching that do not respond to Benadryl. The nurse shouldn't have to call the anesthesiologist because there is almost always an order available for treating this common occurrence. Observing and waiting is not the best choice. It is better to directly inquire regarding the woman's wishes and to let her know that treatment is available.

5. b

   Rationale. Cold is the treatment for breast engorgement when the woman is bottle-feeding. If she were breast-feeding, warmth would be appropriate. It is not appropriate to encourage a woman to breast-feed simply to treat breast engorgement, particularly after she has already made a decision to bottle-feed. It is also not helpful to empty the breasts of milk because this will simply stimulate more milk production.

Critical Thinking: What Would You Do?

1. *Suggested answers:*
   a. Heather probably fainted secondary to postural hypotension after getting up too quickly out of bed. Careful instructions by the nurse that Heather should be accompanied by the nurse the first time up and instructions to dangle her feet at the side of the bed for several minutes before getting up likely could have prevented this fall.
   b. Check her fundus, the lochia, and check for suprapubic distention. The fundus probably will be slightly boggy and deviated to one side. The lochia probably will be moderate to large, and you likely will find suprapubic distention.
   c. Assist Heather to the restroom to void. Run water. If possible have her place her hand in warm water. Give her privacy and time to empty her bladder. If noninvasive measures

don't work, you might have to catheterize her; however, it is best to avoid this if possible because of the increased risk for infection.
   d. You want to do a complete assessment to see if you can find a likely source of infection. Check the breasts for hard, reddened areas. Check the nipples for cracks. Check the lungs for congestion. Check the uterus to see if involution is progressing as expected. Endometritis can interfere with normal involution; it can also make the uterus tender to the touch. Check the lochia. Especially note the odor. A smell like rotting meat is associated with endometrial infection. Check the perineum for signs of infection at the episiotomy site.

2. *Suggested answers:*
   a. Grand multiparity and the difficult, prolonged labor put Marla at risk for uterine atony and subsequent hemorrhage.
   b. She is probably experiencing uterine atony. The first thing you should do is massage the uterus to try to get it to contract. Next you should increase the IV with added Pitocin, if available. Then call for assistance. Someone should take the vital signs. If the bleeding does not come quickly under control, someone needs to call the physician for further orders.

3. *Suggested answers:*
   a. You need to first inquire to find out where Mindy is hurting. There are several potential sources of pain, so you want to find out exactly where she is hurting so that you can better treat her pain.
   b. Incisional pain usually responds well to acetaminophen/narcotic combination products. Gas pain is best relieved by walking, then lying on the left side. Encourage Mindy to release the gas and not hold back because of embarrassment. Mylicon tablets are also helpful. Once you have tried all of these measures without relief, call the physician for an order for a suppository.
   c. First assess to see if there is swelling, redness, and warmth in the leg with the positive Homans' sign. Then report this finding to the RN in charge. This may indicate that there is thrombus formation.

CHAPTER 13

NCLEX-Style Review Questions

1. a

   Rationale. An infant born by cesarean delivery does not have the benefit of passing through the birth canal. Much of the fluid normally present in a fetus' respiratory tract is squeezed out while passing through the birth canal during a vaginal delivery. Surfactant develops in the lungs as the fetus matures. Its presence or absence is not associated with the method of delivery. An infant born by cesarean experiences sensory stimulation during birth, as does the infant born vaginally.

2. c

Rationale. Telling the mother that this is normal and showing how to clean the area reassures the mother and also teaches her how to deal with the leaking fluid. Although it is a normal finding, telling her "not to worry" is too dismissive of her concerns. Deferring to the charge nurse when you don't know is an acceptable strategy, but the nurse should be familiar with "witch's milk." Leaking fluid from the nipples is not a symptom of infection.

3. c

Rationale. The base of the cord should be dry without any redness. This finding could indicate that infection is present. Notify the charge nurse of the finding and carry out any orders that are given. Calling the doctor and asking for IV antibiotics is an over-reaction at this point. Additional assessment is needed. A dressing should not be applied unless the physician orders it. Showing the mother how to wash the area may falsely reassure her that this is a normal finding.

4. d

Rationale. The children running around the bassinet are creating air currents. The baby's blanket is loose, so he has probably lost some heat to convection. The damp T-shirt promotes heat loss by evaporation. Conduction occurs when heat is lost to a cold surface. This scenario does not indicate that the bassinet is cold and the room itself is warm. Radiation occurs when heat is lost to a nearby cold surface. The bassinet is located away from windows and doors, so radiation is not the most likely source of heat loss.

Critical Thinking: What Would You Do?

1. *Suggested answers:*
   a. The mottling and cool extremities indicate that the baby is likely cold. You should immediately wrap the baby in several blankets and make sure he wears a hat.
   b. Instruct the parents on the importance of keeping the baby warm. The baby should be snugly wrapped in blankets, or he should be skin to skin with his parents to avoid cold stress. In addition, the bassinet should be positioned away from windows and doors.

2. *Suggested answers:*
   a. The baby's skin is jaundiced. Jaundice in the newborn is usually caused by breakdown of red blood cells. The immature liver cannot handle the bilirubin released from the red blood cells.
   b. Because the baby's jaundice appeared on day 3 and not in the first 24 hours, it is most likely physiologic jaundice and usually does not indicate illness. However, all jaundice should be evaluated, so explain to Mary that you will report the condition to the pediatrician for follow-up.

3. *Suggested answers:*
   a. Explain to Mary that the baby is giving cues that he is sleepy. He has had enough interaction and needs rest. Reassure her that this does not indicate the baby is rejecting her. Rather, he is communicating a need in the only way he knows how. After he has rested, he will be ready to interact again.
   b. The blue-black spot is most likely a Mongolian spot. It should have been noted and described in the nursery. Reassure Mary that this is a birthmark and does not indicate maltreatment. Tell her that the mark will fade with time.

CHAPTER 14

NCLEX-Style Review Questions

1. b

Rationale. Ovulation can occur in the absence of menstruation and the woman who is exclusively breast-feeding can conceive, therefore she should use some form of contraception. The woman should be offered a nonhormonal type of contraception as a first choice while she is breast-feeding.

2. c

Rationale. Formula does not have the immunologic properties of breast milk. Although it is the woman's choice whether or not she wants to breast-feed, she should be informed before making her decision. The benefits of formula feeding are not equal to those of breast-feeding. The woman's economic status should not determine how the nurse responds to the woman's question.

3. a

Rationale. The position, latch, and sucking of the newborn are the priority assessments to be made during a feeding session. The nurse should assess the woman's support systems, but during a feeding session is not the most appropriate time to do so. An increase in lochia flow is a good indicator for effective newborn sucking. However, checking the woman's perineal pad during a breast-feeding session is inappropriate. The woman can verbalize if her flow has increased or if she has cramping. Before determining the need for a lactation consult, the nurse should first assess the newborn's feeding ability.

Critical Thinking: What Would You Do?

1. *Suggested answers:*
   a. First ask Sally some questions to see if she has had any prior exposure to breast-feeding. Then ask questions about Sally's feelings regarding breast-feeding. Explain to Sally the benefits of breast-feeding for both the woman and the newborn.
   b. Tell Betsy that the woman does not have to stop breast-feeding to return to work or school. She can pump at work, and the newborn's caregiver can feed her newborn the expressed breast milk. If she feels that she would be unable to pump at work, advise Betsy that the newborn gets multiple benefits from breast-feeding, even if it only lasts for several weeks. The baby still gets the antibodies from colostrum. Also, bonding is enhanced.
   c. Teach Elizabeth that the breasts do make milk after delivery in response to hormonal changes. To dry up the milk supply after delivery, she should wear a tight bra and avoid expressing any milk. Teach her to avoid warm water from a shower spraying on her breasts. She may experience some engorgement when the milk comes in, and it may be uncomfortable. Cold packs, a tight bra, and analgesics help to lessen the discomfort, and her body will stop making milk because none is being expressed.
2. *Suggested answers:*
   a. The colostrum that the newborn receives each time he or she breast-feeds provides enough calories. The newborn will not starve, and his frequent feedings will help to establish a good milk supply and help the woman's milk to come in.
   b. Ask Alicia how much the newborn is taking at a feeding and how often the newborn is feeding. She may be overfeeding or spacing the feedings too close together. Ask how much the newborn is spitting up and if it occurs with a burp or not. Also ask if there is a history of cow's milk allergies in Alicia's or the father of the baby's family. The newborn may need a specialty formula, if the pediatrician determines the newborn cannot tolerate a milk-based formula.
   c. Lanya should hold her newborn in the football hold or in the side-lying position. Both of these positions keep the newborn off of her abdomen. She can rest easier in the side-lying position while the newborn breast-feeds.
   d. Teach Tricia the three ways formula is available: ready-to-feed, powder, and concentrate. Ready-to-feed does not need to be mixed, but powder and concentrate need to be mixed according to package directions. She needs to wash all bottles and nipples before the first use and then after each use. Either hand washing or machine washing is acceptable. She does not need to sterilize the bottles.
   e. Breast milk is good at room temperature for as long as 10 hours, in the refrigerator for as long as 8 days, and if frozen in a deep freezer, as long as 6 months. After the milk has been thawed, it should be used within 24 hours.

CHAPTER 15

NCLEX-Style Review Questions

1. c
   Rationale. Baby Boy Alvarez gets a score of 2 for a heart rate greater than 100. All other parameters receive a score of 1 each, for a total score of 6. Apgar scores of 4 to 6 indicate moderate difficulty transitioning. Apgar scores of 1 to 3 indicate severe difficulty making the transition to life outside the womb. Scores of 7 or greater are associated with vigorous newborns.
2. b
   Rationale. The baby is large for gestational age. Although he could have problems in any of the areas listed, hypoglycemia is the likeliest cause of trouble for this baby initially.
3. c
   Rationale. He is most likely to lose heat by evaporation from his head. This situation could be prevented by thoroughly drying the head and putting a cap on the baby. Conductive heat loss occurs with direct contact with a cold surface. Putting him in skin-to-skin contact with his mother prevents this type of heat loss. Convective heat loss occurs through air currents. Covering the baby with a blanket helps prevent this type of heat loss. Radiation of warmth away from the baby to a nearby cold surface is not a likely source of heat loss at this time because the baby is skin to skin with his mother and covered with a blanket.
4. c
   Rationale. It is appropriate to ask to see identification from someone who is not wearing a name

badge. You do not want to provoke a possible kidnapper by threatening her in any way. Stating that the person must be the woman's sister makes an assumption that could very well be erroneous. When nurses make incorrect assumptions, it is easier for kidnappers to carry out their plans.

Critical Thinking: What Would You Do?

1. *Suggested answers:*
   a. Quickly dry the newborn to prevent chilling from evaporation while assessing his respiratory effort. Place him on his mother's bare chest and cover them both with blankets. Be sure to cover his head, as well as his body. In addition to respiratory effort, count the heart rate (taken from feeling the base of the umbilical cord), note muscle tone, reflex irritability, and color. Assign the Apgar score.
   b. The newborn may be suffering from hypoglycemia. He should be put to the breast immediately.
   c. The newborn will need erythromycin ointment placed in both eyes, and he will need a vitamin K injection.
2. *Suggested answers:*
   a. Use the bulb syringe to suction the mouth, then the nose.
   b. Use a suction catheter to suction secretions. Place the catheter down the back of the throat. Apply intermittent suction as you pull the catheter out with a steady motion.
3. *Suggested answers:*
   a. It is likely that the newborn is in pain.
   b. The nurse should try several comfort measures. Swaddling, holding, and rocking may be helpful. Allowing the newborn to suck on a pacifier, especially if a little sweetener is added, is comforting. Check the physician's orders for pain medication. It is appropriate to medicate newborns for pain.
4. *Suggested answers:*
   a. Reassure the mother that the yellow crust is a normal finding after a circumcision and indicates healing. Instruct her not to remove the crust. If redness, swelling, or foul-smelling discharge are noted, the baby should be seen by a physician because these are signs of infection.
   b. Reassure the mother that it is normal for babies to cry. Suggest some ways she might use to try to calm the baby. Walking, rocking, singing, and riding in a car are all good things to try. A pacifier might be helpful. Be sure that she knows it's OK to ask someone to help or for her to take a time out if she begins to feel frustrated.

CHAPTER 16

NCLEX-Style Review Questions

1. b
   Rationale. Most adults do not develop type 2 DM until middle adulthood. Most women who enter pregnancy with DM have type 1 DM.
2. b
   Rationale. Persistent rales in the bases of the lungs are most frequently the first indication of impending heart failure. Blood pressure changes and wheezing are usually not associated with heart failure.
3. a
   Rationale. Infection can trigger a crisis. Staying well hydrated, getting plenty of rest, and avoiding infection can help the pregnant women with sickle cell anemia avoid a crisis.
4. d
   Rationale. Multiple bruises in various stages of healing should raise a strong suspicion of IPV. Typically the woman would display possible suspiciousness or anxiety. Bilateral pedal edema may be a typical discomfort associated with this stage of the woman's pregnancy. A small bruise on the thigh is not highly suggestive of abuse.

Critical Thinking: What Would You Do?

1. *Suggested answers:*
   a. The oral glucose tolerance test. At least two of the following parameters were found: fasting blood sugar greater than 95 mg/dL, 1 hour postprandial blood sugar greater than 180 mg/dL, 2 hour postprandial greater than 155 mg/dL, or 3 hour postprandial greater than 140 mg/dL.
   b. History of a large-for-gestational-age infant, history of GDM, previous unexplained fetal demise, advanced maternal age (greater than 35 years), family history of type 2 DM or GDM, obesity (greater than 200 pounds), non-Caucasian ethnicity, fasting blood glucose of greater than 140 mg/dL, and random blood glucose of greater than 200 mg/dL
   c. Monitoring and maintaining strict blood sugar control, diet and exercise, fetal surveillance, and preventing infection
2. *Suggested answers:*
   a. Pregnancy has variable effects on asthma. Sometimes it gets worse. Sometimes it gets better. And sometimes there is no change.
   b. A teaching plan should include the following points: continuing the use of asthma medications; avoiding over-the-counter medications unless the woman has talked with the physician about using them; identifying and protecting

herself from asthma triggers; avoiding cigarette smoke, exposure to animals, and dusty, damp environments; staying inside in air-conditioned surroundings during pollen seasons and when the pollution or mold index is high; wearing mask or scarf over mouth on excessively cold days to help warm the air; protecting self from colds and flu because respiratory infections can trigger acute asthma attacks (avoiding crowds where viruses may be prevalent; washing hands frequently; and obtaining the flu shot if you have moderate or severe asthma); avoiding foods or chemicals that might have caused a reaction in the past, such as sulfites or MSG; continuing to take allergy shots; monitoring peak expiratory flow rate (PEFR) regularly; developing a crisis management plan in consultation with the physician; and being able to recognize warning signs, such as lack of rapid improvement when taking rescue medications, improvement not sustained, condition worsens, episode is severe, fetal movement decreases, and other warning signs of an impending attack, possibly including headache, itchy throat, sneezing, coughing, or feeling tired.

3. *Suggested answers:*
   a. The most common method of transmission is unprotected sexual intercourse with an infected partner. Risk factors include blood transfusions, sharing needles, and multiple sex partners.
   b. The two priority goals for Rachel's care are to prevent progression of her disease and prevent perinatal transmission to her fetus.
   c. The physician most likely will prescribe oral zidovudine (ZDV) therapy.
   d. The best way to protect an unborn child from HIV (when the mother is HIV-positive) is for the mother to take zidovudine throughout pregnancy, deliver by cesarean section at 38 weeks' gestation, and avoid breast-feeding and administer zidovudine to the newborn infant.
   e. It would be wise for her to have her other children tested. Although she may have tested negative during her last pregnancy, it can take time after exposure for a person to test positive. Having the children tested would relieve her of unnecessary worry.

CHAPTER 17

NCLEX-Style Review Questions

1. d
   Rationale. Although the woman has a history of habitual or recurrent abortion (she has been preg-

nant four times and has never carried a pregnancy to term), the cramps and spotting in the presence of a closed cervix are consistent with a diagnosis of threatened abortion. Symptoms of an ectopic pregnancy often begin before the patient knows for certain that she is pregnant. It is unlikely that she would carry the pregnancy for 12 weeks, if it were not implanted within the uterus (e.g., if it were a tubal pregnancy, the tube already would have ruptured). The pain and closed cervix are inconsistent with a diagnosis of incompetent cervix.

2. c
   Rationale. The woman has an elevated blood pressure. The abdominal pain could be epigastric pain associated with preeclampsia, or it could be pain from a placental abruption. Because her pulse is elevated and she is restless and diaphoretic with dark, red vaginal bleeding, she should first be assessed for signs of placental abruption. This condition presents the greatest immediate danger to mother and baby. The fetal heart tones will give information on the status of the fetus, and palpating the fundus will allow for assessment of uterine irritability, rigidity, tenderness, and/or contractions. Any other assessments would take lower priority.

3. c
   Rationale. The "clumps" in the vaginal discharge probably are pieces of swollen villi being expelled. This finding would be consistent with a molar pregnancy (gestational trophoblastic disease). Bright red painless vaginal bleeding is associated with placenta previa. Brisk deep tendon reflexes occur with preeclampsia, and shoulder pain is most often associated with ectopic pregnancy. Painful uterine contractions occur with labor or placental abruption, and nausea is a nonspecific symptom.

4. b
   Rationale. Limiting fluids with meals will aid in retention of food. The woman with hyperemesis gravidarum should nibble on carbohydrates. Food with high fat content might actually increase feelings of nausea. It is best for a person with nausea to stay away from strong food odors. If possible, someone else should do the cooking, and the food should be served in a pleasant, well-ventilated area. Antiemetics should be given 30 minutes before meals, not after meals.

Critical Thinking: What Would You Do?

1. *Suggested answers:*
   a. The nurse should inquire to see if Maria is experiencing headache, blurred vision, and spots before her eyes, or epigastric pain. Her history of

sudden weight gain and elevated blood pressure raise the suspicion that she is developing preeclampsia. Any woman suspected of having preeclampsia should be asked regarding headache, visual disturbances, and abdominal or epigastric pain. A "yes" answer to any of these parameters is a warning sign that she may soon have a convulsion.

b. Maria's blood pressure should be checked again after lying on her left side for several minutes. Both pressures are recorded. In addition to a complete head-to-toe assessment, Maria's lungs should be auscultated carefully, deep tendon reflexes should be checked for briskness, and the presence of clonus should be determined. The amount of edema is noted and the urine is screened for protein.

c. She is likely to be placed on bed rest in the hospital with orders for a preeclampsia lab workup and a 24-hour urine for protein.

2. *Suggested answers:*
   a. Maria should be placed in a quiet room with the lights dimmed to decrease sensory stimulation. Seizure precautions should be implemented. The side rails should be up and padded with pillows or blankets. Suction and oxygen equipment are set up and checked to see that each is working. These precautions are taken to help prevent seizures or to intervene quickly to prevent injury if a seizure were to occur.

   b. If Maria has preeclampsia, it is likely that the 24-hour urine specimen will have at least 300 grams of protein. She may have a decreased creatinine clearance and an elevated BUN and creatinine, although these findings are usually associated with severe disease. The hematocrit will likely be elevated because of hemoconcentration, and the platelets will be low or on the low side of normal. In mild preeclampsia, liver enzymes should not be elevated and the coagulation profile should be normal. However, if severe disease is present, liver enzymes will be elevated and the bleeding time prolonged.

   c. The private room is ordered and visitors are limited to decrease sensory stimulation. Bright lights, loud noise, and frequent movements associated with frequent visitors may precipitate a seizure.

3. *Suggested answers:*
   a. Fetal kick counts should be done after every meal; NSTs are done at least twice weekly; and biophysical profiles, sonograms, and amniocentesis are done as ordered.

   b. Record FHR and vital signs at least every 4 hours. Auscultate lungs every 2 to 4 hours to detect evidence of developing pulmonary edema. Ask regarding the presence of headache,

visual disturbances, or epigastric pain with each assessment. Check deep tendon reflexes and clonus every 4 hours. Institute seizure precautions. Maintain strict input and output and report output of less than 120 cc every 4 hours.

c. "Mild" is a term used to differentiate two levels of preeclampsia. However, this is a serious condition that requires continuous monitoring. The condition will not go away until the baby is delivered; therefore, hospitalization should continue for the safety of mother and baby. In addition, the disease can progress rapidly. If progression is noted promptly, seizure activity may be averted. The risk is that she could not make it to the hospital in time to prevent seizures if she were to self-monitor at home.

4. *Suggested answers:*
   a. Maria now has signs of severe preeclampsia.
   b. Maria's lungs should be auscultated. She should be asked regarding the presence of epigastric pain. Deep tendon reflexes and clonus are determined. After the assessment, the charge nurse and physician should be immediately notified of the findings.
   c. Maria will now be on strict bed rest. An IV will be inserted, if she does not already have access. A Foley catheter may be ordered to monitor hourly outputs. The nurse should anticipate an order for magnesium sulfate. Labor will probably be induced soon.

CHAPTER 18

NCLEX-Style Review Questions

1. d

   Rationale. Prolonged rupture of membranes, prolonged labor, and maternal fever place the newborn at risk for neonatal pneumonia. ABO incompatibility relates to the woman's and newborn's blood types. You were not given this information in the scenario. Fistula formation and pelvic floor injury are maternal injuries that can result from prolonged or difficult labor.

2. c

   Rationale. Prolonged labor characterized by back pain is most frequently caused by an occiput posterior position of the fetus. Although breech position, fetal macrosomia, and nongynecoid pelvis can cause labor dystocia, the only one characterized by back labor is occiput posterior position.

3. a

   Rationale. Because this woman has a history of preterm birth, she is at very high risk of delivering prematurely again. Although it may be appropriate for her to have hydration and to lie on her left side, she should come into the hospital to be monitored. The sooner she comes in, the sooner treatment can begin. The goal is to delay birth for as long as possible to allow the fetal lungs time to mature.

4. c
Rationale. Flexing the woman's thighs is called McRoberts maneuver. This is an appropriate nursing intervention for shoulder dystocia. Rescue breathing is not appropriate. Fundal pressure is contraindicated. Watching the monitor for signs of fetal distress is not indicated because the fetal head has already been delivered. The priority is assisting the woman to deliver the body. If you had difficulty with this question, review the section Shoulder Dystocia.

Critical Thinking: What Would You Do?

1. *Suggested answers:*
Basically Julia has three options. The physician can attempt to turn the baby using a version procedure; a cesarean delivery can be planned; or, if the physician agrees, Julia can be allowed a trial of labor with a vaginal breech delivery. It is important to remember that not all physicians will perform a vaginal breech delivery. It would be important to know this information before discussing Julia's options with her.

2. *Suggested answers:*
   a. Even though labor is not going to be induced at this time, it is important that Julia and her husband stay in the hospital. Research has shown that women with PROM do better when they are monitored in the hospital versus going home and coming back into the hospital when contractions begin.
   b. Monitor the fetal heart rate as ordered by the primary care practitioner. Be alert for sudden deep variable decelerations of the fetal heart rate that might indicate a prolapsed umbilical cord. Take the woman's temperature at least every 2 hours. Monitor for signs of infection, such as temperature elevation, fetal or maternal tachycardia, and cloudy or foul-smelling amniotic fluid.
   c. Preterm PROM requires expectant management, usually on bed rest, unless there are signs of infection, in which case the fetus will be delivered. Otherwise, administer antibiotics as ordered. Explain pelvic rest to the woman and help her stay on bed rest, as ordered. Do not perform vaginal examinations unless specifically ordered to do so by the primary care practitioner. Instruct the woman to perform fetal kick counts after every meal. Assist the RN to perform daily NSTs, as ordered. Give intramuscular

injections of corticosteroids to hasten fetal lung maturity, as ordered. Other interventions are carried out in the same manner as that used for the woman with term PROM.

3. *Suggested answers:*
Report these findings to the RN right away. The RN will perform a thorough assessment and call report to the physician. An ECG may be ordered. You may have to withhold the next dose of terbutaline, or the physician may decide to try a different tocolytic.

CHAPTER 19

NCLEX-Style Review Questions

1. b
Rationale. The signs and symptoms are those most closely associated with endometritis. Mastitis would involve a localized area of redness on the breast. Subinvolution may occur with endometritis, but the symptoms listed indicate infection. An episiotomy infection probably would not involve such a high fever, and abdominal pain usually is not associated with this diagnosis.

2. c
Rationale. The first action would be to raise the head of the bed. This action may help the woman be able to breathe better. Oxygen should be administered by face mask, not by nasal cannula. Blood gas analysis may be appropriate, but this is not the priority. Telling the woman that she doesn't need to worry is not therapeutic. The woman is in distress.

3. d
Rationale. The only observation of concern is the one in which the woman refers to her baby as "it" and speaks negatively of her crying all the time. These observations may indicate that malattachment is occurring. Actively participating in the newborn's care, comparing the newborn's characteristics with those of a family member, and anticipating discharge indicate positive responses.

4. b
Rationale. A woman who experiences a large amount of bleeding may be experiencing postpartum hemorrhage and is at risk for injury. Changes in vital signs, particularly her blood pressure and pulse, may indicate shock. In this case it would not be appropriate to allow her to ambulate. In addition, complaints of dizziness increase the risk that she might fall. Although it is important to assess attachment, lochia color, degree of responsiveness or level of orientation, fundal location, and support systems, these are not the priority assessments in a

woman experiencing a large amount of vaginal bleeding. Obtaining height would be inappropriate. A complete blood count may be ordered later to evaluate the woman's extent of bleeding.

Critical Thinking: What Would You Do?

1. *Suggested answers:*
   a. Josie is not responding to the baby's cues and is ignoring the crying. These signs along with her age put Josie at risk for malattachment with her baby. You need to evaluate for other signs of malattachment, such as turning away from the baby, not interacting or talking to the baby, or making negative comments.
   b. You should pick up the baby and comfort her. Role model healthy behaviors to Josie and encourage her to interact with the baby. Give her positive feedback when she interacts positively with the baby. Teach Josie how to read the baby's cues. You should involve social services or a clinical psychologist in the discharge planning process.
2. *Suggested answers:*
   a. Tiffany's bladder is probably full. First massage the fundus, and then assist Tiffany to empty her bladder.
   b. If the fundus remains firm and in the midline, but a steady flow of lochia is noted despite fundal massage, Tiffany may have a laceration. Notify the primary care provider of your suspicions because the laceration may require repair. Continue to monitor vital signs and bleeding.
3. *Suggested answers:*
   a. The woman may have an incisional infection. Take the woman's temperature, and then call the primary care provider for additional orders.
   b. Assess any hardened areas for redness, warmth, and tenderness. Instruct the woman to breast-feed frequently and completely empty the affected breast with each feeding. Warm compresses immediately before breast-feeding will help the milk to let down. In addition, it may help to massage the hardened area while the baby is suckling to help unclog the duct. She should use careful handwashing and get plenty of rest.

CHAPTER 20

NCLEX-Style Review Questions

1. d
   Rationale. Based on the Ballard scoring tool, bald areas, plantar creases covering the sole, and 3- to 4-mm breast buds are characteristics found in an older gestational age newborn. Abundant or absent lanugo, flat areola, flat pinna, anterior transverse plantar crease, ear recoil, few scrotal rugae, transparent skin, and prominent clitoris are findings associated with a younger gestational age newborn.
2. c
   Rationale. Maternal diabetes is the most widely known contributing factor for newborns who are LGA. Having no other children and gaining little weight during pregnancy are not associated factors contributing to the size of the newborn. A history of smoking during pregnancy is a contributing factor for newborns who are SGA (small for gestational age).
3. b
   Rationale. The preterm newborn may experience thermoregulation problems (difficulty maintaining body temperature), and as a result, the newborn may develop hypothermia. Therefore, monitoring body temperature would be a priority. Although repositioning every 2 hours, promoting rest between procedures, and recording urinary output would be important, these interventions would not be as high a priority as monitoring the newborn's temperature.
4. c
   Rationale. The newborn of a mother who abused cocaine during pregnancy would most likely experience withdrawal symptoms, including tremors, restlessness, hyperactivity, disorganized or hyperactive reflexes, increased muscle tone, sneezing, tachypnea, vomiting, diarrhea, disturbed sleep patterns, a shrill high-pitched cry, and commonly, feeding problems. Above average weight is not associated with newborns born to cocaine-using mothers. Normally, a newborn sleeps for the majority of hours in a day. However, the newborn of a cocaine-using mother most likely would experience disturbed sleeping patterns. Facial deformities are associated with fetal alcohol syndrome.
5. a, c, d, f
   Rationale. Preterm newborns typically exhibit thin extremities with little muscle or subcutaneous fat, a disproportionately large head and abdomen, visible veins in the abdomen and scalp, and soft, pliable ears with minimal cartilage. In addition, the skin is thin, relatively translucent, and usually wrinkled, and the newborn has plentiful lanugo over the extremities, back, and shoulders.

Critical Thinking: What Would You Do?

1. *Suggested answers:*
   a. The nurse needs to support this mother by listening to her, spending time with her, and answering any questions she has. The nurse

needs to reassure this mother that she did not cause the infant's bilirubin to be elevated and that the condition can be treated.

b. The purpose of the phototherapy is to use special lights to help reduce bilirubin levels.

c. While the infant is under the lights, the infant's eyes will be covered and he will be nude. The infant may have skin rashes; loose, greenish stools; increased temperature; loss of water; and priapism (a perpetual abnormal erection of the penis).

2. *Suggested answers:*

a. No amount of alcohol is believed to be safe, and women should stop drinking at least 3 months before they plan to become pregnant.

b. Fetal alcohol syndrome is often apparent in newborns of mothers with chronic alcoholism and sometimes appears in newborns whose mothers are low to moderate consumers of alcohol.

c. The infant with fetal alcohol syndrome may have low birth weight, smaller length and head circumference, short palpebral fissures (eyelid folds), reduced ocular growth, and a flattened nasal bridge.

d. The child's growth may be slow and his or her mental development may be retarded.

CHAPTER 21

NCLEX-Style Review Questions

1. d

Rationale. The balance of formation and absorption of cerebrospinal fluid found within the ventricles and subarachnoid spaces of the cranial cavity is disturbed in hydrocephalus, thus causing an increase in the head circumference of the child. A sac protruding on the lower back suggests a neural tube defect. Normal respiratory rates for newborns range from 30 to 50 breaths per minute. Gluteal folds higher on one side might suggest developmental hip dysplasia.

2. b

Rationale. The newborn with tetralogy of Fallot has a decreased oxygen saturation and thus has cyanosis, dyspnea, and tachycardia. The child is easily fatigued and often cannot expend enough energy to eat enough to have normal growth and development. Spina bifida, congenital rubella, and hip dysplasia are not associated with these findings.

3. b

Rationale. After repair of a cleft lip and cleft palate, the risk for infection is high. Therefore the nurse's priority would be to monitor the incision and

repair site closely for signs of infection, such as redness or drainage at the incision site, and keep the suture line clean and free of infection, thereby promoting optimal healing without scarring. Although documenting the time period the restraints are on and off, teaching the caregivers about dental care and hygiene, and providing sensory stimulation and age-appropriate toys are important, these are interventions appropriate for any newborn who has had a cleft lip/cleft palate repair but would not be the priority at this time.

4. a

Rationale. Promoting skin integrity and monitoring closely for any signs of skin irritation or breakdown are important in a child with any type of cast, but especially for the child with a spica cast because of the size of the cast and possible soiling from urine or bowel elimination. Changing bedding and clothing every 4 hours, weighing every morning and evening using the same scale, and monitoring temperature and pulse every 2 hours would not necessarily be included in the plan of care for the newborn who has a hip spica cast.

5. a, b, d

Rationale. Antibiotics may be given to prevent possible infection, and the child is monitored closely for any signs of infection. Before surgery, the sac is kept moist and covered to prevent the sac from becoming dry. A prone, not supine, position is maintained to prevent injury to the sac. The dressing is changed every 2 hours to keep it moist.

Critical Thinking: What Would You Do?

1. *Suggested answers:*

a. The nurse offers support and acceptance of this mother by staying with her, putting a hand on her shoulder or gently touching her, and either staying silent or using therapeutic statements to show acceptance of this mother's feelings.

b. The mother might be feeling sadness, guilt, a feeling of loss of having the "perfect" child, and fear of the child's future.

c. The nurse might respond with a comment such as, "this must be difficult for you." After the mother has had time to adjust to the appearance of her child, the nurse can further support her with more information about the correction that can be done.

2. *Suggested answers:*

a. Hydrocephalus occurs when there is an imbalance of the amount of cerebrospinal fluid being formed and the amount being reabsorbed. The child has an excess of cerebrospinal fluid in his cranial cavity. This can happen because of a blockage, an obstruction, or an injury or infection.

b. Cody will have a tube placed just under the skin in his head to drain the excess fluid from his brain into his peritoneal cavity, where it will be absorbed. If untreated, the outcome is poor and can result in death.

c. Cody will need continued follow-up care and shunt revisions, but depending on the cause, treatment, brain damage sustained, and complications, children can lead relatively normal lives.

3. *Suggested answers:*
   a. The infant weighs 4.5 kg.
   b. The low dose would be 4.5 mg.
   c. The high dose would be 9.9 mg.

CHAPTER 22

NCLEX-Style Review Questions

1. a
   Rationale. In the sensorimotor phase, the newborn desires physical satisfaction. The movements are reflex responses, and the infant uses all of the senses. The preoperational phase is typical of the end of the toddler period. The concrete operational phase characterizes the early school-aged child. The formal operational phase characterizes the adolescent stage of growth and development.

2. b
   Rationale. The toddler who is developing autonomy wants to feel in control and to perform tasks independently. This would be indicated by the toddler walking alone around the room. Crying when the caregiver leaves suggest possible separation anxiety. Showing off to gain attention and competing when playing games are not behaviors suggesting autonomy.

3. c
   Rationale. Telling the child that the caregiver would be back after lunch gives the child a reference point with which he or she is familiar. The preschool-aged child does not have a concept of time. To understand when something is going to happen, the preschool child needs a familiar frame of reference. The statements about the child always wanting her own way, not knowing that she has done something wrong, and asking about why the child won't play with others do not reflect the typical developmental aspects associated with preschoolers.

4. d
   Rationale. The child's statement reflects the developmental task of industry. The school-aged child interacts and competes with others and likes activities

he or she can follow through to completion and see tangible results. The development of trust is seen in the infant, autonomy is developed in the toddler, and initiative develops during the preschool age.

5. d
   Rationale. The adolescent develops a sense of being independent but still needs the caregivers to listen and support her or him. Therefore, communication is absolutely essential. Although responding to physical needs, praising the child's actions, and accepting the child's defeats are important responses for the caregiver to give all children, open communication with the adolescent would be *most* important.

6. b, c, d, f
   Rationale. The child who is 4 to 6 years of age is in the phallic stage according to Freud, the stage of initiative versus guilt according to Erikson, the preoperational phase according to Piaget, and the preconventional level according to Kohlberg. The infant is in the oral stage, according to Freud, and the older toddler is in the preoperational stage according to Piaget.

7. Using the growth chart in Appendix G, the child falls into the 75th percentile for height and the 50th percentile for weight.

Critical Thinking: What Would You Do?

1. *Suggested answers:*
   a. The purpose of plotting a child's growth on a growth chart is to provide a concrete measurement of the child's growth, note patterns, and recognize deviations to identify medical issues and concerns.
   b. The child's measurements are taken and plotted each time the child has a well-child or sick-child visit.
   c. As the child is monitored and growth plotted, a pattern of normal growth usually is noted.
   d. Developmental screening offers information regarding any delays in what is considered a standard or normal pattern.

2. *Suggested answers:*
   a. Genetics influences growth and development in that the genetic makeup of each child helps determine characteristics such as the child's gender, race, eye color, height, and weight. Genetics also has a major effect on the overall development of the child.
   b. Nutrition has a major effect on the health and development of the child to resist infection and diseases.
   c. Environmental factors that influence a child's development include family structures, socioeconomic level, supervision of the child, and the use of play in the child's environment.

CHAPTER 23

NCLEX-Style Review Questions

1. b

   Rationale. Typically the infant doubles the birth weight by the age of 6 months and triples it by the age of 1 year.

2. a

   Rationale. At 4 months the infant is able to grasp an object with both hands and bring the object to his or her mouth. Holding a bottle well, trying to pick up a dropped object, and transferring an object from one hand to the other are behaviors typical of an infant older than 4 months of age.

3. a

   Rationale. The posterior fontanel usually closes between the 2nd and 3rd months of life.

4. c

   Rationale. The lower central incisors are the first deciduous teeth to erupt and do so between 6 and 8 months of age. The first molars erupt at approximately 13 to 19 months; upper lateral incisors typically erupt at approximately 9 to 13 months; and the cuspids erupt at about 16 to 23 months.

5. a

   Rationale. Taking the apical pulse with a pediatric stethoscope and counting the rate for a full minute is the most accurate way to obtain the heart rate on an infant.

6. 810 cc

   Rationale. The infant's fluid intake would include: Pedialyte 4 oz (120 cc), dilute apple juice 3 oz (90 cc), iron-fortified formula 8 oz (240 cc), iron-fortified formula 5 oz (150 cc), and iron-fortified formula 7 oz (210 cc). The other items (rice cereal, applesauce, yogurt, and strained vegetables) would be documented as solid food intake but would not be included as fluid intake.

Critical Thinking: What Would You Do?

1. *Suggested answers:*
   a. The 6-month-old will have doubled her birth weight, have lower central incisors or be teething, plays peekaboo, holds a bottle well, sits alone in a high chair, and makes babbling sounds.
   b. The child should receive DTaP, Hib, and IPV immunizations.
   c. At 6 months the child should have begun eating solid baby foods, especially foods that provide iron in the diet.
   d. A review of safety, including the use of car seats, not leaving the child unattended, choosing toys carefully to reduce the possibilities of choking,

and checking the household closely for potential safety concerns would be important to discuss with this father.

2. *Suggested answers:*
   a. The infant should not be permitted to take a bottle of formula, milk, or juice to bed because of the concern of the condition called "bottle mouth."
   b. A bottle of plain water or a pacifier can be used if the child needs the comfort of sucking at bedtime.

3. *Suggested answers:*
   a. The extrusion reflex has the effect of pushing solid food out of the infant's mouth so it may appear the child is spitting out the food. This action decreases as the child learns the skill of eating solid food.
   b. Foods should be given in small amounts, be thin, lukewarm, and bland. One new food at a time should be added to the diet. When teeth begin erupting, foods such as zwieback, specifically made for chewing, are offered.

CHAPTER 24

NCLEX-Style Review Questions

1. c

   Rationale. Each year the toddler gains 5 to 10 pounds.

2. d

   Rationale. The 2-year-old child runs well with little falling, throws and kicks a ball, and walks up and down stairs one step at a time. Turning the pages of a book and drinking from a cup are examples of fine motor skills; using words to explain an object is an example of language development.

3. b

   Rationale. Parallel play occurs when the toddler plays alongside other children but not with them. Sharing stuffed animals, taking turns playing, and feeding one doll and then feeding a second one are examples of other types of play.

4. c

   Rationale. A handful of dry cereal would be most appropriate because the toddler does well with finger foods and likes to self-feed. Yogurt would not be acceptable as a finger food; grapes would be dangerous because of the possibility of choking; and cookies would not be the best source for a nutritional snack.

5. d

   Rationale. Being toilet trained is an example of the toddler developing autonomy or independence.

Wanting to be picked up when falling down, having temper tantrums, and following the same routine at bedtime are not examples of autonomous or independent behaviors.

6. a, b, d, e

Rationale. Accidents are the leading cause of death in the toddler. Most accidents are related to motor vehicles, drowning (regardless of the amount of water), burns, and ingestion of toxic substances (even with child-resistant caps).

Critical Thinking: What Would You Do?

1. *Suggested answers:*
   a. Temper tantrums come from the frustration the toddler experiences in trying to become independent.
   b. Remaining calm and patient will help the child regain control of her behavior.
   c and d. It is important to calmly pick up the child and take her to a quiet, neutral setting. After the child has quieted, talking to her in a calm, controlled manner will help her understand her behavior will not bring about her desired request.

2. *Suggested answers:*
   a. The toddler has a decrease in the number of hours needed for sleep.
   b. Rituals at bedtime provide structure and a feeling of security because the toddler knows what is expected.
   c. Separation anxiety can add to the reluctance of the toddler to go to bed. Gentle, firm consistency, a regular bedtime schedule, and a story or quiet time help the toddler settle at bedtime.

3. *Suggested answers:*
   a. The mother would be asked questions such as does Jed make a connection between the puddle on the floor and something he did, indicate a need to urinate, pull on his wet or soiled diaper, or bring a clean diaper to his caregiver? In addition, the mother might be asked if Jed stays dry for long time periods. Answers of "yes" to any of these questions might indicate a physical readiness for toilet training.
   b. To encourage bowel and bladder training Jed's mother should leave him on the potty chair for only a short time, dress him in clothes that are easily removed, and give praise and approval when the child voids or defecates using the potty chair.
   c. and d. Consistency in putting Jed on the potty chair and using the same terminology, rituals, and praise by all caregivers will have a positive impact on potty training.

CHAPTER 25

NCLEX-Style Review Questions

1. c

   Rationale. The deciduous teeth begin being replaced by permanent teeth toward the end of the preschool period. Between 3 and 5 ½ years, the child would gain 3 to 5 pounds a year and grow about 2½ inches a year. Most preschool and school-age children no longer take a morning nap.

2. a

   Rationale. The preschool child develops an imagination and enjoys pretending and imitating during play. Toddlers play with large balls and blocks; school-age children participate in group activities and collect things.

3. c

   Rationale. Preschool children need guidance in selecting foods and snacks. They should be encouraged to eat nutritiously and eat limited amounts of sugar and sweets in their daily diet. In following normal development, preschool children may call siblings names, have imaginary friends, and play by themselves.

4. d

   Rationale. Masturbation and exploration of the genitalia are natural for the preschooler, and a calm, matter-of-fact response to the child is most effective. Scolding or becoming angry or upset are inappropriate ways to respond when a child masturbates. Masturbation is not unhealthy or dangerous.

5. d

   Rationale. A major cause of accidents in the preschool child occurs when the child is not properly restrained in a motor vehicle. Brushing and flossing teeth after snacks and meals, covering the mouth when coughing or sneezing, and screening for amblyopia are important to reinforce with caregivers of preschool-age children, but safety is the highest priority.

6. a, c, d

   Rationale. Many infections are spread by contact with the causative agent, thus washing hands with warm water and not sharing food, utensils, or tooth brushes will decrease the likelihood of spreading infection. By wiping from front to back there is decreased likelihood of a bacterium entering the urinary tract.

Critical Thinking: What Would You Do?

1. *Suggested answers:*
   a. Caregivers may be concerned that masturbation is an abnormal or dangerous behavior.

b. Exploration of the genitalia is natural for the preschooler and is a way the child learns acceptance of sex as natural and pleasurable.

c. Clara should be encouraged to give the child a calm, matter-of-fact response and explain that this behavior is not appropriate in public.

2. *Suggested answers:*

a. Jenny may be concerned that something serious has happened or is happening to her child.

b. The development of an imagination in the preschool child often leads to a fear of the dark or nightmares.

c. Jenny needs to explain to Krista, "it was only a dream" and offer her love and understanding until the fear has subsided. Giving Krista a small night-light may be reassuring.

3. *Suggested answers:*

a. The preschooler is more independent, aggressive physically and verbally, and enjoys talking, all of which can lead to feelings of frustration in the caregiver.

b. These behaviors often occur because of the child's curiosity about the world around him and his ability to explore that world in greater detail.

c. Consistency in responding to the child, taking away a privilege for misbehavior, and calm reasoning with the child can help the caregiver decrease feelings of frustration.

CHAPTER 26

NCLEX-Style Review Questions

1. a
Rationale. The average annual weight gain of the child from 6 to 10 years of age is about 5 to 6 pounds. The annual height increase is about 2.5 inches. The 6-year-old child has two molars in the lower jaw and an apical pulse of about 70 to 115 beats per minute.

2. c
Rationale. The school-age child enjoys participating in group activities and competitive play. The preschool child pretends during play and enjoys telling stories about themselves. The toddler plays with large balls.

3. b
Rationale. School-aged children who are successful in completing activities during this stage develop a sense of industry. Trying to get up after falling and not crying, following the same bedtime routine, and making up stories are milestones or behaviors seen in other stages of development.

4. d
Rationale. Accidents are a leading cause of death during the school-age years. This age child must be

taught and must follow basic rules of safety, including bicycle and vehicle safety. Encouraging tooth brushing, teaching basic sex education, and screening for scoliosis are important to reinforce with caregivers of school-age children, but safety is the highest priority.

5. a
Rationale. The school-age child needs 10 to 12 hours of sleep each night. Staying up late after taking an after-school nap, not knowing when the child is tired, and sleeping more than a teenager when compared with a school-age child refer to sleep behaviors and needs of children of younger and older ages.

6. a, c, d, f
Rationale. Food jags are common at this age and allowing children to have and express food likes and dislikes is important. Obesity can be a concern at this age, thus snacks high in sugar would not be a nutritionally sound choice. Scoliosis screening is first done at about the age of 10 or 11 years. Sex education taught in the home usually offers the child the most accurate information.

Critical Thinking: What Would You Do?

1. *Suggested answers:*

a. Most school-age children have food "jags," during which they prefer eating certain foods.

b. The child needs foods from all food groups with appropriate numbers of servings in the daily diet.

c and d. Offering Jasmine choices; allowing her to express food likes and dislikes; offering simple, plain foods; setting a good example; and making meal and snack times positive and pleasant will help Jasmine develop good nutritional patterns.

2. *Suggested answers:*

a. Positive attitudes about the body and sexual roles, menstruation and the developing body, reproduction, birth, and nurturing are all topics important to discuss with the school-age child.

b and c. Using books and pamphlets, the school nurse, and female friends and family members might be helpful to Steve in talking with his daughter.

d. Positive, loving family environments are helpful in developing security and family values regarding sex education.

3. *Suggested answers:*

a. School-age children need to be given information regarding the choices they have in regard to decisions about substance abuse and the unhealthy aspects of tobacco, alcohol, and substance use.

b. Open communication and active listening, honest answers to questions, positive role models, and giving correct facts and information are the most effective methods of teaching the school-age child.

   c. The school-age child will ask questions related to cause and effect, especially in relation to how something might affect him and his life.

CHAPTER 27

NCLEX-Style Review Questions

1. c

Rationale. By the age of 12 years, many girls have a broader pelvis, and axillary and pubic hair has begun to grow. The preadolescent between ages 10 and 13 years weighs 77 to 88 pounds, is 56¾ to 59 inches tall, and is just beginning to develop breasts.

2. d

Rationale. The desire to not be different from peers and a concern with body image can lead to unhealthy behaviors and concerns, such as anorexia nervosa in the adolescent. The statements about wanting to be a nurse after finishing college, having money to spend because of a job, and spending time getting ready for school are all statements that indicate behaviors seen in normal adolescent development.

3. a

Rationale. The adolescent girl needs additional iron in her diet, which can be obtained by eating green leafy vegetables, lean meats, dried fruits, and whole-grain and fortified cereals. Milk is not an adequate source of vitamin C; eggs do not supply adequate amounts of calcium; and bread has almost no vitamin A.

4. c

Rationale. The adolescent spends a large amount of time each day with peers and friends of the same and opposite sex. Establishing a career, playing board games with siblings, and volunteering in the community are activities more commonly seen in other stages of growth and development.

5. b

Rationale. Alcohol is the most common mind-altering substance used by adolescents, and its use or use of tobacco or other substances in adolescence can lead to serious concerns.

6. a, d, e

Rationale. The breast exam is done once a month, about a week after having a period. The pads of the fingers are used, and the same pattern is followed to examine the entire breast. The exam is done both lying down and standing in front of a mirror or while in the shower.

Critical Thinking: What Would You Do?

1. *Suggested answers:*

   a. Adolescent girls should do breast self-exams and have routine Pap smears for early detection of health concerns that may need to be monitored or treated.

   b. The breast exam should be done once a month, about a week after your period ends. The sensitive finger pads should be used to feel the breast tissue, using an up-and-down pattern. While standing in front of a mirror, with your hands pressing firmly down on your hips, check the entire breast, looking for any changes. Each underarm should also be examined.

   c. Adolescent girls may feel awkward and uncomfortable talking about their bodies and performing breast self-exams and having Pap smears done. They may also feel concerned about what may be found during these exams, for example a lump in the breast or an STD.

   d. Privacy, confidentiality, and active listening will help decrease the anxiety and concerns of the adolescent girl.

2. *Suggested answers:*

   a. The adolescent athlete might think that eating a carbohydrate-loading diet before an athletic event will enhance his athletic performance.

   b. It would be important to share with Jamal that this diet may hinder the functioning of his heart.

   c. Suggesting that Jamal eat a meal low in fat and high in complex carbohydrates 3 to 4 hours before the event would be more appropriate and healthy.

3. *Suggested answers:*

   a. Adolescent girls and boys need to take responsibility for their own sexual behavior.

   b. Adolescents need to have an understanding of how to protect themselves from pregnancy and STDs.

   c. Adolescents need correct and adequate information and support to make appropriate sexual decisions for themselves. Often adequate and correct information is not received in the home, therefore health education in the high school setting is an alternative means for the adolescent to be informed and taught.

CHAPTER 28

NCLEX-Style Review Questions

1. c

Rationale. The toddler will be safe and feel more secure if allowed to sit on a caregiver's lap during the interview process. Most likely, the child will be somewhat fearful and anxious. Thus, the toddler will feel most secure if in the presence of the caregiver (and not in the playroom or taking a walk with another) and by sitting on the caregiver's lap, instead of in a chair, will feel comforted by physical contact.

2. b

Rationale. The adolescent will feel more comfortable and most likely be more honest about private issues such as sexual history when interviewed in private. The adolescent may not know the details of their early childhood health history. Age-appropriate questions and books and pamphlets may be helpful in working with the adolescent, but promoting privacy is the most important in working with this age group.

3. d

Rationale. A normal pulse average for a 6-month-old infant is 120 to 130 beats per minute (bpm); a temperature of 38.5°C would be considered elevated and a concern for this child. Pulse rates of 90, 114, and 148 bpm, temperatures of 36.9°C, 37.6°C, and 38.0°C, and blood pressure readings of 80/50 mm Hg, 88/60 mm Hg, and 92/62 mm Hg would all be within a normal range for a 6-month-old child.

4. b

Rationale. When doing a physical exam on an infant, aspects of the exam that might be more traumatic or uncomfortable for the child, such as examining the nose, are done last. Examining the heart, extremities, or neurologic status are aspects of the physical exam that are not traumatic or uncomfortable and can be done in any order.

5. a, c, e, f

Rationale. Plotting the measurement on a growth chart gives an indication of how the child is progressing and often indicates wellness. Safety and prevention of infection are important factors, but wearing a gown and mask is not necessary. Wearing the same amount of clothing each time the child is weighed helps to ensure getting an accurate measurement of the child's weight. Allowing the child to sit on the parent's lap would not provide an accurate indication of the child's height and weight.

6.

Critical Thinking: What Would You Do?

1. *Suggested answers:*
   a. In doing an interview with the caregiver the nurse would discuss the chief complaint, history of current health concern, past health and family history, questions regarding allergies, medications, lifestyle, and the child's developmental level.
   b. The nurse would establish a relationship, listen, ask focused questions, and allow the caregiver time to respond.
   c. The preschool child would be included in the interview process, might be seated on the caregiver's lap, asked age-appropriate questions, and given honest answers to their questions. Dolls, stuffed animals, books, and stories might be used to help understand the child's concerns and feelings.

2. *Suggested answers:*
   a. The height and weight are measured because they are helpful indicators of growth, development, and potential health concerns.
   b. The height and weight are recorded and plotted on the growth chart.
   c. Plotting the height and weight gives an indication of the child's health status.

3. *Suggested answers:*
   a. The physical exam is done by examining the body systems of the child.
   b. The physical exam for the child in not necessarily done in a head-to-toe manner, as in the adult. Aspects of the exam that might be more traumatic or uncomfortable for the child are done last.
   c. Safety of the child is the most important consideration in doing a physical exam.

CHAPTER 29

NCLEX-Style Review Questions

1. d

Rationale. Reusable equipment must be cleaned appropriately before using with another patient. Used syringes are disposed of immediately in the appropriate container in the patient room. Gloves must be changed between tasks and procedures after contact with material that may contain microorganisms. Isolation gowns are removed promptly and disposed of properly.

2. d

Rationale. Children as well as adults have pain. The nurse monitors and implements treatment of pain in children after any surgical procedure. The school-age child can be taught how to push the button for the PCA pump. Pain medications may be given by intramuscular injection, and distraction often helps decrease pain levels.

3. c

   Rationale. The 5-year-old child enjoys contact with friends and will feel less lonely and isolated when given the opportunity to visit with friends. Talking with the child about feelings would be appropriate, but it would not decrease the feelings of loneliness. Answering the call light immediately and providing age-appropriate activities for the child to do alone will not decrease the child's feelings of loneliness.

4. c

   Rationale. In response to being separated from caregivers, the child in the denial stage will appear to have accepted the situation, but when the caregiver arrives, the child will show distrust and rejection of the caregiver. During the stage of protest, the child cries, refuses to be comforted, and searches for the caregiver to arrive. In the stage of despair, the child becomes quiet and apathetic.

5. b

   Rationale. The preschool child may show attachment to a toy or blanket and have clinging and demanding behavior upon returning home from hospitalization, most likely not requesting to visit the nurses at the hospital. Upon returning home from a hospitalization, a child may awaken at night or, in the older child, may show anger or jealousy toward siblings.

6. a, b, e, f

   Rationale. Gloves are worn when touching contaminated articles, and hands are washed immediately after gloves are removed. Eye protection is worn to protect eyes during procedures that are likely to generate splashes or sprays of fluids or secretions. Gowns are removed and disposed of immediately if contaminated. Reusable equipment must be sterilized before being reused. Needles should not be removed from syringes or recapped because of the risk of needle-stick injury.

Critical Thinking: What Would You Do?

1. *Suggested answers:*
   a. The child should be given an explanation of the situation in terms and language that she can understand. Her questions should be answered at an appropriate level for her age.
   b. The purpose and benefit of the procedures should be explained. Taking the child to the pediatric unit and giving her a tour of the facility will decrease anxiety and fear. Meeting staff on the unit will decrease anxiety and fear and be helpful to the child.
   c. Simple and complete explanations are important. When explaining to the child what surgery

is, the nurse would talk about the part of the body that is going to be "fixed."

2. *Suggested answers:*
   a. Communication with this child and grandmother is an important aspect of the child's plan of care. The child and caregiver need to be given explanations in their own language when possible.
   b. The use of an interpreter, pictures of objects, or a dictionary with common medical terms in various languages can be helpful. Spending time with the child and caregiver, using objects, pictures, and nonverbal communication will aid in communication.

3. *Suggested answers:*
   a. Using the threat of illness or hospitalization can create concern and fear in a child, especially if at some point the child must be hospitalized.
   b. It is important to encourage caregivers to be positive in the statements and comments they make to children regarding health care and health care providers. Fear is difficult to overcome if inappropriate or incorrect information has been given to a child.
   c. A more appropriate statement might be to express how you feel, your concern for the child and to request the behavior be stopped, for example, "Stop jumping off the slide, I am worried that you might get hurt."

CHAPTER 30

NCLEX-Style Review Questions

1. c

   Rationale. Safety factors such as identifying the patient are always a priority. Although explaining the procedure, gathering supplies, and documenting are important, safety is a priority.

2. a

   Rationale. The mummy restraint keeps the child's hands and legs contained while a procedure is performed. The clove hitch restraint secures an arm or leg, the elbow restraint prevents the child from bending the arm, and the jacket restraint secures the child in the bed or chair.

3. b

   Rationale. Giving a cold bath to a child with an elevated temperature is ineffective, can be dangerous in too rapidly lowering the temperature, and can cause discomfort. Encouraging fluid consumption, administering antipyretic medications such as Tylenol, and not overdressing or heavily covering the child are effective in lowering an elevated temperature.

4. b

   Rationale. Age-appropriate books given to a preschool-age child who has been placed in an oxygen tent would be safe and appropriate. Electric or battery-powered toys and wool or synthetic blankets would not be safe to use in an oxygen tent. Most board games would not be age-appropriate for the preschool child, especially to play alone.

5. d
   Rationale. Monitoring and preventing skin break-down is a priority when caring for a child with an ileostomy. Altered development, ineffective family coping, and bowel incontinence may be appropriate, but they are not as high a priority.

6. Intake of 475 cc and output of 170 cc
   Rationale. To calculate intake: 2 ounces of milk (60 cc), 3 ounce glass of orange juice (90 cc), 120 cc of supplemental feeding, 4 ounces of ice chips (when melted would be measured as 2 ounces of fluid or 60 cc), 25 cc of apple juice, 120 cc gavage feeding. Total 12-hour intake of 475 cc. To calculate output: 75 cc of urine, emesis of 50 cc, 45 cc of urine. Total 12-hour output of 170 cc. Stool would be recorded but not counted in output.

Critical Thinking: What Would You Do?

1. *Suggested answers:*
   a. Caring for the child with an elevated temperature includes encouraging fluid consumption and giving an antipyretic such as acetaminophen. Dressing the child in lightweight clothing, keeping the room cool, and monitoring the temperature closely are methods to reduce fever.
   b. The nurse should explain that it is important to increase hydration and control environmental factors to reduce fever.
   c and d. The highest priority would be to lower the temperature to prevent the child from having a febrile seizure.

2. *Suggested answers:*
   a. The restraints are necessary to keep the child safe and to keep the child from pulling out the intravenous line and feeding tube.
   b. It will be reassuring to the caregiver to explain that the restraints are removed frequently and the child watched closely to prevent any complications or concerns.
   c. Holding the child and removing the restraints at intervals will comfort and support the child.

3. *Suggested answers:*
   a. Oxygen tents allow for movement inside the tent and do not require any device to be put over the child's nose or face.
   b. Electric or battery-powered toys are unsafe to use in an oxygen tent.
   c. Oxygen can be potentially dangerous in the presence of flammable materials, matches or lighters, or wool or synthetic blankets.

CHAPTER 31

NCLEX-Style Review Questions

1. b
   Rationale. Offering the preschool child a choice will increase the likelihood of cooperation from the child in taking the medication. Preschool children can hold the medication cup and often will cooperate when given the opportunity. School-age children might make a poster to schedule medications, and the adolescent can read and understand material printed regarding medications.

2. c
   Rationale. One kilogram is equal to 2.2 pounds. Therefore the child would weigh 7.3 kg.

3. c
   Rationale. The child weighs 34.5 kg, so the dosage range is 37.9 to 62.1 mg per dose. Doses below or above this range would be inappropriate.

4. a
   Rationale. The vastus lateralis is the best and safest injection site for the infant. The deltoid, ventrogluteal, and dorsogluteal sites would be inappropriate for use.

5. a
   Rationale. An infusion pump or volume control device is used to regulate the rate of infusion. Infusion pumps and volume control devices do not change the size of the drops delivered or reduce the rate of infiltration, and they are not used to administer medications.

6.

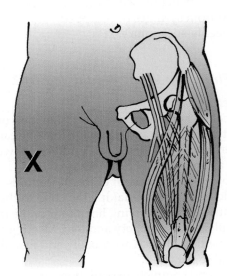

Vastus lateralis muscle

Critical Thinking: What Would You Do?

1. *Suggested answers:*
   a. Following the six rights of medication administration helps to ensure the safe administration of medications to all patients.
   b. The stage of growth and development the child is in must be taken into consideration when medications are given to children.
   c. The child responds to medications in various ways, depending on how the medication is absorbed, metabolized, and excreted in the child.
   d. Medication errors should be acknowledged immediately and steps taken to ensure the safety of the child.
   e. The nurse is legally liable for errors of medication.

CHAPTER 32

NCLEX-Style Review Questions

1. a
   Rationale. Many children with chronic health problems face challenges that interfere with normal growth and development. Helping these children achieve their highest level of growth and development is a goal. Participating in age-appropriate activities, eating at least 75% of each meal, and sharing feelings about changes in body image would most likely be good for children with a chronic illness, but such goals are not always realistic for these children.

2. c
   Rationale. Overprotection occurs when the caregivers of a child with a chronic illness try to protect the child at all costs, which prevents the child from experiencing and growing from success and failures, as well as frustrations. Statements such as, "My child was born with this and it will always be part of our lives," "She should be punished when she breaks things because she knows better," and "My child just isn't what I expected when I decided to become a parent" are examples of statements made by caregivers who are attempting to treat the child in a manner as normal as possible.

3. a
   Rationale. Acceptance occurs when the caregivers of a child with a chronic illness help the child to set realistic goals and encourage the child to achieve social and physical skills within the child's capability. Stating the child should be punished when she breaks things because she knows better, or the child wasn't what the parents expected are examples of statements made by caregivers of a child with a chronic illness which show an understanding of having a chronically ill child. The statement about knowing to let the child try activities but getting frustrated is an example of overprotecting the chronically ill child.

4. b
   Rationale. It is important for families with chronically ill children to openly express their feelings. Refraining from talking about the condition, preventing the child from hearing conversations, and telling stories about themselves do not encourage families to express their feelings and be open about the concerns they encounter living with a child with a chronic illness.

5. a
   Rationale. The siblings of a child with a chronic illness may feel shame or embarrassment, especially if their sibling has a physical disfigurement or cognitive deficit. Siblings of chronically ill children often feel deprived of attention from the caregiver who spends much time caring for the ill child. These siblings may have anger, social withdrawal, and poor school performance.

6. a, b, e
   Rationale. It is important for the nurse to accept without judgment and encourage families to express their feelings. Often by quietly staying with the family, the nurse offers support to these families. Telling the caregivers that it will get better is inappropriate and does not address the caregivers' feelings. Telling the caregivers that anger is inappropriate would be erroneous because anger is part of the grieving process.

Critical Thinking: What Would You Do?

1. *Suggested answers:*
   a. Teach Abby about her diagnosis using age-appropriate level information, encourage her to help remind her caregivers to administer her medications before snacks and meals, and give her fun activities and games to use in her treatment regimen; these actions will be helpful in involving her in caring for herself.
   b. Support Mattie by listening to her concerns, give her explanations about the importance of Abby being involved in her care, and offer ideas that are age-appropriate; these actions will help decrease Mattie's fears and anxieties about Abby.
   c. Caregivers of children with chronic health problems are often overprotective in an attempt to protect their child and prevent the child from feelings of frustration.

2. *Suggested answers:*
   a. Listening and accepting Josh's feelings, giving explanations regarding his brother's diagnosis and behavior, and encouraging Josh to interact with his brother are important in helping to decrease sibling rivalry and anger.
   b. Often the siblings of children with chronic health concerns feel anger, resentment, and jealousy. These may be because of decreased time and attention from their caregiver or from feeling embarrassed or shameful about their sibling.
   c. Encourage caregivers to spend time with each child and to maintain consistent discipline standards for the ill, as well as the healthy, children in the family.
3. *Suggested answers:*
   a. Cassie and her caregivers should be encouraged to each express their feelings and concerns and to communicate openly with each other about the situation.
   b. Encourage the caregivers to recognize the needs of their teenage daughter and support them in dealing with their anxieties.

CHAPTER 33

NCLEX-Style Review Questions

1. a
   Rationale. During the stage of grief known as bargaining, the person or family member attempts to postpone or delay death, especially until after a specific event, such as a holiday. The statement about being mad that the sibling is going to die is an example of the stage of grief known as anger. Thinking that the child will get better because of a new medication is an example of the stage of grief known as denial, in which a person refuses to acknowledge the person is dying. Stating that the child won't be in pain anymore when he dies is an example of the stage of grief known as acceptance, in which the patient or family accepts the person will die.
2. c
   Rationale. During the stage of grief known as denial, the person or family member refuses to acknowledge the person is dying. Wanting the child to come to a birthday party is an example of the stage of grief known as bargaining; the person or family member attempts to postpone or delay death, especially until after a specific event, such as a holiday. Being mad that the sibling is going to die is an example of the stage of grief known as anger. Stating that the child won't be in pain anymore

when he dies is an example of the stage of grief known as acceptance, in which the patient or family accepts the person will die.
3. d
   Rationale. The preschool-age child may view illness or death as a punishment for thoughts and actions. At about age 8 or 9 years, the child gains an understanding that death is irreversible and sometimes thinks or speaks of death as a person, such as a monster or bogeyman. The toddler does not understand the fact that death is irreversible.
4. c
   Rationale. Adolescents understand death but have the feeling that they are immortal and that death will happen to others, not to themselves. School-age children think they can protect themselves from death and understand the sadness that death brings. Preschool children may fear going to sleep because they fear they will go to sleep and not awaken.
5. d
   Rationale. The nurse can best be therapeutic by acknowledging the feelings of the family and supporting them during this time. At the time of a death, giving options or offering advice are not the most therapeutic responses by the nurse. Quietly spending time with the family shows support.
6. a, b, d, e
   Anticipatory grief occurs when a death is expected and the family begins the process of mourning the death of their child. The family may take this time to say and do some of the things they need to do that will help to prepare for and lessen the acute grief when their child dies.

Critical Thinking: What Would You Do?

1. *Suggested answers:*
   a. Financial concerns about costs of hospitalization and nonmedical expenses, stress related to family separations, and loss of control over the care of the child and the life of the family are factors families of terminally ill children must consider.
   b. Feelings of fear, guilt, and anxiety are commonly seen in these families.
2. *Suggested answers:*
   a. Caring for a terminally ill child at home can be rewarding, as well as emotionally and physically difficult. The procedures necessary for the child might be unrealistic for the family to manage.
   b. Offering information, guidance, and choices will be helpful for the family in making decisions regarding the care of their child.

CHAPTER 34

NCLEX-Style Review Questions

1. c

   Rationale. Safety of the child is always the highest priority. Although documenting, teaching, and reassuring are important nursing interventions and should be carried out for the child who has a febrile seizure, they are not the highest priority.

2. c

   Rationale. Sponging the child with cool water is not recommended as a method of lowering an elevated temperature. Additional teaching would be done on ways to lower the child's temperature. Avoiding aspirin, dressing the child lightly, and rechecking the temperature indicate the caregiver has a correct understanding of treating and monitoring a child with a fever.

3. a

   Rationale. Signs of increased intracranial pressure include high-pitched cry, headache, fever, irritability, nuchal rigidity, and arching of the back. Swelling and itching of the eyes, weight gain or loss, and sunken fontanel and decreased head size are not associated with increased intracranial pressure.

4. a, c, e, f

   Rationale. Tonic-clonic seizures begin with an aura, which is a warning that occurs just before the seizure. The child's muscles stiffen and become rigid, followed by generalized jerking muscle movements of the entire body. During the tonic-clonic seizure, the child may lose control of the bowel and bladder. Memory loss and staring do not occur during a tonic-clonic seizure.

5. a, d, f

   Rationale. When working with a blind patient, the nurse must always identify herself upon entering the room and tell the patient when she leaves. The child is encouraged to participate in age-appropriate activities and be as independent as possible. Orienting the child to where foods are on the plate helps encourage independence in eating.

Critical Thinking: What Would You Do?

1. *Suggested answers:*
   a. A tactile tour of the room helps orient the child to the location of furniture and other facilities. The child needs to touch the equipment and have sounds and other sensations explained.
   b. Preparation for a hospital stay will include explanations of what the child will hear, feel, and encounter. Encourage the child to be as independent as possible. Offer finger foods and encourage self-feeding.
   c. It is important the child be involved with as many peers and their activities as possible. The pre-schooler enjoys storytelling and imaginative play.

2. *Suggested answers:*
   a. The caregiver of a child with a hearing impairment is a resource for the nurse. The caregiver can provide information regarding the child's habits and communication patterns.
   b. When caring for the hearing-impaired child, stand or sit face to face on the child's level; be sure the child can see you before you touch her. Demonstrate each procedure, showing the child the equipment or pictures of the equipment to be used. A night light in the child's room is important.

3. *Suggested answers:*
   a. Causes of cerebral palsy may be prenatal, perinatal, or postnatal. They include any process that interferes with the oxygen supply to the brain, maternal infection, nutritional deficiencies, kernicterus (brain damage caused by jaundice), drugs, and radiation. Other causes may be anoxia immediately before, during, and/or birth, intracranial bleeding, anything that interferes with respiratory function, maternal analgesia, birth trauma, or cerebral hemorrhage caused by prematurity. Postnatal causes include head trauma, infection, neoplasms, and cerebrovascular accidents.
   b. Cerebral palsy can possibly be prevented by good prenatal care, perinatal monitoring, postnatal prevention of infection, and protection from trauma.
   c. The child may have spastic type, athetoid type, ataxia type, rigidity type, or mixed type cerebral palsy.

4. *Suggested answers:*
   a. 13.2 pounds is 6 kg
   b. 240 mg will be given in a 24-hour time period (40 mg/kg × 6 kg = 240 mg)
   c. 80 mg per dose, every 8 hours is three doses in a 24-hour time period. (240 mg divided by 3 = 80)
   d. 3 doses per day

5. *Suggested answers:*
   a. 58 pounds is 26.3 kg
   b. 6 mg/kg in 24 hours is a total of 157.8 mg of Dilantin
   c. The medication is given in three divided doses of 52.6 mg each.
   d. Increasing each dose by 20 mg would make each dose 72.6 mg.
   e. After the dose has been increased, the child would receive 217.8 mg of Dilantin in 24 hours.

CHAPTER 35

NCLEX-Style Review Questions

1. d
   Rationale. Bleeding can occur 5 to 7 days after surgery and is often noted by frequent swallowing. This is a concern and should be reported immediately. A sore throat is common for several days after surgery. If an ice collar becomes uncomfortable, it can be removed. Vomiting dark, old blood may be expected within the first 24 hours after a tonsillectomy.

2. b
   Rationale. Dehydration can be a concern for the child with a fever. Therefore the highest priority would be increasing fluid intake to help in the prevention of dehydration. Reducing anxiety, allowing caregivers to talk about their concerns, and promoting adequate caloric intake would be appropriate for the child and caregiver, but they would not be the highest priority.

3. c
   Rationale. Children with asthma should be encouraged to exercise using moderation. They should not become extremely tired, and activities should be spaced to provide for periods of rest. Statements about identifying allergic triggers, using bronchodilator before steroid inhaler, and drinking water to thin secretions indicate that the caregivers have an understanding of treatments important for their child with asthma.

4. c
   Rationale. Postural drainage is performed in the morning and evening to help loosen and move secretions out of the lungs. Maintaining the child in a semi-Fowler's or high Fowler's position will promote lung expansion. High protein snacks will help increase caloric intake. Children with cystic fibrosis need to be protected from infection but do not need to be isolated.

5. a
   Rationale. Cystic fibrosis is a hereditary disease, and when parents are carriers of the disease, one in four children will likely have the disease. Statements about consistent medication administration, play with other children, and salty snacks after exercise indicate that the caregiver has an understanding of the care of the child with cystic fibrosis.

6. a. Total intake = 490 mL
   b. Total output = 400 mL
   Rationale. Intake 3 oz of apple juice (90 cc), 5 oz of milk (150 cc), 1/4 cup of chicken soup (2 oz or 60 cc), 2 oz of gelatin (60 cc), and 130 cc of IV fluid totals 490 cc (or mL). Output equals 400 cc or grams and is determined by adding the weights of the diapers after subtracting the dry diaper weight from each: 87 grams −38 grams (dry weight of diaper) = 49 grams; 124 grams −38 grams (dry weight of diaper) = 86 grams; 138 grams −38 grams (dry weight of diaper) = 100 grams; 146 grams −38 grams (dry weight of diaper) = 108 grams; 95 grams −38 grams (dry weight of diaper) = 57 grams. Add weights minus dry diaper weight 49 + 86 + 100 + 108 + 57 = 400 grams or milliliters of output.

Critical Thinking: What Would You Do?

1. *Suggested answers:*
   a. The caregiver would be asked if Jared had a runny nose or hoarseness before these symptoms, had awakened after a few hours of sleep, was anxious or restless, or had a low-grade fever or symptoms of an upper respiratory infection.
   b. The caregiver should take the child into the bathroom and open the hot water taps with the door closed to provide moist air, and use a cool mist humidifier in the child's bedroom to provide high humidity.
   c. Immediate medical care should be sought if Jared shows symptoms of continuous stridor, use of accessory muscles, labored breathing, lower rib retractions, restlessness, pallor, or rapid respirations.

2. *Suggested answers:*
   a. Often the child with an acute asthmatic attack is totally preoccupied with efforts to breathe and must sit up to do so. The child may be diaphoretic or have cyanosis. Intercostal retractions may be noticed.
   b. Medications used to treat asthma are divided into two categories: quick-relief medications for immediate treatment of symptoms and exacerbations and long-term control medications to achieve and maintain control of the symptoms.
   c. Examples of classifications of drugs that might have been given include bronchodilators, corticosteroids, leukotriene inhibitors, and mast cell stabilizers.
   d. Learning how to recognize early symptoms of an impending attack, control environmental factors, and avoid infections can prevent asthma attacks. Understanding factors related to exercise, drug therapy, and chest physiotherapy also will help to lessen or prevent attacks.

3. *Suggested answers:*
   a. 32 pounds is 14.5 kg
   b. 4 mg x 14.5 kg = 58 mg per dose
   c. A dose every 6 hours will be four doses in 24 hours.
   d. 58 mg per dose x 4 doses = 232 mg in 24 hours

CHAPTER 36

NCLEX-Style Review Questions

1. b
   Rationale. Rheumatic fever is precipitated by a streptococcal infection, which may be undiagnosed or untreated. The disease is not hereditary and is not necessarily seen in family members. Easy bruising and increased urine output are not symptoms seen with rheumatic fever.

2. d
   Rationale. The child with sickle cell disease has severe pain that should be treated promptly. Providing family support, monitoring for skin breakdown, and moving the extremities gently are interventions appropriate for the family and child with sickle cell disease, but they would not be the highest priority.

3. c
   Rationale. When the child with hemophilia has a bleeding episode, the child is placed so the area of bleeding is raised above the level of the heart when possible, therefore additional teaching would be required. Ice and cold packs, keeping pressure on the injury site, and using splints to limit bleeding are all measures used to stop bleeding when the child with hemophilia is injured.

4. a
   Rationale. Low grade fever, bone and joint pain, fatigue, pallor, petechiae, and purpura are signs and symptoms seen in a child with leukemia. High fever; sore throat; swelling around the eyes, ankles, and abdomen; and eyes that are slanted upward and outward are not indicative of leukemia.

5. a
   Rationale. The child with leukemia is susceptible to infection, especially during chemotherapy, and should be monitored closely for signs of infection. Participating in age-appropriate activities, eating at least 60% of each meal, and sharing feelings about changes in body image would be appropriate but not the most important goal.

6. a, c, f
   Rationale. Using a soft, sponge-type brush or gauze will decrease the likelihood of injury when doing oral care. Mouthwash composed of hydrogen peroxide and saline will help in keeping the mucous membranes and mouth clean but will not be irritating to the tissues. Applying pressure to sites of injections or venipunctures will help prevent excess bleeding at these sites. Neutropenic precautions (commonly referred to as reverse isolation) would be important to prevent infection if the child's white blood cell count was extremely low. Wearing a cap or scarf would be appropriate if the child experienced hair loss. Wearing gloves to deliver the child's meal tray would be inappropriate and unnecessary.

Critical Thinking: What Would You Do?

1. *Suggested answers:*
   a. Blood is screened thoroughly for viral contamination, which greatly diminishes the danger of HIV transmission. Individuals treated before the late 1980s were more likely to be exposed to HIV when given blood transfusions.
   b. The cause of the child's illness was in no way related to choices or behaviors the family made.
   c. The nurse often feels empathic and concerned for the child who is HIV positive because of a blood transfusion.

2. *Suggested answers:*
   a and b. Sickle cell disease is a hereditary trait characterized by the production of abnormal hemoglobin that causes the red blood cells to assume a sickle shape. When the sickle cell trait is inherited from both parents, the child has sickle cell disease.
   c. Because sickle cell disease is an inherited disease, there is a chance the second child would have the disease, but in most cases only one in four children in a family has the disease.
   d. Support for the family might be available through the Sickle Cell Disease Association of America (www.sicklecelldisease.org).

3. *Suggested answers:*
   a. 1,000 micrograms (mcg) is 1 milligram
   b. 6.5 pounds is 2.9 kgs
   c. Low dose of 11.6 mcg in a 24-hour time period
   d. High dose of 23.2 mcg in a 24-hour time period
   e. Two doses would be given in a day

4. *Suggested answers:*
   a. 39 pounds is 17.7 kg
   b. 90 mg per 17.7 kg is 1,593 mg per day for the initial dose
   c. If the dose is given every 6 hours, it will be given four times a day, and each dose will be 398.2 mg.
   d. The medication comes in 80-mg tablets, so the dose will be 4.9 tablets.
   e. The antiplatelet dose of 5 mg/kg/day would be 88.5 mg/day.

CHAPTER 37

NCLEX-Style Review Questions

1. b
   Rationale. Children with pyloric stenosis usually have a history of vomiting, which increases with

force and frequency and becomes projectile. Iron deficiency anemia, muscle spasms, and nasal congestion are not commonly seen in the child with pyloric stenosis.

2. d

Rationale. Fever, nausea, and vomiting are common in children with appendicitis. The child with appendicitis may also have abdominal pain but may have a difficult time localizing the pain. Sore throat, bone and joint pain, itching and swelling around the eyes and ankles, convulsions, and weight loss or gain are not signs and symptoms seen in the child with appendicitis.

3. b

Rationale. The caregiver should always call the Poison Control Center immediately when a child has swallowed a known or unknown substance. Depending on the substance swallowed, the Poison Control Center will direct the caregiver as to what steps to take next in treating or obtaining treatment for the child.

4. c

Rationale. The child with type 1 diabetes mellitus will most likely have to take insulin injections to control the disease. Individuals with type 2 diabetes usually are adults, and their disease sometimes can be controlled by taking oral hypoglycemic agents. Most type 1 diabetics will always have to take insulin to control their disease.

5. c, h

Rationale. The goals with the highest priority for the child with a diagnosis of failure to thrive will be to maintain and increase their current intake and weight. Although maintaining good mouth and skin integrity, improving knowledge, increasing daily exercise, decreasing anxiety, satisfying sucking needs, and increasing fluid intake are important, they are not the highest priority for the child with failure to thrive.

Critical Thinking: What Would You Do?

1. *Suggested answers:*
   a. Pinworms are a white, threadlike worm that invades the cecum and may enter the appendix. Articles contaminated with pinworm eggs spread pinworms from person to person.
   b. The infestation is common in children and occurs when the pinworm eggs are swallowed. The eggs hatch in the intestinal tract and grow to maturity in the cecum. Symptoms of a child having pinworms include perianal itching, restlessness, sleeping poorly, and episodes of bedwetting.
   c. The diagnosis is made by using cellophane tape to capture the eggs from around the anus and then examining them under a microscope.
   d. Treatment consists of the use of an anthelmintic medication such as Mebendazole (Vermox).

2. *Suggested answers:*
   a. If the child has collapsed or is not breathing, 911 should be called for emergency help. In cases where the child is conscious and alert and the caregiver suspects poison ingestion, the Poison Control Center should be called.
   b. The antidote used in acetaminophen overdose is N-acetylcysteine (Mucomyst).
   c. The liver can be severely damaged with an acetaminophen overdose.

3. *Suggested answers:*
   a. Symptoms of severe diarrhea include increased frequency of defecation—as many as 12 or more stools per day.
   b. The child may be irritable, experience appetite loss, and have extremely dry skin that loses its turgor. Her fontanel may become sunken and her pulse weak and rapid. Her stools become greenish liquid and may be blood-tinged. She may have an excoriated diaper area, a fever, and sunken eyes.
   c. It is especially important to monitor closely and document the child's intake and output.

4. *Suggested answers:*
   a. 55 pounds is 25 kg
   b. Low dose of 1.0 mg per kg is 25 mg per dose.
   c. High dose of 1.8 mg per kg is 45 mg per dose.
   d. 0.5 mL would be given for a 25-mg dose
   e. 0.9 mL would be given for a 45-mg dose

CHAPTER 38

NCLEX-Style Review Questions

1. c

Rationale. Sponging the child with cool water is not recommended as a method of lowering an elevated temperature. Additional teaching would be done on ways to lower the child's temperature. Avoiding aspiration, dressing the child lightly, and checking temperature frequently indicate the caregiver has a correct understanding of treating and monitoring fever in a child.

2. b

Rationale. The child with nephrotic syndrome is weighed every day using the same scale to accurately monitor the child's fluid gain and loss. The child with nephrotic syndrome is usually on bed rest; fluids may be retained and therefore are not increased; and urine is tested for albumin and specific gravity.

3. b

Rationale. Symptoms of acute glomerulonephritis often appear 1 to 3 weeks after the onset of a streptococcal infection such as strep throat. A sibling with the same disease, hemorrhage or history of easy bruising, or hearing loss with impaired speech are not commonly associated acute glomerulonephritis in a child.

4. a, c, d

Rationale. Dairy products, poultry, processed foods and some grain products are higher in sodium than fruits (apple juice and canned peaches) and fresh vegetables (green beans).

5. a, e

Rationale. The nurse would collect the "clean catch" voided urine specimen before any treatment is started to increase the likelihood of being able to identify the bacterium causing the infection. A priority when giving antibiotics is to always observe for signs of any adverse reaction to the medication. Reporting and recording urinary symptoms and observing for possible sexual abuse would be appropriate but not the priority. Instructing caregivers about avoiding bubble baths and teaching girls to wipe from front to back would be important later in the care of the child.

Critical Thinking: What Would You Do?

1. *Suggested answers:*
   a. It would be important for this caregiver to have her son examined by his care provider. Enuresis may have a physiologic or psychological cause and should be evaluated by a care provider.
   b. The provider most likely will ask the caregiver questions regarding when and if the child has been toilet trained, the child's toilet training experience, and details of the child's current family situation and emotional state.
   c. Physiologic causes may include a small bladder capacity, urinary tract infection, and lack of awareness of the signal to empty the bladder, usually caused by sleeping too soundly.
   d. Psychological causes of enuresis may include rigorous toilet training; resentment toward family caregivers; a desire to regress to an earlier level of development, especially to get attention from a caregiver; emotional stress; and sexual abuse.
2. *Suggested answers:*
   a. Premenstrual syndrome is a group of symptoms women sometimes experience during their monthly hormonal cycle, often just before their period begins.
   b. The cause of PMS is thought to be water retention after progesterone production after ovulation.
   c. Symptoms include edema (resulting in weight gain), headache, increased anxiety, mild depression, and mood swings.
   d. Many times the symptoms of PMS can be relieved by reducing salt intake during the week before menstruation, taking mild analgesics, and applying local heat. In cases in which PMS symptoms are severe, a mild diuretic or oral contraceptive pills may be given.
3. *Suggested answers:*
   a. 44 pounds is 20 kg
   b. 40 mg dose would be a dose of 2 mg per kg
   c. 30 mg dose would be a dose of 1.5 mg per kg

CHAPTER 39

NCLEX-Style Review Questions

1. b

Rationale. The open fracture, also called a compound fracture, penetrates the skin. When the fragments of the bone are separated, the fracture is said to be complete. If the skin is not penetrated, the break is known as a simple or closed fracture, and if the fragments of the bone remain partially joined, the fracture is termed an incomplete fracture.

2. a

Rationale. Any child in traction must be carefully monitored to detect any signs of decreased circulation or neurovascular complications. Cleaning pin sites is appropriate for a child in skeletal traction. Providing age-appropriate activities and monitoring intake and output are important interventions for any ill child but would not be the highest priority interventions for the child in traction.

3. b

Rationale. The brace worn to treat scoliosis is worn day and night and should be removed only very briefly, such as for showering. The child needs to be taught that the brace must be worn at all times, during the day as well as the night.

4. b, c, e

Rationale. Monitoring for signs of pain, decreased circulation, or change or variation in pulses in the extremity is important for the child in a cast. Pain can indicate serious complications, such as compartment syndrome. Wearing a gown or sterile gloves is unnecessary. Checking posterior pulses would be appropriate when a lower extremity is casted.

Critical Thinking: What Would You Do?

1. *Suggested answers:*
   a. Preadolescence is at a sensitive age for children; privacy and being like everyone else are top priorities. The child who must wear a TLSO brace might feel embarrassed, awkward, self-conscious, and even angry.
   b. It is important for the nurse to encourage Carrie to talk about her feelings, encourage her to express what she is concerned about, and offer suggestions as to how she might be able to meet some of the needs she has at her age.
   c. The nurse can support Carrie to select clothing that blends with current styles but is loose enough to hide the brace.

2. *Suggested answers:*
   a. Muscular dystrophy is a hereditary, progressive, degenerative disease of the muscles.
   b. As the disease progresses, physically the child becomes progressively weaker, usually becoming wheelchair-bound by 10 to 12 years of age.
   c. Many times the individual dies, often during young adulthood, of respiratory or heart failure.
   d. The nurse might suggest assistance through the Muscular Dystrophy Association—USA (National Headquarters, 3300 E. Sunrise Drive, Tucson, AZ 85718; 800-572-1717; website: http://www.mdausa.org), through local chapters of this organization, and by talking with other parents who face the same problem.

3. *Suggested answers:*
   a. 17.6 pounds is 8 kg
   b. Low dose of 6.25 mg per kg is 64 mg every 6 hours.
   c. High dose of 12.5 mg per kg is 100 mg every 6 hours.
   d. Every 6 hours is four doses in a 24-hour time period, for a total of 400 mg.

CHAPTER 40

NCLEX-Style Review Questions

1. a
   Rationale. An increase in the respiratory rate after a severe burn may be an indication of possible serious respiratory complications and should be reported immediately in case an endotracheal tube needs to be inserted. A temperature of 38.4°C, hourly urine output of 150 cc, and pain rating of 8 need to be documented and reported but are not as urgent as reporting respiratory concerns.

2. b
   Rationale. Although the sexual partner of the adolescent says she has not had other sexual partners, it is important for the adolescent to protect himself from the possibility of contracting a sexually transmitted disease in the event his partner is not being truthful. The statements about condoms, treatment with antibiotics, and transmission to a fetus indicate the adolescent has an understanding of protection, treatment, and contracting sexually transmitted diseases.

3. a, c, d, e
   Rationale. Preventing the child from scratching the affected areas will help decrease the possibilities of the areas being opened and becoming infected. The nurse monitors for symptoms of infection, gives soothing baths such as Aveeno to help relax the child before sleeping, and encourages fluid consumption to prevent the child from becoming dehydrated. Overdressing could promote heat retention and exacerbate the itching. Using bleach to wash the child's clothes is unnecessary.

4. a, c, d, e
   Rationale. Pediculosis, lice infestation, is passed from child to child by direct or indirect contact. Washing linens, clothing, combs, and brushes and vacuuming carpets, car seats, and furniture will help decrease the spread of pediculosis. Treatment involves the use of pediculicides applied to the affected areas. Wearing gloves is not necessary to prepare food or snacks. However, gloves should be worn if there will be contact with the affected areas or child's clothing or linens.

Critical Thinking: What Would You Do?

1. *Suggested answers:*
   a. HIV cannot be transmitted through casual contact. Transmission of HIV is by contact with infected blood or sexual contact with an infected person.
   b. Following good hygiene habits and avoiding coming in contact with body secretions from the person who is HIV positive will decrease the likelihood of the disease being spread among family members.
   c. To help protect Brian from infectious or opportunistic diseases, the family should practice good handwashing and clean carefully and regularly. Household bleach solutions should be used to clean and when washing Brian's clothes, especially his underwear. Raw fruits and vegetables should be washed and peeled or cooked; meats should be well cooked; and unpasteurized dairy products and foods grown in organic fertilizer should be avoided. Someone other than Brian should care for pets; he should avoid persons

who have any infectious disease; and no live vaccine immunizations should be given to Brian.

2. *Suggested answers:*
   a. Conscientious handwashing is the most important action that can be taken to prevent infection for the child with a burn.
   b. Everyone who comes in contact with Omar should be taught regarding infections and infection control.
   c. An elevated temperature, drainage, unusual odor, and positive cultures all might indicate an infection is present.
   d. When a child is burned, a large portion of the integumentary system, which is the primary defense against infection, has been damaged or destroyed. Detecting signs and symptoms of infection early leads to early treatment and a decreased chance of complications occurring because of infection.

3. *Suggested answers:*
   a. 1,000 mg is 1 gram
   b. 2.5 mL will be given for a 250-mg dose
   c. 100 mg given BID (twice a day) will be 200 mg in a 24-hour period
   d. 200 mg a day for 7 days will be a total of 1,400 mg in 7 days

CHAPTER 41

NCLEX-Style Review Questions

1. d
   Rationale. The adolescent with anorexia nervosa often adheres to a strict routine with regard to schoolwork, exercise, cleanliness, and order in their environment. The adolescent with anorexia usually does well in school, exercises excessively, is very active, and shows little emotion.

2. b
   Rationale. The adolescent with bulimia often has dental caries because of frequent exposure of stomach acids during self-induced vomiting, which causes the teeth to erode. The adolescent with bulimia usually is of normal weight or slightly overweight and often shows few symptoms or clues that she has the condition.

3. b
   Rationale. Fluid and electrolyte imbalances and deficiencies are extremely dangerous and can cause heart conditions and even death in the adolescent with an eating disorder. Verbally expressing positive attitudes and feelings, maintaining fluid and electrolyte balance, and having normal bowel and bladder patterns are important goals for the adolescent with an eating disorder but are not as critical as maintaining a proper fluid and electrolyte balance.

4. c
   Rationale. The adolescent who spends most of his or her time alone may be depressed or even contemplating suicide. Most adolescents spend much of their time with their peers. The statements about fixing all the world problems, being happy about breaking up with the boyfriend, and eating all the time but never wanting to go to sleep are common ideas and concerns of the adolescent and show normal characteristic behaviors of adolescents.

5. Intake = 420 cc; output = 169 cc
   Rationale. To determine intake, the infant had seven feedings of 2 ounces, each for a total of 14 ounces. There are 30 cc in 1 ounce, so the intake is 420 cc. For output, add the amount of emesis (20 + 36 + 28), which totals 84 cc, and the weight of the wet diapers (20 + 18 + 25 + 22), which totals 85 g (cc), for an output of 169 cc. The stool would be documented but not counted in the output total.

Critical Thinking: What Would You Do?

1. *Suggested answers:*
   a. In addition to weight loss, the teen with a diagnosis of anorexia would be observed for an emaciated and almost skeletal appearance, sexual immaturity, dry skin and brittle nails; in addition, such teens often have lanugo (downy hair) over their backs and extremities. Amenorrhea (absence of menstruation), constipation, hypothermia, bradycardia, low blood pressure, and anemia also are seen in teens with anorexia.
   b. Teens with anorexia often are perfectionists and show little emotion. Depression is common; they may deny weight loss and have a rigid program of exercise and rigid schedules for studying and other ritualistic behaviors. They often deny hunger but suffer from fatigue.
   c. In Tanya's nursing care plan, activity intolerance, constipation and diarrhea, skin integrity, noncompliance, and family coping would all be addressed. Nursing interventions to help Tanya meet the goals of these concerns would be included.

2. *Suggested answers:*
   a. Alcohol is the most commonly abused drug among adolescents because drinking alcoholic beverages is considered an acceptable and desirable social behavior, and alcohol, although not legal for the adolescent to use, is available in many homes.
   b. Adolescents are at great risk for becoming substance abusers because they use alcohol to avoid facing their problems, escape and forget the pain of life as they see it, add excitement to social events, and bow to peer pressure. They often use

alcohol as a means of relieving the tensions and pressures of their lives, rather than learning and using appropriate and healthy coping skills.

c. It is important for teens to learn and practice ways to face and deal with their problems and pressures in healthy ways. Learning to have fun without the use of alcohol increases the enjoyment adolescents have with friends and peers.

3. *Suggested answers:*
   a. 75 pounds is 34 kg
   b. Low dose of 0.3 mg per kg would be 10.2 mg.
   c. High dose of 2.0 mg per kg would be 68 mg.
   d. The high dose would not be appropriate for this child because the 68 mg per dose would be higher than the 60 mg dose that should not be exceeded in a day.

Appendix A

Standard and Transmission-Based Precautions

Use Standard Precautions, or the equivalent, for the care of all patients. *Category IB**

A. Handwashing

(1) Wash hands after touching blood, body fluids, secretions, excretions, and contaminated items, whether or not gloves are worn. Wash hands immediately after gloves are removed, between patient contacts, and when otherwise indicated to avoid transfer of microorganisms to other patients or environments. It may be necessary to wash hands between tasks and procedures on the same patient to prevent cross-contamination of different body sites. *Category IB*

(2) Use a plain (nonantimicrobial) soap for routine handwashing. *Category IB*

(3) Use an antimicrobial agent or a waterless antiseptic agent for specific circumstances (e.g., control of outbreaks or hyperendemic infections), as defined by the infection control program. *Category IB* (See Contact Precautions for additional recommendations on using antimicrobial and antiseptic agents.)

B. Gloves

Wear gloves (clean, nonsterile gloves are adequate) when touching blood, body fluids, secretions, excretions, and contaminated items. Put on clean gloves just before touching mucous membranes and nonintact skin. Change gloves between tasks and procedures on the same patient after contact with material that may contain a high concentration of microorganisms. Remove gloves promptly after use, before touching noncontaminated items and environmental surfaces, and before going to another patient, and wash hands immediately to avoid transfer of microorganisms to other patients or environments. *Category IB*

C. Mask, Eye Protection, Face Shield

Wear a mask and eye protection or a face shield to protect mucous membranes of the eyes, nose, and mouth during procedures and patient-care activities that are likely to generate splashes or sprays of blood, body fluids, secretions, and excretions. *Category IB*

D. Gown

Wear a gown (a clean, nonsterile gown is adequate) to protect skin and to prevent soiling of clothing during procedures and patient-care activities that are likely to generate splashes or sprays of blood, body fluids, secretions, or excretions. Select a gown that is appropriate for the activity and amount of fluid likely to be encountered. Remove a soiled gown as promptly as possible, and wash hands to avoid transfer of microorganisms to other patients or environments. *Category IB*

E. Patient-Care Equipment

Handle used patient-care equipment soiled with blood, body fluids, secretions, and excretions in a manner that prevents skin and mucous membrane exposures, contamination of clothing, and transfer of microorganisms to other patients and environments. Ensure that reusable equipment is not used for the care of another patient until it has been cleaned and reprocessed appropriately. Ensure that single-use items are discarded properly. *Category IB*

F. Environmental Control

Ensure that the hospital has adequate procedures for the routine care, cleaning, and disinfection of environmental surfaces, beds, bedrails, bedside equipment, and other frequently touched surfaces, and ensure that these procedures are being followed. *Category IB*

G. Linen

Handle, transport, and process used linen soiled with blood, body fluids, secretions, and excretions in a manner that prevents skin and mucous membrane exposures and contamination of clothing, and that avoids transfer of microorganisms to other patients and environments. *Category IB*

H. Occupational Health and Bloodborne Pathogens

(1) Take care to prevent injuries when using needles, scalpels, and other sharp instruments or devices; when handling sharp instruments after procedures;

(From Recommendations for Isolation Precautions in Hospitals developed by the Centers for Disease Control and Prevention and the Hospital Control Practices Advisory Committee [HICPAC], February 18, 1997.)

*Category IB. Strongly recommended for all hospitals and reviewed as effective by experts in the field and a consensus of HICPAC members on the basis of strong rationale and suggestive evidence, even though definitive studies have not been done.

when cleaning used instruments; and when disposing of used needles. Never recap used needles, or otherwise manipulate them using both hands, or use any other technique that involves directing the point of a needle toward any part of the body; rather, use either a one-handed "scoop" technique or a mechanical device designed for holding the needle sheath. Do not remove used needles from disposable syringes by hand, and do not bend, break, or otherwise manipulate used needles by hand. Place used disposable syringes and needles, scalpel blades, and other sharp items in appropriate puncture-resistant containers, which are located as close as practical to the area in which the items were used, and place reusable syringes and needles in a puncture-resistant container for transport to the reprocessing area. *Category IB*

(2) Use mouthpieces, resuscitation bags, or other ventilation devices as an alternative to mouth-to-mouth resuscitation methods in areas where the need for resuscitation is predictable. *Category IB*

I. Patient Placement

Place a patient who contaminates the environment or who does not (or cannot be expected to) assist in maintaining appropriate hygiene or environmental control in a private room. If a private room is not available, consult with infection control professionals regarding patient placement or other alternatives. *Category IB*

J. Respiratory Hygiene/Cough Etiquette

Instruct symptomatic persons to cover mouth/nose when sneezing/coughing; use tissues and dispose in no-touch receptacle; observe hand hygiene after soiling of hands with respiratory secretions; wear surgical masks if tolerated or maintain spatial separation, >3 feet if possible. *Category IB.*[†]

[†]Guidelines for respiratory hygiene/cough etiquette have been added to the 2004 **DRAFT** *CDC guidelines for isolation precautions: Preventing transmission of infectious agents in healthcare settings. 2004.*
https://www.cdc.gov/nicdod/hip/isoguide.htm

Appendix B

NANDA-Approved Nursing Diagnoses

This list represents the NANDA-approved nursing diagnoses for clinical use and testing.

Domain 1: Health Promotion

Description

The awareness of well-being or normality of function and the strategies used to maintain control of and enhance that well-being or normality of function

Approved Diagnoses

Effective Therapeutic Regimen Management
Ineffective Therapeutic Regimen Management
Ineffective Family Therapeutic Regimen Management
Ineffective Community Therapeutic Regimen Management
Health-Seeking Behaviors (specify)
Ineffective Health Maintenance
Impaired Home Maintenance
Readiness for Enhanced Management of Therapeutic Regimen
Readiness for Enhanced Nutrition

Domain 2: Nutrition

Description

The activities of taking in, assimilating, and using nutrients for the purpose of tissue maintenance, tissue repair, and the production of energy

Approved Diagnoses

Ineffective Infant Feeding Pattern
Impaired Swallowing
Imbalanced Nutrition: Less Than Body Requirements
Imbalanced Nutrition: More Than Body Requirements
Risk for Imbalanced Nutrition: More Than Body Requirements
Deficient Fluid Volume
Risk for Deficient Fluid Volume
Excess Fluid Volume
Risk for Imbalanced Fluid Volume
Readiness for Enhanced Fluid Balance

Domain 3: Elimination

Description

Secretion and excretion of waste products from the body

Approved Diagnoses

Impaired Urinary Elimination
Urinary Retention
Total Urinary Incontinence
Functional Urinary Incontinence
Stress Urinary Incontinence
Urge Urinary Incontinence
Reflex Urinary Incontinence
Risk for Urge Urinary Incontinence
Readiness for Enhanced Urinary Elimination
Bowel Incontinence
Diarrhea
Constipation
Risk for Constipation
Perceived Constipation
Impaired Gas Exchange

Domain 4: Activity/Rest

Description

The production, conservation, expenditure, or balance of energy resources

Approved Diagnoses

Disturbed Sleep Pattern
Sleep Deprivation
Readiness for Enhanced Sleep
Risk for Disuse Syndrome
Impaired Physical Mobility
Impaired Bed Mobility
Impaired Wheelchair Mobility
Impaired Transfer Ability
Impaired Walking
Deficient Diversional Activity
Dressing/Grooming Self-Care Deficit
Bathing/Hygiene Self-Care Deficit
Feeding Self-Care Deficit
Toileting Self-Care Deficit
Delayed Surgical Recovery
Disturbed Energy Field
Fatigue
Decreased Cardiac Output
Impaired Spontaneous Ventilation
Ineffective Breathing Pattern
Activity Intolerance
Risk for Activity Intolerance
Dysfunctional Ventilatory Weaning Response
Ineffective Tissue Perfusion (specify type: Renal, Cerebral, Cardiopulmonary, Gastrointestinal, Peripheral)

Domain 5: Perception/Cognition

Description

The human information-processing system, including attention, orientation, sensation, perception, cognition, and communication

(box continues on page 1080)

Approved Diagnoses
Unilateral Neglect
Impaired Environmental Interpretation Syndrome
Wandering
Disturbed Sensory Perception (specify: Visual,
  Auditory, Kinesthetic, Gustatory, Tactile,
  Olfactory)
Deficient Knowledge (specify)
Readiness for Enhanced Knowledge
Acute Confusion
Chronic Confusion
Impaired Memory
Disturbed Thought Processes
Impaired Verbal Communication
Readiness for Enhanced Communication

Domain 6: Self-Perception
Description
Awareness about the self

Approved Diagnoses
Disturbed Personal Identity
Powerlessness
Risk for Powerlessness
Hopelessness
Risk for Loneliness
Readiness for Enhanced Self-Concept
Chronic Low Self-Esteem
Situational Low Self-Esteem
Risk for Situational Low Self-Esteem
Disturbed Body Image

Domain 7: Role Relationships
Description
The positive and negative connections or associations between persons or groups of persons and
the means by which those connections are
demonstrated

Approved Diagnoses
Caregiver Role Strain
Risk for Caregiver Role Strain
Impaired Parenting
Risk for Impaired Parenting
Readiness for Enhanced Parenting
Interrupted Family Processes
Readiness for Enhanced Family Processes
Dysfunctional Family Processes: Alcoholism
Risk for Impaired Parent/Infant/Child Attachment
Effective Breastfeeding
Ineffective Breastfeeding
Interrupted Breastfeeding
Ineffective Role Performance
Parental Role Conflict
Impaired Social Interaction

Domain 8: Sexuality
Description
Sexual identity, sexual function, and reproduction

Approved Diagnoses
Sexual Dysfunction
Ineffective Sexuality Patterns

Domain 9: Coping/Stress Tolerance
Description
Contending with life events/life processes

Approved Diagnoses
Relocation Stress Syndrome
Risk for Relocation Stress Syndrome
Rape-Trauma Syndrome
Rape-Trauma Syndrome: Silent Reaction
Rape-Trauma Syndrome: Compound Reaction
Post-Trauma Syndrome
Risk for Post-Trauma Syndrome
Fear
Anxiety
Death Anxiety
Chronic Sorrow
Ineffective Denial
Anticipatory Grieving
Dysfunctional Grieving
Impaired Adjustment
Ineffective Coping
Disabled Family Coping
Compromised Family Coping
Defensive Coping
Ineffective Community Coping
Readiness for Enhanced Coping
Readiness for Enhanced Family Coping
Readiness for Enhanced Community Coping
Autonomic Dysreflexia
Risk for Autonomic Dysreflexia
Disorganized Infant Behavior
Risk for Disorganized Infant Behavior
Readiness for Enhanced Organized Infant Behavior
Decreased Intracranial Adaptive Capacity

Domain 10: Life Principles
Description
Principles underlying conduct, thought, and behavior
about acts, customs, or institutions as being true or
having intrinsic worth

Approved Diagnoses
Readiness for Enhanced Spiritual Well-Being
Spiritual Distress
Risk for Spiritual Distress
Decisional Conflict (specify)
Noncompliance (specify)

Domain 11: Safety/Protection
Description
Freedom from danger, physical injury, or immune-
system damage; preservation from loss; and
protection of safety and security

Approved Diagnoses
Risk for Infection
Impaired Oral Mucous Membrane
Risk for Injury
Risk for Perioperative Positioning Injury
Risk for Falls
Risk for Trauma
Impaired Skin Integrity
Risk for Impaired Skin Integrity
Impaired Tissue Integrity
Impaired Dentition
Risk for Suffocation
Risk for Aspiration
Ineffective Airway Clearance
Risk for Peripheral Neurovascular Dysfunction
Ineffective Protection

Risk for Sudden Infant Death Syndrome
Risk for Self-Mutilation
Self-Mutilation
Risk for Other-Directed Violence
Risk for Self-Directed Violence
Risk for Suicide
Risk for Poisoning
Latex Allergy Response
Risk for Latex Allergy Response
Risk for Imbalanced Body Temperature
Ineffective Thermoregulation
Hypothermia
Hyperthermia

Domain 12: Comfort
Description
Sence of mental, physical, or social well-being or ease

Approved Diagnoses
Acute Pain
Chronic Pain
Nausea
Social Isolation

Domain 13: Growth/Development
Description
Age-appropriate increase in physical dimension, organ systems, and/or attainment of developmental milestones

Approved Diagnoses
Risk for Disproportionate Growth
Adult Failure to Thrive
Delayed Growth and Development
Risk for Delayed Development

Appendix C

JCAHO List of "Do Not Use" Abbreviations

The Joint Commission on Accreditation of Healthcare Organizations and the Institute for Safe Medication Practices have listed the following abbreviations as dangerous, due to the potential of medication and other errors being made if these are used.

Abbreviation	Potential Problem	Preferred Term
U (for unit)	Mistaken as zero, four or cc.	Write "unit."
IU (for International Unit)	Mistaken as IV (intravenous) or 10 (ten).	Write "International Unit."
Q.D., Q.O.D (Latin abbreviation for once, and the "O" can be mistaken for "I," daily and every other day)	Mistaken for each other. The period after the Q can be mistaken for an "I."	Write "daily" and "every other day."
Trailing zero (X.0 mg), Lack of leading zero (.X mg)	Decimal point is missed.	Never write a zero by itself after a decimal point (X mg), and always use a zero before a decimal point (0.X mg).
MS MSO$_4$ MgSO$_4$	Confused for one another. Can mean morphine sulfate or magnesium sulfate.	Write "morphine sulfate" or "magnesium sulfate."
μg (for microgram)	Mistaken for mg (milligrams) resulting in 1,000-fold dosing overdose.	Write "mcg."
H.S. (for half-strength or Latin abbreviation for bedtime)	Mistaken for either half-strength or hour of sleep (at bedtime). q.H.S. mistaken every hour. All can result in dosing error.	Write out "half-strength" or "at bedtime."
T.I.W. (for three times a week)	Mistaken for three times a day or twice weekly, resulting in an overdose.	Write "3 times weekly" or "three times weekly."
S.C. or S.Q. (for subcutaneous)	Mistaken as SL for sublingual, or "5 every."	Write "Sub-Q", "subQ", or "subcutaneously."
D/C (for discharge)	Interpreted as discontinue or whatever medications follow (typically discharge meds).	Write "discharge."
c.c. (for cubic centimeter)	Mistaken for U (units) when poorly written.	Write "ml" for milliliters.
A.S., A.D., A.U. (Latin abbreviation for left, right, or both ears)	Mistaken for OS, OD, OU, etc.	Write: "left ear," "right ear," or "both ears."

An abbreviation on the "Do Not Use" list should not be used in any of its forms—upper or lower case, with or without periods. For example, if Q.D. is on your list, you can't use "QD" or "qd." Any of those variations are confusing and can be misinterpreted. Retrieved June 18, 2004, from www.jcaho.org.

Appendix D

Good Sources of Essential Nutrients

Protein	Vitamin A	Vitamin B			Vitamin C	Vitamin D	Minerals		
		Thiamine	Riboflavin	Niacin			Calcium	Iron	Iodine
Meat, poultry, fish, milk products and eggs. Whole wheat grains, nuts, peanut butter, legumes are also good sources of protein, but need to be supplemented by some animal protein, such as meat, eggs, milk, cheese, cottage cheese or yogurt.	Green leafy vegetables, deep yellow vegetables and fruits, whole milk or whole milk products, egg yolk.	Meat, fish, poultry, eggs, whole grain, legumes, potatoes, green leafy vegetables.	Milk (best source), meat, egg yolk, green vegetables.	Meat, fish, poultry, peanut butter, wheat germ, brewer's yeast. Although the amount in milk is small, children whose intake of milk is adequate do not develop pellagra.	Citrus fruits and tomatoes, fresh or frozen citrus fruit juices, strawberries, cantaloupe. Breast milk is an adequate source of vitamin C for young infants only if the mother's diet contains sufficient vitamin C.	Sunlight, fish liver oils, fortified milk and synthetic vitamin D.	Milk and milk products, squash, sweet potatoes, raisins, rhubarb, well-cooked dried beans, turnip greens, Swiss chard, mustard greens.	Green leafy vegetables, liver, meats and eggs, dried fruits, whole grain or enriched bread and cereals.	Seafoods, plants grown on soil near the sea, iodized salt.

Appendix E
Breast-feeding and Medication Use

GENERAL CONSIDERATIONS

- Most medications are safe to use while breast-feeding; however, the woman should always check with the pediatrician, physician, or lactation specialist before taking any medications, including over-the-counter and herbal products.
- Inform the woman that she has the right to seek a second opinion if the physician does not perform a thoughtful risk-versus-benefit assessment before prescribing medications or advising against breast-feeding.
- Most medications pass from the woman's bloodstream into the breast milk. However, the amount is usually very small and unlikely to harm the baby.
- A preterm or other special needs neonate is more susceptible to the adverse effects of medications in breast milk. A woman who is taking medications and whose baby is in the neonatal intensive care unit or special care nursery should consult with the pediatrician or neonatologist before feeding her breast milk to the baby.
- If the woman is taking a prescribed medication, she should take the medication just after breast-feeding. This practice helps ensure that the lowest possible dose of medication reaches the baby through the breast milk.
- Some medications can cause changes in the amount of milk the woman produces. Teach the woman to report any changes in milk production.

LACTATION RISK CATEGORIES (LRC)

Lactation Category	Risk	Rationale
L1	Safest	Clinical research or long-term observation of use in many breast-feeding women has not demonstrated risk to the infant.

Lactation Category	Risk	Rationale
L2	Safer	Limited clinical research has not demonstrated an increase in adverse effects in the infant.
L3	Moderately safe	There is possible risk to the infant; however, the risks are minimal or nonthreatening in nature. These medications should be given only when the potential benefit outweighs the risk to the infant.
L4	Possibly hazardous	There is positive evidence of risk to the infant; however, in life-threatening situations or for serious diseases, the benefit might outweigh the risk.
L5	Contraindicated	The risk of using the medication clearly outweighs any possible benefit from breast-feeding.

POTENTIAL EFFECTS OF SELECTED MEDICATION CATEGORIES ON THE BREAST-FED INFANT

Narcotic Analgesics

- Codeine and hydrocodone appear to be safe in moderate doses. Rarely the neonate may experience sedation and/or apnea. (LRC: L3)
- Meperidine (Demerol) can lead to sedation of the neonate. (LRC: L3)
- Low to moderate doses of morphine appear to be safe. (LRC: L2)

- Trace-to-negligible amounts of fentanyl are found in human milk. (LRC: L2)

Non-narcotic Analgesics and NSAIDs

- Acetaminophen and ibuprofen are approved for use. (LRC: L1)
- Naproxen may cause neonatal hemorrhage and anemia if used for prolonged periods. (LRC: L3 for short-term use and L4 for long-term use)
- The newer COX2 inhibitors, such as celecoxib (Celebrex), appear to be safe for use. (LRC: L2)

Antibiotics

- Levels in breast milk are usually very low.
- The penicillins and cephalosporins are generally considered safe to use. (LRC: L1 and L2)
- Tetracyclines can be safely used for short periods but are not suitable for long-term therapy (e.g., for treatment of acne). (LRC: L2)
- Sulfonamides should not be used during the neonatal stage (the first month of life). (LRC: L3)

Antihypertensives

- A high degree of caution is advised when antihypertensives are used during breast-feeding.
- Some beta blockers can be used.
- Hydralazine and methyldopa are considered to be safe. (LRC: L2)
- ACE inhibitors are not recommended in the early postpartum period.

Sedatives and Hypnotics

- Neonatal withdrawal can occur when antianxiety medications, such as lorazepam, are taken. Fortunately withdrawal is generally mild.
- Phenothiazines, such as Phenergan and Thorazine, may lead to sleep apnea and increase the risk for sudden infant death syndrome.

Antidepressants

- The risk to the baby often is higher if the woman is depressed and remains untreated, rather than taking the medication.
- The older tricyclics are considered to be safe; however they cause many bothersome side effects, such as weight gain and dry mouth, which may lead to noncompliance on the part of the woman.
- The selective serotonin uptake inhibitors (SSRIs) also are considered to be safe and have a lower side effect profile, which makes them more palatable to the woman. (LRC: L2 and L3)

Mood Stabilizers (Antimanic Medication)

- Lithium is found in breast milk and is best not used in the breast-feeding woman. (LRC: L4)
- Valproic acid (Depakote) seems to be a more appropriate choice for the woman with bipolar disorder. The infant will need periodic lab studies to check platelets and liver function.

Corticosteroids

- Corticosteroids do not pass into the milk in large quantities.
- Inhaled steroids are safe to use because they don't accumulate in the bloodstream.

Thyroid Medication

- Thyroid medications, such as levothyroxine (Synthroid), can be taken while breast-feeding.
- Most are in LRC category L1.

MEDICATIONS THAT USUALLY ARE CONTRAINDICATED FOR THE BREAST-FEEDING WOMAN

- Amiodarone
- Antineoplastic agents
- Chloramphenicol
- Doxepin
- Ergotamine and other ergot derivatives
- Iodides
- Methotrexate and immunosuppressants
- Lithium
- Radiopharmaceuticals
- Ribavirin
- Tetracycline (prolonged use—more than 3 weeks)
- Pseudoephedrine (found in many over-the-counter medications)

Material in this Appendix was adapted from information found on the American Academy of Pediatrics website (www.aap.org) and from Riordan, J. (2005). *Breastfeeding and human lactation,* 3rd ed. Jones and Bartlett Publishers: Boston; Hale, T. W. (2004). *Medications and mother's milk,* 11th ed. Amarillo, TX: Pharmasoft Publishing.

Appendix F
Cervical Dilation Chart

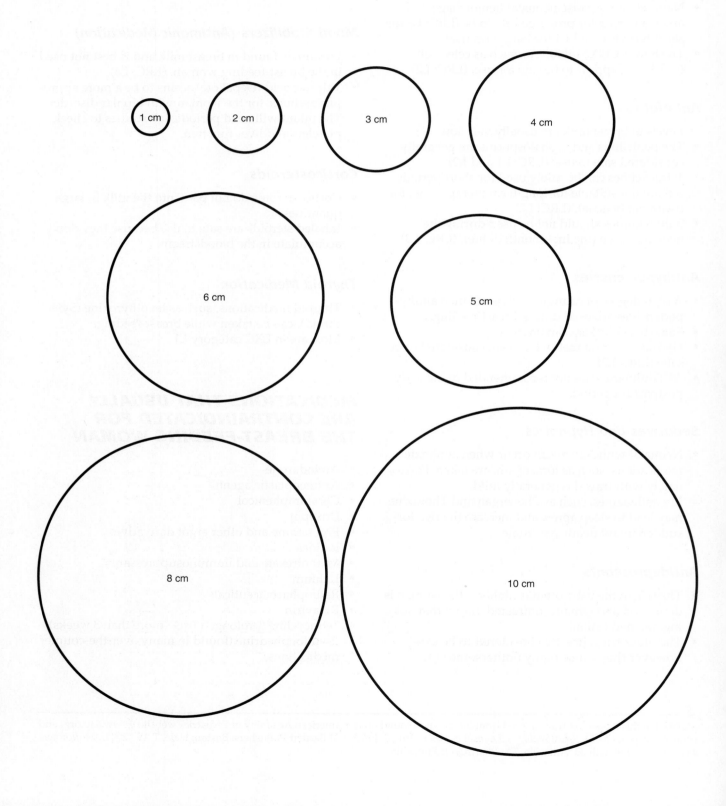

1 cm

2 cm

3 cm

4 cm

6 cm

5 cm

8 cm

10 cm

Appendix G

Growth Charts

Birth to 36 months: Boys
Length-for-age and Weight-for-age percentiles

NAME _____

RECORD# _____

Published May 30, 2000 (modified 4/20/01).
SOURCE: Developed by the National Center for Health Statistics in collaboration with
the National Center for Chronic Disease Prevention and Health Promotion (2000).
http://www.cdc.gov/growthcharts

CDC
SAFER·HEALTHIER·PEOPLE™

Birth to 36 months: Boys
Head circumference-for-age and
Weight-for-length percentiles

NAME _____

RECORD# _____

Published May 30, 2000 (modified 10/16/00).
SOURCE: Developed by the National Center for Health Statistics in collaboration with
   the National Center for Chronic Disease Prevention and Health Promotion (2000).
   http://www.cdc.gov/growthcharts

SAFER · HEALTHIER · PEOPLE™

Birth to 36 months: Girls
Length-for-age and Weight-for-age percentiles

NAME _____

RECORD# _____

Mother's Stature _____
Father's Stature _____

Gestational
Age: _____ Weeks

Comment

Date	Age	Weight	Length	Head Circ.	
	Birth				

Published May 30, 2000 (modified 4/20/01).

SOURCE: Developed by the National Center for Health Statistics in collaboration with
the National Center for Chronic Disease Prevention and Health Promotion (2000).
http://www.cdc.gov/growthcharts

SAFER · HEALTHIER · PEOPLE™

Birth to 36 months: Girls
Head circumference-for-age and
Weight-for-length percentiles

NAME _____

RECORD# _____

Published May 30, 2000 (modified 10/16/00).
SOURCE: Developed by the National Center for Health Statistics in collaboration with
the National Center for Chronic Disease Prevention and Health Promotion (2000).
http://www.cdc.gov/growthcharts

SAFER·HEALTHIER·PEOPLE™

2 to 20 years: Boys
Stature-for-age and Weight-for-age percentiles

NAME _____

RECORD# _____

*To Calculate BMI: Weight (kg) ÷ Stature (cm) ÷ Stature (cm) x 10,000
or Weight (lb) ÷ Stature (in) ÷ Stature (in) x 703

Published May 30, 2000 (modified 11/21/00).
SOURCE: Developed by the National Center for Health Statistics in collaboration with
the National Center for Chronic Disease Prevention and Health Promotion (2000).
http://www.cdc.gov/growthcharts

SAFER · HEALTHIER · PEOPLE™

2 to 20 years: Girls
Stature-for-age and Weight-for-age percentiles

NAME _____

RECORD# _____

Published May 30, 2000 (modified 11/21/00).
SOURCE: Developed by the National Center for Health Statistics in collaboration with
the National Center for Chronic Disease Prevention and Health Promotion (2000).
http://www.cdc.gov/growthcharts

SAFER · HEALTHIER · PEOPLE™

Appendix H

Pulse, Respiration, and Blood Pressure Values for Children

Normal Pulse Ranges in Children

Age	Normal Range	Average
0–24 hours	70–170 bpm	120 bpm
1–7 days	100–180 bpm	140 bpm
1 month	110–188 bpm	160 bpm
1 month–1 year	80–180 bpm	120–130 bpm
2 years	80–140 bpm	110 bpm
4 years	80–120 bpm	100 bpm
6 years	70–115 bpm	100 bpm
10 years	70–110 bpm	90 bpm
12–14 years	60–110 bpm	85–90 bpm
14–18 years	50–95 bpm	70–75 bpm

bpm, beats per minute.

Normal Blood Pressure Ranges

Age	Systolic (mm Hg)	Diastolic (mm Hg)
Newborn–12 hr (less than 1,000 g)	39–59	16–36
Newborn–12 hr (3,000 g)	50–70	24–45
Newborn–96 hr (3,000 g)	60–90	20–60
Infant	74–100	50–70
Toddler	80–112	50–80
Preschooler	82–110	50–78
School-Age	84–120	54–80
Adolescent	94–140	62–88

Variations in Respirations with Age

Age	Rate per Minute
Newborn	40–90
1 year	20–40
2 years	20–30
3 years	20–30
5 years	20–25
10 years	17–22
15 years	15–20
20 years	15–20

Appendix I

Temperature and Weight Conversion Charts

Conversion of Pounds to Kilograms

Pounds	0	1	2	3	4	5	6	7	8	9
0	—	0.45	0.90	1.36	1.81	2.26	2.72	3.17	3.62	4.08
10	4.53	4.98	5.44	5.89	6.35	6.80	7.25	7.71	8.16	8.61
20	9.07	9.52	9.97	10.43	10.88	11.34	11.79	12.24	12.70	13.15
30	13.60	14.06	14.51	14.96	15.42	15.87	16.32	16.78	17.23	17.69
40	18.14	18.59	19.05	19.50	19.95	20.41	20.86	21.31	21.77	22.22
50	22.68	23.13	23.58	24.04	24.49	24.94	25.40	25.85	26.30	26.76
60	27.21	27.66	28.12	28.57	29.03	29.48	29.93	30.39	30.84	31.29
70	31.75	32.20	32.65	33.11	33.56	34.02	34.47	34.92	35.38	35.83
80	36.28	36.74	37.19	37.64	38.10	38.55	39.00	39.46	39.91	40.37
90	40.82	41.27	41.73	42.18	42.63	43.09	43.54	43.99	44.45	44.90
100	45.36	45.81	46.26	46.72	47.17	47.62	48.08	48.53	48.98	49.44
110	49.89	50.34	50.80	51.25	51.71	52.16	52.61	53.07	53.52	53.97
120	54.43	54.88	55.33	55.79	56.24	56.70	57.15	57.60	58.06	58.51
130	58.96	59.42	59.87	60.32	60.78	61.23	61.68	62.14	62.59	63.05
140	63.50	63.95	64.41	64.86	65.31	65.77	66.22	66.67	67.13	67.58
150	68.04	68.49	68.94	69.40	69.85	70.30	70.76	71.21	71.66	72.12
160	72.57	73.02	73.48	73.93	74.39	74.84	75.29	75.75	76.20	76.65
170	77.11	77.56	78.01	78.47	78.92	79.38	79.83	80.28	80.74	81.19
180	81.64	82.10	82.55	83.00	83.46	83.91	84.36	84.82	85.27	85.73
190	86.18	86.68	87.09	87.54	87.99	88.45	88.90	89.35	89.81	90.26
200	90.72	91.17	91.62	92.08	92.53	92.98	93.44	93.89	94.34	94.80

Conversion of Pounds and Ounces to Grams For Newborn Weights

Pounds	Ounces															
	0	1	2	3	4	5	6	7	8	9	10	11	12	13	14	15
0	—	28	57	85	113	142	170	198	227	255	283	312	340	369	397	425
1	454	482	510	539	567	595	624	652	680	709	737	765	794	822	850	879
2	907	936	964	992	1021	1049	1077	1106	1134	1162	1191	1219	1247	1276	1304	1332
3	1361	1389	1417	1446	1474	1503	1531	1559	1588	1616	1644	1673	1701	1729	1758	1786
4	1814	1843	1871	1899	1928	1956	1984	2013	2041	2070	2098	2126	2155	2183	2211	2240
5	2268	2296	2325	2353	2381	2410	2438	2466	2495	2523	2551	2580	2608	2637	2665	2693
6	2722	2750	2778	2807	2835	2863	2892	2920	2948	2977	3005	3033	3062	3090	3118	3147
7	3175	3203	3232	3260	3289	3317	3345	3374	3402	3430	3459	3487	3515	3544	3572	3600
8	3629	3657	3685	3714	3742	3770	3799	3827	3856	3884	3912	3941	3969	3997	4026	4054
9	4082	4111	4139	4167	4196	4224	4252	4281	4309	4337	4366	4394	4423	4451	4479	4508
10	4536	4564	4593	4621	4649	4678	4706	4734	4763	4791	4819	4848	4876	4904	4933	4961
11	4990	5018	5046	5075	5103	5131	5160	5188	5216	5245	5273	5301	5330	5358	5386	5415
12	5443	5471	5500	5528	5557	5585	5613	5642	5670	5698	5727	5755	5783	5812	5840	5868
13	5897	5925	5953	5982	6010	6038	6067	6095	6123	6152	6180	6209	6237	6265	6294	6322
14	6350	6379	6407	6435	6464	6492	6520	6549	6577	6605	6634	6662	6690	6719	6747	6776
15	6804	6832	6860	6889	6917	6945	6973	7002	7030	7059	7087	7115	7144	7172	7201	7228

Conversion of Fahrenheit to Celsius

Celsius	Fahrenheit	Celsius	Fahrenheit	Celsius	Fahrenheit
34.0	93.2	37.0	98.6	40.0	104.0
34.2	93.6	37.2	99.0	40.2	101.4
34.4	93.9	37.4	99.3	40.4	104.7
34.6	94.3	37.6	99.7	40.6	105.2
34.8	94.6	37.8	100.0	40.8	105.4
35.0	95.0	38.0	100.4	41.0	105.9
35.2	95.4	38.2	100.8	41.2	106.1
35.4	95.7	38.4	101.1	41.4	106.5
35.6	96.1	38.6	101.5	41.6	106.8
35.8	96.4	38.8	101.8	41.8	107.2
36.0	96.8	39.0	102.2	42.0	107.6
36.2	97.2	39.2	102.6	42.2	108.0
36.4	97.5	39.4	102.9	42.4	108.3
36.6	97.9	39.6	103.3	42.6	108.7
36.8	98.2	39.8	103.6	42.8	109.0

$(°C) \times (9/5) + 32 = °F$

$(°F - 32) \times (5/9) = °C$

Appendix J

Communicating With Children and Family Caregivers

OVERVIEW

- Communication occurs during well-child visits and focuses on immunizations, anticipatory guidance, and development assessment. Communicating with children and family caregivers is a primary source of data collection during a health crisis.
- Information about the child is derived from the child, the caregivers, and the nurse's observations of the child and family.
- Understanding the developmental level of the child and influences on the child and caregiver communication (e.g., family, culture, community, age, and personality) are important.
- Communication includes the spoken and written words as well as the body language, facial expressions, voice intonations, and emotions behind the words.
- Listening is one of the most important aspects of communication. Listening includes more than hearing. It includes tuning into the other person, being sensitive to the person's feelings, and concentrating on what the other person is trying to express. When listening, think about what the person is saying and *not* about how you are going to respond.
- Listening includes attending (giving the other person physical signs that you are listening) and following (encouraging the speaker to fully express what it is he or she needs to say).
- Silence is also a form of communication. It might indicate that the person is thinking, is unclear about what is being said, is having difficulty responding, is angry, etc.
- It is always important to clarify statements and feelings expressed by caregivers and children. Reflective statements help indicate what you believed was expressed. For example you might state, "You seem worried about Maria's loss of appetite."
- Good strategies when communicating with children include: maintaining eye contact, playful engagement, and talking about what interests the child or caregiver.
- One of the biggest challenges when several people are present is deciding to whom you should direct your questions. Although eventually you'll need information from the child and caregivers, start with the child if he/she can talk. Even at age 3 some children can tell you about the specific problem.
- To direct the focus of a conversation, use open-ended questions followed by guided statements.
- Some nurses have difficulty accepting their own feelings while working with children. Nurses might feel anxious or inadequate when starting new relationships and beginning to communicate with children. Nurses need to accept the fact that this is normal and okay.
- Play is an important form of communication for children and can be an effective technique in communicating with children.
- Avoid communication blocks, which include socializing, giving unasked for advice, providing false assurances, being defensive, giving pat or clichéd responses, being judgmental or stereotyping, not allowing issues to be fully explored, interrupting, and not allowing the person to finish a response.
- Sometimes it is necessary to communicate through an interpreter because of language barriers or hearing impairments. A medical interpreter trained in the language of the child is preferable but not always available. When using an interpreter, ensure the interpreter understands the goal of the conversation; allow the interpreter and family to become acquainted; communicate directly with the family and child, observing nonverbal responses; pose questions to elicit one answer at a time; do not interrupt the conversation between the interpreter and family; do not talk about the family and child to the interpreter in English because family might understand some information; avoid medical jargon; respect cultural differences; follow up with the interpreter regarding his impression of the interaction; arrange for the interpreter to meet with the family on subsequent visits.

- Time management is an important aspect of communication. You should communicate in a calm and unhurried manner; however, work demands and time constraints often make this difficult. It is important to gain skill in balancing communication needs of children and families with other nursing responsibilities.

COMMUNICATING WITH INFANTS

- Infants evaluate only actions and respond to only sensory cues. Infants cannot realize the nurse who handles them abruptly and hurriedly may be rushed or insecure; they feel only that the nurse is frightening and unloving. To comfort the infant hold, cuddle, and soothe him, or allow caregivers to do so. Spending time in the beginning of an interaction to calm down and connect with the infant is helpful.
- It is important to establish a relationship with the caregiver upfront. Begin by recognizing and praising the hard work of parenting. Allow the caregiver to hold the infant as you initiate conversation, and begin observing the infant, caregiver, and their interactions. When appropriate, ask the caregiver for permission to hold the infant yourself or to place him/her on an examination table or bed.
- Sensory play activities, such massaging the infant, stretching the arms/legs, looking at a colorful/moving object, peek-a-boo, and "this little piggy," can ease the child and convey information.

COMMUNICATING WITH YOUNG CHILDREN

- Allow the caregiver to hold the young child as you initiate conversation, and begin observing the child, caregiver, and their interactions. When appropriate, ask the caregiver permission to hold the child yourself or to place him/her on an examination table or bed.
- Young children are egocentric. Explain to them how they will feel or what they can do. Experiences of others have no relevance. Use short sentences, positive explanations, familiar and nonthreatening terms, and concrete explanations.
- Young children tend to be frightened of strangers. Sudden abrupt or noisy approaches signal danger. The child needs time to evaluate the situation while still in the arms of the caregiver. Do not rush

the situation, but allow time for the child to initiate the relationship. Spending time calming down or connecting with the child is helpful. Conversation might be started through a doll, toy, or puppet. "What's doll's name?" "How does doll feel?" A casual approach with reluctant children is most effective. Games that pique the younger child's curiosity ("Which hand has the car?") might also help put him or her at ease. Children who show rejecting or aggressive behavior are putting up a defense. Ignore these behaviors unless they are harmful to the child or someone else.

- Allow young children to handle or explore equipment that will come in contact with them. For example, have them touch the bell of a stethoscope, listen to their teddy bear's heart, etc. Or play a simple game with these objects.
- Do not stand over children and talk down to them. Get down to eye level. Speak in a slow, clear, positive voice. Use simple words. Keep sentences short. Express statements and questions positively. Listen to the child's fears and worries. Be honest in answers.
- Choices should be simple and limited. Only offer choices if they exist. Do not ask "Do you want medicine now?" if that's not an option. Do ask "Would you like the red cup or the blue cup for your medicine?" Consult with the caregiver about which choices are reasonable.
- Young children tend to be literal and cannot separate fantasy from reality. Do not use analogies. For example, "This will be a little bee sting." Young children visualize a bee sting, which might be traumatic.
- Because verbal skills are limited, pay particular attention to nonverbal clues such as pushing an object away, covering the eyes, crying, kicking, pointing, clinging, exploring an object with the fingers, etc.

COMMUNICATING WITH SCHOOL-AGE CHILDREN

- Remember to begin by calming down or connecting with the child. If caregivers are present, briefly acknowledge them. Then, focus on the child. Include the child in the plan of care.
- School-age children are interested in knowing the "what" and "why" of things. They will ask more questions if their curiosity is not satisfied. Provide simple, concrete responses using age-appropriate vocabulary. Complex or detailed explanations are not necessary. Provide explanations that help them understand how equipment works. Explain what is going to happen and why it is being done to *them*

specifically. Charts, diagrams, and metaphors might be helpful.

- Elicit the child's cooperation by offering reasonable and limited choices.

- Be sensitive to the child's concern about body integrity. Children are particularly concerned about anything that poses a threat of injury to their bodies. Help reduce their anxieties by allowing them to voice concerns and by providing reassurances.

- Play, reenactment, or artwork can give insight into how well a child understands a procedure or experience. These also can reveal the child's perception of interpersonal relationships. Subsequent play can provide clues to the child's progress or changing feelings.

COMMUNICATING WITH ADOLESCENTS

- Communicating with adolescents might be challenging. Adolescents waiver between thinking like an adult and thinking like a child. Behavior is related to their developmental stage not necessarily to chronologic age or physical maturation. Their age and appearance may fool you into assuming that they are functioning on a different level.

- Adolescents respond positively to individuals who show a genuine interest in them. Show interest early and sustain a connection. Focus the interview on them rather than the problem. Build rapport by opening with informal conversation about friends, school, hobbies, and family. Once you have established rapport, return to more open-ended questions.

- Adolescents might need to relate information they do not wish others to know. Adolescents might not reveal much with caregivers present. A discussion about confidentiality with both parent and adolescent might set concerns at ease. Explain to both that some degree of independence will improve health care. Encourage adolescents to discuss sensitive issues with parents.

- If adolescents and caregivers are to be interviewed, it might help to first interview the adolescent (thereby establishing relationship), then both the adolescent and caregivers, then the caregivers separately. Remember, confidentiality must be discussed—why it is important, what will not be shared with caregivers, and what must be shared with caregivers (i.e., what the adolescent states is confidential unless the adolescent indicates that he/she intends to harm him/herself or somebody else.)

- Adolescents and caregivers might not always agree. In this case more clearly define the problem so an agreement might be reached.

- Let adolescents know that you will listen in an open-minded, nonjudgmental way. Do not impose your values on adolescents or give unwanted advice; they will likely reject you.

- Do not ask prying or embarrassing questions. Phrase questions regarding sensitive information in a way that encourages the adolescent to respond without feeling embarrassed.

- When feeling threatened, adolescents might not respond or only respond with monosyllabic answers. Reduce anxiety by confining conversations to nonthreatening topics until the adolescent feels at ease. Be aware of clues that he or she is ready to talk.

- Make contracts with adolescents so that communication can remain open and honest and the plan of care may be more closely followed.

COMMUNICATING WITH CAREGIVERS

- Identify the child's family caregivers (not always mom or dad) and clarify roles. When the family structure is not immediately clear, you may avoid embarrassment by asking directly about other family members. "Who else lives in the home?" "Who is Jimmy's father?" "Do you live together?" Don't assume that because parents are separated that the other parent isn't actively involved in care of the child.

- Much of the information you obtain comes from the family. In general, family members provide most of the care and are allies in promoting the health of the child. View the parents as experts in the care of their child and you as their consultant.

- Include parents in providing information, problem solving, and planning of care. Keep caregivers well informed of what is going on. Make the caregiver feel welcome and important.

- Encourage conferences/meetings between family caregivers and members of the health care team. By doing so, parents form a clearer picture of the child, his behavior, condition, and health needs, and have an opportunity to consider different types of treatments and relationships.

- Pay attention to the verbal and nonverbal clues a parent uses to convey concerns, worries, and anxieties about the child. Worries might be conveyed in an off-handed manner or referenced frequently. Remember the chief complaint might not relate to the real reason the parent has brought the child to the health care facility. Create a trusting atmosphere that allows parents to be open about all of their concerns. Ask facilitating questions: "Do you have any other concerns about Richie that you would like to tell me about?" "What did you hope I would be able to do for you today?" Was there anything else that you wanted to tell or ask me about today?"

- When a parent introduces a concern or offers information without prompting, follow up with clarifying questions. Other times it might be necessary to direct the conversation based on observations.

- When communicating with the parent, provide positive reinforcement and ask open-ended questions. This approach is nonthreatening and encourages description. Be supportive, not judgmental. "Why didn't you bring him sooner?" or "What did you do that for?" does not improve the relationship. Rather, acknowledge the hard work of parenting and praise successes.

- To elicit information, it might be useful to compare what is actually happening with what the parent expects to be happening. Mom: "My 2-year-old son barely eats anything". Nurse: "What do you think your child should be eating? Mom: "Three full meals a day, including green vegetables."

- Explain procedures and invite caregivers to help. Do not force them to participate if they are not comfortable doing so.

- Each individual in the room, including the health care provider, might have a different idea about the nature of the problem. Discover as many of these perspectives as possible. Family members who are not present may also have concerns. It is a good idea to ask about those concerns: "If Sally's father were here today, what questions or concerns would he have?" Agreement about a problem might not be mutual. Sometimes parents might not perceive a problem the nurse sees; other times parents might perceive a problem that the nurse does not see. Explore what's behind the parents' perception and work toward a mutual agreement. Other members of the health care team might be needed.

- Parents' concerns, anxieties, and negative attitudes might be conveyed to the child, which sometimes causes negative reactions from the child. Be alert to negative attitudes. Provide caregivers with opportunities to discuss and explore their anxieties, concerns, or problems. Demonstrate genuine care and concern to help ease these feelings.

- Some children might feel self-sufficient and view the caregivers' presence as being treated like a baby. However, it is often normal for the child to regress during illness, in which case the caregivers' presence may offer support.

- When talking with caregivers, observe how they interact with the child and how the child interacts with the environment. Watch how parents set limits or fail to set limits.

- Provide anticipatory guidance related to normal growth and development, nurturing childcare practices, and safety and injury prevention. In addition to providing information, help parents in using the information.

INDEX

Page numbers followed by an *f* indicate figures; those followed by *t* indicate tables.